FOR INSTRUCTORS

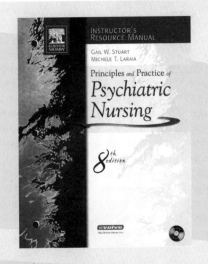

Instructor's Resource Manual ISBN 0-323-03298-2

The print Instructor's Resource Manual for *Principles and Practice of Psychiatric Nursing, 8th Edition*, is designed to help instructors develop lectures and student assignments and evaluate student comprehension. The *Instructor's Manual* includes sample course outlines as well as critical thinking questions and activities and research topics for each chapter of the text. The *Test Bank*, featuring over 1,000 test items, includes an answer key that lists the following categories of information for each question: correct answer, rationale, cognitive level, corresponding stage of the nursing process, appropriate NCLEX label, and corresponding text page reference. The Instructor's Resource Manual is available free to instructors on adoption of the textbook.

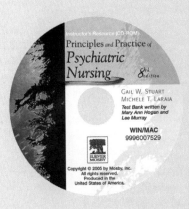

Instructor's Resource (CD-ROM)

The Instructor's Resource (CD-ROM) for *Principles and Practice of Psychiatric Nursing, 8th Edition*, is an additional tool designed to help instructors develop lectures and student assignments and evaluate student comprehension. The *Instructor's Manual* includes sample course outlines as well as critical thinking questions and activities and research topics for each chapter of the text. The *Computerized Test Bank*, featuring over 1,000 test items, can generate tests and also allows instructors to customize tests and perform online testing. An answer key is included, along with the rationale, cognitive level of each question, corresponding stage of the nursing process, appropriate NCLEX label, and corresponding text page reference. *PowerPoint Slides* offer presentations with more than 200 slides, including four-color images from the text. The Instructor's Resource (CD-ROM) is available free to instructors on adoption of the textbook.

Evolve Course Management System

http://evolve.elsevier.com/Stuart/principles/

Evolve is an interactive learning environment that works in coordination with *Principles and Practice of Psychiatric Nursing, 8th Edition*, providing Internet-based course content that reinforces and expands on the concepts instructors deliver in class. In addition to the resources available to students, instructors are able to access all of the components of the Instructor's Resource, including sample course outlines, a syllabus conversion guide, the Computerized Test Bank, and the PowerPoint Slides.

Instructors can also use Evolve to: publish class syllabi, outline and lecture notes; set up "virtual office hours" and e-mail communication; share important dates and information through the online class *Calendar*; and encourage student participation through *Chat Rooms* and *Discussion Boards*. Instructors are encouraged to contact their sales representative for more information about integrating Evolve into their curriculum.

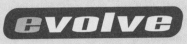

http://evolve.elsevier.com

CONTENTS

The Stuart Stress Adaptation Model of Psychiatric Nursing Care

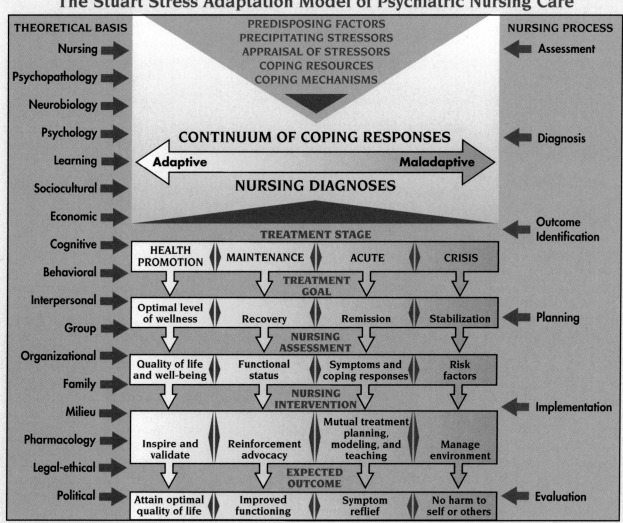

Principles and Practice of
Psychiatric Nursing

8th edition

GAIL WISCARZ STUART, PhD, APRN, BC, FAAN

DEAN AND PROFESSOR, COLLEGE OF NURSING
PROFESSOR, COLLEGE OF MEDICINE
DEPARTMENT OF PSYCHIATRY AND BEHAVIORAL SCIENCES
MEDICAL UNIVERSITY OF SOUTH CAROLINA
CHARLESTON, SOUTH CAROLINA

MICHELE T. LARAIA, PhD, RN, CS

ASSOCIATE PROFESSOR
DIRECTOR, ADVANCED PRACTICE NURSING PROGRAMS
SCHOOL OF NURSING
OREGON HEALTH AND SCIENCE UNIVERSITY
PORTLAND, OREGON

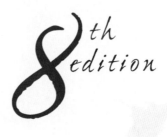

ELSEVIER
MOSBY

ELSEVIER
MOSBY
An Affiliate of Elsevier

11830 Westline Industrial Drive
St. Louis, Missouri 63146

NOTICE

Nursing is an ever-changing field. Standard safety precautions must be followed, but as new research and clinical experience broaden our knowledge, changes in treatment and drug therapy become necessary or appropriate. Readers are advised to check the most current product information provided by the manufacturer of each drug to be administered to verify the recommended dose, the method and duration of administration, and the contraindications. It is the responsibility of the treating licensed prescriber, relying on experience and knowledge of the patient, to determine dosages and the best treatment for the patient. Neither the publisher nor the editor assumes any liability for any injury and/or damage to persons or property arising from this publication.

Previous editions copyrighted 2001, 1998, 1995, 1991, 1987, 1983, 1979 by Mosby, Inc. ·

International Standard Book Number 0-323-02608-7

Acquisitions Editor: Tom Wilhelm
Developmental Editor: Jill Ferguson
Publishing Services Manager: Deborah Vogel
Senior Project Manager: Mary Drone
Senior Book Designer: Julia Dummitt

Printed in China

ABOUT THE AUTHORS

Dr. Gail Stuart is dean and a tenured professor in the College of Nursing and a professor in the College of Medicine in the Department of Psychiatry and Behavioral Sciences at the Medical University of South Carolina. She received her Bachelor of Science degree in nursing from Georgetown University, her Master of Science degree in psychiatric nursing from the University of Maryland, and her doctorate in behavioral sciences from Johns Hopkins University, School of Hygiene and Public Health. She is Board Certified by the American Credentialing Center as a Clinical Specialist in Adult Psychiatric and Mental Health Nursing, a fellow in the American Academy of Nursing, a member of Sigma Theta Tau, president of the American College of Mental Health Administration, a Distinguished Practitioner in the National Academies of Practice, and a past president of the American Psychiatric Nurses Association. She has also been a van Ameringen fellow at the Beck Institute of Cognitive Therapy and Research and is a visiting professor at King's College, Institute of Psychiatry, at the Maudsley in London.

Dr. Stuart's current position at the Medical University of South Carolina is dean of the College of Nursing. Prior to that appointment she was the director of Doctoral Studies and coordinator of the Psychiatric-Mental Health Nursing Graduate Program. She was previously the associate director of the Center for Health Care Research where she worked as a member of an interdisciplinary research team focusing on issues of access, resource utilization, and health care delivery systems. She was also the administrator and chief executive officer of the Institute of Psychiatry at the Medical University, where she was responsible for all clinical, fiscal, and human operations across the continuum of psychiatric care. Dr. Stuart has taught in undergraduate, graduate, and doctoral programs in nursing. She serves on numerous academic, pharmaceutical, and government boards and represents nursing on a variety of National Institute of Mental Health policy and research panels. She is a strong advocate for the specialty and is in great demand to speak and consult both nationally and internationally. She is a prolific writer and has published numerous articles, textbooks, and media productions. She has received many awards, including the American Nurses Association Distinguished Contribution to Psychiatric Nursing Award and the Psychiatric Nurse of the Year Award from the American Psychiatric Nurses Association. Dr. Stuart's clinical and research interests involve the study of depression, anxiety disorders, clinical outcomes, and mental health delivery systems.

Dr. Michele Laraia is an associate professor and director of Advanced Practice Nursing Programs in the School of Nursing at Oregon Health and Science University, Portland, Oregon. She received her Bachelor of Science degree in nursing from D'Youville College, Buffalo, New York; her Master of Science degree in psychiatric mental health nursing from the University of Virginia, Charlottesville, Virginia; and her doctorate in public health at the University of South Carolina, Columbia, South Carolina. Dr. Laraia has more than 25 years' experience in psychiatric mental health nursing, including teaching, conducting research, and treating persons with psychiatric disorders. She has taught at the undergraduate, master's, and doctoral levels of nursing education. She is the Project Director of a grant for the education of psychiatric mental health nurse practitioners in rural Oregon. Her particular areas of expertise include psychobiology and psychopharmacology, for which she has a national reputation in the field. Her research has a focus in the areas of panic and other anxiety disorders, depression, and health services. She specializes in the treatment of persons with mood and anxiety disorders. She is certified as a cognitive therapist from the Beck Institute for Cognitive Therapy and Research. She is also certified as an advanced practice registered nurse by the American Nursing Credentialing Center. Dr. Laraia presents at a variety of psychiatric nursing conferences throughout the United States and has published and produced teaching materials for the psychiatric mental health nursing specialty. She received the American Psychiatric Nurses Association Award for Excellence in Research and has held several national and local consultant and advisory positions. Most notably, Dr. Laraia chaired the American Nurses Association Psychopharmacology Task Force for Psychiatric Mental Health Nurses.

ABOUT THE ARTIST

My life's work is from an aerial perspective, a view of the earth I choose to transcribe onto silk using dyes in the ancient medium of batik. Photographing from the open cockpit of my grandfather's '46 Ercoupe plane with my father or brother as pilot, we explore the natural wonders unaltered by man. Satellite photographs, maps, and charts are often referenced. I observe the health of our planet as an environmental landscape artist.

With appreciation to my patrons whose batiks are shown in this book: Daniel M. Roach, Jr., Gail Stuart, Seth Koch, Marjory S. Aronson, Jeffery L. Prebluda, Pamela and Stan Kaplan, and Karen Lehman.

For more information on Mary Edna Fraser's batiks, go to www.maryedna.com. The artist lives in Charleston, South Carolina.

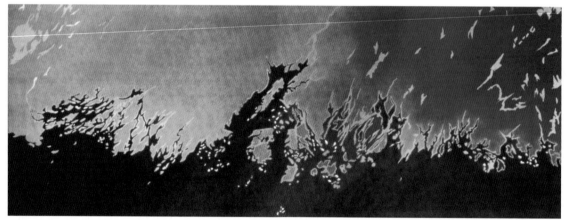

Cover art:
Maine Coastline
41" x 112" batik on silk
1994
Mary Edna Fraser
www.maryedna.com

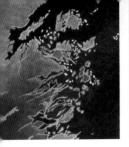

CONTRIBUTORS

Sandra E. Benter, DNSc, ARNP, CS
Psychiatric Nurse Practitioner
Private Practice and Consultation
Boca Raton, Florida

Carol M. Burns, MSN, RN, CS
Electroconvulsive Therapy (ECT) Program Coordinator
Institute of Psychiatry
Medical University of South Carolina
Charleston, South Carolina

Jacquelyn C. Campbell, PhD, RN, FAAN
Anna D. Wolf Endowed Professor
Associate Dean for Faculty Affairs
Johns Hopkins University School of Nursing
Baltimore, Maryland

Penelope Chase, MEd, APRN, BC
Psychiatric Consultation Liaison Nurse
Medical University of South Carolina
Charleston, South Carolina

Carolyn E. Cochrane, PhD, RN, CS
Assistant Professor of Psychiatry
Baylor University College of Medicine;
Director, Eating Disorder Program
Menniger Clinic
Houston, Texas

Victoria Conn, MN, MA, RPRP
Curriculum Consultant
NAMI PA Training Institute
Philadelphia, Pennsylvania

Nancy Fishwick, PhD, APRN, BC
Associate Professor
University of Maine School of Nursing
Orono, Maine;
Family Nurse Practictioner
The Acadia Hospital
Bangor, Maine

Janet A. Grossman, DNSc, CS, RN, FAAN
Associate Professor
College of Nursing
Medical University of South Carolina
Charleston, South Carolina

Christine Diane Hamolia, MS, RN, CS
Advanced Practice Nurse
Institute of Psychiatry
Medical University of South Carolina
Charleston, South Carolina

Therese K. Killeen, PhD, APRN, BC
Assistant Professor
Clinical Neuroscience Division
Institute of Psychiatry
Medical University of South Carolina
Charleston, South Carolina

Arthur J. LaSalle, EDD, LCPC
Consultant, Trainer
Ellicott City, Maryland

Paula M. LaSalle, MSN, RN-P, CS, LCPC
Psychotherapist, Consultant, Trainer
Ellicott City, Maryland

Elizabeth G. Maree, MSN, RN, CS
Director, Behavioral Health Services
Hamilton Medical Center
Dalton, Georgia

Mary D. Moller, MSN, RN, ARNP, BC, CPRP
Clinical Director
Suncrest Wellness Center
Nine Mile Falls, Washington;
Adjunct Instructor of Nursing
Washington State University College of Nursing
Spokane, Washington;
CEO, Psychiatric Resource Network
Nine Mile Falls, Washington;
President, NurSeminars, Inc.
Nine Mile Falls, Washington

Linda D. Oakley, PhD, PMH-NP
Associate Professor
University of Wisconsin—Madison
Madison, Wisconsin

Barbara Parker, PhD, RN, FAAN
Professor and Director of the Doctoral Program
University of Virginia School of Nursing
Charlottesville, Virginia

Susan G. Poorman, PhD, RN, CS
Professor
Department of Nursing and Allied Health Professions
Indiana University of Pennsylvania
Indiana, Pennsylvania

Sally Raphel, MS, APRN/PMH, FAAN
Deputy Director, PAHO/WHO Collaborating Centre for
    Mental Health Nursing
Project Coordinator for Child and Adolescent Graduate
    Nursing
School of Nursing
University of Maryland
Baltimore, Maryland

Audrey Redston-Iselin, MA, RN, CS
Clinical Specialist in Private Practice
White Plains, New York;
Senior Nurse Clinician
Children's Services
Soundview Throgs Neck Community Mental Health Center
Albert Einstein College of Medicine of Yeshiva University
Bronx, New York

Georgia L. Stevens, PhD, APRN, BC
Geropsychiatric Consultant and Therapist
Aftercare Coordinator, Maryland Mental Hygiene
    Administration
Washington, DC

Sandra J. Sundeen, MS, RN
Program Director
Systems Evaluation Center
Mental Health Systems Improvement Collaborative
Department of Psychiatry
University of Maryland School of Medicine
Baltimore, Maryland

REVIEWERS

Florence P. Best, BSN, MEd, RN
Psychiatric Instructor
School of Nursing
Firelands Regional Medical Center
Sandusky, Ohio

Judy A. Glaister, PhD, RN, CS, LMFT, BCETS
Associate Professor
School of Nursing
University of Texas Medical Branch
Galveston, Texas

Mary Ann Glendon, PhD, RN
Associate Professor
Southern Connecticut State University
New Haven, Connecticut

Coleen L. Heckner, MS, APRN, BC
Acadia Hospital
Bangor, Maine

Connie S. Heflin, MSN, RN
Professor
Paducah Community College
Paducah, Kentucky

Rita Butchko Kerr, PhD, RN
Professor of Nursing
Capital University
Columbus, Ohio

Marina Martinez-Kratz, MS, RNC
Assistant Professor of Nursing
Jackson Community College
Jackson, Mississippi

Ann W. Ryan, MSN, RN, C, MPH
Associate Professor
Chesapeake College/MGW Nursing Program
Wye Mills, Maryland

Mary-Margaret Sinclair, MSN, RNC
Instructor
Abilene Intercollegiate School of Nursing
Abilene, Texas

Harriet Wichowski, PhD, RN
Associate Professor of Nursing
University of Tennessee at Chattanooga
Chattanooga, Tennessee

PREFACE

Amazing! It is amazing that the first edition of this textbook was published over 25 years ago in 1979. So what makes a textbook stand the test of time as evident in this 8th edition of *Principles and Practice of Psychiatric Nursing*? We believe such "staying power" is due to clear organization, comprehensive content, engaging format, and contemporary relevancy. Synthesizing the wealth of information in the mental health field gets more challenging with each edition, but the consistent use of the Stuart Stress Adaptation Model and a deliberate focus on evidence-based practice sets this text apart from all others.

This new edition builds on this legacy of excellence. It integrates a holistic biopsychosocial approach to psychiatric nursing care, emphasizing the full continuum of preventive, crisis, and rehabilitative nursing activities and the strong partnerships that psychiatric nurses form with patients and their families. In this edition there is an expanded discussion of stigma, values, and ethical issues, consistent with the movement in the field to a recovery model of psychiatric care. To these elements we have added the latest scientific knowledge on neurobiology, genetics, and psychopharmacology and new information on families, treatment settings, and care of patients with life-threatening illness. The text weaves this content together, providing the reader with the foundation of both contemporary and future psychiatric nursing practice. Once again with this new edition, our goal is to help psychiatric nurses and nursing students stay abreast with state-of-the-art knowledge to foster competent caring in their work with patients and families.

■ CONTENT ORGANIZATION

This book is divided into six units. Unit 1 presents psychiatric nursing principles that are fundamental to practice. First, the contemporary psychiatric nurse's roles and functions are addressed, followed by a chapter on therapeutic relationship skills. Conceptual models of psychiatric treatment, including the Stuart Stress Adaptation Model of Psychiatric Nursing Care, are then presented, as well as an important chapter describing evidence-based psychiatric nursing practice. These are followed by chapters devoted to the biological, psychological, social, cultural, spiritual, environmental, legal, and ethical contexts of practice. Finally, the two ending chapters in this unit focus on families as resources, caregivers, and collaborators and on implementing the nursing process using the American Nurses Association (ANA) professional practice and performance standards.

Unit 2 addresses the continuum of care, including mental health promotion and illness prevention, crisis intervention, and psychiatric rehabilitation and recovery. These topics, unique to this textbook, are more important than ever because health care reform is shifting focus to a public health model of care that is consumer and family driven, using nontraditional settings and a wide range of treatment strategies.

Unit 3 applies psychiatric nursing principles to specific clinical disorders, based on a continuum of adaptive-maladaptive coping responses, the six-step nursing process, the diagnoses of the *Diagnostic and Statistical Manual of Mental Disorders (DSM-IV-TR)* and North American Nursing Diagnosis Association (NANDA), and the Nursing Interventions Classification (NIC) and Nursing Outcomes Classification (NOC) systems. There are separate chapters on anxiety, somatoform and sleep, dissociative, mood, psychotic, personality, substance abuse, eating, sexual, and organic mood disorders, as well as suicidal behavior. The information in this unit has been completely updated and includes all *DSM-IV-TR* diagnostic categories.

Unit 4 describes evidence-based modalities of psychiatric treatment, including chapters on psychopharmacology, somatic therapies, complementary and alternative therapies, preventing and managing aggressive behavior, and cognitive behavioral therapy. Each of these areas is of importance in the field, and together they join with chapters on therapeutic groups and family interventions to round out the repertoire of psychiatric nursing practice.

Unit 5 includes chapters on hospital- and community-based psychiatric nursing care that reflect the most recent developments and current practice in these settings. Although most psychiatric nurses work in hospital settings, the majority of mental health care is provided in the community. Thus knowledge of both settings is critical to the practicing nurse.

Unit 6 concludes the text with a discussion of the unique issues and concerns in the psychiatric treatment of special populations and includes revised chapters on children, adolescents, the elderly, survivors of abuse and violence, and a new chapter on the psychological care of patients with life threatening illness.

■ SPECIAL FEATURES

We hope you are excited about embarking with us on a fascinating journey through the art and science of psychiatric nursing. On the way, look for other signposts and special features that we have included to illuminate your journey. These features are described in the "Special Features" preface that follows.

We wish to communicate our respect for individuals and the roles they enact, regardless of their gender. To that end, we have attempted to avoid pronouns that express bias and to give recognition and support for the commitment of both men and women to the nursing profession. However, this sometimes creates difficult and tedious language for the reader. Therefore, for clarity and simplicity, the nurse is referred to in the third person, female gender, and the patient in the third person, masculine gender, when necessary. It should also be noted that Ms. is used instead of Miss or Mrs. in examples used in the text.

With age comes wisdom. We hope that this 8th edition will add to your growing understanding of mental health and psychiatric care. We invite you now to open the pages beneath your fingers and join us in a world of new ideas, challenging beliefs, and expanding competencies.

GAIL WISCARZ STUART
MICHELE T. LARAIA

SPECIAL FEATURES

Learning Objectives and a **Topical Outline** introduce the basic concepts and organization of the chapter.

Chapter Review Questions assist in mastery of the chapter's content. Answers are provided in Appendix D.

Important information is bolded throughout the text, and new **Chapter Focus Points** at the end of each chapter emphasize critical concepts.

Key Terms are highlighted in color throughout the text, listed at the end of each chapter with page number references, and included in the glossary at the back of the book.

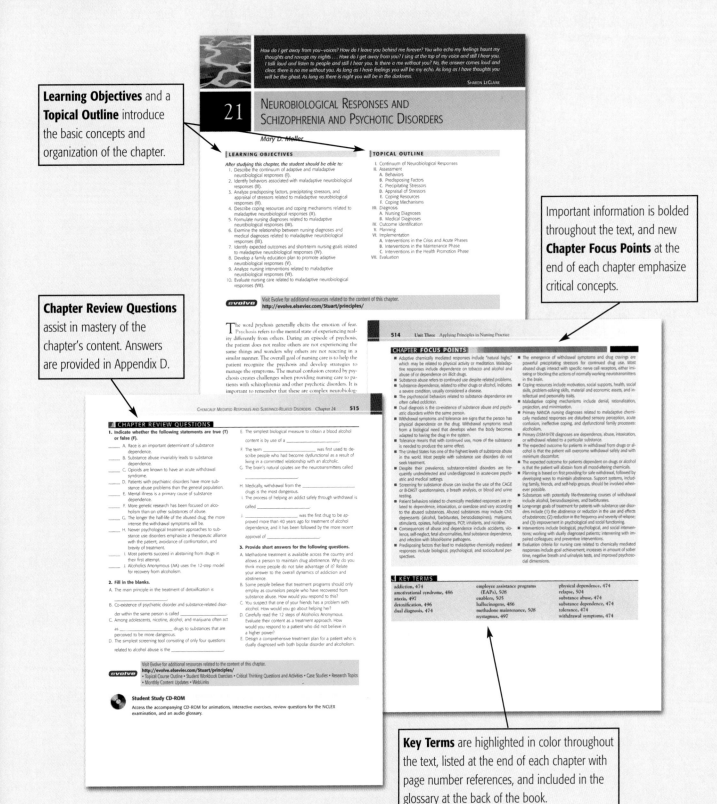

Therapeutic Dialogue boxes provide specific examples of nurse-patient interactions, demonstrating the difference between therapeutic and nontherapeutic communication.

Summarizing the Evidence boxes review treatments that have proven effective for specific disorders.

Critical Thinking About Contemporary Issues boxes present discussions about current, sometimes controversial issues.

Citing the Evidence boxes summarize the background, results, and implications for practice of the latest clinical research studies.

Medical and Nursing Diagnoses boxes and **Detailed Diagnoses** tables present examples of NANDA diagnoses applicable for a specific disorder and describe the essential features of related *DSM-IV-TR* diagnoses.

Patient Education Plans and **Family Education Plans** guide the education of the patient and family about important treatment issues.

The six steps of the nursing process—**Assessment, Diagnosis, Outcome Identification, Planning, Implementation, Evaluation**—are highlighted with special headings in clinical chapters.

Nursing Treatment Plan Summaries guide nursing care related to the treatment of major disorders.

A Patient Speaks and **A Family Speaks** boxes offer a better understanding of the patient's and family's perspectives on treatment.

Critical Thinking Questions throughout each chapter promote independent clinical reasoning and encourage integration of the text material with an individual's understanding of the world and nursing.

Clinical Examples are taken from actual clinical situations. Many provide samples of nursing diagnoses related to the particular clinical situation.

Competent Caring: A Clinical Exemplar of a Psychiatric Nurse are featured boxes written by practicing psychiatric nurses who share their clinical experiences and personal insights.

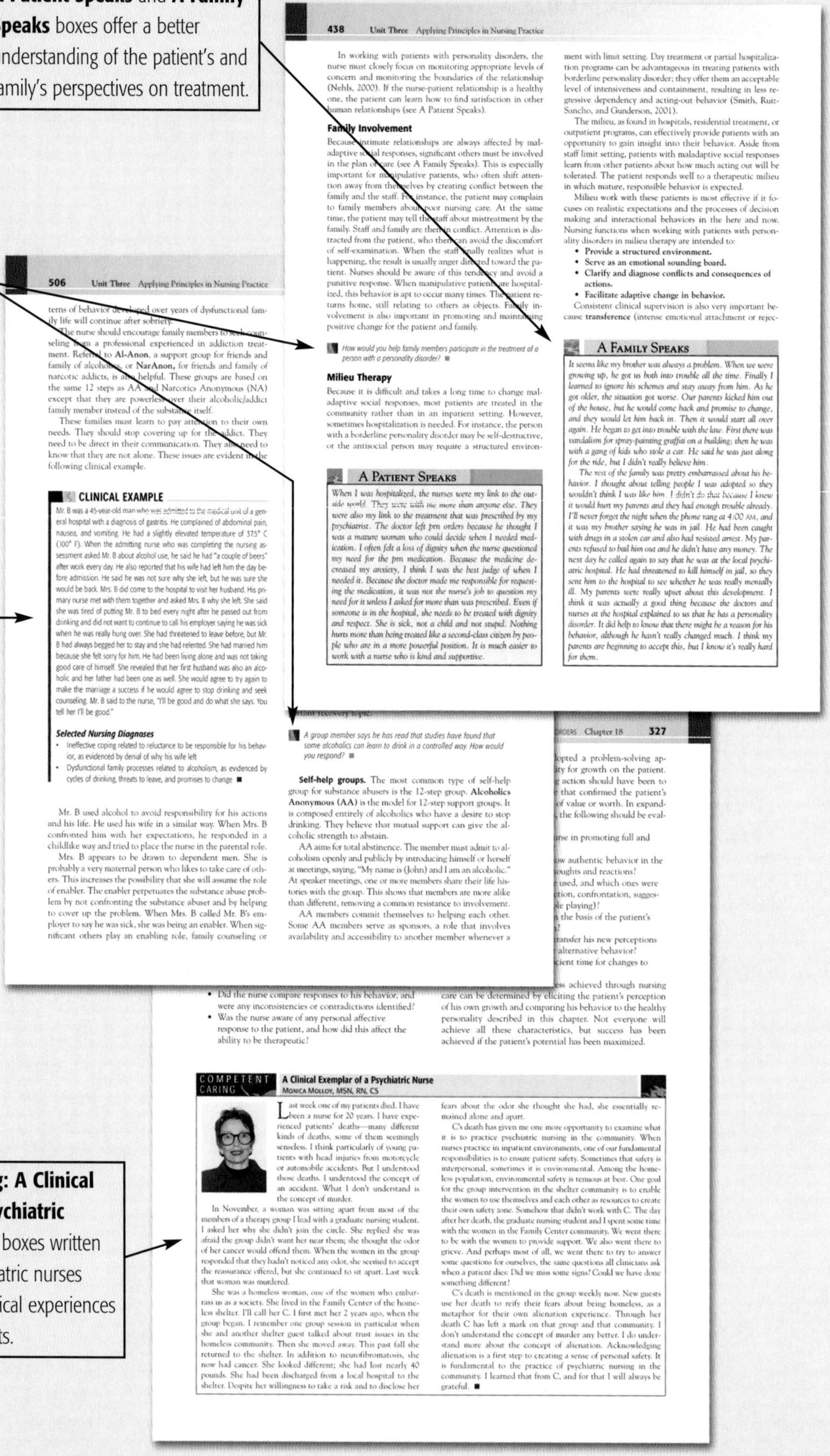

---

438 Unit Three Applying Principles in Nursing Practice

In working with patients with personality disorders, the nurse must closely focus on monitoring appropriate levels of concern and monitoring the boundaries of the relationship (Nehls, 2000). If the nurse-patient relationship is a healthy one, the patient can learn how to find satisfaction in other human relationships (see A Patient Speaks).

Family Involvement

Because intimate relationships are always affected by maladaptive social responses, significant others must be involved in the plan of care (see A Family Speaks). This is especially important for manipulative patients, who often shift attention away from themselves by creating conflict between the family and the staff. For instance, the patient may complain to family members about poor nursing care. At the same time, the patient may tell the staff about mistreatment by the family. Staff and family are then in conflict. Attention is distracted from the patient, who then can avoid the discomfort of self-examination. When the staff readily realizes what is happening, the result is usually anger directed toward the patient. Nurses should be aware of this tendency and avoid a punitive response. When manipulative patients are hospitalized, this behavior is apt to occur many times. The patient returns home, still relating to others as objects. Finally, involvement is also important in promoting and maintaining positive change for the patient and family.

How would you help family members participate in the treatment of a person with a personality disorder? ■

Milieu Therapy

Because it is difficult and takes a long time to change maladaptive social responses, most patients are treated in the community rather than in an inpatient setting. However, sometimes hospitalization is needed. For instance, the person with a borderline personality disorder may be self-destructive, or the antisocial person may require a structured environ-

ment with limit setting. Day treatment or partial hospitalization programs can be advantageous in treating patients with borderline personality disorder; they offer them an acceptable level of intensiveness and containment, resulting in less regressive dependency and acting-out behavior (Smith, Ruiz-Sancho, and Gunderson, 2001).

The milieu, as found in hospitals, residential treatment, or outpatient programs, can effectively provide patients with an opportunity to gain insight into their behavior. Aside from staff limit setting, patients with maladaptive social responses learn from other patients about how much acting out will be tolerated. The patient responds well to a therapeutic milieu in which mature, responsible behavior is expected.

Milieu work with these patients is most effective if it focuses on realistic expectations and the processes of decision making and interactional behaviors in the here and now. Nursing functions when working with patients with personality disorders in milieu therapy are intended to:

- **Provide a structured environment.**
- **Serve as an emotional sounding board.**
- **Clarify and diagnose conflicts and consequences of actions.**
- **Facilitate adaptive change in behavior.**

Consistent clinical supervision is also very important because **transference** (intense emotional attachment or rejec-

A FAMILY SPEAKS

It seems like my brother was always a problem. When we were growing up, he got us both into trouble all the time. Finally I learned to ignore his schemes and stay away from him. As he got older, the situation got worse. Our parents kicked him out of the house, but he would come back and promise to change, and they would let him back in. Then it would start all over again. He began to get into trouble with the law. First there was vandalism for spray-painting graffiti on a building; then he was with a gang of kids who stole a car. He said he was just along for the ride, but I didn't really believe him.

The rest of the family was pretty embarrassed about his behavior. I thought about telling people I was adopted so they wouldn't think I was like him. I didn't do that because I knew it would hurt my parents and they had enough trouble already. I'll never forget the night when the phone rang at 4:00 AM, and it was my brother saying he was in jail. He had been caught with drugs in a stolen car and also had resisted arrest. My parents refused to bail him out and he didn't have any money. The next day he called again to say that he was at the local psychiatric hospital. He had threatened to kill himself in jail, so they sent him to the hospital to see whether he was really mentally ill. My parents were really upset about this development. I think it was actually a good thing because the doctors and nurses at the hospital explained to us that he has a personality disorder. It did help to know that there might be a reason for his behavior, although he hasn't really changed much. I think my parents are beginning to accept this, but I know it's really hard for them.

---

506 Unit Three Applying Principles in Nursing Practice

terms of behavior developed over years of dysfunctional family life will continue after sobriety.

The nurse should encourage family members to seek counseling from a professional experienced in addiction treatment. Referral to Al-Anon, a support group for friends and family of alcoholics, or NarAnon, for friends and family of narcotic addicts, is also helpful. These groups are based on the same 12 steps as AA and Narcotics Anonymous (NA) except that they are powerless over their alcoholic/addict family member instead of the substance itself.

These families must learn to pay attention to their own needs. They should stop covering up for the addict. They need to be direct in their communication. They also need to know that they are not alone. These issues are evident in the following clinical example.

CLINICAL EXAMPLE

Mr. B was a 45-year-old man who was admitted to the medical unit of a general hospital with a diagnosis of gastritis. He complained of abdominal pain, nausea, and vomiting. He had a slightly elevated temperature of 37.5° C (100° F). When the admitting nurse was completing the nursing assessment asked Mr. B about alcohol use, he said he had "a couple of beers" after work every day. He also reported that his wife had left him the day before admission. He said he was not sure why she left, but he was sure she would be back. Mrs. B did come to the hospital to visit her husband. His primary nurse met with them together and asked Mrs. B why she left. She said she was tired of putting Mr. B to bed every night after he passed out from drinking and did not want to continue to call his employer saying he was sick when he was really hung over. She had threatened to leave before, but Mr. B had always begged her to stay and she had relented. She had married him because she felt sorry for him. He had been living alone and was not taking good care of himself. She revealed that her first husband was also an alcoholic and her father had been one as well. She would agree to try again to make the marriage a success if he would agree to stop drinking and seek counseling. Mr. B said to the nurse, "I'll be good and do what she says. You tell her I'll be good."

Selected Nursing Diagnoses

- Ineffective coping related to reluctance to be responsible for his behavior, as evidenced by denial of why his wife left
- Dysfunctional family processes related to alcoholism, as evidenced by cycles of drinking, threats to leave, and promises to change ■

Mr. B used alcohol to avoid responsibility for his actions and his life. He used his wife in a similar way. When Mrs. B confronted him with her expectations, he responded in a childlike way and tried to place the nurse in the parental role. Mrs. B appears to be drawn to dependent men. She is probably a very maternal person who likes to take care of others. This increases the possibility that she will assume the role of enabler. The enabler perpetuates the substance abuse problem by not confronting the substance abuser and by helping to cover up the problem. When Mrs. B called Mr. B's employer to say he was sick, she was being an enabler. When significant others play an enabling role, family counseling or

A PATIENT SPEAKS

When I was hospitalized, the nurses were my link to the outside world. They were with me more than anyone else. They were also my link to the treatment that was prescribed by my psychiatrist. The doctor left prn orders because he thought I was a mature woman who could decide when I needed medication. I often felt a loss of dignity when the nurse questioned my need for the prn medication. Because the medicine decreased my anxiety, I think I was the best judge of when I needed it. Because the doctor made me responsible for requesting the medication, it was not the nurse's job to question my need for it unless I asked for more than was prescribed. Even if someone is in the hospital, she needs to be treated with dignity and respect. She is sick, not a child and not stupid. Nothing hurts more than being treated like a second-class citizen by people who are in a more powerful position. It is much easier to work with a nurse who is kind and supportive.

A group member says he has read that studies have found that some alcoholics can learn to drink in a controlled way. How would you respond? ■

Self-help groups. The most common type of self-help group for substance abusers is the 12-step group. **Alcoholics Anonymous (AA)** is the model for 12-step support groups. It is composed entirely of alcoholics who have a desire to stop drinking. They believe that mutual support can give the alcoholic strength to abstain.

AA aims for total abstinence. The member must admit to alcoholism openly and publicly by introducing himself or herself at meetings, saying, "My name is (John) and I am an alcoholic." At speaker meetings, one or more members share their life histories with the group. This shows that members are more alike than different, removing a common resistance to involvement.

AA members commit themselves to helping each other. Some AA members serve as sponsors, a role that involves availability and accessibility to another member whenever a

---

DISORDERS Chapter 18 **327**

adopted a problem-solving approach for growth on the patient. action should have been to that confirmed the patient's of value or worth. In expanding, the following should be evaluated:

nse in promoting full and

in the for authentic behavior in the thoughts and reactions? be used, and which ones were ction, confrontation, suggesle playing?

n the basis of the patient's

ransfer his new perceptions alternative behavior? ient time for changes to

sss achieved through nursing

care can be determined by eliciting the patient's perception of his own growth and comparing his behavior to the healthy personality described in this chapter. Not everyone will achieve all these characteristics, but success has been achieved if the patient's potential has been maximized.

- Did the nurse compare responses to his behavior, and were any inconsistencies or contradictions identified?
- Was the nurse aware of any personal affective response to the patient, and how did this affect the ability to be therapeutic?

A Clinical Exemplar of a Psychiatric Nurse
MONICA MOLLOY, MSN, RN, CS

Last week one of my patients died. I have been a nurse for 20 years. I have experienced patients' deaths—many different kinds of deaths, some of them seemingly senseless. I think particularly of young patients with head injuries from motorcycle or automobile accidents. But I understood those deaths. I understood the concept of an accident. What I don't understand is the concept of murder.

In November, a woman was sitting apart from most of the members of a therapy group I lead with a graduate nursing student. I asked her why she didn't join the circle. She replied she was afraid the group didn't want her near them; she thought the odor of her cancer would offend them. When the women in the group responded that they hadn't noticed any odor, she seemed to accept the reassurance offered, but she continued to sit apart. Last week that woman was murdered.

She was a homeless woman, one of the women who embarrass us as a society. She lived in the Family Center of the homeless shelter. I'll call her C. I first met her 2 years ago, when the group began. I remember one group session in particular when she and another shelter guest talked about trust issues in the homeless community. Then she moved away. This past fall she returned to the shelter. In addition to neurofibromatosis, she now had cancer. She looked different; she had lost nearly 40 pounds. She had been discharged from a local hospital to the shelter. Despite her willingness to take a risk and to disclose her

fears about the odor she thought she had, she essentially remained alone and apart.

C's death has given me one more opportunity to examine what it is to practice psychiatric nursing in the community. When nurses practice in inpatient environments, one of our fundamental responsibilities is to ensure patient safety. Sometimes that safety is interpersonal, sometimes it is environmental. Among the homeless population, environmental safety is tenuous at best. One goal for the group intervention in the shelter community is to enable the women to see themselves and each other as resources to create their own safety zone. Somehow that didn't work with C. The day after her death, the graduate nursing student and I spent some time with the women in the Family Center community. We went there to be with the women to provide support. We also went there to grieve. And perhaps most of all, we went there to try to answer some questions for ourselves, the same questions all clinicians ask when a patient dies: Could we have done something different?

C's death is mentioned in the group weekly now. New guests use her death to reify their fears about being homeless, as a metaphor for their own alienation experience. Through her death C has left a mark on that group and that community. I don't understand the concept of murder any better. I do understand more about the concept of alienation. Acknowledging alienation is a first step to creating a sense of personal safety. It is fundamental to the practice of psychiatric nursing in the community. I learned that from C, and for that I will always be grateful. ■

CONTENTS

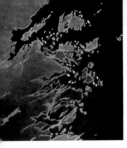

Unit Four

Treatment Modalities

Unit Six

Special Populations in Psychiatry

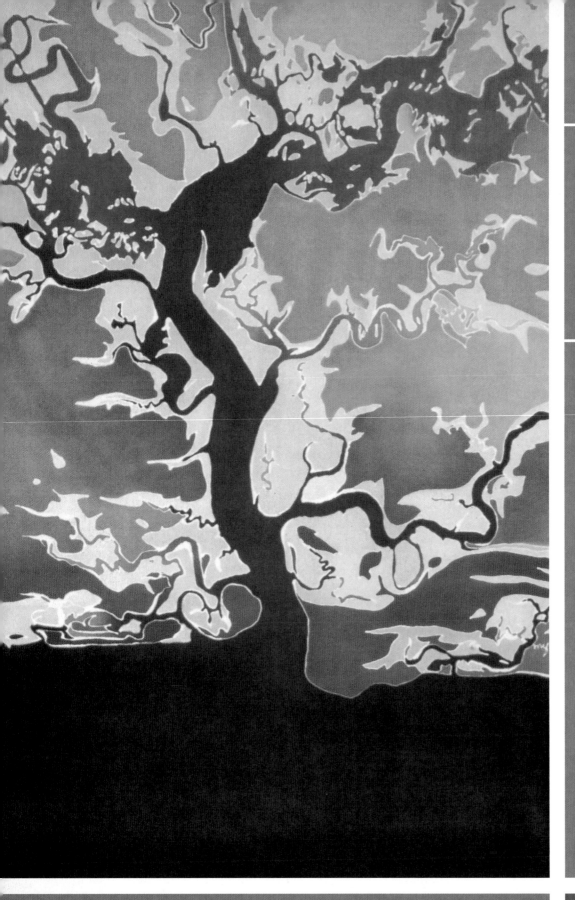

Unit One

North Edisto (SC)
39" × 36" batik on silk, 1996

Artist's Note: This was a commission for a wedding gift from the bride for her future husband. After a good bit of interrogative conversation, she and I knew we had found the landscape closest to his heart. Patience and prayers for their new life together are part of this batik designed from a nautical chart.

Principles of Psychiatric Nursing Care

You are about to begin a voyage to places you have never been before: the world of psychiatric and mental health nursing. In the old days of nursing, students learned about pieces of people—an infected toe, a congested lung, a troubling twitch, or maybe even a broken heart—but pieces nonetheless. Today, students learn about the wholeness of people: a physically ill child struggling to find safety in an abusive family, an adolescent coping with eating problems and self-esteem, a young adult grieving over the diagnosis of HIV/AIDS, or an elder, living alone, feeling confused and disoriented at times and yet frightened at the thought of going to a nursing home. This is the exciting world of today's psychiatric nurse. It integrates the biological, psychological, sociocultural, environmental, legal, and ethical realities of life and weaves them together in a rich tapestry called *psychiatric nursing practice*.

This unit introduces you to parts of this world that may be new to you. It will help you explore how patients think, feel, and behave. It will help you learn how to talk with patients and families as partners in the caregiving process. It will suggest that you think about people in terms of their overall functioning and adaptation rather than by the symptoms of their specific illness. Most importantly, it will define for you the responsibilities you have as a professional health care provider. We hope you are ready to begin your journey, and we wish you curiosity about human nature, openness to new ways of thinking, and delight in the process of learning.

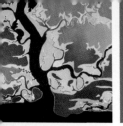

To be what we are, and to become what we are capable of becoming, is the only end of life.

ROBERT L. STEVENSON

1 ROLES AND FUNCTIONS OF PSYCHIATRIC NURSES: COMPETENT CARING

Gail W. Stuart

LEARNING OBJECTIVES

After studying this chapter, the student should be able to:

1. Describe the evolution of the psychiatric nursing role and functions (I).
2. Discuss the nature, settings, and functions of contemporary psychiatric nursing practice (II).
3. Analyze the factors that influence the psychiatric nurse's level of performance (III).
4. Critique areas of importance for psychiatric nursing's future agenda (IV).

TOPICAL OUTLINE

 Visit Evolve for additional resources related to the content of this chapter.
http://evolve.elsevier.com/Stuart/principles/

Nursing, or caring for the sick, has existed since the beginning of civilization. Before 1860 the emphasis in psychiatric institutions was on custodial care, and attendants were hired to maintain control of the patients. Often these attendants were little more than jailers who had little training, and the psychiatric care was poor. Nursing as a profession began to emerge in the late nineteenth century, and by the twentieth century it had evolved into a specialty with unique roles and functions.

■ HISTORICAL PERSPECTIVES

In 1873 Linda Richards graduated from the New England Hospital for Women and Children in Boston. She developed better nursing care in psychiatric hospitals and organized nursing services and educational programs in state mental hospitals in Illinois. For these activities, **Linda Richards** is called the first American psychiatric nurse. Basic to Richards' theory of care was her statement, "It stands to reason that the mentally sick should be at least as well cared for as the physically sick" (Doona, 1984).

The first school to prepare nurses to care for the mentally ill opened at McLean Hospital in Waverly, Massachusetts, in 1882. It was a 2-year program and the care was mainly custodial, focused on the patients' physical needs, such as medica-

tions, nutrition, hygiene, and ward activities. Until the end of the nineteenth century, little changed in the role of psychiatric nurses. They had limited training in psychiatry, and they primarily applied the principles of medical-surgical nursing to the psychiatric setting. At that time, psychological care consisted of kindness and tolerance toward the patients.

One of Linda Richards' more important contributions was her emphasis on assessing both the physical and emotional needs of the patients. In this early period of nursing history, nursing education separated these two needs; nurses were taught either in the general hospital or in the psychiatric hospital. In 1913 Johns Hopkins became the first school of nursing to include a fully developed course for psychiatric nursing in the curriculum. Other schools soon followed. It was not until the late 1930s that nursing education recognized the importance of psychiatric knowledge in general nursing care for all illnesses (Box 1-1).

An important factor in the development of psychiatric nursing was the emergence of various somatic therapies, including insulin shock therapy (1935), psychosurgery (1936), and electroconvulsive therapy (1937). These techniques all required the medical-surgical skills of nurses. Although these therapies did not help the patient understand his or her problems, they did control behavior and make the patient more amenable to psychotherapy. Somatic therapies also increased

Evolutionary Timeline in Psychiatric Nursing

SOCIAL ENVIRONMENT	DATE	PSYCHIATRIC NURSING
	1873	Linda Richards graduated from New England Hospital for Women and Children
	1882	First school to prepare nurses to care for the mentally ill opened at McLean Hospital in Massachusetts
American Journal of Nursing first published	1900	
Florence Nightingale died	1910	
	1913	Johns Hopkins was first school of nursing to include a course on psychiatric nursing in its curriculum
Electroconvulsive therapy developed	1937	
National Mental Health Act passed by Congress, creating National Institute of Mental Health (NIMH) and providing training funds for psychiatric nursing education	1946	
	1950	National League for Nursing (NLN) required that to be accredited schools of nursing must provide an experience in psychiatric nursing
	1952	Hildegard Peplau published *Interpersonal Relations in Nursing*
Maxwell Jones published *The Therapeutic Community*	1953	
Development of major tranquilizers	1954	
Community Mental Health Centers Act passed	1963	*Perspectives in Psychiatric Care* published; *Journal of Psychiatric Nursing and Mental Health Services* published
	1973	*Standards of Psychiatric–Mental Health Nursing Practice* published; certification of psychiatric–mental health nurse generalist established by American Nurses Association (ANA)
Report of the President's Commission on Mental Health	1978	
	1979	*Issues in Mental Health Nursing* published; certification of psychiatric–mental health nurse specialists established by ANA First edition of *Principles and Practice of Psychiatric Nursing* published (Stuart and Sundeen)
Nursing: A Social Policy Statement published by ANA	1980	
National Center for Nursing Research created in National Institutes of Health (NIH)	1985	*Standards of Child and Adolescents Psychiatric and Mental Health Nursing Practice* published by ANA
	1986	American Psychiatric Nurses Association (APNA) established
	1987	*Archives of Psychiatric Nursing* published; *Journal of Child and Adolescent Psychiatric and Mental Health Nursing* published
	1988	*Standards of Addictions Nursing Practice* published by ANA
	1990	*Standards of Psychiatric Consultation Liaison Nursing Practice* published by ANA
Center for Mental Health Services created	1992	
	1994	
		Revised Standards of Psychiatric–Mental Health Clinical Nursing Practice published by ANA *Psychopharmacology Guidelines for Psychiatric–Mental Health Nurses* published by ANA
Revised *Nursing Social Policy Statement* published by ANA	1995	*Journal of the American Psychiatric Nurses Association (JAPNA)* published
Report of the Surgeon General on Mental Health	1999	Hildegard Peplau died
	2000	
		Revised Scope and Standards of Psychiatric–Mental Health Clinical Nursing Practice published by ANA
	2001	
Report of the President's New Freedom Commission on Mental Health	2003	Certification of Psychiatric Nurse Practitioners by ANA

A Nurse Speaks

We do not hesitate to emphasize the need of some psychiatric training in the life of every nurse who would represent her profession on the basis of modern standards. The psychiatrically trained nurse must remember, on the other hand, that all symptoms are not of mental origin. This fact has been long recognized, so nurses trained in mental hospitals have wisely requested affiliation in general hospitals, thus avoiding the danger of overspecialization. Does it not seem rational, therefore, that the general hospital shall guarantee its nurse an equivalent knowledge of the workings of the patient's mind as the psychiatric nurse has of the workings of his body? Modern psychology reveals the close interrelation of the two; it recognizes the ceaseless interaction of one on the other. Should we not then more consistently work toward the ideal that every hospital shall graduate nurses trained in preventive and curative methods of caring for the inevitably associated physically and mentally ill?

Annie L. Crawford, RN, BS
South Carolina Nurses' Association
Annual Convention Presentation
October 6, 1934

A Physician Speaks

I have spent all of my professional career in close association with, and close dependency on, nurses, and like many of my faculty colleagues, I've done a lot of worrying about the relationship between medicine and nursing.

The doctors worry that nurses are trying to move away from their historical responsibilities to medicine (meaning, really, to the doctors' orders). The nurses assert that they are their own profession, responsible for their own standards, coequal colleagues with physicians, and they do not wish to become mere ward administrators or technicians.

My discovery as a patient is that the institution is held together, *glued* together, enabled to function as an organism, by the nurses and by nobody else.

The nurses make it their business to know everything that is going on. They spot errors before errors can be launched. They know everything written on the chart. Most important of all, they know their patients as unique human beings, and they soon get to know the close relatives and friends. Because of this knowledge, they are quick to sense apprehensions and act on them. The average sick person in a large hospital feels at risk of getting lost, with no identity left beyond a name and a string of numbers on a plastic wristband, in danger always of being whisked off on a litter to the wrong place to have the wrong procedure done, or worse still, *not* being whisked off at the right time. The attending physician or the house officer, on rounds and usually in a hurry, can murmur a few reassuring words on his way out the door, but it takes a confident, competent, and cheerful nurse, there all day long and in and out of the room on one chore or another through the night, to bolster one's confidence that the situation is indeed manageable and not about to get out of hand.

Knowing what I know, I am all for the nurses. If they are to continue their professional feud with the doctors, if they want their professional status enhanced and their pay increased, if they infuriate the doctors by their claims to be equal professionals, if they ask for the moon, I am on their side.

Lewis Thomas, MD
The Youngest Science
New York, 1983, Viking Press

the demand for improved psychological treatment for patients who did not respond.

As nurses became more involved with somatic therapies, they began the struggle to define their role as psychiatric nurses. An editorial in the *American Journal of Nursing* in 1940 described the conflict between nurses and physicians as nurses tried to implement what they saw as appropriate care for psychiatric patients. This conflict continues to demand attention in current nursing practice (Box 1-2).

The period after World War II was one of major growth and change in psychiatric nursing. Because of the large number of military service–related psychiatric problems and the increase in treatment programs offered by the Veterans Administration, psychiatric nurses with advanced preparation were in demand. The content of psychiatric nursing had by then become an integral part of the generic nursing curriculum. Its principles were applied to other areas of nursing practice, including general medical, pediatric, and public health nursing. By 1947 eight graduate programs in psychiatric nursing had been started.

Role Emergence

The role of psychiatric nursing began to emerge in the early 1950s. In 1947 Weiss published an article in the *American Journal of Nursing* that reemphasized the shortage of psychiatric nurses and outlined the differences between psychiatric and general duty nurses. She described "attitude therapy" as the nurse's directed use of attitudes that contribute to the patient's recovery. In implementing this therapy, the nurse observes the patient for small and fleeting changes; demonstrates acceptance, respect, and understanding of the patient; and promotes the patient's interest and participation in reality.

An article by Bennett and Eaton in the *American Journal of Psychiatry* in 1951 identified the following problems affecting psychiatric nurses:

1. Scarcity of qualified psychiatric nurses
2. Underuse of their abilities
3. The fact that "very little real psychiatric nursing is carried out in otherwise good psychiatric hospitals and units"

These psychiatrists believed that the psychiatric nurse should join mental health societies, consult with welfare agencies, work in outpatient clinics, practice preventive psychiatry, engage in research, and help educate the public. They supported the nurse's participation in individual and group psychotherapy and stated, "Despite the fact that most psychiatrists seem to ignore the role of the psychiatric nurse in psychotherapy, all nurses in psychiatric wards do psychotherapy of one kind or another by their contacts with patients" (Bennett and Eaton, 1951). Many of the issues raised in the article were debated years later.

Do you think that the problems affecting psychiatric nurses described by Bennett and Eaton in 1951 continue to exist in the specialty today? ■

Also in 1951 Mellow wrote of the work she did with schizophrenic patients. She called these activities "nursing therapy." A year later, Tudor (Tudor, 1952) published a study in which she described the nurse-patient relationships she established, which were characterized by unconditional care, few demands, and the anticipation of her patients' needs. These articles were some of the earliest descriptions by psychiatric nurses of the nurse-patient relationship and the nature of its therapeutic process.

As nurses engaged in these kinds of activities, many questions arose. Are these activities therapeutic or are they therapy? What is a therapeutic relationship or a one-to-one nurse-patient relationship? How does it differ from psychotherapy? These questions were addressed by Dr. Hildegard Peplau, a dynamic nursing leader whose ideas and beliefs shaped psychiatric nursing.

In 1952 Peplau published a book, *Interpersonal Relations in Nursing,* in which she described the first theoretical framework for psychiatric nursing and the specific skills, activities, and roles of psychiatric nurses. Peplau defined nursing as a "significant, therapeutic process." While she studied the nursing process, she saw nurses emerge in various roles: as a resource person; a teacher; a leader in local, national, and international situations; a surrogate parent; and a counselor. She wrote, "Counseling in nursing has to do with helping the patient remember and to understand fully what is happening to him in the present situation, so that the experience can be integrated with rather than dissociated from other experiences in life" (Peplau, 1952).

Compare the roles of psychiatric nurses identified by Hildegard Peplau in 1952 with your observations of contemporary psychiatric nursing practice. ■

Two other significant developments in psychiatry in the 1950s also affected nursing's role for years to come. The first was Jones' publication of *The Therapeutic Community: A New Treatment Method in Psychiatry* in 1953. This method encouraged using the patient's social environment to provide a therapeutic experience. The premise of the therapeutic community was that each patient was to be an active participant in care, become involved in the daily problems of the unit, and help solve problems, plan activities, and develop the required unit rules. Therapeutic communities became the preferred environment for psychiatric patients.

The second significant development in psychiatry in the early 1950s was the use of **psychotropic drugs.** With these drugs more patients became treatable, and fewer environmental constraints such as locked doors and straitjackets were required. Also, more personnel were needed to provide therapy, and the roles of various psychiatric practitioners were expanded, including the nurse's role.

Evolving Functions

In 1958 the following functions of psychiatric nurses were described (Hays, 1975):

- Dealing with patients' problems of attitude, mood, and interpretation of reality
- Exploring disturbing and conflicting thoughts and feelings
- Using the patient's positive feelings toward the therapist to bring about psychophysiological homeostasis
- Counseling patients in emergencies, including panic and fear
- Strengthening the well part of patients

The nurse-patient relationship was referred to by a variety of terms, including "therapeutic nurse-patient relationship," "psychiatric nursing therapy," "supportive psychotherapy," "rehabilitation therapies," and "nondirective counseling." The distinction between these terms and the exact nature of the nurse's role remained hazy.

Once again Peplau clarified psychiatric nursing's position and directed its future growth. In *Interpersonal Techniques: the Crux of Psychiatric Nursing,* published in 1962, Peplau identified the heart of psychiatric nursing as the role of **counselor** or psychotherapist. In her article, she differentiated between general practitioners who were staff nurses working on psychiatric units and psychiatric nurses who were specialists and expert clinical practitioners with graduate degrees in psychiatric nursing. Thus from an undefined role involving primarily physical care, psychiatric nursing was evolving into a role of clinical competence based on interpersonal techniques and use of the nursing process. For her considerable contributions to the specialty, **Hildegard Peplau** is often called the mother of psychiatric nursing.

In the 1960s the focus of psychiatric nursing began to shift to **primary prevention** and implementation of **care and consultation in the community.** Representative of these changes was the shift in the name of the field from "psychiatric nursing" to "psychiatric and mental health nursing." This focus was stimulated by the Community Mental Health Centers Act of 1963, which made federal money available to states to plan, construct, and staff community mental health centers. This legislation was prompted by growing awareness of the value of treating people in the community and preventing hospitalization whenever possible. It also encouraged the formation of multidisciplinary treatment teams by combining the skills of many professions to alleviate illness and promote mental health. This team approach continues to be negotiated. The issues of territoriality, professionalism, authority structure, consumer rights, and the use of paraprofessionals are still being debated.

The 1970s gave rise to the further development of the specialty. Psychiatric nurses became the pacesetters in specialty nursing practice. They were the first to:

- Develop standards and statements on scope of practice.
- Establish generalist and specialist certification.

At this same time, the nursing profession was defining caring as a core element of all nursing practice, and the contributions of psychiatric nurses were embraced by nurses of all specialty groups.

Partly as a result of this broader definition of psychiatric nursing and the perceived skills of psychiatric nurses, nursing education reorganized its curriculum and began to integrate psychiatric nursing content into nonpsychiatric courses. This blending of content was evident in the second change in the name of the field in the 1970s from "psychiatric and mental health nursing" to "psychosocial nursing." Clinical rotations focusing on the psychiatric illnesses of patients in psychiatric settings were often replaced by clinical rotations integrating psychosocial aspects of the care of physically ill patients in general medical-surgical units. Unfortunately, this trend often did not provide students with an opportunity to care for patients with psychiatric illnesses and learn about new information that was emerging in the field of psychiatry and the broader behavioral sciences.

It has been suggested that psychiatric nursing content can be learned by taking care of patients in medical-surgical settings because patients in these settings have depression, anxiety, and other psychiatric problems as well. How do the problems of these patients differ from those experienced by psychiatric patients? Patients in psychiatric settings have diabetes, cancer, heart disease, and other medical problems, the same as patients in medical-surgical settings. If there are no differences, why couldn't medical-surgical nursing content be learned by taking care of psychiatric patients? ■

The 1980s were years of exciting scientific growth in the area of psychobiology. New focus was placed on:

- Brain imaging techniques.
- Neurotransmitters and neuronal receptors.
- Psychobiology of emotions.
- Understanding the brain.
- Molecular genetics related to psychobiology.

Although this information explosion advanced knowledge in the field, it lacked integration and was often of limited clinical usefulness. It was also noted that psychiatric nurses in the 1980s were slow to make the shift away from primarily psychodynamic models of the mind to more balanced psychobiological models of psychiatric care (Pothier et al, 1990; Abraham, Fox, and Cohen, 1992).

Psychiatric nurses thus entered the 1990s faced with the challenge of integrating the expanding bases of neuroscience into the holistic biopsychosocial practice of psychiatric nursing. Advances in understanding the relationships of the brain, behavior, emotion, and cognition offered new opportunities for psychiatric nursing (Hayes, 1995). Psychiatric nurses saw the need to become realigned with care and car-

ing, which represent the art of psychiatric nursing and complement the high technology of current health care practices (McBride, 1996).

The new millennium brought with it issues of balance, differentiation, and integration, along with the understanding that the knowledge base of the specialty is based on the integration of the biological, psychological, spiritual, social, and environmental realms of the human experience. As Flaskerud and Wuerker (1999) note: "The philosophical and ethical challenge to nursing is to integrate the biological and behavioral concepts into the nursing care of mentally ill people while remaining centered in the nursing domain and maintaining our focus on caring and our sensitivity to the human condition."

Compare the length of your clinical rotation in psychiatric nursing with your "clinicals" in medicine, surgery, and pediatrics. Given the high prevalence of mental health problems such as depression and substance abuse, do you feel your educational opportunities provide sufficient learning time in psychiatric nursing? ■

■ CONTEMPORARY PRACTICE

Psychiatric nursing is an interpersonal process that promotes and maintains patient behavior that contributes to integrated functioning. The patient may be an individual, family, group, organization, or community. The American Nurses Association *Scope and Standards of Psychiatric–Mental Health Nursing Practice* defines psychiatric nursing as "a specialized area of nursing practice, employing the wide range of explanatory theories of human behavior as its science and purposeful use of self as its art" (American Nurses Association, 2000). The Center for Mental Health Services officially recognizes psychiatric nursing as one of the five core mental health disciplines. The other four disciplines are marriage and family therapy, psychiatry, psychology, and social work.

The current practice of psychiatric nursing is based on a number of underlying premises or beliefs. The philosophical beliefs of psychiatric nursing practice on which this text is based are described in Box 1-3. The psychiatric nurse uses knowledge from the psychosocial and biophysical sciences and theories of personality and human behavior. From these sources the nurse derives a theoretical framework on which to base nursing practice. Various models of psychiatric treatment are described in Chapter 3. Chapter 4 presents the Stuart Stress Adaptation Model of psychiatric nursing care that is used as the organizing framework for this text.

The contemporary practice of psychiatric nursing occurs within a social and environmental context (see Critical Thinking About Contemporary Issues). Thus the "nurse-patient relationship" has evolved into a "nurse-patient partnership" that expands the dimensions of the professional psychiatric nursing role. These elements include **clinical competence, patient-family advocacy, fiscal responsibility, interdisciplinary collaboration, social accountability,** and **legal-ethical parameters** (Figure 1-1).

BOX 1-3

Philosophical Beliefs of Psychiatric Nursing Practice

The individual has intrinsic worth and dignity and each person is worthy of respect.

The goal of the individual is one of growth, health, autonomy, and self-actualization.

Every individual has the potential to change.

Each person functions as a holistic being who acts on, interacts with, and reacts to the environment as a whole person.

All people have common, basic human needs. These needs include physical requirements, safety, love, belonging, esteem, and self-actualization.

All behavior of the individual is meaningful. It arises from personal needs and goals and can be understood only from the person's internal frame of reference and within the context in which it occurs.

Behavior consists of perceptions, thoughts, feelings, and actions. From one's perceptions thoughts arise, emotions are felt, and actions are conceived. Disruptions may occur in any of these areas.

Individuals vary in their coping capacities, which depend on genetic endowment, environmental influences, nature and degree of stress, and available resources. All individuals have the potential for both health and illness.

Illness can be a growth-producing experience for the individual.

All people have a right to an equal opportunity for adequate health care regardless of gender, race, religion, ethics, sexual orientation, or cultural background.

Mental health is a critical component of comprehensive health care services.

The individual has the right to participate in decision making regarding physical and mental health.

The person has the right to self-determination, including the decision to pursue health or illness.

The goal of nursing care is to promote wellness, maximize integrated functioning, and enhance self-actualization. Nursing care is based on health care needs and expected treatment outcomes mutually determined with individuals, families, groups, and communities.

An interpersonal relationship can produce change and growth within the individual. It is the vehicle for the application of the nursing process and the attainment of the goal of nursing care.

Critical Thinking *About* Contemporary Issues

Are Psychiatric Nurses Vulnerable or Valuable as Mental Health Care Providers?

One question that is often raised when nurses talk about the health care environment is whether psychiatric nurses will be vulnerable to being replaced as expensive and outdated providers or be valued as competent clinicians who can function in a world of changing needs, processes, and structures. Potential areas of vulnerability have been identified and include the following (Halter, 2002; McCabe, 2002; Puskar and Bernardo, 2003; Stuart, 2001):

- Fewer nurses are attracted to psychiatric nursing as compared with other specialty areas.
- Content devoted to understanding psychiatric illnesses and working with psychiatric patients in nursing education programs has decreased steadily during the past decade.
- Graduate programs are moving toward the preparation of nurse practitioners who have significantly less course work related to the diagnosis and treatment of psychiatric illnesses.
- Biopsychosocial skills and expertise of psychiatric nurses are often underused in mental health care systems.
- Psychiatric nurses often are viewed as expensive health care providers who can be replaced by two or more less costly personnel.
- Threats to nursing autonomy are increasing as state boards of nursing and other regulatory bodies attempt to establish separate advanced practice licensure and examinations, and require advanced practice nurses to be under the full supervision of physicians.

- Few outcome studies have been done that document the nature, extent, and effectiveness of care delivered by psychiatric nurses.
- Psychiatric nurses have difficulty receiving direct reimbursement for services, despite the 1997 achievement of Medicare reimbursement.
- The specialty is struggling with the education and certification of advanced practice psychiatric–mental health nurses in clinical nurse specialist, nurse practitioner, and combined roles.
- Role differentiation for psychiatric nurses based on education and experience is often lacking in the position descriptions, job responsibilities, and reward programs of the health care systems in which nurses practice.
- APRNs-PMH are underused in managed care and primary care delivery systems.
- Stigmatizing attitudes and negative perceptions of psychiatric nursing exist among other nursing specialties, other health care professionals, the public, nurse educators, and nursing students.

Each of these issues must be addressed if psychiatric nursing is to continue to develop as a specialty area. Nurses need to move into the continuum of care and clearly articulate and actively market their skills, functions, and abilities. They also must demonstrate their cost effectiveness and establish differentiated levels of practice based on education, experience, and credentials. Such strategies will position psychiatric nurses as visible, interdependent, central, and collaborating professionals who have much to offer a reformed health care system.

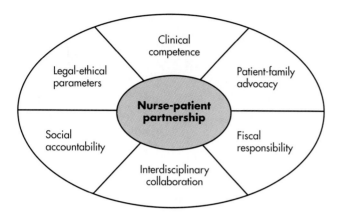

Figure 1-1   Elements of the psychiatric nursing role.

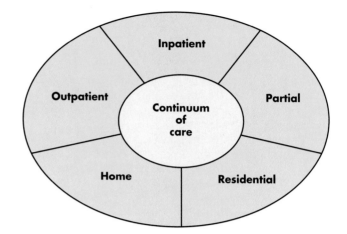

Figure 1-2   Continuum of mental health care settings.

No longer can psychiatric nurses focus exclusively on bedside care and the immediacy of patient needs. Today, they must broaden the context of their care and the responsibility and understanding they bring to the caregiving situation. The current practice of psychiatric nursing requires greater sensitivity to the social environment and the advocacy needs of patients and their families. It also requires thoughtful consideration of complex legal and ethical dilemmas that arise from a delivery system that often discriminates against those with mental illness. New models of mental health care also require greater skill in interdisciplinary collaboration that is built on the psychiatric nurse's clinical competence and professional self-assertion and balanced by a clear understanding of the costs of psychiatric care in general and psychiatric nursing care in particular. Each of these elements must influence the education, research, and clinical aspects of contemporary psychiatric nursing practice.

Continuum of Care

Traditional settings for psychiatric nurses include psychiatric facilities, community mental health centers, psychiatric units in general hospitals, residential facilities, and private practice. Many psychiatric hospitals also have become integrated clinical systems that provide inpatient care, partial hospitalization or day treatment, residential care, home care, and outpatient or ambulatory care (Figure 1-2).

Psychiatric nurses who continue to work within inpatient units have seen the goals, processes, and structures of care change drastically. In addition, community-based treatment settings have expanded to include foster care or group homes, hospices, visiting nurse associations, home health agencies, emergency departments, nursing homes, shelters, primary care clinics, schools, prisons, industrial settings, managed care facilities, and health maintenance organizations.

Psychiatric nurses are also moving into the domain of primary care and working with other nurses and physicians to diagnose and treat psychiatric illness in patients with somatic complaints (Saur et al, 2002). Cardiovascular, gynecological, respiratory, gastrointestinal, and family practice settings are appropriate for assessing patients for anxiety, depression, and substance abuse disorders. As health care initiatives continue

to move into schools and other community settings, psychiatric nurses are assuming leadership roles in providing expertise through consultation and evaluation.

Psychiatric nurses are very well suited to provide comprehensive health care to patients in both psychiatric settings and primary care environments. In particular, advanced practice psychiatric nurses acting as consultants to nonpsychiatric providers in hospital-based or outpatient clinics are in a unique position to assess and triage these patients. Early assessment and triage can minimize the length of time between psychiatric referral and intervention and enhance the efficacy of treatment.

Psychiatric nurses are also providing medical and medication management for selected groups of patients in collaborative practices. For example, patients who are having difficulty becoming stabilized on their medications or who have comorbid medical illnesses are seen in a psychiatric nursing clinic in which nurses and physicians collaborate to provide high-quality patient care. Psychiatric nurses who obtain prescriptive authority can further expand the services they provide and deliver cost-effective psychiatric care to communities that do not have access to a psychiatrist.

The new opportunities for psychiatric nursing practice that are emerging throughout the continuum of mental health care are very exciting. They allow psychiatric nurses to be proactive in demonstrating their expertise in designing interventions, planning programs, implementing treatment strategies, and managing staff in a variety of traditional and nontraditional settings. Psychiatric nurses also must continue to demonstrate flexibility, accountability, and self-direction as they move into these expanding areas of practice.

Competent Caring

There are three domains of contemporary psychiatric nursing practice: **direct care**, **communication**, and **management**. Within these overlapping domains of practice, the **teaching**, **coordinating**, **delegating**, and **collaborating** functions of the nursing role are expressed (Figure 1-3). Often the communication and management domains of practice are overlooked when discussing the psychiatric nursing role. However, these integrating activities are critically important and very time-

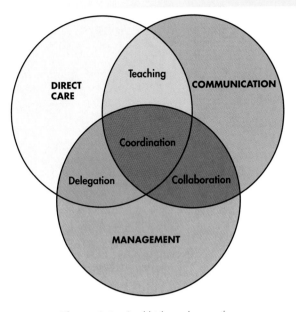

Figure 1-3 Psychiatric nursing practice.

consuming aspects of a nurse's role. They have become even more important in a reformed health care system that places emphasis on efficient patient triage and management.

Box 1-4 lists specific psychiatric nursing activities that reflect the current nature and scope of competent caring functions performed by psychiatric nurses. Not all nurses perform all of these activities. Psychiatric nurses participate in these activities based on their education and experience. In addition, psychiatric nurses are able to:

- Make culturally sensitive biopsychosocial health assessments.
- Design and implement treatment plans for patients and families with complex health problems and comorbid conditions.
- Engage in case management activities such as organizing, accessing, negotiating, coordinating, and integrating services and benefits for individuals and families.
- Provide a "health care map" for individuals, families, and groups to guide them to community resources for

---

BOX **1-4**

Domains of Psychiatric Nursing Practice

Direct Care Activities
Activity therapy
Advocacy
Aftercare follow-up
Behavioral treatments
Case consultation
Case management
Cognitive treatments
Community assessment
Community-based care
Community education
Complementary interventions
Compliance counseling
Counseling
Crisis intervention
Discharge planning
Environmental change
Environmental safety
Family interventions
Group work
Health maintenance
Health promotion
Health teaching
High-risk assessment
Holistic interventions
Home health care
Individual counseling
Informed consent acquisition
Intake screening and evaluation
Interpreting diagnostic and laboratory tests
Medication administration
Medication management
Mental health promotion
Mental illness prevention
Milieu therapy
Nutritional counseling
Ordering diagnostic and laboratory tests

Direct Care Activities—cont'd
Parent education
Patient triage
Physical assessment
Physiological treatments
Play therapy
Prescription of medications
Promotion of self-care activities
Provision of environmental safety
Psychiatric rehabilitation
Psychobiological interventions
Psychoeducation
Psychosocial assessment
Psychotherapy
Rehabilitation counseling
Relapse prevention
Research implementation
Social action
Social skills training
Somatic treatments
Stress management
Support of social systems
Telehealth

Communication Activities
Clinical case conferences
Development of treatment plans
Documentation of care
Forensic testimony
Interagency liaison
Peer review
Professional nurse networking
Report preparation
Staff meetings
Transcription of orders
Treatment team meetings
Verbal reports of care

Management Activities
Budgeting and resource allocation
Clinical supervision
Collaboration
Committee participation
Community action
Consultation/liaison
Contract negotiation
Coordination of services
Delegation of assignments
Grant writing
Marketing and public relations
Mediation and conflict resolution
Mentorship
Needs assessment and forecasting
Organizational governance
Outcomes management
Performance evaluations
Policy and procedure development
Practice guidelines formulation
Professional presentations
Program evaluation
Program planning
Publications
Quality improvement activities
Recruitment and retention activities
Regulatory agency activities
Risk management
Software development
Staff scheduling
Staff and student education
Strategic planning
Unit governance
Utilization review

CITING THE EVIDENCE ON

Psychiatric Nurses in Practice

BACKGROUND: This study examined the professional, work, and organizational characteristics and the actual and preferred work activities of 330 nurses employed in a state mental health system.

RESULTS: The nurses had varied educational preparation and work characteristics but responded similarly to almost every measure of their work including job satisfaction, work autonomy, commitment to the organization, and nursing participation in organizational decision making. On all of these items they had neutral ratings or negative ratings. Nurses with higher levels of education had more negative responses. There were two areas of difference. First, most inpatient nurses (92%) were supervised by a nurse, whereas most community-based nurses (31%) were not. This was seen as a problem by the community nurses. Second, the salaries of inpatient nurses were significantly higher than the community-based nurses, regardless of education or experience. All the nurses identified the need for better wages and 51% expressed interest in pursuing a higher degree in nursing. The

most important findings relate to their specific work activities. Although nursing functions did vary by education, nurses in inpatient settings reported providing less direct clinical care but more communication and management activities. Nurses in community settings spent most of their time delivering direct clinical care. Nurses in both settings wished to increase their direct care activities and reduce by half the amount of time they spent doing clerical tasks.

IMPLICATIONS: Psychiatric nurses possess a complex set of biological, psychological, and sociocultural skills that they use on a daily basis. In order to capitalize on these nurses as a resource for the mental health system, a better understanding of their role capacity and full use of their skills needs to be developed. The salary structure for psychiatric nurses must be competitive with both the work performed and the overall health care marketplace. Finally, nurses need greater participation in the governance structures and administrative posts of mental health agencies and organizations if they are to fully contribute to improving the mental health care system.

Stuart G et al: *Adm Policy Ment Health* 27:423, 2000.

mental health, including the most appropriate providers, agencies, technologies, and social systems.
- Promote and maintain mental health and manage the effects of mental illness through teaching and counseling.
- Provide care for the physically ill with psychological problems and the psychiatrically ill with physical problems.
- Manage and coordinate systems of care integrating the needs of patients, families, staff, and regulators.

Psychiatric nurses need to be able to explain both the general and the specific aspects of their practice to patients, families, other professionals, administrators, and legislators. Only when such skills are identified will psychiatric nurses be able to ensure their appropriate roles, adequate compensation for the nursing care provided, and the most efficient use of scarce human resources in the delivery of mental health care (see Citing the Evidence).

■ LEVELS OF PERFORMANCE

Psychiatric nursing roles and activities include a wide variation in levels of performance. Not all psychiatric nurses perform each of these functions. Individual nurses have primary responsibility and accountability for their own practice. Four major factors—laws, qualifications, setting, and personal initiative—play a part in determining the roles engaged in by each nurse.

Laws

Laws are the primary factor affecting the level of nursing practice. Each state has its own nursing practice act, which regulates entry into the profession and defines the legal lim-

its of nursing practice that must be adhered to by all nurses. Nurse practice acts also address aspects of advanced practice, including prescriptive authority (Haber et al, 2003). Nurses must be familiar with the nursing practice act of their state and define and limit their practice accordingly.

Qualifications

A nurse's qualifications include **education**, **work experience**, and **certification**. Two levels of psychiatric–mental health clinical nursing practice, basic and advanced, have been identified (American Nurses' Association, 2000).

1. **Basic Level: Psychiatric–Mental Health Registered Nurse.** Registered nurses at the basic level have completed a nursing program and passed the state licensure examination. Registered nurses, who practice in psychiatric–mental health nursing, care for mental health patients in various settings. Basic level nurses work as staff nurses, case managers, nurse managers, and other nursing roles in the psychiatric–mental health field.

2. **Advanced Level: Advanced Practice Registered Nurse—Psychiatric–Mental Health.** The Advanced Practice Registered Nurse in Psychiatric–Mental Health (APRN-PMH) is a licensed Registered Nurse (RN) who is educationally prepared at least at the master's degree level in the specialty. The nurse's graduate level preparation is distinguished by a depth of knowledge of theory and practice, validated experience in clinical practice, and competence in advanced clinical nursing skills. The APRN-PMH focuses clinical practice on persons with diagnosed psychiatric disorders or those at risk of mental health disorders and applies knowledge, skills, and experi-

ence autonomously to complex mental health problems. The term *APRN-PMH* applies to either the **clinical nurse specialist** or the **nurse practitioner** whose education and experience in psychiatric nursing practice meets criteria established by the profession (Bjorklund, 2003).

Another qualification is the nurse's work experience. Although work experience does not replace education, it does provide an added and necessary dimension to the nurse's level of competence and ability to function therapeutically.

Practice Setting

Psychiatric nurses may practice in settings that vary widely in purpose, type, location, and administration. They may be employed by an organization or self-employed in private practice. Nurses employed by an organization are paid for their services on a salaried or fee-for-service basis. Most nurses work in such organized settings. The administrative policies of these organizations can either foster or limit full use of the psychiatric nurse's potential. Nurses who are self-employed are paid for their services through third-party payment and direct patient fees. Some self-employed advanced practice psychiatric nurses maintain staff privileges with institutional facilities.

The role of a nurse in any psychiatric mental health setting depends on the following:

- Philosophy, mission, values, and goals of the treatment setting
- Definitions of mental health and mental illness that prevail in the setting
- Needs of the consumers of the mental health services
- Number of clinical staff available and the services they are able to provide
- Organizational structure and reporting relationships in the setting
- Consensus reached by the mental health care providers regarding their respective roles and responsibilities
- Resources and revenues available to offset the cost of care needed and provided
- Presence of strong nursing leadership and mentorship

A supportive environment for psychiatric nurses is one in which there is open and honest communication among staff, interdisciplinary respect, recognition of nurses' contributions, nursing involvement in decision making about both clinical care and the work environment, delegation of nonessential nursing tasks, opportunity to expand into new roles and responsibilities, and the encouragement that comes from being involved in professional psychiatric nursing activities and organizations.

What specific characteristics would you look for in an organization to determine whether it promotes professional psychiatric nursing practice? ■

Personal Initiative

The personal competence and initiative of the psychiatric nurse also influence the roles and activities of the nurse. This is a very important factor. One strategy psychiatric nurses can

Table 1-1	Psychiatric Nursing Support Groups	
Purpose	**Related Activities**
Provide practical help and professional feedback	Review clinical cases Evaluate documentation methods Analyze staff interactions and performance Develop nursing practice guidelines Discuss changes in one's role and work setting Describe successful interventions Share difficult work experiences
Exchange information and stimulate ideas	Report on conferences attended Distribute articles for reading and discussion Update on new developments in psychiatric nursing Review nursing practice legislative issues Share organizational policies and procedures Suggest resources for new information and problem solving

use to enhance their personal growth and competence is joining and participating in support groups. Examples of the purposes and possible activities of a professional support group are described in Table 1-1.

Psychiatric nurses also benefit from networking. Networks are groups of people drawn together by common concerns to support and help one another. Networks range from informal friendships and small groups providing contacts to larger open groups providing emotional support and local and national organizations representing one's specialty. Forming networks can help nurses unite and learn the value of their profession. Networking at the staff nurse level is crucial to the unity and survival of the profession. It helps nurses care for one another and influences their work environment.

What support networks do you have in your life at this time and how do they help you? How might professional networks help you when you graduate? ■

■ PSYCHIATRIC NURSING AGENDA

Psychiatric nursing will continue to grow and evolve in the years ahead. More than 82,000 registered nurses are working in mental health organizations in the United States, and over 17,000 of them have graduate degrees (Manderscheid and Henderson, 2001). Health care reform, patient and family needs, scientific developments, economic realities, and societal expectations will shape the future roles and functions of psychiatric nurses. To best meet the challenges of the next decade, psychiatric nurses need to focus their energies on three areas: outcome evaluation, leadership skills, and political action.

Outcome Evaluation

Psychiatric nurses need to identify, describe, measure, and explain the process and outcomes of the care they provide patients, families, and communities. Outcome studies documenting the quality, cost, and effectiveness of psychiatric nursing practice are an important part of the psychiatric nursing agenda. Focusing on ways to critically evaluate the outcomes of psychiatric nursing activities is a task for every psychiatric nurse regardless of role, qualifications, or practice setting. Psychiatric nurse clinicians, educators, administrators, and researchers all must assume responsibility for answering the question, "What difference does psychiatric nurse caring make?"

Leadership Skills

Psychiatric nurses need knowledge and strategies that enable them to exercise leadership and management in their work. Such leadership has a direct effect on the care patients receive. It also strengthens and expands the contribution of psychiatric nursing to the larger health care system (Gebbie, Wakefield, and Kerfoot, 2000). Psychiatric nurses should use their leadership skills and work as change agents to advocate for the mental health needs of patients, families, and communities. Mental health consumers need adequate, humane, and socially acceptable care. To this end nurses can initiate change; help by supporting, participating, or implementing change; engage in joint ventures for planned change; and evaluate completed change.

Another form of leadership is demonstrated by nurses who join their specialty organization. The American Psychiatric Nurses Association (APNA), located in Washington, D.C., is the largest organization of psychiatric nurses in the United States, representing more than 4000 registered nurses in both basic and advanced psychiatric nursing practice. Mental health nurses in Canada belong to the Canadian Federation of Mental Health Nurses (CFMHN). Nurses in Australia and New Zealand belong to the Australian & New Zealand College of Mental Health Nurses (ANZ-PSYCH). Organizations such as APNA, CFMHN, and ANZ-PSYCH also can provide informational networks to psychiatric nurses that are essential for consumer advocacy, continuing education, and effective political action.

Talk with some of the staff nurses who work in psychiatry and ask whether they know about APNA. Are they members? If not, what would it take for them to join? ■

Political Action

Psychiatric nurses can be a significant force in shaping the future of health care. To do so, they must learn to use their power and resources in the political arena—one of the most important targets for nursing action. Increasing psychiatric nurses' political awareness and skills is necessary to bring about needed changes in the mental health care delivery system. The political empowerment of nursing involves the following dimensions:

- Raising consciousness of sociocultural realities
- Building coalitions
- Developing positive self-esteem
- Adopting feminist theory as empowering rather than threatening
- Acquiring proactive political skills

These dimensions are overlapping and interactive and form the basis of political action by psychiatric nurses that is respectful of others, confirming of self, and directed toward the common good.

It is essential that psychiatric nurses recognize the value and legitimacy of their own voices. Nurses must become educated in legislative and regulatory processes, get involved in political campaigns, and testify in legislative hearings. Psychiatric nurses can then assert their right to an equitable share of the resources, given the value of the services they provide. Passive acceptance of decisions made by legislators, insurers, managed care companies, and other professionals should be replaced with proactive strategies. In this way the psychiatric nursing agenda of the next decade will advance nursing's commitment to caring in a mental health delivery system that is fair, sensitive, and responsible in meeting the biopsychosocial needs of patients, families, and communities.

CHAPTER FOCUS POINTS

- Psychiatric nursing began to emerge as a profession in the late nineteenth century, and by the twentieth century it had evolved into a specialty with unique roles and functions.
- Linda Richards and Hildegard Peplau were early leaders in the specialty.
- Psychiatric nursing was also influenced by the concept of the therapeutic community and the development of psychotropic drugs.
- The role of counselor or therapist was identified as the basis of psychiatric nursing practice.
- The 1980s were years of exciting scientific growth in the area of psychobiology.
- The current knowledge base of the specialty is based on the integration of the biological, psychological, spiritual, social, and environmental realms of the human experience.
- Psychiatric nursing is an interpersonal process that promotes and maintains behaviors that contribute to integrated functioning. The patient may be an individual, family, group, organization, or community.

- The "nurse-patient relationship" has evolved into a "nurse-patient partnership," which includes the elements of clinical competence, patient-family advocacy, fiscal responsibility, interdisciplinary collaboration, social accountability, and legal-ethical parameters.
- Psychiatric nurses work throughout the continuum of care in settings ranging from hospital based to community based with growing interest in providing psychiatric care in primary care settings.
- The three primary domains of psychiatric nursing practice are direct care, communication, and management with overlapping teaching, coordinating, delegating, and collaborating functions.
- Four factors that help to determine the level of a psychiatric nurse's performance are the law, the nurse's qualifications, the practice setting, and the nurse's personal initiative.
- To best meet the challenges of the next decade, psychiatric nurses need to focus their energies on three areas: outcome evaluation, leadership skills, and political action.

KEY TERMS

psychiatric nursing, 6
therapeutic community, 5

CHAPTER REVIEW QUESTIONS

1. Fill in the blanks.

A. _____ is known as the first American psychiatric nurse.

B. The book *Interpersonal Relations in Nursing* was written by

_____.

C. The three domains of contemporary psychiatric nursing practice are _____, _____,

and _____.

D. The two levels of psychiatric–mental health clinical practice

are _____ and _____.

E. The largest professional organization of psychiatric nurses in

the United States is the _____.

2. Identify whether the following statements are true (T) or false (F).

_____ A. The psychiatric nursing role evolved from primarily physical care to clinical competence based on interpersonal techniques and use of the nursing process.

_____ B. Psychiatric nursing was the first specialty to establish generalist and specialty certification.

_____ C. Many psychiatric hospitals are integrated clinical systems that provide the full continuum of psychiatric care.

_____ D. Each state has its own nursing practice act that regulates entry into the profession and defines the legal limits of nursing practice.

_____ E. Fewer than 50,000 registered nurses work in mental health organizations in the United States.

_____ F. Numerous studies have been published on the nature and outcome of psychiatric nursing care.

3. Provide short answers for the following questions.

A. Why was the development of psychotropic drugs so important in the treatment of people with mental illness?

B. List the five core mental health disciplines.

C. Identify the six dimensions of the nurse-patient partnership that characterize today's psychiatric nursing role.

D. Access APNA on the World Wide Web at http://www.apna.org. Do you think that having information about this nursing organization on the Internet is a service to psychiatric nurses?

Visit Evolve for additional resources related to the content of this chapter.
http://evolve.elsevier.com/Stuart/principles/
• Topical Course Outline • Student Workbook Exercises • Critical Thinking Questions and Activities • Case Studies • Research Topics
• Monthly Content Updates • WebLinks

Student Study CD-ROM

Access the accompanying CD-ROM for animations, interactive exercises, review questions for the NCLEX® examination, and an audio glossary.

REFERENCES

Abraham IL, Fox JC, Cohen BT: Integrating the bio into the biopsychosocial understanding and treating biological phenomena in psychiatric–mental health nursing, *Arch Psychiatr Nurs* 6:296, 1992.

American Nurses' Association: *Scope and standards of psychiatric–mental health clinical nursing practice*, Washington, DC, 2000, The Association.

Bennett A, Eaton J: The role of the psychiatric nurse in the newer therapies, *Am J Psychiatry* 108:167, 1951.

Bjorklund P: The certified psychiatric nurse practitioner: advanced practice psychiatric nursing reclaimed, *Arch Psychiatr Nurs* 17:77, 2003.

Doona M: At least as well cared for . . . Linda Richards and the mentally ill, *Image* 16:51, 1984.

Editorial, *Am J Nurs* 40:23, 1940.

Flaskerud JH, Wuerker AK: Mental health nursing in the 21st century, *Issues Ment Health Nurs* 20:5, 1999.

Gebbie KM, Wakefield M, Kerfoot K: Nursing and health policy, *J Nurs Sch* 32:307, 2000.

Haber J et al: Advanced practice psychiatric nurses: 2003 legislature update, *J Am Psychiatr Nurs Assoc* 9:205, 2003.

Halter M: Stigma in psychiatric nursing, *Perspect Psychiatr Care* 38: 23, 2002.

Hayes A: Psychiatric nursing: what does biology have to do with it? *Arch Psychiatr Nurs* 9:216, 1995.

Hays D: Suggested clinical practice of psychiatric nurses recorded in the literature between 1946 and 1958. In *Psychiatric nursing 1946 to 1974: a report on the state of the art*, New York, 1975, American Journal of Nursing.

Jones M: *The therapeutic community: a new treatment method in psychiatry*, New York, 1953, Basic Books.

Manderscheid R, Henderson M, editors: *Mental health United States, 2000*, Washington, DC, 2001, Department of Health and Human Services, Center for Mental Health Services.

McBride A: Psychiatric–mental health nursing in the twenty-first century. In McBride A, Austin J, editors: *Psychiatric–mental health nursing: integrating the behavioral and biological sciences*, Philadelphia, 1996, WB Saunders.

McCabe S: The nature of psychiatric nursing: the intersection of paradigm, evolution, and history, *Arch Psychiatr Nurs* 16:51, 2002.

Mellow J: Nursing therapy, *Am J Nurs* 68:2365, 1968.

Peplau H: *Interpersonal relations in nursing,* New York, 1952, GP Putnam's Sons.

Peplau H: Interpersonal techniques: the crux of psychiatric nursing, *Am J Nurs* 62:53, 1962.

Pothier PC et al: Dilemmas and directions for psychiatric nursing in the 1990s, *Arch Psychiatr Nurs* 4:284, 1990.

Puskar K, Bernardo L: Psychiatric nursing in crisis: strategies for recruitment, *J Am Psychiatr Nurs Assoc* 9:29, 2003.

Saur et al: Treating depression in primary care: an innovative role for mental health nurses, *J Am Psychiatr Nurs Assoc* 8:159, 2002.

Stuart G: Recent changes and current issues in psychiatric nursing. In McCloskey J, editor: *Current issues in nursing,* St Louis, 2001, Mosby.

Tudor G: Sociopsychiatric nursing approach to intervention in a problem of mutual withdrawal on a mental hospital ward, *Psychiatry* 15:193, 1952.

Weiss MO: The skills of psychiatric nursing, *Am J Nurs* 47:174, 1947.

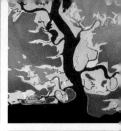

When we treat man as he is, we make him worse than he is. When we treat him as if he already were what he potentially could be, we make him what he should be.

JOHANN WOLFGANG VON GOETHE

THERAPEUTIC NURSE-PATIENT RELATIONSHIP

2

Gail W. Stuart

LEARNING OBJECTIVES

After studying this chapter the student should be able to:

1. State the goals of the therapeutic nurse-patient relationship (**I**).
2. Discuss six personal qualities a nurse needs to be an effective helper (**II**).
3. Describe the nurse's tasks and possible problems in the four phases of the relationship process (**III**).
4. Examine the levels of communication, two models of the communication process, and therapeutic communication techniques (**IV**).
5. Analyze how the nurse uses each of the responsive dimensions in a therapeutic relationship (**V**).
6. Analyze how the nurse uses each of the action dimensions in a therapeutic relationship (**VI**).
7. Evaluate therapeutic impasses, and identify nursing interventions to deal with them (**VII**).
8. Demonstrate increasing effectiveness in using therapeutic relationship skills to produce a therapeutic outcome (**VIII**).

TOPICAL OUTLINE

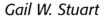 Visit Evolve for additional resources related to the content of this chapter.
http://evolve.elsevier.com/Stuart/principles/

The therapeutic nurse-patient relationship is a mutual learning experience and a corrective emotional experience for the patient. It is based on the underlying humanity of nurse and patient, with mutual respect and acceptance of ethnocultural differences. In this relationship the nurse uses personal attributes and clinical techniques in working with the patient to bring about insight and behavioral change.

■ CHARACTERISTICS OF THE RELATIONSHIP

The goals of a therapeutic relationship are directed toward achieving the patient's optimal growth and include the following dimensions:

- Self-realization, self-acceptance, and an increased genuine self-respect

- A clear sense of personal identity and an improved level of personal integration
- An ability to form intimate, interdependent, interpersonal relationships with a capacity to give and receive love
- Improved functioning and increased ability to satisfy needs and achieve realistic personal goals

To achieve these goals, various aspects of the patient's life experiences are explored. The nurse allows the patient to express thoughts and feelings and relates these to observed and reported behaviors, clarifying areas of conflict and anxiety. The nurse identifies and maximizes the patient's ego strengths and encourages socialization and family relatedness. Together the patient and nurse correct communication problems and modify maladaptive behavior patterns by testing new patterns of behavior and more adaptive coping mechanisms.

In the nurse-patient relationship, differing values are respected. The two communicate through a dialogue, or discussion, not a monologue, affirming the patient's reality and worth and allowing the patient to more fully define ego identity. Rogers (1961) summarizes the characteristics of a helping relationship that facilitate growth (Box 2-1). All nurses working with patients should ask themselves these questions. One's answers will determine the progress of the relationship.

The therapeutic nurse-patient relationship is complex (Sundeen et al, 1998). Evidence exists that the therapeutic alliance in the context of psychotherapy has a positive effect on patient outcomes. This chapter examines the personal qualities of the nurse as helper, the phases of the relationship, facilitative communication, responsive and action dimensions, therapeutic impasses, and the therapeutic outcome (Figure 2-1). Each of these factors influences the nurse's effectiveness.

BOX 2-1

Characteristics That Facilitate Growth in Helping Relationships

Can I behave in some way that will be perceived by the other person as trustworthy, as dependable, or consistent in some deep sense?

Can I be expressive enough as a person that what I am will be communicated unambiguously?

Can I let myself experience positive attitudes toward this other person—attitudes of warmth, caring, liking, interest, and respect?

Can I be strong enough as a person to be separate from the other?

Am I secure enough within myself to permit him his separateness?

Can I let myself enter fully into the world of his feelings and personal meaning and see these as he does?

Can I be acceptant of each facet of the other person that he presents to me? Can I receive him as he is?

Can I communicate this attitude? Or can I only receive him conditionally, acceptant of some aspects of his feelings and silently or openly disapproving of others?

Can I act with sufficient sensitivity in the relationship that my behavior will not be perceived as a threat?

Can I free him from the threat of external evaluation?

Can I meet this other individual as a person who is in the process of *becoming,* or will I be bound by his past and my past?

From Rogers C: *On becoming a person,* Boston, 1961, Houghton Mifflin.

■ PERSONAL QUALITIES OF THE NURSE

The key therapeutic tool of the psychiatric nurse is the **use of oneself**. Thus self-analysis is the first building block in providing quality nursing care.

> Now, if a nurse is afraid or even ignorant of her own self, she is highly likely to be threatened by a patient's real-self expressions. . . . A nurse who is more aware of the breadth and depth of her own real self is in a much better position to empathize with her patients and to encourage (or at least not block) their self-disclosures (Jourard, 1971).

Research suggests that some essential qualities are needed if one is to help others. These qualities are necessary for all nurses who wish to be therapeutic. They also help the nurse set goals for future growth.

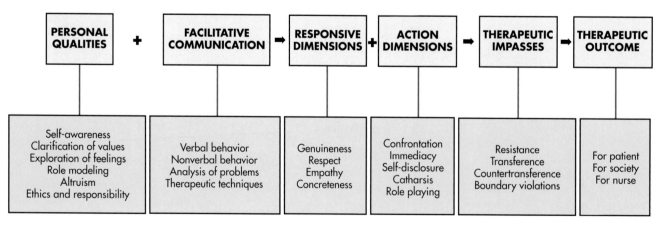

Figure 2-1   Elements affecting the nurse's ability to be therapeutic.

Awareness of Self

Effective helpers must be able to answer the question, Who am I? Nurses who care for the biological, psychological, and sociocultural needs of patients see a broad range of human experiences. They must learn to deal with anxiety, anger, sadness, and joy in helping patients throughout the health-illness continuum.

Self-awareness is a key part of the psychiatric nursing experience, and the nurse's goal is to achieve authentic, open, and personal communication. The nurse must be able to examine personal feelings, actions, and reactions. A good understanding and acceptance of self allow the nurse to acknowledge a patient's differences and uniqueness (Eckroth-Bucher, 2001).

Campbell (1980) has identified a holistic nursing model of self-awareness that consists of four interconnected components: psychological, physical, environmental, and philosophical.

1. The **psychological** component includes knowledge of emotions, motivations, self-concept, and personality. Being psychologically self-aware means being sensitive to feelings and outside events that affect those feelings.
2. The **physical** component is the knowledge of personal and general physiology, as well as of bodily sensations, body image, and physical potential.
3. The **environmental** component consists of the sociocultural environment, relationships with others, and knowledge of the relationship between humans and nature.
4. The **philosophical** component is the sense of life having meaning. A personal philosophy of life and death may or may not include a spiritual being, but it does take into account responsibility to the world and the ethics of behavior.

Together these components provide a model that can be used to promote the self-awareness and self-growth of nurses and the patients for whom they care.

Increasing Self-Awareness. No one ever completely knows the inner self, as shown in the Johari window (Figure 2-2). Quadrant 1 is the open quadrant; it includes the behaviors, feelings, and thoughts known to the individual and others. Quadrant 2 is the blind quadrant; it includes all the things that others know but the individual does not know. Quadrant 3 is the hidden quadrant; it includes the things about the self that only the individual knows. Quadrant 4 is the unknown quadrant, containing aspects of the self that are unknown to the individual and to others. Taken together, these quadrants represent the total self. The following three principles help explain how the self functions:

1. A change in any one quadrant affects all other quadrants.
2. The smaller quadrant 1, the poorer the communication.
3. Interpersonal learning means that a change has taken place, so quadrant 1 is larger and one or more of the other quadrants is smaller.

The goal of increasing self-awareness is to enlarge the area of quadrant 1 while reducing the size of the other three quadrants. To increase self-knowledge, it is necessary to **listen to the self**. This means the individual allows genuine emotions to be experienced; identifies and accepts personal needs; and moves the body in free, joyful, and spontaneous ways. It includes exploring personal thoughts, feelings, memories, and impulses.

The next step in the process is to reduce the size of quadrant 2 by **listening to and learning from others**. Knowledge of self is not possible alone. As we relate to others, we broaden our perceptions of self, but such learning requires active listening and openness to the feedback others provide.

The final step involves reducing the size of quadrant 3 by **self-disclosing**, or revealing to others important aspects of the self. Self-disclosure is both a sign of personality health and a means of achieving healthy personality.

Compare A and B of Figure 2-3. A represents a person with little self-awareness whose behaviors and feelings

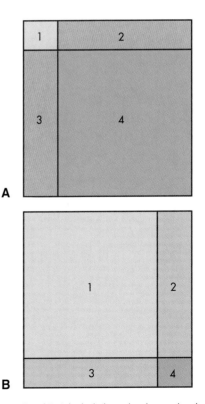

Figure 2-3   **A** and **B,** Johari windows showing varying degrees of self-awareness.

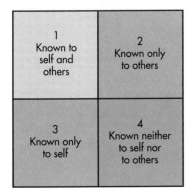

Figure 2-2   Johari window. Each quadrant, or windowpane, describes one aspect of the self.

are limited. *B,* however, shows an individual with great openness to the world. Much of this person's potential is being developed and realized. *B* represents an individual who has an increased capacity for experiences of all kinds: joy, hate, work, and love. This person also has few defenses and can interact more spontaneously and honestly with others. This configuration is a worthy goal for the nurse to pursue.

Draw your own Johari window. What changes would you like to make to any of the quadrants? ■

The Nurse and Self-Growth.

Nurses need time to explore and define the many parts of their personalities. If their nursing experiences involve perceiving, feeling, and thinking, then nursing students should be given the time and opportunity to study these experiences. Authenticity in relationships must be learned, and nurses must first experience openness and authenticity in relationships with instructors and supervisors. The student and instructor can participate in a relationship that accepts and respects their individual differences. Instructors can help students by facilitating students' self-awareness, increasing their level of functioning, stimulating more self-direction, and enabling students to cope more effectively with stressors.

Authenticity involves being open to self-exploration of thoughts, needs, emotions, values, defenses, actions, communications, problems, and goals. Nursing students have many new experiences that provide opportunities for self-learning. The student will be faced with disease, bizarre behavior, complex problems, and even death. Feelings related to these experiences should be focused on and discussed. Students might enter clinical settings with high ideals and unrealistic images. Perhaps they view nurses as all-knowing, all-caring "miracle workers." During initial encounters, students may feel fearful, anxious, and inadequate, wondering how a nurse gains the necessary knowledge. Nursing students might devalue their abilities and feel like an imposition on patients. At another time, nurses may identify closely with patients and feel anger toward the impersonal system and unresponsive personnel. The feelings involved in all of these situations should be identified, discussed, and analyzed. Only then can nurses resolve them in a constructive manner.

Throughout the growing process the student needs the support and guidance of a noncritical but challenging instructor. Together they can analyze the student's behavior, and the student can assess personal strengths and limitations. Also, it is often helpful if students share these experiences with a peer group. Students can empathize, critique, and support each other as they learn more about themselves.

Finally, objective self-examination is not easy or pleasant, particularly when findings conflict with self-ideals. However, like many painful experiences, discovering self-awareness presents a challenge—that of accepting self-limitations or changing the behaviors that support them.

Think back over the courses you have taken as a student. How much time and emphasis were placed on developing your self-awareness as a person and a nurse? ■

Clarification of Values

Nurses should be able to answer the question, What is important to me? Awareness of one's own values helps the nurse to be honest, to better accept difference in others, and to avoid the unethical use of patients to meet personal needs. Nurses should avoid the temptation to use patients for the pursuit of personal satisfaction or security. If nurses do not have sufficient personal fulfillment, they should realize that fact. Their sources of dissatisfaction should then be clarified to prevent them from interfering with the success of the nurse-patient relationship.

Value Systems.

Values are concepts that are formed as a result of life experiences with family, friends, culture, education, work, and relaxation. The word value has positive connotations because it denotes worth or significance. Yet values also imply negatives. If we value honesty, then it follows that we do not value dishonesty. People are likely to hold strong values related to religious beliefs, family ties, sexual preferences, other ethnic groups, and gender role beliefs.

One of the many challenges facing psychiatric nurses today is the need to provide care for patients from many different ethnocultural backgrounds. Because the goals of treatment are determined greatly by beliefs and values, establishing a therapeutic relationship with patients from different ethnocultural backgrounds requires particular skill and sensitivity (see Chapter 8).

Value systems provide the framework for many daily decisions and actions. By being aware of their value systems, nurses can identify situations in which value systems are in conflict. Clarification of values also provides some insurance against the tendency to project values onto other people. Many therapeutic relationships test the nurse's values. For example, a patient may describe a sexual behavior that the nurse finds unacceptable; a patient may talk about divorce, whereas the nurse may strongly believe that marriage contracts should not be broken; or a patient may be a "born-again" Christian, but the nurse may not believe in God or religion.

Can a nurse empathize with and help a patient solve a problem while maintaining personal values that are different from the values of the patient? ■

Value Clarification Process.

The value clarification process allows individuals to discover their values by assessing, exploring, and determining what those values are and how they influence their own thoughts, attitudes, and behaviors. Value clarification does not determine what the individual's values should be or what values should be followed. To prevent the imposition of values, value clarification focuses exclusively on the process of valuing, or on how people come to have the values they hold.

Steps in the Value Clarification Process	
CHOOSING	Freely
↓	From alternatives
	After thoughtful consideration of the consequences of each alternative
PRIZING	Cherishing, being happy with the choice
↓	Willing to affirm the choice publicly
ACTING	Doing something with the choice
	Repeatedly, in some pattern of life

Seven criteria are used to determine a value. These criteria should be considered in relation to a person's strongest value and tested against the person's own definition of a value. The seven criteria are broadly grouped into the three steps listed in Box 2-2.

The three criteria of **choosing** rely on the person's **cognitive abilities**, the two criteria of **prizing** emphasize the emotional or **affective level**, and the two criteria of **acting** have a **behavioral focus**.

A change takes place when certain contradictions are perceived in the person's value system. To eliminate the distress that follows such a realization, the person realigns values to coincide with the new view of self.

The Mature Valuing Process. The valuing process in the mature person is complex, and the choices are often difficult. There is no guarantee that the choice made will be self-actualizing. The valuing process in the mature person has the following characteristics (Kirschenbaum and Simon, 1973):

- It is fluid and flexible, based on the particular moment and the degree to which the moment is enhancing, enriching, and actualizing. Values are continually changing.
- The valuing experience is tied to a particular time and experience.
- Personal experience provides the value information. Although the person is open to all evidence obtained from other sources, outside evidence is not considered as important as subjective responses. The psychologically mature adult trusts and uses personal wisdom.
- In the valuing process the person is open to the immediacy of experience, trying to sense and clarify all its complex meanings. However, the immediate impact of the moment is colored by experiences from the past and conjecture about the future.

Exploration of Feelings

It is often assumed that helping others requires complete objectivity and detachment. This is definitely not true. Complete objectivity and detachment describe someone who is unresponsive, false, unapproachable, impersonal, and self-alienated—qualities that block the establishment of a therapeutic relationship.

Rather, nurses should be open to, aware of, and in control of their feelings so that they can be used to help patients. The feelings that nurses have serve an important purpose as barometers for feedback about themselves and their relationships with others. In helping others, nurses have many feelings: elation at seeing a patient improve, disappointment when a patient regresses, distress when a patient refuses help, anger when a patient is demanding or manipulative, and power when a patient expresses strong dependence on the nurse.

Nurses who are open to their feelings understand how they are responding to patients and how they appear to patients. The nurse's feelings are valuable clues to the patient's problems. For example, despite the patient's statement that "things are going real well," the nurse might perceive a strong sense of despair or anger. So too, nurses should be aware of the feelings they convey to the patient. Is the nurse's mood one of hopelessness or frustration? If nurses view feelings as barometers and feedback instruments, their effectiveness as helpers will improve.

Serving As Role Model

Formal helpers have a strong influence on those they help, and nurses function as role models for their patients. Research has shown the power of role models in molding socially adaptive, as well as maladaptive, behavior. Thus a nurse has an obligation to model adaptive and growth-producing behavior. If a nurse has a chaotic personal life, it will show in the nurse's work with patients, thereby decreasing the effectiveness of care. The nurse's credibility as a helper also will be questioned. The nurse may object, saying that it is possible to separate one's personal life from one's professional life, but in caring for patients this is not possible because psychiatric nursing *is* the therapeutic use of self.

This is not to suggest that the nurse must conform totally to local community norms or must live a happy, fully contented life. What is suggested is that the effective nurse has a fulfilling and satisfying personal life that is not dominated by conflict, distress, or denial and that the nurse's approach to life conveys a sense of growing, hopefulness, and adapting.

Who have been role models in your life, and what qualities did you most admire about them? ■

Altruism

It is important for nurses to have an answer to the question, Why do I want to help others? An effective helper is interested in people and tends to help out of a deep love for humanity. It also is true that everyone seeks a certain amount of personal satisfaction and fulfillment from work. The goal is to maintain a balance between these two needs. Helping motives can become destructive tools in the hands of naive or zealous users.

Another danger lies in adopting an extreme view of altruism. Altruism is concern for the welfare of others. It does not mean that an altruistic person should not expect adequate compensation and recognition or must practice denial or self-sacrifice. Only if personal needs have been appropriately met can the nurse expect to be maximally therapeutic.

Finally, a sense of altruism also can apply to changing social conditions to meet human welfare needs. One goal of all helping professionals should be to create a people-serving and growth-facilitating society. Thus a legitimate and necessary role for the nurse is to work to change the larger structure and process of society in ways that will promote the individual's health and well-being.

Ethics and Responsibility

Personal beliefs about people and society can serve as conscious guidelines for action. The Code for Nurses reflects common values regarding nurse-patient relationships and responsibilities and serves as a frame of reference for all nurses in their judgments about patient welfare and social responsibility. For psychiatric nurses, decisions are a part of daily functioning. Responsible ethical choice involves accountability, risk, commitment, and justice.

Related to the nurse's sense of ethics is the need to assume responsibility for behavior. This involves knowing limitations and strengths and being accountable for them. As a member of a health care team, the nurse has ready access to the knowledge and expertise of other people and these resources should be used appropriately.

■ PHASES OF THE RELATIONSHIP

A vital characteristic of the nurse-patient relationship is the sharing of behaviors, thoughts, and feelings. As such, it is important to distinguish between social support and professional support. In social support, two people are part of a natural social network, and the relationship is based on reciprocal trust and congruent expectations. In contrast, the relationship between a professional and a patient is based on clear role expectations. The support requested and ultimately provided should be within the domain of the nurse's role as a professional caregiver. It also is important to remember that the elements of a therapeutic nurse-patient relationship apply to all clinical settings. Thus nurses working in medical, surgical, obstetrical, oncological, and other specialty areas also need to understand and be able to use therapeutic nurse-patient relationship skills.

Four phases of the nurse-patient relationship have been identified: preinteraction phase; introductory, or orientation, phase; working phase; and termination phase. Each phase builds on the preceding one and is characterized by specific tasks.

Preinteraction Phase

Concerns of New Nurses. The preinteraction phase begins before the nurse's first contact with the patient. The nurse's initial task is one of **self-exploration**. This is no small task because the psychiatric nursing clinical experience can bring both stress and challenge to the student. In the first experience of working with psychiatric patients, the nurse brings the misconceptions and prejudices of the general public, in addition to feelings and fears common to all novices (Box 2-3).

BOX 2-3

Common Concerns of Psychiatric Nursing Students

- Acutely self-conscious
- Afraid of being rejected by the patients
- Anxious because of the newness of the experience
- Concerned about personally overidentifying with psychiatric patients
- Doubtful of the effectiveness of skills or coping ability
- Fearful of physical danger or violence
- Insecure in therapeutic use of self
- Suspicious of psychiatric patients stereotyped as "different"
- Threatened in nursing role identity
- Uncertain about ability to make a unique contribution
- Uncomfortable about the lack of physical tasks and treatments
- Vulnerable to emotionally painful experiences
- Worried about hurting the patient psychologically

An overriding one usually is anxiety or nervousness, which is common to new experiences of any kind. A related feeling is ambivalence or uncertainty because nurses may see the need for working with these patients but feel unclear about their ability to do so.

The informal nature of psychiatric settings also may threaten the nurse's role identity. A common first reaction among students is a feeling of panic when they realize that they "can't tell the patients from the staff." It also is unsettling for many students to give up their uniforms, stethoscopes, and scissors. Doing so dramatically emphasizes that, in this nursing setting, the most important tools are the ability to communicate, empathize, and solve problems. Without a tangible physical illness to care for, new students are likely to feel acutely self-conscious and hesitant about introducing themselves to a patient and starting a conversation.

Many nurses express feelings of inadequacy and fears of hurting or exploiting the patient. They worry about saying the wrong thing, which might drive the patient "over the brink." With their limited knowledge and experience, they doubt that they will be of any value. They wonder how they can help or whether they can really make a difference. Some nurses perceive the plight of psychiatric patients as hopeful; others perceive it as hopeless.

A common fear of nurses is related to the stereotype of psychiatric patients being violent. Because this is the picture portrayed by the media, many nurses are afraid of being physically hurt by a patient's outburst of aggressive behavior. Some nurses fear being psychologically hurt by a patient through rejection or silence. A final fear is related to nurses' questioning their own mental health status. Nurses may fear mental illness and worry that exposure to psychiatric patients might cause them to lose their own grasp on reality. Nurses who are working on their own crises of identity and intimacy may fear overidentifying with patients and using patients to meet their own needs.

The following clinical example contains many of the feelings and fears expressed by one nursing student in the preinteraction phase of self-analysis, as reported in the notes from her diary of her psychiatric rotation.

CLINICAL EXAMPLE

When first told that I would have a clinical psychiatric nursing experience, I received this information with a blank mind. Mental overload, denial, repression, or whatever it was made me hear the words but put off dealing with it. Then, when given a chance to sort through my thoughts and feelings, I thought more about what this experience would entail. Having never been personally involved with any people who were psychiatrically ill before, I was unable to rely on past personal experiences. I did, however, have quite a "pseudo knowledge base" from my novels, television, and movie encounters. Do places like the hospitals in *One Flew Over the Cuckoo's Nest* or *Frances* really exist? Was the portrayal of *Sybil* accurate? How could I possibly help someone who has so many problems, like the boy in *Ordinary People* or the young women in *Girl, Interrupted*? After all, I have problems myself. I'm afraid these thoughts have raised more questions in me than they have answered.

Three things scare me the most about this experience. First, I feel that the behavior of a psychiatric patient is quite unpredictable. Would they get violent or aggressive without any warning? Would this aggression be directed toward me? If so, would I be hurt? Did I provoke them, and was I wrong in my actions that caused this sudden shift?

The second, related to the first, is my feeling of inadequacy. I've been exposed to physically ill people and have learned how to respond to them. But, the psychiatrically ill are almost totally alien to me. How can I help? What if I do, or say, or infer something they could take offense to? Will I have the patience to persevere? I just don't know, and my not knowing makes me even more nervous.

My third fear is how seeing and being in contact with the psychiatrically ill will affect me. Although I know it's not contagious, the more exposure and knowledge I acquire in this area, the more I may begin to doubt my own stability and sanity. I mean, adolescence hasn't been easy for me, and I feel like I'm just now beginning to see things more clearly and feel better about myself. Will this experience stir up any past fears and doubts and, if so, how will I handle it? I am beginning to realize that there is a fine line between health and illness and that the psychiatric patients we'll meet have been unable to gather enough resources from within to cope with their problems. Help, reassurance, and understanding are their needs. I'm hoping I can help them . . . but I'm just not sure. ■

What feelings, fears, and fantasies do you have about working with psychiatric patients? ■

Self-Assessment. Experienced nurses benefit by asking themselves the following questions:

- Do I label patients with the stereotype of a group?
- Is my need to be liked so great that I become angry or hurt when a patient is rude, hostile, or uncooperative?
- Am I afraid of the responsibility I must assume for the relationship, and do I therefore limit my independent functions?
- Do I cover feelings of inferiority with a front of superiority?
- Do I require sympathy, warmth, and protection so much that I become too sympathetic or too protective toward patients?
- Do I fear closeness so much that I am indifferent, rejecting, or cold?
- Do I need to feel important and keep patients dependent on me?

The self-analysis of the preinteraction phase is a necessary task. To be effective, nurses should have a reasonably stable self-concept and an adequate amount of self-esteem. They should engage in positive relationships with others and face reality to help patients do the same. If they are aware of and in control of what they convey to their patients verbally and nonverbally, nurses can function as role models. To do this, however, some nurses abandon their personal strengths and assume a facade of "professionalism" that alienates their authentic self. This facade immobilizes them and acts as a barrier to establishing mutuality with patients.

Other tasks of this phase include **gathering data** about the patient if information is available and **planning for the first interaction** with the patient. The nursing assessment is begun, but most of the work related to it is done with the patient in the second phase of the relationship. Finally, nurses review general goals of a therapeutic relationship and consider what they have to offer patients.

Introductory, or Orientation, Phase

It is during the introductory phase that the nurse and patient first meet. One of the nurse's primary concerns is to find out **why the patient sought help** (Table 2-1). The reason for seeking help and whether or not it was voluntary forms the basis of the nursing assessment and helps the nurse focus on the patient's problem and determine the patient's motivation for treatment.

Formulating a Contract. The tasks in this phase of the relationship are to establish a climate of trust, understanding, acceptance, and open communication and formulate a contract with the patient. Box 2-4 lists the elements of a nurse-patient contract. The contract begins with the introduction of the nurse and patient, exchange of names, and explanation of roles. An explanation of roles includes the responsibilities and expectations of the patient and nurse, with a description of what the nurse can and cannot do. This is followed by a discussion of the purpose of the relationship, in which the nurse emphasizes that the focus of it will be the patient and the patient's life experiences and areas of conflict. Because establishing the contract is a mutual process, it is a good opportunity to clarify misperceptions held by either the nurse or patient.

Once the "who" and the "why" are determined, the "where, when, and how long" can be discussed. Where will they meet? How often and how long will the meetings be? The conditions for termination should be reviewed and may include a specified length of time, reaching mutual goals, or the discharge of the patient from the treatment setting. The issue of confidentiality is an important one to discuss with the patient at this time. Confidentiality involves the disclosure of certain information only to another specifically authorized person (see Chapter 10). This means that information about the patient will be shared only with people who are directly involved in the patient's care in the form of verbal reports

Table 2-1	Analysis of Why Patients Seek Psychiatric Help	
REASONS FOR PATIENTS' SEEKING PSYCHIATRIC CARE	APPROPRIATE NURSING APPROACH	SAMPLE RESPONSE
Environmental Change From Home to Treatment Setting		
They desire protection, comfort, rest, and freedom from demands of their home and work environments.	Emphasize the ability of the environment to provide protection and comfort while the healing process of the mind occurs.	"Tell me what it was at home/on the job that made you feel so overwhelmed."
Nurturance		
They wish for someone to care for them, cure their illness, and make them feel better.	Acknowledge their nurturance needs and assure them that help and caring are available.	"I'm here to help you feel better."
Control		
They are aware of their destructive impulses directed toward themselves or others but lack internal control.	Offer sources of internal control such as medication, if prescribed; reinforce external controls available through the staff.	"We're not going to let you hurt yourself. Tell us when these thoughts come to mind, and someone will stay with you."
Psychiatric Symptoms		
They describe symptoms of depression, nervousness, or crying spells and actively want to help themselves.	Ask for clarification of symptoms and strive to understand life experiences of the patient.	"I can see that you're nervous and upset. Can you tell me about how things are at home/on the job so I can better understand?"
Problem Solving		
They identify a specific problem or area of conflict and express desire to reason it out and change.	Help patient look at problem objectively; use problem-solving process.	"How has drinking affected your life?"
Advised to Seek Help		
Family member, friend, or health professional has convinced them to get treatment. They may feel angry, ambivalent, or indifferent.	Confirm facts surrounding seeking of help and set appropriate limits.	"I see that you're angry about being here. I hope that after we talk you might feel differently."

Modified from Burgess A, Burns J: Why patients seek care, *Am J Nurs* 73:314, 1973.

BOX 2-4

Elements of a Nurse-Patient Contract

- Names of individuals
- Roles of nurse and patient
- Responsibilities of nurse and patient
- Expectations of nurse and patient
- Purpose of the relationship
- Meeting location and time
- Conditions for termination
- Confidentiality

---

and written notes. This is important in providing for the continuity and comprehensiveness of patient care and should be clearly explained to the patient.

Establishing a contract is a mutual process in which the patient participates as fully as possible. In some cases, such as with the psychotic or severely withdrawn patient, the patient may be unable to fully participate, and the nurse must take the initiative in establishing the contract. As the patient's contact with reality increases, the nurse should review the elements of the contract when appropriate and strive to make it mutual.

Exploring Feelings. Both the nurse and patient may experience some degree of discomfort and nervousness in the introductory phase. Reasons that patients may have difficulty receiving help are listed in Box 2-5. The nurse may be well aware of personal anxieties and fears, but the patient's difficulty in receiving help may be overlooked.

Other tasks of the nurse in the orientation phase of the relationship are:
- To explore the patient's perceptions, thoughts, feelings, and actions.
- To identify pertinent patient problems.
- To define mutual, specific goals with the patient.

Patients also may display manipulative or testing behavior during this phase as they explore the nurse's consistency and intent. They may show temporary regressions as reactions to a large amount of self-disclosure in a previous meeting or to the anxiety created by a particular topic.

Finally, nurses need to be flexible in anticipating the length of time required for the orientation phase, particularly for patients who have a serious and persistent mental illness. Nurses might expect that more time will be required for patients who have had many or lengthy hospitalizations in the past. Also, staff changes affect the patient's ability to progress in the therapeutic relation-

BOX **2-5**

Reasons Patients Have Difficulty Seeking Help

- It may be difficult to see or admit one's difficulties, first to oneself and then to another.
- It is not easy to trust or be open with strangers.
- Sometimes problems seem too large, too overwhelming, or too unique to share them easily.
- Sharing personal problems with another person can threaten one's sense of independence, autonomy, and self-esteem.
- Solving a problem involves thinking about some things that may be unpleasant, viewing life realistically, deciding on a plan of action, and then, most important, following through with whatever it takes to bring about a change. These activities place great demands on the patient's energy and commitment.

BOX **2-6**

Criteria for Determining Patient Readiness for Termination

- The patient experiences relief from the presenting problem.
- The patient's functioning has improved.
- The patient has increased self-esteem and a stronger sense of identity.
- The patient uses more adaptive coping responses.
- The patient has achieved the planned treatment outcomes.
- An impasse has been reached in the nurse-patient relationship that cannot be resolved.

ship and should be taken into account when planning nursing care.

Talk with a friend or family member who has sought counseling. Why did they do so? Did anything make them uncomfortable about asking for help? What did the clinician do to put them at ease? ■

Working Phase

Most of the therapeutic work is carried out during the working phase. The nurse and the patient explore stressors and promote the development of **insight** in the patient by linking perceptions, thoughts, feelings, and actions. These insights should be translated into action and a **change in behavior**. They can then be integrated into the individual's life experiences. The nurse helps the patient master anxieties, increase independence and self-responsibility, and develop constructive coping mechanisms. Actual behavioral change is the focus of this phase.

Patients often display resistance behaviors during this phase because it involves the greater part of the problem-solving process. As the relationship develops, the patient begins to feel close to the nurse and responds by clinging to old defenses and resisting the nurse's attempts to move forward. An impasse or plateau in the relationship can result. Because overcoming resistance behaviors is crucial to the progress of the therapeutic relationship, these behaviors are discussed in greater detail later in this chapter.

Termination Phase

Termination is one of the most difficult but most important phases of the therapeutic nurse-patient relationship. During this phase, learning is maximized for both the patient and the nurse. Termination is a time to exchange feelings and memories and to evaluate mutually the patient's progress and goal attainment. Levels of trust and intimacy are heightened, reflecting the quality of the relationship and the sense of loss experienced by both nurse and patient. Box 2-6 lists criteria that can be used to determine whether the patient is ready to terminate.

Although agreement between the patient and the nurse is desirable in deciding when to terminate, this is not always possible. Nonetheless, the nurse's tasks during this phase revolve around establishing the reality of the separation. Together the nurse and the patient review the progress made in treatment and the attainment of specified goals. Feelings of rejection, loss, sadness, and anger are expressed and explored. It may be helpful to prepare the patient for termination by decreasing the number of visits, incorporating others into the meetings, or changing the location of the meetings. The reasons behind a change should be clarified so that the patient does not interpret it as rejection by the nurse. It also may be appropriate to make referrals at this time for continued care or treatment.

Successful termination requires that the patient work through feelings related to separation from emotionally significant people. The nurse can help by allowing the patient to experience and feel the effects of the anticipated loss, to express the feelings generated by the impending separation, and to relate those feelings to former symbolic or real losses.

Reactions to Termination. Patients react to termination in different ways. They may deny the separation or deny the significance of the relationship, perhaps causing the inexperienced nurse to feel rejected by the patient. Patients may express anger and hostility, either overtly and verbally or covertly through lateness, missed meetings, or superficial talk. These patients may view the termination as personal rejection, which reinforces their negative self-concept. Patients who feel rejected by the nurse may terminate prematurely by rejecting the nurse before the nurse rejects them. It also is common to see the patient regress to an earlier behavior pattern, hoping to convince the nurse not to terminate because of the need for further help.

The nurse should be aware of these possible reactions and discuss them with the patient if they occur. For some patients, termination is a critical therapeutic experience because many of their past relationships were terminated in a negative way that left them with unresolved feelings of abandonment, rejection, hurt, and anger.

All these patient reactions have a similar goal: to cope with the anxiety concerning the separation and to delay the termination process. The patient's response will be signifi-

Table 2-2	Nurse's Tasks in Each Phase of the Relationship Process
PHASE	TASK
Preinteraction	Explore own feelings, fantasies, and fears
	Analyze own professional strengths and limitations
	Gather data about patient when possible
	Plan for first meeting with patient
Introductory, or orientation	Determine why patient sought help
	Establish trust, acceptance, and open communication
	Mutually formulate a contract
	Explore patient's thoughts, feelings, and actions
	Identify patient's problems
	Define goals with patient
Working	Explore relevant stressors
	Promote patient's development of insight and use of constructive coping mechanisms
	Overcome resistance behaviors
Termination	Establish reality of separation
	Review progress of therapy and attainment of goals
	Mutually explore feelings of rejection, loss, sadness, and anger and related behaviors

cantly affected by the nurse's ability to remain open, sensitive, empathic, and responsive to the patient's changing needs. Helping the patient work and grow through the termination process is an essential goal of each relationship. It is important that the nurse not deny the reality of it or allow the patient to repeatedly delay the process. Particularly in this phase of the relationship, as in the orientation phase, the patient will be testing the nurse's judgment, and the issues of trust and acceptance will again arise.

The impending termination can be as difficult for the nurse as for the patient. Nurses who can begin reviewing their thoughts, feelings, and experiences will be more aware of personal motivation and more responsive to patients' needs. Learning to bear the sorrow of the loss while integrating positive aspects of the relationship into one's life is the goal of termination for both the nurse and the patient. At the end of the relationship, students can be helped to gain insight into their psychiatric nursing clinical experience and to better appreciate the roles of psychiatric nurses. The major tasks of the nurse during each phase of the nurse-patient relationship are summarized in Table 2-2.

Watch the movies The Dream Team *and* Girl, Interrupted *and discuss how staff-patient relationships are portrayed.* ■

■ FACILITATIVE COMMUNICATION

Communication can either facilitate the development of a therapeutic relationship or serve as a barrier to it. Everyone communicates constantly from birth until death. **All behavior is communication, and all communication affects be-**

havior. This reciprocity is central to the communication process. Communication is critical to nursing practice because of the following:

- Communication is the vehicle used to establish a therapeutic relationship.
- Communication is the means by which people influence the behavior of another, leading to the successful outcome of nursing intervention.
- Communication is the relationship itself because without it, a therapeutic nurse-patient relationship is impossible.

Communication takes place on two levels: verbal and nonverbal.

Verbal Communication

Verbal communication occurs through words, spoken or written. Taken alone, verbal communication can convey factual information accurately and efficiently. It is a less-effective means of communicating feelings or nuances of meaning, and it represents only a small part of total human communication.

Another limitation of verbal communication is that words can change meaning with different cultural groups or subgroups because words have both denotative and connotative meanings. The **denotative** meaning of a word is its actual or concrete meaning. For example, the denotative meaning of the word "bread" is "a food made of a flour or grain dough that is kneaded, shaped, allowed to rise, and baked." The **connotative** meaning of a word, in contrast, is its implied or suggested meaning. Thus the word "bread" can conjure up many different connotative or personalized meanings. Depending on a person's experiences, preferences, and present frame of reference, he or she may think of French bread, rye bread, a sesame seed roll, or perhaps pita bread. When used as slang, "give me some bread" may be understood to mean "give me some money." Thus the characteristics of the speaker and the context in which the phrase is used influence the specific meaning of verbal language.

When communicating verbally, many people assume that they are "on the same wavelength" as the listener. But because words are only symbols, they seldom mean precisely the same thing to two people. And if the word represents an abstract idea such as "depressed" or "hurt," the chance of misunderstanding or misinterpretation may be great. In addition, many feeling states or personal thoughts cannot be put into words easily. Nurses should try to overcome these problems by checking their interpretation and incorporating information from the nonverbal level as well.

Today more than ever before, nurses need to be prepared to communicate effectively with people from a variety of ethnocultural backgrounds. For example, psychiatric patients may be evaluated in their second language, yet competence in a second language varies depending on the individual and the stage of illness. In addition, cultural nuances in language often are not conveyed in translation, even when the patient uses similar words in the second language. Patients also may use a second language as a form of resistance to avoid intense feelings or conflicting thoughts, and events that may have occurred before a person learned English, if that is the second language, may not be easily communicated.

The effective psychiatric nurse uses verbal communication sensitively to promote mutual respect based on understanding and acceptance of cultural differences. The nurse also may communicate respect for the patient's dialect by adapting to the patient's linguistic style by using fewer words, more gestures, or more expressive facial behaviors.

Think of someone you know whose cultural background is different from your own. How does this difference influence your verbal and nonverbal communication? ■

Nonverbal Communication

Nonverbal communication includes all relayed information that does not involve the spoken or written word, including cues from all of the five senses. It has been estimated that about 7% of meaning is transmitted by words, 38% is transmitted by paralinguistic cues such as voice, and 55% is transmitted by body cues. Nonverbal communication is often unconsciously motivated and may more accurately indicate a person's meaning than the words being spoken. People tend to say what they think the receiver wants to hear, whereas less acceptable or more honest messages may be communicated by the nonverbal route.

Types of Nonverbal Behaviors. There are various types of nonverbal behaviors. Each of these is greatly influenced by sociocultural background. Following are brief descriptions of five categories of nonverbal communication.

Vocal cues include all the nonverbal qualities of speech. Some examples include pitch; tone of voice; quality of voice; loudness or intensity; rate and rhythm of talking; and unrelated nonverbal sounds such as laughing, groaning, nervous coughing, and sounds of hesitation ("um," "uh"). These are particularly vital cues of emotion and can be powerful conveyors of information.

Action cues are body movements, sometimes referred to as *kinetics*. They include automatic reflexes, posture, facial expression, gestures, mannerisms, and actions of any kind. Facial movements and posture can be particularly significant in interpreting the speaker's mood.

Object cues are the speaker's intentional and nonintentional use of all objects. Dress, furnishings, and possessions all communicate something to the observer about the speaker's sense of self. These cues often are consciously selected by the individual, however, and therefore may be chosen specifically to convey a certain look or message. Thus they can be less accurate than other types of nonverbal communication.

Space provides another clue to the nature of the relationship between two people. It must be examined based on sociocultural norms and customs. The following four zones of space are evident interpersonally in typical North American culture:

- **Intimate space**: up to 18 inches. This small degree of separation between people allows for maximum interpersonal sensory stimulation.
- **Personal space**: 18 inches to 4 feet. This zone is used for close relationships and when touching distance is desired. Visual sensation is improved over that of the intimate range.
- **Social-consultative space**: 9 to 12 feet. This zone is less personal and less dependent; it requires that speech be louder.
- **Public space**: 12 feet and more. This is used in speech giving and other public occasions.

Observation of seating arrangements and use of space by patients can yield valuable information to the nurse, with implications that inform both the nurse's assessment of the patient and how the nursing intervention should be implemented.

Touch involves both personal space and action. It is possibly the most personal of the nonverbal messages. A person's response to it is influenced by setting, cultural background, type of relationship, gender of communicators, ages, and expectations. Touch can express a desire to connect with another person, as a way of meeting them or relating to them. It can be a way of expressing or conveying something to another, such as concern, empathy, or caring. Touch also can be used as a way of sensing or perceiving another person or can allow someone to leave an imprint on another person. Finally, there is the concept of therapeutic touch, or the nurse's laying hands on or close to the body of an ill person for the purpose of helping or healing. Touch continues to be the imprimatur of nursing, and the therapeutic, comforting effects of touch are often overlooked. Thus touch is a universal and basic aspect of all nurse-patient relationships. It is often described as the first and most fundamental means of communication.

Interpreting Nonverbal Behavior. All types of nonverbal messages are important, but interpreting them correctly can present problems for the nurse. It is impossible to examine nonverbal messages out of context, and sometimes the individual's body reveals a number of different and perhaps conflicting feelings at the same time.

Sociocultural background also is a major influence on the meaning of nonverbal behavior. In the United States, with its diverse ethnic communities, messages between people of different upbringing can easily be misinterpreted. For instance, Arab Americans tend to stand closer together when speaking, and Asian Americans tend to touch more; touching in the United States is often minimized because of perceived sexual overtones. Because the meaning attached to nonverbal behavior is so subjective, it is essential that the nurse check and evaluate its meaning carefully.

Nurses should take note of and respond to the variety of nonverbal behaviors displayed by the patient, particularly voice inflections, body movements, gestures, facial expression, posture, and physical energy levels. Incongruent behavior and contradictory messages are especially significant communications. The nurse should refer to the specific behavior observed and try to confirm its meaning and significance with the patient. The nurse may use the following three kinds of responses to the patient:

1. Questions or statements intended to increase the patient's awareness
2. Statements that reflect content
3. Statements suggesting the nurse's responsiveness

These possible responses are illustrated in the following interaction.

■ THERAPEUTIC DIALOGUE

PATIENT *(Shifting nervously in his chair, eyes scanning the room and avoiding the nurse)* What . . . what do you want to talk about today?

NURSE RESPONSE NO. 1 *I sense that you are uncomfortable talking to me. Could you describe to me how you are feeling?*

NURSE RESPONSE NO. 2 *You're not sure what we should be talking about, and you want me to start us off?*

NURSE RESPONSE NO. 3 *You look very nervous, and I can feel those same feelings in me as I sit here with you.*

The nurse's first possible response is a reflection of and an attempt to validate the patient's feelings. The purpose is to communicate to the patient the nurse's awareness of his feelings, to show acceptance of those feelings, and to request that he focus on them and elaborate on them. The nurse's second possible response deals with the content of the patient's message. The nurse clarifies what the patient is trying to say. The third possible response shares both the nurse's perception of her patient's feelings and the personal disclosure that she has some of those same feelings. This type of response may help the patient feel that the nurse accepts and understands him.

Implications for Nursing Care. Besides responding to patients' nonverbal behavior, nurses should incorporate aspects of it into patient care (Raingruber, 2001). For example, patients who resist closeness will be disturbed by entry into their intimate space. The nurse can assess the patient's level of spatial tolerance by observing the distance the patient maintains with other people. The nurse also can be alert to the patient's response during their interaction. If the nurse sits next to the patient on the sofa, does the patient get up and move to a chair? If the nurse moves closer to the patient does the patient move away to reestablish the original space? Sometimes increasing the space between the nurse and an anxious patient can reduce the anxiety enough to allow the interaction to continue. A decrease in the distance the patient chooses to maintain from others may indicate a decrease in interpersonal anxiety.

Height may communicate dominance and submission. Communication is made easier when both participants are at similar levels. Orientation of the participants' body positions also is significant. Face-to-face confrontation is more threatening than oblique (sideways) body positions. The physical setting also has spatial meaning. Control issues are minimized when communication takes place in a neutral area that belongs to neither participant. However, people quickly identify their own turf, even in unfamiliar settings, and then begin to exert ownership rights over this area. A common example of this can be seen in most classroom settings. At the beginning of the semester, people sit randomly, but the arrangement usually solidifies after a couple of classes. Students then feel vaguely annoyed if they arrive in class to find another person in "their seat." They are experiencing an invasion of personal space.

Touch also should be used carefully. Patients who are sensitive to issues of closeness may experience a casual touch as an invasion or an invitation to intimacy, which may be even more frightening. Physical contact with a person of the same gender may be experienced by the patient as a homosexual advance and may precipitate a panic reaction. If procedures requiring physical contact must be carried out, careful explanations should be given both before and during the procedure. In addition, the nurse should always be aware of the potential for touch to be interpreted in a sexual way, thus creating problems related to the sexual conduct of the nurse within the nurse-patient relationship.

Despite these issues, touch is a significant part of psychiatric nursing practice. Reasons that nurses use touch include the following:

- Establishing contact with the patient
- Enhancing communication
- Communicating caring, interest, and recognition
- Providing reassurance and comfort

Nurses also must be aware not only of patients' nonverbal cues but also of their own. The nurse's nonverbal cues can communicate interest, respect, and genuineness or disinterest, lack of respect, and an impersonal facade. Affiliative nonverbal behaviors include smiles, positive head nods, gestures, eye contact, and a forward body lean.

Follow the treatment team making patient rounds and observe body positions. Are staff and patients at eye level? What personal space is maintained? Is touch used at all? ■

The Communication Process

The three elements of the communication process are perception, evaluation, and transmission. **Perception** occurs when the sensory end organs of the receiver are activated. The impulse is then transmitted to the brain. Human beings mostly rely on visual and auditory stimuli for communications.

When the sensory impulse reaches the brain, evaluation takes place. Personal experience allows for the evaluation of the new experience. If the person encounters a new experience for which there is no frame of reference, confusion results. **Evaluation** results in two responses: a cognitive response related to the informational part of the message and an affective response related to the relationship aspect of the message. Most messages stimulate both types of responses.

When the evaluation of the message is complete, **transmission** takes place that is perceived by the sender as feedback. This feedback influences the continued course of the communication cycle. It is impossible not to transmit some kind of feedback. Even lack of any visible response is feedback to the sender that the message did not get through, was considered unimportant, or was an undesirable interruption. Feedback stimulates perception, evaluation, and transmission by the original sender. The cycle continues until the participants agree to end it or one participant physically leaves the setting.

Theoretical models of the communication process show visual relationships more clearly and can aid in finding and correcting communication breakdowns or problems. Two models, the structural and the transactional analysis models, are presented here because each gives a valuable but different perspective on the communication process.

Structural Model. The structural model has five functional components in communication: the sender, the message, the receiver, the feedback, and the context (Figure 2-4):

1. The **sender** is the originator of the message.
2. The **message** is the information that is transmitted from the sender to the receiver.
3. The **receiver** is the perceiver of the message.
4. The **feedback** is the verbal or behavioral response of the receiver to the sender.
5. The **context** is the setting in which the communication takes place.

Knowledge of context is necessary to understand the full meaning of the communication. For example, the phrase "I don't understand what you mean" may have different meanings in the context of a classroom or a courtroom. Context involves more than the physical setting for communication, however. It also includes the psychosocial setting, which includes the relationship between the sender and the receiver, their past experiences with each other, their past experiences with similar situations, and cultural values and norms. Consider again the meaning of "I don't understand what you mean" in the following contexts: two college students discussing a philosophy assignment, a wife responding to her husband's accusation of infidelity, and a Japanese tourist asking directions in San Francisco. Although the content of the message is the same, its meaning is different, depending on the context in which the communication takes place.

In evaluating communication from the perspective of the structural model, specific problems can be identified (Table 2-3).

Sender. If the sender is communicating the same message on both the verbal and nonverbal levels, it is called congruent communication. However, if the levels are not in agreement, it is called incongruent communication, which can be problematic. Incongruent, or double-level, messages produce a dilemma for the listener, who does not know to which level to respond, the verbal or nonverbal. Because both levels cannot be responded to, the listener is likely to feel frustrated, angry, or confused. Obviously, both patients and nurses can display incongruent communication if they are not aware of their internal feeling states and the nature of their communication.

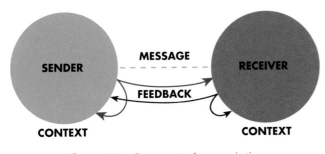

Figure 2-4   Components of communication.

■ THERAPEUTIC DIALOGUE

CONGRUENT COMMUNICATION
VERBAL LEVEL *I'm pleased to see you.*
NONVERBAL LEVEL *Warm tone of voice, continuous eye contact, smile.*
INCONGRUENT COMMUNICATION
VERBAL LEVEL *I'm pleased to see you.*
NONVERBAL LEVEL *Cold and distant tone of voice, little eye contact, neutral facial expression.*

Another problem initiated by the sender is inflexible communication that is either too rigid or too permissive. A rigid

Table 2-3	Problems With the Structural Elements of the Communication Process	
STRUCTURAL ELEMENT	**COMMUNICATION PROBLEM**	**DEFINITION**
Sender	Incongruent communication	Lack of agreement between the verbal and nonverbal levels of communication
	Inflexible communication	Exaggerated control or permissiveness by the sender
Message	Ineffective messages	Messages that are not goal directed or purposeful
	Inappropriate messages	Messages not relevant to the progress of the relationship
	Inadequate messages	Messages that lack a sufficient amount of information
	Inefficient messages	Messages that lack clarity, simplicity, and directness
Receiver	Errors of perception	Various forms of listening problems
	Errors of evaluation	Misinterpretation due to personal beliefs and values
Feedback	Misinformation	Communication of incorrect information
	Lack of validation	Failure to clarify and ratify understanding of the message
Context	Constraints of physical setting	Noise, temperature, or various distractions
	Constraints of psychosocial setting	Impaired previous relationship between the communicators

approach by the nurse does not allow for spontaneous expression by the patient, nor does it allow the patient to contribute to the flow or direction of the interaction. Exaggerated permissiveness, on the other hand, refers to the lack of a direction and mutuality in the interaction established by the nurse. The patient may interpret the nurse's behavior as incompetence or lack of interest.

Message. The message of the communication process also can pose problems. Messages can be ineffective, inappropriate, inadequate, or inefficient. Ineffective messages serve at least to distract and at most to prevent the objectives of the nurse-patient relationship from being met. Inappropriate messages are not relevant to the progress of the relationship. They may include failures in timing, stereotyping the receiver, or overlooking important information. Inadequate messages lack sufficient information. In this case, senders assume that receivers know more than they actually do. Inefficient messages lack clarity, simplicity, and directness. Using more energy than is necessary, these messages confuse or complicate the information.

Receiver. The third element, the receiver, may experience errors of perception. The receiver may miss nonverbal cues, respond only to content and ignore messages of affect, be selectively inattentive to the speaker's message because of physical or psychological discomfort, be preoccupied with other thoughts, or have a physiological hearing impairment. These errors are problems of listening. The receiver also may have problems in evaluating the message. The meaning of the message may be misinterpreted because the receiver views it in terms of the receiver's value system rather than that of the speaker.

Feedback. Errors in the feedback element include all of those that apply to the message. Feedback also can convey to the sender incorrect information about the message. Another serious error occurs when the receiver fails to use feedback to validate understanding of the message. Although feedback is the last step, it has the potential for correcting previous errors and clarifying the nature of the communication.

Context. The fifth element, context, also can contribute to communication problems. The setting may be physically noisy, cold, or distracting to one or both parties. The psychosocial context, or past relationship between the communicators, may be one of mistrust or harbored resentment.

This analysis shows the complexity of the communication process. It may seem surprising that successful communication can occur, given all of these vulnerable areas. However, it does occur among people who understand the process and use appropriate techniques.

Transactional Analysis Model. Transactional analysis is the study of the communication or transactions that take place between people. It uncovers the sometimes unconscious and destructive ways ("games") in which people relate to each other. This approach to personality was developed by Eric Berne (1964), a psychiatrist who made transactional analysis a popular theory through his classic book, *Games People Play: The Psychology of Human Relationships*. It is a method of therapy as well as a model of communication.

The cornerstone of this theory is that each person's personality is made up of three distinct components called *ego*

states. An ego state is a consistent pattern of feeling, experiencing, and behaving. The three ego states that make up personality are the parent ego state, adult ego state, and child ego state. It is as though three people reside in each person:

1. The "parent" incorporates all the attitudes and behaviors the individual was taught (directly or indirectly) by parents.
2. The "child" contains all the feelings the individual had as a child.
3. The "adult" deals with reality in a logical, rational, realistic manner.

The parent and child ego states are made up of the feelings, attitudes, and behaviors that are remnants of the past but can be reexperienced under certain conditions. The parent ego state consists of all the nurturing, critical, and prejudicial attitudes, behaviors, and experiences learned from other people, especially parents and teachers. The adult ego state is the reality-oriented part of the personality. It gathers and processes information about the world and is objective, emotionless, and intelligent in its approach to problem solving. The child ego state is the feeling part of the personality. In it resides feelings of happiness, joy, sadness, depression, and anxiety.

Berne's model of communication makes it possible to diagram transactions using these ego states. A transaction or communication between two people can be complementary, crossed, or ulterior. In a complementary transaction (Figure 2-5), the arrows in the ego state diagram are parallel, and the communication flows smoothly.

■ THERAPEUTIC DIALOGUE
COMPLEMENTARY TRANSACTION
PATIENT *I know that when I get mad at my boss, I take it out on my wife and kids.*

NURSE *Are you ready to think about some other ways you can handle your anger?*

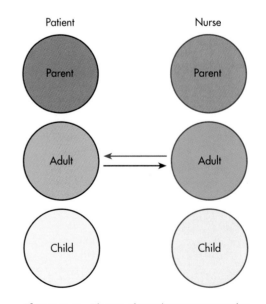

Figure 2-5   Diagram of complementary transaction.

If the arrows in the ego state diagram cross, however, communication breaks down (Figure 2-6).

■ **THERAPEUTIC DIALOGUE**

CROSSED TRANSACTION

PATIENT *I know that when I get mad at my boss, I take it out on my wife and kids.*

NURSE *Men always think that's OK, but the women have to suffer for it.*

The third type of transaction is ulterior transaction (Figure 2-7). It takes place on two levels: the social, or overt, level and the psychological, or covert, level. These transactions tend to be destructive because the communicators conceal their true motivations. One of the best known examples of this is the "Why Don't You . . . Yes But" game. This game involves one person asking for a solution to a problem; however, every suggested solution is negated, until the helper is silenced. On the surface, the interaction is two adults problem solving; in reality, one person is using the child ego state to show what a bad parent the other person is.

■ **THERAPEUTIC DIALOGUE**

ULTERIOR TRANSACTION

PATIENT *I know that when I get mad at my boss, I take it out on my wife and kids, but I don't know what else to do.*

NURSE *Do you think you could let your boss know how you're feeling?*

PATIENT *He'll fire me for sure.*

NURSE *Perhaps you could talk it over with a co-worker.*

PATIENT *I don't have time to chat on the job like that. Besides, no one cares about someone else's beefs.*

NURSE *Sometimes physical exercise helps people get rid of their anger. Have you ever tried it?*

PATIENT *Sure. I work out a lot, but it doesn't help.*

NURSE *Perhaps you can explain all this to your family.*

PATIENT *My wife's tired of "all my talk" as she puts it. She says she wants some action.*

The transactional analysis model of communication provides a framework for the nurse to use in exploring the patient's recurrent behaviors, identifying patterns, thinking about causes, and planning alternative ways to respond. Thus nonproductive communication patterns can be stopped and new, healthier ones learned.

Using the transactional analysis model, diagram three recent conversations you have had: one with a friend, one with your instructor, and one with a patient. ■

Therapeutic Communication Techniques

There are two requirements for therapeutic communication:
1. All communication must be aimed at preserving the self-respect of both individuals.
2. The communication of understanding should come before any suggestions or advice giving.

The collection of data and the planning, implementation, and evaluation activities are carried out *with* the patient, not *for* the patient, when the nurse uses therapeutic communication skills. Although seemingly simple on the surface, these techniques are difficult and require practice. Because they are techniques, they are only as effective as the person using them. If they are used appropriately, they can enhance the nurse's effectiveness. If they are used as automatic responses, they will block the formation of a therapeutic relationship, negate both the nurse's and the patient's individuality, and deprive them of their dignity.

To ensure that the nurse is using these skills effectively, the nurse needs to record interactions with the patient in some way and then analyze them (Festa et al, 2000). The nurse also should seek feedback from others. The nurse can benefit from maintaining a diary of thoughts, feelings, and

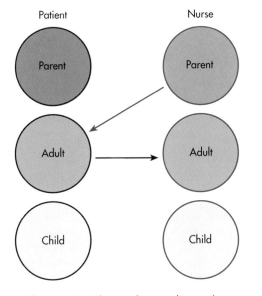

Figure 2-6 Diagram of a crossed transaction.

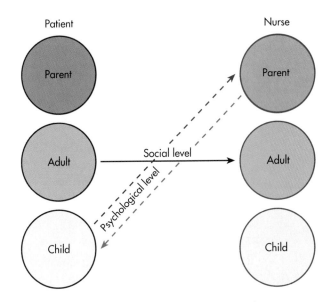

Figure 2-7 Diagram of an ulterior transaction.

impressions in relation to clinical work. An example of part of a process recording is shown in Table 2-4.

Only by analyzing the interaction can the nurse evaluate the degree of success achieved in using therapeutic communication techniques. Descriptions of some of the most helpful techniques follow.

Listening. Listening is essential to understanding the patient. The only person who can tell the nurse about the patient's feelings, thoughts, and perception of the self is the patient. Therefore the first rule of a therapeutic relationship is to listen to the patient. It is the foundation on which all other therapeutic skills are built (Nichols, 1995).

Inexperienced nurses often find it difficult not to talk. This may be caused by their anxiety, the need to prove themselves, or their usual way of social interaction. It is helpful to remember that the patient should be talking more than the nurse during the interaction; the task of the nurse is to listen.

Real listening is difficult. It is an active, not a passive, process. The nurse should give complete attention to the patient and should not be preoccupied. The nurse should suspend thinking of personal experiences and problems and making personal judgments of the patient. Listening is a sign of respect for the patient and is a powerful reinforcer.

Broad Openings. Broad openings such as, "What are you thinking about?" "Can you tell me more about that?" and "What shall we discuss today?" encourage the patient to select topics to discuss. Broad openings let the patient know that the nurse is there, listening to and following what the patient says. Also serving in this way are acceptance responses, such as "I understand," "And then what happened?" "Uh huh," or "I follow you."

Restating. Restating is the nurse's repeating of the main thought the patient has expressed. Sometimes only a part of the patient's statement is repeated. Restating also indicates that the nurse is listening, and it can be a reinforcer or bring attention to something important that might otherwise have been passed over.

Clarification. Clarification occurs when the nurse attempts to put into words vague ideas or thoughts that are implicit or explicit in the patient's talking. It is necessary because state-

Table 2-4	Process Recording		
PATIENT VERBAL (NONVERBAL)	**NURSE VERBAL (NONVERBAL)**	**NURSE ANALYSIS**	**SUPERVISOR'S COMMENTS**
Sometimes I think that life isn't worth living, and that my family would be better off without me. (Looking down, with sad expression and twirling the tassel on her belt)	You sound very "down" today. I can feel a sense of hopelessness. Am I right about that? (Using a low voice)	I was trying to express empathy and mirror her sense of sadness.	Very good in reflecting, promoting the therapeutic alliance and asking for clarification.
Yes, when I found out that my husband was having an affair, it triggered a whole range of feelings. (Looks up at me as she finishes the sentence)	Tell me more about them. (Maintaining eye contact)	I was shocked by her disclosure and really wasn't sure what to say.	I understand, but you handled it well. Asking for more information was a good response, and it encouraged the patient's emotional catharsis.
Well, I began to feel that I'm not smart enough, not pretty enough, not accomplished enough....and so he found someone else who is everything I'm not. (She looks uncomfortable but also as if she is looking for some confirmation from me)	Are these feelings that you've had in the past or are they new—a reaction to what is going on in your life now? (Trying to be objective)	I didn't feel like I could reassure her so I tried to learn more about her.	Again, a good approach. You did not make automatic assumptions, nor did you give false reassurance.
No...actually I have always felt pretty good about myself. I have been a good wife and mother and thought that I had something to contribute. (Seemed brighter as she was talking)	So let's put things in perspective. You're still that same person. Maybe something is going on with your husband. Have you talked with him about all this? (Using direct eye contact)	I thought she should explore what was going on, particularly with her husband, to confirm or discount her perceptions. I thought I could help her with this.	Examining the evidence is a useful strategy. Your approach was supportive and helpful.
No, I've not had the courage to do it. (Looks down again, frowning and twirls her wedding ring)	That's silly. You're a very strong person. (Said with animation)	I guess this wasn't as helpful as I had wanted it to be. I think it might have come across as a bit demeaning.	Perhaps. I think your intentions were good but your choice of expression did not effectively confirm her sense of self-efficacy.

ments about emotions and behaviors are rarely straightforward. The patient's verbalizations, especially if the patient is upset or overwhelmed with feelings, are not always clear and obvious. Nothing should be allowed to pass that the nurse does not hear or understand. Because of this uncertainty, clarification responses often are tentative or phrased as questions, such as "I'm not sure what you mean. Are you saying that . . .?" or "Could you go over that again?" This technique is important because two functions of the nurse-patient relationship are to help clarify feelings, ideas, and perceptions and to provide an explicit link between them and the patient's actions.

Reflection. Reflection can signify understanding, empathy, interest, and respect for the patient. It increases the level of involvement between the nurse and patient. Reflection of content is also called validation, which lets the patient know that the nurse has heard what was said and understands the content. It consists of repeating in fewer and different words the essential ideas of the patient and is like paraphrasing. Sometimes it helps to repeat a patient's statement, emphasizing a key word.

■ THERAPEUTIC DIALOGUE

PATIENT *When I walked into the room, I felt like I was going to faint. I knew I had tried to do too much too quickly, and I just wasn't ready for it.*

NURSE *You thought you were ready to put yourself to the test, but when you got there, you realized it was too much too soon.*

Reflection of feelings consists of responses to the patient's feelings about the content. These responses let the patient know that the nurse is aware of what the patient is feeling. Broad openings, restatements, clarifications, and reflections of content may not communicate empathic understanding. The purpose of reflecting feelings is to focus on feeling rather than content to bring the patient's vaguely expressed feelings into clear awareness. It helps the patient accept or own those feelings. The steps in reflection of feelings are to determine what feelings the patient is expressing, describe these feelings clearly, observe the effect, and judge by the patient's reaction whether the reflection was correct. Sometimes even inaccurate reflections can be useful be-

Table 2-4	Process Recording—cont'd		
PATIENT VERBAL (NONVERBAL)	NURSE VERBAL (NONVERBAL)	NURSE ANALYSIS	SUPERVISOR'S COMMENTS
Maybe you're right. Maybe it's not that I am a failure, but maybe it has more to do with the both of us. I guess I really do need to talk with him…if I can do it right. (Speaks tentatively)	What do you mean by "do it right"? (Moved body slightly toward her while looking interested)	I wanted to see what she was thinking here. Use of clarification.	That was worth following up on and clarification is good. You did miss an opportunity to confirm her sense of self and the fact that her husband was also responsible for his actions.
Well…not make him mad or not cry like a baby. (Shifted in her seat and seemed uncomfortable)	It sounds like you feel responsible for his responses. (Moved back in chair and said firmly)	I hope I did not come across as not approving. I thought she was assuming all the guilt and she needed to separate her feelings and behaviors from those of her husband. She also reminded me of my mother and how she assumed all the responsibility for my father's behavior.	Your intentions were appropriate. Good use of confrontation and sharing perceptions. Also your body language was responsive to her. This is also an example of how our personal issues come to the surface with our patients and how we need to be constantly vigilant about separating our own issues from those of our patients.
Yes, I guess that's the over-responsible part of me. It really hasn't worked though. It's only made me feel bad. (Looked up expectantly)	So what's an alternative? (Eye contact with hopeful expression)	I was trying to help her with problem solving.	Very appropriate and well timed.
I guess I can just let him know how I feel as truthfully as possible and then see how he reacts. (Said somewhat tentatively)	Are you willing to try that?	I wanted to move her into taking action.	Exactly—because insight alone does not result in resolving life issues.
Yes, I think I can. Maybe we can talk about how it goes? (She moved forward in her chair and seemed eager to have someone to process this with)	Absolutely. It's always good to problem solve together. (Using positive eye contact)	I was a bit surprised that she agreed so readily and also pleased that it seemed like she wanted to share how things went with me. Did I sound too eager?	Positive feedback is important to us as nurses as well. Your response let her know that she had a partner in this process and that no matter how the discussion went, she had someone with whom to share and analyze it. Isn't that similar to how we use this process recording? Well done.

cause the patient may correct the nurse and then state feelings more clearly.

■ THERAPEUTIC DIALOGUE

PATIENT *It's not so much that I mind changing jobs. It's just that I let down all the people working for me . . . relying on me.*
NURSE *You feel responsible for your employees, and so you're both sad and guilty about what has happened at work.*
PATIENT *Yes—sad, guilty . . . and pretty angry now that we're talking about it.*

Although reflecting techniques are some of the most useful, it is possible for the nurse to use them incorrectly. One common error is stereotyping of responses; that is, the nurse begins reflections in the same monotonous way, such as "You think" or "You feel." A second error involves timing. Reflecting back almost everything the patient says provokes feelings of irritation, anger, and frustration in the patient because the nurse appears to be insincere and fails to be therapeutic.

Other nurses may have trouble interrupting patients who continue talking in long monologues. It is difficult to capture a feeling after it has passed, and by not interjecting comments, the nurse is failing to be a responsible, active partner in the relationship. Interruptions may at times be productive and necessary. Another error is responding with an inappropriate depth of feeling. The nurse fails by being either too superficial or too deep in assessing the patient's feelings. The final error is use of language that is inappropriate to the patient's sociocultural experience and educational level. Effective language is language that is natural to the nurse and readily understood by the patient.

Focusing. Focusing helps the patient expand on a topic of importance. Effectively used, it can help the patient become more specific, move from vagueness to clarity, and focus on reality.

By avoiding abstractions and generalizations, focusing helps the patient face problems and analyze them in detail. It helps a patient talk about life experiences or problem areas and accept the responsibility for improving them. If the goal is to change thoughts, feelings, or beliefs, the patient must first identify and own them.

■ THERAPEUTIC DIALOGUE

PATIENT *Women always get put down. It's as if we don't count at all.*
NURSE *Tell me how you feel as a woman.*

Encouraging a description of the patient's perceptions, encouraging comparisons, and placing events in time sequence are focusing techniques that promote specificity and problem analysis.

Sharing Perceptions. Sharing perceptions involves asking the patient to verify the nurse's understanding of what the patient is thinking or feeling. The nurse can ask for feedback from the patient while possibly providing new information. Perception checking can consist of paraphrasing what the patient is saying or doing, asking the patient to confirm the nurse's understanding, and allowing the patient to correct that perception if necessary. Perception checking also can note the implied feelings of nonverbal language. It is best to describe the observed behavior first and then reflect on its meaning.

■ THERAPEUTIC DIALOGUE

PATIENT *She was such a good girl . . . and really seemed to care about other people. I don't know what's happened to her . . . what I could have done differently.*
NURSE *You seem to be very disappointed with your daughter, and maybe with yourself. Am I right about that?*

Perception checking is a way to explore incongruent or double-blind communication. "You're smiling, but I sense that you're really angry with me." Perception checking conveys understanding to the patient and clears up confusing communication.

Theme Identification. Themes are underlying issues or problems experienced by the patient that emerge repeatedly during the course of the nurse-patient relationship. Once the nurse has identified the patient's basic themes, he or she can better decide which of the patient's many feelings, thoughts, and beliefs to respond to and pursue. Important themes tend to be repeated throughout the relationship. They can relate to feelings (depression or anxiety), behavior (rebelling against authority or withdrawal), experiences (being loved, hurt, or raped), or combinations of all three.

Silence. Silence on the part of the nurse has varying effects, depending on how the patient perceives it. To a vocal patient, silence on the part of the nurse may be welcome, as long as the patient knows the nurse is listening. When patients pause, they often expect and want the nurse to respond. If the nurse does not, patients may perceive this as rejection, hostility, or disinterest. With a depressed or withdrawn patient, the nurse's silence may convey support, understanding, and acceptance. In this case, verbalization by the nurse may be perceived as pressure or frustration.

Silence can prompt the patient to talk. Some introverted people find out that they can be quiet but still be liked. Silence allows the patient time to think and to gain insights. Finally, silence can slow the pace of the interaction. In general, the nurse should allow the patient to break a silence, particularly when the patient has introduced it. Obviously, sensitivity is called for in this regard, and silence should not develop into a contest. However, if the nurse is unsure how to respond to a patient's comments, a safe approach is to maintain silence. If the nurse's nonverbal behavior communicates interest and involvement, the patient often will elaborate or discuss a related issue.

As a general technique, direct questioning has limited usefulness in the therapeutic relationship. Repetitive questioning takes on the tone of an interrogation and negates the element of mutuality. "Why" questions are particularly ineffective and are to be avoided, as are questions that can be answered yes or no. One consequence of these types of questions is that patients do not take the initiative and are discouraged or prevented from engaging in the process of exploration.

Humor. Humor is a basic part of the personality and has a place within the therapeutic relationship. As a part of interpersonal relationships, it is a constructive coping behavior. By learning to express humor, a patient may be able to learn to express other feelings. As a planned approach to nursing intervention, humor can promote insight by making conscious repressed issues. A change in the expression of humor and the quality of interpersonal relationships may be indicators of significant change in the patient.

Humor can serve many functions within the nurse-patient relationship (Box 2-7). These can be either positive or negative. There are no rules for determining how, when, or where humor should be used in the therapeutic relationship. It depends on the nature and quality of the relationship, the patient's receptivity to such themes, and the relevance of the tale or witticism. Humor may be of therapeutic value in the following situations:

- When the patient is experiencing mild to moderate levels of anxiety, humor serves as a tension reducer. It is inappropriate if a patient has severe or panic anxiety levels.
- When it helps a patient cope more effectively, facilitates learning, puts life situations in perspective, decreases social distance, and is understood by the patient for its therapeutic value. It is inappropriate when it promotes maladaptive coping responses, masks feelings, increases social distance, or allows the individual to avoid dealing with difficult situations.
- When it is consistent with the social and cultural values of the patient and when it allows the patient

to laugh at life, the human situation, or a particular set of stressors. It is inappropriate when it violates a patient's values, ridicules people, or belittles others.

The nurse also must be aware of the dangerous ways humor can be used to hide conflicts, ward off anxiety, manipulate the patient, and serve the nurse's own need to be liked and admired (Sayre, 2001). If it is used indiscriminately, humor meets only the nurse's needs and may be destructive to the relationship and frightening to the patient.

Informing. Informing, or information giving, is an essential nursing technique in which the nurse shares simple facts or information with the patient. It is a skill used by nurses in health teaching or patient education, such as explaining to a patient when to take medication, what precautions should be taken, and what side effects may occur. Giving information is not the same as giving suggestions or advice.

Suggesting. Suggesting is the presentation of alternative ideas. As a therapeutic technique, it is a useful intervention in the working phase of the relationship when the patient has analyzed the problem area and is exploring alternative coping mechanisms. At that time, suggestions by the nurse will increase the patient's perceived options.

Suggesting, or giving advice, also can be nontherapeutic. Some patients who seek help expect some pronouncement from the health care professional on what to do. Likewise, nursing students often perceive their function as giving "common sense" advice. In these instances giving advice shifts responsibility to the nurse and reinforces the patient's dependence.

Another limitation is that the patient may take the nurse's advice and still have an unsuccessful outcome. The patient then returns to blame the nurse for failure. Most commonly, though, patients do not follow the advice offered by others, as in the transactional analysis model. The request for advice is often a child's expression of dependency; when in reality, the patient already knows what to do. The nurse who falls into the trap and responds with advice receives the patient's anger and contempt. A more productive strategy is for the nurse to deal with the patient's feelings first—feelings of indecision, dependence, and perhaps fear. Then the request for advice can be looked at and responded to in its proper perspective.

Suggesting also is nontherapeutic if it occurs early in the relationship before the patient has analyzed personal conflicts or if it is a technique the nurse uses frequently. Then it negates the possibility of mutuality and implies that the patient is incapable of assuming responsibility for thoughts and actions. Likewise, suggestion by the nurse is nontherapeutic when it is actually covert coercion, as when the nurse tells patients how they should be living their lives.

The nurse's intent in using the suggesting technique should be to provide feasible alternatives and allow the pa-

---

BOX 2-7

Functions of Humor

• Establishes relationships	• Expresses emotion
• Reduces stress and tension	• Facilitates learning
• Promotes social closeness	• Reinforces self-concept
• Provides social control	• Voices social conflict
• Permits cognitive reframing	• Avoids conflict
• Reflects social change	• Facilitates enculturation
• Provides perspective	• Instills hope

tient to explore their value in his or her unique life situation. The nurse can then focus on helping the patient explore the advantages and disadvantages and the meaning and implications of the alternatives. In this way suggestions can be offered in a nonauthoritarian manner with such phrases as "Some people have tried. . . . Do you think that would work for you?" When using the technique of suggesting, nurses must be careful about both the timing of their intervention and their underlying motivation.

The therapeutic communication techniques presented in this chapter are summarized in Box 2-8.

Which therapeutic communication techniques listed in Box 2-8 are you skilled in using? Which techniques are more difficult for you? ■

BOX 2-8

Therapeutic Communication Techniques

Listening
Definition: An active process of receiving information and examining reaction to the messages received
Example: Maintaining eye contact and receptive nonverbal communication
Therapeutic value: Nonverbally communicates to the patient the nurse's interest and acceptance
Nontherapeutic threat: Failure to listen

Broad Openings
Definition: Encouraging the patient to select topics for discussion
Example: "What are you thinking about?"
Therapeutic value: Indicates acceptance by the nurse and the value of the patient's initiative
Nontherapeutic threat: Domination of the interaction by the nurse; rejecting responses

Restating
Definition: Repeating the main thought the patient expressed
Example: "You say that your mother left you when you were 5 years old."
Therapeutic value: Indicates that the nurse is listening and validates, reinforces, or calls attention to something important that has been said
Nontherapeutic threat: Lack of validation of the nurse's interpretation of the message; being judgmental; reassuring; defending

Clarification
Definition: Attempting to put into words vague ideas or unclear thoughts of the patient to enhance the nurse's understanding or asking the patient to explain what he or she means
Example: "I'm not sure what you mean. Could you tell me about that again?"
Therapeutic value: Helps to clarify feelings, ideas, and perceptions of the patient and provide an explicit correlation between them and the patient's actions
Nontherapeutic threat: Failure to probe; assumed understanding

Reflection
Definition: Directing back the patient's ideas, feelings, questions, or content
Example: "You're feeling tense and anxious, and it's related to a conversation you had with your husband last night?"
Therapeutic value: Validates the nurse's understanding of what the patient is saying and signifies empathy, interest, and respect for the patient

Nontherapeutic threat: Stereotyping the patient's responses; inappropriate timing of reflections; inappropriate depth of feeling of the reflections; inappropriate to the cultural experience and educational level of the patient

Humor
Definition: The discharge of energy through the comic enjoyment of the imperfect
Example: "That gives a whole new meaning to the word *nervous,*" said with shared kidding between the nurse and patient.
Therapeutic value: Can promote insight by making conscious repressed material, resolving paradoxes, tempering aggression, and revealing new options; a socially acceptable form of sublimation
Nontherapeutic threat: Indiscriminate use; belittling patient; screen to avoid therapeutic intimacy

Informing
Definition: The skill of information giving
Example: "I think you need to know more about how your medication works."
Therapeutic value: Helpful in health teaching or patient education about relevant aspects of patient's well-being and self-care
Nontherapeutic threat: Giving advice

Focusing
Definition: Questions or statements that help the patient expand on a topic of importance
Example: "I think that we should talk more about your relationship with your father."
Therapeutic value: Allows the patient to discuss central issues and keeps the communication process goal-directed
Nontherapeutic threat: Allowing abstractions and generalizations; changing topics

Sharing Perceptions
Definition: Asking the patient to verify the nurse's understanding of what the patient is thinking or feeling
Example: "You're smiling, but I sense that you are really very angry with me."
Therapeutic value: Conveys the nurse's understanding to the patient and has the potential for clearing up confusing communication
Nontherapeutic threat: Challenging the patient; accepting literal responses; reassuring; testing; defending

BOX **2-8**

Therapeutic Communication Techniques—cont'd

Theme Identification
Definition: Underlying issues or problems experienced by the patient that emerge repeatedly during the course of the nurse-patient relationship
Example: "I've noticed that in all of the relationships that you have described, you've been hurt or rejected by the man. Do you think this is an underlying issue?"
Therapeutic value: Allows the nurse to best promote the patient's exploration and understanding of important problems
Nontherapeutic threat: Giving advice; reassuring; disapproving

Silence
Definition: Lack of verbal communication for a therapeutic reason
Example: Sitting with a patient and nonverbally communicating interest and involvement

Therapeutic value: Allows the patient time to think and gain insights, slows the pace of the interaction, and encourages the patient to initiate conversation, while conveying the nurse's support, understanding, and acceptance
Nontherapeutic threat: Questioning the patient; asking for "why" responses; failure to break a nontherapeutic silence

Suggesting
Definition: Presentation of alternative ideas for the patient's consideration relative to problem solving
Example: "Have you thought about responding to your boss in a different way when he raises that issue with you? For example, you could ask him whether a specific problem has occurred."
Therapeutic value: Increases the patient's perceived options or choices
Nontherapeutic threat: Giving advice; inappropriate timing; being judgmental

■ RESPONSIVE DIMENSIONS

The nurse must possess certain skills or qualities to establish and maintain a therapeutic relationship. Specific core conditions for facilitative interpersonal relationships can be divided into responsive dimensions and action dimensions (Carkhoff, 1969; Carkhoff and Berenson,1967; Carkhoff and Truax, 1967).

The responsive dimensions include genuineness, respect, empathic understanding, and concreteness. One study reports that patients had much anxiety when interacting with psychiatric nurses, although they found them to be friendly and caring. However, they also experienced psychiatric nurses as lacking in empathy and intimacy and thought that they related to patients in stereotypical ways, acting as custodians and enforcers of rules (Muller and Poggenpoel, 1996). The helping process can therefore impede the patient's growth rather than enhance it, depending on the level of the nurse's responsive and facilitative skills.

The responsive dimensions are crucial in a therapeutic relationship to establish trust and open communication. The nurse's goal is to understand the patient and to help the patient gain self-understanding and insight. These responsive conditions then continue to be useful throughout the working and termination phases.

Genuineness

Genuineness means that the nurse is an open, honest, sincere person who is actively involved in the relationship. Genuineness is the opposite of self-alienation, which occurs when many of an individual's real, spontaneous reactions to life are suppressed. Genuineness means that the nurse's response is sincere, that the nurse is not thinking and feeling one thing and saying something different. It is an essential quality because nurses cannot expect openness, self-acceptance, and personal freedom in patients if they lack these qualities themselves. Whatever the nurse shows must be real and not merely a "professional" response that has been learned and repeated. In focusing on the patient, much of the nurse's personal needs are put aside, as well as some of the usual ways of relating to others.

Following is an example of genuineness.

■ THERAPEUTIC DIALOGUE

PATIENT *I'd like my parents to give me my freedom and let me do my own thing. If I need them or want their advice, I'll ask them. Why don't they trust what they taught me? Why do parents have to make it so hard—like it's all or nothing?*

NURSE *I know what you mean. My parents acted the same way. They offered advice, but what they expected was obedience. When they saw I could handle things on my own and used good judgment, they began to accept me as an individual. There are still times when they slip back into their old ways, but we understand each other better now. Do you think you and your parents need to share more openly and honestly your feelings and ideas?*

Respect

Respect is also called *nonpossessive warmth* or *unconditional positive regard*. It does not depend on the patient's behavior. Caring, liking, and valuing are other terms for respect. The patient is regarded as a person of worth and is respected as such. The nurse's attitude is nonjudgmental; it is without criticism, ridicule, or reservation. This does not mean that the nurse condones or accepts all aspects of the patient's behavior as desirable or likable. Patients are accepted for who they are, as they are. The nurse does not demand that the patient change or be perfect to be accepted. Imperfections are accepted along with mistakes and weaknesses as part of the human condition. The inexperienced nurse may have difficulty accepting the patient without transferring feelings about the patient's thoughts or actions. However, acceptance means viewing the patient's actions as coping behaviors that will change as the patient becomes less threatened and learns more adaptive ways. It involves viewing the patient's behavior as natural, normal, and expected, given the circumstances.

Although the nurse should have a basic respect for the patient simply as a person, respect is increased with understanding of the patient's uniqueness. Respect can be communicated in many different ways: by sitting silently with a patient who is crying, by exhibiting genuine laughter along with the patient in response to a particular event, by accepting the patient's request not to share a certain experience, by apologizing for the hurt unintentionally caused by a particular phrase, or by being open enough to communicate anger or hurt caused by the patient. Being genuine with and listening to the patient also are signs of respect.

When nurses communicate conditional warmth, they foster feelings of dependency in patients because nurses become the evaluator and superior in the relationship, making mutuality impossible. If dependency feelings arise in patients, nurses can effectively deal with them by acknowledging and exploring these feelings with patients.

There is a common expression that "respect needs to be learned." How does this idea affect the lives of psychiatric patients? ■

Empathic Understanding

Empathy is the ability to enter into the life of another person, to accurately perceive his or her current feelings and their meanings, and to communicate this understanding to the patient. It is an essential part of the therapeutic process (Bohart and Greenberg, 1997). When communicated, it forms the basis for a helping relationship between nurse and patient. Rogers (1975) described it as "to sense the client's private world as if it were your own, but without losing the 'as if' quality. A high degree of empathy is one of the most potent factors in bringing about change and learning—one of the most delicate and powerful ways we have of using ourselves."

Accurate empathy involves more than knowing what the patient means. It also involves sensitivity to the patient's current feelings and the verbal ability to communicate this understanding in a language attuned to the patient. It means frequently confirming with the patient the accuracy of personal perceptions and being guided by the patient's responses. It requires that the nurse put aside personal views and values to enter another's world without prejudice. New approaches are needed to facilitate the development of empathy in nursing students, as well as to more fully explore the concept of empathy as a nursing phenomenon (Reynolds, 2000; Walker and Alligood, 2001).

Development of Empathy. Empathic understanding consists of a number of stages. If patients allow nurses to enter

their private world and attempt to communicate their perceptions and feelings, nurses must be receptive to this communication. Next, nurses must understand the patient's communication by putting themselves in the patient's place. Nurses must then step back into their own role and communicate understanding to the patient. It is not necessary or even desirable for nurses to feel the same emotion as the patient. Neither should empathy be confused with sympathy, which is feeling sorry for the patient. Instead, it is an appreciation and awareness of the patient's feelings. A good deal of research has been conducted on empathy. The findings presented in Box 2-9 underscore its importance in counseling.

Rogers (1975) expands on the profound consequences empathy can have in promoting constructive learning and change. In the first place, it dissolves the patient's sense of alienation by connecting the patient on some level to a part of the human race. The patient can perceive that "I make sense to another human being . . . so I must not be so strange or alien. . . . And if I am in touch with someone else, I am not so alone." On the other hand, if not responded to empathically, the patient may believe, "If no one understands me, if no one can see what I'm experiencing, then I must be very bad off. . . . I'm sicker than even I thought." Another benefit of empathy is that the patient can feel valued, cared for, and accepted as a person. Then perhaps he or she will come to think, "If this other person thinks I'm worthwhile, maybe I could value and care for myself. . . . Maybe I am worthwhile after all."

Empathic responses. First, the nurse needs to be consistently genuine when interacting with the patient and give unconditional positive regard for the patient. Then the understanding conveyed to the patient through empathy gives him or her personhood or identity. The patient incorporates these aspects into a new, changing self-concept. Once self-concept changes, behavior also changes, thus producing the positive clinical outcome of therapy.

BOX 2-9

Research Findings About Empathy

- Empathy is related to positive clinical outcome.
- The ideal therapist is first of all empathic.
- Empathy is correlated with self-exploration and self-acceptance.
- Empathy early in the relationship predicts later success.
- Understanding is provided by, not drawn from, the therapist.
- More experienced therapists are more likely to be empathic.
- Empathy is a special quality in a relationship, and therapists offer more of it than even helpful friends.
- The better self-integrated the therapist, the higher the degree of empathy.
- Experienced therapists often fall far short of being empathic. Brilliance and diagnostic skill are unrelated to empathy.
- An empathic way of being can be learned from empathic people.

Nursing research has demonstrated a connection between nurse-expressed empathy and positive patient outcomes (Olson, 1995). One nursing study identified the following specific verbal and nonverbal behaviors that conveyed high levels of empathy to the patient (Mansfield, 1973):

- Having nurses introduce themselves to patients
- Head and body positions turned toward the patient and occasionally leaning forward
- Verbal responses to the patient's comments and responses that focus on the patient's strengths and resources
- Consistent eye contact and response to the patient's nonverbal cues such as sighs, tone of voice, restlessness, and facial expressions
- Conveyance of interest, concern, and warmth by the nurse's own facial expressions
- A tone of voice consistent with facial expression and verbal response
- Mirror imaging of body position and gestures between the nurse and patient

Empathic functioning scale. Kalisch (1973) devised the Nurse-Patient Empathic Functioning Scale, which describes five categories of empathy. High levels of empathy (categories 3 and 4) communicate "I am with you;" the nurse's responses fit perfectly with the patient's current feelings and content. The nurse's responses also serve to expand the patient's awareness of hidden feelings through the use of clarification and reflection. Such empathy is communicated by the language used, voice qualities, and nonverbal behavior, all of which reflect the nurse's seriousness and depth of feeling.

At low levels of empathy (categories 0 and 1), the nurse ignores the patient's feelings, goes off on a tangent, or misinterprets what the patient is feeling. The nurse at this level may be uninterested in the patient or concentrating on the "facts" of what the patient says rather than on current feelings and experiences. The nurse is doing something other than listening, such as evaluating the patient, giving advice, sermonizing, or thinking about personal problems or needs. A middle level of empathy (category 2) shows that the nurse is making an effort to understand the patient's feelings.

Empathic responses must be properly timed within the nurse-patient relationship. Category 4 responses in the orientation phase may be viewed as too intense and intrusive. Usually a number of category 2 responses are required initially to build an atmosphere of trust and openness. In the later stages of the orientation phase and most particularly in the working phase, categories 3 and 4 responses are appropriate and most effective. Responses from categories 0 and 1 are nontherapeutic at all times and block the development of the relationship.

The various levels of empathy are evident in the following example:

■ THERAPEUTIC DIALOGUE

PATIENT *I'm really jittery today, and I hope I can get things out right. It started when I saw Bob on Friday, and it's been building up since then.*

NURSE *You're feeling tense and anxious, and it's related to a talk you had with Bob on Friday. (Category 2.)*

PATIENT *Yes. He began putting pressure on me to have sex with him again.*

NURSE *It sounds like you resent it when he pressures you for sex. (Category 3.)*

PATIENT *I do. Why does he think things always have to be his way? I guess he knows I'm a pushover.*

NURSE *It makes you angry when he wants his way even though he knows you feel differently. But you usually give in and then you wind up disappointed in yourself and feeling like a failure. (Category 4.)*

PATIENT *It happens just like that over and over. It's as if I never learn.*

NURSE *So when the incident's all over, you're left blaming yourself and wallowing in self-pity. (Category 4.)*

PATIENT *I guess that's right.*

Finally, sociocultural differences between nurses and patients can be barriers to empathy if nurses are not sensitive to them. Differences in gender, age, income, belief systems, education, and ethnicity can block the development of empathic understanding. However, the greater the nurse's cultural sensitivity and the greater the openness to the world view of others, the greater will be the potential for understanding people.

Identical or similar experiences are not essential for empathy. No man can really experience what it is like to be a woman; no white person can experience what it is like to be a black person. It is not necessary to be exactly like another, but it is desirable for nurses to prepare themselves in any way they can to understand potential patients. It also is important for nurses to realize that empathy can be learned and enhanced in a variety of ways, including staff development programs.

Evaluate a recent interaction you had with a patient based on the empathy scale described. Use it again at the end of your psychiatric nursing experience and note any differences. ■

Concreteness

Concreteness involves using specific terminology rather than abstractions when discussing the patient's feelings, experiences, and behavior. It avoids vagueness and ambiguity and is the opposite of generalizing, labeling, and making assumptions about the patient's experiences. It has three functions: to keep the nurse's responses close to the patient's feelings and experiences, to foster accuracy of understanding by the nurse, and to encourage the patient to attend to specific problem areas.

The level of concreteness should vary during the various phases of the nurse-patient relationship (Figure 2-8). In the orientation phase, concreteness should be high; at that time it can contribute to empathic understanding. It is essential for the formulation of specific goals and plans. As patients explore various feelings and perceptions related to their problems in the working phase of the relationship, concreteness

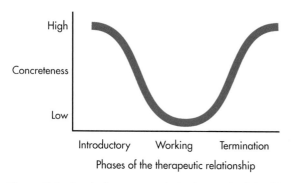

Figure 2-8   Levels of concreteness in the therapeutic relationship.

should be at a low level to facilitate a thorough self-exploration. High levels of concreteness are again desirable at the end of the working phase, when patients are engaging in action, and during the termination phase.

Concreteness is evident in the following examples:

■ THERAPEUTIC DIALOGUE

EXAMPLE 1

PATIENT *I wouldn't have any problems if people would quit bothering me. They like to upset me because they know I'm high strung.*

NURSE *What people try to upset you?*

PATIENT *My family. People think being from a large family is a blessing. I think it's a curse.*

NURSE *Could you give me an example of something someone in your family did that upset you?*

EXAMPLE 2

PATIENT *I don't know what the problem is between us. My wife and I just don't get along anymore. We seem to disagree about everything. I think I love her, but she isn't affectionate or caring—hasn't been for a long time.*

NURSE *You say you're not sure what the problem is, and you think you love your wife. But the two of you argue often and she hasn't given you any sign of love or affection. Have you felt affectionate toward her, and when was the last time you let her know how you felt?*

■ ACTION DIMENSIONS

The action-oriented conditions for facilitative interpersonal relationships are confrontation, immediacy, therapist self-disclosure, catharsis, and role playing. The separation of these therapeutic conditions into two groups—the understanding, or responsive, conditions and the initiating, or action, conditions—is not a distinct separation. To some extent all the dimensions are present throughout the therapeutic relationship. The action dimensions must have a context of warmth and understanding. This is important for inexperienced nurses to remember because they may be tempted to move into high levels of action dimensions without having established adequate understanding, empathy, warmth, or

respect. The responsive dimensions allow the patient to achieve insight, but this is not enough. With the action dimensions, the nurse moves the therapeutic relationship upward and outward by identifying obstacles to the patient's progress and the need for specific behavior change.

Confrontation

Confrontation often implies venting anger and engaging in aggressive behavior. However, confrontation as a therapeutic action dimension is an assertive rather than aggressive action. Confrontation is an expression by the nurse of perceived discrepancies in the patient's behavior. Three categories of confrontation include the following (Carkhoff, 1969):

- Discrepancies between the patient's expression of what he or she is (self-concept) and what he or she wants to be (self-ideal)
- Discrepancies between the patient's verbal self-expression and nonverbal behavior
- Discrepancies between the patient's expressed experience of himself or herself and the nurse's experience of him or her

Confrontation is an attempt by the nurse to make the patient aware of incongruence in his or her feelings, attitudes, beliefs, and behaviors. It also may lead to the discovery of ambivalent feelings in the patient. Confrontation is not limited to negative aspects of the patient. It includes pointing out discrepancies involving resources and strengths that are unrecognized and unused. It requires that the nurse collect sufficient data about the patient's history and accumulate sufficient perceptions and observations of verbal and nonverbal communication so that validation of reality is possible.

The nurse must have developed an understanding of the patient to perceive discrepancies, inconsistencies in word and deed, distortions, defenses, and evasions. The nurse must be willing and able to work through the crisis after confronting the patient. Without this commitment the confrontation lacks therapeutic potential and can be damaging to both nurse and patient. Without question, the effects of confrontation are challenge, exposure, risk, and the possibility for growth.

Timing in Relationships. Before confrontation, nurses should assess the following factors:

- Trust level in the relationship
- Timing
- Patient's stress level
- Strength of the patient's defense mechanisms
- Patient's perceived need for personal space or closeness
- Patient's level of rage and tolerance for hearing another perception

Patients have the capacity to deny or accept nurses' observations, and their response to the confrontation can serve as a measure of its success or failure. Acceptance indicates appropriate timing and patient readiness. Denial serves to allay any threat that the confrontation posed to the patient. It provides nurses with additional information; it tells them that

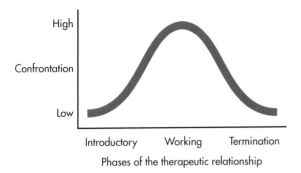

Figure 2-9 Levels of confrontation in the therapeutic relationship.

patients are resisting change and are unwilling to enlarge their view of reality at this time.

Confrontation also must be appropriately timed to be effective (Figure 2-9). In the orientation phase of the relationship, the nurse should use confrontation infrequently and pose it as an observation of incongruent behavior. A simple mirroring of the discrepancy between a patient's actions and words is the most nonthreatening type of confrontation. The nurse might say, "You seem to be saying two different things." This type of confrontation closely resembles clarification at this time. Nurses also might identify discrepancies between how they and patients are experiencing their relationship, point out unnoticed patient strengths or untapped resources, or provide patients with objective but perhaps different information about their world. Finally, to be effective, confrontation requires high levels of empathy and respect.

In the working phase of the relationship, more direct confrontations may focus on specific patient discrepancies. The nurse may confront the patient with areas of weakness or shortcomings or may focus on the discrepancy between the nurse's perception of the patient and the patient's self-perception. This expands the patient's awareness and helps the patient move to higher levels of functioning. Confrontation is especially important in pointing out when the patient has developed insight but has not changed behavior. This encourages the patient to act in a reasonable and constructive manner, rather than assuming a dependent and passive stance toward life.

Research indicates that effective counselors use confrontation frequently, confronting patients with their assets more often in earlier interviews and with their limitations in later interviews. In the initial interview, these confrontations were based on attempts to clarify the relationship, eliminate misconceptions, give patients more objective information about themselves and their world, and emphasize patient strengths and resources.

Inexperienced nurses often avoid confrontation. It can be nontherapeutic when it is not associated with empathy or warmth or when it is used to vent the nurse's feelings of anger, frustration, and aggressiveness. However, carefully monitored confrontation can be viewed as an extension of genuineness and concreteness. It is a useful therapeutic intervention that can further the patient's growth and progress.

Following are examples of confrontation:

■ THERAPEUTIC DIALOGUE

EXAMPLE 1
NURSE *I see you as someone who has a lot of strength. You've been able to give a tremendous amount of emotional support to your children at a time when they needed it very much.*

EXAMPLE 2
NURSE *You say you want to feel better and go back to work, but you're not taking your medicine, which will help you to do that.*

EXAMPLE 3
NURSE *The fact that Sue didn't accept your date for Friday night doesn't necessarily mean she never wants to go out with you. She could have had another date or other plans with her family or girlfriends. But if you don't ask her, you'll never find out why she refused you or if she'll accept in the future.*

EXAMPLE 4
NURSE *You tell me that your parents don't trust you and never give you any responsibility, but each week you also tell me how you stayed out beyond your curfew or had friends over when your parents weren't home. Do you see a connection between the two?*

EXAMPLE 5
NURSE *We've been talking for 3 weeks now about your need to get out and try to meet some people. We even talked of different ways to do that. But so far you haven't made any effort to join aerobics, take a class, or act on any of the other ideas we had.*

Your friend tells you that she feels uncomfortable using confrontation with patients. Why do you think this might be and what advice would you give her? ■

Immediacy

Immediacy involves focusing on the current interaction of the nurse and the patient in the relationship. It is a significant dimension because the patient's behavior and functioning in the relationship are indicative of functioning in other interpersonal relationships. Most patients experience difficulty in interpersonal relationships; thus the patient's functioning in the nurse-patient relationship must be evaluated. The nurse has the opportunity to intervene directly with the patient's problem behavior, and the patient has the opportunity to learn and change behavior.

Immediacy involves sensitivity to the patient's feelings and a willingness to deal with these feelings rather than ignore them. This is particularly difficult when the nurse must recognize and respond to negative feelings the patient expresses toward the nurse. The difficulty is compounded by the fact that patients often express these messages indirectly and conceal them in references to other people.

It is not possible or appropriate for the nurse to focus continually on the immediacy of the relationship. It is most appropriate to do so when the relationship seems to be stalled or is not progressing. It also is helpful to look at immediacy when the relationship is progressing particularly well. In both instances the patient is actively involved in describing what is helping or hindering the relationship.

As with the other dimensions, high-level immediacy responses should not be presented suddenly to the patient. The nurse must first know and understand the patient and must have developed a good, open relationship. The nurse's initial expressions of immediacy should be tentatively phrased, such as, "Are you trying to tell me how you feel about our relationship?" As the relationship progresses, observations related to immediacy can be made more directly, and as communication improves, the need for immediacy responses may decrease.

Following are two examples of immediacy:

■ THERAPEUTIC DIALOGUE

EXAMPLE 1

PATIENT *I've been thinking about our meetings, and I'm really too busy now to keep coming. Besides, I don't see the point in them, and we don't seem to be getting anywhere.*

NURSE *Are you trying to say you're feeling discouraged and you feel our meetings aren't helping you?*

EXAMPLE 2

PATIENT *The staff here couldn't care less about us patients. They treat us like children instead of adults.*

NURSE *I'm wondering if you feel that I don't care about you or perhaps I don't value your opinion?*

Nurse Self-Disclosure

Self-disclosures are subjectively true, personal statements about the self, intentionally revealed to another person. The nurse may share experiences or feelings that are similar to those of the patient and may emphasize both the similarities and differences. This kind of self-disclosure is an index of the closeness of the relationship and involves a particular kind of respect for the patient. It is an expression of genuineness and honesty by the nurse and is an aspect of empathy.

The research literature provides significant evidence that therapist self-disclosure increases the likelihood of patient self-disclosure. Patient self-disclosure is necessary for a successful therapeutic outcome. However, the nurse must use self-disclosure carefully, and this is determined by the quality, quantity, and appropriateness of the disclosures (Deering, 1999, Psychopathology Committee, 2001). Criteria for self-disclosure include the following:

- To model and educate
- To foster the therapeutic alliance
- To validate reality
- To encourage the patient's autonomy

The number of self-disclosures appears to be crucial to the success of the therapy. Too few nurse self-disclosures may fail to produce patient self-disclosures, whereas too many may decrease the time available for patient disclosure or may alienate the patient. The problem for the nurse is knowing where the middle ground is. Clinical experience is necessary to determine the optimum therapeutic level.

BOX 2-10

Guidelines for Self-Disclosure

Cooperation: Will the disclosure enhance the patient's cooperation, which is necessary to the development of a therapeutic alliance?

Learning: Will the disclosure assist the patient's ability to learn about himself or herself, to set short- and long-term goals, and to deal more effectively with life's problems?

Catharsis: Will the disclosure assist the patient to express formerly held or suppressed feelings, important to the relief of emotional symptoms?

Support: Will the disclosure provide the patient with support or reinforcement for attaining specific goals?

The appropriateness or relevance of the nurse's self-disclosure also is important. The nurse should self-disclose in response to statements made by the patient. If the nurse's disclosure is far from what the patient is experiencing, it can distract the patient from the problem or cause feelings of alienation. A patient who is experiencing severe anxiety may feel threatened or frightened by the nurse's self-disclosure. In these cases the nurse must be careful not to burden a patient with self-disclosures. Above all, disclosure by the nurse is always for the patient's benefit. When self-disclosing, the nurse should have a particular therapeutic goal in mind. The nurse does not disclose to meet personal needs or to feel better.

Guidelines that nurses can use to evaluate the potential usefulness of their self-disclosure are listed in Box 2-10. These guidelines govern the "dosage" and timing of self-disclosures and help the nurse assess the appropriateness, effectiveness, and anticipated response of the patient to the disclosure.

Self-disclosure by the nurse is evident in the following example:

■ THERAPEUTIC DIALOGUE

PATIENT *When he told me he didn't want to see me again, I felt like slapping him and hugging him at the same time. But then I knew the problem was really me and no one could ever love me.*

NURSE *When I broke off with a man I had been seeing, I felt the anger, hurt, and bitterness you just described. I remember thinking I would never date another man.*

In this example the nurse self-disclosed to emphasize that the patient's feelings were natural. She also reinforced the external cause for the separation (boyfriend's decision to leave versus the patient's inadequacy) and implied that, with time, the patient will be able to resolve the loss.

Emotional Catharsis

Catharsis occurs when the patient is encouraged to talk about things that are most bothersome. Catharsis brings fears, feelings, and experiences out into the open so that they can be examined and discussed with the nurse. The expression of feelings can be very therapeutic in itself, even if behavioral change does not result. The previously described responsive dimensions create an atmosphere within the nurse-patient relationship in which emotional catharsis is possible. The patient's responsiveness depends on the confidence and trust the patient has in the nurse.

The nurse must be able to recognize cues from the patient concerning readiness for discussion of problems. It is important that the nurse proceed at the rate chosen by the patient and provide support during discussion of difficult areas. Forcing emotional catharsis on the patient could bring about a panic episode because the patient's defenses are attacked without sufficient alternative coping mechanisms being available.

Patients are often uncomfortable expressing their feelings. Nurses may be equally uncomfortable with expressing feelings, particularly sadness or anger. Nurses often assume that they know the patient's feelings and do not attempt to specifically validate them. The dimensions of empathy and immediacy require the nurse to notice and express emotions. Unresolved feelings and feelings that are avoided can cause stalls or barriers in the nurse-patient relationship. Specific examples are transference and countertransference phenomena, which are discussed later in the chapter.

If patients have difficulty in expressing feelings, nurses may help by suggesting how they or others might feel in the patient's specific situation. Some patients respond directly to the question, "How did that make you feel?" Others intellectualize and avoid the emotional element in their answer. When patients realize they can express their feelings within an accepting relationship, they expand their awareness and potential acceptance of themselves.

The following example illustrates emotional catharsis:

■ THERAPEUTIC DIALOGUE

NURSE *How did you feel when your boss corrected you in front of all those customers?*

PATIENT *Well, I understood that he needed to set me straight, and he's the type that flies off the handle pretty easily anyhow.*

NURSE *It sounds like you're defending his behavior. I was wondering how you felt at that moment.*

PATIENT *Awkward . . . uh . . . upset, I guess. (pause)*

NURSE *That would have made me pretty angry if it had happened to me.*

PATIENT *Well, I was. But you can't let it show, you know. You have to keep it all in because of the customers. But he can let it out. Oh sure! (emphatically) He can tell me anything he wants. Just once I'd like him to know how I feel.*

Role Playing

Role playing involves acting out a particular situation. It increases the patient's insight into human relations and can deepen the ability to see the situation from another person's point of view. The purpose of role playing is to closely represent real-life behavior that involves individuals holistically, to focus attention on a problem, and to permit individuals to see themselves in action in a neutral situation. It provides a bridge between thought and action in a safe environment in which the patient can feel free to experiment with new behavior. It is action oriented and provides immediate information. Role playing consists of the following steps:

1. Defining the problem
2. Creating a readiness for role playing
3. Establishing the situation
4. Casting the characters
5. Briefing and warming up
6. Acting
7. Stopping
8. Analyzing and discussing
9. Evaluating

When role playing is used to facilitate attitude change, one key element of the exercise is role reversal. The patient may be asked to assume the role of a certain person in a specific situation or to play the role of someone with opposing beliefs. Role reversal can help a person reevaluate another person's intentions and become more understanding of the other person's position. After experiencing role reversal, patients may be more receptive to modifying their own attitudes.

Used as a method of promoting self-awareness and conflict resolution, role playing may help the patient "experience" a situation, which can be more helpful than just talking about it. Role playing can elicit feelings in the patient that are similar to those that would be experienced in the actual situation. It provides an opportunity for the patient to develop insight and to express affect. These attributes of role playing can heighten a patient's awareness of feelings related to a specific situation.

One of the specific ways in which role playing can be used to resolve conflicts and increase self-awareness is through a dialogue that requires the patient to take turns speaking for each person or each side of a problem. If the conflict is internal, the dialogue occurs in the present tense and alternates between the patient's conflicting selves until one part of the conflict outweighs the other. If the conflict involves a second person, the patient is instructed to "imagine that the other person is sitting in the chair across from you." The patient is told to begin the dialogue by directing comments to the other person. Then the patient changes chairs, assumes the role of the other person, and responds to what was just said. The patient assumes the first role again and responds to the other person. Using dialogue in this way not only serves as practice for the patient in expressing feelings and opinions but also provides a reality base from which the probable response from the other party involved in the conflict can be explored. Often this can eliminate the barrier that is keeping the patient from making a decision and acting on it.

Role playing is included as an action dimension because in addition to helping patients develop insight, it also can help patients practice new and more adaptive behaviors. For example, role playing can help patients develop better social,

Table 2-5	Responsive and Action Dimensions for Therapeutic Nurse-Patient Relationships	
DIMENSION	**DESCRIPTION**
Responsive	
Genuineness	Implies that the nurse is an open person who is self-congruent, authentic, and transparent
Respect	Suggests that the patient is regarded as a person of worth who is valued and accepted without qualification
Empathic understanding	Views the patient's world from the patient's internal frame of reference, with sensitivity to the patient's current feelings and the verbal ability to communicate this understanding in a language attuned to the patient
Concreteness	Involves the use of specific terminology rather than abstractions in the discussion of the patient's feelings, experiences, and behavior
Action	
Confrontation	Nurse expresses perceived discrepancies in the patient's behavior to expand the patient's self-awareness
Immediacy	Occurs when the current interaction of the nurse and patient is focused on for the purpose of learning about the patient's functioning in other interpersonal relationships
Nurse self-disclosure	Nurse reveals personal information, ideas, values, feelings, and attitudes to the patient to facilitate the patient's cooperation, learning, or catharsis or to indicate support of the patient
Emotional catharsis	Takes place when the patient is encouraged to talk about the things that are most bothersome to him or her
Role playing	Patient acts out a particular situation to increase insight into human relations and enhance the ability to see a situation from another point of view; it also allows the patient to experiment with new behaviors in a safe environment

assertiveness, and anger management skills. Role playing can be particularly effective when an impasse has been reached in the patient's progress or when it is difficult for the patient to translate insight into action. In these instances it can reduce tension and give the patient the opportunity to practice or test new behaviors for future use.

Table 2-5 summarizes the responsive and action dimensions for therapeutic nurse-patient relationships. It is important to remember that the nurse's effectiveness is based on openness to learning what works best with particular kinds of patients in particular situations. Both the use of communication techniques and the therapeutic conditions must be individualized to the nurse's personality and the patient's needs. The nurse needs to be willing to try other approaches that can be helpful if the current approach proves to be ineffective.

■ THERAPEUTIC IMPASSES

Therapeutic impasses are blocks in the progress of the nurse-patient relationship. They come about for a variety of reasons, but all impasses create stalls in the therapeutic relationship. Impasses provoke intense feelings in both the nurse and the patient, which may range from anxiety and apprehension to frustration, love, or intense anger. Four specific therapeutic impasses and ways to overcome them are discussed here: resistance, transference, countertransference, and boundary violations.

Resistance

Resistance is the patient's reluctance or avoidance of verbalizing or experiencing troubling aspects of oneself. The term *resistance* was initially introduced by Freud to mean the patient's unconscious opposition to exploring or recognizing unconscious or even preconscious material. Resistance is often caused by the patient's unwillingness to change when the need for change is recognized. Patients usually display resist-

ance behaviors during the working phase of the relationship, because the greater part of the problem-solving process occurs during this phase.

Resistance also may be a reaction by the patient to the nurse who has moved too rapidly or too deeply into the patient's feelings or who has intentionally or unintentionally communicated a lack of respect. It also may simply be the result of a patient working with a nurse who is an inappropriate role model for therapeutic behavior.

Secondary gain may be another cause of resistance. Secondary gain is a related benefit that a patient experiences as a result of his or her illness. For example, the development of the illness may result in the patient experiencing favorable environmental, interpersonal, monetary, or situational changes. Specific types of secondary gain include financial compensation, avoiding unpleasant situations, increased sympathy or attention, escape from work or other responsibilities, attempted control of people, and lessening of social pressures. Secondary gain can become a powerful force in perpetuating an illness because it makes the environment more comfortable and change less desirable.

Resistance may take many forms. Box 2-11 lists some of the forms of resistance that patients display.

Transference

Transference is an unconscious response in which the patient experiences feelings and attitudes toward the nurse that were originally associated with other significant figures in his or her life. They may be triggered by a superficial similarity, such as a facial feature or manner of speech, or by a personality style or trait. These reactions are the patient's attempt to reduce anxiety. The important trait defining transference is the inappropriate intensity of the patient's response.

Transference reduces self-awareness by allowing the patient to maintain an inaccurate view of the world in which all people are seen in similar terms. Thus the nurse may be

BOX **2-11**

Forms of Resistance Displayed by Patients

- Suppression and repression of pertinent information
- Intensification of symptoms
- Self-devaluation and a hopeless outlook on the future
- Forced flight into health in which a sudden, but short-lived recovery is experienced by the patient
- Intellectual inhibitions, which may be evident when the patient says she has "nothing on her mind" or that she is "unable to think about her problems" or when she breaks appointments, is late for sessions, or is forgetful, silent, or sleepy
- Acting out or irrational behavior
- Superficial talk
- Intellectual insight in which the patient verbalizes self-understanding with correct use of terminology yet continues destructive behavior or uses the defense of intellectualization in which no insight is verbalized
- Contempt for normality, which is evident when the patient has developed insight but refuses to assume the responsibility for change on the grounds that normality "isn't so great"
- Transference reactions

viewed as an authority figure from the past, such as a parent figure, or as a lost loved person, such as a former spouse. Transference reactions are harmful to the therapeutic process only if they remain ignored and unexamined.

Two types of transference are particularly problematic in the nurse-patient relationship. The first is the **hostile transference**. If the patient internalizes anger and hostility, this resistance may be expressed as depression and discouragement. The patient may ask to terminate the relationship on the grounds that there is no chance of getting well. If the hostility is externalized, the patient may become critical, defiant, and irritable and may express doubts about the nurse's training, experience, or competence. The patient may attempt to compete with the nurse by reading books on psychology and debating intellectual issues rather than working on real life problems.

Hostility also may be expressed by the patient as detachment, forgetfulness, irrelevant chatter, or preoccupation with childhood experiences. An extreme form of uncooperativeness and negativism is evident in prolonged silences. Some of the most frustrating moments for the nurse are those spent in total silence with a patient. This is not the therapeutic silence that communicates mutuality and understanding. Rather, it is the silence that seems to be hostile, oppressive, and eternal. It is particularly disturbing for the nurse in the orientation phase, before a relationship has been established. The nurse's task is to understand the meaning of the patient's silence and decide how to deal with it despite feeling somewhat awkward and uncertain.

A second difficult type of transference is the **dependent reaction transference**. This resistance is characterized by patients who are submissive, subordinate, and ingratiating and who regard the nurse as a godlike figure. The patient over-

values the nurse's characteristics and qualities, and their relationship becomes jeopardized because the patient views it as magical. In this reaction the nurse must live up to the patient's overwhelming expectations, which is impossible because these expectations are completely unrealistic. The patient continues to demand more of the nurse, and when these needs are not met, the patient is filled with hostility and contempt.

Overcoming Resistance and Transference. Resistances and transferences can be difficult problems for the nurse. The psychiatric nurse must be prepared for being exposed to powerful negative and positive emotional feelings coming from the patient—feelings that often have an irrational basis. The relationship can become stalled and nonbeneficial if the nurse is not prepared to deal with the patient's feelings.

Sometimes resistances occur because the nurse and patient have not arrived at mutually acceptable goals or plans of action. This may occur if the contract was not clearly defined in the orientation stage of the relationship. The appropriate action then is to return to clarifying the goals, purposes, and roles of the nurse and patient in the relationship.

Whatever the patient's motivations, the analysis of the resistance or transference is geared toward the patient gaining awareness of these motivations and learning about being completely responsible for all actions and behavior. The first thing the nurse must do is listen. When the nurse recognizes the resistance, clarification and reflection of feeling can be used. Clarification gives the nurse a more focused idea of what is happening. Reflection of content may help patients become aware of what has been going on in their own minds. Reflection of feeling acknowledges the resistance and mirrors it to the patient. The nurse may say, "I sense that you're struggling with yourself. Part of you wants to explore the issue of your marriage and another part says 'No—I'm not ready yet.'"

However, it is not sufficient to merely identify that resistance is occurring. The behavior must be explored and possible reasons for its occurrence analyzed. The depth of exploration and analysis engaged in by nurse and patient is related to the nurse's experience and knowledge base.

Countertransference

Countertransference is a therapeutic impasse created by the nurse's specific emotional response to the qualities of the patient. This response is inappropriate to the content and context of the therapeutic relationship and inappropriate in the degree of intensity of emotion. Countertransference is transference applied to the nurse. Inappropriateness is the important element of this impasse, just as it is with transference. It is natural, for example, that the nurse will feel a warmth toward or liking for some patients more than others, and the nurse also will be genuinely angry at times in regard to the actions of certain patients. But in the case of countertransference, the nurse's responses are not justified by reality. In such cases, nurses identify the patient with individuals from their past, and personal needs interfere with their therapeutic effectiveness.

Countertransference reactions are usually of the following three types:

1. Reactions of intense love or caring
2. Reactions of intense disgust or hostility
3. Reactions of intense anxiety, often in response to resistance by the patient

Through the use of immediacy, the nurse can identify countertransference in one of its various forms (Box 2-12). These reactions can be powerful tools for exploring and uncovering inner states. They are destructive only if they are ignored or not taken seriously (Ens, 1999).

If studied objectively, these reactions can lead to learning further information about the patient. The ability to remain objective does not mean that the nurse may not at times become irritated or dislike what the patient says. The patient's resistance to acquiring insight and transforming it into action and the refusal to change maladaptive and destructive coping mechanisms can be frustrating. However, the nurse's ability to understand these feelings helps to maintain a working relationship with the patient.

Countertransference also can be a group phenomenon. Psychiatric staff members can become involved in countertransference reactions when they overreact to a patient's aggressive behavior, ignore available patient data that would promote understanding, or become locked in a power struggle with a patient. Other types of countertransference might include ignoring patient behavior that does not fit the staff's diagnosis, minimizing a patient's behavior, joking about or criticizing a patient, or becoming caught up in intimidation.

The experienced nurse is constantly on the lookout for countertransference, becomes aware of it when it occurs, and works with it to promote the therapeutic goals. In identifying a countertransference, the nurse applies the same standards of honest self-appraisal personally that are expected of the patient. The nurse should use self-examination throughout the course of the relationship, particularly when the patient attacks or criticizes. Asking oneself the following questions may be helpful:

- How do I feel about the patient?
- Do I look forward to seeing the patient?
- Do I feel sorry for or sympathetic toward the patient?
- Am I bored with the patient and believe that we are not progressing?
- Am I afraid of the patient?
- Do I get extreme pleasure out of seeing the patient?
- Do I want to protect, reject, or punish the patient?
- Do I dread meeting the patient and feel nervous during the sessions?
- Am I impressed by or try to impress the patient?
- Does the patient make me very angry or frustrated?

If the answer to any of these questions suggests a problem, the nurse should pursue it: What is the patient doing to provoke these feelings? Who does the patient remind me of? The nurse must discover the source of the problem. Because countertransference can be harmful to the relationship, it should be dealt with as soon as possible. When it is recognized, the nurse can exercise control over it. If the nurse needs help in

---

BOX **2-12**

Forms of Countertransference Displayed by Nurses

- Difficulty empathizing with the patient as concerns certain problem areas
- Feelings of depression during or after the session
- Carelessness about implementing the contract, such as being late, running overtime, etc.
- Drowsiness during the sessions
- Feelings of anger or impatience because of the patient's unwillingness to change
- Encouragement of the patient's dependency, praise, or affection
- Arguments with the patient or a tendency to push before the patient is ready
- Attempts to help the patient in matters not related to the identified nursing goals
- Personal or social involvement with the patient
- Dreams about or preoccupation with the patient
- Sexual or aggressive fantasies toward the patient
- Recurrent anxiety, unease, or guilt related to the patient
- Tendency to focus on only one aspect or way of looking at information presented by the patient
- Need to defend nursing interventions used with the patient to others

---

dealing with countertransference, individual or group supervision can be most helpful.

Problem Patients. Countertransference problems are most evident when a patient is labeled a *problem* or *difficult patient.* Usually such a patient elicits strong negative feelings such as anger, fear, and helplessness and is often described by nurses as manipulative, dependent, inappropriate, and demanding. The label **problem patient** implies that the patient's behavior should change for the sake of the helper rather than for the patient's own benefit. This labeling often causes the patient and nurse to become adversaries, and the nurse avoids contact.

It is more productive for a nurse to view a problem patient rather as one who poses problems for the nurse. This turns the responsibility for action back onto the nurse (see Citing the Evidence). It forces the nurse to explore responses to the patient that reinforce the patient's unproductive behavior. In this way the nurse also makes patients responsible for their behavior. By stepping back and reviewing again the patient's needs and problems, the nurse can become aware of failing to use the responsive dimensions of genuineness, respect, empathic understanding, and concreteness. Without this groundwork, a therapeutic outcome is impossible.

Boundary Violations

A final but very important therapeutic impasse is that of boundary violations, which occur when a nurse goes outside the boundaries of the therapeutic relationship and establishes a social, economic, or personal relationship with a patient. As a general rule, whenever the nurse is doing or thinking of doing something special, different, or unusual for a patient,

CITING THE EVIDENCE ON

Problem Patients

BACKGROUND: Although recognition of the existence of "difficult" patients who present particular challenges to mental health nurses is increasing, no research has been conducted into their perceptions of services and their experience of care. This study had three aims: first, to identify people currently using services who mental health nurses defined as "difficult;" second, to explore the experiences of these patients; and third, to develop an understanding of the "difficult" nurse-patient relationship, which might suggest a therapeutic approach acceptable to both parties.

RESULTS: "Difficult" patients were found to be those who challenged nurses' competence and control. Despite their different roles, both nurses and "difficult" patients were aware of the struggle to gain or retain a notion of control. Feelings of anger were reduced in instances where nurses were perceived to demonstrate respect, time, skilled care, and a willingness to give patients some control and choice in their own care.

IMPLICATIONS: The external validity of the study is limited by the small sample size. Nonetheless, study findings suggest that "difficult" patients engender feelings of powerlessness in the nurse. In return, the nurse increases control over the patient and engages in a struggle with him or her. Skills that need to be present in order for nurses to empower patients are trust, knowledge, concern, communication, caring, respect, and courtesy. It is suggested that control is linked to the concept of "power over," whereas competence can be seen as "power to." Psychiatric nurses need to minimize the former and maximize the latter.

Breeze J, Repper J: *J Adv Nurs* 28:1301, 1998.

often a boundary violation is involved. A nurse should consider the possibility of a boundary violation if he or she encounters the following:

- Receives feedback that his or her behavior is intrusive with patients or their families
- Has difficulty setting limits with a patient
- Relates to a patient like a friend or family member
- Has sexual feelings toward a patient
- Feels that he or she is the only one who understands the patient
- Receives feedback that he or she is too involved with a patient or family
- Feels that other staff are too critical of a particular patient
- Believes that other staff members are jealous of his or her relationship with a patient

Specific examples of possible boundary violations are listed in Box 2-13.

Boundary violations can occur in the following categories (Baron, 2001; Gallop, 1998; Norris, Gutheil, and Strasburger, 2003; Reid, 1999; Simon and Williams, 1999):

- **Role boundaries:** These are related to the psychiatric nurse's role. They are reflected in the question, Is this what a professional psychiatric nurse does? Problems with role boundaries require the insight of the nurse and the setting of firm therapeutic limits with the patient.
- **Time boundaries:** These relate to the time of day that the nurse implements treatment. Odd and unusual treatment hours that have no therapeutic necessity must be evaluated as potential boundary violations.
- **Place and space boundaries:** These are related to where treatment takes place. An office or hospital unit is the usual locale for most treatment. Treatment outside of the office usually merits special scrutiny. Most often treatment provided over lunch, in the car, or in the patient's home must have a good therapeutic

BOX 2-13

Possible Boundary Violations Related to Psychiatric Nurses

- The patient takes the nurse out to lunch or dinner.
- The professional relationship turns into a social relationship.
- The nurse attends a party at a patient's invitation.
- The nurse regularly reveals personal information to the patient.
- The patient introduces the nurse to family members, such as a son or daughter, for the purpose of a social relationship.
- The nurse accepts free gifts from the patient's business.
- The nurse agrees to meet the patient for treatment outside of the usual setting without therapeutic justification.
- The nurse attends social functions that include the patient.
- The patient gives the nurse an expensive gift.
- The nurse routinely hugs or has physical contact with the patient.
- The nurse does business with or purchases services from the patient.

rationale and be related to explicit treatment goals. In an inpatient setting, any time spent by a nurse in a patient's room should be done so only if indicated and with appropriate action taken to respect boundary concerns, such as leaving the door open and being sure other staff are present nearby.

- **Money boundaries:** These relate to evaluating the compensation for treatment between the nurse and patient. Bartering or seeing an indigent patient for free should be carefully reviewed for potential boundary violations.
- **Gifts and services boundaries:** Gift giving is a controversial issue in nursing (see Critical Thinking about Contemporary Issues). Gifts that are obvious boundary violations place undue obligations on the

patient for the benefit of the nurse. Gifts can be divided into the following five types (Morse, 1991):

- Gifts to reciprocate for care given
- Gifts intended to manipulate or change the quality of care given or the nature of the nurse-patient relationship
- Gifts given as perceived obligation by the patient
- Serendipitous gifts or gifts received by chance
- Gifts given to the organization to recognize excellence of care received

- **Clothing boundaries:** These pertain to the nurse's need to dress in an appropriate therapeutic manner. Suggestive or seductive clothing of the nurse is unacceptable, and limits should be set on inappropriate dress by patients as well.

- **Language boundaries:** This boundary raises questions of when patients should be addressed by their first or last names, the tone that the nurse uses when talking with the patient, and the nurse's choice of words in implementing care. Too familiar, sexual, off-color, or leading language constitutes a boundary violation.

- **Self-disclosure boundaries:** Inappropriately timed self-disclosure by the nurse and nurse self-disclosure

that lacks therapeutic value are suspect for boundary violations, as discussed previously in this chapter.

- **Postdischarge social boundaries:** Postdischarge social contact of a patient by the nurse always raises questions of boundary violation. Such contacts confuse social support with professional support, can place the patient at risk, and disregard the basic tenets of the professional role.

- **Physical contact boundaries:** All physical contact with a patient must be evaluated for possible boundary violations. **Sexual contact of any kind is never therapeutic and never acceptable within the nurse-patient relationship.**

The nurse must carefully consider how to respond to each of these categories based on the possibility of boundary violations. Clinical supervision can be helpful in anticipating and heading off possible boundary violations (Walker and Clark, 1999).

What unique situations and customs may complicate the task of maintaining treatment boundaries in small communities and rural areas? How should they be handled? ■

Critical Thinking *About* Contemporary Issues

Is Gift Giving Acceptable Behavior in the Therapeutic Nurse-Patient Relationship?

Gift giving is a controversial issue in nursing. The taboo against nurses accepting gifts from patients has been long accepted. However, some have questioned the theoretical rationale for this position and suggest that gift giving can sometimes serve discrete therapeutic purposes.

Gifts can take many forms. They can be tangible or intangible, lasting or temporary. Tangible gifts may include such items as a box of candy, a bouquet of flowers, a hand-knit scarf, or a hand-painted picture. Intangible gifts can be the expression of thanks to a nurse by a patient who is about to be discharged or a family member's sense of relief and gratitude at being able to share an emotional burden with another caring person. The underlying element of all of these gifts is that something of value is voluntarily offered to another person, usually to convey gratitude.

Because gifts can be so varied, it is inappropriate to lump them all together in deciding upon a nursing action. Rather, the nurse's response to gift giving and the role it plays in the therapeutic relationship depends on the timing of the particular situation, the intent of the giver, and the meaning of the giving of the gift. Occasionally it may be most appropriate and therapeutic for the nurse to accept a patient's gift; on other occasions it may be quite inappropriate and detrimental to the relationship.

The timing of the gift giving is an important consideration. In the introductory, or orientation, phase of the relationship, nurses may be asked, "Do you have a cigarette I can borrow?" or "Will you buy me a cup of coffee?" These seemingly minor requests may make the nurse feel uncomfortable about refusing them. The nurse may rationalize compliance by thinking that it indicates interest in the patient and may help win his or her trust. However, these responses indicate the nurse's failure to examine the patient's underlying need and the nurse's own needs in complying with it. Also, in this early phase of the relationship, the nurse may be the one to initiate gift giving by giving the patient a book, plant, or some other item that expresses interest in the patient.

In the orientation phase of the relationship, gift giving can be harmful if it meets personal needs rather than therapeutic goals. By giving a gift, the patient may be trying to manipulate the nurse and control the relationship. In contrast, by giving gifts to the patient, the nurse may be attempting to relate through objects instead of the therapeutic use of self and to avoid exploring possible feelings of inadequacy or frustration.

As the relationship progresses, gift giving may take on a different significance. In the working phase, for example, the patient may one day offer to buy the nurse a cup of coffee. This can be a sign of the patient's respect for the nurse and in their work together. As an isolated incident, the nurse's acceptance of it can enhance the patient's confidence, self-esteem, and sense of responsibility.

Gift giving most often arises in the termination phase of the relationship, and it is in this phase that the meaning behind it can be the most complex and difficult to determine. At this time, gift giving can be tangible or intangible and can reflect a patient's need to make the nurse feel guilty, delay the termination process, compensate for feelings of inadequacy, or attempt to transform the therapeutic nurse-patient relationship into a social one that can possibly go on indefinitely. The nurse can initiate gift giving for similar reasons. The feelings evoked during the termination process can be very powerful, and they must be acknowledged and explored if termination is to be a learning experience for both participants. If feelings are identified and clarified, then a small gift that reflects gratitude and remembrance can be exchanged, accepted, and valued.

■ THERAPEUTIC OUTCOME

The nurse's effectiveness in working with psychiatric patients is related to knowledge base, clinical skills, and capacity for introspection and self-evaluation. The nurse and patient, as participants in an interpersonal relationship, are joined in a pattern of reciprocal emotions that directly affect the therapeutic outcome. The nurse conveys feelings to the patient. Some of these are in response to the patient; others arise from the nurse's personal life and are not necessarily associated with the patient.

Many painful feelings arise within the nurse because of the nature of the therapeutic process, which can be quite stressful. These "normal" stresses are caused by a variety of factors. Although it is necessary to be a skilled listener, it is inappropriate for the nurse to discuss personal conflicts or responses, except when they may help the patient. This bottling up of emotions can be painful. The nurse is expected to empathize with the patient's emotions and feelings. At the same time, however, the nurse is expected to retain objectivity and not be caught up in a sympathetic response. This can create a kind of double bind.

Termination poses another stress when the nurse must separate from a patient she or he has come to know well and care for deeply. It is common to experience a grief reaction in response to the loss. Many nurses find it emotionally draining when a patient communicates a prolonged and intense expression of emotion, such as sadness, despair, or anger. Discomfort also arises when the nurse feels unable to help a patient who is in great distress. Suicide dramatizes this situation. Treating suicidal individuals can arouse intense and prolonged anxiety in the nurse.

The painful nature of these emotional responses makes the practice of psychiatric nursing challenging and stressful. The therapeutic use of self involves the nurse's total personality, and total involvement is not an easy task. It is essential that the nurse be aware of personal feelings and responses and receive guidance and support as needed.

CHAPTER **FOCUS POINTS**

- The therapeutic nurse-patient relationship is a mutual learning experience and a corrective emotional experience for the patient. The nurse uses personal attributes and specified clinical techniques in working with the patient to bring about behavioral change.
- The qualities needed by nurses to be effective helpers include awareness of self, clarification of values, exploration of feelings, ability to serve as a role model, altruism, and a sense of ethics and responsibility.
- The four phases of the nurse-patient relationship are preinteraction phase; introductory, or orientation, phase; working phase; and termination phase. Each phase builds on the preceding one and is characterized by specific tasks.
- In the preinteraction phase the nurse's initial task is one of self-exploration. Other tasks of this phase include gathering data about the patient if information is available and planning for the first interaction with the patient.
- In the introductory, or orientation, phase, one of the nurse's primary concerns is to find out why the patient sought help. Other tasks in this phase of the relationship are to establish a climate of trust, understanding, acceptance, and open communication; to formulate a contract with the patient; to explore the patient's perceptions, thoughts, feelings, and actions; to identify pertinent patient problems; and to define mutual, specific goals with the patient.
- In the working phase, the nurse and the patient explore stressors and promote the development of insight in the patient by linking perceptions, thoughts, feelings, and actions. These insights should be translated into action and a change in behavior.

- In the termination phase, learning is maximized for both the patient and the nurse as they exchange feelings and memories and evaluate mutually the patient's progress and goal attainment.
- Communication can take place on two levels—verbal and nonverbal—and both are critical to the success of the nurse-patient relationship. Types of nonverbal communication include vocal cues, action cues, object cues, space, and touch.
- The communication process involves perception, evaluation, and transmission. Structural and transactional analysis models can be used to examine components of the communication process and to identify common problems.
- Therapeutic communication techniques include listening, broad openings, restating, clarification, reflection, focusing, sharing perceptions, theme identification, silence, humor, informing, and suggesting.
- Responsive dimensions of a therapeutic relationship include genuineness, respect, empathic understanding, and concreteness.
- Action dimensions of a therapeutic relationship include confrontation, immediacy, nurse self-disclosure, emotional catharsis, and role playing.
- Therapeutic impasses such as resistance, transference, countertransference, and boundary violations are roadblocks in the progress of the nurse-patient relationship.
- The therapeutic outcome in working with psychiatric patients is related to the nurse's knowledge base, clinical skills, and capacity for introspection and self-evaluation.

◀ KEY TERMS

CHAPTER REVIEW QUESTIONS

1. For each of the activities described below, write in the correct phase of the therapeutic relationship:

Orientation   Termination
Preinteraction   Working

_____ A. Analyze own feelings and fears
_____ B. Define goals with the patient
_____ C. Determine why the patient sought help
_____ D. Explore feelings of loss and separation
_____ E. Evaluate patient stressors
_____ F. Formulate a contract
_____ G. Gather data about the patient
_____ H. Overcome resistance
_____ I. Promote insight and behavioral change
_____ J. Review goal attainment

2. Fill in the blanks.

A. When a person sends double messages or verbal and nonverbal messages that do not agree, it is called _____ communication.

B. Reflection of the content of a patient's communication back to him is called _____.

C. The responsive dimension of _____ is the ability to see the patient's world from her point of view and to communicate this to the patient.

D. A _____ occurs when a nurse goes outside the limits of the therapeutic relationship and establishes a social, economic, or personal relationship with a patient.

3. Provide short answers for the following questions.

A. Identify four guidelines that should be used to evaluate the potential usefulness of nurse self-disclosure.

B. List elements that should be included in a nurse-patient contract.

C. Describe how the items listed below apply to a social relationship and a therapeutic relationship.
Use of feelings
Content of interaction
Confidentiality
Termination

D. Think of a patient you recently cared for as a nurse. Evaluate how well you demonstrated each of the responsive dimensions of the therapeutic nurse-patient relationship described in this chapter.

E. Have you observed any boundary violations among your nursing colleagues? If so, have you talked with them about it? If not, why not?

4. Match each of the terms in Column A with the correct example in Column B.

Column A
_____ Altruism
_____ Catharsis
_____ Confrontation
_____ Countertransference
_____ Resistance
_____ Role playing
_____ Transference

Column B
A. Dependency by a patient on the nurse for getting better and coping with life.

B. Encouraging a patient to talk about her feelings related to her brother's death.

C. Having the patient assume the part of her husband when talking with the nurse about her marital problems.

D. Irritation and disgust evidenced by a nurse toward a patient who is not responding to the treatment plan.

E. Refusal by a patient to discuss early events as they relate to her current depression.

F. Sharing the observation with a patient that he asks to be treated as a responsible adult but has not been able to keep his last three jobs longer than a month.

G. Volunteering to prepare and serve meals at a local homeless shelter.

Visit Evolve for additional resources related to the content of this chapter.
http://evolve.elsevier.com/Stuart/principles/
• Topical Course Outline • Student Workbook Exercises • Critical Thinking Questions and Activities • Case Studies • Research Topics
• Monthly Content Updates • WebLinks

Student Study CD-ROM

Access the accompanying CD-ROM for animations, interactive exercises, review questions for the NCLEX examination, and an audio glossary.

REFERENCES

Baron S: Boundaries in professional relationships, *J Am Psych Nurs Assoc* 7:32, 2001.

Berne E: *Games people play: the psychology of human relationships*, New York, 1964, Grove Press.

Bohart A, Greenberg L: *Empathy reconsidered*, Washington, DC, 1997, American Psychological Association.

Campbell J: The relationship of nursing and self-awareness, *Adv Nurs Sci* 2:15, 1980.

Carkhoff R: *Helping and human relations*, vols 1 and 2, New York, 1969, Holt, Rinehart & Winston.

Carkhoff R, Berenson B: *Beyond counseling and therapy*, New York, 1967, Holt, Rinehart & Winston.

Carkhoff R, Truax C: *Toward effective counseling and psychotherapy*, Chicago, 1967, Aldine Publishing.

Deering CG: To speak or not to speak? Self-disclosure with patients, *Am J Nurs* 99:34, 1999.

Eckroth-Bucher M: Philosophical basis and practice of self-awareness in psychiatric nursing, *J Psychosoc Nurs*, 39:32, 2001.

Ens I: The lived experience of countertransference in psychiatric/mental health nurses, *Arch Psychiatr Nurs* 13:321, 1999.

Festa L et al: Maximizing learning outcomes by videotaping nursing students' interaction with a standardized patient, *J Psychosoc Nurs*, 38: 37, 2000.

Gallop R: Postdischarge social contact: a potential area for boundary violation, *J Am Psychiatr Nurs Assoc* 4:105, 1998.

Jourard S: *The transparent self*, New York, 1971, Litton Educational Publishing.

Kalisch BJ: What is empathy? *Am J Nurs* 73:1548, 1973.

Kirschenbaum H, Simon S, editors: *Readings in values clarification*, Minneapolis, 1973, Winston Press.

Mansfield E: Empathy: concept and identified psychiatric nursing behavior, *Nurs Res* 22:525, 1973.

Morse JM: The structure and function of gift giving in the patient-nurse relationship, *West J Nurs Res* 13:597, 1991.

Muller A, Poggenpoel M: Patients' internal world experiences of interacting with psychiatric nurses, *Arch Psychiatr Nurs* 10:143, 1996.

Nichols M: *The lost art of listening*, New York, 1995, The Guilford Press.

Norris D, Gutheil TG, Strasburger LH: This couldn't happen to me: boundary problems and sexual misconduct in the psychotherapy relationship, *Psychiatr Serv* 54: 517, 2003.

Olson JK: Relationships between nurse-expressed empathy, patient-perceived empathy and patient distress, *Image J Nurs Sch* 27:317, 1995.

Psychopathology Committee of the Group for the Advancement of Psychiatry: Reexamination of therapist self-disclosure, *Psychiatr Serv* 52: 1489, 2001.

Raingruber B: Settling into and moving in a climate of care: styles and patterns of interaction between nurse psychotherapists and clients, *Perspect Psychiatr Care*, 37: 15, 2001.

Reid W: Boundary issues and violations, *J Pract Psychiatr Behav Health* 4:173, 1999.

Reynolds W: *The measurement and development of empathy in nursing*, United Kingdom, 2000, Ashgate Publishing Co.

Rogers C: *On becoming a person*, Boston, 1961, Houghton Mifflin.

Rogers C: Empathic: an unappreciated way of being, *J Counsel Psychol* 5:2, 1975.

Sayre J: The use of aberrant medical humor by psychiatric unit staff, *Issues Ment Health Nurs* 22: 669, 2001.

Simon RI, Williams IC: Maintaining treatment boundaries in small communities and rural areas, *Psychiatr Serv* 50:1440, 1999.

Sundeen S et al: *Nurse-client interaction: implementing the nursing process*, ed 6, St Louis, 1998, Mosby.

Walker K, Alligood M: Empathy from a nursing perspective: moving beyond borrowed theory, *Arch Psychiatr Nurs* 15:140, 2001.

Walker R, Clark JK: Heading off boundary problems: clinical supervision as risk management, *Psychiatric Serv* 50:1435, 1999.

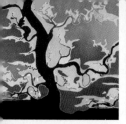

Though this be madness, yet there is method in't.

WILLIAM SHAKESPEARE *HAMLET*, ACT II

3 CONCEPTUAL MODELS OF PSYCHIATRIC TREATMENT

Gail W. Stuart

LEARNING OBJECTIVES

After studying this chapter, the student should be able to:
1. Analyze the psychoanalytical model, including its view of behavioral deviations, the therapeutic process, and roles of the patient and therapist (**I**).
2. Analyze the interpersonal model, including its view of behavioral deviations, the therapeutic process, and roles of the patient and therapist (**II**).
3. Analyze the social model, including its view of behavioral deviations, the therapeutic process, and roles of the patient and therapist (**III**).
4. Analyze the existential model, including its view of behavioral deviations, the therapeutic process, and roles of the patient and therapist (**IV**).
5. Analyze the supportive therapy model, including its view of behavioral deviations, the therapeutic process, and roles of the patient and therapist (**V**).
6. Analyze the medical model, including its view of behavioral deviations, the therapeutic process, and roles of the patient and therapist (**VI**).

TOPICAL OUTLINE

I. Psychoanalytical Model
  A. View of Behavioral Deviations
  B. Psychoanalytical Therapeutic Process
  C. Roles of Patient and Psychoanalyst
  D. Other Psychoanalytical Theorists
II. Interpersonal Model
  A. View of Behavioral Deviations
  B. Interpersonal Therapeutic Process
  C. Roles of Patient and Interpersonal Therapist
III. Social Model
  A. View of Behavioral Deviations
  B. Social Therapeutic Process
  C. Roles of Patient and Social Therapist
IV. Existential Model
  A. View of Behavioral Deviations
  B. Existential Therapeutic Process
  C. Roles of Patient and Existential Therapist
V. Supportive Therapy Model
  A. View of Behavioral Deviations
  B. Supportive Therapeutic Process
  C. Roles of Patient and Supportive Therapist
VI. Medical Model
  A. View of Behavioral Deviations
  B. Medical Therapeutic Process
  C. Roles of Patient and Medical Therapist

 Visit Evolve for additional resources related to the content of this chapter.
http://evolve.elsevier.com/Stuart/principles/

Mental health professionals should base their practice on a conceptual model of psychiatric treatment. A model is a way of organizing a complex body of knowledge, such as concepts related to human behavior. Models help clinicians by suggesting:
- Reasons for observed behavior.
- Therapeutic treatment strategies.
- Appropriate roles for patient and therapist.

Models also provide for the organization of data. Organization allows the clinician to measure the effectiveness of the treatment process and facilitates research into human behavior.

This chapter presents an overview of some of the conceptual models used by mental health professionals, including the psychoanalytical, interpersonal, social, existential, supportive, and medical models. Other models often used by nurses are discussed in other chapters of this text, including cognitive behavioral (Chapter 31), group (Chapter 32), and

family (Chapter 33). Finally, the Stuart Stress Adaptation Model of psychiatric nursing, which is the organizing conceptual framework for this text, is presented in detail in Chapter 4.

■ PSYCHOANALYTICAL MODEL

Psychoanalytical theory was developed by **Sigmund Freud** (Figure 3-1) in the late nineteenth and early twentieth centuries (1974). It focused on the nature of deviant behavior and proposed a new perspective on human development. Many of Freud's ideas were controversial, particularly in the Victorian society of that time. Objective observation of human behavior was a great contribution of the psychoanalysts, as was the identification of a mental structure. Such concepts as id, ego, superego, and ego defense mechanisms are still widely used. Most people also accept the existence of an un-

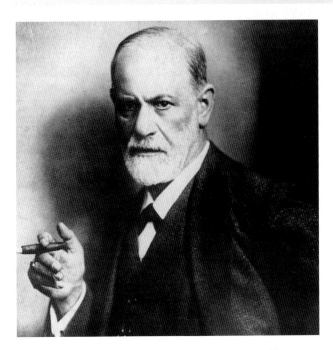

Figure 3-1   Sigmund Freud. (From the Bettman Archive.)

conscious level of mental functioning, first introduced by Freud.

View of Behavioral Deviations

Psychoanalysts trace disrupted behavior in the adult to earlier developmental stages. Each stage of development has a task that must be accomplished. If too much emphasis is placed on any stage or if unusual difficulty arises in dealing with the associated conflicts, psychological energy (libido) becomes fixated in an attempt to deal with anxiety.

Psychoanalysts believe that neurotic symptoms arise when so much energy goes into controlling anxiety that it interferes with the individual's ability to function. They believe that everyone is neurotic to some extent. Everyone carries the burden of childhood conflicts and is influenced in adulthood by childhood experiences. Psychoanalysts in training must undergo personal analysis so that their own neurotic behavior does not hinder their objectivity as therapists.

According to psychoanalytic theory, symptoms are symbols of the original conflict. For instance, compulsive hand washing may represent the person's attempt to cleanse the self of impulses that a parent labeled unclean during the anal stage of development. However, the meaning of the behavior is hidden from the conscious awareness of the person, who usually is upset about these uncontrollable feelings.

Freud developed most of his theories around neurotic symptoms. His theory is less well developed in the area of psychosis. However, other psychoanalytical theorists such as Frieda Fromm-Reichmann (1950) have successfully worked with patients with psychosis. They believe that the psychotic symptom arises when the ego must invest most or all of the libido in defending against primitive id impulses. This leaves little energy to deal with external reality and leads to the lack of reality testing seen in psychosis.

Psychoanalytical Therapeutic Process

Psychoanalysis is a therapeutic approach based on the belief that behavioral disorders are related to unresolved, anxiety-provoking childhood experiences that are repressed into the unconscious. Its goal is to bring repressed experiences into conscious awareness and to learn healthier means of coping with the anxiety. It uses free association and dream analysis to reconstruct the personality. Free association is the verbalization of thoughts as they occur, without any conscious screening or censorship. Of course, unconscious censorship of thoughts and impulses that threaten the ego is always at work in the mind. The psychoanalyst searches for patterns in the areas that are unconsciously avoided. Conflicting areas that the patient does not discuss or recognize are identified as resistances. Analysis of the patient's dreams can provide additional insight into the nature of the resistances because dreams symbolically communicate areas of intrapsychic conflict.

The therapist helps the patient recognize intrapsychic conflicts by using interpretation. Interpretation involves explaining to the patient the meaning of dream symbolism and the significance of the issues that are discussed or avoided. However, the process is complicated by transference, which occurs when the patient develops strong positive or negative feelings toward the analyst. These feelings are unrelated to the analyst's current behavior or characteristics; they represent the patient's past response to a significant other, usually a parent. Strong positive transference causes the patient to want to please the therapist and to accept the therapist's interpretations of the patient's behavior. Strong negative transference may impede the progress of therapy as the patient actively resists the therapist's interventions. Countertransference, or the therapist's response to the patient, also can interfere with therapy if the analyst is unaware of it or unable to deal with it.

Because the therapist can temporarily replace the significant other of the patient's early life, previously unresolved conflicts can be brought into the therapeutic situation. These conflicts can be worked through to achieve a healthier resolution and more mature adult functioning. Psychoanalytical therapy is usually long term. Often the patient is seen five times a week for several years. This approach is therefore time consuming and expensive.

Roles of Patient and Psychoanalyst

The roles of the patient and the psychoanalyst were defined by Freud. The patient was to be an active participant, freely revealing all thoughts exactly as they occurred and describing all dreams. The patient often lies down during therapy to induce relaxation, which facilitates free association.

The psychoanalyst is a shadow person. The patient is expected to reveal all private thoughts and feelings, and the analyst reveals nothing personal. The analyst usually is out of the patient's sight during therapy sessions, to ensure that nonverbal responses do not influence the patient. The analyst keeps his or her verbal responses brief and noncommittal in order to prevent interference with the associative flow. For instance, the analyst might respond with "Uh huh," "Go on," or "Tell me more."

The therapist changes this communication style when interpreting behavior. Interpretations are presented for the patient to accept or reject, but rejections suggest resistance. Likewise, frustration that the patient expresses toward the analyst is interpreted as transference. By the end of therapy, the patient should be able to view the analyst realistically, having worked through conflicts and dependency needs.

 Do you think that roles of the patient and psychoanalyst support patient empowerment or patient dependency? ■

Other Psychoanalytical Theorists

Much of Freud's theory is still used by psychotherapists. The theorists who followed him have modified and built on the original psychoanalytical theories. Box 3-1 lists several other psychoanalytical theorists and gives a brief statement identifying the major contributions of each.

BOX 3-1

Contemporary Psychoanalytical Theorists

Erik Erikson (1963): Expanded Freud's theory of psychosocial development to encompass the entire life cycle
Anna Freud (1966): Expanded psychoanalytical theory in the area of child psychology
Melanie Klein (1949): Extended the use of psychoanalytical techniques to work with young children through development of play therapy
Karen Horney (1950): Focused on psychoanalytical theory in terms of cultural and interpersonal factors; rejected Freud's view of feminine sexuality
Frieda Fromm-Reichmann (1950): Used psychoanalytical techniques with psychotic patients
Karl Menninger (1963): Applied the concepts of dynamic equilibrium and coping to mental functioning

---

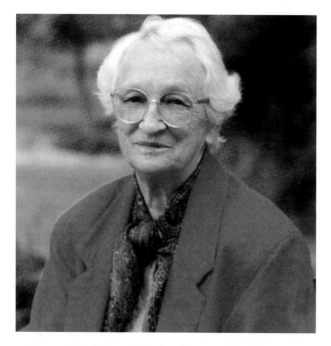

Figure 3-2   Hildegard E. Peplau. (Courtesy Hildegard E. Peplau.)

■ INTERPERSONAL MODEL

Interpersonal therapy has been found to be an effective form of treatment for patients with a wide variety of psychiatric disorders (see Citing the Evidence). The theorist who originated the interpersonal model is **Harry Stack Sullivan**, a twentieth-century American therapist (1953, 1954). Since then it has been further developed and refined by **Gerald Klerman** (1993). Attention is also given to the interpersonal nursing theory of **Hildegard Peplau** (1952) (Figure 3-2). Her work on the psychotherapeutic role of the nurse in the interpersonal relationship is a milestone in the field.

The goal of interpersonal therapy is to reduce symptoms, improve social functioning, and assist the person in developing more adaptive ways of relating to others. It is particularly effective with issues related to grief, role disputes, role transitions, and interpersonal deficits.

View of Behavioral Deviations

Interpersonal theorists believe that behavior evolves around interpersonal relationships. Whereas Freudian theory emphasizes a person's intrapsychic experience, interpersonal theory emphasizes social or interpersonal experience (Evans, 1996). Sullivan, like Freud, traces a progression of psychological development. Sullivan's theory states that the person bases behavior on two drives: the drive for satisfaction and the drive for security. Satisfaction includes the basic human drives of hunger, sleep, lust, and loneliness. Security relates to culturally defined needs such as conformity to the social norms and the value system of the individual's reference group. Sullivan states that when a person's self-system interferes with the ability to

---

■ CITING THE EVIDENCE ON
Interpersonal Therapy

BACKGROUND: Antenatal depression is a significant risk factor for postpartum depression, with a 10% to 12% prevalence in all pregnancies. Rates of depression are higher for pregnant women with chronic stressors, financial and housing problems, and inadequate social support. Furthermore, treatment of depression during pregnancy has been identified as a health care priority. This controlled clinical trial compared a group receiving interpersonal psychotherapy for antepartum depression to a parenting education control group.

RESULTS: The interpersonal psychotherapy treatment group showed significant improvement compared to the parenting education control program on all measures of mood. A significant correlation between maternal mood and mother-child interaction was noted.

IMPLICATIONS: Interpersonal psychotherapy is an effective treatment for depression during pregnancy and should be considered a first-line treatment for antepartum depression. Given that depressed mothers negatively impact their newborns, timely and effective assessment and treatment by nurses and other health care providers is essential.

Spinelli M, Endicott J: *Am J Psychiatry* 160:555, 2003.

meet the need for satisfaction or security, the person becomes mentally ill.

When Peplau defined nursing as an interpersonal process, she also discussed the importance of basic human needs. Needs must be met if a healthy state is to be achieved and maintained. For Peplau, the two interacting components of health are physiological demands and interpersonal conditions. These components may be seen as parallel to the drives of satisfaction and security identified by Sullivan, as is evident in the following clinical example.

CLINICAL EXAMPLE

Ms. Y, an attractive 26-year-old woman, appeared at a psychiatric outpatient clinic requesting therapy. She said, "I can't get close to people." She said that her childhood was happy and that she had loving parents and liked her sister. Her family were devout members of a fundamentalist Protestant church, so most of her activities were church related. She had many friends during childhood and then one close girlfriend in early adolescence. She thought that her fear of closeness began when she slept over at her friend's house. During the night her friend began to fondle her in a way that she interpreted as sexual. She became very frightened and felt guilty. She did not tell her parents because of her feelings of guilt and, in fact, had told no one before entering therapy. Although she attended college, she never dated and participated only in superficial social contacts. She realized that this was not healthy young adult behavior and, because the behavior continued into her twenties, Ms. Y decided to seek help. ■

From an interpersonal perspective, Ms. Y was unable to fulfill her needs for friendship and sexual love. Interpersonal theorists would view the unfulfilled sexual love dynamism as a lack of satisfaction, and her fear that she had deviated from the norm as a lack of security. Her anxiety stemmed from her conviction that her parents would disown her if they heard what had happened. This belief was based on their earlier responses to childhood sexual play. The therapist decided that Ms. Y first needed to experience intimacy on a nonsexual level. This need was approached in therapy. After Ms. Y began to feel comfortable sharing closeness with the therapist, she gradually explored friendships and later began dating.

Interpersonal Therapeutic Process

The interpersonal therapist focuses on the "here and now," uses exploratory and behavioral change techniques, and encourages the expression of affect. The crux of the therapeutic process is the corrective interpersonal experience. The idea is that by experiencing a healthy relationship with the therapist, the patient can learn to have more satisfying interpersonal relationships. The therapist actively encourages the development of trust by relating authentically to the patient and sharing feelings and reactions with the patient. The process of therapy is a process of reeducation.

The therapist helps the patient identify interpersonal problems and then encourages attempts at more successful styles of relating. For example, patients often have a fear of intimacy. The therapist allows the patient to become close while showing him or her that there is no threat of sexual in-

volvement. It is believed that closeness within the therapeutic relationship builds trust, facilitates empathy, enhances self-esteem, and fosters growth toward healthy behavior. Peplau describes this process as "psychological mothering," which includes the following steps:

1. The patient is accepted unconditionally as a participant in a relationship that satisfies needs.
2. There is recognition of and response to the patient's readiness for growth, as initiated by the patient.
3. Power in the relationship shifts to the patient, as the patient is able to delay gratification and to invest energy in goal achievement.

Therapy is complete when the patient can establish satisfying human relationships, thereby meeting basic needs. Termination is a significant part of the relationship that must be shared by the therapist and the patient. The patient learns that leaving a significant other involves pain but also can be an opportunity for growth.

Do you think that "psychological mothering" promotes maternalism or mutuality in the patient-therapist relationship? ■

Roles of Patient and Interpersonal Therapist

The patient-therapist dyad is viewed as a partnership in interpersonal therapy. Sullivan describes the therapist as a "participant observer" whose role is to engage the patient, establish trust, and empathize. An active effort is put forth to help the patient realize that other people have similar perceptions and concerns. An atmosphere of uncritical acceptance encourages the patient to speak openly. The therapist interacts as a real person who also has beliefs, values, thoughts, and feelings. The patient's role is to share concerns with the therapist and to participate as fully as possible in the relationship. The relationship itself serves as a model of adaptive interpersonal relationships. While the patient matures in the ability to relate, life experiences with people outside the therapeutic situation are enhanced.

Interpersonal nursing roles have been identified by Peplau and are listed in Box 3-2. These roles may be assumed by the

---

BOX 3-2

Interpersonal Nursing Roles Identified by Peplau

Stranger: The role assumed by both nurse and patient when they first meet
Resource person: Provides health information to a patient who has assumed the consumer role
Teacher: Helps the patient grow and learn from experience with the health care system
Leader: Helps the patient participate in a democratically implemented nursing process
Surrogate: Assumes roles that have been assigned by the patient, based on significant past relationships, as in the psychoanalytical phenomenon of transference
Counselor: Helps the patient integrate the facts and feelings associated with an episode of illness into the patient's total life experience

nurse or assigned to others. The therapist helps the patient meet the goals of therapy: need satisfaction and personal growth. In addition, through role performance the nurse also experiences growth and self-discovery. Self-awareness is essential to success as an interpersonal therapist.

SOCIAL MODEL

The two preceding models focused on the individual and intrapsychic processes and interpersonal experiences. The social model moves beyond the individual to consider the social environment as it affects the person and the person's life experience (see Chapter 8). Psychoanalytical theory has been criticized for not extending to other cultures and times. For example, Freud's view of women has been repeatedly challenged, particularly by feminists. Some theorists such as **Thomas Szasz** (1961, 1987, 1993, 2002) and **Gerald Caplan** (1964) believe that the culture itself is useful in defining mental illness, prescribing therapy, and determining the patient's future. Others contend that the social realm is intrinsic to concepts of mind and mental illness and can complement or correct the prevailing assumptions of purely biological models (Cohen, 2000). In addition, the community mental health movement is an example of a government effort to respond to the philosophy of the social theorists (see Chapter 35).

View of Behavioral Deviations

According to the social theorists, social conditions are largely responsible for deviant behavior. Deviance is culturally defined. Behavior considered normal in one cultural setting may be eccentric in another and psychotic in a third. An example is the African exchange student described in the following clinical example.

CLINICAL EXAMPLE

Early in the fall semester a black male exchange student from Africa was brought to the psychiatric emergency room. He had been walking around the campus carrying a spear and had been apprehended by the university security patrol. His speech was heavily accented and they could not understand his explanation of his behavior. Later evaluation revealed that in his native culture one never went walking at night without a spear to defend against attack by wild beasts or hostile neighboring tribes. He was sent back to his dormitory after being convinced that his spear was not appropriate to the culture of the American college campus. ■

From this point of view, Szasz (1961) writes of the "myth of mental illness." He believes that society must find a way to manage "undesirables," so it labels them as mentally ill. People who are so labeled usually are unable or unwilling to conform to social norms, and their behavior usually leads to confinement. If these people then conform to social expectations, they are considered to have recovered and are allowed to return to the community. Confinement performs the dual function of removing deviant members from the community at large and exerting social control over their behavior.

Szasz believes that people are responsible for their own behavior. Each person has control over whether to conform to social expectations. Those labeled as mentally ill may be scapegoats, but they participate in the scapegoating process by inviting it or by allowing it to occur. Szasz objects to describing deviant behavior as illness. He believes that illness can occur and that diseases of the body (such as brain tumors) can influence behavior, but that no physiological disruption can be demonstrated to cause most deviancy. He distinguishes between the biological condition that is central to illness and the social role that is the focus of deviance.

Caplan also has studied deviant behavior from a social perspective. He has extended the public health model of primary, secondary, and tertiary prevention to the mental health field. He has focused particularly on primary prevention because much attention has been given to the secondary and tertiary levels. Lack of understanding of the cause of deviant behavior has hindered the development of primary prevention techniques.

Caplan believes that social situations can predispose a person to mental illness. Such situations include poverty, family instability, and inadequate education. Deprivation throughout the life cycle results in limited ability to cope with stress. The person has few environmental supports. The result is a predisposition to maladaptive coping responses.

How do you distinguish between social deviance and psychiatric illness? How do your friends and family define them? ■

Social Therapeutic Process

Szasz advocates freedom of choice for psychiatric patients. People should be allowed to select their own therapeutic modalities and therapists. This freedom requires a well-informed consumer who can base this decision on knowledge of effective modes of psychotherapy (see Critical Thinking About Contemporary Issues). Szasz does not believe in involuntary hospitalization of people with mental illness. He questions whether any psychiatric hospitalization is truly voluntary. Szasz disapproves of the community mental health movement to place mental health care within the reach of every American. He questions government involvement in what he views as a private concern.

Caplan, on the other hand, supports community psychiatry. He sees the mental health professional using consultation to combat societal problems. He believes that future psychiatric patients would benefit indirectly from positive social change.

Roles of Patient and Social Therapist

Szasz believes that a therapist can help the patient only if the patient requests help. The patient initiates therapy and defines the problem to be solved. The patient also has the right to approve or reject the recommended therapeutic intervention. Therapy is successfully completed when the patient is satisfied with the changes in his or her life. The therapist collaborates with the patient to promote change. This change includes making recommendations about possible means of effecting behavioral adjustment, but it does not include any

■ **Critical Thinking** *About* **Contemporary Issues**

What Kind of Psychotherapy Works Best, for Whom, Under What Circumstances, and at What Cost?

Competition among the various models of psychiatric treatment has tended to distract attention from questions about what model of psychotherapy works best, for what type of patient, under what life conditions, and at what cost. Answering these questions has been difficult, but characteristics of effective treatments have been identified (O'Donohue et al, 2000; Stone, 2001). These include having a specific problem focus, using continuous assessment of the patient's progress, and the presence of a strong patient-therapist therapeutic alliance. It also has been suggested that using an approach that integrates a number of treatments and a range of interventions may have an advantage over a unidimensional approach (Winston and Winston, 2001). Although evaluating the outcomes of treatment is a current topic of research interest, studies in this area have proven to be less exact and more subjective because of the following factors:

- The therapist's evaluation of changes that have occurred
- The patient's report of changes
- Reports from the patient's family and friends
- Comparison of pretreatment and posttreatment behavioral rating scale scores
- Measures of changes in selected symptoms or behaviors

Unfortunately, each of these sources has serious limitations, and they may even conflict with each other. In addition, these studies often fail to measure other important aspects of treatment, such as the nature of the therapeutic alliance, health belief systems of the patient and therapist, cost of treatment, and impact of treatment on the patient's overall biopsychosocial functioning and quality of life. What is needed is greater specificity about the people and problems for which psychotherapy can provide the greatest benefit, the methodology that would be most useful in providing these data, and the comprehensive and accurate measurement of the indications for, cost of, and outcomes of psychotherapy.

element of coercion, particularly the threat of hospitalization if the patient does not agree with the therapist's recommendations. The therapist's role also may involve protecting the patient from social demands for coercive treatment.

Caplan believes that society has a moral obligation to provide a wide range of therapeutic services covering all three levels of prevention. The patient has a consumer role and selects the appropriate level of help from a wide array of services. Ideally, effective primary preventive services decrease the need for secondary or tertiary care.

According to this model, therapists may be professionals or nonprofessionals with professional consultation skills. People such as clergy, police, bartenders, and beauticians can be trained to listen and to refer people who need professional help to appropriate resources. The therapist in the social context is not tied to the office but is involved in the community. Activities may include home visits, lectures to community groups, or consultation with other agencies. The rationale for this approach is that the more involved therapists are in the community, the greater the impact on the community's mental health. Community involvement also enhances the therapist's understanding of patients who live in that environment.

Do you think bartenders and salon staff can be effective therapists? Why or why not? ■

■ **EXISTENTIAL MODEL**

The existential model focuses on the person's experience in the here and now, with much less attention focused on the person's past than is the case in other theoretical models.

View of Behavioral Deviations

Existentialist theorists believe that behavioral deviations result when one is out of touch with oneself or the environment. This alienation is caused by self-imposed restrictions.

The individual is not free to choose from among all alternative behaviors. Deviant behavior often is a way of avoiding more socially acceptable or more responsible behavior.

The person who is self-alienated feels helpless, sad, and lonely. Self-criticism and lack of self-awareness prevent participation in authentic, rewarding relationships with others. Theoretically, the person has many choices in terms of behavior. However, existentialists believe that people tend to avoid being real and instead surrender to the demands of others.

Existential Therapeutic Process

Existential therapy focuses on the importance of experience in the present and the belief that humans find meaning through their experiences. Existential therapies assume that the patient must be able to choose freely from what life has to offer. Examples include rational-emotive therapy by **Albert Ellis** (1989), reality therapy by **William Glasser** (1965), and gestalt therapy by **Frederick Perls** (1969). Although the approaches are somewhat different, the goal of each is to return the patient to an authentic awareness of being.

The existential therapeutic process focuses on the encounter. The encounter is not merely the meeting of two or more people; it also involves their appreciation of the total existence of each other. Through the encounter the patient is helped to accept and understand personal history, to live fully in the present, and to look forward to the future.

Roles of Patient and Existential Therapist

Existential theorists emphasize that the therapist and the patient are equal in their common humanity. The therapist acts as a guide to the patient, who has gone astray in the search for authenticity. The therapist is direct in specifying areas where the patient should consider changing, but caring and warmth are also emphasized. The therapist and the patient are to be open and honest. The therapeutic experience is a model for the patient; new behaviors can be tested before risks are taken in daily life.

The patient is expected to assume and accept responsibility for behavior. Dependence on the therapist generally is not encouraged. The patient is treated as an adult. Often, illness is deemphasized. The patient is viewed as a person who is alienated from the self and others but for whom there is hope if he or she trusts the therapist and follows directions. The patient is always active in therapy, working to meet the challenge presented by the therapist.

■ SUPPORTIVE THERAPY MODEL

Supportive therapy is a mode of psychotherapy that is widely used in hospital and community-based psychiatric treatment settings. It differs from other models in that it does not depend on any overriding concept or theory. Instead, it uses many psychodynamic theories to understand how people change. The aims of supportive psychotherapy as described by **Lawrence Rockland** (1989) include the following:

- Promote a supportive patient-therapist relationship
- Enhance patient's strengths, coping skills, and ability to use coping resources
- Reduce the patient's subjective distress and maladaptive coping responses
- Help the patient achieve the greatest independence possible based on the specific psychiatric or physical illness
- Foster the greatest amount of autonomy in treatment decisions with the patient

Controlled studies have shown supportive therapy to be effective in treating schizophrenia, borderline conditions, and affective, anxiety, posttraumatic stress, eating, and substance abuse disorders, as well as the psychological component of many physical illnesses (Rockland, 1993).

View of Behavioral Deviations

Supportive therapists are psychodynamically based, and they describe behavioral deviations as neurotic, borderline, or psychotic. They believe in the concepts of id, ego, and superego and emphasize the important role of psychological defenses in adaptive functioning. Compared with those of other therapists, however, their focus is more behavior oriented. They emphasize current biopsychosocial coping responses and the person's ability to use available coping resources.

Supportive Therapeutic Process

Supportive therapy is an eclectic form of psychotherapy; that is, it is not based on a particular theory of psychopathology. Rather, it can draw as needed from other models and may address different symptoms with different therapeutic methods. Supportive therapy is equally applicable to high-functioning patients in crisis and low-functioning patients with psychosis or persistent mental illness. Its emphasis is on improving behavior and subjective feelings of distress rather than on achieving insight or self-understanding.

Principles of supportive therapy include the following:

- Immediate help to the patient, which may include a variety of treatment modalities
- Family and social support system involvement
- Focus on the present
- Anxiety reduction through supportive measures and medication if necessary
- Clarification and problem solving using a variety of approaches including advice, supportive confrontation, limit setting, education, and environmental change
- Helping the patient to avoid future crises and seek help early when under stress

Roles of Patient and Supportive Therapist

In supportive therapy the therapist plays an active and directive role in helping the patient improve social functioning and coping skills. The setting for supportive therapy should allow for a moderate to high level of activity by both the patient and the therapist. Communication is seen as an active two-way process, and the use of medications or other therapies is encouraged.

The therapist builds a therapeutic alliance with the patient. Expressing empathy, concern, and nonjudgmental acceptance of the patient are important therapist qualities. The therapist supports the patient's healthy adaptive efforts, conveys a willingness to understand, respects the patient as a unique human being, and takes a genuine interest in the patient's life activities and well-being. The therapist regards the patient as a partner in treatment and encourages the patient's autonomy to make treatment and life decisions. In turn, the patient is expected to show a willingness to talk about life events, accept the therapist's supportive role, participate in the therapeutic program, and adhere to the therapeutic structure.

What aspects of supportive therapy are similar to those of the therapeutic nurse-patient relationship? In what ways are they different? ■

■ MEDICAL MODEL

The medical model refers to psychiatric care that is based on the traditional physician-patient relationship. It focuses on the diagnosis of a mental illness, and subsequent treatment is based on this diagnosis. Somatic treatments, including pharmacotherapy and electroconvulsive therapy, are important parts of the treatment process. The interpersonal aspect of the medical model varies widely, from intensive insight-oriented intervention to brief sessions involving management of medications. Many physicians are associated with this model including **Allen Frances** and **Robert Spitzer**.

The medical model dominates modern psychiatric care. Other health professionals may be involved in interagency referrals, family assessment, and health teaching, but physicians are seen as the leaders of the team under this model. Elements of other models of care may be used in conjunction with the medical model. For instance, a patient with schizophrenia may be treated with phenothiazine medication. This patient also may be in supportive therapy to develop adaptive social skills.

One contribution of the medical model is the continuous search for causes of mental illness using the scientific process. Great strides have been made in learning about the functioning of the brain and nervous system (see Chapter 6). This progress has led to greater understanding of the physiological components of many behavioral disorders and thus more effective psychiatric treatments.

> *What problems might the medical model pose for interdisciplinary collaboration in psychiatric treatment?* ■

View of Behavioral Deviations

The medical model proposes that all mental processes, even the most complex psychological processes, derive from operations of the brain, and deviant behavior is a symptom of a brain disorder. Several types of brain disorders could lead to mental illness: loss of nerve cells, excesses or deficits in chemical transmission, abnormal patterns of brain circuitry, problems in the command centers, and disruptions in the movement of messages along nerve pathways. In addition, the medical model proposes that genes, and combinations of genes, exert significant control over behavior.

Medical Therapeutic Process

The medical process of therapy is well defined and familiar to most patients. The examination of the patient includes the history of the present illness, social history, medical history, review of body systems, physical examination, and mental status examination. Additional data may be collected from significant others, and medical records are reviewed if available. A preliminary diagnosis is then formulated, pending further diagnostic studies and observation of the patient's behavior. This process may take place on an ambulatory or an inpatient basis, depending on the patient's condition.

The diagnosis is classified according to the *Diagnostic and Statistical Manual of Mental Disorders*, fourth edition, text revision (*DSM-IV-TR*) of the American Psychiatric Association (2000). The names of the illnesses are accompanied by a description of diagnostic criteria, associated general medical and psychiatric features, diagrams showing the longitudinal course of the disorder, and specific gender, age, and cultural aspects of each illness. Changes in this manual reflect changes in the medical model of psychiatric care. *DSM-I* was first published in 1952 (Grob, 1991), and *DSM-IV-TR*, published in 2000, is the most up-to-date edition.

After the diagnosis is made, treatment begins. The physician-patient relationship is developed to foster trust in the physician and compliance with the treatment plan. Other health team members may contribute their expertise. Response to treatment is evaluated on the basis of the patient's subjective assessment and the physician's objective observations of symptomatic behavior. Therapy is terminated when the patient's symptoms have remitted. For instance, most people who experience depression are able to return to their usual lifestyles after a course of medication and supportive therapy. Other patients may require long-term therapy, often including pharmacotherapy and periodic laboratory studies.

Roles of Patient and Medical Therapist

The roles of physician and patient have been well defined by tradition. The physician, as the healer, identifies the patient's illness and formulates a treatment plan. The patient may have some say about the plan, but the physician prescribes the therapy.

The role of the patient involves admitting being ill, which can be a problem in psychiatry. Patients sometimes are not aware of their disturbed behavior and may actively resist treatment. This is not congruent with the medical model. The patient is expected to comply with the treatment program and try to get well. If observable improvement does not occur, caregivers and significant others often suspect that the patient is not trying hard enough. This can be frustrating to a patient who is trying to get well and is disappointed with the lack of progress. The patient also may have difficulty letting people extend care while still being self-sufficient.

> *How would each conceptual model described in this chapter view the issue of patient nonadherence to the psychiatric treatment plan?* ■

CHAPTER **FOCUS POINTS**

MODEL (MAJOR THEORISTS)	VIEW OF BEHAVIORAL DEVIATION	THERAPEUTIC PROCESS	ROLES OF PATIENT AND THERAPISTS
■ **Psychoanalytical** (S. Freud, Erikson, A. Freud, Klein, Horney, Fromm-Reichmann, Menninger)	Based on inadequate resolution of developmental conflicts. Ego defenses unable to control anxiety. Symptoms result in effort to deal with anxiety and are related to unresolved conflicts.	Uses techniques of free association and dream analysis. Identifies problem areas through interpretation of patient's resistances and transferences.	Patient verbalizes all thoughts and dreams; considers therapist's interpretations. Therapist remains remote to encourage development of transference and interprets patient's thoughts and dreams.
■ **Interpersonal** (Sullivan, Klerman, Peplau)	Anxiety arises and is experienced interpersonally. Basic fear is fear of rejection. Person needs security and satisfaction that result from positive interpersonal relationships.	Relationship between therapist and patient builds feeling of security. Therapist helps patient experience trusting relationship and gain interpersonal satisfaction.	Patient shares anxieties and feelings with therapist. Therapist uses empathy to perceive patient's feelings, and uses relationship as a corrective interpersonal experience.

CHAPTER **FOCUS POINTS**—cont'd

Model (Major Theorists)	View of Behavioral Deviation	Therapeutic Process	Roles of Patient and Therapists
■ **Social** (Szasz, Caplan)	Social and environmental factors create stress, which causes anxiety and symptoms. Unacceptable (deviant) behavior is socially defined.	Patient helped to deal with social system. May use crisis intervention, environmental manipulation, and social supports.	Patient presents problem to therapist, works with therapist and uses community resources. Therapist explores patient's social system and resources available.
■ **Existential** (Perls, Glasser, Ellis)	Life is meaningful when the person can fully experience and accept the self. The self can be experienced through authentic relationships with other people.	Person aided to experience authenticity in relationships. Therapy often conducted in groups. Patient encouraged to accept self and to assume control of behavior.	Patient participates in meaningful experiences to learn about real self. Therapist helps patient recognize value of self, clarify realities of situation, and explore feelings.
■ **Supportive therapy** (Rockland)	Problems are a result of biopsychosocial factors. Emphasis on current maladaptive coping responses.	Reality testing and self-esteem–enhancing measures. Social supports are enlisted and adaptive coping responses are reinforced.	Patient actively involved in treatment. Therapist is warm, empathic, and allied with patient.
■ **Medical** (Frances, Spitzer)	Behavioral disruptions result from a biological disease process. Symptoms result from a combination of physiological, genetic, environmental, and social factors.	Treatment is related to diagnosis and includes somatic therapies and various interpersonal techniques. Treatment approach adjusted depending on symptomatic response.	Patient complies with prescribed therapy and reports effects of therapy to therapist. Therapist diagnoses illness and prescribes therapeutic approach.

KEY TERMS

existential therapy, 55
free association, 51
psychoanalysis, 51

CHAPTER REVIEW QUESTIONS

1. **Match each of the theorists in Column A with the corresponding model of psychiatric treatment in Column B.**

Column A
_____ Freud
_____ Rockland
_____ Ellis
_____ Spitzer
_____ Sullivan
_____ Szasz

Column B
A. Existential
B. Interpersonal
C. Medical
D. Psychoanalytical
E. Social
F. Supportive

2. **Fill in the blanks.**

A. Psychoanalysts believe that behavior problems in adulthood are caused by _____.

B. _____ is the verbalization of thoughts as they occur without any conscious screening or censorship.

C. Interpersonal theorists believe that behavior problems arise from _____.

D. The drives for _____ and _____ are critical to a person's psychological health according to the interpersonal model.

E. Social theorists believe that deviant behavior is caused by _____.

F. The community mental health movement is an example of the _____ model of psychiatric treatment.

G. Existential theorists believe that behavior problems arise when _____.

H. The existential therapeutic process focuses on the _____.

I. Supportive therapy theorists believe that behavior problems arise from _____.

J. In supportive therapy a therapist plays an _____ role and regards the patient as a _____ in the treatment process.

K. Medical model theorists believe that behavior problems arise from _____.

L. A significant contribution of the medical model has been _____.

M. The classification system used in the medical model to diagnose psychiatric illness is the _____.

3. **Provide short answers for the following questions.**

A. What purposes do dreams serve in psychoanalysis and how are dreams perceived by people today?

B. Describe the six nursing roles identified by Peplau.

C. What model of psychiatric treatment do you think is most culture-bound? Which is the most culture-free? Defend your answer.

D. On a scale of 1 to 5, rank in order your preference for the five models of psychiatric treatment described in this chapter. Explain your ranking.

Visit Evolve for additional resources related to the content of this chapter.

http://evolve.elsevier.com/Stuart/principles/
• Topical Course Outline • Student Workbook Exercises • Critical Thinking Questions and Activities • Case Studies • Research Topics
• Monthly Content Updates • WebLinks

Student Study CD-ROM

Access the accompanying CD-ROM for animations, interactive exercises, review questions for the NCLEX examination, and an audio glossary.

REFERENCES

American Psychiatric Association: *Diagnostic and statistical manual of mental disorders*, ed 4, text revision, Washington, DC, 2000, American Psychiatric Association.

Caplan G: *Principles of preventive psychiatry*, New York, 1964, Basic Books.

Cohen CI: Overcoming social amnesia: the role of a social perspective in psychiatric research and practice, *Psychiatr Serv* 51:72, 2000.

Ellis A: *Inside rational emotive therapy*, San Diego, 1989, Academic Press.

Erikson E: *Childhood and society*, ed 2, New York, 1963, WW Norton.

Evans F: *Harry Stack Sullivan: interpersonal theory and psychotherapy*, New York, 1996, Routledge.

Freud A: *The ego and the mechanisms of defense*, New York, 1966, International Universities Press.

Freud S. In Strachey J, editor: *The standard edition of the complete psychological works of Sigmund Freud*, London, 1953-1974, Hogarth Press.

Fromm-Reichmann F: *Principles of intensive psychotherapy*, Chicago, 1950, University of Chicago Press.

Glasser W: *Reality therapy: a new approach to psychiatry*, New York, 1965, Harper & Row.

Grob GN: Origins of DSM-I: a study in appearance and reality, *Am J Psychiatry* 148:421, 1991.

Horney K: *The collected works of Karen Horney*, vols 1 and 2, New York, 1950, WW Norton.

Klein M: *The psychoanalysis of children*, London, 1949, Hogarth Press.

Klerman G, Weissman M: *New applications of interpersonal psychotherapy*, Washington, DC, 1993, American Psychiatric Press.

Menninger KA: *The vital balance*, New York, 1963, Viking Press.

O'Donohue W et al: Characteristics of empirically supported treatments, *J Psychother Pract Res* 9: 69, 2000.

Peplau HE: *Interpersonal relations in nursing*, New York, 1952, GP Putnam.

Perls FS: *In and out of the garbage pail*, Lafayette, Calif, 1969, Real People Press.

Rockland LH: *Supportive therapy: a psychodynamic approach*, New York, 1989, Basic Books.

Rockland LH: A review of supportive psychotherapy, 1986-1992, *Hosp Community Psychiatry* 44:1053, 1993.

Stone AA: Psychotherapy in the managed care health market, *J Psychiatr Pract* 7:238, 2001.

Sullivan HS: *The interpersonal theory of psychiatry*, New York, 1953, WW Norton.

Sullivan HS: *The psychiatric interview*, New York, 1954, WW Norton.

Szasz T: *The myth of mental illness*, New York, 1961, Hoeber-Harper.

Szasz T: *Insanity: the idea and its consequences*, New York, 1987, Wiley.

Szasz T: *A lexicon of lunacy*, New Brunswick, NJ, 1993, Transactional Publishers.

Szasz T: *Liberation by oppression*, London, 2002, Transactional Publishers.

Winston A, Winston B: Toward an integrated brief psychotherapy, *J Psychiatr Pract* 7: 377, 2001.

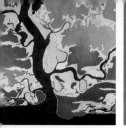

Much madness is Divinest Sense—To a discerning eye.

EMILY DICKINSON

4 THE STUART STRESS ADAPTATION MODEL OF PSYCHIATRIC NURSING CARE

Gail W. Stuart

LEARNING OBJECTIVES

After studying this chapter, the student should be able to:
1. Discuss the theoretical assumptions underlying the Stuart Stress Adaptation Model of psychiatric nursing care (I).
2. Describe criteria of mental health and dimensions of mental illness in the United States (II).
3. Analyze the biopsychosocial components of the Stuart Stress Adaptation Model of psychiatric nursing care (III).
4. Compare coping responses, nursing diagnoses, health problems, and medical diagnoses (IV).
5. Evaluate nursing activities appropriate to the various stages of psychiatric treatment (V).

TOPICAL OUTLINE

evolve Visit Evolve for additional resources related to the content of this chapter.
http://evolve.elsevier.com/Stuart/principles/

Models have many purposes. They can help clarify relationships, generate hypotheses, and give perspective to an abstract idea. They also can provide a structure for thinking, observing, and interpreting what is seen. Conceptual nursing models are frames of reference within which patients, their environments and health states, and nursing activities are described. They explain in general terms why individuals respond to stress as they do and help provide an understanding of the process and desired outcomes of nursing interventions. Psychiatric nurses can enhance their practice if their actions are based on a model of psychiatric nursing care that is inclusive, holistic, and relevant to the needs of patients, families, groups, and communities.

This textbook is based on the Stuart Stress Adaptation Model of psychiatric nursing care, which integrates biological, psychological, sociocultural, environmental, and legal-ethical aspects of patient care into a unified framework for practice. It was originally developed by Gail Stuart in the 1980s as a synthesis of diverse bodies of knowledge from the perspective of psychiatric nursing and, equally important, as an application of this knowledge to clinical practice. Since then the model has been revised and expanded to include

emerging theoretical and scientific discoveries, as well as a clearer and more complete reflection of the process, content, and context of contemporary psychiatric nursing care. This model is based on five theoretical assumptions.

■ THEORETICAL ASSUMPTIONS

The first assumption of the Stuart Stress Adaptation Model is that nature is ordered as a **social hierarchy** from the simplest unit to the most complex (Figure 4-1). Each level of this hierarchy is an organized whole with distinct properties. Each level also is a part of the next higher level, so nothing exists in isolation. Thus the individual is a part of family, group, community, society, and the larger biosphere. Material and information flow across levels, and each level is influenced by all the others. For this reason, one level of organization, such as the individual, cannot be seen as a dynamic system without incorporating the other levels of the social hierarchy. The most basic level of nursing intervention is the individual. However, in working with the individual, the nurse must consider how the individual relates to the whole because wholeness is the essence of psychiatric nursing practice.

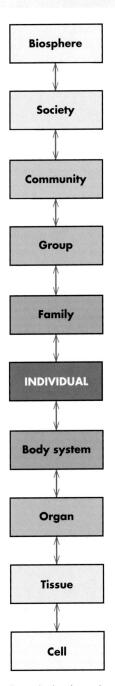

```
Biosphere
   ↕
Society
   ↕
Community
   ↕
Group
   ↕
Family
   ↕
INDIVIDUAL
   ↕
Body system
   ↕
Organ
   ↕
Tissue
   ↕
Cell
```

Figure 4-1   Levels of organization that make up the social hierarchy.

The second assumption of the model is that nursing care is provided within a **biological, psychological, sociocultural, environmental,** and **legal-ethical context.** Each of these aspects of care is described in detail in Chapters 6 to 10. The nurse must understand each of them in order to provide competent, holistic psychiatric nursing care. The theoretical basis for psychiatric nursing practice is derived from nursing science as well as from the behavioral, social, and biological sciences. The range of theories used by psychiatric nurses includes nursing, developmental psychology, neurobiology, pharmacology, psychopathology, learning, sociocultural, cognitive, behavioral, economic, organizational, political, legal-ethical, interpersonal, group, family, and milieu. Psychiatric nursing practice requires the use of many theories because of the variation in patients' responses, the philosophical backgrounds of psychiatric nurses, and the various settings in which nurses work. No one theory is universally applicable to all patients. Rather, the appropriate theory should be selected for its relevance to a particular patient, the presenting problem, and the environment of caregiving.

The third assumption of the model is that health/illness and adaptation/maladaptation are two distinct continuums. **The health/illness continuum comes from a medical world view. The adaptation/maladaptation continuum comes from a nursing world view.** This means that a person with a medically diagnosed illness may be adapting well to it. An example of this is the adaptive coping responses used by some people who have chronic physical or psychiatric illnesses. In contrast, a person without a medically diagnosed illness may have many maladaptive coping responses. This can be seen in the adolescent whose problematic behaviors reflect poor coping responses to the many issues that must be resolved during adolescence. These two continuums thus reflect the complementary nature of the nursing and medical models of practice.

The fourth assumption is that the model includes the **primary, secondary,** and **tertiary levels of prevention by describing four discrete stages of psychiatric treatment: crisis, acute, maintenance,** and **health promotion.** For each stage of treatment the model suggests a treatment goal, a focus of the nursing assessment, the nature of nursing interventions, and the expected outcome of nursing care. This aspect of the model is particularly useful in organizing one's practice, as well as in creating a structure for documenting both the process and outcome of psychiatric nursing care. Since it includes the full continuum of psychiatric care, it can direct nursing practice in hospital, community, and home settings.

The fifth assumption of the Stuart Stress Adaptation Model is that it is based on the use of the **nursing process and the standards of care and professional performance for psychiatric nurses** (see Chapter 12). Psychiatric nursing care is provided through assessment, diagnosis, outcome identification, planning, implementation, and evaluation. Each step of the process is important, and the nurse assumes full responsibility for all nursing actions implemented and the enactment of a professional nursing role.

In summary, the Stuart Stress Adaptation Model is unique in that it:
- Views nature as ordered on a social hierarchy.
- Assumes a holistic biopsychosocial approach to psychiatric nursing practice.
- Regards adaptation/maladaptation as distinct from health/illness.
- Incorporates elements of primary, secondary, and tertiary levels of prevention.
- Identifies four stages of psychiatric treatment and related nursing activities.
- Can be used across psychiatric settings throughout the continuum of care.
- Is based on standards of psychiatric nursing care and professional performance.

■ DESCRIBING MENTAL HEALTH AND ILLNESS

The standards of mental health are less clear than those of mental illness. Viewing mental health as the average or mean mental state of a group is problematic because what is average is not necessarily healthy. It is also dangerous to equate social alternatives with illness, such as when an unusual lifestyle is regarded as sick or when aberrant behavior is taken to be a sign of personal abnormality. These problems can be avoided if one thinks of health/illness and conformity/deviance as independent variables. Combining them creates four patterns: the healthy conformist, the healthy deviant, the unhealthy conformist, and the unhealthy deviant (Figure 4-2). Psychiatric nurses must carefully consider the meaning of an individual's behavior and its context because it may reflect an adaptation to realistic forces in the individual's life or conformity to group norms.

Defining Mental Health

Mental health is often spoken of as a state of well-being associated with happiness, contentment, satisfaction, achievement, optimism, or hope. These terms are difficult to define, and their meanings change as they relate to a particular person and life situation. Some have suggested that mental health cannot be confined to a simple concept or a single aspect of behavior. Instead, mental health incorporates a number of criteria that exist on a continuum with gradients or degrees. These criteria form the basis of the optimum of mental health. However, they are not absolute, and each person has limits. Although no one reaches the ideal in all the criteria, most people can approach the optimum.

Do you think that a person with diabetes that is controlled with medication can still be regarded as healthy? How does this compare with a person who has schizophrenia that is controlled with medication? ■

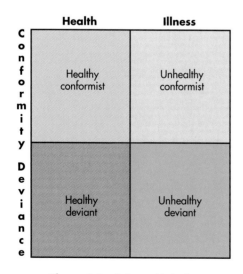

	Health	**Illness**
C o n f o r m i t y	Healthy conformist	Unhealthy conformist
D e v i a n c e	Healthy deviant	Unhealthy deviant

Figure 4-2   Patterns of behavior.

Criteria of Mental Health. The following six criteria are indicators of mental health:
1. Positive attitudes toward self
2. Growth, development, and self-actualization
3. Integration
4. Autonomy
5. Reality perception
6. Environmental mastery

Positive attitudes toward self include an acceptance of self and self-awareness. A person must have some objectivity about the self and realistic aspirations that necessarily change with age. A healthy person also must have a sense of identity, wholeness, belongingness, security, and meaningfulness.

Growth, development, and **self-actualization** mean that the individual seeks new experiences to more fully explore aspects of oneself. Maslow (1958) and Rogers (1961) (e.g., developed theories on the realization of the human potential). Maslow describes the concept of self-actualization, and Rogers emphasizes the fully functioning person. Both theories focus on the entire range of human adjustment. They describe a self as being engaged in a constant quest, always seeking new growth, development, and challenges. These theories focus on the total person and whether the person has the following characteristics:
- Is adequately in touch with one's self and able to use the resources one has
- Has free access to personal feelings and can integrate them with thoughts and behaviors
- Can interact freely and openly with the environment
- Can share with other people and grow from such experiences

Integration is a balance between what is expressed and what is repressed, between outer and inner conflicts. It includes the regulation of emotional responses and a unified philosophy of life. This criterion can be measured at least in part by the person's ability to withstand stress and cope with anxiety. A strong but not rigid ego allows the person to handle change and grow as a result of it.

Autonomy involves self-determination, a balance between dependence and independence, and acceptance of the consequences of one's actions. It implies that the person is self-responsible for decisions, actions, thoughts, and feelings. As a result, the person can respect autonomy and freedom in others.

Reality perception is the individual's ability to test assumptions about the world by empirical thought. The mentally healthy person can change perceptions in light of new information. This criterion includes empathy or social sensitivity, a respect for the feelings and attitudes of others.

Environmental mastery enables a mentally healthy person to feel success in an approved role in society. The person can deal effectively with the world, work out personal problems, and obtain satisfaction from life. The person should be able to cope with loneliness, aggression, and frustration without being overwhelmed. The mentally healthy person can respond to others, love and be loved, and cope with reciprocal relationships. This individual can build new friendships and have satisfactory social group involvement.

Finally, a person should not be assessed against some vague or ideal notion of health. Rather, each person should be seen in both a **group and an individual context**. The issue is not how well someone fits an arbitrary sociocultural standard, but rather what is reasonable for a particular person. Is there continuity or discontinuity with the past? Does the person adapt to changing needs throughout the life cycle? Such a view incorporates the concept of resilience, which proposes that humans must weather periods of stress and change throughout life. Successfully weathering each period of disruption and reintegration leaves the person better able to deal with the next life change (Dyer and McGuinness, 1996; Humphreys, 2003; Paris, 2000; Rew et al, 2001).

Dimensions of Mental Illness

Mental disorders are a major contributor to the burden of illness in the United States. Nearly 50% of all people ages 15 to 54 have had a psychiatric or substance abuse disorder in their lifetimes, and close to 30% have had one of these disorders in the past year (Figure 4-3). Most importantly, more than half of all lifetime disorders occur in the 14% of the population who have a history of three or more co-existing disorders (Kessler et al, 1994). This group includes most of the people with severe psychiatric illness and represents a very vulnerable portion of the population.

The seriousness and persistence of some disorders cause great strain on affected individuals, their families and communities, and the larger health care system. In addition, the increased risk of premature death from natural and unnatural causes for people with common mental disorders is well known (Dembling, Chen, and Vachon, 1999). Other key facts about mental illness are presented in Box 4-1.

Identify two key facts about mental illness presented in Box 4-1 that you did not know. How will these facts change your views about needed health care reform in this country? ■

In 1996 the Global Burden of Disease Study examined the disabling outcomes of 107 diseases around the world. Of the 15 specific leading causes of disability in developed countries, five are mental health problems: (1) unipolar major depressive disorder, (2) alcohol use, (3) schizophrenia, (4) self-inflicted injuries, and (5) bipolar disorder (Murray and Lopez, 1996). With regard to years lived with disability, depressive disorders as a single diagnostic category were the leading cause of disability worldwide.

The Global Burden of Disease Study thus showed the true magnitude of the long underestimated impact of mental health problems. Furthermore, by the year 2020, mental disorders are projected to increase, and major depression is predicted to become the second leading cause in disease burden worldwide. The Global Burden of Disease Study has thus been eye-opening in regard to public health in terms of mainstreaming mental health and highlighting the public significance of mental disorders (Neugebauer, 1999; Ustun, 1999).

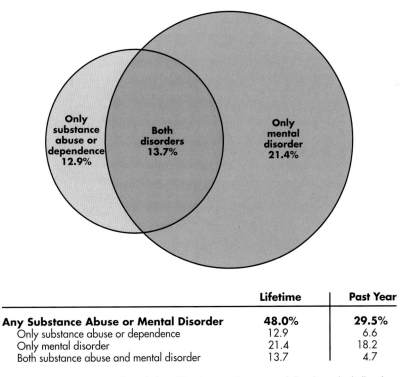

	Lifetime	Past Year
Any Substance Abuse or Mental Disorder	**48.0%**	**29.5%**
Only substance abuse or dependence	12.9	6.6
Only mental disorder	21.4	18.2
Both substance abuse and mental disorder	13.7	4.7

Figure 4-3   Percentage of population with substance abuse, mental disorder, or both disorders, ages 15 to 54. (Redrawn from Kessler et al: *Arch Gen Psychiatry* 51:8, 1994.)

BOX **4-1**

Key Facts About Mental Illness

Extent and Severity of the Problem

The full spectrum of mental disorders affects 25% of the adult population in a given year. This figure refers to *all* mental disorders and is comparable to rates for "physical disorders" when similarly broadly defined (for example, respiratory disorders affect 50% of adults, and cardiovascular diseases affect 20%).

Severe mental disorders, such as schizophrenia, manic-depressive illness and severe forms of depression, panic disorder, and obsessive-compulsive disorder affect 2.8% of the adult population (approximately 5 million people) and account for 25% of all federal disability payments.

About one in five children in the United States younger than 18 years have a mental health problem severe enough to require treatment.

Approximately 18 million people in the United States 18 years of age and older have problems as a result of alcohol use; 10.6 million of these suffer from alcoholism.

An estimated 23 million people in the United States currently use illicit drugs.

At least two thirds of elderly nursing home residents have a diagnosis of a mental disorder, such as major depression.

Nearly one third of the nation's estimated 600,000 homeless people are believed to be adults with severe mental illness.

More than one in four jail inmates has a mental disorder.

Routinely, 29% of the nation's jails hold people who have a mental illness but have not been charged with a crime.

Cost of Mental Disorders

In 1990 the nation's health care bill was $670 billion; the direct cost of treating all mental disorders was 10% of this amount, or $67 billion. Treatment plus indirect costs for all mental disorders was $148 billion in 1990, compared with $159 billion for the total cost of cardiovascular system diseases in 1990.

The total direct treatment costs for severe mental disorders are $20 billion per year plus $7 billion for long-term nursing home care. Indirect and related costs bring the total for severe mental disorders to $74 billion per year.

It has been estimated that drug and alcohol abuse contribute to more than $163.6 billion in health care costs, lost productivity, and crime. Estimates of hospital beds occupied by patients whose physical condition is complicated by alcohol and drug problems range from 25% to 50%.

Alcohol or mental illness is involved in 94% of all suicides, and suicide ranks as the second leading cause of death among people ages 15 to 24 years.

Alcoholism is the third leading cause of illness and disability in the United States and accounts for 10% of all deaths.

Treatment Efficacy

How effective are treatments for severe mental disorders as compared with treatments for physical illness?

DISORDER	TREATMENT SUCCESS RATE (%)
Panic	80
Bipolar	80
Major depression	65
Schizophrenia	60
Obsessive compulsive	60
Cardiovascular treatments	
Atherectomy	52
Angioplasty	41

The majority of alcoholics improve through treatment, and evidence suggests that alcoholism treatment is effective in containing costs throughout the health care system and increasing worker productivity.

Reimbursement

People who need help often do not receive it. Approximately 30% of the 2.8 million people with severe mental illness receive active treatment in a given year; 70% to 80% of children needing mental health treatment do not receive appropriate services.

Only 15% of all drug and alcohol abusers are in treatment. Only 150,000 of an estimated 1.4 million intravenous drug abusers are currently in treatment.

Under insurance plans offering full, comprehensive, and equitable coverage for mental disorders, the percentage of cost represented by these disorders plateaus at about 10% to 11%. Inpatient care for treatment of severe psychiatric disorders has grown less rapidly than inpatient care for all health conditions.

Under health care reform, making mental health coverage for the severely mentally ill commensurate to other health care coverage would do the following:

- Add only $6.5 billion in new mental health care costs—10% more than is currently spent
- Produce a 10% decrease in the cost and use of general medical services by people with severe mental disorders
- Yield a $2.2 billion net saving for the United States

From National Advisory Mental Health Council: *Am J Psychiatry* 150:1447, 1993.

■ BIOPSYCHOSOCIAL COMPONENTS

The Stuart Stress Adaptation Model of psychiatric nursing care views human behavior from a holistic perspective that integrates biological, psychological, and sociocultural aspects of care. For instance, a man who has had a myocardial infarction also may be severely depressed because he fears he will lose his ability to work and to satisfy his wife sexually. He also may have a family history of depression. Likewise, a patient who seeks treatment for a major depression also may have gastric ulcers that are exacerbated by her depression. The holistic nature of psychiatric nursing practice examines all aspects of the individual and his or her environment. The

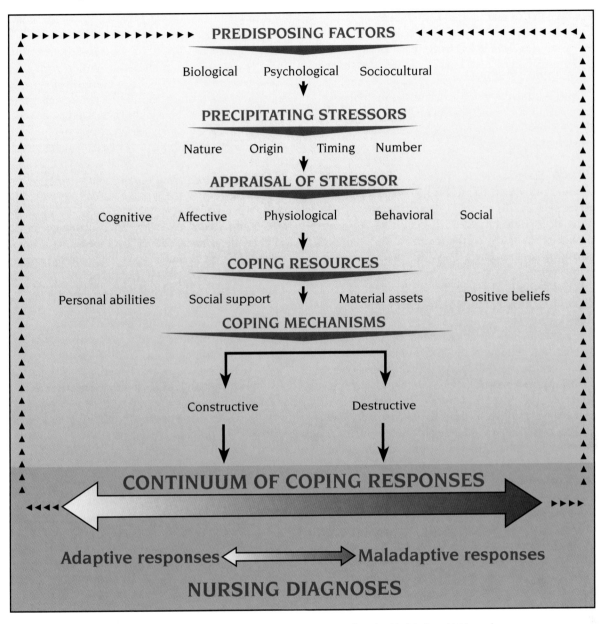

Figure 4-4   Biopsychosocial components of the Stuart Stress Adaptation Model of psychiatric nursing care.

specific biopsychosocial components of the Stuart Stress Adaptation Model are shown in Figure 4-4.

Predisposing Factors

Predisposing factors are risk factors that influence both the type and amount of resources the person can use to handle stress and are biological, psychological, and sociocultural in nature. Together these factors provide a link to higher and lower levels of the social hierarchy and a backdrop against which all the experiences of a person are given meaning and value.

- **Biological** predisposing factors include genetic background, nutritional status, biological sensitivities, general health, and exposure to toxins.
- **Psychological** predisposing factors include intelligence; verbal skills; morale; personality; past experiences; self-

concept, motivation; psychological defenses; and locus of control, or a sense of control over one's own fate.
- **Sociocultural** predisposing factors include age, gender, education, income, occupation, social position, cultural background, religious upbringing and beliefs, political affiliation, socialization experiences, and level of social integration or relatedness.

Explain why predisposing factors are also sometimes called risk factors. ■

Precipitating Stressors

Precipitating stressors are stimuli that are challenging, threatening, or demanding to the individual. They require excess energy and produce a state of tension and stress (Cohen, 2000). They may be biological, psychological, or sociocultural in **nature**, and they may **originate** either in the person's internal or external environment. Besides describing the nature and origin of a stressor, it is important to assess the **timing** of the stressor. Timing has many dimensions, such as when the stressor occurs, how long one is exposed to the stressor, and the frequency with which it occurs. A final factor to be considered is the **number** of stressors an individual experiences within a certain time period because stressful events may be more difficult to deal with when many of them occur close together.

Stressful Life Events. The relationship of stressful life events to the cause, onset, course, and outcomes of psychiatric illnesses, such as schizophrenia, depression, and anxiety, has been the focus of much research. Recent issues related to life events as stressors focus on the nature of the event and the amount of change it requires. There are three ways of categorizing life events:

1. **By social activity.** This includes family, work, educational, social, health, financial, legal, or community crises.
2. **By social field.** These events are defined as entrances and exits. An entrance is the introduction of a new person into the individual's social field; an exit is the departure of a significant other from the person's social field.
3. **By social desirability.** In terms of the currently shared values of American society, one group of events can be considered generally desirable, such as promotion, engagement, and marriage. A larger group of events can generally be viewed unfavorably, such as death, financial problems, being fired, and divorce.

Unfortunately, it is hard to draw conclusions about the exact role played by stressful life events. Although they have been correlated with the onset of anxiety and disease symptoms, the methodological and theoretical aspects of research in this area have been criticized. Intervening or moderating variables often are not taken into account in the research studies. Also, the particular events listed on a stressful life event scale may not be the most relevant to certain groups, such as students, working mothers, the elderly, the poor, or the persistently mentally ill. Finally, the life-events approach provides no clues to the specific way in which the events affect physical or mental health.

It may be more helpful, therefore, to suggest that stressful life events act along a continuum to influence the development of psychiatric illness. At one end of the continuum, they may act as triggers that precipitate an illness in people who would have developed the illness eventually for one reason or another. At the other end of the continuum, stressful life events may have a vulnerability effect and reduce an individual's resistance and coping resources and thus greatly advance or bring about psychiatric illness (see Citing the Evidence).

What sociocultural norms and values must be considered in evaluating the impact of potentially stressful life events? ■

Life Strains and Hassles. Stressful life-events theory is built on the idea of change in response to major episodic events. However, much stress also can arise from more chronic conditions including continuing family tension, job dissatisfaction, and loneliness. Such life strains commonly occur in four areas:

1. Strife associated with marital relations
2. Parental challenges associated with teenage and young adult children
3. Strains associated with household economics
4. Overloads and dissatisfactions associated with the work role

In fact, small daily hassles or strains may have a greater effect on a person's moods and health than do major misfortunes. Hassles are irritating, frustrating, or distressing incidents that occur in everyday life. Such incidents may include disagreements, disappointments, and unpleasant occurrences such as losing a wallet; getting stuck in a traffic jam; or arguing with a family member—a teenage son or daughter or spouse. Research suggests that daily hassles may be better predictors of psychological and physical health than major life events. The more frequent and intense the hassles people reported, the poorer their overall mental and physical health. Major events did have some long-term effects, but these effects may be accounted for by the daily hassles they bring with them. A study of the specific hassles and their frequency among people with severe mental illness found that loneliness and boredom were serious concerns. Finances, crime, self-expression, and upward mobility also were important (Segal and VanderVoort, 1993).

▐ CITING THE EVIDENCE ON
Negative Life Events

BACKGROUND: One of the most controversial questions is, Do the stressful events of ordinary life, such as the death of a parent, unemployment, and divorce definitely cause physical or psychological impairment? This study investigated whether negative life events experienced by adult men affected these subjects' long-term physical and mental health.

RESULTS: Negative life events were found to affect men's psychological health more than their physical health. Negative life events were significantly associated with affective disorders. In addition, a family history of depression, a bleak childhood environment, mood fluctuations in college, death of the maternal grandmother, and poor psychosocial adjustment in youth all predicted the occurrence of affective disorders before age 52.

IMPLICATIONS: This study supports the evidence that biological factors (heredity), psychological factors (unstable personality), and social factors (negative life events) are all etiologically related to depression. It offers clear support for a biopsychosocial model of health and illness.

Cui X, Vaillant G: *Am J Psychiatry* 153:21, 1996.

It is true that a certain amount of stress is necessary for survival, and degrees of it can challenge the individual to grow in new ways. However, too much stress at inappropriate times can place excessive demands on the individual and interfere with integrated functioning. Stress is not inherent within the particular life event itself or within the individual. Rather, it is in the interaction between the individual and situation. The questions that emerge are these: How much stress is too much and what is a stressful life event? These questions lead the nurse to explore the significance of the event as it relates to the individual's value system.

Appraisal of Stressor

Appraisal of a stressor involves determining the meaning of and understanding the impact of the stressful situation for the individual. It includes cognitive, affective, physiological, behavioral, and social responses. Appraisal is an evaluation of the significance of an event in relation to a person's well-being. The stressor assumes its meaning, intensity, and importance as a consequence of the unique interpretation and significance given to it by the person at risk.

Cognitive Response. Cognitive appraisal is a critical part of this model (Monat and Lazarus, 1991). Cognitive factors play a central role in adaptation. They account for the impact of the stressful event; the choice of coping patterns used; and the person's emotional, physiological, behavioral, and social reactions. Cognitive appraisal mediates psychologically between the person and the environment in any stressful encounter; that is, damage or potential damage is evaluated according to the person's understanding of the situation's power to produce harm and the resources the person has available to neutralize or tolerate the harm.

There are three types of primary cognitive appraisals of stress:

1. **Harm/loss** that has already occurred
2. **Threat** of anticipated or future harm
3. **Challenge** that focuses on potential gain, growth, or mastery rather than on the possible risks

The perception of challenge may play an important role in psychological hardiness or resistance to stress. This theory suggests that psychologically hardy people are less likely than nonhardy people to fall ill as a result of stressful life events. It has been found that hardy people are high in the following (Tartasky, 1993):

- **Commitment**—the ability to involve oneself in whatever one is doing
- **Challenge**—the belief that change rather than stability is to be expected in life, so events are seen as stimulating rather than threatening
- **Control**—the tendency to feel and believe that one is influencing events, rather than feeling helpless in the face of life's problems

In summary, stress-resistant people have a specific set of attitudes toward life, an openness to change, a feeling of involvement in whatever they are doing, and a sense of control over events. Those who view stress as a challenge are more likely to transform events to their advantage and thus reduce their level of stress. In contrast, if a person uses passive, hostile, avoidant, or self-defeating tactics, the source of stress is not likely to go away.

What is your level of hardiness as measured by the elements of commitment, challenge, and control? How will it influence your effectiveness as a nurse?

Affective Response. An affective response is the arousal of a feeling. In the appraisal of a stressor, the major affective response is a nonspecific or generalized anxiety reaction, which becomes expressed as emotions. These may include joy, sadness, fear, anger, acceptance, distrust, anticipation, or surprise. Emotions also may be described according to their type, duration, and intensity—characteristics that change over time and as a result of events. For example, when an emotion continues over a long period of time, it can be classified as a mood; when prolonged over an even longer time, it can be considered an attitude. It has been suggested that an insightful, optimistic, and positive attitude in dealing with life events can lead to greater feelings of well-being and perhaps even a longer life (Danner et al, 2001; Lazarus, 1991; Seligman, 2000).

Physiological Responses. Physiological responses reflect the interaction of several neuroendocrine axes involving growth hormone, prolactin, adrenocorticotropic hormone (ACTH), luteinizing and follicle-stimulating hormones, thyroid-stimulating hormones, vasopressin, oxytocin, insulin, epinephrine, norepinephrine, and a variety of other neurotransmitters in the brain. The fight-or-flight physiological response stimulates the sympathetic division of the autonomic nervous system and increases activity of the pituitary-adrenal axis. Additionally, stress has been shown to affect the body's immune system, affecting one's ability to fight disease.

Behavioral Responses. Behavioral responses are the result of emotional and physiological responses, as well as one's cognitive analysis of the stressful situation. Caplan (1981) described four phases of an individual's behavioral responses to a stressful event:

- *Phase 1* is behavior that changes the stressful environment or allows the individual to escape from it.
- *Phase 2* is behavior that allows the individual to change the external circumstances and their aftermath.
- *Phase 3* is intrapsychic behavior that serves to defend against unpleasant emotional arousal.
- *Phase 4* is intrapsychic behavior that helps one come to terms with the event and its sequelae by internal readjustment.

Social Responses. Finally, the possible social responses to stress and illness are many. The precise nature of a person's response is based on three activities (Mechanic, 1977):

1. **Search for meaning,** in which people seek information about their problem. This is necessary for devising a coping strategy because only through having some idea of what is occurring can one come up with a reasonable response.

2. **Social attribution,** in which the person tries to identify the factors that contributed to the situation. Patients who see their problems as resulting from their own negligence may be "blocked" and not able to activate a coping response. They may see their problems as a sign of their personal failure and engage in self-blame and passive, withdrawn behavior. Thus the way patients and health professionals view cause can greatly affect successful coping.
3. **Social comparison,** in which people compare skills and capacities with those of others with similar problems. A person's self-assessment depends very much on those with whom comparisons are made. The outcome is an evaluation of the need for support from the person's social network or support system. Predisposing factors such as age, developmental level, and cultural background, as well as the characteristics of the precipitating stressor, determine the perceived need for social support.

In summary, the way a person appraises an event is the psychological key to understanding coping efforts and the nature and intensity of the stress response. Unfortunately, many nurses and other health professionals ignore this fact when they presume to know how certain stressors will affect a patient and thus provide "routine" care. This practice not only depersonalizes the patient but also undermines the basis of nursing care. The patient's appraisal of life stressors, with its cognitive, affective, physiological, behavioral, and social components, must be an essential part of the psychiatric nurse's assessment.

How might social attribution influence a nurse's response to a rape victim, a person with a substance abuse disorder, or a patient with HIV?

Coping Resources

Coping resources are options or strategies that help determine what can be done, as well as what is at stake. They take into account which coping options are available, the likelihood that a given option will accomplish what it is supposed to, and the likelihood that the person can apply a particular strategy effectively.

Coping resources include economic assets, abilities and skills, defensive techniques, social supports, and motivation. They incorporate all levels of the social hierarchy represented in Figure 4-1. Relationships between the individual, family, group, and society are critically important at this point of the model. Other coping resources include health and energy, spiritual supports, positive beliefs, problem solving and social skills, social and material resources, and physical well-being.

Spiritual beliefs and viewing oneself positively can serve as a basis of hope and can sustain a person's coping efforts under the most adverse circumstances. Problem-solving skills include the ability to search for information, identify the problem, weigh alternatives, and implement a plan of action. Social skills facilitate the solving of problems involving other people, increase the likelihood of getting cooperation and support from others, and give the individual greater social control. Finally, material assets refer to money and the goods and services that money can buy. Obviously, monetary resources greatly increase a person's coping options in almost any stressful situation.

Knowledge and intelligence are other coping resources that allow people to see different ways of dealing with stress. Finally, coping resources also include a strong ego identity, commitment to a social network, cultural stability, a stable system of values and beliefs, a preventive health orientation, and genetic or constitutional strength.

Coping Mechanisms

It is at this point in the model that coping mechanisms emerge. This is an important time for nursing activities directed toward primary prevention. Coping mechanisms are any efforts directed at stress management. There are three main types of coping mechanisms:

1. **Problem-focused** coping mechanisms, which involve tasks and direct efforts to cope with the threat itself. Examples include negotiation, confrontation, and seeking advice.
2. **Cognitively focused** coping mechanisms, by which the person attempts to control the meaning of the problem and thus neutralize it. Examples include positive comparison, selective ignorance, substitution of rewards, and the devaluation of desired objects.
3. **Emotion-focused** coping mechanisms, by which the patient is oriented to moderating emotional distress. Examples include the use of ego defense mechanisms such as denial, suppression, or projection. A detailed discussion of coping and defense mechanisms appears in Chapter 16.

Coping mechanisms can be constructive or destructive. They are **constructive** when anxiety is treated as a warning signal and the individual accepts it as a challenge to resolve the problem. In this respect anxiety can be compared to a fever: Both serve as warnings that the system is under attack. Once used successfully, constructive coping mechanisms modify the way past experiences are used to meet future threats. **Destructive** coping mechanisms ward off anxiety without resolving the conflict, using evasion instead of resolution.

■ PATTERNS OF RESPONSE

According to the Stuart Stress Adaptation Model, an individual's response to stress is based on specific predisposing factors, the nature of the stressor, the perception of the situation, and an analysis of coping resources and mechanisms. Coping responses of the patient are then evaluated on a continuum of adaptation/maladaptation (see Figure 4-4). **Responses that support integrated functioning are seen as adaptive.** They lead to growth, learning, and goal achievement. **Responses that block integrated functioning are seen as maladaptive.** They prevent growth, decrease autonomy, and interfere with mastery of the environment.

Nursing Diagnoses

Responses to stress, whether actual or potential, are the subject of nursing diagnoses. A nursing diagnosis is a clinical judgment about individual, family, or community responses to stress (see Critical Thinking About Contemporary Issues). It is a statement of the patient's problem from a nursing perspective that includes both the adaptive and maladaptive responses and contributing stressors. These responses may be overt, covert, existing, or potential and may lie anywhere on the continuum from adaptive to maladaptive. Formulating the diagnosis and implementing treatment are nursing functions for which the nurse is accountable. NANDA-approved nursing diagnoses are listed in Appendix A.

Relationship to Medical Diagnoses

Medical diagnosis is the health problem or disease state of the patient. In the medical model of psychiatry, these health problems are mental disorders or mental illnesses. It is important for psychiatric nurses to distinguish between nursing and medical models of care, as shown in Figure 4-5. In particular, the following differences should be noted:

- **Nurses** assess **risk factors** and look for **vulnerabilities.**
- **Physicians** assess **disease states** and look for **causes.**
- **Nursing diagnoses** focus on the **adaptive/maladaptive coping continuum of human responses.**
- **Medical diagnoses** focus on the **health/illness continuum of health problems.**
- **Nursing intervention** consists of **caregiving activities.**
- **Medical intervention** consists of **curative treatments.**

A nurse may implement the nursing process for maladaptive responses based on the Stuart Stress Adaptation Model whether or not a physician has diagnosed the presence of a medical or psychiatric illness. Also, patients with a persistent psychiatric illness may be adapting well to it. People can successfully adapt to an illness without recovering from it. This is an important aspect of the Stuart Stress Adaptation Model because it suggests that psychiatric nurses can promote their patients' adaptive responses regardless of their health or illness state.

Classifying Mental Disorders

Mental illnesses can be broadly differentiated as neurotic or psychotic. Neuroses have the following characteristics:

- A symptom or group of symptoms is distressing and is recognized as unacceptable and alien to the individual.
- Reality testing is grossly intact.

- Behavior does not violate major social norms (although functioning may be significantly impaired).
- The disturbance is enduring or recurrent without treatment and is not merely a transitory reaction to stressors.
- No demonstrable organic cause or factor is present.

However, in situations of severest conflict, the person may distort reality, as in psychosis. Psychosis consists of the following characteristics:

- Regressive behavior
- Personality disintegration
- A significant reduction in level of awareness
- Great difficulty in functioning adequately
- Gross impairment in reality testing

This last characteristic is critical. When people demonstrate gross impairment in reality testing, they incorrectly

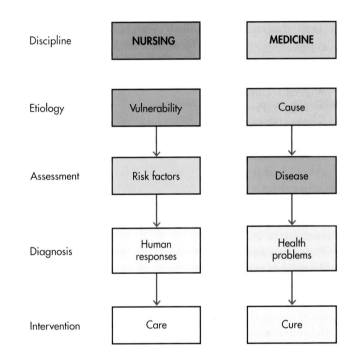

Figure 4-5   Comparison of nursing and medical models of care.

Critical Thinking *About* Contemporary Issues

How Does Mind-Body Dualism Influence the Way Nurses Think About Patients and Their Illnesses?

In formulating diagnoses, psychiatric nurses must be careful to avoid the mind-body dualism that dominates the diagnosis, treatment, and use of health care services in the United States. In most other cultures this division between mind and body does not exist. A wide range of behavior exists for expressing emotion and psychological disorders, and in America many people express their distress somatically and attribute their problems to physical illness rather than to psychological, social, or spiritual dilemmas. This can create a variety of problems.

One problem is that nurses can respond to patients' somatic complaints and treat them as problems of physical illness without questioning them about possible psychosocial causes. Many patients often want a somatic explanation and treatment, and react with fear or anger to the suggestion that there may be a psychological component to their problem. These patients may re-

ceive treatment that results in harm to themselves or not receive treatment that is needed to resolve their underlying psychological problem. Conversely, a physical illness with affective or cognitive symptoms might be misdiagnosed and inappropriately treated as a psychological problem. Another mistake is for nurses to believe that if a patient's problem is psychiatric, then physical symptoms can be discounted or ignored.

As a consequence of mind-body dualism, patients are separated according to whether their illnesses are deemed to be psychological or physical. They are then sent to different hospitals and are seen by different kinds of health care providers. The practical consequence of this dualistic thinking is that it can interfere with a nurse's ability to holistically understand people's reactions to events in their lives and the ways in which they cope and adapt.

The synthesis of all of the elements of the Stuart Stress Adaptation Model of psychiatric nursing care is displayed in Figure 4-7. These elements also are summarized in Table 4-3. On the far left side of Figure 4-7 one can see the many theories that contribute to psychiatric nursing care. On the far right side are the six steps of the nursing process. In the middle of the figure, the top portion shows the impact of predisposing factors, precipitating stressors, appraisal of stressors, coping resources, and coping mechanisms, all of which lead to either adaptive or maladaptive coping responses and

Table 4-3	Summary of the Elements of the Stuart Stress Adaptation Model	
ELEMENT	DEFINITION	EXAMPLES
Predisposing factors	Risk factors that influence both the type and amount of resources the person can elicit to cope with stress	Genetic background, intelligence, self-concept, age, ethnicity, education, gender, belief systems
Precipitating stressors	Stimuli that the person perceives as challenging, threatening, or demanding and that require excess energy for coping	Life events, injury, hassles, strains
Appraisal of stressor	An evaluation of the significance of a stressor for a person's well-being, considering the stressor's meaning, intensity, and importance	Hardiness, perceived seriousness, anxiety, attribution
Coping resources	An evaluation of a person's coping options and strategies	Finances, social support, ego integrity
Coping mechanisms	Any effort directed at stress management	Problem solving, compliance, defense mechanisms
Continuum of coping responses	A range of adaptive or maladaptive human responses	Social changes, physical symptoms, emotional well-being
Treatment stage activities	Range of nursing functions related to treatment goal, nursing assessment, nursing intervention, and expected outcome	Environment management, patient teaching, role modeling, advocacy

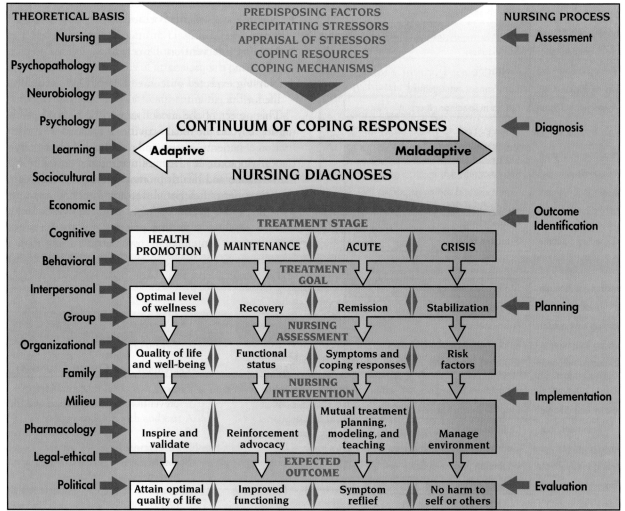

Figure 4-7   The Stuart Stress Adaptation Model of psychiatric nursing care.

related nursing diagnoses. Also in the middle of the figure one sees each treatment stage with its related treatment goal, nursing assessment, nursing intervention and expected outcome of care.

Chapters 16 through 26 of this text explore various maladaptive coping responses and related medical diagnoses. The phases of the nursing process are described for patients with maladaptive responses. Each chapter begins with a continuum of coping responses, followed by a discussion of behaviors, predisposing factors, precipitating stressors, appraisal of stressor, coping resources, coping mechanisms, nursing diagnoses, and related interventions. Through consistent application of the Stuart Stress Adaptation Model, the art and science of psychiatric nursing practice emerges.

CHAPTER FOCUS POINTS

- The Stuart Stress Adaptation Model assumes that nature is ordered as a social hierarchy; that psychiatric nursing care is provided through the nursing process within a biological, psychological, sociocultural, environmental, and legal-ethical context; that health/illness and adaptation/maladaptation are distinct concepts; and that primary, secondary, and tertiary levels of prevention are included in the four discrete stages of psychiatric treatment.
- Criteria of mental health include positive attitudes toward self; growth, development and self-actualization; integration; autonomy; reality perception; and environmental mastery.
- Nearly one of every two people in the United States has had a psychiatric illness or substance abuse disorder in his or her lifetime.

- The biopsychosocial components of the model include predisposing factors, precipitating stressors, appraisal of stressor, coping resources, and coping mechanisms (see Table 4-3).
- Patterns of response include the individual's coping responses, which are the subject of NANDA nursing diagnoses, and health problems, which are the subject of medical diagnoses described by Axes I to V of the *DSM-IV-TR*. In addition, the *DSM-IV-TR* has an outline for cultural formulation designed to help in evaluating the person's cultural and social reference group and ways in which the cultural context is relevant to clinical care.
- Psychiatric nursing goals, assessment, intervention, and expected outcome can be identified for each of the four stages of treatment: crisis, acute, maintenance, and health promotion.

KEY TERMS

appraisal of a stressor, 67
coping mechanisms, 68
coping resources, 68
culture-bound syndromes, 70
hardiness, 67

medical diagnosis, 69
mental health, 62
neuroses, 69
nursing diagnosis, 68
precipitating stressors, 65

predisposing factors, 65
psychosis, 69
resilience, 63

CHAPTER REVIEW QUESTIONS

1. Indicate whether the following statements are true (T) or false (F).

_____ A. The standards of mental health are less clear than those of mental illness.

_____ B. Approximately one of every three people will experience a psychiatric or substance abuse problem in his or her lifetime.

_____ C. The treatment for depression is more effective than that for cardiovascular illness.

_____ D. The parasympathetic division of the autonomic nervous system is stimulated by the fight-or-flight response.

_____ E. A coping mechanism is considered to be constructive when it treats anxiety as a warning signal and the person accepts it as a challenge to solve the problem.

_____ F. Psychotic health problems reflect the most severe level of illness.

2. Fill in the blanks.

A. A person's ability to test assumptions about the world by empirical thought is called _____.

B. The concept of _____ proposes that humans must weather periods of stress and change throughout life.

C. Intelligence, morale, and self-concept are examples of _____ predisposing factors.

D. _____ is when a person tries to identify the unique factors that contributed to one's particular situation.

E. The three types of primary cognitive appraisals of stress are _____, _____, and _____.

F. Personality disorders are identified on Axis _____ of the *DSM-IV–TR.*

G. Recurrent, locality-specific patterns of aberrant behavior and troubling experience that may be linked to a particular *DSM-IV-TR* diagnostic category are called _____.

3. Provide short answers for the following questions.

A. Describe the three parts of a hardy personality and the way in which they help a person cope with stress.

B. List the three types of coping mechanisms, and give an example of each.

C. Compare the nursing and medical models of care. Which model do you think currently receives more health care resources, research funding, and professional status? Defend your answer.

D. Identify the four stages of psychiatric treatment and the level of prevention related to each one.

Visit Evolve for additional resources related to the content of this chapter.

http://evolve.elsevier.com/Stuart/principles/

• Topical Course Outline • Student Workbook Exercises • Critical Thinking Questions and Activities • Case Studies • Research Topics • Monthly Content Updates • WebLinks

Student Study CD-ROM

Access the accompanying CD-ROM for animations, interactive exercises, review questions for the NCLEX examination, and an audio glossary.

REFERENCES

American Psychiatric Association: *Diagnostic and statistical manual of mental disorders*, ed 4, text revision, Washington, DC, 2000, American Psychiatric Association.

Caplan G: Mastery of stress: psychosocial aspects, *Am J Psychiatry* 138:41, 1981.

Cohen J: Stress and mental health: a biobehavioral perspective, *Issues Ment Health Nurs* 21:185, 2000.

Danner D et al: Positive emotions in early life and longevity: findings from the nun study, *J Personal Soc Psychol* 80: 804, 2001.

Dembling BP, Chen DT, Vachon L: Life expectancy and causes of death in a population treated for serious mental illness, *Psychiatr Serv* 50:1036, 1999.

Dyer JG, McGuinness TM: Resilience: analysis of concept, *Arch Psychiatr Nurs* 10:276, 1996.

Humphreys J: Resilience in sheltered battered women, *Issues Ment Health Nurs* 24: 137, 2003.

Kessler R et al: Lifetime and 12-month prevalence of DSM-III-R psychiatric disorders in the United States, *Arch Gen Psychiatry* 51:8, 1994.

Lazarus R: *Emotion and adaptation*, New York, 1991, Oxford University Press.

Maslow A: *Motivation and personality*, New York, 1958, Harper & Row.

Mechanic D: Illness behavior, social adaptation, and the management of illness: a comparison of educational and medical models, *J Nerv Ment Dis* 165:79, 1977.

Monat A, Lazarus R: *Stress and coping*, New York, 1991, Columbia University Press.

Murray C, Lopez A: *The global burden of disease: a comprehensive assessment of mortality and disability from disease, injuries, and risk factors in 1990 and projected to 2020*, Cambridge, Mass, 1996, Harvard University Press.

Neugebauer R: Mind matters: the importance of mental disorders in public health's 21st century mission, *Am J Public Health* 89:1309, 1999.

Paris J: The primacy of early experience: a critique, an alternative, and some clinical implications, *J Psychiatr Pract* 6:147, 2000.

Rew L et al: Correlates of resilience in homeless adolescents, *Image J Nurs Sch* 33:33, 2001.

Rogers C: *On becoming a person*, Boston, 1961, Houghton Mifflin.

Segal SP, VanderVoort DJ: Daily hassles of persons with severe mental illness, *Hosp Community Psychiatry* 44:276, 1993.

Seligman M: Optimism, pessimism, and mortality, *Mayo Clinic Proceed* 75:133, 2000.

Tartasky DS: Hardiness: conceptual and methodological issues, *Image J Nurs Sch* 25:225, 1993.

Tucker GJ: Putting DSM-IV in perspective, *Am J Psychiatry* 155:159, 1998.

Ustun TB: The global burden of mental disorders, *Am J Public Health* 89:1315, 1999.

> *Everything has changed but our ways of thinking, and if these do not change we drift toward unparalleled catastrophe.*
>
> ALBERT EINSTEIN

EVIDENCE-BASED PSYCHIATRIC NURSING PRACTICE   5

Gail W. Stuart

LEARNING OBJECTIVES

After studying this chapter, the student should be able to:
1. Define evidence-based practice (**I**).
2. Describe the activities necessary for providing evidence-based psychiatric nursing care (**I**).
3. Analyze practice guidelines and their contribution to clinical care (**II**).
4. Examine the importance of outcome measurement in psychiatric and mental health nursing practice (**III**).
5. Evaluate the evidence base for psychiatric nursing practice and an agenda for psychiatric nursing research (**IV**).

TOPICAL OUTLINE

 Visit Evolve for additional resources related to the content of this chapter.
http://evolve.elsevier.com/Stuart/principles/

Currently, "evidence-based practices" have become a priority in the delivery of health care, including care to those with psychiatric and substance abuse disorders. In 1999, the *Report of the Surgeon General on Mental Health* (USDHHS, 1999) emphasized the great gap that existed between the kind of mental health care that research found to be most effective and the kind of care most Americans receive. In 2003 this finding was reinforced in *Achieving the Promise: Transforming Mental Health Care in America*, the report of the New Freedom Commission on Mental Health (2003).

Despite extensive evidence and agreement on what are effective mental health care practices for persons with mental illness, research shows that most mental health programs do not provide evidence-based practices for most patients with psychiatric disorders (Drake et al, 2001). Thus increasing national attention has been focused on evidence-based treatments. In psychiatry these treatments include the following:
- The use of specific medications prescribed in the range of effective dosages
- Specialized psychotherapies
- Self-help and peer supports
- Family psychoeducation
- Psychosocial rehabilitation and supported employment
- Case management based on the principles of assertive community treatment

- Substance abuse treatment that is integrated with mental health treatment
- Multisystemic therapy for children and adolescents
- Therapeutic foster care

For psychiatric nurses, the movement to use evidence-based practices poses three questions:
1. Do psychiatric nurses know the efficacy of the treatments and interventions they provide?
2. Are they practicing evidence-based psychiatric nursing?
3. Are they documenting the nature and outcomes of the care they provide?

The answers to these questions will be important in determining the contributions that nurses can make to mental health care. They will shape the present and future role nurses have in a specialty area that is growing in its understandings of molecular and cell biology and genetics, as well as understanding of the cognitive and behavioral sciences.

This textbook uses an **evidence-based approach** to psychiatric nursing practice. It examines the research that supports psychiatric nursing care and highlights findings in the field by including **Citing the Evidence boxes** in each chapter, and **Summarizing the Evidence boxes** in Unit 3. It also provides primary sources of evidence in the references of each chapter. Another aspect of evidence-based practice requires that the nurse continue to access current findings in the field. The website for this textbook will be a useful resource to nurses who wish to stay abreast with new research findings and ongoing developments in psychiatric and mental health care.

EVIDENCE-BASED PRACTICE

Accountability for patient care outcomes is a basic responsibility of professional nurses. Central to this accountability is the ability to examine nursing practice patterns, evaluate the nature of the data supporting them, and demonstrate sound clinical decision making in a way that can be empirically supported. This approach is the essence of evidence-based practice.

In the current health care environment, psychiatric nurses can no longer rely on opinion-based processes or unproven theories (see Critical Thinking About Contemporary Issues). They need to question their current practices and find better alternatives to improve patient care. To do so, nurses must learn to search the research literature, critically synthesize research findings, and apply relevant evidence to practice.

Evidence-based practice is the conscientious, explicit, and judicious use of the best evidence gained from systematic research for the purpose of making informed decisions about the care of individual patients (Sackett et al, 1996). It blends a nurse's clinical expertise with the best available research evidence. It is also a method of self-directed, career-long learning in which the nurse continuously seeks the best possible outcomes for patients and implements effective interventions based on the most current research evidence. The evidence-based paradigm for nursing is based on the following assumptions:

- It is risky to generalize from a small sample of patients or a single case to the universe of patients.
- It is not possible to rule out other aspects of the situation that may have caused the observed patient behavior but that are not known to the nurse.
- Information gathered from one's own clinical practice tends to involve unsystematic observations.
- All clinicians have biases that influence clinical care.
- Even theories from respected colleagues must give rise to testable hypotheses and evidence of efficacy in order to be useful to clinical practice.
- Knowing that conclusions were reached through scientific methodology permits a higher level of confidence in one's nursing actions.
- Replication of findings increases confidence in their validity.
- Randomized controlled clinical trials are the gold standard of research methodologies.
- Nurses who are able to critically review the research literature related to a specific clinical question will be able to provide better nursing care.

Bases for Nursing Practice

There are four bases for nursing practice (Stetler et al, 1998):

1. The lowest level is the **traditional basis** for practice, which includes rituals, unverified rules, anecdotes, customs, opinions, and unit culture.
2. The second level is the **regulatory basis** for practice, which includes state practice acts and reimbursement and other regulatory requirements.
3. The third level is the **philosophical or conceptual basis** for practice, which includes the mission, values, and vision of the organization; professional practice models; untested conceptual frameworks; and ethical frameworks and professional codes.
4. The fourth and highest level is **evidence-based practice,** which includes research findings, performance data, and consensus recommendations of recognized experts.

Apart from situations requiring a philosophical or regulatory basis, the best basis for substantiating clinical practice is the evidence of well-established research findings. Such evidence reflects verifiable, replicable facts and relationships that have been exposed to stringent scientific criteria. This research has less potential for bias than the other bases for practice, most particularly the traditional "that's how we've always done it" basis for practice.

It is also important to remember, however, that not all clinical practice is based on science. Many aspects will not or can-

---

Critical Thinking *About* Contemporary Issues

How Effective are Mental Health Services and Providers?

Some believe that society has lost confidence in the mental health industry to deliver cost-effective services. This loss of confidence may result from a number of "myths" in the field including (Bickman, 2000):

- Clinicians improve with experience.
- Advanced-degree programs produce more effective clinicians.
- Continuing education improves the effectiveness of clinicians.
- Licensing helps ensure effective clinicians.
- Accreditation of health delivery organizations improves outcomes for consumers.
- Clinical supervision results in more effective clinicians.

Existing research does not support any of these commonly held beliefs. In fact, it appears that training and education are failing the field at all levels. Specifically, it is noted that most clinicians are not taught evidence-based assessment and treatment as a standard and that proficiency and competency standards do not reflect current thinking in the field, particularly its increasing scientific basis (Hoge, 2002).

Thus there has been a "call to action" issued to examine and reform the current accrediting and credentialing organizations and the academic training community to implement teaching evidence-based practice and developing responsive competency standards (ACMHA, 2000). Other recommendations call for additional research and training on manualized treatments and practice guidelines and the implementation of comprehensive outcome measurement and quality improvement systems. Failure to implement these recommendations may jeopardize the credibility and availability of mental health services for those who need them.

not be adequately tested empirically. Clinical experience is invaluable in these situations. Furthermore, clinical acumen or intuition is also important, particularly with respect to certain patient problems (Benner, Hooper-Hyriakidis, and Stannard, 1999). For example, if a patient situation is very complex, scientific inquiry will not be able to give clear guidance on many of the variables related to clinical decisions, so the judgment developed from experience is essential to psychiatric nursing practice. Finally, biases may be present in the analysis and interpretation of research data. Thus the nurse needs to critically evaluate studies from both a methodological and clinical perspective.

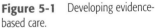 *Think of one or two examples of psychiatric nursing interventions that have been "handed down" from colleague to colleague without empirical validation. Compare these to one or two nursing interventions that do have a research basis.* ■

Developing Evidence-Based Care

Evidence-based psychiatric nursing practice involves the following series of activities (Figure 5-1).

Defining the clinical question is the first step in the process. Clear answers require clear questions. The formulation of a precise clinical question involves defining the patient's problems, identifying the existing nursing interven-

tion, and specifying the expected outcome. This process should be completed in partnership with the patient and family, and in collaboration with other health care providers.

Finding the evidence is the next step. Most nurses rely on textbooks, journal articles, and drug booklets to help guide their practice. However, each of these poses a problem for the practicing psychiatric nurse who wants to stay abreast of findings in the field. For example, textbooks become outdated, and nurses need to purchase the new editions of their favorite textbooks to stay current. Journal articles may produce contradictory findings and suffer from poor design, whereas drug booklets may be laden with promotional material. Thus finding the evidence can be challenging.

However, recent advances in information technology have made it easier now to search the health care literature. Access to electronic databases such as MEDLINE is now widespread. Increasingly journals offer World Wide Web pages on the Internet, displaying tables of contents, abstracts, and some full-text articles. Another strategy is that of using **systematic reviews** prepared by others. A systematic reviewer uses explicit methods of searching for and critically appraising the primary studies. If these are comparable, the reviewer may then perform a formal quantitative synthesis, called *meta-analysis*, of the results. A **meta-analysis** summarizes the findings from a

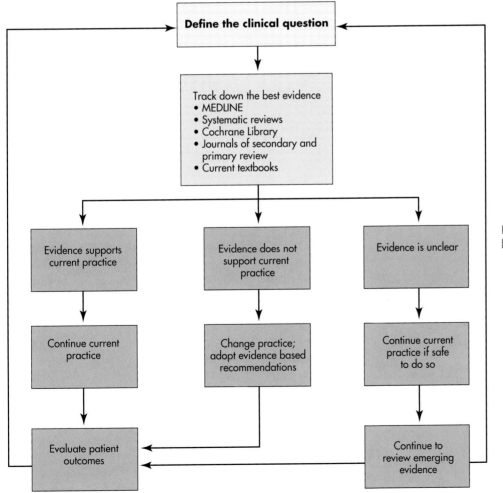

Figure 5-1 Developing evidence-based care.

number of studies in order to arrive at an objective and authoritative guide to treatment for a given condition.

A particularly useful source of systematic reviews of health care interventions is the **Cochrane Library** (2003), a regularly updated electronic library that is available on computer disk and the Internet. It contains a unique, cumulative collection of systematic reviews that are valuable, not only because of their rigorous methodology but also because they are regularly updated as new research evidence is published. A new type of journal also is available that specializes in reviewing articles that conform to rigorous methodological standards before they are subject to informed comment and summaries by seasoned clinicians. They are published in the United Kingdom; examples include *Clinical Evidence, Evidence-Based Nursing,* and *Evidence-Based Mental Heath.*

Analyzing the evidence requires that nurses develop the ability to understand and use appropriate research findings. In so doing, they will be confident that the evidence selected is of high quality and is based on rigorous and systematic study. Evidence needs to be critically evaluated for its reliability and application to the particular clinical problem. Implicit in the process of evaluating the evidence is the idea that there is a hierarchy in the quality of research evidence. A commonly used hierarchy (with 1 indicating the best) for research designs is presented in Box 5-1.

Systematic reviews or meta-analyses of randomized controlled trials (RCTs) are the most reliable study design for the evaluation of treatments. RCTs are considered to be the "gold standard" of research design. However, for many interventions, RCTs may not exist, and the nurse needs to use evidence from the next level of the hierarchy. The idea being that the nurse selects the intervention that is supported by the best available evidence.

Using the evidence means that the nurse has to be able to apply research in a practical way. In fact, translating research findings into clinically usable information is one of the most challenging aspects of evidence-based practice. One development in the field that can help with this process is the development of practice guidelines based on sound evidence about best practices. It is clear, however, that interpreting the evidence and translating it into health care decisions is a complex process. Evidence is helpful but not sufficient for clinical

decision making. The key aspect of evidence-based practice is that it ensures the best use is made of the available evidence.

Evaluating the outcome is the final activity of evidence-based practice. Here the nurse asks whether the application of evidence leads to an improvement in care. This inquiry requires that psychiatric nursing practice incorporate ways of demonstrating effectiveness by ongoing evaluation of clearly specified outcomes. This process involves the use of outcome measurement and reevaluation.

Ask some practicing nurses how they stay current with the latest developments in the field. How will you stay current after graduation?

■ PRACTICE GUIDELINES

Practice guidelines in psychiatric care are strategies for mental health care delivery that are developed to facilitate clinical decision making and provide patients with critical information about their treatment options. They have arisen over the past decade in direct response to the greater number of empirically validated treatments that have been identified (Nathan and Gorman, 2002). Although they vary widely in format, all practice guidelines are designed to provide detailed specification of methods and procedures to ensure effective treatment for each disorder.

More than 30 groups have developed practice guidelines in the mental health or substance abuse field, addressing the child, adolescent, adult, and geriatric populations. Experts agree that practice guidelines are valuable tools when developed, modified, and implemented in a collaborative, scientifically valid, and pragmatic manner.

The goals of practice guidelines are as follows:
- Document preferred practices
- Increase consistency in care
- Facilitate outcome research
- Enhance the quality of care
- Improve staff productivity
- Reduce costs

Practice guidelines can be developed in a variety of ways. The best mental health practice guidelines are based on a scientific review of the available clinical research literature to establish which treatments are safe and effective for particular psychiatric disorders. Guidelines also have been developed by professional associations, managed care companies, and academic centers using techniques such as expert consensus and data analysis. Regardless of how they are developed, it is essential that they be updated regularly to keep up with the latest findings in the field.

Guidelines can vary in several ways:
- *Clinical orientation*—whether the focus is on a clinical condition, technology, or process
- *Clinical purpose*—whether information is presented on screening and prevention, evaluation or diagnosis, or various aspects of treatment
- *Complexity*—whether the guideline is relatively straightforward or presented with detail, complicated logic, or lengthy narrative

---

BOX **5-1**

Hierarchy of Research Evidence

1. A systematic review (meta-analysis) of all relevant randomized controlled trials (RCTs)
2. At least one properly designed randomized controlled trial
3. Well designed controlled trials without randomization
4. Well designed cohort, case-controlled, or other quasi-experimental study
5. Nonexperimental descriptive studies, such as comparative studies
6. Expert committee reports and opinions of respected authorities based on clinical experience

- *Format*—whether the guideline is presented as free text, tables, algorithms, critical pathways, or decision pathways
- *Intended audience*—whether the guideline is intended for practitioners, patients, regulators, or payers

Much variability is also to be found in how guidelines are used. One of the major limitations to their use is that they may not adequately take into account all four variables that influence treatment outcome: (1) patient characteristics, (2) the nature of the therapeutic relationship, (3) treatment interventions, and (4) the placebo effect.

Another limitation is that practice guidelines are often developed in isolation by only one discipline and may therefore contain treatment biases reflective of that discipline's model of practice. Other concerns are that they may be based on insufficient evidence or be too rigid or inflexible. Box 5-2 lists questions that can be helpful in judging the potential usefulness of a practice guideline.

The American College of Mental Health Administration (ACMHA) (Stuart, Rush, and Morris, 2002) has created a taxonomy of building blocks for informed decision making in behavioral health assessment and treatment. This taxonomy identifies treatment options from the most general to the most specific (Figure 5-2). Those at the top of the triangle provide maximum choice and flexibility, whereas those at the bottom of the triangle provide for maximum accountability. Thus **best practices** are broad consensus statements of a general nature; **practice guidelines** have greater specificity; and **algorithms** or **protocols** are the most specific with the strongest evidence base.

This taxonomy is a useful way of informing decision making in the practice setting. It is also unique in that it incorporates prevention as well as treatment options, which is an underdeveloped area in most practice guidelines. ACMHA also has identified 10 characteristics of good behavioral health practice guidelines. These are listed in Box 5-3.

Should each profession develop its own guidelines or should guidelines cross disciplines and treatment settings? ■

BOX **5-2**

Questions to Ask When Evaluating a Practice Guideline

- Who wrote the guideline? Is it a guild document created by one professional discipline or does it reflect an interdisciplinary point of view?
- Who sponsored the guideline? Where did the money come from that supported its creation and distribution?
- When was the guideline written? Does it reflect the latest developments in the field?
- What methodology was used? Was it based on scientific evidence? Does it differentiate between research findings and clinical opinion?
- Do the treatments recommended in the guideline respect consumer rights?
- Are the treatments recommended in the guideline affordable and accessible? Can the treatments be provided by a variety of clinicians in various settings or are they limited in some way?
- Was the guideline reviewed by a variety of groups, including nurses and consumers?
- How does the guideline compare with other guidelines in the field?

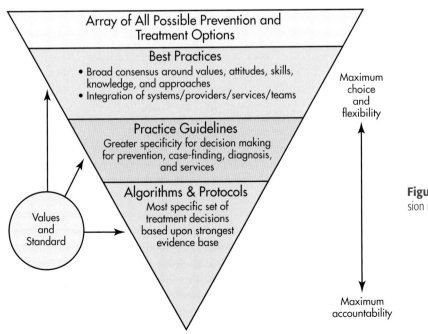

Figure 5-2   Taxonomy of building blocks for informed decision making in behavioral health assessment and treatment.

BOX **5-3**

Characteristics of Good Behavioral Health Practice Guidelines

1. Practice guidelines should be developed in partnership with recipients, consumers, family members, people in recovery, and a wide range of disciplines and organizations.
2. Practice guidelines should be clear, educational, and fully available to recipients, consumers, families, people in recovery, all mental health providers, and all payers.
3. Practice guidelines should be a toolbox of options, and not prescriptive in nature.
4. Practice guidelines should be flexible and accommodate consumer choice as well as consumer values, goals, and desired outcomes.
5. Practice guidelines should be sensitive and responsive to the individual's environment, ethnicity, culture, gender, sexual orientation, and socioeconomic status.
6. Practice guidelines should be based on scientific evidence of efficacy, effectiveness, and established best practices in the field.
7. Practice guidelines should be reviewed and updated regularly.
8. A prevention framework and public health paradigm should be incorporated into every practice guideline.
9. Practice guidelines should identify process and outcome measures, including engagement in the treatment process, adherence to treatment, continuity of care, symptom reduction, enhanced quality of life, improved functional ability, integration of medical, psychiatric, and substance abuse treatment, and improved social status related to employment, housing, or school.
10. Practice guidelines should produce positive clinical outcomes that are sensitive to time for quality improvement.

From Stuart GW, Rush AJ, Morris JA: *Adm Policy Ment Health* 30:21, 2002.

Clinical Pathways

Many health care organizations have undertaken the creation of clinical pathways, which identify the key clinical processes and corresponding timelines involved in patient care as a means to achieve standard outcomes within a specific period of time. These pathways provide one way in which not only the rationale for mental health care but also the patient's progress and response to care can be documented.

A clinical pathway is a written plan that serves as both a map and a timetable for the efficient and effective delivery of health care. Valid clinical pathways are developed over time by a multidisciplinary team. They can be constructed around *DSM-IV-TR* diagnoses, North American Nursing Diagnosis Association (NANDA) diagnoses, clinical conditions, treatment stages, clinical interventions, or targeted behaviors.

They are most often used in inpatient settings, serve as a shortened version of the multidisciplinary plan of care for a patient, and require high levels of team cooperation and quality monitoring. Some clinical settings have computerized their paths to enhance the consistency and efficiency of care provided.

The key elements of the clinical pathway are (1) the identification of a target population; (2) the expected outcome of treatment described in a measurable, realistic, and patient-centered way; (3) specified treatment strategies and interventions; and (4) documentation of patient care activities, variances, and goal achievement. The development of a clinical pathway involves reviewing for efficiency and necessity the many activities that occur from the time the patient enters the health care facility through discharge and aftercare. These activities include preadmission work-ups, tests, consultations, treatments, activities, diet, and health teaching.

Many health care providers believe that clinical pathways are more difficult to develop in psychiatry than in other specialty areas. What problems would be particularly challenging in designing clinical pathways for psychiatric treatment? ■

Clinical Algorithms

Clinical algorithms, focusing on treatment or medications, take practice guidelines to a greater level of specificity by providing step-by-step recommendations on issues such as treatment options, treatment sequencing, preferred dosage, and progress assessment. They thus provide clinicians with a framework that can enhance treatment planning and decision making for individual patients. Algorithms help the clinician select from large databases of information relevant to decision making. They are cognitive tools for the clinician, intended to assist and not limit clinical decision making.

A clinical algorithm can be represented by a flowchart that identifies what clinical process is likely to follow based on a patient's current clinical status and response to prior treatments, thereby providing a more specific statement of priority, or what to do next if the treatment is not effective.

Algorithms in psychiatry have grown in popularity for a number of reasons. First, they reduce unnecessary variation in clinical practice. They also can help facilitate the decision making process for clinicians who cannot integrate into their daily practice all of the published data concerning new knowledge and treatments. Algorithms make explicit the "art" of diagnostic reasoning; algorithm-based treatment should reduce symptoms and improve a patient's psychosocial functioning faster than nonalgorithm-guided treatment. This approach also should reduce the cost of treatment. Finally, algorithms provide a way to compare a patient's actual progress with expected progress and allow for important feedback about what works best for which patients and under what circumstances.

Most recently, computerized medication algorithms have been developed (Trivedi et al, 2000). They can facilitate clinician decision making by integrating patient information such as drug allergies, age, weight, laboratory results, and clinical and prescription history with up-to-date treatment guidelines for a primary condition. They are also helpful in tracking patient follow-up and preventive care. As such, they can be a great asset to clinical practice.

Clinical algorithms are presented simply as drawn diagrams. What advantages does such a display have over practice guidelines that can be as many as 50 pages long? ■

■ OUTCOME MEASUREMENT

In the past, although mental health clinicians tried to give the best care possible to their patients, they did this most often without the benefit of reliable data that compared their work with that of others in the field. Increasing emphasis is now placed on providing the most effective care in the most appropriate setting. To accomplish this goal and demonstrate the effectiveness of clinical programs, outcome measurement is needed (Speer, 1998; Berman et al, 1998).

Outcomes are the extent to which health care services are cost-effective and have a favorable effect on the patient's symptoms, functioning, and well-being. They include all the things that affect the patient and his or her family while they are in the health care system, such as health status, functional status, quality of life, the presence or absence of illness, type of coping response, and satisfaction with treatment. They include both positive (well-being) and negative (illness state) dimensions.

Outcome measurement can focus on a clinical condition, an intervention, or a caregiving process (Coughlin, 2001). It is important to measure both short-term and long-term outcomes when providing psychiatric care. These data are then used to make decisions affecting staffing levels, program development, and financial support. Outcomes that can be examined include **clinical**, **functional**, **satisfaction**, and **financial indicators** related to the provision of psychiatric care (Box 5-4). The specific purposes of outcome measurement are to:

- Evaluate the outcomes of care.
- Suggest changes in treatment.
- Analyze program effectiveness.
- Profile the practice pattern of providers.
- Determine the most appropriate level of care.
- Predict the path of a patient's illness and recovery.
- Contribute to quality improvement programs.

Implementing outcome measurement is no simple task, however. Many scientific and practical problems are involved in knowing what to measure and how to measure it. One of the most difficult aspects is selecting an appropriate scale or measurement tool (see Appendix C for a list of behavioral rating scales commonly used in psychiatry). Other difficulties involved in outcome measurement include the following:

- Resistance of clinicians to completing the rating scales
- High rates of spontaneous remission and placebo effect among psychiatric patients
- Wide variety of therapeutic approaches and interventions used by mental health clinicians
- Many interacting biological, psychological, and sociocultural factors that affect a patient's improvement
- Lack of clarity regarding when to measure outcomes (before, during, or after treatment or during long-term follow-up)
- Validity and reliability problems with patient report and clinical report scales
- Lack of correlation between measures of patient satisfaction and clinical assessment of improvement
- Practical problems of administering, collecting, and analyzing the outcome data.

BOX 5-4

Categories of Outcome Indicators

Clinical Outcome Indicators
High-risk behaviors
Symptomatology
Coping responses
Relapse
Recurrence
Readmission
Number of treatment episodes
Medical complications
Incidence reports
Mortality

Functional Outcome Indicators
Functional status
Social interaction
Activities of daily living
Occupational abilities
Quality of life
Family relationships
Housing arrangement

Satisfaction Outcome Indicators
Patient and family satisfaction with:
Outcomes
Providers
Delivery system
Caregiving process
Organization

Financial Outcome Indicators
Cost per treatment episode
Revenue per treatment episode
Length of inpatient stay
Use of health care resources
Costs related to disability

In spite of these problems, psychiatric nurses should routinely use rating scales to assess their patients to determine their state at baseline (before beginning treatment), their progress during treatment, and the clinical progress they have made at the end of treatment. In this way nurses will be able to document the effectiveness of the care they provide. Table 5-1 presents issues that should be considered in selecting outcome measures in psychiatric nursing practice.

 One of your nursing colleagues complains about having to complete clinical rating scales on each new admission. She says she "doesn't have time for such busywork." How would you respond? ■

Patient Satisfaction

Measurement of patient satisfaction in mental health services has received increasing attention because of clinicians' and researchers' desire to measure outcomes that reflect the patient's unique perspective. The growing recognition of the importance of patient satisfaction is also reflected in the requirements of regulatory and certification agencies that man-

Table 5-1	Considerations in Selecting Outcome Measures in Psychiatric Nursing Practice
CONSIDERATION	**DESIRED ATTRIBUTE**
Applicable	Measures should address an important aspect of the structure, process, and/or outcome of care
Acceptable	Measures should be brief and easy to administer
Practical	Measures should be simple to use and interpret and inexpensive to implement
Integrity	Measures should have established reliability and validity and have been tested on the population to be assessed
Sensitive to change	Measures should be able to detect even small changes in a patient's status over time

date that treatment facilities collect and use patient satisfaction data in their quality assurance activities.

However, controversy exists regarding the methods used to measure patient satisfaction and the meaning and importance of patient satisfaction data in mental health services. For example, patients may report high levels of satisfaction with services because of a variety of factors, some unrelated to the actual treatment, including their relationship with the interviewing staff.

Patient satisfaction is also multidimensional. This means that patients can be satisfied with the treatment staff but not with other aspects of the treatment process, such as the environment or timeliness in which the treatment was provided. Thus although patient satisfaction is an important outcome measure to consider in evaluating mental health services, more research is needed before its relation to the structure, process, and outcome of psychiatric care can be fully evaluated.

Quality Report Cards

Another type of outcome measure is related not to the patient, but to the performance of the behavioral health care organization itself. Like their academic counterparts, report cards for mental health and substance abuse services are intended to provide feedback on achievements and problems. At least three dimensions must be considered when discussing these report cards: content, point of view, and intended audience (Manderscheid, 2001).

Content refers to the topics that are addressed. In school, content would be the courses being graded. Generally, report cards for behavioral health care services cover one or more of the following domains of care: access, appropriateness, cost, and outcomes. Access and cost are the domains most commonly covered.

Point of view refers to the perspective taken. In school, the perspective is that of the teacher. In a behavioral service setting, the perspective might be that of the payer, the managed care company, the provider, the consumer, or the family member. Most often the perspective is that of the managed care company.

Intended audience can be both explicit and implicit. In schools, the explicit audience of a report card is the parent;

an implicit audience may be a future employer. In behavioral service settings, the explicit audience could be the payer, the managed care entity, the provider, the consumer, or the family member. Most often, the explicit audience is the payer, whereas the implicit audience is often the media.

Most discussions about report cards focus on their content. Why do you think the point of view and intended audience are often ignored? What are the implications of not attending to these other domains? ■

■ THE EVIDENCE BASE FOR PSYCHIATRIC NURSING PRACTICE

Psychiatric nurses are being asked to describe what they do and how they add value to the health care organization. Their responses should be couched with sensitivity regarding the issues of effectiveness, cost, and quality. Currently the mysteries of mental illness are closer to being understood than ever before. New findings are emerging almost daily about their causes and most effective treatments. Nurses need to keep abreast of these developments and base their interventions on the evidence of emerging research rather than on the untested notions of tradition.

Psychiatric nurses need to educate consumers, other health professionals, the business community, and managed care companies regarding the services they can provide, including prevention and rehabilitation, and the ways in which they are able to deliver high-quality, cost-effective care. Nurses must then support this position with data from outcome studies that reflect clinical, functional, satisfaction, and financial indicators. This research is the essence of evidence-based psychiatric nursing practice (Newell and Gournay, 2000).

Much of current psychiatric nursing practice does not meet the ideals of evidence-based care. For example, many advanced practice psychiatric nurses have reported that they do not use clinical rating scales or outcome measures in their practice (Barrell, Merrwin, and Poster, 1997). Yet the use of measurement or rating scales should be viewed as an essential part of psychiatric nursing practice.

Furthermore, much of what psychiatric nurses do is based on untested theories or cherished traditions rather than on scientifically based evidence. There is no literature that describes the use of practice guidelines by psychiatric nurses, and very few studies of the clinical, functional, satisfaction, or financial outcomes of psychiatric nursing care have been conducted. In addition, most psychiatric nursing textbooks use secondary references instead of primary references, thus creating ambiguity about the evidence base for the nursing practice.

Nurses need to research the impact of their activities on focused patient outcomes (see Citing the Evidence). They also need to know how to access, interpret, and use findings from outcome research before they can engage in evidence-based psychiatric nursing care.

An Agenda for Psychiatric Nursing Research

The relationship between practice, theory, and research is interactive and reciprocal. For theory to be useful, it must have implications for practice, and for practice to be tested and

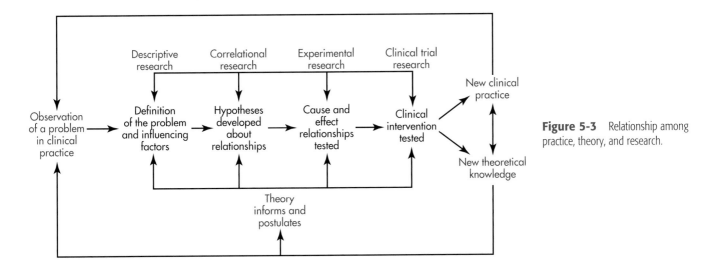

Figure 5-3 Relationship among practice, theory, and research.

CITING THE EVIDENCE ON

Patient Outcomes

BACKGROUND: Although many studies demonstrate the cost-effectiveness and clinical outcomes of and satisfaction with the services of nurse practitioners and nurse midwives, few studies report the cost-effectiveness and clinical outcomes of and patient satisfaction with psychotherapy provided by psychiatric clinical nurse specialists (CNSs). This prospective study was designed to examine the following questions: (1) Were there improvements in clinical symptoms and quality of life between initiation and termination of psychotherapy? (2) Were improvements in clinical symptoms and quality of life maintained 6 months after psychotherapy? (3) What level of patient satisfaction was reported 6 months after termination of psychotherapy? Instruments used were the Profile of Mood States–Short Form, Quality of Life, and the Patient Satisfaction Survey.

RESULTS: Patients reported significant improvement in clinical symptoms and quality of life at termination. Improvements were maintained 6 months after termination for clinical symptoms and quality of life, with the exception of the job domain. Patients reported a very high level of satisfaction with the care provided by psychiatric clinical nurse specialists.

IMPLICATIONS: Mental health care provided by psychiatric CNSs can improve the quality of life and the level of patient satisfaction for consumers of health care services. Data support the inclusion of psychiatric CNSs as providers in the rapidly changing health care system. The data from this study lend further support to psychotherapy as an autonomous role for psychiatric CNSs.

Baradell J, Bordeaux B: *J Am Psychiatr Nurs Assoc* 7:77, 2001.

validated, it must be based in theory (Stetler, 2001). Theory that arises out of practice is validated by research, which rebounds to direct practice and inform clinical care.

This cyclical relationship is seen in Figure 5-3. It shows how the observation of a problem in practice can lead to a more systematic observation and definition of terms, including the nature of the problem and influencing factors. Descriptive and exploratory research can further define a problem. Hypotheses may then be developed concerning relationships between identified variables, which may be tested in correlational or survey research designs. Cause-and-effect relationships between the variables might then be tested in various experiments with natural or controlled settings. Only after establishing cause and effect can specific interventions aimed at changing the clinical problem be prescribed and tested in randomized controlled clinical trials. In this way studies feed knowledge back into practice to improve health care. **This progression of observing from practice, theorizing, testing in research, and subsequently modifying practice is an essential part of psychiatric nursing.**

At this time psychiatric nursing research is mostly descriptive, correlational, and qualitative in nature (Cutcliffe and

Goward, 2000). Relatively few outcome studies exist that test the effectiveness of psychiatric nursing care. Most of the studies that do exist do not meet the criteria of the highest scientific evidence as represented by randomized controlled clinical trials.

A review of the psychiatric nursing journals leads one to conclude that the field has many small scale studies and theory-rich insights, but little of the evidence necessary to direct care practices. Most studies in the field are qualitative, which provide detailed experiences at an individual level. In contrast, relatively few quantitative studies with the rigorous methodology needed to answer questions about the efficacy and effectiveness of psychiatric nursing interventions have been conducted. Psychiatric nurse researchers need to move beyond this basic level of study and be guided by a national-international research agenda that meets the level of scientific inquiry set by the current research community.

One evolving framework for measuring nursing outcomes is the Iowa Nursing Intervention Project, which developed Nursing Intervention Classification (NIC) codes (Dochterman and Bulecheck, 2004) and Nursing Outcome Classification (NOC) codes (Moorhead, Johnson, and Maas, 2004). These codes lay out a taxonomy for nursing interventions and out-

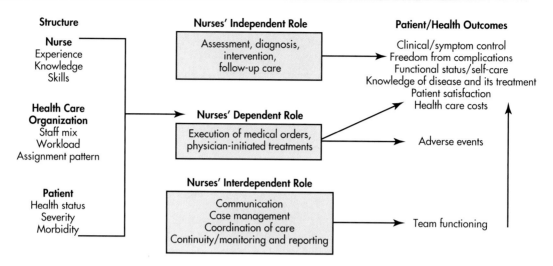

Figure 5-4   Model for testing nursing role effectiveness.

comes from a biopsychosocial perspective. They are a fertile area of potential nursing research that can document the nature and outcomes of psychiatric nursing practice.

Another model identifying areas for nursing research is seen in Figure 5-4. It proposes relationships between the different roles nurses assume in health care and outcomes expected of nursing care (Irvine, Sidani, and Hall, 1998). Psychiatric nurses can use such a model to formulate theories, test interventions, and evaluate their impact on patient care outcomes, thus moving the specialty forward toward evidence-based practice.

Beyond Evidence-Based Practice

New ways of thinking take the field beyond evidence-based practice. It has been suggested that there is evidence-supported, evidence-informed, and evidence-suggested prac-tice. Also, the notion of **practice-based evidence** suggests that much is to be gained from gathering good data from routine practices.

Although clearly the movement toward evidence-based practice has been very beneficial for all of health care, it does reflect the fact that research to date has largely been focused on **programs of care**. Another focus for the future research agenda will be on studying the **processes of care** occurring between patients and providers. Specifically, future studies might focus on such processes as collaborative goal setting, the nature of the therapeutic alliance, family engagement, providing environmental accommodations, and coaching. It is likely that only by coming to understand how evidence-based processes complement evidence-based practices will the true value of psychiatric care emerge.

CHAPTER FOCUS POINTS

- Evidence-based practice is the conscientious, explicit, and judicious use of the best evidence gained from systematic research to make decisions about the care of individual patients.
- Evidence-based practice blends the nurse's clinical experience with the best available research evidence. It is the best basis for practice and involves defining the clinical question, finding the evidence, analyzing the evidence, using the evidence, and evaluating the outcome.
- The four bases for nursing practice are traditional, regulatory, philosophical, and evidence-based. The best basis for clinical nursing practice is evidence-based.
- The four steps to developing evidence-based care are defining the clinical question, finding the evidence, analyzing the evidence, and evaluating the outcome.
- Practice guidelines are developed to help clinical decision making and provide patients information about their treatment options. The best practice guidelines are based on scientific review of the available clinical research literature to establish which treatments are safe and effective for particular psychiatric disorders.

- Clinical pathways identify the key clinical processes and corresponding timelines necessary for a patient to achieve standard outcomes within a specific period of time.
- Clinical algorithms or protocols provide step-by-step recommendations on issues such as treatment options, treatment sequencing, preferred dosage, and progress assessment.
- Outcome measurements provide important data about the clinical program and include clinical, functional, satisfaction, and financial indicators.
- Patient satisfaction indicators and quality report cards are used to measure the performance of the behavioral health care organization.
- Much of current psychiatric nursing practice does not meet the ideals of evidence-based practice. Nurses need to use outcome measurements, test theories and interventions through randomized controlled clinical trials, and measure the clinical, functional, satisfaction, and financial outcomes of the care they provide.
- It is likely that only by coming to understand how evidence-based processes complement evidence-based practices will the true value of psychiatric care emerge.

KEY TERMS

clinical algorithms, 80
clinical pathways, 80
evidence-based practice, 76

outcomes, 81
practice guidelines, 78

CHAPTER REVIEW QUESTIONS

1. Indicate whether the following statements are true (T) or false (F).

_____ A. Evidence-based practice is a method of self-directed, career-long learning.

_____ B. Descriptive studies are the gold standard of research methodologies.

_____ C. A key aspect of evidence-based practice is that it ensures the best use is made of the available evidence.

_____ D. Practice guidelines are similar in format and design.

_____ E. Controversy exists regarding the methods used to measure patient satisfaction and the meaning and importance of patient satisfaction data in mental health services.

_____ F. Psychiatric nurses routinely use behavioral rating scales in their practice.

2. Fill in the blanks.

A. The gap identified by the report of the Surgeon General is that between the kind of mental health care that

_____ found to be most effective and

the kind of care most Americans _____.

B. The five steps for developing evidence-based care are:

1. _____,

2. _____,

3. _____,

4. _____, and

5. _____.

C. A _____ summarizes the findings from a number of studies to arrive at an objective and authoritative guide to treatment.

D. Strategies that have been developed to facilitate clinical decision making and provide patients with information about their

treatment options are called _____.

E. _____ take practice guidelines to a greater level of specificity by providing step-by-step recommendations on issues such as treatment options, treatment sequencing, preferred dosage, and progress assessment.

F. Four categories of outcome indicators that can be

used by nurses are _____,

_____, _____,

and _____.

3. Provide short answers for the following questions.

A. What activities are central to the psychiatric nurse's accountability for patient care?

B. Discuss the four bases for nursing practice. Which one is best and why?

C. View Figure 5-4. Is anything missing from this model of nursing? How would you begin to test it out?

Visit Evolve for additional resources related to the content of this chapter.

 http://evolve.elsevier.com/Stuart/principles/
• Topical Course Outline • Student Workbook Exercises • Critical Thinking Questions and Activities • Case Studies • Research Topics
• Monthly Content Updates • WebLinks

Student Study CD-ROM

Access the accompanying CD-ROM for animations, interactive exercises, review questions for the NCLEX examination, and an audio glossary.

REFERENCES

American College of Mental Health Administration (ACMHA): Sounding a call to action, *Behav Healthcare Tomorrow* 9:43, 2000.

Barrell LM, Merrwin EI, Poster EC: Patient outcomes used by advanced practice psychiatric nurses to evaluate effectiveness of practice, *Arch Psychiatr Nurs* 11:184, 1997.

Benner P, Hooper-Hyriakidis P, Stannard D: *Clinical wisdom and interventions in critical care: a thinking-in-action approach*, Philadelphia, 1999, WB Saunders.

Berman WH et al: Toto, we're not in Kansas anymore: measuring and using outcomes in behavioral health care, *Clin Psychol Sci Pract* 5:115, 1998.

Bickman L: Our quality-assurance methods aren't so sure, *Behav Healthcare Tomorrow* 9:41, 2000.

Cochrane Library (quarterly CD-ROM *and database online*). Oxford, 2003, Update Software.

Coughlin KM, editor: 2001 *Behavioral outcomes & guidelines sourcebook*, New York, 2001, Faulkner and Gray.

Cutcliffe JR, Goward P: Mental health nurses and qualitative research methods: a mutual attraction? *J Adv Nurs* 31:590, 2000.

Dochterman J, Bulechek G: *Nursing interventions classification (NIC)*, ed 4, St Louis, 2004, Mosby.

Drake R et al: Implementing evidence-based practices in routine mental health service settings, *Psychiatr Serv* 52:179, 2001.

Hoge MA: The training gap: an acute crisis in behavioral health education, *Adm Policy Ment Health* 29:305, 2002.

Irvine D, Sidani S, Hall LM: Linking outcomes to nurses' roles in health care, *Nurs Econ* 16:58, 1998.

Manderscheid RW: Assessing performance at the millennium. In Coughlin KM, editor: *2001 Behavioral outcomes & guidelines sourcebook*, New York, 2001, Faulkner and Gray.

Moorhead S, Johnson M, Maas M: *Nursing outcomes classification (NOC)*, ed 3, St Louis, 2004, Mosby.

Nathan P, Gorman J, editors: *A guide to treatments that work*, ed 2, New York, 2002, Oxford University Press.

New Freedom Commission on Mental Health, *Achieving the promise: transforming mental health care in America, final report*, DHHS Pub. No. SMA-03-3832, Rockville, Md, 2003, USDHHS.

Newell R, Gournay K: *Mental health nursing: an evidence-based approach*, London, 2000, Churchill Livingstone.

Sackett D et al: Evidence-based medicine: what it is and what it isn't, *BMJ* 312:71,1996.

Speer DC: *Mental health outcome evaluation*, San Diego, 1998, Academic Press.

Stetler CB et al: Evidence-based practice and the role of nursing leadership, *J Nurs Adm* 28:45, 1998.

Stetler CB: Updating the Stetler model of research utilization to facilitate evidence-based practice, *Nurs Outlook* 49:272, 2001.

Stuart GW, Rush AJ, Morris JA: Practice guidelines in mental health and addiction services: contributions from the American College of Mental Health Administration, *Adm Policy Ment Health* 30:21, 2002.

Trivedi MH et al: Computerizing medication algorithms and decision support systems for major psychiatric disorders, *J Psychiatr Pract* 6:237, 2000.

U.S. Department of Health and Human Services: *Mental health: a report of the surgeon general*, Rockville, Md, 1999, National Institute of Mental Health.

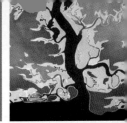

> *We must recollect that all our provisional ideas in psychology will some day be based on an organic substructure. This makes it probable that special substances and special chemical processes control the operation.*
> SIGMUND FREUD

BIOLOGICAL CONTEXT OF PSYCHIATRIC NURSING CARE 6

Michele T. Laraia

LEARNING OBJECTIVES

After studying this chapter, the student should be able to:

1. Apply knowledge about the structure and function of the brain to psychiatric nursing practice (**I**).
2. Describe neuroimaging techniques used in psychiatry (**II**).
3. Examine the impact of biological rhythms and sleep on a person's abilities and moods (**III**).
4. Describe how psychoneuroimmunology relates to mental health and illness (**IV**).
5. Discuss genetics and the impact of the Human Genome Project on the understanding of mental illness (**V**).
6. Assess patients from a biological perspective (**VI**).

TOPICAL OUTLINE

 Visit Evolve for additional resources related to the content of this chapter.
http://evolve.elsevier.com/Stuart/principles/

Although interest in the brain and human behavior has a history as old as the human race, the explosion of new-found scientific information during the 20th century has been unprecedented. The 1990s were named by the U.S. Congress the "Decade of the Brain," and what has been learned during this time from study of the neurosciences has changed forever how the brain and behavior, health and illness, and thus human experience itself are understood. The year 1990 was also the year the Human Genome Project began its 13 years of intensive work. The information gained from this project has ushered in the 21st century with a focus on the biology of the brain. Genes are the keys to the doorways through which a new understanding of not only humans but also all living cells can be realized. Unlocking these doorways will open up the realm of potential manipulation of all living things.

Research that has focused on how the brain is structured, how the nervous system functions, how these systems affect health, how they are affected by disease, and how new treatments are designed and delivered has changed psychiatric nursing in significant ways. The field of neuroscience encompasses many disciplines (Figure 6-1). They come together to provide a more complete understanding of the human brain and how it is integrated with the body and with the human environment. The neurosciences present new paradigms and great challenges that psychiatric nurses can embrace and thus can help them take a significant step forward in further defining their scope of practice, their research interests, and the measure of outcomes associated with psychiatric nursing care.

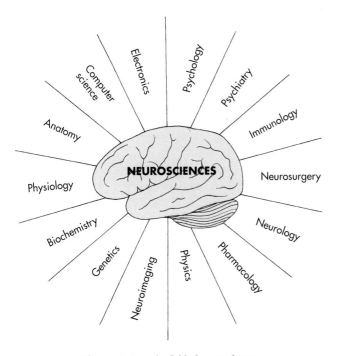

Figure 6-1 The field of neurosciences.

STRUCTURE AND FUNCTION OF THE BRAIN

All nurses should have a working knowledge of the normal structure and function of the brain in association with mental health and neuropsychiatric illness, just as all nurses

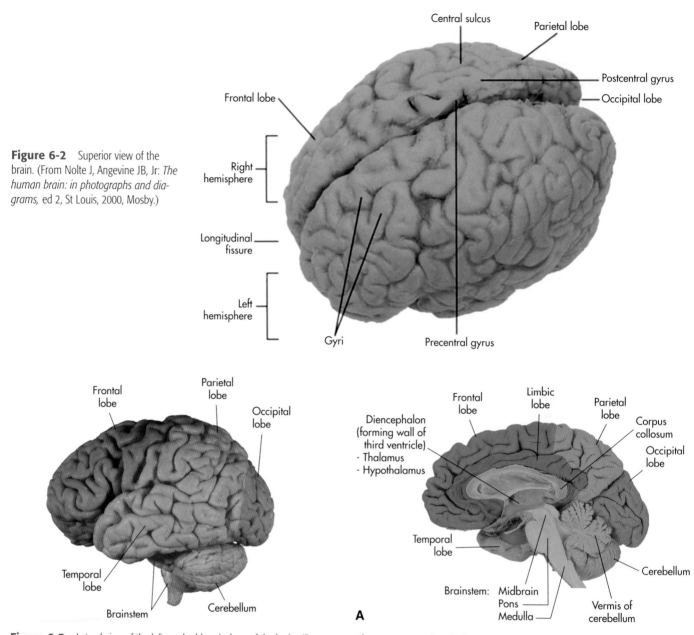

Figure 6-2   Superior view of the brain. (From Nolte J, Angevine JB, Jr: *The human brain: in photographs and diagrams,* ed 2, St Louis, 2000, Mosby.)

Figure 6-3   Lateral view of the left cerebral hemisphere of the brain. (From Nolte J, Angevine JB, Jr: *The human brain: in photographs and diagrams,* ed 2, St Louis, 2000, Mosby.)

Figure 6-4   When the brain is cut between the two hemispheres down the middle (a midsagittal section), the main divisions can be clearly seen, as in **A** and **C**, which are schematic representations. (**A** from Nolte J, Angevine JB, Jr: *The human brain: in photographs and diagrams,* ed 2, St Louis, 2000, Mosby.)

should know the structure and function of the heart. Much is known about various brain structures and how they are linked to some of the symptoms of mental illness. The reader is encouraged to review texts on basic anatomy and physiology or neurophysiology to learn more about these areas (Nolte, 2002; Thibodeau and Patton, 2002). A brief review of key brain regions is presented in Figures 6-2 to 6-6 and in Box 6-1. This information can be used as a reference for topics discussed in this chapter.

The brain weighs about 3 pounds. It is composed of trillions of groups of cells that have formed highly specific structures and sophisticated communication pathways that have changed over millions of years of evolution. The brain continues to develop and change **(neural plasticity)** in utero and

throughout the life span. During adolescence, efficiency of the brain is refined by eliminating unneeded circuits **(synaptic pruning)** and strengthening others. This process allows humans to have a brain that accommodates both its genetic potential and the environmental influences surrounding it.

The changing brain reacts to a variety of influences that can support health or promote illness, both before birth and across the life span. About 100 billion brain cells **(neurons)** form groups, or structures, that are highly specialized. Neurotransmission is the process by which neurons communicate with each other through electrical impulses and chemical messengers. This communication between neurons is carried out by chemical "first" messengers called neurotransmitters and gives rise to human activity, body functions, conscious-

Text continued on p. 93.

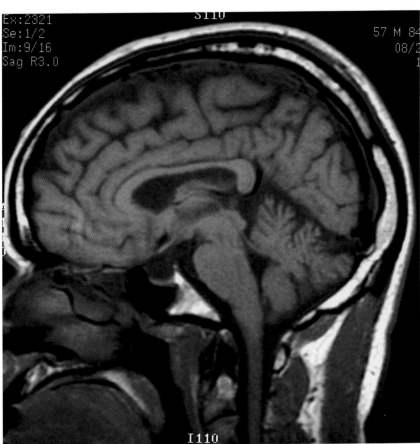

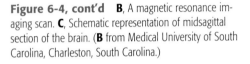

Figure 6-4, cont'd   B, A magnetic resonance imaging scan. **C**, Schematic representation of midsagittal section of the brain. (**B** from Medical University of South Carolina, Charleston, South Carolina.)

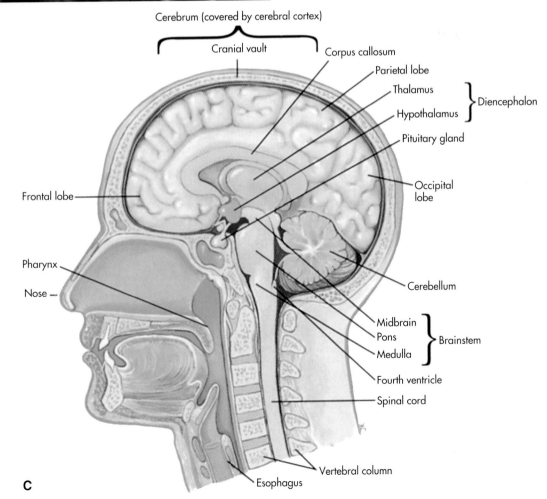

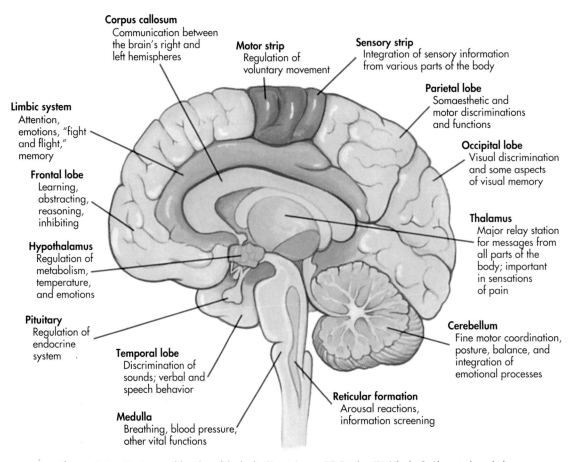

Corpus callosum
Communication between the brain's right and left hemispheres

Motor strip
Regulation of voluntary movement

Sensory strip
Integration of sensory information from various parts of the body

Parietal lobe
Somaesthetic and motor discriminations and functions

Occipital lobe
Visual discrimination and some aspects of visual memory

Limbic system
Attention, emotions, "fight and flight," memory

Frontal lobe
Learning, abstracting, reasoning, inhibiting

Hypothalamus
Regulation of metabolism, temperature, and emotions

Pituitary
Regulation of endocrine system

Temporal lobe
Discrimination of sounds; verbal and speech behavior

Medulla
Breathing, blood pressure, other vital functions

Thalamus
Major relay station for messages from all parts of the body; important in sensations of pain

Cerebellum
Fine motor coordination, posture, balance, and integration of emotional processes

Reticular formation
Arousal reactions, information screening

Figure 6-5 Structure and function of the brain. (From Carson RC, Butcher JN, Mineka S: *Abnormal psychology and modern life,* ed 11, Boston, 2000, Allyn and Bacon.)

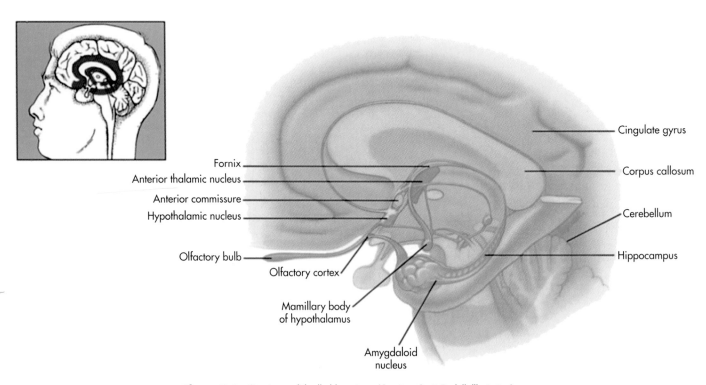

Fornix
Anterior thalamic nucleus
Anterior commissure
Hypothalamic nucleus

Olfactory bulb

Olfactory cortex

Mamillary body of hypothalamus

Amygdaloid nucleus

Cingulate gyrus

Corpus callosum

Cerebellum

Hippocampus

Figure 6-6 Structures of the limbic system. (Courtesy Scott Bodell, illustrator.)

BOX **6-1**

Structure and Function of the Brain

Cerebrum
Largest portion of the brain

Responsible for conscious perception, thought, and motor activity

Governs muscle coordination and the learning of rote movements

Can override most other systems

Divided into two hemispheres, each of which is divided into four lobes

Dominant hemisphere
Left side is dominant in most people (in 95% of right-handed and more than 50% of left-handed people)

Responsible for the production and comprehension of language, mathematical ability, and the ability to solve problems in a sequential, logical fashion

Nondominant hemisphere
Right side is nondominant in most people

Responsible for musical skills, recognition of faces, and tasks requiring comprehension of spatial relationships

Corpus callosum
Largest fiber bundle in the brain

Connects the two cerebral hemispheres and passes information from one to the other, welding the two hemispheres together into a unitary consciousness, allowing the "right hand to know what the left hand is doing"

Cerebral cortex
A few millimeters thick and about 2.5 square feet in area

Sheet of gray matter containing 30 billion neurons interconnected by almost 70 miles of axons and dendrites

Forms the corrugated surface of the four lobes of the cerebral hemispheres

Connected to various structures of the brain and has a great deal to do with the abilities we think of as uniquely human, such as language and abstract thinking, as well as basic aspects of perception, movement, and adaptive response to the outside world

Functional areas have been mapped by imaging technology

Damage to certain cortical areas usually results in predictable deficits, depending on the area affected

Frontal lobes
Aid in planning for the future, motivation, control of voluntary motor function, and production of speech

Play an important part in emotional experience and expression of mood

Clinical example: Aphasia (absent or defective speech or comprehension) results from a lesion in the language areas of the cortex. The several types of aphasia depend on the site of the lesion. Damage to Broca's area, which contains the motor programs for the generation of language, results in expressive, or motor, aphasia, with difficulty producing either written or spoken words but no difficulty comprehending language.

Parietal lobes
Reception and evaluation of most sensory information (excluding smell, hearing, and vision)

Concerned with the initial processing of tactile and proprioceptive (sense of position) information, complex aspects of spacial orientation and perception, and the comprehension of language (share Wernicke's area with the temporal lobes)

Central sulcus
Groove or fissure on the surface of the brain that divides the frontal and parietal lobes

Temporal lobes
Receive and process auditory information, involved in higher order processing of visual information, involved in complex aspects of memory and learning, and are important in the comprehension of language

Associated with functions such as abstract thought and judgment

Clinical example: Damage to Wernicke's area, which contains the mechanisms for the formulation of language, results in receptive, or sensory, aphasia, in which words are produced but their sequence is defective in linguistic content, resulting in paraphasia (word substitutions), neologisms (insertion of new and meaningless words), or jargon (fluent but unintelligible speech), and a general deficiency in the comprehension of language is noted. If the lesion occurs in the connection between Broca's area and Wernicke's area, conduction aphasia results, in which a person has poor repetition but good comprehension.

Lateral fissure
Separates the temporal lobe from the rest of the cerebrum

Occipital lobes
Reception and integration of visual input

Damage to the occipital lobes can result in blindness

Diencephalon
Constitutes only 2% of the central nervous system (CNS) by weight

Has extremely widespread and important connections; the great majority of sensory, motor, and limbic pathways involve the diencephalon

Thalamus
Composes 80% of the diencephalon

All sensory pathways and many other anatomical loops relay in the thalamus

Takes sensory information and relays it to areas throughout the cortex

Influences prefrontal cortical functions such as affect and foresight

Influences mood and general body movements associated with strong emotions, such as fear or rage

Pineal gland
Endocrine gland involved in reproductive cycles

During darkness it secretes an antigonadotropic hormone called *melatonin*, which decreases during light, thus increasing gonadal function

Important in mammals with seasonal sexual cycles; its effects in humans are not yet clear, although tumors of the pineal gland affect human sexual development

Also may be involved in the sleep-wake cycle

Continued

BOX 6-1

Structure and Function of the Brain—cont'd

Diencephalon—cont'd

Hypothalamus

Weighs only 4 g

Major control center for the pituitary gland; for maintaining homeostasis; and for regulating autonomic, endocrine, emotional, and somatic functions

Controls various visceral functions and activities involved in basic drives and is very important in a number of functions that have emotional and mood relationships

Directly involved in stress-related and psychosomatic illnesses and with feelings of fear and rage

Regulates feeding and drinking behavior, temperature regulation, cardiac function, gut motility, and sexual activity

Coordinates responses for the sleep-wake cycle to other areas of the body

Contains the mamillary bodies, which are involved in olfactory reflexes and emotional responses to odors

Brainstem

Connects the spinal cord to the brain

Location of cranial nerve nuclei

Controls automatic body functions such as breathing and cardiovascular activity

Midbrain

Contains ascending and descending nerve tracks

Visual cortex center

Part of auditory pathway

Regulates the reflexive movement of the eyes and head

Aids in the unconscious regulation and coordination of motor activities

Contains the part of the basal ganglia, the substantia nigra, that manufactures dopamine

Pons

Contains ascending and descending nerve tracks

Relays between cerebrum and cerebellum

Reflex center

Contains the locus ceruleus, which manufactures most of the brain's norepinephrine

Medulla oblongata

Conduction pathway for ascending and descending nerve tracks

Conscious control of skeletal muscles

Involved in functions such as balance, coordination, and modulation of sound impulses from the inner ear

Center for several important reflexes: heart rate, breathing, swallowing, vomiting, coughing, sneezing

Reticular formation

Central core of the brainstem

Controls cyclic activities such as the sleep-wake cycle (called the *reticular activating system,* or *RAS*)

Plays an important role in arousing and maintaining consciousness, alertness, and attention

Contributes to the motor system, respiration, cardiac rhythms, and other vital body functions

Clinical example: Damage to the RAS can result in coma. General anesthetics function by suppressing this system. It also may be the target of many tranquilizers. Ammonia (smelling salts) stimulate the RAS, resulting in arousal.

Basal Ganglia

Several deep gray matter structures that are related functionally and are located bilaterally in the cerebrum, diencephalon, and midbrain

Control muscle tone, activity, and posture

Coordinate large-muscle movements

Major effect is to inhibit unwanted muscular activity

Cause extrapyramidal syndromes when dysfunctional

Clinical example: Parkinson's disease (characterized by muscular rigidity; a slow, shuffling gait; and a general lack of movement) is associated with a dysfunction of the basal ganglia, probably a destruction of the dopamine-producing neurons of the substantia nigra (part of the basal ganglia but located in the midbrain).

Limbic System

Forms the limbus, or border, of the temporal lobes and is intimately connected to many other structures of the brain

Concerned both with subjective emotional experiences and with changes in bodily functions associated with emotional states

Particularly involved in aggressive, submissive, and sexual behavior and with pleasure, memory, and learning

Associated with mood, motivation, and sensations, all central to preservation

Clinical example: Klüver-Bucy syndrome develops when the entire limbic system is removed or destroyed. Symptoms include fearlessness and placidity (absence of emotional reactions), an inordinate degree of attention to sensory stimuli (ceaseless and intrusive curiosity), and visual agnosia (the inability to recognize anything).

Hippocampus

Consolidates recently acquired information about facts and events, somehow turning short-term memory into long-term memory

Contains large amounts of neurotransmitters

Clinical example: Surgical removal of the hippocampus results in the inability to form new memories of facts and events (names of new acquaintances, day-to-day events, inability to remember why a task was begun), although long-term memory, intelligence, and the ability to learn new skills are unaffected. A similar memory problem is Korsakoff's syndrome, in which patients have intact intelligence but cannot form new memories. They typically confabulate (make up answers to questions), which occurs when the hippocampus and surrounding areas are damaged by chronic alcoholism. This also is seen in Alzheimer's disease, in which the memory loss is profound, and extensive cellular degeneration in the hippocampus is noted.

Amygdala

Generates emotions from perceptions and thoughts (presumably through its interactions with the hypothalamus and prefrontal cortex)

Contains many opiate receptors

Clinical example: Electrical stimulation of the amygdala in animals causes responses of defense, raging aggression, or fleeing. In humans the most common response is fear and its related autonomic responses (dilation of the pupils, increased heart rate, and release of adrenalin).

BOX 6-1

Structure and Function of the Brain—cont'd

Limbic System—cont'd

Amygdala—cont'd

Conversely, bilateral destruction of the amygdala causes a great decrease in aggression, and animals become tame and placid. This is thought to be another kind of memory dysfunction that impairs the ability to learn or remember the appropriate emotional and autonomic responses to stimuli.

Fornix

Two-way fiber system that connects the hippocampus to the hypothalamus

Cerebellum

"Little brain"

Full range of sensory inputs finds its way here and in turn projects to various sites in the brainstem and thalamus.

Although it is extensively involved with the processing of sensory information, it also is part of the motor system and is involved in equilibrium, muscle tone, postural control, and coordination of voluntary movements.

It is thought that, because of connections to other brain regions, the cerebellum may be involved in cognitive, behavioral, and affective functions.

Clinical example: The malnutrition often accompanying chronic alcoholism causes a degeneration of the cerebellar cortex, resulting in the anterior lobe syndrome in which the legs are primarily affected, and the most prominent symptom is a broad-based, staggering gait and a general incoordination, or ataxia, of leg movements.

Ventricles

Each cerebral hemisphere contains a large cavity, the lateral ventricle.

A smaller midline cavity, the third ventricle, is located in the center of the diencephalon, between the two halves of the thalamus.

The fourth ventricle is in the region of the pons and medulla oblongata and connects with the central canal of the spinal cord, which extends nearly the full length of the spinal cord.

Clinical example: Although the clinical significance of these findings is uncertain, imaging techniques have shown enlargement of the ventricles in many psychiatric disorders, suggesting an atrophy of the many critical structures in the brain with these illnesses.

Spinal Fluid

Cerebral spinal fluid (CSF) is procured from the blood choroid plexuses, located in the ventricles, and fills the ventricles, subarachnoid space (between the brain and the skull), and the spinal cord.

CSF bathes the brain with nutrients, cushions the brain within the skull, and exits through the blood stream.

Approximately 140 ml of spinal fluid within the CNS travels from its point of origin to the blood stream at approximately 0.4 ml/min.

Clinical example: Neurotransmitters and their metabolites can be measured in the CSF, plasma, and urine and give an approximation of neurotransmitter production and metabolism in the brain. This provides clues to abnormal neurotransmission in some mental illnesses.

Blood-Brain and Blood-CSF Barriers

Neuronal function requires a microenvironment that is protected from changes elsewhere in the body that may have an adverse effect.

Blood-brain and blood-CSF barriers protect the CNS in several ways: Large molecules, such as plasma proteins, present in the blood, are excluded from the CSF and nervous tissue. The brain and spinal cord are protected from neurotransmitters in the blood, such as epinephrine produced by the adrenal gland. Neurotransmitters produced in the CNS are prevented from precipitously leaking into the general circulation. Toxins are excluded either because of their molecular size (too big) or because of their solubility (only substances soluble in water and cell-membrane lipids can pass these barriers), so many drugs are not able to enter the brain and spinal cord.

---

ness, intelligence, creativity, memory, dreams, and emotion. **Neurotransmission** is a key factor in understanding how various regions of the brain function and how interventions, such as medications and other therapies, affect brain activity and human behavior.

Neurotransmitters are manufactured in the neuron and released from the axon, or presynaptic cell, into the synapse, which is the space between neurons. From there the neurotransmitters are received by the dendrite, or postsynaptic cell, of the next neuron. This neurotransmission process makes communication between brain cells possible (Figure 6-7). Like a key inserted into a lock, each of these chemicals fits precisely into specific receptor cells (made of protein) embedded in the membranes of the axons and dendrites. These receptor cells then either open or close doors (**ion channels**) into the cell, allowing for the interchange of chemicals, such as ions like sodium (NA^+), potassium (K^+), and calcium (Ca^+), which changes the electrical charge of the cell (**depolarization**). This change then triggers a cascade of chemical and electrical processes that are caused by a variety of chemicals (**second messengers**) within the cell itself. The second messengers regulate the function of the ion channels, the production of neurotransmitters and their release into the synapse, and continue the process of neurotransmission.

Depending on the chemical makeup of the neurotransmitter, the signal it gives either excites the receiving cells, causing them to produce an action, or inhibits the receiving cells, which slows or stops an action. After release into the synapse and communication with receptor cells, the neurotransmitters are transported back from the synapse into the axon in a process called reuptake, where they are stored for future use or are inactivated (**metabolized**) by enzymes.

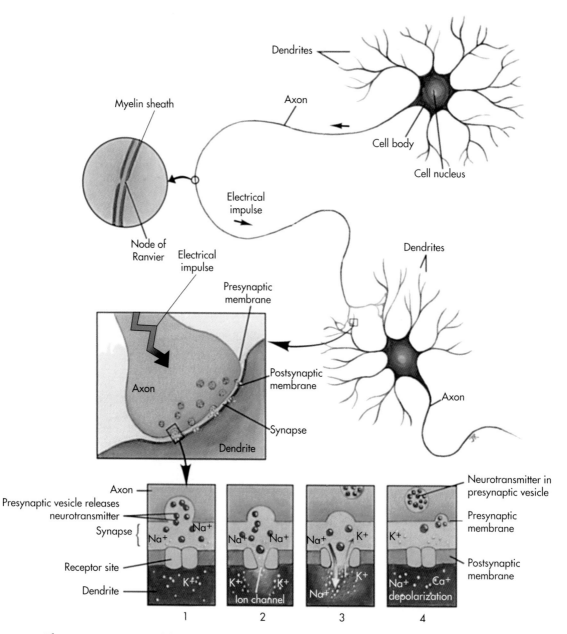

Figure 6-7   Neurotransmission. *Bottom:* 1, Neurotransmitter is released from presynaptic cell into synapse. 2, Neurotransmitter, recognized by receptor cell, causes channel to open, and ions are exchanged. 3, Exchange of ions causes impulse, which causes reaction in receptor cell. 4, Neurotransmission has taken place, receptor channel closes, and neurotransmitter returns to presynaptic membrane (reuptake).

The nervous system cells are surrounded by myelin sheaths formed by specialized groups of cells called glial cells. These are support cells that insulate neurons, remove excess transmitters and ions from the extracellular spaces in the brain, provide glucose to some nerve cells, and direct the flow of blood and oxygen to various parts of the brain.

Several chambers (**ventricles**) within the brain carry fluid (**cerebral spinal fluid, CSF**). The CSF cushions and protects and bathes the brain and spinal cord, carrying chemicals, nutrients, and wastes to and from the blood stream.

From this basic explanation it is evident that neurons are very specialized, and neurotransmitters perform vital functions in the normal working brain. Their absence or excess can play a major role in brain disease and behavioral disorders. A single neurotransmitter can affect other brain chemicals as well as several different subtypes of receptor cells, each located along tracks connecting different regions of the brain. Thus the same neurotransmitter can have one effect in one part of the brain and different effects in another part of the brain.

Nearly all of the known neurotransmitters fall into one of two categories: small amine molecules (monoamines, acetylcholine, and amino acids) and peptides (Coleman and Kay, 2000). These are described in Table 6-1.

One clinical implication of this process is that abnormalities in the structure of the brain or in its ability to communi-

Table 6-1	Neurotransmitters and Neuromodulators in the Brain	
SUBSTANCE	LOCATION	FUNCTION

Amines

Amines are neurotransmitters that are synthesized from amino molecules such as tyrosine, tryptophan, and histidine. Found in various regions of the brain, amines affect learning, emotions, motor control, and other activities.

Monoamines		
Norepinephrine (NE)	Derived from tyrosine, a dietary amino acid. Located in the brainstem (particularly the locus ceruleus). *Effect:* Can be excitatory or inhibitory.	Levels fluctuate with sleep and wakefulness. Plays a role in changes in levels of attention and vigilance. Involved in attributing a rewarding value to a stimulus and in the regulation of mood. Plays a role in affective and anxiety disorders. Antidepressants block the reuptake of NE into the presynaptic cell or inhibit monoamine oxidase from metabolizing it.
Dopamine (DA)	Derived from tyrosine, a dietary amino acid. Located mostly in the brainstem (particularly the substantia nigra). *Effect:* Generally excitatory.	Involved in the control of complex movements, motivation, and cognition and in regulating emotional responses. Many drugs of abuse (such as cocaine and amphetamines) cause DA release, suggesting a role in whatever makes things pleasurable. Involved in the movement disorders seen in Parkinson's disease and in many of the deficits seen in schizophrenia and other forms of psychosis. Antipsychotic drugs block DA receptors in the postsynaptic cell.
Serotonin (5-HT)	Derived from tryptophan, a dietary amino acid. Located only in the brain (particularly in the raphe nuclei of the brainstem). *Effect:* Mostly inhibitory.	Levels fluctuate with sleep and wakefulness, suggesting a role in arousal and modulation of the general activity levels of the CNS, particularly the onset of sleep. Plays a role in mood and probably in the delusions, hallucinations, and withdrawal of schizophrenia. Involved in temperature regulation and the pain-control system of the body. LSD (the hallucinogenic drug) acts at 5-HT receptor sites. Plays a role in affective and anxiety disorders. Antidepressants block its reuptake into the presynaptic cell.
Melatonin	A further synthesis of serotonin produced in the pineal gland. *Effect:* Implicated in seasonal affective disorder and the sleep-wake cycle.	Induces pigment lightening effects on skin cells and regulates reproductive function in animals. Role in humans is unclear.
Acetylcholine	Synthesized from choline. Located in the brain and spinal cord but is more widespread in the peripheral nervous system, particularly the neuromuscular junction of skeletal muscle. *Effect:* Can have an excitatory or inhibitory effect.	Plays a role in the sleep-wakefulness cycle. Signals muscles to become active. Alzheimer's disease is associated with a decrease in acetylcholine-secretin neurons. Myasthenia gravis (weakness of skeletal muscles) results from a reduction in acetylcholine receptors.
Amino acids		
Glutamate	Found in all cells of the body, where it is used to synthesize structural and functional proteins. Also found in the CNS, where it is stored in synaptic vesicles and used as a neurotransmitter. *Effect:* Excitatory.	Implicated in schizophrenia; glutamate receptors control the opening of ion channels that allow calcium (essential to neurotransmission) to pass into nerve cells, propagating neuronal electrical impulses. Its major receptor, NMDA, helps regulate brain development. This receptor is blocked by drugs (such as PCP) that cause schizophrenic-like symptoms. Overexposure to glutamate is toxic to neurons and may cause cell death in stroke and Huntington's disease.
Gamma-aminobutyric acid (GABA)	A glutamate derivative; most neurons of the CNS have receptors. *Effect:* Major transmitter for postsynaptic inhibition on the CNS.	Drugs that increase GABA function, such as the benzodiazepines, are used to treat anxiety and to induce sleep.

Continued

Table 6-1 Neurotransmitters and Neuromodulators in the Brain—cont'd

SUBSTANCE	LOCATION	FUNCTION
Peptides		
Peptides are chains of amino acids found throughout the body. About 50 have been identified to date, but their role as neurotransmitters is not well understood. Although they appear in very low concentrations in the CNS, they are very potent. They also appear to play a "second messenger" role in neurotransmission; that is, they modulate the messages of the nonpeptide neurotransmitters.		
Endorphins and enkephalins	Widely distributed in the CNS. *Effect:* Generally inhibitory.	The opiates morphine and heroin bind to endorphin and enkephalin receptors on presynaptic neurons, blocking the release of neurotransmitters and thus reducing pain.
Substance P	Spinal cord, brain, and sensory neurons associated with pain. *Effect:* Generally excitatory.	Found in pain transmission pathway. Blocking the release of substance P by morphine reduces pain.

CNS, Central nervous system; *LSD*, lysergic acid diethylamide; *NMDA*, N-methyl-D-asparate; *PCP*, phencyclidine hydrochloride.

cate in specific locations can cause or contribute to neuropsychiatric disorders. For example, a communication problem in one small part of the brain can cause widespread dysfunction, because brain communication is like a chain reaction causing changes from one cell to the next and thus from one structure to the next.

The following are examples of networks of nuclei, groups of brain cells, that control cognitive, behavioral, and emotional functioning and thus are of particular interest in the study of psychiatric disorders:

- **Cerebral cortex:** Critical in decision making and higher-order thinking, such as abstract reasoning
- **Limbic system:** Involved in regulating emotional behavior, memory, and learning
- **Basal ganglia:** Coordinate involuntary movements and muscle tone
- **Hypothalamus:** Regulates pituitary hormones; temperature; and behaviors such as eating, drinking, and sex
- **Locus ceruleus:** Makes norepinephrine, a neurotransmitter involved in the body's response to stress
- **Raphe nuclei:** Make serotonin, a neurotransmitter involved in the regulation of sleep, behavior, and mood
- **Substantia nigra:** Makes dopamine, a neurotransmitter involved in complex movements, thinking, and emotions

A second clinical implication is related to the use of therapeutic interventions, such as psychotropic medications (see Chapter 27), electroconvulsive therapy (ECT) (see Chapter 28), alternative therapies (see Chapter 29) and cognitive therapy (see Chapter 31). All of these therapies work ultimately by regulating neurotransmission, either with a chemical, electricity, or thoughts. The ultimate goal is to facilitate normal brain communication, thus decreasing "symptoms" of illness and enhancing "normal" behavior.

To date many interventions effect changes too broadly; thus they lack **specificity.** They not only cause desired changes but also cause changes that are not wanted (**side effects**). As the understanding of the structure and function of the brain increases, and as techniques such as **gene therapy** get perfected, research continues to provide more refined interventions, resulting in treatments that are more specific in where they are directed, are safer, and have fewer side effects.

By understanding the neurobiological processes underlying psychiatric symptoms and the actions of interventions, the psychiatric nurse can make a correct diagnosis; select effective treatments; maximize positive effects; minimize unwanted effects; and predict, measure, and refine the outcomes of psychiatric nursing care.

How would you respond to a nursing colleague who says that psychiatric nurses do not need to know much about anatomy and physiology because what they do primarily is talk to people? ■

■ NEUROIMAGING TECHNIQUES

Until the last few decades the only way to directly study the brain was through brain surgery, open head trauma, or autopsy. Brain imaging techniques allow direct viewing of the structure and function of the intact, living brain. These techniques not only help in diagnosing some brain disorders but also in mapping the regions of the brain, measuring the activity or function in these regions, and correlating this activity with the effects of interventions. These images are pictures of the working brain. Table 6-2 describes some of the imaging techniques used in brain research, and Figure 6-8 shows positron emission tomography (PET) scans of the normal brain.

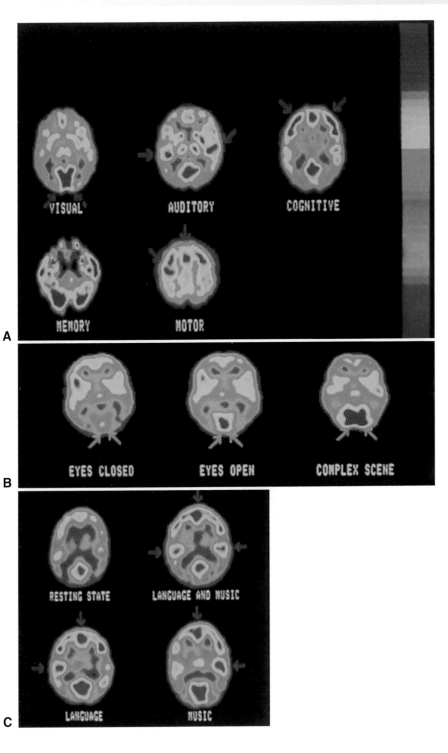

Figure 6-8   Positron emission tomography (PET) scan shows varying patterns of glucose consumption during different tasks. The color scale ranges from 2 *(violet)* to 45 *(red)*. **A**, Different kinds of tasks cause increased glucose consumption in distinct areas of the brain. A checkerboard visual stimulus activates the occipital lobes. An auditory stimulus causes increased glucose consumption in the temporal lobes. When an individual is engaged in an active, cognitive task rather than passive perception of stimuli, glucose consumption increases in the frontal lobes. Subjects trying to remember information from a verbal stimulus (a story) show increased glucose consumption in the temporal lobes. Sequential movements of the fingers of the right hand activate motor cortex on the left and the supplementary motor arc *(vertical arrow)*. **B**, Increasing complexity of a particular kind of task causes increased glucose consumption in progressively larger areas of the cortex. With the subject blindfolded ("eyes closed"), there is relatively little glucose consumption in the occipital lobes. With the eyes open, looking at a plain white light source activates the primary visual cortex of the occipital lobes. Looking at an outdoor scene ("complex scene") activates the visual association cortex in additional areas of the occipital lobes. **C**, The left hemisphere usually plays a dominant role in language functions, the right hemisphere is involved in musical and certain other functions. When a subject listens simultaneously to a Sherlock Holmes story and a Brandenberg concerto, both superior temporal lobes and both frontal lobes are activated. Listening to just the story activates predominately the left hemisphere. Musical chords alone activate predominantly the right hemisphere. (**A** and **C** from Phelps ME, Mazziotta JC: *Science* 228:779, 1985; **B** courtesy Dr. ME Phelps and Dr. JC Mazziotta, University of California School of Medicine.)

Computed tomography (CT) and magnetic resonance imaging (MRI) permit visualization of **brain structures**. They can detect structural abnormalities, changes in the volume of brain tissue, and enlargement of the cerebral ventricles.

Brain function can be studied using other imaging techniques to determine both normal activity and malfunctioning in specific regions. Techniques that show brain function include brain electrical activity mapping (BEAM), which measures sensory input; PET; and single photon emission computed tomography (SPECT), which permits the study of brain metabolism and cerebral blood flow.

PET, SPECT, and the newer functional magnetic resonance imaging (fMRI) techniques can measure the use of **glucose** (glucose utilization) and the amount of **blood flowing** in a region of the brain (regional cerebral blood flow). These are the two basic indicators of brain activity. The more active a region of the brain is, the more blood will flow through it, the more glucose it will use, and the brighter (yellow, orange, and red) the imaging scan looks.

When these techniques are coupled with neuropsychological test results, deficits in a person's performance, such as language or cognitive and sensory information processing, can be linked to the activity of the region of the brain responsible for those functions (see Figure 6-8).

> *Do you think there is a gene responsible for alcohol dependence, aggressive behavior, or sexual preference? How would your belief affect the nursing care you give patients?* ■

■ BIOLOGICAL RHYTHMS

In humans biological clocks keep track of time and govern timed activities such as hormonal surges. They also account for the dysregulation characteristic of jet lag and the winter blues. Biological rhythms affect every aspect of health and well-being, including lifestyle, sleep, mood, eating, drinking, fertility, body temperature, and menses.

These rhythms can fluctuate in fractions of a second, such as those recorded in an electroencephalogram; or in a day, such as the 24-hour circadian rhythm; or in seasonal rhythms that span months or even years, such as those seen in migratory animals, birds, and insects; or in the billion years of evolutionary events (Table 6-3). A variety of internal pacemakers set these clocks and underlie the simple to the most sophisticated human tasks. For this reason, timing mechanisms offer insights into aging and disease. Cancer, Parkin-

Table 6-2   Brain Imaging Techniques

TECHNIQUE	HOW IT WORKS	WHAT IT IMAGES	ADVANTAGES/DISADVANTAGES
Computed tomography (CT)	Series of radiographs that are computer-constructed into "slices" of the brain that can be stacked by the computer, giving a three-dimensional image	Brain structure	Provides clearer pictures of the brain than radiographs alone
Magnetic resonance imaging (MRI)	A magnetic field surrounding the head induces brain tissues to emit radio waves that are computerized to provide clear and detailed construction of sectional images of the brain	Brain structure; newer functional MRI (fMRI) techniques show brain activity	Avoids the use of harmful radiation, although MRI can be adapted to use radioactive materials also
Brain electrical activity mapping (BEAM)	Uses computed tomographic techniques to display data derived from electroencephalographic (EEG) recordings of brain electrical activity that can be sensory-evoked by specific stimuli, such as a flash of light or a sudden sound, or cognitive-evoked by specific mental tasks	Brain activity/function	Reflects the cumulative activity of broad areas of the brain, usually near the surface, making it difficult to locate areas of possible pathological states
Positron emission tomography (PET)	An injected radioactive substance travels to the brain and shows up as a bright spot on the scan; different substances are taken up by the brain in different amounts, depending on the type of tissues and the level of activity	Brain activity/function	Allows the injection of labeled drugs for the study of neurotransmitter receptor activity or concentration in the brain
Single photon emission computed tomography (SPECT)	Similar to PET but uses more stable substances and different detectors to visualize blood flow patterns	Brain activity/function	Useful in diagnosing cerebrovascular accidents and brain tumors

Table 6-3   Time: an Instant to Eternity

MEASUREMENT	DESCRIPTION
1 Nanosecond	A billionth of a second; the microprocessor inside a personal computer will typically take 2 to 4 nanoseconds to execute a single instruction, such as adding two numbers.
One tenth of a second	The duration of the fabled "blink of an eye," the time it takes the human ear to distinguish between an echo and the original sound; a hummingbird can beat its wings 7 times in a tenth of a second.
1 Minute	The brain of a newborn baby grows 1 to 2 milligrams in 1 minute; a person can speak about 150 words or read about 250 words in a minute.
1 Day	In 1 day's time the human heart beats about 100,000 times, whereas the lungs inhale about 11,000 liters of air; the baby blue whale gains 200 pounds; the earth turns once on its axis in 1 day.
1 Year	Earth circles the sun and spins on its axis 365.26 times in a year; North America moves about 3 centimeters away from Europe in 1 year; ocean surface currents travel 1/4 of the way around the globe in a year.
1 Million years	A spaceship moving at the speed of light, traveling to the Andromeda galaxy 2.3 million light years away, would be only half way there after 1 million years; Los Angeles will creep about 40 kilometers northwest of its present location in the next million years.
1 Billion years	The newly formed earth cooled, developed oceans, gave birth to single-celled life, and developed an oxygen-rich atmosphere in 1 billion years.

Modified from Labrador D: *Sci Am* 287:56, 2002.

son's disease, seasonal depression, and attention deficit disorder have all been linked to defects in biological clocks (Wright, 2002).

The **interval timer** acts as the brain's stopwatch, marking seconds, minutes, and sometimes hours, and helps one judge how fast to run to catch a ball or how long to lounge in bed after the alarm rings. It helps tap a foot to the music, dodge an oncoming car, and know how long the traffic light will stay yellow before turning red. The interval timer is flexible, and can easily be turned on and off, but acts as the brain's stopwatch, contributing to the seamless execution of every-day moment to moment activities.

Rao, Mayer, and Harrington (2001) used fMRI technology to show that when research subjects listened to two pairs of tones and were asked to decide whether the interval between the second pair was shorter or longer than the interval between the first pair, the cerebral cortex, the brain center that governs perception, memory, and conscious thought, and the basal ganglia, particularly the striatum, long associated with movement, consumed more oxygen, and thus were more active during this interval timing task.

According to one model, the onset of an event lasting a familiar amount of time, such as the timing of the yellow traffic light, activates the start button of the interval timer by evoking two brain responses: (1) it induces a particular set of cortical nerve cells that usually fire at different rates to instead momentarily act together, and (2) it prompts neurons of the substantia nigra to release the neurotransmitter dopamine. Both activities stimulate the striatum to monitor these patterns of impulses, until after the cells resume their normal nonsynchronous firing rates. Thus the cortical cells act in synchrony at the start of the interval. The subsequent patterns occur in the same sequence every time until the end of the familiar interval is reached. Then the striatum sends a "time's up" signal through other parts of the brain to the decision-making cortex, and the brain remembers such brief timed intervals for next time, increasing the likelihood of getting through intersections before the light turns red (Wright, 2002).

Circadian Rhythms

Circadian rhythm is like a network of internal clocks that coordinate events in the body according to a 24-hour cycle (Figure 6-9). This cycle corresponds to the time it takes the earth to spin on its axis, exposing all of life to daily rhythms of light, darkness, and temperature.

Because the body's fluids and tissues function according to circadian rhythms, physical and mental abilities and moods may vary widely from one time of day to another. To run according to the 24-hour clock, the circadian system must have a time cue from the external environment. That cue is usually sunlight, which resets the clock each day and synchronizes the body's complex set of rhythms.

Light enters the retina of the eye, which acts like an antenna of the brain. From the retina, specialized nerve cells send signals of light and dark through special pathways to the hypothalamus and other regions of the brain (Figure 6-10). One of the most important internal timekeepers is located in the hypothalamus. It consists of two clusters of nerve cells called the suprachiasmatic nuclei (SCN). A direct track leads from the retina to these two clusters of cells, which in turn respond to the light signals from the retina (Young, 2000).

The SCN is the pacemaker of circadian rhythm; it sends electrical and chemical messages to other parts of the brain, including the hypothalamus, pituitary, pineal gland, and parts of the brainstem. These brain structures send hormonal messages to other control systems in the body, such as the heart, adrenal glands, liver, kidney, and intestines, keeping them regulated to the internal clock and modulating thoughts, moods, body functions, and human activities.

Sleep

According to most surveys, people sleep between 6 to 9 hours a night, with 8 hours reported most often. Few people normally sleep fewer than 5 or more than 10 hours. Usually, people sleep in one nightly phase, although in some cultures and during some times of life, a siesta, or afternoon nap, is common. Studies show that the sleep cycle is related to the tim-

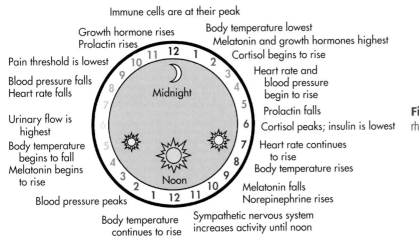

Figure 6-9   The day within: a sample of the body's daily rhythms.

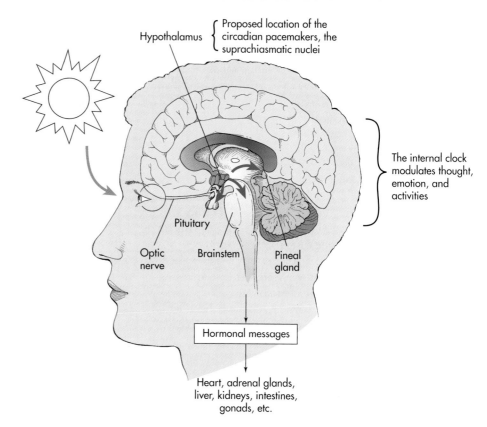

Hypothalamus { Proposed location of the circadian pacemakers, the suprachiasmatic nuclei

The internal clock modulates thought, emotion, and activities

Pituitary

Optic nerve   Brainstem   Pineal gland

Hormonal messages

Heart, adrenal glands, liver, kidneys, intestines, gonads, etc.

Figure 6-10   From the sun to the brain.

ing of circadian rhythms, changes in light and darkness, and temperature changes.

Generally, each night a person's sleep passes through a repeated sequence of five stages. The first stage is that of "falling asleep," which is called stage 1 sleep. A person then progresses into sleep itself (stage 2), followed by deep sleep, also called delta sleep (stages 3 and 4). After a brief return to stage 2 sleep, the person moves into stage 5, or rapid eye movement (REM), sleep. Stages 2 through REM repeat themselves several times a night, with deep sleep becoming briefer in the course of a night and REM sleep becoming progressively longer (Figure 6-11).

REM sleep occupies approximately 20% to 25% of the sleep time of adults, stage two about 50%, and stages three and four about 15%. Stages three and four occur primarily in the first half of the sleep period. The lighter stages of sleep and longer REM periods typically occur in the second half.

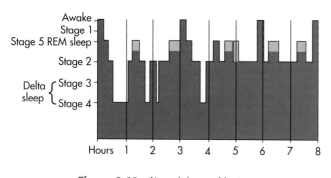

Figure 6-11   Normal sleep architecture.

Usually, during REM sleep the individual has vivid dreams, and the eyes show bursts of rapid movement beneath the closed lids.

It is important for optimal health that people progress through the normal stages of sleep each night. Studies show that in depressed persons, REM sleep is excessive, the deeper stages of sleep are decreased, and dreams may be unusually intense. Thus, although they may sleep 6 to 9 hours each night, people with depression frequently report fatigue, poor concentration, and irritability associated with sleep deprivation.

How much sleep do you need each night? How does it effect your functioning if you have less sleep, or more sleep? ■

■ PSYCHONEUROIMMUNOLOGY

Psychosocial factors can have a profound effect on a person's immune system. The brain and the immune system continuously signal each other, often along the same pathways, which may explain how state of mind influences health. The job of the immune system is to bar foreign pathogens from the body and to recognize and destroy those that penetrate its shield.

The immune system also must neutralize dangerous toxins, facilitate the repair of damaged or worn tissues, and dispose of normal cells, all while it is being regulated to ensure its activity is not excessive or directed at its own body, which would cause autoimmune diseases (Sternberg and Gold, 2002). In particular, psychosocial stressors and the mental state associated with them may depress immune function to the point of enhancing vulnerability to almost any antigen to which the person is exposed. The central nervous system (CNS) is involved in mediating any such effects.

Psychoneuroimmunology is a relatively new field that explores the interactions between the CNS, the endocrine system, and the immune system; the impact of behavior/stress on these interactions; and how psychological and pharmacological interventions may modulate these interactions. Communication between these systems is accomplished by a feedback loop of chemical messengers from each system: neurotransmitters produced by nerve cells, hormones secreted by endocrine glands, and cytokines and other peptides secreted by immune cells.

Research has demonstrated the suppression of white blood cell reproduction and increased susceptibility to illness following sleep deprivation, marathon running, space flight, death of a spouse, and during the course of depression. Another example is that of natural killer (NK) cells, which are believed to play a role in tumor surveillance and the control of viral infections. These cells seem to decrease in number with increasing levels of stress.

■ THE NEW GENETICS

The history of biology was altered forever at the end of the 20th century by the launching of the Human Genome Project, a research program that has characterized the complete set of genetic instructions of the human being. Science is uncovering information showing that the complexity of human emotions and behavior is governed by a variety of genes and their interplay with each other, environmental factors, personality, and life experiences. Begun in 1990 by the U.S. Department of Energy, and supported by dozens of collaborators around the world, the Human Genome Project had several goals, including the following:

- Identifying all human genes
- Providing a high quality reference DNA sequence for the human gene
- Building computer models to support future research and commercial applications
- Exploring human gene function through animal comparisons
- Studying human gene variation
- Training future scientists in genomics

The high quality reference DNA sequence for the human gene was completed in April of 2003, marking the end of the Human Genome Project, 2 years ahead of time. This provides an unprecedented biological resource that will serve throughout the century as a basis for research and discovery and will provide many practical applications. Perhaps one of the most daunting challenges remaining is that of understanding how all the parts of cells—genes, proteins, and many other molecules—work together to create complex living organisms in health and illness (U.S. DOE, 2003). Some of the highlights of what has been learned thus far are listed in Box 6-2.

DNA from all organisms is made up of the same chemical and physical components. The DNA sequence is the partic-

---

BOX 6-2

Insights Gained From the Human DNA Sequence

- The human genome contains 3 billion chemical nucleotide bases (A, C, T, and G), combinations of which comprise all genetic codes. The average gene contains 3000 bases. Humans contain about 30,000 genes (1/3 as many as previously thought), as does the laboratory mouse.
- The functions of more than 50% of the discovered genes are still unknown.
- The human genome sequence is almost (99.9%) exactly the same in all people.
- Slight variations in DNA sequences can have a major impact on whether a disease is developed and on responses to environmental factors such as the presence of microbes, toxins, and drugs.
- Single nucleotide polymorphisms (SNPs) are sites in the human genome where individuals differ in their DNA sequence, often only by a single base. Sets of SNPs on the same chromosome are inherited in blocks and may provide the answers to what causes disease and what new treatments would be beneficial.

---

ular side-by-side arrangement of bases along the DNA strand (e.g., ATTCCGGA). This order spells out the exact instructions required to create a particular organism with its own unique traits. The genome, an organism's complete set of DNA instructions, is organized into chromosomes, which contain many genes, the basic physical and functional units of heredity. Genes are specific sequences of bases that encode instructions on how to make proteins, large, complex molecules made up of amino acids. It is the proteins that perform most life functions and make up the majority of cellular structures. The constellation of all proteins in a cell is called its proteome. The proteome is a dynamic molecular machine that constantly changes as a result of the many environmental signals within a cell, and communities of cells make up the hundred trillion cells in a human being (Figure 6-12). Studies designed to explore protein structure and activities, known as proteomics, will be the focus of research in the future and will help discover the molecular basis of health and illness (Human Genome Project Information, 2003).

Genetic mapping, also called linkage mapping, is the first step in isolating a gene. It can offer firm evidence that a disease transmitted from parent to child is linked to one or more genes, and it provides clues as to which chromosome contains the gene and where the gene is on the chromosome. Although genetic maps have helped successfully identify single genes responsible for some rare diseases (see gene testing), the maps also have become useful as a guide by which scientists can identify the many genes that are believed to interact to cause more common disorders such as asthma, heart disease, diabetes, and psychiatric disorders.

Genetic testing is among the first commercial medical applications of the new genetic discoveries. It can be used to diagnose disease, confirm a diagnosis, provide prognostic informa-

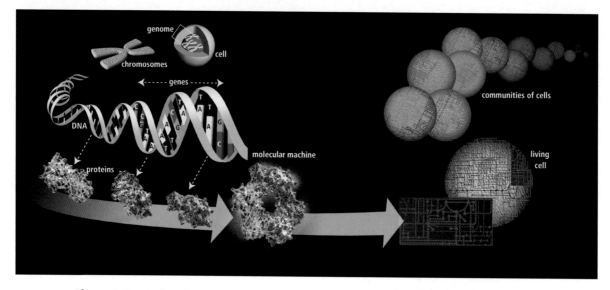

Figure 6-12   A primer: from DNA to life. Cells contain DNA—the hereditary material of all living things. The genome is an organism's complete set of DNA and is organized into chromosomes. DNA contains genes whose sequence specifies how and when to build proteins. Proteins perform most essential life functions, often working together as molecular machines. Molecular machines interact through complex, interconnected pathways and networks to make the cell come alive. Communities of cells range from associations of microbes (each a single cell) to the hundred trillion cells in a human being. (Courtesy U.S. Department of Energy Genome Programs, website: doegenomes.org/.)

tion about the course of a disease, confirm the existence of a disease in asymptomatic individuals, and also detect predispositions to disease in healthy individuals and their offspring. Currently, several hundred genetic tests are in clinical use for illnesses such as muscular dystrophies, cystic fibrosis, sickle cell anemia, Huntington's disease, and breast, ovarian, and colon cancers.

The new field of pharmacogenetics, the discipline that blends pharmacology with genomic capabilities, will eventually allow researchers to match DNA variants with individual responses to medical treatments. This will allow for the design of custom drugs based on individual genetic profiles. These drugs will be specific for the targeted causes of the illness and will avoid nonillness targets in the body, thereby eliminating unwanted drug effects.

Gene therapy, still an experimental field, holds potential for treating or even curing genetic and acquired diseases such as cancer and AIDS by using normal genes to supplement or replace defective genes or bolster a normal function such as immunity (U.S. DOE, 2003). It is not likely to be clinically applicable in psychiatry in the near future (Sapolsky, 2003). However, as of 2002, more than 600 clinical gene therapy trials involving about 3500 patients were identified worldwide (Journal of Gene Medicine website, 2003).

Although having relevant genetic information can help patients and their health care providers manage illnesses more effectively, there are drawbacks as well. These can include emotional and psychological effects on individuals and their families, confusion about the meaning of the information from an ethical or moral perspective, discrimination at work or by insurance companies, the use of genetic information in reproductive decision making, and lack of privacy and confidentiality regarding genetic information, which may lead to stigmatization.

Geneticists (a medical specialty) and genetic counselors (a graduate level specialty) are trained to diagnose and explain disorders from a genetic perspective. They can review available options for testing and treatment and provide emotional support to individuals or families who have genetic disorders or are at risk for them or need information about risks to their offspring.

Genetics of Mental Illness

The search for the genes that cause mental illness has been difficult and inconclusive to date but has stimulated significant scientific, political, and clinical debate (see Critical Thinking About Contemporary Issues). Although research involving the genetics of mental illness has been complex and challenged many past assumptions, genetic investigations have continued to demonstrate that familial and genetic factors underlie most of the major psychiatric illnesses.

An example of a genetically heterogeneous (caused by more than one gene) disorder is the rare form of Alzheimer's disease (AD) that affects people before age 65. Early onset AD affects only about 10% of cases and seems to be linked to mutations in any of three specific genes responsible for amyloid-beta, causing excess deposits of this substance in the brains of persons with AD. The search for the genes responsible for the more common late-onset AD and for other neuropsychiatric illness is ongoing and has captured the attention of the political, scientific, and lay communities.

Several issues make research on the inheritance of mental illness difficult (Merikangas and Risch, 2003). These include:

- The psychiatric diagnostic classification system continues to change.
- The psychiatric diagnostic system is organized by symptom clusters, an increasingly confusing approach

because abnormalities in different brain systems often cause similar and overlapping symptoms.

- A gene that sometimes produces a psychiatric disorder may not always do so.
- The presence of several different genes may be necessary to produce psychiatric disorders.
- Nongenetic factors also contribute to the development of a disorder.

Critical Thinking *About* Contemporary Issues

Are the Mentally Ill Particularly Vulnerable to Attempts at Genetic Engineering?

In Nazi Germany and in the United States during the early 20th century, people with mental disorders were among the first targets of society's attempt to minimize the transmission of disease-causing genes by reducing or preventing reproduction by people who might be carrying them. People with psychiatric illness were subject to immigration restrictions, involuntary sterilization, and extermination. Today's more sophisticated technology and increased knowledge of genetics have led to speculation about the susceptibility of the mentally ill to future attempts to control their reproductive choices. For example, sterilization laws still stand in many states, as does the 1927 Supreme Court ruling that such sterilization is constitutional.

Eugenics, the science of selective breeding, is probably not a major concern for most people at this time. Furthermore, current understanding of the cause of psychiatric disorders suggests that they do not have a simple genetic base and that nongenetic factors play an important role. This country's emphasis on human rights also makes the practice of eugenics unlikely here. However, it is not difficult to see how indirect pressure not to have children may be placed on people who seem to have a greater risk for mental illness and how society may label them as irresponsible or immoral for transmitting illnesses to their children. When technology advances to the point that the developing fetus can be tested for genes that cause mental illnesses, some questions that may arise include: Will the parents be more inclined to abort that pregnancy? Will that child be able to get health insurance if that genetic potential is considered a pre-existing condition? Will a person with genes for mental illness be considered a poor risk for certain jobs, for expensive educations, for parenthood? Given the direct and indirect costs of mental illness to society and the stigma surrounding these disorders, future scientific advances may revive these and other eugenics issues.

- It is difficult to generalize from animal to human behavior (transgenic research).
- Ethical dilemmas arise from human breeding and genetic engineering experiments.

Although the search for the genes of neuropsychiatric illness continues to hold promise, current information regarding the transmission of mental illness is based primarily on investigations into human inheritance such as family, twin, and adoption studies (see Citing the Evidence). The study designs for inheritance and genetic research on mental disorders are listed in Table 6-4.

There are several other proposed uses of genetics in psychiatry. These include:

- Developing new drugs that will target molecular regulators of gene expression that control neuroproteins and neuroenzymes in brain regions shown to be abnormal in a particular psychiatric illness.

CITING THE EVIDENCE ON
Family Study of Affective Spectrum Disorder

BACKGROUND: Certain psychiatric disorders commonly occur together in individuals (co-occurrence) and in families (co-aggregation), suggesting that such disorders may share common causal factors. The hypothesis of this study was that major depressive disorder shares a causal factor or set of factors with seven other psychiatric and medical disorders. The hypothesis was based on the fact that each of the seven disorders responded to treatment with antidepressants. Two predictions were tested: That affective spectrum disorder (ASD), taken as a single entity, would aggregate in families and that major depressive disorder (MDD) would co-aggregate with other forms of ASD in families. Patients with and without MDD were interviewed with their first-degree relatives and familial aggregation and co-aggregation were analyzed.

RESULTS: In the 178 interviewed relatives of 64 probands with MDD and 152 relatives of 58 probands without MDD, the estimated odds ratio (95% confidence interval) for the familial aggregation of ASD as a whole was significant.

IMPLICATIONS: Affective spectrum disorder aggregates strongly in families, and MDD displays a significant familial co-aggregation (occurs) with other forms of ASD, suggesting that forms of ASD may share heritable pathophysiological features.

Hudson J et al: *Arch Gen Psychiatry* 60:170, 2003.

Table 6-4   Study Designs for Inheritance and Genetic Research on Mental Disorders

TYPE OF STUDY	WHO IS STUDIED	GOAL OF THIS STUDY DESIGN
Population	Subjects in the general population	Establish lifetime incidence
Family	First- and second-degree relatives (pedigree) of the affected person (proband)	Establish familiarity; estimate mode of transmission and risk to relative cases
Twin	Monozygotic (identical—share all of their genes) and dizygotic (fraternal—share half of their genes) twins	Distinguish genetic from environmental effects
Adoption	Adoptees and their adoptive and biological relatives	Distinguish genetic from environmental effects
Linkage	Nuclear and/or extended families	Establish chromosomal location of a disease susceptibility gene
Association	Unrelated affected persons and controls	Identify a specific disease susceptibility gene
Transgenic	Gene expression and function in animals	Specify developmental outcomes/pathways

- Conducting gene therapy—the introduction of genes into existing cells to prevent or cure disease—which is expected to one day be commonplace for the treatment of psychiatric illness.
- Implementing studies that use "candidate genes" (cloned human genes that are functionally related to the disease of interest) in research procedures in the laboratory. These are becoming more available for psychiatric research.

The nurse is often in the position to answer questions from patients and their families about the genetics of mental illness (Lea et al, 2000; Pestka, 2003). The nurse can objectively share the evidence to date while reminding people that this information is preliminary. Also, this information must be conveyed with the highest respect for the patient's and family's autonomy. Referral to a genetic counselor should be considered when the questions are persistent and complex.

Impact of the Human Genome Project

The information gained from the Human Genome Project has thus far provided little clinical relevance for the treatment of neuropsychiatric disorders. However, there are reasons to feel optimistic about the future. Each new investigation leading to a better understanding of genes and the proteins that make each cell come alive brings science closer to the time when significantly increased understanding of the role of inheritance, environment, and social influences and their interactions on mental health and illness will be a reality.

Gene therapies will become commonplace, and the tools for prevention of mental illness will be available. Gaining understanding of the significance of genetic risk factors and learning proper interpretation of their meaning for patients and their families will ultimately become part of clinical practice. Clinicians will be involved more than ever in helping patients comprehend the meaning and potential impact of genetic risk factors for these disorders (Merikangas and Risch, 2003).

■ BIOLOGICAL ASSESSMENT OF THE PATIENT

Psychiatric nurses are faced with the challenge of integrating the latest neuroscientific information with the long-standing biopsychosocial model of psychiatric nursing care. In doing so, they need to apply this new information and still provide holistic, evidence-based, and individualized psychiatric nursing care. This begins with a thorough biological assessment of the patient.

Several steps are necessary in the assessment of psychiatric patients from a biological perspective. Brain disorders can be physical or "neurological" and can include many different diagnoses such as stroke, head and spinal cord injury, brain tumors, multiple sclerosis, Parkinson's disease, and Huntington's disease. Schizophrenia, depression, anxiety disorders, and Alzheimer's disease also are brain disorders, although they are classified as psychiatric disorders.

The symptoms of psychiatric versus neurological illnesses can overlap and can even mimic each other. The treatments can be very different, and treatments for one disorder may make another disorder worse. Thus the ability to screen for both undiagnosed physical and psychiatric disorders has important implications for the psychiatric nurse in the assessment of the presenting symptoms, treatment selection, and possible need for referral to a specialist in another discipline.

Undiagnosed physical illness, particularly organic brain disorders, can be costly and dangerous if treated incorrectly. Physical illnesses such as brain tumors and endocrine disorders can cause psychiatric symptoms and exacerbate an existing psychiatric illness as well, and patients who are psychiatrically ill may be misdiagnosed in nonpsychiatric settings. Thus for these reasons, psychiatric nurses need to include a thorough biological assessment in their evaluation of psychiatric patients.

The psychiatric nurse is well suited for the task of screening patients for the major signs of physical or organic disorders that may complicate a patient's psychiatric status. The purpose of such screening is to identify physical illnesses that may have been overlooked and then to refer the patient for a thorough medical diagnostic work-up if indicated. In fact, this is one of the unique areas of expertise that the psychiatric nurse brings to the mental health treatment team, and it is essential that psychiatric nurses continue to demonstrate their competence in all aspects of their biopsychosocial assessment.

A complete health care history of the patient, including lifestyle review, physical examination, analysis of laboratory values, and discussion of presenting symptoms and coping responses, is an essential element of a baseline biological assessment (Box 6-3). The nurse should be able to perform a basic physical examination to assess for gross abnormalities and be able to interpret the results of more complex physical examinations. Appearance, gait, coordination, bilateral strength, tremors and tics, speech, and symptoms such as headaches, blurred vision, dizziness, vomiting, motor weakness, disorientation, confusion, and memory problems should be assessed in detail.

Obtaining permission from the patient to access other people and documents that will help the nurse and health care team gain a thorough view of the patient is an important step in the screening process. Particularly when brain disorders, whether physical or psychiatric, are suspected, the nurse should pay close attention to inconsistencies in the patient's account, between those of other people, and in previous health care records. Throughout the course of the screening, the nurse should be alert for any indications of head trauma at any time in the patient's life as a result of incidents such as accidents, fevers, surgery, or seizures.

Why is a history of psychiatric medications taken from a patient's first-degree relatives an important part of the psychiatric nurse's biological assessment? ■

Biological Assessment of the Psychiatric Patient

Health Care History
General health care
Regular and specialty health care provider
Frequency of health care visits
Date of last examination
Any unusual circumstances of birth, including mother's preterm habits and condition
Allergies
Immunizations
Papanicolaou smear and mammogram
Chest x-ray and ECG
TB test
Hospitalizations, surgeries, and medical procedures
When, why indicated, treatments, outcome
Brain impairment
Diagnosed brain problem
Head trauma
Details of accidents or periods of unconsciousness for any reason: blows to the head, electrical shocks, high fevers, seizures, fainting, dizziness, headaches, falls
Cancer
Full history, particularly consider metastases (lung, breast, melanoma, gastrointestinal tract, and kidney are most likely to metastasize)
Results of treatments (chemotherapy and surgeries)
Lung problems
Details of any condition or event that restricts the flow of air to the lungs for more than 2 minutes or adversely affects oxygen absorption (the brain uses 20% of the oxygen in the body), such as with chronic obstructive pulmonary disease, near drowning, near strangulation, high-altitude oxygen deprivation, and resuscitation events
Cardiac problems
Childhood illnesses such as scarlet fever or rheumatic fever
History of heart attacks, strokes, or hypertension
Arteriosclerotic conditions
Diabetes
Stability of glucose levels
Endocrine disturbances
Thyroid and adrenal function particularly
Menstrual history
Age at occurrence of first menstrual period
Regularity of menstrual periods, impact on lifestyle
Date of last menstrual period, duration
Menopausal history
Assess for premenstrual syndromes
Sexual history
Assess sexual function and activity
Screen for sexual dysfunction
Safe-sex practices and sexually transmitted diseases
Reproductive history
Number of pregnancies, births, children and their ages
Assess birth control methods

Lifestyle
Eating
Details of unusual or unsupervised diets, appetite, weight changes, cravings, and caffeine intake

Medications
Full history of current and past psychiatric medications in self and first-degree relatives
Full history of current use of nonpsychiatric prescription medicines, over-the-counter medicines, and herbal and other alternative remedies
Substance use
Alcohol, drug, caffeine, and tobacco use
Toxins
Overcome by automobile exhaust or natural gas
Exposure to lead, mercury, insecticides, herbicides, solvents, cleaning agents, lawn chemicals
Fetal alcohol syndrome
Occupation (current and past)
Chemicals in the workplace (e.g., pesticides used in farming, solvents used in painting)
Work-related accidents (e.g., construction, mining)
Military experiences
Stressful job circumstances
Injury
Contact sports and sports-related injuries
Exposure to violence or abuse
Rape or molestation
Impact of culture, race, ethnicity, and gender

Physical Examination
Review of physiological systems
Integumentary: skin, nails, hair, and scalp
Head: eyes, ears, nose, mouth, throat, and neck
Breast
Respiratory
Cardiovascular
Hematolymphatic
Gastrointestinal tract
Urinary tract
Genital
Neurological, soft signs, and cranial nerves
Musculoskeletal
Nutritive
Restorative: sleep and rest
Endocrine
Allergic and immunological
Gait, coordination, and balance

Laboratory Values
Hematology: CBC and sedimentation rate, screen for anemia
Chemistry, BUN, glucose, thyroid, adrenal, liver and kidney function, etc.
Serology, especially syphilis screen, HIV, hepatitis
Urinalysis, screen for drugs
Stool tests for occult blood

Presenting Symptoms and Coping Responses
Description: nature, frequency, and intensity
Threats to safety of self or others
Functional status
Quality of life
Support system

BUN, Blood urea nitrogen; *CBC*, complete blood count; *ECG*, electrocardiogram; *HIV*, human immunodeficiency virus; *TB*, tuberculosis.

Only after a patient has been carefully screened can the nurse determine which of the patient's problems are primarily psychiatric and amenable to psychiatric intervention and which may need the attention of a consultant in another specialty. The identified problems that can be treated appropriately by psychiatric intervention then become the target symptoms of specific interventions, and progress toward expected outcomes can be measured throughout the course of treatment.

CHAPTER FOCUS POINTS

- All nurses should have a working knowledge of the normal structure and function of the brain related to mental health and neuropsychiatric illness, just as all nurses should know the structure and function of the heart.
- Neurotransmission is a key factor in understanding how various regions of the brain function and how interventions, such as medications and other therapies, affect brain activity and human behavior.
- One clinical implication of the neurotransmission process is that abnormalities in the structure of the brain or in its ability to communicate in specific locations can cause or contribute to neuropsychiatric disorders.
- Brain imaging techniques allow direct viewing of the structure and function of the intact, living brain. These techniques not only help in diagnosing some brain disorders but also in mapping the regions of the brain, measuring the activity or function in these regions, and correlating this activity with the effects of interventions.
- Biological rhythms affect every aspect of health and well-being, including lifestyle, sleep, mood, eating, drinking, fertility, body temperature, and menses.
- Circadian rhythm is like a network of internal clocks that coordinate events in the body according to a 24-hour cycle.
- Studies show that the sleep cycle is related to the timing of circadian rhythms, changes in light and darkness, and temperature changes. For optimal health, it is important that people progress through the normal stages of sleep each night.
- Psychoneuroimmunology is a relatively new field that explores the interactions between the CNS, the endocrine system, and the immune system; the impact of behavior/stress on these interactions; and how psychological and pharmacological interventions may modulate these interactions.
- Science is uncovering information showing that the complexity of human emotions and behavior is governed by a variety of genes and their interplay with each other, environmental factors, personality, and life experiences.
- Although research involving the genetics of mental illness has been complex and challenged many past assumptions, genetic investigations have continued to demonstrate that familial and genetic factors underlie most of the major psychiatric illnesses.
- Psychiatric nurses are faced with the challenge of integrating the latest neuroscientific information with the long-standing biopsychosocial model of psychiatric nursing care. This begins with a thorough biological assessment of the patient.
- The psychiatric nurse is well-suited for the task of screening patients for the major signs of physical or organic disorders that may complicate a patient's psychiatric status. The purpose of such screening is to identify physical illnesses that may have been overlooked and then to refer the patient for a thorough medical diagnostic work-up if indicated.

KEY TERMS

axon, 93
brain electrical activity mapping (BEAM), 97
chromosomes, 101
circadian rhythm, 99
computed tomography (CT), 97
dendrite, 93
DNA sequence, 101
eugenics, 103
gene therapy, 102
genes, 101

genetic mapping, 101
genetic testing, 101
genome, 101
glial cells, 94
Human Genome Project, 101
magnetic resonance imaging (MRI), 97
myelin sheaths, 94
neurotransmission, 88
neurotransmitters, 88
pharmacogenetics, 102

positron emission tomography (PET), 96
proteins, 101
proteome, 101
proteomics, 101
psychoneuroimmunology, 101
reuptake, 93
single photon emission computed tomography (SPECT), 97
synapse, 93

CHAPTER REVIEW QUESTIONS

1. Match each of the terms in Column A with the best description from Column B.

Column A

_____ Basal ganglia
_____ Eugenics
_____ Hippocampus
_____ Hypothalamus
_____ Locus ceruleus
_____ PET
_____ REM
_____ Synapse
_____ Tryptophan

Column B

A. Homeostasis
B. Memory
C. Space between brain cells
D. Dream sleep
E. Manufactures norepinephrine
F. Neurotransmitter precursor
G. Functional neuroimaging technique
H. Movement
I. Selective breeding

2. Fill in the blanks.

A. The microenvironment that protects the central nervous system (CNS) from large molecules, toxins, and peripheral chemicals is the _____ and _____ barriers.

B. Communication between neurons in the brain is called _____.

C. The scientific field made up of many disciplines that has revolutionized our understanding of mental illness is called _____.

D. The network of internal clocks that times and coordinates events within the body according to a 24-hour cycle is called _____.

3. Indicate whether the following statements are true (T) or false (F).

_____ A. The interval timer helps the body stay in synchrony with the 24-hour cycle of the earth's rotation on its axis.

_____ B. Family, adoption, and twin studies suggest that the pattern of inherited vulnerability to mental illness probably results from the interaction of genes with the environment.

_____ C. Proteins perform most life functions and make up the majority of cellular structures.

_____ D. Brain imaging techniques have generally found smaller ventricles in some people with schizophrenia, depression, and anxiety disorders than in nonaffected people.

_____ E. When neurotransmission has taken place, the process by which neurotransmitters travel from the synapse back into the presynaptic axon is called reuptake.

4. Provide short answers for the following questions.

A. Briefly describe the role of each of the following components in brain communication:
Axon
Dendrite
Receptor cell
Second messengers
Reuptake
Enzymatic degradation

B. Discuss how the limbic system is involved in feelings, emotion, and self-preservation.

C. List the stages of sleep and define REM latency and decreased REM latency.

Visit Evolve for additional resources related to the content of this chapter.

http://evolve.elsevier.com/Stuart/principles/

• Topical Course Outline • Student Workbook Exercises • Critical Thinking Questions and Activities • Case Studies • Research Topics • Monthly Content Updates • WebLinks

Student Study CD-ROM

Access the accompanying CD-ROM for animations, interactive exercises, review questions for the NCLEX examination, and an audio glossary.

REFERENCES

Coleman F, Kay J: The biology of the brain. In Kay J, Tasman A, editors: *Psychiatry: behavioral science and clinical essentials*, Philadelphia, 2000, WB Saunders.

Hudson JI et al: Family study of affective spectrum disorder, *Arch Gen Psychiatry* 60:170, 2003.

Human Genome Project Information: The Science Behind the Human Genome Project, 2003, www.ornl.gov/TechResources/Human_Genome/project/info.html

Journal of Gene Medicine: www.wiley.co.uk/genetherapy, accessed March 2003.

Lea D et al: Genetic health care: creating partnerships with nursing in clinical practice, *Natl Acad Pract Forum* 2:177, 2000.

Merikangas KR, Risch N: Will the genomics revolution revolutionize psychiatry? *Am J Psychiatry* 160:625, 2003.

Nolte J: *The human brain: an introduction to its functional anatomy*, ed 5, St Louis, 2002, Mosby.

Pestka E: Genetic core competencies: exploring the implications for psychiatric nursing, *J Am Psychiatr Nurs Assoc* 9:1, 2003.

Rao SM, Mayer AR, Harrington DL: The evolution of brain activation during temporal processing, *Nat Neurosci* 4:317, 2001.

Sapolsky RM: Gene therapy for psychiatric disorders, *Am J Psychiatry* 160:208, 2003.

Sternberg EM, Gold PW: The mind-body interaction in disease. In *The Hidden Mind*, New York, Spring 2002, Scientific American Inc.

Thibodeau G, Patton K: *The human body in health and disease*, ed 3, 2002, Mosby.

US Department of Energy (US DOE): Genomics and its impact on science and society, Washington, DC, 2003, US Department of Energy Genome Programs, www.doegenomes.org/

Wright K: Times of our lives, *Sci Am* 287:58, 2002.

Young MW: The tick-tock of the biological clock, *Sci Am* 282:64, 2000.

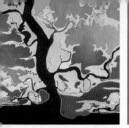

Information is of no value for its own sake, but only because of its personal significance.

ERIC BERNE

7 PSYCHOLOGICAL CONTEXT OF PSYCHIATRIC NURSING CARE

Gail W. Stuart

Visit Evolve for additional resources related to the content of this chapter.
http://evolve.elsevier.com/Stuart/principles/

Holistic psychiatric nursing care requires the nurse to complete an assessment of the patient's biological, psychological, and sociocultural health status. The assessment of the patient's psychological well-being should include a mental status examination. All nurses, regardless of the clinical setting, should be proficient in administering the mental status examination and be able to incorporate findings from it into the nursing care plan for the patient.

The mental status examination is a cornerstone in the evaluation of any patient with a medical, neurological, or psychiatric disorder that affects thought, emotion, or behavior (American Psychiatric Association, 1995). It is used to detect changes or abnormalities in a person's intellectual functioning, thought content, judgment, mood, and affect and can be used to identify possible lesions in the brain. The mental status examination is to psychiatric nursing what the physical examination is to general medical nursing.

■ MENTAL STATUS EXAMINATION

The mental status examination represents a cross section of the patient's psychological life and the sum total of the nurse's observations and impressions at the moment. It involves observing the patient's behavior and describing it in an objective, nonjudgmental manner. The elements of the examination depend on the patient's clinical presentation, as well as on his or her educational and cultural background. It also serves as a basis for future comparison to facilitate tracking the patient's progress over time.

The examination itself is usually divided into several parts. They can be arranged in different ways, as long as the nurse covers all the areas. Much of the information needed for the mental status examination can be gathered during the course of the routine nursing assessment. It should be integrated into the nurse's assessment in a smooth manner. Some parts of the mental status examination are completed through simple observation of the patient, such as by noting the patient's clothing or facial expressions. Other aspects require asking specific questions, such as those related to memory or attention span. Most of all, the nurse should remember that the mental status examination does not reflect how the patient was in the past or will be in the future; it is an **evaluation of the patient's current state**.

Information obtained during the mental status examination is used along with other objective and subjective data. These include findings from the physical examination, laboratory test results, patient history, description of the presenting problem, and information obtained from family, caregivers, and other health professionals. With these data, the nurse is able to formulate nursing diagnoses and design the plan of care with the patient.

Do nurses on medical-surgical units routinely assess a patient's psychological status? Explain your findings given that all nurses should be providing holistic, biopsychosocial nursing care. ■

Eliciting Clinical Information

The mental status examination requires a clinical rather than social approach to the patient (Wiger and Huntley, 2002). The nurse listens closely to what is said and reflects on what is not said, structuring the process in a way that allows for broad exploration of many areas for the purpose of uncovering potential problems and for facilitating a more in-depth exploration of obvious symptoms or maladaptive coping responses. The patient is critically observed. Behaviors that the nurse might not normally attend to in more general situations must be carefully observed and described. Global and judgmental statements are not acceptable.

The skilled nurse attends to both the content and the process of the patient's communication. **Content** is the overtly communicated information. **Process** is how the communication occurs and includes feelings, intuition, and behaviors that accompany speech and thought. The content and process may not always be congruent. For example, a patient may deny feeling depressed and yet appear sad and cry. In this case, the stated message does not match the process, and the nurse should record this incongruity.

It is also important for nurses to monitor their own feelings and reactions while implementing the mental status examination. A nurse's gut reactions may reflect subtle emotions being expressed by the patient. For example, a depressed patient may make the nurse feel sad, and a hostile patient may make the nurse feel threatened and angry. The nurse's feelings are useful information to consider in formulating the mental status assessment of a patient.

The nurse needs to be aware of these feelings and respond in a therapeutic manner toward the patient, regardless of the nature of such feelings. The nurse should remain calm throughout the interview and simply reflect observations back to the patient. These observations should be related in an objective and nonthreatening manner, as in "You are obviously quite upset about this," or "It seems like you don't feel safe here." By conveying a sense of calm, the nurse also demonstrates being in control, even if the patient is not.

The nurse should try to blend specific questions into the general flow of the interview. For example, questions about orientation, arithmetic problems, or proverbs may be introduced by soliciting patient comments about potential problems with concentration, memory, or understanding of written material. The nurse might then suggest that the patient try answering a few questions to determine whether such problems exist.

Finally, as with any other skill, nurses need to practice performing the mental status examination to gain proficiency and be comfortable with the process. The nurse might start by observing a colleague conduct the examination. Videotapes of patient interviews are a particularly effective teaching-learning tool. A colleague or supervisor should then observe the nurse administering the mental status examination. The colleague can provide helpful feedback and identify ways to further enhance the nurse's competency.

■ CONTENT OF THE EXAMINATION

The mental status examination includes information in a number of categories (Box 7-1). It is one part of a complete psychiatric nursing assessment tool. In completing this examination, it is critically important to be aware that sociocultural factors can greatly influence the outcome of the examination (Box 7-2). In addition, biological expressions of psychiatric illness also may be evident during the interview. The content, observations, and some of the clinical implications associated with each category are described below (Robinson, 2002).

Appearance

When conducting the mental status examination, the nurse takes note of the patient's appearance. This part of the examination is intended to provide an accurate mental image of the patient in general, as in the following clinical example.

BOX 7-1

Categories of the Mental Status Examination

General Description	**Thinking**
Appearance	Thought content
Speech	Thought process
Motor activity	
Interaction during interview	**Sensorium and Cognition**
	Level of consciousness
Emotional State	Memory
Mood	Level of concentration and
Affect	calculation
	Information and intelligence
Experiences	Judgment
Perceptions	Insight

BOX 7-2

Clinical Judgment or Sociocultural Bias?

In completing the mental status examination clinicians need to be aware of the possibility that they may be using subconscious and culturally determined criteria when judging a patient. Examples of potential sociocultural clinician bias include the following:

- How is the manner of dress judged (that is, what is unusual or expected dress)?
- Do all cultures accept the American norm of direct eye contact?
- What are the clinician's values about personal hygiene, and how do these values influence assessment?
- Does a person's speech and use of language vary based on social class and lifestyle?
- How does body language and use of personal space vary by ethnicity and social group?
- Given that 20 to 30 million American adults lack basic educational skills, what is the expected "norm" regarding reading, writing, or problem-solving tasks?
- How familiar are common proverbs? Which interpretations of them are truly correct?

CLINICAL EXAMPLE

Mr. W is a middle-aged white man of average weight who appears older than his stated age. He was disheveled, dressed in a torn shirt and jeans, and was unshaven. He was slightly jaundiced and had a prominent red nose and a scar on his left cheek. He sat slumped in the chair and made little eye contact with the interviewer. ■

OBSERVATIONS

The following physical characteristics should be included in the assessment:

- Apparent age
- Manner of dress
- Cleanliness
- Posture
- Gait
- Facial expressions
- Eye contact
- Pupil dilation or constriction
- General state of health and nutrition

CLINICAL IMPLICATIONS

- Dilated pupils are sometimes associated with drug intoxication.
- Pupil constriction may indicate narcotic addiction.
- Stooped posture is often seen in patients with depression.
- Manic patients may dress in colorful or unusual attire.

Speech

Speech is usually described in terms of rate, volume, amount, and distinct characteristics. Rate is the speed of the patient's speech, and volume is how loud a patient talks.

OBSERVATIONS

Speech can be described as follows:

- Rate: Rapid or slow
- Volume: Loud or soft
- Amount: Paucity, muteness, pressured speech
- Characteristics: Stuttering, slurring of words, or unusual accents

CLINICAL IMPLICATIONS

- Speech disturbances are often caused by specific brain disturbances. For example, mumbling may occur in patients with Huntington's chorea, and slurring of speech may occur in intoxicated patients.
- Manic patients often show pressured speech.
- People suffering from depression often are reluctant to speak at all.

Motor Activity

Motor activity describes the patient's physical movement.

OBSERVATIONS

The nurse should record the following:

- Level of activity: Lethargic, tense, restless, or agitated
- Type of activity: Tics, grimaces, or tremors
- Unusual gestures or mannerisms: Compulsions

CLINICAL IMPLICATIONS

- Excessive body movement may be associated with anxiety, mania, or stimulant abuse.
- Little body activity may suggest depression, organicity, catatonic schizophrenia, or drug-induced stupor.
- Tics and grimaces may suggest medication side effects (see Chapter 27).
- Repeated motor movements or compulsions may indicate obsessive-compulsive disorder.
- Repeated picking of lint or dirt off of clothing is sometimes associated with delirium or toxic conditions.

Which category of psychotropic medications is most often associated with tics and grimaces? ■

Interaction During the Interview

Interaction describes how the patient relates to the nurse during the interview, as in this clinical example.

CLINICAL EXAMPLE

The patient was interviewed in her room on the second day of hospitalization. She was a white woman, slightly overweight, neatly dressed in jeans and a sweater, and appeared younger than her 36 years of age. Although she was cooperative, her guarded responses to all questions seemed excessively self-centered. She gave the interviewer the feeling that she didn't trust anyone and was preoccupied during the interview. When asked how other people treated her, she responded angrily, "I'd rather not say!" ■

Because this part of the examination relies heavily on nurses' emotional subjectivity, nurses must carefully examine their responses based on their own personal and sociocultural biases. They must guard against overinterpreting or misinterpreting patients' behavior because of social or cultural differences between patients and nurses (see Chapter 8).

OBSERVATIONS

Is the patient hostile, uncooperative, irritable, guarded, apathetic, defensive, suspicious, or seductive? The nurse may explore the nature of the observed behavior by asking, "You seem irritated about something. Is that an accurate observation?"

CLINICAL IMPLICATIONS

- Suspiciousness may be evident in patients with paranoia.
- Irritability may suggest an anxiety disorder.

Mood

Mood is the patient's self-report of the prevailing emotional state and reflects the patient's life situation.

OBSERVATIONS

Mood can be evaluated by asking a simple, nonleading question such as "How are you feeling today?" Does the patient report feeling sad, fearful, hopeless, euphoric, or anxious? Asking the patient to rate his or her mood on a scale of 0 to 10 can help provide the nurse with an immediate reading. It also can be valuable for comparing changes that occur during treatment.

If the potential for suicide is suspected, the nurse should inquire about the patient's thoughts about self-destruction (see Chapter 20). Suicidal and homicidal thoughts must be addressed directly. Has the patient felt the desire to harm himself or herself or someone else? Have any previous attempts been made to cause harm, and if so, what events surrounded the attempts? To judge a patient's suicidal or homicidal risk, the nurse should assess the **patient's plans, ability to carry out those plans** (such as the availability of guns), **the patient's attitude about death,** and **support systems available to the patient.** Such assessments would be warranted in the following clinical example.

CLINICAL EXAMPLE

The patient responded to most of the questions in a flat, dull manner. Although he stated that he felt sad about the recent changes in his life, his lifeless posture and tone of voice did not convey any emotional response. He denied any current suicidal or homicidal plans. He related having made two suicidal gestures in the past year by "taking pills." ■

CLINICAL IMPLICATIONS

- Most people with depression describe feeling hopeless, and 25% of those with depression have suicidal ideation.
- Suicidal ideation is also common in patients with anxiety disorders and schizophrenia.
- Elation is most common in those with mania.

Affect

Affect is the patient's apparent emotional tone. The patient's statements of emotions and the nurse's empathic responses provide clues to the appropriateness of the affect.

OBSERVATIONS

Affect can be described in terms of the following:
- Range
- Duration
- Intensity
- Appropriateness

Flat affect is the absence of emotional expression, as seen by a patient who reports significant life events without exhibiting any emotional response. A patient's response also may appear to be restricted or blunted in some way. Other patients may demonstrate great **lability** in expression by shifting from one affect to another quickly. Finally one should assess whether the patient's emotional response is congruent with the speech content. For example, it would be **incongruent** if a patient reports being persecuted by the police and then laughs.

CLINICAL IMPLICATIONS

- Labile affect is often seen in patients with mania.
- Flat affect and incongruent affect are often evident in those with schizophrenia.

Perceptions

The two major types of perceptual problems are hallucinations and illusions. Hallucinations are defined as false sensory impressions or experiences. Illusions are false perceptions or false responses to a sensory stimulus.

OBSERVATIONS

Hallucinations may occur in any of the five major sensory modalities:
- Auditory (sound)
- Visual (sight)
- Tactile (touch)
- Gustatory (taste)
- Olfactory (smell)

Auditory hallucinations are the most common. Command hallucinations are those that tell the patient to do something, such as to kill oneself, harm another, or join someone in afterlife. The nurse might inquire about the patient's perceptions by asking "Do you ever see or hear things?" or "Do you have strange experiences as you fall asleep or upon awakening?"

CLINICAL IMPLICATIONS

- Auditory hallucinations suggest schizophrenia.
- Visual hallucinations suggest organicity.
- Tactile hallucinations suggest organic mental disorders, cocaine abuse, and delirium tremors.

You see in the chart that a nursing order has been written placing a patient with command hallucinations on one-to-one observation. What is the rationale for this nursing intervention? ■

Thought Content

Thought content is the specific meaning expressed in the patient's communication. It refers to the "what" of the patient's thinking.

⚡ OBSERVATIONS

Although the patient may talk about a variety of subjects during the interview, several specific content areas should be noted in the mental status examination (Box 7-3). They may be complicated and are often concealed by the patient, as in this clinical example.

⚡ CLINICAL EXAMPLE

The patient's speech was rapid, and he acknowledged feeling as if his thoughts were coming too fast, saying, "My mind is racing ahead." The rapidity of his speech compounded the difficulty of understanding him as he quickly moved from one topic to another in what appeared to be an unrelated manner. He denied any visual or auditory hallucinations; however, he believed that he could talk with God if he needed a consultant on his life situation. He felt this was a special blessing given to him over others. ■

Tactful questioning by the nurse is needed to explore these areas. Does the patient have recurring, persistent thoughts? Is the patient afraid of certain objects or situations, or does the patient worry excessively about body and health issues? Does the patient ever feel that things are strange or unreal? Has the patient ever experienced being outside of his or her body? Does the patient ever feel singled out or watched or talked about by others? Does the patient think that thoughts or actions are being controlled by an outside person or force? Does the patient claim to have psychic or other special powers or believe that others can read the patient's mind? Throughout this part of the interview it is important that the nurse only obtain information and not dispute the patient's beliefs.

⚡ CLINICAL IMPLICATIONS

- Obsessions and phobias are symptoms associated with anxiety disorders.
- Delusions, depersonalization, and ideas of reference suggest schizophrenia and other psychotic disorders.

Thought Process

Thought process is the "how" of the patient's self-expression. A patient's thought process is observed through speech. The patterns or forms of verbalization rather than the content are assessed.

⚡ OBSERVATIONS

A number of problems in a patient's thinking can be assessed (Box 7-4). The nurse might ask questions to evaluate the patient's thought process. Does the patient's thinking proceed in a systematic, organized, and logical manner? Is the patient's self-expression clear? Is it easy for the patient to move from one topic to another?

BOX 7-3

Thought Content Descriptors

Delusion: False belief that is firmly maintained even though it is not shared by others and is contradicted by social reality

Religious delusion: Belief that one is favored by a higher being or is an instrument of that being

Somatic delusion: Belief that one's body or parts of one's body are diseased or distorted

Grandiose delusion: Belief that one possesses greatness or special powers

Paranoid delusion: Excessive or irrational suspicion and distrust of others, characterized by systematized delusions that others are "out to get them" or spying on them

Thought broadcasting: Belief that one's thoughts are being aired to the outside world

Thought insertion: Belief that thoughts are being placed into one's mind by outside people or influences

Depersonalization: The feeling of having lost self-identity and that things around the person are different, strange, or unreal

Hypochondriasis: Somatic overconcern with and morbid attention to details of body functioning

Ideas of reference: Incorrect interpretation of casual incidents and external events as having direct personal references

Magical thinking: Belief that thinking equates with doing, characterized by lack of realistic relationship between cause and effect

Nihilistic ideas: Thoughts of nonexistence and hopelessness

Obsession: An idea, emotion, or impulse that repetitively and insistently forces itself into consciousness, although it is unwelcome

Phobia: A morbid fear associated with extreme anxiety

BOX 7-4

Thought Process Descriptors

Circumstantial: Thought and speech associated with excessive and unnecessary detail that is usually relevant to a question, and an answer is eventually provided

Flight of ideas: Overproductive speech characterized by rapid shifting from one topic to another and fragmenting ideas

Loose associations: Lack of a logical relationship between thoughts and ideas that renders speech and thought inexact, vague, diffuse, and unfocused

Neologisms: New word or words created by the patient, often a blend of other words

Perseveration: Involuntary, excessive continuation or repetition of a single response, idea, or activity; may apply to speech or movement, but most often verbal

Tangential: Similar to circumstantial but the person never returns to the central point and never answers the original question

Thought blocking: Sudden halt in the train of thought or in the middle of a sentence

Word salad: Series of words that seem totally unrelated

CLINICAL IMPLICATIONS

- Circumstantial thinking may be a sign of defensiveness or paranoid thinking.
- Loose associations and neologisms suggest schizophrenia or other psychotic disorders.
- Flight of ideas indicates mania.
- Perseveration is often associated with brain damage and psychotic disorders.
- Word salad represents the highest level of thought disorganization.

Level of Consciousness

Mental status examinations routinely assess a patient's orientation to the current situation. Deciding whether a patient is oriented involves evaluating some basic cognitive functions.

OBSERVATIONS

A variety of terms can be used to describe a patient's level of consciousness, such as **confused, sedated,** or **stuporous.** In addition, the patient should be questioned regarding orientation to **time, place,** and **person.** Typically the nurse can determine this by evaluating the patient's answers to three simple questions:

- **Person:** What is your name?
- **Place:** Where are you today (such as in what city or in what particular building)?
- **Time:** What is today's date?

BOX 7-5

Questions Useful in Determining Orientation

Questions Related to Time
Have you been keeping track of the time lately?
What is the date today? (If patient claims not to recall, ask for an estimate. Estimates can help assess level of disorientation.)
What month (or year) is it?
How long have you been here?

Questions Related to Place
There's been a lot happening these past few days (or hours); I wonder if you can describe for me where you are?
Do you recall what city we're in?
What is the name of the building we're in right now?
Do you know what part of the hospital we're in?

Questions Related to Person
What is your name?
Where are you from?
Where do you currently live?
What kinds of activities do you engage in during your free time?
Are you employed? If so, what do you do for a living?
Are you married? If so, what is your spouse's name?
Do you have any children?

If the patient answers correctly, the nurse can note "oriented times three." Level of orientation can be pursued in greater depth, but this area may be confounded by sociocultural factors.

Fully functioning patients may be offended by questions about orientation, so the skilled nurse should integrate questions pertaining to this area in the course of the interview and develop other ways of assessing this category. For example, the nurse could use some of the approaches listed in Box 7-5.

CLINICAL IMPLICATIONS

- Patients with organic mental disorders may give grossly inaccurate answers, with orientation to person remaining intact longer than orientation to time or place.
- Patients with schizophrenic disorders may say that they are someone else or somewhere else or reveal a personalized orientation to the world.

Memory

A mental status examination can provide a quick screen of potential memory problems but not a definitive answer to whether a specific impairment exists. Neuropsychological assessment is required to specify the nature and extent of memory impairment. Memory is broadly defined as the ability to recall past experiences.

OBSERVATIONS

The following areas must be tested:

- **Remote memory:** Recall of events, information, and people from the distant past
- **Recent memory:** Recall of events, information, and people from the past week or so
- **Immediate memory:** Recall of information or data to which a person was just exposed

Recall of remote events involves reviewing information from the patient's history. This part of the evaluation can be woven into the history-taking portion of the nursing assessment. This involves asking the patient questions about time and place of birth, names of schools attended, date of marriage, ages of family members, and so forth. The problem with an evaluation of the patient's remote memory is that the nurse is often unable to tell whether the patient is reporting events accurately. This situation raises the possibility that confabulation is being used, as when the patient makes up stories to recount situations or events that cannot be remembered. The nurse may need to call on past records or the report of family or friends to confirm this historical information.

Recent memory can be tested by asking the patient to recall the events of the past 24 hours or past week. A reliable informant may be needed to verify this information.

Immediate recall can be tested by asking the patient to repeat a series of numbers either forward or backward within a 10-second interval. The nurse should begin with a short series of numbers and proceed to longer lists. Another test of recent memory is asking the patient to remember three words (an object, a color, and an address) and then repeat them 15 minutes later in the interview.

CLINICAL IMPLICATIONS

- Loss of memory occurs with organicity, dissociative disorder, and conversion disorder.
- Patients with Alzheimer's disease retain remote memory longer than recent memory.
- Anxiety and depression can impair immediate retention and recent memory.

Level of Concentration and Calculation

Concentration is the patient's ability to pay attention during the course of the interview. Calculation is the person's ability to do simple math. These and other areas of cognitive functioning may vary in expected and unexpected ways (Box 7-6).

BOX 7-6

Gender Differences in the Brain

Women and men differ in physical attributes and in the way they think. The effect of sex hormones on brain organization appears to occur early in life, so the effects of the environment are secondary to the effects of biology. Behavioral, neurological, and endocrinological studies help explain the processes giving rise to gender differences in the brain. Major gender differences in intellectual functioning seem to lie in patterns of ability rather than in the overall level of intelligence. For example, the problem-solving tasks favoring women and men are shown below.

PROBLEM-SOLVING TASKS FAVORING WOMEN

Women tend to perform better than men on tests of perceptual speed, in which subjects must rapidly identify matching items, as in pairing the house on the far left with its twin.

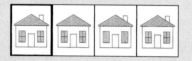

In addition, women remember whether an object or a series of objects has been displaced or rearranged.

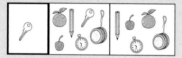

On some tests of ideational fluency, such as those in which subjects must list objects that are the same in color, and on tests of verbal fluency, in which participants must list words that begin with the same letter, women also outperform men.

L _ _ _ Limp, Livery, Love, Laser, Liquid, Low, Like, Lag, Live, Lug, Light, Lift, Liver, Lime, Leg, Load, Lap, Lucid ...

Women do better on precision manual tasks—that is, those involving fine motor coordination—such as placing the pegs in holes on a board.

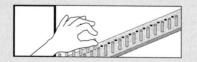

And women do better than men on mathematical calculation tests.

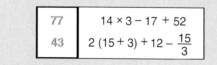

| 77 | $14 \times 3 - 17 + 52$ |
| 43 | $2(15 + 3) + 12 - \dfrac{15}{3}$ |

PROBLEM-SOLVING TASKS FAVORING MEN

Men tend to perform better than women on certain spatial tasks. They do well on tests that involve mentally rotating an object or manipulating it in some fashion, such as imagining turning this three-dimensional object

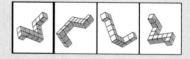

or determining where the holes punched in a folded piece of paper will fall when the paper is unfolded.

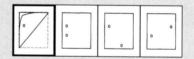

Men also are more accurate than women in target-directed motor skills, such as guiding or intercepting projectiles.

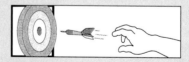

Men do better on disembedding tests, in which they have to find a simple shape, such as the one on the left, hidden within a more complex figure.

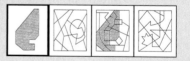

And men tend to do better than women on tests of mathematical reasoning.

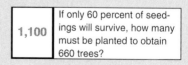

| 1,100 | If only 60 percent of seedings will survive, how many must be planted to obtain 660 trees? |

From Kimura D: *Sci Am* 267:120, 1992. Illustrated by Jared Schneidman.

OBSERVATIONS

The nurse should note the patient's level of distractibility. Calculation can be assessed by asking the patient to do the following:

- Count from 1 to 20 rapidly
- Do simple calculations, such as 2×3 or $21 + 7$
- Serially subtract 7 from 100

If patients have difficulty subtracting 7 from 100, they can be asked to subtract 3 from 20 in the same way. Finally, more functional calculation skills can be assessed by asking practical questions such as "How many nickels are there in $1.35?"

CLINICAL IMPLICATIONS

- Many psychiatric illnesses impair the ability to concentrate and complete simple calculations.
- It is particularly important to differentiate between organic mental disorder, anxiety, and depression.

Critical Thinking *About* Contemporary Issues

Can a Person's Intellectual Functioning Be Validly Assessed in the Mental Status Examination?

The evaluation of a person's intellectual functioning during the mental status examination is a subject of controversy, given the brief nature of the interview and the sociocultural biases that may be brought to it. Nonetheless, knowing a patient's intellectual capacity is important to the nurse in evaluating the patient's coping resources and designing an effective treatment plan.

Furthermore, it has been suggested that there is more than one type of intelligence. Rather, there are seven different types of intelligence (Gardner, 1993).

1. Linguistic intelligence
2. Logical-mathematical intelligence
3. Spatial intelligence
4. Musical intelligence
5. Bodily-kinesthetic intelligence
6. Interpersonal intelligence
7. Intrapersonal intelligence

The last two intelligences taken together (interpersonal and intrapersonal) can be described as forming one's personal intelligence or "emotional quotient" (Goleman 1995, 1998).

This expanded view of intelligence takes into account the talents people express in the arts, athletics, the ability to work cooperatively with people, and self-definition, as well as the more traditional verbal and mathematical skills usually assessed in standard intelligence tests. For example, a patient may have excellent spatial and mathematical intelligence but may lack formal education and interpersonal intelligence, and thus have difficulty obtaining a job. Such a person could be successful at a job that involved minimal contact with people but close work with designs and visual layouts. Nurses should take a broad approach to the assessment of intellectual functioning. This approach will allow them to identify the intellectual strengths, skills, and abilities of patients that may otherwise be overlooked.

Information and Intelligence

Information and intelligence are controversial areas of assessment, and the nurse should be cautious about judging intelligence after a brief and limited contact typical of the time it takes to conduct a mental status examination (see Critical Thinking About Contemporary Issues). The nurse also should remember that information in this category is highly influenced by sociocultural factors of the nurse, the patient, and the treatment setting.

OBSERVATIONS

The nurse should assess the patient's last grade of schooling completed, general knowledge, and use of vocabulary. It is also critically important to assess the patient's level of literacy. The ability to conceptualize and abstract can be tested by having the patient explain a series of proverbs. The patient can be given an example of a proverb and its interpretation and then be asked to explain what several other proverbs mean. Common proverbs include the following:

- When it rains, it pours.
- A stitch in time saves nine.
- A rolling stone gathers no moss.
- The proof of the pudding is in the eating.
- People who live in glass houses shouldn't throw stones.
- A bird in the hand is worth two in the bush.

Most adults are able to interpret proverbs as being symbolic of human behavior or events. However, sociocultural background should be considered when assessing a patient's information and intelligence.

If the patient's educational level is below the eighth grade, asking the patient to list similarities between a series of paired objects may better help the nurse assess the ability to abstract. The following paired objects are often used for this purpose:

- Bicycle and bus
- Apple and pear
- Television and newspaper

A higher-level reply addresses function, whereas a description of structure indicates more concrete thinking. To assess a patient's general knowledge, the nurse can ask the patient to name the last five presidents, the mayor, five large cities, or the occupation of a well-known person.

CLINICAL IMPLICATIONS

- The patient's educational level and any learning disabilities should be carefully evaluated.
- Mental retardation should be ruled out whenever possible.
- The patient's level of literacy may be part of a general assessment, but it is also an important factor in any health teaching or didactic information presented to the patient.

Judgment

Judgment involves making decisions that are constructive and adaptive. It involves the ability to understand facts and draw conclusions from relationships.

OBSERVATIONS

Judgment can be evaluated by exploring the patient's involvement in activities, relationships, and vocational choices. For example, is the patient regularly involved in illegal or dangerous activities or engaged in destructive relationships with others? It is also useful to determine whether the judgments are deliberate or impulsive. Finally, several hypothetical situations can be presented for the patient to evaluate:

- What would you do if you found a stamped, addressed envelope lying on the ground?
- How would you find your way out of a forest in the daytime?
- What would you do if you entered your house and smelled gas?
- If you won $10,000, what would you do with it?

CLINICAL IMPLICATIONS

- Judgment is impaired in organic mental disorders, schizophrenia, psychotic disorders, intoxication, and borderline or low IQ.
- It also may be impaired in manic patients and those with personality disorders.

What factors would you consider in evaluating the judgment of a man who engages in bungee jumping, rock climbing, and skydiving? How would this compare with a woman who has been in many relationships with abusive men? ■

Insight

Insight is the patient's understanding of the nature of the problem or illness.

OBSERVATIONS

It is important for the nurse to determine whether the patient accepts or denies the presence of a problem or illness. In addition, the nurse should ask whether the patient blames the problem on someone else or some external factors. Several questions may help to determine the patient's degree of insight. What does the patient think about the current situation? What does the patient want others, including the nurse, to do about it? The following clinical example illustrates a patient's level of insight.

CLINICAL EXAMPLE

The patient described several problems he was having at work. He reluctantly stated that he might have to change, but really thought his difficulties were because of his wife's drinking. He believed he could do nothing until she changed. ■

CLINICAL IMPLICATIONS

- Insight is impaired in those with many psychotic illnesses, including organic mental disorders, psychosis, substance abuse, eating disorders, personality disorders, and borderline or low IQ.

- Whether a patient sees the need for treatment also critically affects the therapeutic alliance, setting of mutual goals, implementation of the treatment plan, and future adherence to it.

Documenting Clinical Information

Information from the mental status examination may be recorded in various ways. Some clinicians write a descriptive report such as the one presented in the Case Study. Written reports should be brief, clear, and concise and address all categories of information. Others use an outline format that is completed with short answers. Still others use a format that is compatible with computerized information systems. Regardless of the format, important findings should be documented, and verbatim responses by the patient should be recorded whenever they add important information and support the nurse's assessment.

Mini-Mental State Examination

At times it is not practical or desirable to complete a full mental status examination. On these occasions, nurses may find it helpful to use the Mini-Mental State Examination (Folstein, Folstein, and McHugh, 1975). It is a simplified scored form of the cognitive mental status examination. It consists of 11 questions, requires only 5 to 10 minutes to administer, and can therefore be used quickly and routinely. It is "mini" because it concentrates on only the cognitive aspects of mental functions and excludes questions concerning mood, abnormal psychological experiences, and the content or process of thinking.

■ PSYCHOLOGICAL TESTS

Psychological tests are of two types: those designed to evaluate intellectual and cognitive abilities and those designed to describe personality functioning. Commonly used **intelligence tests** are the Wechsler Adult Intelligence Scale (WAIS) and the Wechsler Intelligence Scale for Children (WISC). Although intelligence tests often are criticized as being culturally biased, their ability to determine a person's strengths and weaknesses within the culture provides important therapeutic information.

Material obtained from **projective tests** reflects aspects of a person's personality function, including reality testing ability, impulse control, major defenses, interpersonal conflicts, and self-concept. A battery of tests is usually administered to provide comprehensive information. The Rorschach Test, Thematic Apperception Test (TAT), Bender Gestalt Test, and Minnesota Multiphasic Personality Inventory (MMPI) are commonly used by the clinical psychologist.

Psychological tests have typically been standardized on white, middle class populations. What implications does this have on the validity and reliability of these tests when used with individuals from other cultural backgrounds? ■

■ BEHAVIORAL RATING SCALES

The psychological context of psychiatric nursing care goes beyond the important assessment of a patient's mental status. Neither mental health nor mental illness can be meas-

CASE STUDY

Ms. T was a stylishly dressed, neatly groomed, slender woman in apparent good physical health who appeared to be her stated 22 years of age. She was cooperative during the interview but had difficulty expressing herself in specific terms. Her vague responses left the interviewer feeling perplexed about the difficulties she was describing.

The patient was alert and awake and oriented to person, place, and time. Immediate recall and recent memory were intact, demonstrated by her ability to recall three unrelated objects immediately and again 15 minutes later. Some of the historical information given was inconsistent with historical facts reported by her father. Although the vocabulary used by Ms. T and her knowledge of general information was congruent with her twelfth-grade education and past employment, she had difficulty completing the serial sevens but performed serial threes with ease. She stated that she was "nervous," which may be a factor related to performance. She was able to abstract two of three proverbs presented.

Proverb	Interpretation
Don't cry over spilled milk.	"If something happens, then forget about it. Maybe things will get better."
A rolling stone gathers no moss.	"A good person gathers no enemies. If a person stays active, he won't get depressed."
People who live in glass houses shouldn't throw stones.	"The glass will break."

Her responses to hypothetical situations were appropriate; however, the manner in which she coped with difficulties at work and home showed impaired judgment about personal issues.

Ms. T's speech was clear, coherent, and of normal rate and tone. Except for the vague, tangential manner in which she discussed her concern for her aunt, her communication was goal directed. There were no apparent delusions, hallucinations, or illusions. She denied any obsessions, compulsions, or phobias.

The central theme during the interview was her fear of being irresponsible and hurting her aunt. Her sadness and concern about her behavior in relation to the aunt pervaded the interview. She appeared nervous (looking away, fidgeting) and cried whenever she talked about her aunt. She described her mood as "low" and rated it as a 4 on a scale of 1 to 10. She denied having any suicidal or homicidal ideas or plan either previously or at the present time.

Her insight was questionable because she debated her need for treatment, but she agreed to return. She knew that a problem existed but was unaware of the causes of her behavior.

ured directly. Rather, its measurement depends on gathering a number of behavioral indicators of adaptive or maladaptive responses, which together represent the overall concept.

Behavioral rating scales and measurement tools have been designed to help clinicians:

- Measure the extent of the patient's problems.
- Make an accurate diagnosis.
- Track patient progress over time.
- Document the efficacy of treatment.

Each of these points is very important to the psychiatric nurse. The knowledge base for psychiatric care is expanding rapidly, and increased emphasis is being placed on clearly describing the nature of the patient's problems and the extent of the patient's progress toward attaining the expected outcomes of treatment (American Psychiatric Association, 2000; Coughlin et al, 2001). Thus nurses must be able to demonstrate in a valid and reliable way what problems they are treating and what effect their nursing care is having on attaining the treatment goals (see Citing the Evidence).

CITING THE EVIDENCE ON
Clinical Assessment and Patient Outcomes

BACKGROUND: Because of the increasing demands in the mental health care environment, providers are called upon to demonstrate the efficacy of treatment. Few studies have examined the relationship between symptoms at admission and level of functioning, involvement in treatment, and rehospitalization rates. The purposes of this study were to (a) examine the relationship between symptoms at admission, level of functioning, and exposure to activities for patients with depression and anxiety disorders and (b) examine the association between inpatient exposure to activities and rehospitalization rates. The Global Assessment Scale (GAS) and Beck Depression Inventory (BDI) were used to assess functioning and symptoms. The Nursing Record of Patient Daily Activities was used to record patient activities.

RESULTS: Higher GAS scores at time of admission were positively related to independent patient activities. No relationship was found between depression scores and patient daily activities. Readmitted patients were more likely to have the diagnosis of depression and be taking anxiolytics at the time of admission.

IMPLICATIONS: More studies are needed to examine the relationship between admission and posthospitalization symptoms, level of functioning in patients, and treatment components to determine which aspects of treatment are most effective for patients with specific symptoms, level of functioning, and diagnoses. Patients' symptoms and level of functioning at the time of admission should help guide the development of appropriate treatment plans.

Cronin J et al: *J Am Psychiatr Nurs Assoc* 7:145, 2001.

Nurses should become familiar with the many standardized rating scales that are available to enhance each stage of the nursing process. Many of the commonly used behavioral rating scales are listed by category in Appendix C. Nurses with training can use any of these scales. If the scales are to be used by a group of nurses, such as nurses working together in a specific treatment program or facility, interrater reliability among the nurses should be established.

These tools do not replace required nursing documentation. Rather, they are used to complement nursing care and provide measurable indicators of treatment outcome. For example, if the nurse is caring for a patient with depression, it would be helpful to use one of the depression rating scales with the patient at the beginning of treatment to establish a baseline profile of the patient's symptoms and help confirm the diagnosis. The nurse might then administer the same scale at various times during the course of treatment to measure the patient's progress. Finally, completing the rating scale at the end of treatment would document the efficacy of the care provided.

Computer Technology

Computerized clinical information systems that provide on-line support for assessment, diagnosis, treatment planning and implementation, and outcome evaluation are becoming widely available to mental health providers. When used with established ethical guidelines, computers offer a reliable, inexpensive, accessible, and time-efficient way of assessing psychiatric symptoms.

Computer-administered versions of clinician-administered rating scales are now available for the assessment of a number of psychiatric illnesses including depression, anxiety, obsessive-compulsive disorder, and social phobia. Patient reaction has been positive, with patients being generally more honest with their responses and often expressing a preference for the computer-administered assessments of sensitive areas such as suicide, alcohol and drug use, sexual behavior, or HIV-related symptoms.

Use of Interactive Voice Response (IVR) technology can help monitor patients by use of the telephone and do not require office visits to collect data. With an IVR system, the person dials a central phone number, listens to questions generated by a computer but asked by a human voice, and then responds to the questions by pressing numbers on a touch-tone telephone. Such a system can provide useful, timely information to clinicians. However, not all patients like the use of such technology, and it is important to match expressed patient preferences with assessment and treatment strategies (Stuart et al, 2003).

Give examples of some potential ethical problems that could arise from the use of computers in psychiatric care. How could these be safeguarded against? ■

CHAPTER FOCUS POINTS

- All nurses, regardless of the clinical setting, should be proficient in administering the mental status examination and be able to incorporate findings from it into the nursing care plan for the patient.
- The mental status examination represents a cross section of the patient's psychological life at that moment in time. It requires the nurse to observe the patient's behavior and describe it in an objective, nonjudgmental manner.
- Nurses should attend to both the content and process of the patient's communication.
- It is also important for the nurse to monitor his or her own feelings and reactions during the mental status examination.
- The nurse should blend specific questions into the general flow of the interview.
- The categories assessed in the mental status examination include the patient's appearance, speech, motor activity, mood, affect, interaction during the interview, perceptions, thought content, thought process, level of consciousness, memory, level of concentration and calculation, information and intelligence, judgment, and insight.
- The nurse should know what observations to make in each of the above categories and what the clinical implications of the findings would be.
- Psychological tests evaluate intellectual and cognitive abilities and describe personality functioning.
- Behavioral rating scales help clinicians measure the extent of the patient's problem, make an accurate diagnosis, track patient progress over time, and document the efficacy of treatment. These scales should be used by psychiatric nurses to complement nursing care and provide measurable indicators of treatment outcome.
- Computerized clinical information systems provide on-line support for assessment, diagnosis, treatment planning and implementation, and outcome evaluation.

KEY TERMS

affect, 111
circumstantial, 112
command hallucinations, 111
confabulation, 113
delusion, 112
depersonalization, 112
flat affect, 111
flight of ideas, 112
hallucinations, 111

hypochondriasis, 112
ideas of reference, 112
illusions, 111
loose associations, 112
magical thinking, 112
mental status examination, 108
mood, 111
neologisms, 112
nihilistic ideas, 112

obsession, 112
perseveration, 112
phobia, 112
tangential, 112
thought blocking, 112
thought broadcasting, 112
thought insertion, 112
word salad, 112

CHAPTER REVIEW QUESTIONS

1. **Match each of the terms in Column A with its correct description in Column B.**

Column A

_____ Affect
_____ Delusion
_____ Flight of ideas
_____ Hallucinations
_____ Illusions
_____ Insight
_____ Loose associations
_____ Mood

Column B

A. False belief not shared by others or confirmed by reality
B. False perception or response to a sensory stimulation
C. Feeling, mood, or emotional tone
D. Lack of a logical relationship between thoughts and ideas, resulting in unfocused speech
E. Overproductive speech with rapid shifting of topics and ideas
F. Perceptual distortion arising from any of the five senses
G. Self-report by patient of his or her prevailing emotional state
H. Understanding by the patient of the nature of his or her problem or illness

2. **Fill in the blanks.**

A. A patient who describes the death of a younger brother without any emotional response is said to have

_____.

B. _____ are false sensory impressions that tell the patient to do something he or she would not ordinarily do.

C. The most common type of hallucination involves the sense of

_____.

D. When a patient makes up stories in response to questions about situations or events that cannot be remembered, it is

called _____.

3. **Provide short answers for the following questions.**

A. What are the five major categories of information that should be included in a mental status examination?
B. What three questions have been asked when a patient is described as oriented times three?
C. Identify four reasons why psychiatric nurses should use behavioral rating scales in their practice.
D. Identify four reasons why psychiatric nurses do not use behavioral rating scales in their practice.
E. What impact do you think computer technology could have on improving mental health care for currently underserved populations?

Visit Evolve for additional resources related to the content of this chapter.

http://evolve.elsevier.com/Stuart/principles/

• Topical Course Outline • Student Workbook Exercises • Critical Thinking Questions and Activities • Case Studies • Research Topics • Monthly Content Updates • WebLinks

---

Student Study CD-ROM

Access the accompanying CD-ROM for animation, interactive exercises, review questions for the NCLEX examination, and an audio glossary.

REFERENCES

American Psychiatric Association: *Handbook of psychiatric measures,* Washington DC, 2000, American Psychiatric Association.
American Psychiatric Association: Practice guideline for psychiatric evaluation of adults, *Am J Psychiatry* 152(11):67, 1995 (suppl).
Coughlin KM et al, editors: *2001 Behavioral outcomes & guidelines sourcebook,* New York, 2000, Faulkner & Gray.
Folstein MF, Folstein SE, McHugh PR: "Mini-mental state": a practical method for grading the cognitive state of patients for the clinician, *J Psychiatr Res* 12:189, 1975.

Gardner HE: *Multiple intelligences: the theory in practice,* New York, 1993, Basic Books.
Goleman D: *Emotional intelligence,* New York, 1995, Bantam.
Goleman D: *Working with emotional intelligence,* New York, 1998, Bantam.
Robinson DJ: *The mental status exam explained,* New York, 2002, Rapid Psychler Press.
Stuart G et al: An interactive voice response system to enhance antidepressant medication compliance, *Top Health Inf Manage* 24:15, 2003.
Wiger DE, Huntley DK: *Essentials of interviewing,* New York, 2002, John Wiley & Sons.

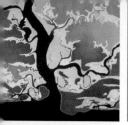

We know what we belong to, where we come from, and where we are going. We may not know it with our brains, but we know it with our roots.

NOEL COWARD, *THIS HAPPY BREED*

8 SOCIAL, CULTURAL, AND SPIRITUAL CONTEXT OF PSYCHIATRIC NURSING CARE

Linda D. Oakley

LEARNING OBJECTIVES

After studying this chapter, the student should be able to:
1. Describe the qualities of cultural competency in psychiatric nursing care (I).
2. Discuss the importance of social, cultural, and spiritual risk factors and protective factors in developing, experiencing, and recovering from psychiatric illness (II).
3. Apply knowledge of social, cultural, and spiritual contexts to psychiatric nursing assessment and diagnosis (III).
4. Examine the treatment implications of culturally competent psychiatric nursing care (IV).

TOPICAL OUTLINE

I. Cultural Competency
II. Risk Factors and Protective Factors
  A. Age
  B. Ethnicity
  C. Gender
  D. Education
  E. Income
  F. Beliefs
III. Nursing Assessment and Diagnosis
IV. Treatment Implications
  A. Service Utilization
  B. Therapeutic Nurse-Patient Interactions
  C. Psychopharmacology

 Visit Evolve for additional resources related to the content of this chapter.
http://evolve.elsevier.com/Stuart/principles/

Disparities are widespread in the diagnosis and treatment of mental illness, as in other areas of health care. In 2001 the Surgeon General of the United States issued a report titled *Mental Health: Culture, Race, and Ethnicity* (USDHHS, 2001) that emphasized the significant role that cultural factors play in mental health. Its main message was that culture counts. The report underscored the following points:

- Mental illnesses are real, disabling conditions that affect all populations, regardless of race or ethnicity.
- Striking disparities in mental health care are found for racial and ethnic minorities.
- Disparities impose a greater disability burden on minorities.
- Racial and ethnic minorities should seek help for mental health problems and illnesses.

In effect, the report was a call to understand and appreciate the diversity of all cultures and the impact sociocultural factors have on the mental health of all people. This was reinforced by the report of the New Freedom Commission on Mental Health, *Achieving the Promise: Transforming Mental Health Care in America* (2003). One of the goals identified in this report was to see that "Disparities in mental health services are eliminated." This was followed by two recommendations:

1. Improve access to quality care that is culturally competent.
2. Improve access to quality care in rural and geographically remote areas.

Holistic psychiatric nursing care must take into consideration a wide range of patient characteristics in the assessment, diagnosis, treatment, and recovery process. Human beings live within social, cultural, and spiritual contexts that shape and give meaning to their lives. Typically expressed as beliefs, norms, and values, these characteristics can have both direct and indirect influences on patients' perceptions of health and illness, their help-seeking behavior, and treatment outcomes. They are strong determinants of actual and potential coping resources and coping responses and influence all phases of an illness, including treatment effectiveness.

Specifically, these social, cultural, and spiritual characteristics can impact a person's **access to mental health care, risk for or protection against developing a certain psychiatric disorder, how symptoms will be experienced and expressed, the ease or difficulty of participating in psychiatric treatment,** and **one's ability to achieve recovery.** Thus quality psychiatric nursing care must incorporate the unique aspects of the individual into every element of practice and be based on an understanding of the importance of culture, as outlined in Box 8-1.

Table 8-1	Cultural Competence: Have You "ASKED" the Right Questions?
COMPETENCE CONSTRUCT	QUESTION TO ASK YOURSELF TO ASSESS COMPETENCY
Awareness	Are you aware of your personal biases and prejudices toward cultures different than your own?
Skill	Do you have the skill to conduct a cultural assessment and perform a culturally based physical assessment?
Knowledge	Do you have the knowledge of the patient's worldview, cultural-bound illnesses, and the field of biocultural ecology?
Encounters	How many face-to-face encounters have you had with patients from diverse cultural backgrounds?
Desire	What is your desire to "want to be" culturally competent?

From Campinha-Bacote J: *J Am Psychiatr Nurs Assoc* 8:183, 2002.

BOX 8-1

The Functions of Culture

Perception: Perception of reality is based on a cultural interpretation and understanding of events.
Motives: Motives for behavior are conditioned by the values assumed by a culture.
Identity: Individual and group identity is fostered by the oral, written, and social constructs defining a culture.
Values: Concepts of ethics and morality are conditioned by cultural background.
Communication: Language, music, and dance are the external expressions of culture.
Emotions: Emotions are significantly enabled and shaped by cultural ideas, practices, and institutions.

■ CULTURAL COMPETENCY

Advocates of cultural competency in psychiatric care believe that increased use of health care services and improved treatment outcomes are due to the purposeful consideration of a patient's social, cultural, and spiritual attributes. Culturally competent practice requires far more than recording the patient's age, sex, ethnicity, and religion. As a practice skill, cultural competency is the ability to view each patient as a unique individual, fully considering the patient's cultural experiences within the context of the common developmental challenges faced by all people. The nurse applies this information in nursing interventions that are consistent with the life experiences and values of each patient.

Cultural competence is actually nursing competence and is an essential psychiatric nursing skill (Dreher and MacNaughton, 2002; Warren, 2000, 2002). For example, the culturally competent nurse recognizes that different persons with identical psychiatric symptoms might be tolerated by some sociocultural groups, ignored by others, and sanctioned by still others. There are a number of reasons for this. First, if a behavior or symptom is widespread in a social group, it may be considered normal. Second, if the behavior fits in with social values, it may similarly be accepted. If the behavior does not fit in, it may be seen as a sign of deviancy or illness.

For example, hallucinations in Western society are considered a sign of serious illness because the social values emphasize rationality and control. In contrast, visions, hexes, and hearing voices are not necessarily considered signs of psychosis among other cultures, nor is communicating with the dead. In addition, some cultural groups would view symptoms typically associated with mental illness as signs of normality, meanness, laziness, sin, or spiritual distress. So too, patients' personal reactions to their symptoms can range from self-hate to self-acceptance to striving for self-actualization. Patients' responses and the responses of important others also influence whether professional treatment is likely to be desired, offered, accepted, or rejected.

Campinha-Bacote proposed a model of cultural competence based on five constructs: awareness, skill, knowledge, encounters, and desire. She suggests that culturally competent psychiatric nursing care implies cultural awareness rather than unawareness, cultural abilities rather than inabilities, cultural knowledge rather than illiteracy, cultural comfort rather than discomfort, and cultural interest rather than apathy (Campinha-Bacote, 2002).

Questions that the nurse can ask to assess one's cultural competency are identified in Table 8-1. Nurses who achieve cultural competency work *with* patients and are more effective in their care of them. Nurses who work *on* patients are less likely to truly interact with patients and risk creating superficial nurse interactions that communicate cultural unawareness, inability, discomfort, disrespect, or apathy.

Culturally competent nurses remain in touch with their own cultural beliefs, values, and norms. They are willing to challenge their own assumptions and to alter unintentional actions when shown how these actions can be offensive or ineffective. The culturally competent nurse understands the importance of social, cultural, and spiritual forces, recognizes the uniqueness of each patient, respects nurse-patient differences, and incorporates sociocultural information into psychiatric nursing care. This chapter provides a conceptual framework for the practice of cultural competency in psychiatric nursing that is based on common sociocultural influences and patient characteristics.

Challenge the evidence for one of your own cultural biases that is a result of your upbringing or personal experiences. ■

■ RISK FACTORS AND PROTECTIVE FACTORS

As a result of being influenced by personal, social, cultural, and spiritual development, every patient has unique risk factors and protective factors that can change with age and personal circumstances. The culturally competent psychiatric nurse strives to incorporate these risk and protective factors throughout the assessment, diagnosis, and treatment process.

The concept of **risk and protective factors** is important to understanding how people acquire, experience, and recover from illness. These factors are the same as the **predisposing factors** that nurses assess in the Stuart Stress Adaptation Model of psychiatric nursing (see Chapter 4).

Understanding the risk and protective factors involved in health and illness is essential in the prevention, early detection, and effective treatment of physiological illnesses such as cardiac, pulmonary, and hepatic diseases. Identifying risk and protective factors is also valuable in providing psychiatric care.

Risk factors for psychiatric disorders are characteristics of a person that can significantly increase the potential for developing a psychiatric disorder, decrease the potential for recovery, or both. Protective factors are characteristics of a person that can significantly decrease the potential for developing a psychiatric disorder, increase the potential for recovery, or both. Perhaps the most important outcome of the inclusion of risk factors and protective factors in nursing practice is the development of individualized, culturally competent, and socially relevant mental health care.

Six patient characteristics, influenced by social norms, cultural values, and spiritual beliefs, are known to act as risk factors, protective factors, or both. These are patient age, ethnicity, gender, education, income, and beliefs. They influence the patient's exposure to stressors, appraisal of stressors, coping resources, and coping responses, as described in the Stuart Stress Adaptation Model (Figure 8-1) (Donnelly, 2002).

The sociocultural factors of age, ethnicity, gender, education, income, and beliefs are predisposing or conditioning factors that influence the amount and type of coping resources available to a person. Any single risk factor or protective factor or a combination of factors can have multiple effects or may have little or no effect, depending on the individual and the circumstances. They also interact, so that different ones become important at different times. For this reason, assessment and diagnosis of patient risk and protective factors is a continuous process.

For example, being female increases the risk of depressive disorders in women, but decreases their risk of alcohol abuse disorders. Being male is associated with less risk of depression, but a significantly higher risk of suicide. Poverty increases the risk of a range of stress disorders, but the circumstance of poverty itself also can occur as a *result* of a severe thought disorder, such as schizophrenia. Spiritual faith or the practice of cultural traditions can sustain hopeful and positive coping in the face of overwhelming adversity, whereas the loss of faith can increase the risk of depressive or anxiety disorders.

Social and cultural group membership promotes the adoption of specific values, beliefs, and behavioral norms intended to benefit the health and well being of the group and its members. However, characteristics of an individual can still differ significantly from the characteristics of the group in general. Thus a culturally competent nurse does not assume knowledge of a patient based on casual observations of age, ethnicity, or gender.

Neither should a nurse draw generalizations about groups based upon these factors. Literature that describes and summarizes the values or beliefs of specific populations such as blacks, Hispanics, and Asians often creates new stereotypes, and these generalizations can further depersonalize nursing care. In contrast, the sociocultural view is based on the assessment of social, cultural, spiritual, and environmental factors that are individualized and that change over time.

It is true that some group differences in psychiatric risk and protective factors have been observed. For example, regardless of age, ethnicity, education, or income, more females than males are diagnosed and treated for depression (Piccinelli and Wilkinson, 2000). However, it is not known whether the different prevalence of a psychiatric disorder between groups is an indicator of clinical differences, cultural differences, or both.

Specifically, it is not known whether the prevalence of depression among females is greater than that among males because the two groups are clinically different or because females are exposed more often to social and cultural stressors that can precipitate depression. If the latter were true, it would suggest that if males were exposed to the same stressors and were taught the same coping style as females, the rate of depression for the two groups would be equal.

Thus, while understanding that being female is a risk factor for depression, the culturally competent nurse would not assume that all female patients are at equal risk for depression; that depression in females is normal; or that depression in males is rare. Rather, the culturally competent nurse would understand that no two women are likely to have the same risk of depression, and that an individual woman's risk for depression changes over time and with life circumstances.

Some findings about each of these risk and protective factors and their possible effects on holistic psychiatric nursing care are described in the following sections. Box 8-2 lists some sociocultural trends and their influence on the health care system.

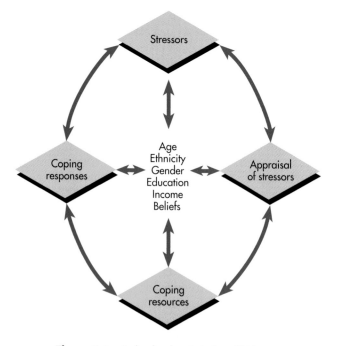

Figure 8-1 Sociocultural context of psychiatric care.

Think of a group you belong to based on one of your sociocultural characteristics. What stereotypes exist about this group? Do you fit these stereotypes? ■

Sociocultural Diversity and the Health Care System

Current U.S. data suggest that the following sociocultural trends will influence the health care system and the way health care is provided:

- The population will increase by 60% to almost 400 million by the year 2050.
- Growth will be concentrated at the two ends of the age spectrum. By 2050 the number of people in the population ages 65 and older will more than double, and those ages 85 years and older will be the fastest-growing age-group.
- The U.S. population is becoming more diverse by race and ethnicity. By 2050 Hispanics will be about 25% of the population; blacks about 14%; Asian and Pacific Islanders about 8%; Native American Indians, Eskimo, and Aleut about 1%; and whites about 53%.
- The United States has become a predominantly urban nation, with the population occupying only 2.5% of the land mass.

These trends will have a profound impact on the health care system for the following reasons:

- As the aging population grows, an increase in chronic conditions and chronic diseases related to behavior will occur that will exact a greater toll on the health care system.
- A rise in the number of young people will bring new waves of problems typically committed by the young, such as murder, rape, robbery, and assault. Almost half of all violent crimes are committed by people under age 24, with those 15 to 19 years of age responsible for the most crime. The overall crime rate has increased 500% since 1960.
- Minority populations are currently underserved, a problem that may only intensify. In addition, an increase in low-birth-weight babies among minority populations is expected.
- Minority populations are underrepresented in all health care professions, causing concern about whether health care providers will understand health problems within a cultural context and be able to provide culturally sensitive care.

From Center for Mental Health Services, *Cultural competence standards*, Rockville, Md, 1998, Center for Mental Health Services.

Age

Age-related variations in life stressors, support resources, and coping skills are common. It has been reported that the frequency of seeking psychiatric care peaks between 25 and 44 years of age, then declines with increasing age. Age-related increases and decreases in the use of mental health services tend to occur as a reflection of various social, cultural, developmental, and spiritual changes associated with aging.

Aging, income, and education also interact strongly. For example, among the elderly, the prevalence of depression is decreased among those with high socioeconomic status and more education. In terms of support resources, African-American, Hispanic, and white elderly people often find church attendance to be a positive and adaptive coping resource.

Evidence of age as a protective factor also has been observed across cultures (McCrae et al, 1999). For example, the rate of depression among aging adults is lower than the rate in younger age-groups. Compared with younger age-groups, depressed elderly people tend to recover more quickly and are less likely to suffer recurrence.

Age as a protective factor interacts with socioeconomic status in that the elderly who are socially and economically stable are often more resilient to the life experiences that are likely to lead to depression. Compared with younger age-groups, the elderly have had more time and experience with life stress and may have developed better coping strategies or adopted less demanding social roles.

Ethnicity

The term ethnicity, as used in this chapter, includes a person's racial, national, tribal, linguistic, and cultural origin or background. Ethnic groups typically include a variety of specific cultures. For example, Latin American, Hispanic, and Hispanic American are terms used to represent native Spanish speakers. Yet the racial, national, language, and cultural backgrounds of Hispanic people are as diverse as Mexico, the Caribbean islands (including Puerto Rico, Cuba, and the Dominican Republic), Central and South America, and Spain. Each group has its own distinct history, customs, beliefs, and traditions.

Similarly, the terms Asian and Asian American refer to 40 different ethnic groups with 30 different languages. As a census category, Native American includes Alaskan and Hawaiian natives, but both groups have hundreds of tribes, each with their own history, languages, and traditions. Black Americans living in the United States also represent highly diverse countries, as do white Americans. Although there may be similarities in physical characteristics for each of these groups, differences in ethnic and cultural heritage may be immense.

For ethnic and racial minority groups, personal protective factors often are embedded in a tightly shared social identity. Such groups often have well-defined healing practices and traditions that are important positive resources for the nurse to consider when providing care. In contrast, patient ethnicity also can have direct and indirect negative effects on the development of and recovery from psychiatric disorders and access to health care services.

Members of minorities often have difficulty gaining access to appropriate mental health services. For example, studies have found that Latino youths were significantly less likely than white youths to use specialty mental health services regardless of diagnosis, gender, or age (Hough et al, 2002; Yeh et al, 2002). So too, there is greater unmet need for alcoholism and drug abuse treatment and mental health care among black Americans and Hispanics as compared to whites (Wells et al, 2001).

Many minority individuals lack medical insurance or access to primary care clinicians who could assist with the referral process. Difficulty with language and communication or lack of knowledge in how to negotiate the mental health care system also limits their ability to receive needed care.

A number of studies have identified specific barriers to effective mental health care for minority populations (Hines-Martin et al, 2003; Husaini et al, 2003; Johnson and Cameron, 2001; Leong and Lau, 2001; Snowden, 2001; Vega and Lopez, 2001; Weinick, Zuvekas, and Cohen, 2000). Such research suggests that members of minority groups delay seeking help until their problems are intense, chronic, and at a difficult-to-treat stage and until community and family support systems have been exhausted. Delays in accessing care and early termination from care create a cyclical reliance on more costly health care services.

Ethnicity also has been shown to influence the development of and recovery from psychiatric disorders. Significant differences exist in the prevalence of certain disorders among various ethnic groups and in their use of mental health services. Misdiagnosis is a problem that creates inappropriate admissions to state hospitals. For example, blacks and Hispanics have been reported to be diagnosed on admission with severe mental illness at a rate almost twice as high as individuals from other groups. In addition, the most severe types of psychopathology tend to be diagnosed in black patients, with blacks being underrepresented in the count of patients with affective disorders and overdiagnosed in regard to schizophrenia (Trierweiler et al, 2000).

In terms of hospitalization, members of ethnic groups are admitted to psychiatric institutions three times more often than the general population. In addition, blacks, Native Americans, and Hispanics have higher rates of admission to state and county mental hospitals than to community and private psychiatric hospitals. Other studies have found that blacks were more likely to use emergency mental health services and less likely to use individual or group treatment. In contrast, Asians have extremely low admission rates to state hospitals and low utilization of mental health services in general (Shin, 2002).

Studies also have examined racial differences in relation to treatment and have found that nonpsychotic black patients had shorter lengths of stay in inpatient facilities than white patients with similar disorders. White patients were more likely to be on one-to-one observational status, and clinicians were more likely to order urine drug screens for black patients with high socioeconomic status than for comparable white patients (Baker and Bell, 1999).

Other studies have found that black patients with schizophrenia are less likely to receive atypical antipsychotics and more likely to receive depot anitpsychotics (Kreyenbuhl et al, 2003) and blacks seen in primary care settings were less likely to be provided a psychotropic medication (Snowden and Pingitore, 2002). These studies point to the importance of engaging patients from diverse ethnic groups in the treatment process and the need for clinical skills and training in bridging cultural differences.

How might ethnicity influence the coping responses and the specific symptoms expressed by a patient? Give a specific example. ■

Gender

As a predisposing factor, gender is similar to ethnicity in that at first glance there appears to be distinctive male and female patterns of risk and protection (Horsfall, 2001). However, when all psychiatric disorders are included, the prevalence of mental illness among males and females is roughly equal.

The actual difference between the two groups is in the type of disorder that is most commonly diagnosed. Substance abuse and antisocial personality disorder are the most prevalent psychiatric disorders among males, whereas affective disorders and anxiety disorders are most prevalent among females. In contrast, the prevalence of schizophrenia and manic episodes for males and females is about equal.

These findings support the idea that male and female role socialization in contemporary American society is a significant determinant of the perception of health and illness and that the risk of psychiatric disorders may be sex typed by sociocultural factors. Specifically, it has been proposed that males are taught to aggressively externalize their psychological experiences, whereas females are taught to passively internalize their social experiences.

Only recently have advances in the study of human genes and psychiatric disorders made cause and effect studies of biological sex and psychiatric disorders possible. Nevertheless, gender-typed social learning effects have been observed even with severe psychiatric disorders such as schizophrenia.

For example, gender differences exist in both symptom presentation and in the course of illness. Specifically, with schizophrenia the age of onset is later for women, and they tend to have greater preillness social functioning. Men, on the other hand, are more likely to be aggressive, to be self-destructive, and to spend more time in jail and are more likely to commit suicide. In terms of treatment, women have a better response to both pharmacological and psychosocial treatments, but they are much more vulnerable to negative psychosocial outcomes such as victimization and substance abuse (Gearon and Tamminga, 2000).

Such evidence suggests that the treatment approach for men and women with schizophrenia should be tailored to the gender differences. Specifically, women should have lower doses of medicine over shorter periods of time. They should have access to focused psychosocial treatments aimed at reducing substance abuse and the occurrence of violent sexual and physical violence. Men, in contrast, should have more aggressive pharmacological treatments and psychosocial treatments aimed at improving interpersonal skills and controlling aggression.

The following clinical example demonstrates the interaction of ethnicity and gender and the way in which they can affect a person's response to stress.

■ ⸤ CLINICAL EXAMPLE

Jose Rodriguez is a 36-year-old Hispanic man. Jose planned to graduate from an MBA program in May and marry his fiancée, Lisa, in June. The couple met in class 2 years ago and have dated for 1 year. Jose visited Lisa's family for the first time during spring break. Lisa's parents are of German descent, and they were shocked when Lisa told them she planned to marry Jose in

3 months. Lisa's father informed her that if she goes through with her wedding plans he will disown her. He said that her mother and brothers agreed with him and that she had to choose between Jose and her family. When she told Jose about her father's reaction, he felt they should leave immediately, but Lisa said she could not go with him if it meant going against her family.

Jose drove back to school and on the way was cited twice for speeding. When he returned to his room, he spent 2 days alone drinking beer. He did not shave, shower, or change his clothes. On the third day he went out for more beer, and as he walked past a group of men, one of them called him a "dirty wetback." When Jose got home, he destroyed his room and everything in it, including his completed master's thesis, which he needed to hand in the next day in order to graduate in May. ■

Finally, similar to age and ethnicity, gender, as a risk or protective factor, interacts with other patient characteristics. Younger women, older women, women of color, highly educated women, and women with high incomes are likely to vary significantly from their counterparts, male or female. Cultural competency thus requires a consideration of the potential impact of both a patient's sex (male, female) and gender (masculinity, femininity).

How might a psychiatric nurse's view of gender-appropriate behavior influence his or her diagnosis and treatment of male and female patients? ■

Education

Numerous studies identify the importance of education as a coping resource in protecting against the development of and promoting recovery from mental illness. For example, it has been found that education is more important than income in determining use of mental health services, with those with the highest educational level using mental health services most often. Patients with less education are often less likely to seek psychiatric care and are somewhat more at risk for dropping out of treatment. Less informed individuals may not fully understand psychiatric care, believing it to be little more than talking. Few people are likely to make much of an effort to obtain or participate in care they know little about or cannot understand.

Experts point out that patients with less education often also have little income and thus are required to spend most of their time and energy solving financial problems. Ironically, low-income persons may be more likely to view psychiatric care both as a middle-income luxury item and as something for people who have something seriously "wrong" with their mind. Public education programs have helped to correct some of these misconceptions, but far more work is needed.

Finally, mental status examinations are often used to determine diagnosis and treatment for various psychiatric disorders (see Chapter 7). Yet questions have been raised about the cultural context of such evaluations. It also has been noted that patients who are not proficient in English are often misdiagnosed. Therefore, programs need to adapt to the needs of people with limited English proficiency by providing either

clinicians who speak native languages or skilled translators and interpreters who can facilitate communication between patients and care providers. Written materials and forms also need to be printed in the native languages of the patients and at the literacy levels of the populations being served.

The clinical example that follows illustrates the effect ethnicity, gender, and education can have on a person's ability to interact with others effectively.

◁ CLINICAL EXAMPLE

Ms. Wong is a 22-year-old Chinese-American woman. She is employed at a university computer center and is a part-time law student. Her roommate is a second-year English major and has an active social life. Because her courses are demanding and her family expects her to be successful, Ms. Wong spends all of her free time studying. While Ms. Wong was studying one Friday afternoon, her roommate came home with several friends, including a young man from Ms. Wong's law class that she thought was very attractive. She was excited about seeing him and acted very friendly toward him until she realized that he was her roommate's date for the evening. Ms. Wong felt humiliated by her behavior and abruptly left the apartment. While she was leaving, she heard her roommate say, "Now that Miss Perfect is gone, we can party."

Ms. Wong did not know what to do or in whom to confide. She walked around town for hours. Although she was becoming exhausted, she did not stop to rest, eat, or drink. She continued to walk and smiled at the romantic couples she passed but became sad again when they did not smile back at her. Ms. Wong noticed a wig store across the street from where she stood and went in and bought a curly blonde wig that she immediately put on. She then wore this wig every day and insisted that everyone call her Patty, her new American name. ■

Income

The profound negative impact of poverty as a risk factor for psychiatric illness is evident regardless of age, ethnicity, gender, or education. The relationship of poverty and severe financial stressors with poor health has been well documented (Cattell, 2001; Hoffman and Hatch, 2000). Although the impact of poverty can be generalized to all social and cultural groups, higher prevalence rates of poverty are consistently found among women, the elderly, and ethnic and racial minorities (Alegria et al, 2002).

Some experts argue that the impact of poverty is so great that most observed group differences in the risk for developing a psychiatric disorder is the result of the social stratification of poverty. The more commonly held view is that the impact of all other risk factors is multiplied by poverty.

The obvious benefits of income as a protective factor generally have to do with being better able to avoid life events associated with the development of severe psychiatric disorders and faster and easier access to psychiatric services. However, the highly publicized mental health and substance abuse problems of the celebrated and the wealthy suggest that the actual protective impact of higher income may not be as great as is commonly believed.

The following clinical example describes the effect of ethnicity and income on self-esteem.

CLINICAL EXAMPLE

John Willis is a 20-year-old black man. He has been looking for work since he graduated from high school 2 years ago and has had several job interviews with local employers. Over the phone, all of these employers seemed very interested in hiring John, but he never received a job offer. Each time he called back after an interview, he was told that the position had been filled and that his application would be kept on file. Last fall, John obtained an interview for an entry-level position at a local bank. He felt that his luck had changed and this would be the perfect job for him.

He arrived early for his interview, and after waiting an hour to meet with the interviewer, John was told that the position had been filled. John was very surprised to hear this. He felt that he had not been treated fairly and that the interviewer just wanted to look him over and decided that he did not like what he saw. John asked the interviewer, "Did the position get filled before or after I got here, or don't you know that either?" The interviewer alerted security and asked John to leave. John was angry and embarrassed and asked the interviewer why he was being treated like a criminal when he came here to apply for a job. Before the interviewer could answer, John left the building. Since then, John has refused to look for work or go to another interview. He has been unemployed for 2 years and continues to live with his parents, sleeping until noon everyday and spending all of his time "hanging out" with his male friends. ■

Most single-parent households in this country are headed by women, and many of them are below the poverty level. How might this affect the mental health of the children living in these homes? ■

Beliefs

Personal beliefs touch all aspects of life. A person's belief system, worldview, religion, or spirituality can have a positive or negative effect on mental health. People have a psychological need to make sense out of and explain their experiences. This need is especially important when they are suffering or in distress.

In this quest for meaning, belief systems play a vital role in determining whether a particular explanation and associated treatment plan will have meaning for the patient and others in the patient's social network. The degree of compatibility between the patient's and provider's belief systems often determines the patient's satisfaction with treatment, medication compliance, and treatment outcome. The true importance of patient beliefs is evident by the impasse that can be created when beliefs of the patient and provider conflict.

Adaptive belief systems can enhance well being, improve quality of life, and support recovery from psychiatric disorders. Maladaptive belief systems may contribute to poor adjustment to changes in health status, refusal of necessary treatment, nonadherence with treatment recommendations, or even self-injury.

For example, certain religious belief systems stress avoidance of alcohol, illicit drugs, and cigarette smoking. Spiritually based intervention programs, such as 12-step programs, which encourage the individual to surrender control to an external supreme being, are commonly used treatments for addictive disorders (Galanter, 2002).

The role of religion in mental health and mental illness remains understudied. The concepts of religion, religiosity, and spirituality are complex. However, it appears that some dimensions of religiosity are related to reduced risk of some psychiatric disorders (Kendler et al, 2003) and that religious beliefs and practices may be related to greater life satisfaction, happiness, positive affect, morale, and general well-being (Koenig et al, 2001).

The religious person often lives in a world perceived as having purpose and meaning. Religion can provide the basis for self-esteem and a personal identity rooted both within the individual and within the faith community and its shared traditions. It can thus instill in the individual a sense of hope and optimism, as well as promote social support, transcendent connection, and adaptive coping (see Citing the Evidence).

Patient beliefs can take on incredible complexity, touching every aspect of daily life. Beliefs are shaped by formal systems such as family networks or organized religion, as well as informal systems such as peer groups and popular media. Beliefs change slowly if at all, but they are nevertheless constantly under construction.

For example, a patient who is profoundly depressed but does not believe in taking psychiatric medications can, over time, become open to questioning and testing such beliefs. Life experiences routinely lead to serious questioning of one's social, cultural, religious, and spiritual beliefs. These experiences include being diagnosed and treated for a psychiatric disorder.

Think about two patients you took care of last week. Did you discuss with them their beliefs about their health and current illnesses? Did you ask about their worldview, religion, or spirituality? If not, how might this information have influenced your nursing interventions with them? ■

In summary, age, ethnicity, gender, education, income, and beliefs can be risk or protective factors for psychiatric illness.

CITING THE EVIDENCE ON
Religious Coping

BACKGROUND: The purpose of this study was to examine the prevalence of religious coping among persons with persistent mental illness and to gain a preliminary understanding of the relationship between religious coping, symptom severity, and overall functioning.

RESULTS: More than 80% of the participants in the study used religious beliefs or activities to cope with daily difficulties or frustrations. A majority devoted as much as half of their total coping time to religious practices, with prayer being the most frequent activity. Specific religious coping strategies such as prayer or reading the Bible were associated with having more severe symptoms and with greater functional impairment.

IMPLICATIONS: Religious activities and beliefs may be particularly compelling for persons who are experiencing more severe symptoms. Religion may serve as a pervasive and potentially effective method of coping for persons with mental illness, thus suggesting the potential importance of integrating religion into clinical practice.

Tepper L et al: *Psychiatr Serv* 52: 660, 2001.

As such, they can significantly impact treatment effectiveness and treatment outcome and must be an essential element of a culturally competent nurse's ongoing care of all patients.

NURSING ASSESSMENT AND DIAGNOSIS

Self-assessment is essential in the delivery of culturally competent psychiatric nursing care. Nurses should explore their responses to the following questions:

- Does the patient's appearance or language make me think that what I am seeing or hearing is pathological?
- What labels am I subconsciously applying to this patient, and how did I learn them?
- What socioeconomic status am I assuming for the patient, and what are my assumptions about that socioeconomic group?
- What other explanations might account for the patient's behavior?
- What personal characteristics of the patient have I noted, and what are my reactions, positive and negative, to those characteristics?
- What differences do I think may exist between the patient and myself, and what assumptions have I made based on them?
- Have I given the patient the opportunity to express his or her treatment beliefs, values, norms, expectations, and concerns?

So too, the nurse should be aware of sociocultural stressors that can hinder the delivery of psychiatric care (Barbee, 2002; Banks-Wallace and Parks, 2001). These are listed in Box 8-3. Disadvantagement creates profound problems in the prevention, diagnosis, and treatment of psychiatric disorders. In addition to lacking basic resources, people who are poor and poorly educated are often stereotyped in society as being freeloaders or lazy. Such people are often the focus of bias and other negative attitudes and behaviors such as intolerance, stigma, prejudice, discrimination, and racism (Snowden, 2003).

Social, cultural, and spiritual assessment of the patient, including personal risk and protective factors, greatly enhances the nurse's ability to establish a therapeutic alliance, identify the patient's problems, and develop a treatment plan that is accurate, appropriate, and culturally relevant. Box 8-4 presents questions the nurse might ask related to each of the factors described in this chapter.

BOX 8-3

Sociocultural Stressors

Disadvantagement: The lack of socioeconomic resources that are basic to biopsychosocial adaptation

Discrimination: Differential treatment of individuals or groups not based on actual merit

Intolerance: Unwillingness to accept different opinions or beliefs from people of different backgrounds

Prejudice: A preconceived, unfavorable belief about individuals or groups that disregards knowledge, thought, or reason

Racism: The belief that inherent differences among the races determine individual achievement and that one race is superior

Stereotype: A depersonalized conception of individuals within a group

Stigma: An attribute or trait deemed by the person's social environment as unfavorable

---

BOX 8-4

Questions Related to Sociocultural Risk and Protective Factors

Age
Questions
What is the patient's current stage of development?
What are the developmental tasks of the patient?
Are those tasks age-appropriate for the patient?
What are the patient's attitudes and beliefs regarding the patient's age-group?
With what age-related stressors is the patient coping?
What impact does the patient's age have on mental and physical health?

Example
Assessment. Jim is 38 years old and trying to come to terms with balancing his need for intimacy with that of finding his own identity and sense of purpose in life. He describes feelings of anxiety along with waves of hopelessness. He states, "At my age I should stop acting like I'm twenty-something and accept myself, but I just can't seem to do that."

Evaluation. Jim is worried that he will never settle down into an adult lifestyle, but he is more afraid of the high stress and loss of social attractiveness that he associates with being middle-aged.

Ethnicity
Questions
What is the patient's ethnic background?
What is the patient's ethnic identity?
Is the patient traditional, bicultural, multicultural, or culturally alienated?
What are the patient's attitudes, beliefs, and values regarding his or her ethnic group?
With what ethnicity-related stressors is the patient coping?
What impact does the person's ethnicity have on mental and physical health?

Example
Assessment. Landa is a black woman. She strongly endorses African-American values and considers herself to be culturally traditional. Landa believes that African-American values are superior to Western values and that there would be less poverty and crime in black communities if all black people shared her beliefs. She spends much of her time reading about traditional African ways and has become isolated from her friends and family.

Continued

BOX 8-4

Questions Related to Sociocultural Risk and Protective Factors—cont'd

Ethnicity—cont'd
Example—cont'd
Evaluation. Landa lacks the social support she needs to feel good about her ethnicity without having to idealize or reject members of her own or other ethnic groups. She is having difficulty integrating her values with those of her family and friends.

Gender
Questions
What is the patient's gender?

What is the patient's gender identity?

How does the patient define gender-specific roles?

What are the patient's attitudes and beliefs regarding males and females and masculinity and femininity?

With what gender-related stressors is the patient coping?

What impact does the person's gender have on mental and physical health?

Example
Assessment. Kelly is male, and enacting the male role is very important to him. As a man, he feels he must provide for his family by working hard, making money, and being smart. Kelly feels that his wife should respect how hard he works and support his plans for providing for her. Recently, he and his wife have had increasing marital conflict. He states, "I am doing what is right for both of us. All my wife has to do is help me." Yet Kelly states that his wife does not want him to work 7 days a week and that she does not want to wait until he builds their house before she can go to college. He reports drinking more in the past couple of months and admits that it is difficult for him to express his emotional needs or to respond to those of his wife.

Evaluation. Kelly defines masculinity as authority, and it is extremely important to his self-image. He is unable to express feelings and is struggling to maintain a self-ideal that is in conflict with his wife's needs for her own growth as an individual and as a spouse.

Education
Questions
What is the patient's education level?

What were the patient's educational experiences like?

What are the patient's attitudes and beliefs regarding education in general and the patient's own education in particular?

With what education-related stressors is the patient coping?

What impact does the patient's education have on mental and physical health?

Example
Assessment. Ron completed eighth grade and then dropped out of school. He learned to be a plumber by working with a family friend who owned a plumbing business. Recently the friend retired and sold the business to Ron. Ron wants his son to work with him and learn the business, but his son wants to go to college. Ron and his son have been having violent fights about this issue, and Ron has told him, "College is what you do when you don't know anything. Do you think that by going to college you'll be better than me?"

Evaluation. Ron feels bad about his lack of formal education and the negative stereotypes people hold about plumbers. His insecurity makes him unable to support his son's desire to attend college because he fears that his relationship with his son will suffer and that his son will think less of him in the future.

Income
Questions
What is the patient's income?

What is the source of the patient's income?

How does the patient describe his or her income group?

What are the patient's attitudes and beliefs regarding personal socioeconomic status?

With what income-related stressors is the patient coping?

What type of health insurance does the patient have, if any?

What impact does the patient's income have on mental and physical health?

Example
Assessment. Amanda is unemployed. She has always believed that people who are in good health should work; however, Amanda has never been employed. She married a wealthy, older man when she was 19 years old, and for 10 years he supported her. Then with no warning, her husband left the country with a younger woman and filed for divorce. Amanda states, "He left me. I'm penniless. I'm homeless. I'm nothing." Her family is middle-income and is willing to help her if she gets a job, but she is unwilling to interview for a job because the concept of paid employment conflicts with her self-concept of being a wealthy wife.

Evaluation. Amanda's self-concept and self-esteem were based on her marriage and financial status. She never imagined being without these things, and she feels unprepared and resentful of the changes she needs to make.

Beliefs
Questions
What are the patient's beliefs about health and illness?

What was the patient's religious or spiritual upbringing?

What are the patient's current religious or spiritual beliefs?

Who is the patient's regular health care provider?

With what belief system–related stressors is the patient coping?

What impact does the patient's belief system have on mental and physical health?

Example
Assessment. Xiao believes that illness of the mind is correct punishment. Since her mother's death 2 months ago, she has experienced insomnia, fatigue, and weight loss. She and her mother argued frequently, including the morning her mother had a fatal car accident on her way to work. Xiao now avoids her family and for the last week has been unable to go to work. Xiao states, "I did not love my mother and now I am being punished. No one can help me."

Evaluation. Xiao is unable to resolve her feelings about her mother and to grieve her loss adaptively. She feels guilt about her arguments with her mother and welcomes depression as a correct punishment. Because of this belief, seeking help is unacceptable.

A culturally competent psychiatric nursing diagnosis appropriately considers relevant social, cultural, and spiritual characteristics of the patient. Often, nurses exclude sociocultural information in their analysis because they want to avoid stereotyping the patient, feel that the patient's health care problems are not related to the patient's age, ethnicity, gender, income, education, or beliefs or incorrectly assume that the patient shares their worldview.

However, social, cultural, and spiritual information must be included in each phase of the nursing process because it has a significant influence on the patient's coping responses. Conversations with patients about their values, norms, and beliefs are not likely to require substantial increases in nursing time, effort, or skill; but not having these conversations could needlessly undermine care.

Do you think it is possible that two patients displaying the same symptoms could receive two different diagnoses based on the sociocultural factors of age, ethnicity, and gender of either the patient or the clinician? ■

■ TREATMENT IMPLICATIONS

Awareness that the psychotherapeutic treatment process is influenced by the cultural and ethnic context of both the patient and the health care provider is growing (see Critical Thinking About Contemporary Issues). Yet few studies are available that document the successful outcomes of mental health intervention among multicultural populations.

However, it has been suggested that the following aspects of care can help to reduce racial and ethnic health disparities:

Critical Thinking *About* Contemporary Issues

Should Ethnic Minority Patients Be Treated by White Therapists?

The effectiveness of psychotherapy for ethnic minority patients, especially when treated by white therapists, is controversial. Some researchers and practitioners believe that ethnic minority patients are less likely to benefit from treatment. Others maintain that ethnic minority patients are just as likely as whites to show favorable outcomes from treatment and that studies of ethnic or racial matching of patients have failed to show different outcomes on the basis of the race or ethnicity of the patients and clinicians.

It is likely that ethnicity or race by itself tells very little about the values, attitudes, and experiences of patients and clinicians who engage in the treatment process. Thus ethnic matches can result in cultural mismatches, as patients and clinicians from the same ethnic group may show markedly different values. Conversely, ethnic mismatches may be cultural matches because patients and clinicians from different ethnic groups may share similar values, lifestyles, and expectations. Thus sociocultural sensitivity includes respect for individual differences regardless of one's age, ethnicity, gender, education, income, or belief system. The consideration of all of these characteristics and the ability to individualize patient care appear to be the best predictors of treatment outcome.

interpreter services, recruitment and retention of minority staff, cultural competency training programs, coordination with traditional healers, use of community health workers, culturally competent health promotion, inclusion of family and community members, immersion into another culture, and administrative and organizational accommodations (Brach and Fraser, 2000).

In terms of treatment planning, it is clear that the psychiatric nurse needs to be sensitive to sociocultural issues but also must transcend them. Together, the nurse and patient need to agree on the nature of the patient's coping responses, the means for solving problems, and the expected outcomes of treatment. A central responsibility of the nurse is to understand what the illness means to the patient and the way in which the patient's beliefs can help to mediate the stressful events or make them easier to bear by redefining them as opportunities for personal growth.

Considered central to the delivery of effective psychiatric nursing care, cultural competency improves the quality of nurse-patient interactions and patient satisfaction, two aspects of treatment that can have significant treatment outcome implications. Treatment outcome research that includes comparisons of different cultural competency practice strategies is needed to help determine best practice guidelines. Informed by such data, psychiatric nurses will be better able to reduce disparities in psychiatric service utilization rates and improve nurse-patient interactions and treatment outcomes.

Service Utilization

An important first consideration for effective treatment is the design of a culturally competent mental health service delivery system. Patients desire accessible, affordable, psychiatric care delivered by skilled professionals who reflect important social, cultural, and spiritual characteristics of their communities. To successfully deliver such services, mental health providers have to make a major commitment to building community relationships, receiving continuing education training in cultural competency, and translating research into action (Aguilar-Gaxiola et al, 2002). Mental health care programs need to find ways to ensure the active participation of patient community representatives in the design, delivery, and evaluation of psychiatric services.

A culturally competent mental health care system acknowledges the importance of culture and incorporates this value into all levels of care. To do this requires the assessment of cross-cultural relations, an understanding of the dynamics of cultural differences, an expansion of knowledge about different cultures, and a commitment to adapt services to meet culturally based needs. In this way, culturally competent mental health care provides better access to more appropriate, effective care and the opportunity for improved outcomes.

Specifically, service delivery can be improved through cultural and clinical consultation by experts in the care of all populations, including ethnic and cultural minorities and those with physical disabilities. Service use can be improved by the standardization of clinical assessment and treatment guidelines that address patients' cultural issues.

In addition, delivery systems should be sensitive to the fact that if a mental health service operates under the auspices of a dominant ethnic, socioeconomic, or religious group, people not of that group may feel uncomfortable or unable to access that service. Staffing also has been shown to affect service use by minorities in that use of diverse staff who understand the language and culture of patients enhances service use.

Finally, an administrative environment must be created that places importance on the role of culture in understanding mental illness and treatment. Criteria should be established that holds clinicians accountable for practicing in culturally appropriate ways and provides them with the necessary tools, training, and performance measurements (Siegel et al, 2000).

The Center for Mental Health Services funded a report (1998) urging that all public and private mental health agencies be staffed with culturally competent and appropriately qualified bicultural and bilingual personnel. Specific standards, along with 16 guiding principles, form the basis of the report and are complemented by guidelines for implementation. Despite efforts such as these and public campaigns promoting more accessible and more appropriate mental health care services, low treatment utilization rates among vulnerable patient population groups continues to be a major concern.

Look around at the furniture, pictures, and other aspects of the environment in one of your clinical settings. What does it express about culture? Would an African-American, Asian, or Latino feel comfortable in this setting? ■

Therapeutic Nurse-Patient Interactions

Culturally responsive counseling strategies should consider ethnic identity and acculturation, family influences, sex-role socialization, religious and spiritual influences, and immigration experiences. In addition, sociocultural differences between the nurse and patient can be a source of misunderstanding by the nurse and resistance by the patient.

Expert nurses have learned the importance and treatment value of nurse-patient interactions, as well as their endless potential for problems such as patient misperceptions of nurse disinterest, disapproval, or disrespect. Many vulnerable sociocultural groups are wary of psychiatric care and fear that the costs of treatment may include their dignity. Alternatively, healthy recognition of nurse-patient sociocultural differences can enrich the health care experience for both the nurse and patient (Hines-Martin, 2002; Mahoney and Engebretson, 2000; Thorton and Tuck, 2000).

Family systems, friends, and community groups can be major sources of strength for people with mental illness. Nurses should view them as allies and integral components of the treatment process. Families can provide an important economic and emotional buffer against the burden imposed by the patient's illness and give the patient a supportive environment for recovery. Support networks also are sources of economic, social, and emotional relief from the many personal and social burdens of psychiatric disorders.

Religion also can be a core social and spiritual resource. Patients with religious, faith-based, or spiritual networks may wish to have their network serve as an active component of their psychiatric care and the sociocultural context for their recovery (Tuck, Pullen, and Warren, 2001). They also may look to their religious and spiritual relationships for guidance with psychiatric disorders. African-American and Latino communities are two examples of the many population groups that have church- and faith-based sociocultural traditions.

As with any network, membership offers collective support, opportunities for self-expression, and the ability to help others, which can give meaning to life. Supernatural belief systems also may provide a natural support system for people with mental illness, as well as a culturally based way of understanding how the illness fits into the patient's life. For example, some people believe they are looked after by a protective "angel." Whatever the context, culturally competent nurses should support adaptive patient beliefs and strive to incorporate them into their nurse-patient interactions.

Psychopharmacology

Patients' social, cultural, and spiritual attributes can have obvious and subtle effects on their attitudes and behaviors regarding psychiatric medications (Lutz and Warren, 2001). Specifically, a patient's ethnicity, gender, beliefs, and age can impact medication pharmacokinetics, pharmacodynamics, effectiveness, and side-effect risks. For example, ethnicity is one of the most important variables that contribute to variations in patients' biological responses to medications (Flaskerud, 2000). Racial and ethnic differences in response to psychotropic drugs include the following:

- Extrapyramidal effects at lower dosage levels for Asians
- Lower effective dosage levels and a lower side-effect threshold for antidepressants among Hispanics
- Higher red blood cell plasma-lithium ratio in blacks

Gender differences also may result in the need for different doses of psychotropic drugs. For example, women secrete 40% less stomach acid than men, so drugs such as tricyclic antidepressants, benzodiazepines, and certain antipsychotic drugs are more likely to be absorbed before they can be neutralized by the acid, thus requiring a lower dose of the drug. In addition, over time, women accumulate more of a drug in their bodies than men do because fatty tissue stores psychotropic drugs longest.

Whereas ethnicity and gender can have direct and indirect psychopharmacology effects, cultural and spiritual beliefs can have somewhat unpredictable effects. Some religious tenants reject the consumption of drugs for any purpose despite the trend of medications becoming the first line of treatment for an increasing number of psychiatric disorders.

The social stigma attached to all psychiatric medications is yet another powerful influence that must be considered. People who view psychiatric disorders as personal failings rather than disorders may have great ambivalence about taking psychiatric medications and stop taking recommended medications despite full symptom relief and meaningful improvement in psychosocial functioning.

Some patients may seriously question taking any medication designed to alter brain functioning for sociocultural reasons. Secondhand stories of the medication experiences of others, reports found on Internet websites, media articles, and direct marketing are just a few of the formidable patient information sources that nurses must understand. Black American patients may have undisclosed mistrust of all prescription medications, and persistent health disparities among blacks and a sad history of racial exploitation

may account for their sometimes fatalistic attitude towards illness.

Equally important is that indigenous systems of health beliefs and practices persist in all societies, including those exposed to modern Western medicine. The nurse should keep in mind that, despite the availability of Western medicine, traditional herbal medicines continue to be used extensively by many different cultural groups living in the United States, and some of these drugs have active pharmacological properties that may interfere with other medications. Dramatic increases in the availability of herbal medicines and remedies from around the world ensure that public interest in and use of such products will continue.

CHAPTER FOCUS POINTS

- Social, cultural, and spiritual characteristics can impact a person's access to mental health care, risk for or protection against developing a certain psychiatric disorder, how symptoms will be experienced and expressed, the ease or difficulty of participating in psychiatric treatment, and one's ability to achieve recovery.
- Cultural competency is the ability to view each patient as a unique individual, fully considering the patient's cultural experiences within the context of the common developmental challenges faced by all people.
- The culturally competent nurse understands the importance of social, cultural, and spiritual forces, recognizes the uniqueness of each patient, respects nurse-patient differences, and incorporates sociocultural information into psychiatric nursing care.
- Risk factors for psychiatric disorders are characteristics of a person that can significantly increase the potential for developing a psychiatric disorder, decrease the potential for recovery, or both. Protective factors are characteristics of a person that can significantly decrease the potential for developing a psychiatric disorder, increase the potential for recovery, or both.
- The culturally competent nurse does not assume knowledge of a patient based on casual observations of age, ethnicity, or gender. Neither should a nurse draw generalizations about groups based on these factors.
- Age-related variations in life stressors, support resources, and coping skills are common.
- For ethnic and racial minority groups, personal protective factors often are embedded in a tightly woven social identity. Members of minorities often have difficulty gaining access to appropriate mental health services. Ethnicity also has been shown to influence the development of and recovery from psychiatric disorders.
- When all psychiatric disorders are included, the prevalence of mental illness among males and females is roughly equal. The actual

difference between the two groups is in the type of disorder that is most commonly diagnosed.
- Numerous studies identify the importance of education as a coping resource in protecting against the development of and promoting recovery from mental illness.
- The profound negative impact of poverty as a risk factor for psychiatric illness is evident regardless of age, ethnicity, gender, or education.
- Adaptive belief systems, worldview, religion, or spirituality can enhance well-being, improve quality of life, and support recovery from psychiatric disorders. Maladaptive belief systems may contribute to poor adjustment to changes in health status, refusal or nonadherence with needed treatment, or even self-injury.
- Social, cultural, and spiritual assessment of the patient, including personal risk and protective factors, greatly enhances the nurse's ability to establish a therapeutic alliance, identify the patient's problems, and develop a treatment plan that is accurate, appropriate, and culturally relevant. Together, the nurse and patient need to agree on the nature of the patient's coping responses, the means for solving problems, and the expected outcomes of treatment.
- A culturally competent mental health care system assesses cross-cultural relations, understands the dynamics of cultural differences, expands knowledge about different cultures, and is committed to adapt services to meet culturally based needs.
- Culturally responsive counseling strategies should consider ethnic identity and acculturation, family influences, sex-role socialization, religious and spiritual influences, and immigration experiences.
- A patient's ethnicity, gender, beliefs, and age can impact medication pharmacokinetics, pharmacodynamics, effectiveness, and side-effect risks.

KEY TERMS

cultural competency, 121
disadvantagement, 127
discrimination, 127
ethnicity, 123

intolerance, 127
prejudice, 127
protective factors, 122
racism, 127

risk factors, 122
stereotype, 127
stigma, 127

CHAPTER REVIEW QUESTIONS

1. Match each term in Column A with the correct definition in Column B.

Column A

_____ Disadvantagement
_____ Discrimination
_____ Intolerance
_____ Prejudice
_____ Racism
_____ Stereotype
_____ Stigma

Column B

A. A depersonalized conception of individuals within a group
B. A preconceived, unfavorable belief about individuals or groups that disregards knowledge, thought, or reason
C. An attribute or trait deemed by the person's social environment as unfavorable
D. Differential treatment of individuals or groups not based on actual merit
E. The belief that inherent differences among the races determine individual achievement and that one race is superior
F. The lack of socioeconomic resources that are basic to biopsychosocial adaptation
G. Unwillingness to accept different opinions or beliefs from people of different backgrounds

2. Fill in the blanks.

A. The main message of the Surgeon General's report on culture and mental health is that _____.

B. The term _____ is used to describe a person's racial, national, tribal, linguistic, or cultural origin or background.

C. _____ and _____ disorders are the most prevalent psychiatric disorders among males.

D. _____ and _____ disorders are the most prevalent psychiatric disorders among females.

E. The prevalence of _____ and _____ disorders is about equal for males and females.

F. Risk factors are characteristics of an individual that can significantly _____ a person's potential for developing a psychiatric disorder or significantly _____ the potential for recovery, or both.

G. The five constructs of cultural competency identified by Campinha-Bacote are (1) _____, (2) _____, (3) _____, (4) _____, and (5) _____.

3. Indicate whether the following statements are true (T) or false (F).

_____ A. Evidence that age can be a protective factor is consistent across cultures.
_____ B. Ethnicity only serves as a risk factor for psychiatric illness.
_____ C. Education is a protective factor and contributes to adaptive coping.
_____ D. Poverty compounds the impact of all other risk factors.

4. Provide short answers for the following questions.

A. Define cultural competency.
B. Give an example of how your cultural background influences your perceptions, motives, individual identity, group identity, values, and communication.
C. Think about the facility in which you are having your psychiatric nursing experience. Evaluate whether it meets the criteria of a culturally competent mental health delivery system as described in this chapter.

Visit Evolve for additional resources related to the content of this chapter.

http://evolve.elsevier.com/Stuart/principles/
• Topical Course Outline • Student Workbook Exercises • Critical Thinking Questions and Activities • Case Studies • Research Topics
• Monthly Content Updates • WebLinks

Student Study CD-ROM

Access the accompanying CD-ROM for animations, interactive exercises, review questions for the NCLEX examination, and an audio glossary.

REFERENCES

Alegria M et al: Inequalities in use of specialty mental health services among Latinos, African Americans, and non-Latino whites, *Psychiatr Serv* 53:1547, 2002.

Aguilar-Gaxiola AA et al: Translating research into action: reducing disparities in mental health care for Mexican Americans, *Psychiatr Serv* 53:11563, 2002.

Baker FM, Bell CC: Issues in the psychiatric treatment of African Americans, *Psychiatr Serv* 50:362, 1999.

Banks-Wallace J, Parks L: "So that our souls don't get damaged": the impact of racism on maternal thinking and practice related to the protection of daughters, *Issues Ment Health Nurs* 22:77, 2001.

Barbee E: Racism and mental health, *J Am Psychiatr Nurs Assoc* 8:194, 2002.

Brach C, Fraser I: Can cultural competency reduce racial and ethnic health disparities? A review and conceptual model, *Med Care Res and Rev* 57(Suppl 1):181, 2000.

Campinha-Bacote J: Cultural competence in psychiatric nursing: Have you asked the right questions? *J Am Psychiatr Nurs Assoc* 8:183, 2002.

Cattell V: Poor people, poor places, and poor health: the mediating role of social networks and social capital, *Soc Sci Med* 52:1501, 2001.

Center for Mental Health Services, *Cultural competence standards*, Rockville, Md, 1998, Center for Mental Health Services.

Donnelly TT: Contextual analysis of coping: implications for immigrants' mental health care, *Issues Ment Health Nurs* 23:715, 2002.

Dreher M, MacNaughton N: Cultural competence in nursing: foundation or fallacy? *Nurs Outlook* 50: 181, 2002.

Flaskerud JH: Ethnicity, culture and neuropsychiatry, *Issues Ment Health Nurs* 21:5, 2000.

Galanter M: Healing through social and spiritual affiliation, *Psychiatr Serv* 53:1072, 2002.

Gearon J, Tamminga C: Gender differences in schizophrenia, *J Calif Alliance Mentally Ill* 10(4):11, 2000.

Hines-Martin V: African American consumers: what should we know to meet their mental health needs? *J Am Psychiatr Nurs Assoc* 8:188, 2002.

Hines-Martin V et al: Barriers to mental health care access in an African American population, *Issues Ment Health Nurs* 24:237, 2003.

Hoffman S, Hatch MC: Depressive symptomatology during pregnancy: evidence for an association with decreased fetal growth in pregnancies of lower social class women, *Health Psychol* 19:535, 2000.

Horsfall J: Gender and mental illness: an Australian overview, *Issues Ment Health Nurs* 22:421, 2001.

Hough RL et al: Mental health services for Latino adolescents with psychiatric disorders, *Psychiatr Serv* 53:1556, 2002.

Husaini BA et al: Racial differences in the diagnosis of dementia and in its effects on the use and costs of health care services, *Psychiatr Serv* 54:92, 2003.

Johnson JL, Cameron MC: Barriers to providing effective mental health services to American Indians, *Ment Health Serv Res* 3:215, 2001.

Kendler KS et al: Dimensions of religiosity and their relationship to lifetime psychiatric and substance use disorders, *Am J Psychiatry* 160:496, 2003.

Koenig HG et al: *Handbook of religion and health*, Oxford, 2001, University Press.

Kreyenbuhl J et al: Racial disparity in the pharmacological management of schizophrenia, *Schizophr Bull* 29:183, 2003.

Leong FT, Lau AS: Barriers to providing effective mental health services to Asian Americans, *Ment Health Serv Res* 3:201, 2001.

Lutz W, Warren B: Symptomatology and medication monitoring for public mental health consumers: a cultural perspective, *J Am Psychiatr Nurs Assoc* 7:115, 2001.

McCrae RR et al: Age differences in personality across the adult life span: parallels in five cultures, *Dev Psychol* 35:466, 1999.

Mahoney JS, Engebretson J: The interface of anthropology and nursing guiding culturally competent care in psychiatric nursing, *Arch Psychiatr Nurs* 14:183, 2000.

New Freedom Commission on Mental Health, *Achieving the promise: transforming mental health care in America, final report*, DHHS Pub. No. SMA-03-3832, Rockville, Maryland, 2003, USDHHS.

Piccinelli M, Wilkinson G: Gender difference in depression, *Br J Psychiatry* 177:486, 2000.

Shin J: Help seeking behaviors by Korean immigrants for depression, *Issues Ment Health Nurs* 23:461, 2002.

Siegel C et al: Performance measures of cultural competency in mental health organizations, *Adm Policy Ment Health* 28:91, 2000.

Snowden LR: Barriers to effective mental health services for African Americans, *Ment Health Serv Res* 3:181, 2001.

Snowden LR: Bias in mental health assessment and intervention: theory and evidence, *Am J Public Health* 93:239, 2003.

Snowden LR, Pingitore D: Frequency and scope of mental health service delivery to African Americans in primary care, *Ment Health Serv Res* 4:123, 2002.

Thorton K, Tuck I: Promoting the mental health of elderly African Americans: a case illustration, *Arch Psychiatr Nurs* 14:191, 2000.

Trierweiler SJ et al: Clinician attributions associated with the diagnosis of schizophrenia in African-American and non-African American patients, *J Consult Clin Psychol* 68:171, 2000.

Tuck I, Pullen L, Wallace D: A comparative study of the spiritual perspectives and interventions of mental health and parish nurses, *Issues Ment Health Nurs* 22:593, 2001.

US Dept Health and Human Services: *Mental health: culture, race and ethnicity*, Rockville Md, 2001, Office of the Surgeon General.

Vega WA, Lopez SR: Priority issues in Latino mental health services research, *Ment Health Serv Res* 3:189, 2001.

Warren B: Cultural competence: a best practice process for psychiatric-mental health nursing, *J Am Psychiatr Nurs Assoc* 66:135, 2000.

Warren B: The interlocking paradigm of cultural competence: a best practice approach, *J Am Psychiatr Nurs Assoc* 8:209, 2002.

Weinick R, Zuvekas S, Cohen J: Racial and ethnic differences in access to and use of health care services, 1977 to 1996, *Med Care Res Rev* 57(Suppl 1):36, 2000.

Wells K et al: Ethnic disparities in unmet need for alcoholism, drug abuse, and mental health care, *Am J Psychiatry* 158:2027, 2001.

Yeh M et al: Referral sources, diagnoses, and service types in youth in public outpatient mental health care: a focus on ethnic minorities, *J Behav Health Serv Res* 29:45, 2002.

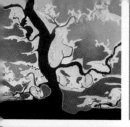

There is a tide in the affairs of men, Which, when taken at the flood, leads on to fortune; Omitted, all the voyage of their life Is bound in shallows and in miseries. On such a full sea are we now afloat. And we must take the current when it serves, Or lose our ventures.

WILLIAM SHAKESPEARE, ACT IV, SCENE III, *JULIUS CAESAR*

9 ENVIRONMENTAL CONTEXT OF PSYCHIATRIC NURSING CARE

Gail W. Stuart

LEARNING OBJECTIVES

After studying this chapter, the student should be able to:

1. Describe global and national perspectives on psychiatric care (I).
2. Analyze the current mental health delivery system, including the characteristics of managed behavioral health care and payment and cost-control mechanisms (II).
3. Examine problems and opportunities in accessing behavioral health services (III).
4. Discuss clinical appropriateness and medical necessity in the provision of psychiatric services (IV).
5. Evaluate issues of accountability in relation to patients, providers, and service settings (V).
6. Apply knowledge about the environment of psychiatric care to psychiatric nursing practice (VI).

TOPICAL OUTLINE

I. Environmental Perspectives
   A. The Global View
   B. The National View
II. Mental Health Delivery System
   A. Managed Behavioral Health Care
III. Access to Services
   A. Employee Assistance Programs
   B. Treatment Parity
   C. Telepsychiatry
IV. Clinical Appropriateness
   A. Medical Necessity
V. Accountability Issues
   A. Consumer Empowerment
   B. Provider Concerns
   C. Service Settings
VI. Impact on Psychiatric Nursing
   A. Roles in Managed Care
   B. Threats and Opportunities

 Visit Evolve for additional resources related to the content of this chapter.
http://evolve.elsevier.com/Stuart/principles/

The environment affects every aspect of a person's life and well-being. Physical aspects of the environment, such as chemicals and contaminants, have a direct impact on health. Equally as important are the structural aspects of the environment. This would include the way a society organizes its health care system, how it finances it, the priorities of care it establishes, and the resources it makes available to individuals, families, and communities to promote and preserve health.

To be an effective caregiver, a nurse must be knowledgeable about the structural aspects of the environment as it relates to health care. The best interventions and most advanced technology will be of little benefit to patients if they cannot gain access to them, cannot afford them, or find them unacceptable.

Nowhere is this more important than in the area of mental health care. Each day, environmental forces shape, support, challenge, block, and defeat how well the mental health needs of individuals, families, and communities are met. Competent psychiatric nurses need to understand mental health–related policies, the way mental health care is organized and delivered, how mental health care is paid for, and the role of psychiatric nurses in the broader mental health care environment.

ENVIRONMENTAL PERSPECTIVES

The environmental context of psychiatric care can be viewed from a global and a national perspective. As citizens of the world, both views are important contexts of care for the psychiatric nurse.

The Global View

The World Bank, the World Health Organization, and several private foundations funded a major study that assessed premature death and disability from diseases and injuries around the world (Murray and Lopez, 1996). It compared a range of physical and mental disorders to determine their contribution to the burden of disease. The data showed that:

- Depression was the number one psychiatric cause of disability in the world.
- Four other psychiatric disorders were among the top 10: alcohol use, bipolar disorder, schizophrenia, and obsessive-compulsive disorder.
- Depression ranked second in the United States as a cause of disability.
- Depression was projected to rank second in the world as a cause of disability by 2020.

This study raised a global awareness of the impact that psychiatric disorders have on the lives of people around the world each and every day.

The National View

Three important reports compiled in the United States also promise to impact the delivery of psychiatric care. The most recent one is the report of the New Freedom Commission on Mental Health, *Achieving the Promise: Transforming Mental Health Care in America* (NFCMH, 2003). The commission, which was established by Executive Order on April 29, 2002, was formed to address the problems in the mental health service delivery system that allow Americans to fall through the system's "cracks."

The commission found that the current system is unintentionally focused on managing disabilities associated with mental illness rather than promoting recovery. This is because of fragmentation, gaps in care, and uneven quality in mental health services. Instead, the commission recommends a focus on promoting recovery and building resilience—the ability to withstand stresses and life challenges (see Chapter 15).

The commission identified six goals and a series of recommendations for federal agencies, states, communities, and providers nationwide. These are listed in Box 9-1. It is hoped, that working together with the public and private sectors, these recommendations will achieve the needed transformation in mental health care and put the country's limited resources to their best use.

BOX 9-1

Goals and Recommendations in a Transformed Mental Health System

Goal 1   Americans Understand That Mental Health Is Essential to Overall Health.
Recommendations
1.1 Advance and implement a national campaign to reduce the stigma of seeking care and a national strategy for suicide prevention.
1.2 Address mental health with the same urgency as physical health.

Goal 2   Mental Health Care Is Consumer and Family Driven.
Recommendations
2.1 Develop an individualized plan of care for every adult with a serious mental illness and every child with a serious emotional disturbance.
2.2 Involve consumers and families fully in orienting the mental health system toward recovery.
2.3 Align relevant Federal programs to improve access and accountability for mental health services.
2.4 Create a Comprehensive State Mental Health Plan.
2.5 Protect and enhance the rights of people with mental illness.

Goal 3   Disparities in Mental Health Services Are Eliminated.
Recommendations
3.1 Improve access to quality care that is culturally competent.
3.2 Improve access to quality care in rural and geographically remote areas.

Goal 4   Early Mental Health Screening, Assessment, and Referral to Services Are Common Practice.
Recommendations
4.1 Promote the mental health of young children.
4.2 Improve and expand school mental health programs.
4.3 Screen for co-occurring mental and substance use disorders and link with integrated treatment strategies.
4.4 Screen for mental disorders in primary health care, across the life span, and connect to treatment and supports.

Goal 5   Excellent Mental Health Care Is Delivered and Research Is Accelerated.
Recommendations
5.1 Accelerate research to promote recovery and resilience and, ultimately, to cure and prevent mental illness.
5.2 Advance evidence-based practices using dissemination and demonstration projects and create a public-private partnership to guide their implementation.
5.3 Improve and expand the workforce providing evidence-based mental health services and supports.
5.4 Develop the knowledge base in four understudied areas: mental health disparities, long-term effects of medications, trauma, and acute care.

Goal 6   Technology Is Used to Access Mental Health Care and Information.
Recommendations
6.1 Use health technology and telehealth to improve access and coordination of mental health care, especially for Americans in remote areas or in underserved populations.
6.2 Develop and implement integrated electronic health record and personal health information systems.

From New Freedom Commission on Mental Health: *Achieving the promise: transforming mental health care in America. Final report*, DHHS Pub. No. SMA-03-3832, Rockville, Md, 2003, USDHHS.

The commission's report follows the first report ever issued by a U.S. Surgeon General on the topic of mental health and mental illness, *Mental Health: A Report of the Surgeon General* (USDHHS, 1999). This report, issued in 1999, was based on an extensive review of the scientific literature and on consultations with mental health providers and consumers. This landmark document concluded that:

- Mental health is fundamental to health.
- Mental disorders are real health conditions that have an immense impact on individuals and families.
- The efficacy of mental health treatments is well documented.
- A range of treatments exists for most mental disorders.

On the strength of the findings in the report, the one explicit recommendation is that people should seek help if they have a mental health problem or think that they have symptoms of a mental disorder.

A third notable report is *Healthy People 2010*, which identified a list of leading health indicators that reflect the major public health concerns in the United States (USDHHS, 2000). These include the following:

- Physical activity
- Overweight and obesity
- Tobacco use
- Substance abuse
- Responsible sexual behavior
- Mental health
- Injury and violence
- Environmental quality
- Immunization
- Access to health care

For each of the leading health indicators, specific objectives derived from *Healthy People 2010* have been identified. The objectives related to mental health are presented in Box 9-2. This set of measures will provide a snapshot of the mental health of the United States and should have a significant impact on psychiatric care in the next decade.

These studies and reports underscore the critical importance of mental health care, and they help advocate for a more effective and efficient mental health delivery system.

Given the recognized importance of mental health problems, why do you think so much stigma surrounds them? ■

■ MENTAL HEALTH DELIVERY SYSTEM

The interface between mental health care and the environment has become increasingly complex. In the past, the mental health care delivery system had only two parts: mental health providers and patients. Now, however, the system has grown to include six forces, each of which must be taken into account when trying to provide psychiatric care (Figure 9-1).

BOX 9-2

Healthy People 2010 Objectives Related to Mental Health

- Reduce the suicide rate.
- Reduce the rate of suicide attempts by adolescents.
- Reduce the proportion of homeless adults who have serious mental illness.
- Increase the proportion of persons with serious mental illnesses who are employed.
- Reduce the relapse rates for persons with eating disorders, including anorexia nervosa and bulimia nervosa.
- Increase the number of persons seen in primary health care who receive mental health screening and assessment.
- Increase the proportion of children with mental health problems who receive treatment.
- Increase the proportion of juvenile justice facilities that screen new admissions for mental health problems.
- Increase the proportion of adults with mental disorders who receive treatment.
- Increase the proportion of persons with co-occurring substance abuse and mental disorders who receive treatment for both disorders.
- Increase the proportion of local governments with community-based jail diversion programs for adults with serious mental illnesses.
- Increase the number of states and the District of Columbia that track consumers' satisfaction with the mental health services they receive.
- Increase the number of states, territories, and the District of Columbia with an operational mental health plan that addresses cultural competence.
- Increase the number of states, territories, and the District of Columbia with an operational mental health plan that addresses mental health crisis interventions, ongoing screening, and treatment services for elderly persons.

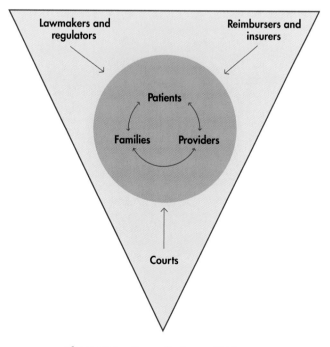

Figure 9-1 Forces affecting psychiatric care.

These groups have related but slightly different interests. For example, **patients** are concerned that appropriate services are available when and where they are needed, and they want to be involved in establishing treatment priorities. **Families** want what is best for their members and are concerned about issues related to quality of life, support, education, and empowerment. **Providers** have clinical and professional biases. If outside controls must exist, providers want them applied fairly, with responsibilities and liabilities clearly defined. **Lawmakers and other regulators** want citizens to have high-quality care at the lowest cost and want providers to be accountable for their care. **Reimbursers and insurance companies** are concerned about paying for covered services by licensed and credentialed professionals and making a profit. Finally, the **courts** want to protect patients' constitutional rights regarding access to care and treatment received. The changing priorities and interactions of these six forces have a direct and sometimes dramatic impact on the quality, availability, and responsiveness of mental health services.

Managed Behavioral Health Care

The phrase "managed care" describes a variety of systems and arrangements for planning, managing, and paying for health services. Some of these systems bring quality to the care setting. Others limit consumer choice and access without supplying the appropriate balances. Managed care means a defined group of people receive treatment services that are clinically necessary, medically appropriate, within defined benefit parameters, for a set amount of time, in compliance with quality standards, and with outcomes that are anticipated and measurable. The term behavioral health is used to describe both mental health and addiction services as one set of health problems. The term *managed behavioral health care* combines the elements of managed care with a focus on psychiatric and addictive disorders (Mechanic, 1999).

Some people support the use of the term behavioral health care, *believing that it helps to reduce the stigma associated with mental illness. Others oppose the term, believing that it discounts the biological basis of mental disorders. What is your position on this issue?* ◼

Managed care differs in some significant ways from the traditional fee-for-service health care delivery system. These differences are outlined in Table 9-1. Each of the characteristics on the left side of the table is described in relation to the traditional fee-for-service health delivery system and a managed care health delivery system. As can be seen from this table, managed care involves a major shift away from the **person-as-customer** to the **population-as-customer**.

It deemphasizes high-cost, episodic inpatient admissions and procedures in favor of creating a full continuum of care and then selecting the correct level of care and treatment setting.

Table 9-1	**Comparison of Traditional and Managed Care Delivery Systems**	
CHARACTERISTIC	TRADITIONAL SYSTEM	MANAGED CARE SYSTEM
Provider focus	Specialized care of individual patient	Total care of member population
Pricing	Separate physician and hospital fee schedules	Discounts, case rate, and capitation
Market share	Number of admissions Number of procedures Number of visits	Number of covered lines
Management focus	High inpatient occupancy rate	Low inpatient occupancy rate Correct level of care
Service line	Acute care programs as drivers: Inconsistent integration Physician dependents Individual services	Continuum of care: Inpatient Partial hospitalization Outpatient Residential Home
Cost management	Payers assume admission rate risk; provider assumes length-of-stay risk	Provider networks assume both admission rate and length-of-stay risk
Costs	Cost per procedure Cost per hospitalization	Cost per life Inpatient days per 1000 Visits per 1000
Competition	Multiple hospitals for communities Duplication of services and technology	Increased consolidation and network formation as occupancy declines Closure of beds Alternative use of hospitals
Outcomes	Qualitative measures: Reputation Facilities	Quantitative measures: Quality Cost
Referral base	Focus on high-tech capabilities and separate physician and hospital marketing efforts	Ability to form primary care networks Mutual goals/strategies of providers and hospitals

Whereas the traditional system fostered duplication of services and technology among hospitals, managed care encourages the consolidation of services, formation of networks, and use of primary care networks for referral and gatekeeping functions.

Managed care is not a single entity. Rather, it has various forms. The most common are health maintenance organizations (HMOs), independent practice associations (IPOs), preferred provider organizations (PPOs), and point-of-service organizations (POSs). Each of these is described in Box 9-3. **Managed competition** is a purchasing strategy in which managed care organizations contract with several hospitals that provide cost-effective, comprehensive services. Consumers are then informed about the hospitals from which they may receive services, even though the facility may not be the patient's preferred choice.

One of your nursing colleagues complains that managed care is really only "managed costs." Based on the characteristics of managed care described in this chapter, how might you respond? ■

In a managed care system, there are three major payment mechanisms: discounted fee-for-service, case rate, and capitation. Under a **discounted fee-for-service** payment plan, clinicians are paid for all services that have been authorized and provided to a consumer. The payment rate is discounted or is less than the clinician's standard fee and often requires that a co-payment be collected from the consumer at the time of each visit.

Under a **case rate** system, the clinician is paid a flat fee for a predefined episode of care. The best known case rate system is Medicare's Diagnostic Related Groups (DRGs). With DRGs, Medicare pays a flat fee for a particular hospitalization episode regardless of how many days the person is hospitalized. This system shifts the financial risk to the provider because the provider receives a flat fee regardless of the actual cost of care.

Under a **capitation** system, the consumer pays a fixed fee or per-member-per-month (PMPM) premium. In return, the managed care company that receives the PMPM fee agrees to provide all medically necessary health care for all covered people. In this case, most of the financial risk lies with the managed care company, which must deliver all necessary health care within the premiums received by their population pool. HMOs are the best-known examples of capitated payment systems.

Managed care exerts cost control measures through, gatekeeping, preadmission certification, utilization review, and case management. These are described in Box 9-4.

BOX 9-3

Types of Managed Care

Health Maintenance Organizations (HMOs):
HMOs are organized delivery systems that provide care to a defined population, usually for a predetermined fixed amount (capitation rate). Consumers enrolled in HMOs are limited to using HMO providers.

Independent Practice Associations (IPOs):
IPOs are plans in which a network of providers serve the enrollees. The insurance plan is capitated, and the providers are free to participate in other types of managed care plans.

Preferred Provider Organizations (PPOs):
PPOs are plans that contract with a limited number of clinicians, most often physicians, and hospitals that provide care at discounted rates. Members of these plans are given financial incentives to use the preferred providers but are not prevented from using other providers. Insurers or employers select the providers to be included in their preferred plan.

Point-of-Service Plans (POSs):
POSs allow consumers to choose between delivery systems at the time they seek care. In a triple-option plan, for example, people can choose among an HMO, PPO, or fee-for-service plan. Financial incentives are usually provided to encourage people to use the least expensive option.

BOX 9-4

Cost Control Strategies of Managed Care

Gatekeeping
Gatekeeping is a process that limits direct access to specialists, hospitals, and expensive procedures. Patients select a primary care provider who manages everyday care and is a gatekeeper for referral to other health care providers. The primary care providers have incentives to be judicious in making referrals.

Preadmission Certification
Preadmission certification takes into account the patient's medical and psychiatric status, level of functioning, socioenvironmental factors, and procedural issues related to treatment. It is the role of the managed care reviewer to determine the most appropriate form of treatment and the proper treatment setting. In this way, the reviewer monitors issues of cost and quality.

Utilization Review
Utilization review evaluates the appropriateness and necessity of health care services and procedures. It is a way of monitoring the care and services administered, and it has the most immediate impact on patient care. The patient's treatment plan, diagnostic and therapeutic interventions, and discharge plan are continuously monitored by a third party. Determination for reimbursement of treatment is made by this third party based on current standards of care. The review and approval can be done before providing the services (precertification review), at the time the service is rendered (concurrent review), or after the service has been provided (retrospective review), which may be used to retroactively deny payment.

Case Management
Case management typically is targeted to patients who have treatment complications, have high-expense episodes of care, or who need alternative, less expensive treatments or settings. This target group often includes those with serious and persistent mental illness. Case management focuses on the achievement of desirable patient outcomes, appropriate lengths of stay, efficient use of resources, and patient involvement and satisfaction.

Today the U.S. government is the largest buyer of health care. Through Medicaid and Medicare and numerous other public programs, it is the single most important purchaser of health care in the United States. It is here where health care reform is taking place and where future action will continue.

Medicaid is a health care entitlement program for Aid to Families with Dependent Children (AFDC) recipients; Supplemental Security Income (SSI) recipients; low-income, disabled, elderly people; low-income pregnant women, infants, and children; and medically needy recipients. The serious and persistently mentally ill are often recipients of Medicaid. The states and the federal government share the costs of this program. Although all states are required to provide a basic set of services, other services can be included or excluded at the discretion of the individual state.

> *Managed behavioral health care companies often employ nurses as utilization reviewers and case managers. Identify the special skills and expertise psychiatric nurses can bring to these roles.* ▪

▪ ACCESS TO SERVICES

Access is the degree to which services and information about health care are easily obtained. It is a critically important part of an effective mental health care delivery system. An ideal comprehensive health care system would provide multiple points of entry for treatment, including direct access through self-referral, by a wide variety of providers.

Today two thirds of the people who seek mental health care are treated by primary care practitioners. However, many who need care do not receive it, either from a primary care or specialty provider. It is also known that when access to mental health care is made difficult, the overall costs of general medical care increase because those with behavioral health care problems are frequent users of medical services. For example, people suffering from panic disorder typically are seen by 10 different health care providers before they are properly diagnosed.

Some access problems apply to the entire health care system, such as the lack of providers in rural areas and care for people who lack health insurance. Other problems are unique to mental health care. These include the stigma associated with seeking care, the lack of knowledge about how to find the right clinician for a highly personal problem, and the lack of general medical settings to adequately respond to mental health and substance abuse disorders.

> *Why do you think that most mental health care is given in primary care settings? Do you think primary care providers are prepared to give this type of care?* ▪

Employee Assistance Programs

Employee assistance programs (EAPs) are worksite-based programs designed to help identify and resolve behavioral, health, and productivity problems that may affect employees' well-being or job performance. Their focus is wide ranging, covering alcohol and other drug abuse; physical and emotional health; and marital, family, financial, legal, and other personal concerns. As such, they are important points of access to behavioral health care.

EAPs have developed from first being primarily alcoholism assessment and referral centers to being specialized behavioral health programs. Many cost-effectiveness studies document the value of these programs in providing workplace education, skill development, and policy and environmental changes.

Comprehensive EAPs are defined by six major components: identification of problems based on job performance, consultation with supervisors, constructive confrontation, evaluation and referral, liaison with treatment providers, and substance abuse expertise. They thus represent a rich foundation on which other services may be added to promote access to mental health and substance abuse treatment.

Treatment Parity

Many of the people who need treatment for mental and chemical dependency disorders do not receive it because their insurance policies deny or restrict coverage for the treatment of these illnesses. Historically, insurers and employers have been cautious about offering mental health and substance abuse coverage, often believing that mental disorders were not treatable or were too expensive to treat. In recent years, mental health advocates and professionals have placed increased emphasis on parity in insurance coverage between physical and mental health services.

There have been some wins and losses in that struggle in the United States. A loss for the field was reflected in a law passed by Congress in 1996. It ended the cash benefits as well as Medicare and Medicaid coverage for people whose disability is based on drug addiction or alcoholism. A win for mental health treatment was the adoption of treatment parity legislation in many states and passage of The National Mental Health Parity Act in 1996 and its extension through 2003. The law requires parity in annual and lifetime dollar limits only. Thus it still does not ensure true parity of mental health with physical health coverage.

Evidence suggests that this law did not broaden access to mental health services as intended. As of 2002, 34 states had some degree of mental health parity. State laws differ from each other in conditions served, specificity of parity, minimum benefits, approved providers, managed care usage, exemptions, and populations covered (Peck and Scheffler, 2002).

Both economics and stigma have been cited as reasons for the lack of parity between coverage for mental and physical illnesses (Barry and Frank, 2002). Yet a government-sponsored study on the costs and effects of parity for mental health and substance abuse insurance benefits found that (Sing et al, 1998):

- Most state parity laws are limited in scope or application.
- State parity laws have had a small effect on premiums.
- Employers have not attempted to avoid parity laws by becoming self-insured, and they do not tend to pass on the costs of parity to employees.
- Costs for mental health and substance abuse services have not shifted from the public to the private sector.

Furthermore, a Mental Health Parity Survey conducted by the National Mental Health Association in 2002 found that 83% of Americans believe that it is unfair for health insurance companies to limit mental health benefits and require people to pay more out-of-pocket for mental health care than for any other medical care; and 79% said they support parity legislation even if it increases their health insurance premium by $1 a month.

Ideally, parity would include insurance coverage for mental and addictive disorders that is equal to that provided for any physical disease or illness in terms of service, dollar limits, deductibles, and co-payments. Yet most current parity provisions are much narrower (Druss and Rosenheck, 1998).

For example, equal coverage may be provided only for medically necessary services to people with severe mental disorders that are biologically based. Even more problematic, the federal parity law allows for the use of a wide range of cost control mechanisms for mental health services, such as higher deductibles or co-payments and limits on services or hospital days that differ from those used for physical health services.

In addition, current exemptions in many state insurance regulations severely limit the number of people covered by parity laws as well as the services they may receive. Parity that covers only "medical treatment" of a particular mental illness may minimize or exclude preventive services and psychosocial treatments that are necessary to maintain a person's functional capacities. Sadly, little attention is given to preventive, rehabilitative, and chronic care services. Thus although progress is being made in mandating behavioral health benefits, much additional work remains to be done (see Citing the Evidence).

CITING THE EVIDENCE ON
The Public's Knowledge of Mental Health Benefits

BACKGROUND: This study explored knowledge of mental health benefits and preferences for providers among the general public.

RESULTS: A large proportion of the respondents were uninformed about their mental health benefits; 25% were unsure whether their health plan even included mental health benefits; 43% believed that their mental health benefits were equal to those provided for general medical services; and 25% of the older respondents said they would not seek care even when needed. The majority said they would initially seek care from their primary care provider for a mental health problem.

IMPLICATIONS: The general public lacks information about important mental health benefits, and this lack of information may represent a barrier in their seeking care when needed. Given the overriding preference for primary care providers to treat mental health problems, mental health issues should be given more attention at all levels of primary care education.

Mickus M et al: *Psychiatr Serv* 51:199, 2000.

Do you know what coverage your insurance provides for mental and chemical dependency disorders? Check your policy for inpatient, outpatient, partial hospitalization, and home care benefits. Compare these benefits with those you receive for medical and surgical illnesses. If the coverages are not similar, write a letter bringing this disparity to the attention of your insurance company and requesting a response.

Telepsychiatry

An exciting development in the field that may have important implications for access to care issues is the emergence of telepsychiatry. Telepsychiatry connects people by audiovisual communication and is seen as one means of providing expert health care services to patients distant from a source of care. It is suggested for the diagnosis and treatment of patients in remote locations or where psychiatric expertise is scarce.

The high cost of providing the needed technology, particularly by public mental health systems with limited resources, has hampered its widespread use. Also issues of reliability of diagnosis, effectiveness of treatment, confidentiality, liability, reimbursement, and patient satisfaction all need further study (Frueh et al, 2000; Jenkins and White, 2001).

■ CLINICAL APPROPRIATENESS

Clinical appropriateness is the degree to which the type, amount, and level of clinical services are delivered to promote the best clinical outcomes. A basic premise of managed behavioral health care is that more is not always better.

To meet managed care's criteria of clinical appropriateness, behavioral health care organizations are developing diversified but fully integrated continuums of care by expanding their own services, contracting with other health care organizations, or affiliating with area providers. These continuums of care must be capable of providing services and alternative levels of care to children, adolescents, adults, and elderly people requiring psychiatric and substance abuse services.

The goal is to provide "one-stop shopping" for managed behavioral care and to secure market dominance in a particular geographic area. The levels of care for each stage of treatment expected in an integrated continuum of care are listed in Table 9-2.

Medical Necessity

To comply with issues of clinical appropriateness of care, managed behavioral care companies, government agencies, professional associations, and treatment facilities have each established criteria for the medical necessity of the various levels of care. Criteria are strongest for hospitalization; consensus regarding outpatient therapy is less strong.

General criteria for admission to psychiatric services used in one psychiatric setting are presented in Table 9-3. This setting uses additional criteria to assess suicide risk, self-injury risk, risk for violence assaultiveness, acute psychosis, impaired judgment, substance detoxification, substance abuse rehabilitation, need for electroconvulsive therapy, need for medication monitoring, regulation, initiation or withdrawal, and need for diagnostic evaluation or treatment. In this way, psychiatric facilities can both document and justify the medical appropriateness of the level of psychiatric care selected for a particular patient.

> One way to provide cost-effective behavioral health care in a primary care setting is to have an advanced practice registered nurse (APRN) in psychiatric and mental health care available on site to work with patients with psychiatric and substance abuse problems. What do you think would be the advantages and disadvantages of such an arrangement? ■

■ ACCOUNTABILITY ISSUES

Driven by the demand to demonstrate quality and reduce costs, the behavioral health care environment is confronted by new issues of accountability. Areas of concern range from restrictions on patient autonomy in choice of treatment and service setting to the relationship between the patient and provider, to collaborative treatment planning between patients and providers, to patient responsibility for complying with treatment recommendations, and to the denial, curtailment, or restriction of access to treatment.

Consumer Empowerment

Consumer empowerment has been an emerging movement over the past decade. The term **consumer** is one in a long list of labels that users of psychiatric services have applied to themselves. Other terms include **client, customer, patient, ex-patient,** and **survivor.** The term consumer is most often used when it applies to empowerment.

Consumer empowerment is the situation in which psychiatric patients (Geller et al, 1998):
- Form their own independent networks not dependent on professionals for support.
- Use professionals for technical assistance to make better decisions themselves in environments where they exercise full participation in decisions affecting their lives.

Table 9-2	Levels of Care for Each Stage of Treatment in an Integrated Behavioral Continuum of Care			
STAGES OF TREATMENT	CRISIS	ACUTE	MAINTENANCE	HEALTH PROMOTION
GOAL	Stabilization	Remission	Recovery	Optimal level of wellness
EXPECTED OUTCOME	No harm to self or others	Symptom relief	Improved functioning	Attain optimal quality of life
LEVEL OF CARE	• Inpatient hospitalization • 24-hour mobile emergency intervention • Crisis stabilization unit and beds • 23-hour observation beds • Outpatient detoxification • Telephone access and triage	• Partial hospitalization • Intensive remission-oriented outpatient • Assertive community treatment • Intensive in-home intervention • 23-hour respite beds • Telepsychiatry	• Rehabilitative day treatment • Multimodal recovery-oriented outpatient • Relapse prevention • Rehabilitation-oriented residential • Supported independent living	• Education • Respite care • Drop-in centers • Peer support • Social activities • School • Employment • Housing

Table 9-3	General Criteria for Psychiatric Admission Across the Continuum of Care			
	LEVEL OF CARE			
INPATIENT	PARTIAL HOSPITALIZATION	INTENSIVE OUTPATIENT	OUTPATIENT
Imminent risk for acute medical status deterioration caused by the presence of an active psychiatric or substance abuse condition Unsafe at a less intensive level of service	High risk for acute medical status deterioration caused by the presence of an active psychiatric or substance abuse condition Unsafe at a less intensive level of service Needs intensive therapeutic intervention with physician availability Adequate support system to maintain safety overnight/weekend Reasonable expectation that the patient will form a treatment alliance Unresponsive to treatment or deterioration of usual level of functioning despite participation in a less intensive level of service	Requires frequent therapeutic intervention to improve functioning Unsafe at or inappropriate for a less intensive level of service Adequate support system or coping skills to maintain stability and safety between therapeutic visits Reasonable expectation that the patient will form a treatment alliance Unresponsive to treatment, intensification of symptoms, or deterioration of usual level of functioning despite participation in a less intensive level of service	Outpatient therapy required to alleviate acute symptoms Demonstrates intent to form treatment alliance Adequate support system to maintain safety between therapeutic visits

- Participate in their treatment in collaboration with professionals and paraprofessionals, and not behaving passively as people merely receiving treatment, but instead acting as the primary informants concerning what treatment is wanted and needed from providers.
- Are respected for the legitimacy of their points of view, which are not written off as just a product of their illness.
- Are using resources from the entire community and not just from the formal mental health system.
- Are operating within a health-promoting system.
- Have significant input, beyond that of their individual treatment, into decision making at program, agency, community, state, and federal levels.
- Achieve a sense of self-responsibility.
- Are sure that consumer empowerment is more than just a buzzword.

As such, empowered consumers are asking mental health delivery systems for greater accountability and responsiveness to the people they are intended to serve (see Critical Thinking About Contemporary Issues).

Also important are questions about the extent to which patients' rights are compromised. With managed care, limits are placed on patients' choice of providers, service settings, and sometimes even treatment options. If only a limited number of options are available, patients may be unable to take advantage of newer treatments that could help them.

Partly in response to these concerns, a number of different groups have identified essential principles for managed mental health care systems. For example, the Center for Mental Health Services has developed a set of principles that emphasizes the need for comprehensive services, continuity of care, and responsiveness to the needs of service recipients (Center for Mental Health Services, 1998).

Also, a number of mental health organizations, including the American Psychiatric Nurses Association, have endorsed a Bill of Rights for managed care. All of these initiatives reflect a focused effort to protect patients and balance the issues of cost and quality in the current psychiatric care environment.

Provider Concerns

Providers are increasingly aware of their responsibility to provide cost-effective care in an environment of shrinking psychiatric resources. New dilemmas arise for clinicians who must balance their responsibility to both an individual patient and a population of patients. Also, the tension between patient advocacy and resource allocation has been heightened by the introduction of managed care, because providers may feel the need to serve the bottom line of the organization and, in so doing, jeopardize the interests of the patient (Wolff and Schlesinger, 2002). For nurses, this focus on resource allocation can mean that staffing levels are often reduced as a cost-cutting measure, while patient census and acuity levels increase.

Providers also struggle with the ambiguity of many of the rules, regulations, and expectations of this new health care environment. They complain about the overreliance of managed care on treatment protocols that limit professional judgment and minimize individual patient or clinical factors, and they cite reduced clinician productivity because of administrative burdens and excessive documentation.

So too, the designated roles and functions of care providers can be confusing, as seen in the example of case managers. From one setting to another the activities, educational preparation, and expertise of case managers vary greatly. These

---

Critical Thinking *About* Contemporary Issues

Is the Internet Helpful or Hazardous to Your Health?

Many people are now seeking information over the Internet, including behavioral health information. People are learning about the latest or recommended treatments, entering chat rooms, and participating in support groups. A smaller number are even undergoing counseling and psychotherapy on-line and accessing their employee assistance plans. All this raises a pertinent question: Is the Internet good for one's health?

Clearly, a number of benefits can be gained from the use of this new technology. The first is that many people accessing the Internet causes a shift in the expanding power and control of health information, making it no longer accessible to just a privileged few. This shift provides opportunities for new power dynamics, a shift away from the provider as the authoritative figure and toward a patient-empowered partnership (Dickerson and Brennan, 2002). It also begins to reverse the stigma surrounding mental illness and results in a quicker exchange of information among patients and providers, which ultimately improves practice. The Internet is an intermediate bridge that allows people to get information, take self-tests, and make inquiries. It is self-directed and private. All of these aspects are very compelling reasons to promote Internet use.

But Internet access also may be hazardous to one's health. One problem is the "digital divide," in which people choose not to or are unable to access the Internet. This puts those groups at a distinct disadvantage. Another reason is that not all the information on the web is reliable. It may be of poor quality and even potentially harmful. For example, depression is one of the health-related topics most searched for on-line. But two studies of web-based information on the treatment of depression raise serious questions about what consumers are learning by way of the Internet (Belcher and Holdcraft, 2001; Griffiths and Christensen, 2000). Both studies found some very good websites with clear, accurate information. Sites owned by organizations that had full disclosure of their editorial boards had better quality information. Other sites, however, provided confusing, overwhelming, or superficial information. Still other sites contained erroneous, unsafe, or hazardous information. Many did not cite scientific evidence to support their conclusions.

The Internet cannot be underestimated as an increasingly popular source of information. However, consumers and health care providers alike need to carefully evaluate the quality of the information being presented. With the Internet, as in other areas of health care, it is *caveat emptor*—let the buyer beware—your health is at stake.

managers may fill a cost-containment function, a coordination function, or a direct care function. Some have college or professional degrees; others have little higher education.

Finally, the realities of the new environment often increase conflict among disciplines rather than enhancing interdisciplinary collaboration. This heightened tension occurs because when economic resources become scarcer, disciplines revert to protecting and expanding their professional turf as a way of ensuring survival.

> *Many mental health providers and managed care companies are hotly debating which of them should decide what is best for the patient. But where is the patient in all this? Contact a managed care company in your area and ask them how they involve patients in their decision-making processes.* ■

Service Settings

Service settings may experience the greatest number of challenges to accountability. These challenges can occur on many fronts. For example, mental health facilities have been criticized for denying inpatient care or transferring patients to another facility for economic reasons when it is not in the patient's best interests.

Another effect of managed care has been the layoffs of staff and downsizing of inpatient facilities. The resulting shortage of staff and the increased work the remaining staff must assume may adversely affect the care provided. Just as the staff size is decreasing in many service settings, the severity of inpatients' problems is on the rise, which requires an adequate number of well-trained staff to deliver quality patient care.

Challenges also arise in the area of information management. Computerization of health care information is radically changing how behavioral health care services are managed and delivered. Computerized patient records now provide standardized formats for easier data collection and analysis. Clinical, financial, and administrative information systems are being integrated so that outcomes related to quality and costs of care can be measured. Information system connections are being made between service units within an organization and also among organizations, so that for many activities, electronic data communication is replacing the paper documentation used in the past (Unutzer et al, 2002).

This new information technology presents both opportunities and risks. Important accountability issues are confidentiality, appropriate uses of data, protection of data, and compliance with HIPAA regulations, particularly in areas as sensitive as psychiatric and substance abuse disorders. Data are being shared within and among organizations, which increases the risk of problems with misrouting, mishandling, misinterpreting, and generally misusing sensitive and potentially stigmatizing data (see Chapter 10).

> *Each night, a secretary on your surgical unit pulls up the list of psychiatric patients on his computer. When you ask him about it, he says that he wants to see whether anyone he knows has been admitted so that he can visit. How would you respond to him, and what actions would you take?* ■

■ IMPACT ON PSYCHIATRIC NURSING

The environment in which psychiatric nurses practice is changing every day. To thrive in this environment, psychiatric nurses need to be knowledgeable about current developments and focus their talents on services, programs, and systems of care, with patients and families being in the center of their vision. They must continue to be patient advocates and help to create an environment that is ethical and respectful of consumers and their psychiatric and mental health needs. Over 82,000 psychiatric nurses are employed in mental health facilities in the United States (Manderscheid and Henderson, 2002). Working together, they can have a significant impact on the behavioral health care delivery system.

Roles in Managed Care

Nurses bring great value to the managed care arena through their rich blend of skills and expertise. In part because the variability of nursing activity based on service setting and geographic location is diverse, psychiatric nurses have assumed a number of roles:

Psychiatric–mental health clinician: Nurses with various backgrounds are currently employed as direct care providers in managed care settings. They function as staff nurses in inpatient and partial hospitalization programs, nurse clinicians in home and community settings, primary care providers, and advanced practice nurses, including nurse practitioners and clinical nurse specialists.

Case manager: In the role of case manager, psychiatric nurses assess patient needs, develop treatment plans, allocate resources, and supervise the care given by other providers.

Evaluation and triage nurse: Many psychiatric nurses evaluate patients, either in person or over the telephone, and are responsible for triaging the patient to the most appropriate level of care (Kevin, 2002).

Utilization review nurse: Many managed care companies employ psychiatric nurses to function as utilization reviewers who review aspects of the patient's care and influence decisions about treatment assignment. In this role, they serve as "gatekeepers" to mental health services.

Patient educator: Some settings hire nurses who are given responsibility for patient and family education. This role of patient educator has grown as greater emphasis has been placed on patient compliance and disease management programs.

Risk manager: Nurses who work as risk managers are charged with the task of decreasing the probability of adverse outcomes related to patient care. They engage in identifying risk factors, individual and system-wide problems, corrective actions, and the implementation of strategies to reduce risk.

Quality improvement officer: Nurses have assumed primary responsibility for formulating and implementing quality improvement plans for managed care companies. They train other staff on-site and synthesize data related to improvement activities across the organization.

Marketing and development specialist: Some psychiatric nurses work in the managed care growth areas of marketing and development. In this role they interact with consumers, employers, providers, and regulators and make recommendations for furthering the mission and goals of the managed care organization.

Corporate managers and executives: Psychiatric nurses are also present in the boardrooms of some behavioral managed care organizations, where they influence corporate policy and strategic planning.

Threats and Opportunities

Every threat also represents an opportunity. To take advantage of the opportunities, psychiatric nurses must stay knowledgeable about the environmental context of mental health care in their own communities and across the United States, and then integrate and apply this information to their practices.

For example, Figure 9-2 shows how the current context of mental health care interacts with the activities of the nursing process. Nurses must master computer technology and refine their business and accounting skills. In this way, they can use new developments in the environment to deliver better patient care. Finally, the current environment mandates that

nurses market their skills to ensure they will be included among the mental health providers of the future.

One last but critically important fact is that whatever the environment, individuals, families, and communities will continue to experience significant mental health problems. Thus the need for psychiatric nurses to be competent and caring professionals also will continue.

Nurses must be proactive in realigning their positions within the changing environment. As psychiatric hospitals continue to downsize, more nurses will be needed in primary care, in the community, and in home settings. Many of the programs needed by patients in the community are only beginning to be designed. Psychiatric nurses can assume a leadership role in this arena. They also must keep their practice knowledge current with the realities of the mental health delivery system, doing so by learning new skills in the areas of evidence-based therapies, group interventions, psychopharmacology, and disease management.

Psychiatric nurses are in an ideal position to work closely with primary care providers to improve access and quality of care for patients with behavioral health problems. Finally, they should continue their commitment to working with underserved populations, the elderly, children, and the seriously mentally ill, because they have much to offer in regard to the care and well-being of these vulnerable groups.

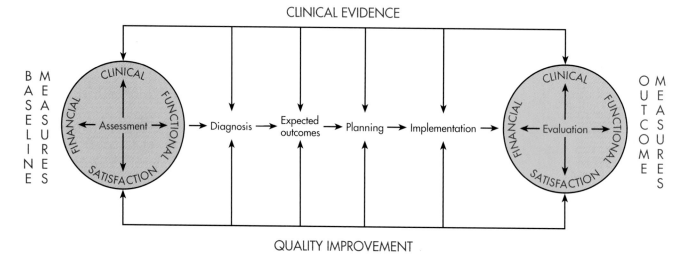

Figure 9-2 Interaction between the current context of mental health care and the nursing process.

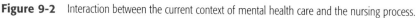

CHAPTER FOCUS POINTS

- Competent psychiatric nurses need to understand mental health–related policies, the way mental health care is organized and delivered, how mental health care is paid for, and the role of psychiatric nurses in the broader mental health care environment.
- Three important reports in the United States promise to impact the delivery of psychiatric care: (1) the report of the New Freedom Commission on Mental Health, *Achieving the Promise: Transforming Mental Health Care in America;* (2) the first report ever issued by a U.S. Surgeon General on the topic of mental health and mental illness, *Mental Health: A Report of the Surgeon General;* and

(3) *Healthy People 2010,* which identified a list of leading health indicators that reflect the major public health concerns in the United States.
- Managed care means a defined group of people receive treatment services that are clinically necessary, medically appropriate, and within defined benefit parameters for a set amount of time, in compliance with quality standards, and with outcomes that are anticipated and measurable. Behavioral health is used to describe both mental health and addiction services as one set of health problems.

CHAPTER FOCUS POINTS—cont'd

- In a managed care system there are three major payment mechanisms: discounted fee-for-service, case rate, and capitation.
- Today the U.S. government is the largest buyer of health care. Through Medicaid and Medicare and numerous other public programs, it is the single most important purchaser of health care in the United States.
- Today two thirds of the people who seek mental health care are treated by primary care practitioners. However, many who need care do not receive it, either from a primary care or a specialty provider.
- Employee assistance programs (EAPs) are worksite-based programs designed to help identify and resolve behavioral, health, and productivity problems that may affect employees' well-being or job performance.
- Many of the people who need treatment for mental and chemical dependency disorders do not receive it because their insurance policies deny or restrict coverage for the treatment of these illnesses.
- Ideally, parity would include insurance coverage for mental and addictive disorders that is equal to that provided for any physical disease or illness in terms of service, dollar limits, deductibles, and co-payments.

- Telepsychiatry connects people by audiovisual communication and is seen as one means of providing expert health care services to patients who live a great distant from a source of care.
- To meet managed care's criteria of clinical appropriateness, behavioral health care organizations are developing diversified but fully integrated continuums of care by expanding their own services, contracting with other health care organizations, or affiliating with area providers.
- To comply with issues of clinical appropriateness of care, managed behavioral care companies, government agencies, professional associations, and treatment facilities have each established criteria for the medical necessity of the various levels of care.
- Areas of concern related to accountability range from restrictions on patient autonomy in choice of treatment and service setting to the relationship between the patient and provider, to collaborative treatment planning between patients and providers, to patient responsibility for complying with treatment recommendations, and to the denial, curtailment, or restriction of access to treatment.
- To thrive in this environment, psychiatric nurses need to be knowledgeable about current developments and focus their talents on services, programs, and systems of care with patients and families in the center of their vision.

KEY TERMS

access, 139
behavioral health, 137
clinical appropriateness, 140

employee assistance programs
   (EAPs), 139
managed care, 137

Medicaid, 139
telepsychiatry, 140

CHAPTER REVIEW QUESTIONS

1. Match each term in Column A with the correct definition in Column B.

Column A

_____ Access
_____ Capitation
_____ Case rate
_____ Clinical appropriateness
_____ Outcomes
_____ Utilization review

Column B

A. Degree to which services and information about care are conveniently and easily obtained
B. Degree to which the type, amount, and level of clinical services are delivered to promote positive outcomes for the patient
C. Evaluates the appropriateness and necessity of health care services and procedures
D. Extent to which services are cost-effective and have a favorable effect on the patient's symptoms, functioning, and well-being
E. Payment system in which the clinic is paid a flat fee regardless of the cost of care
F. Payment system in which the consumer pays a flat fee and in return receives all medically necessary health care

2. Fill in the blanks.

A. The term _____ is used in managed care to describe the combination of mental and substance abuse disorders.
B. Managed care involves a major shift away from the

   _____ as customer to the

   _____ as customer.
C. The serious and persistently mentally ill are often recipients of

   the government entitlement program called _____.
D. Two thirds of people who seek mental health care are treated

   by _____.
E. Worksite-based programs designed to help identify and facilitate the resolution of behavioral, health, and productivity problems that may adversely affect an employee's well-being

   or job performance are called _____.
F. Ideally, parity would include insurance coverage for mental

   and addictive disorders that is _____ to that provided for any physical disease or illness.

G. _____ is the term used to describe audiovisual communication between people geographically apart that allows for psychiatric diagnosis and treatment.

3. Provide short answers for the following questions.

A. Describe the four forms of managed care organizations. If you belong to a managed care organization, identify which type of managed care plan you have.

B. Discuss how stigma associated with substance abuse may have contributed to the law passed in 1996 that ended Medicaid and Medicare coverage for people whose disability is based on drug addiction or alcoholism.

C. Some people believe that we should limit care to people with brain-based mental disorders or the major mental illnesses and not reimburse less serious or minor mental health problems. What position would you take on this issue? Compare this issue to reimbursement policies for major and minor physical illnesses.

Visit Evolve for additional resources related to the content of this chapter.

 http://evolve.elsevier.com/Stuart/principles/
• Topical Course Outline • Student Workbook Exercises • Critical Thinking Questions and Activities • Case Studies • Research Topics
• Monthly Content Updates • WebLinks

Student Study CD-ROM

Access the accompanying CD-ROM for animations, interactive exercises, review questions for the NCLEX examination, and an audio glossary.

REFERENCES

Barry CL, Frank RG: Economic grand rounds: economics and the surgeon general's report on mental health, *Psychiatr Serv* 53:409, 2002.

Belcher J, Holdcraft C: Web-based information for depression: helpful or hazardous? *J Am Psychiatr Nurs Assoc* 7:61, 2001.

Center for Mental Health Services: *Mental health, United States, 1998,* Washington, DC, 1998, US Government Printing Office.

Dickerson SS, Brennan PF: The Internet as a catalyst for shifting power in provider-patient relationships, *Nurs Outlook* 50:195, 2002.

Druss BG, Rosenheck RA: Mental disorders and access to medical care in the United States, *Am J Psychiatry* 155:1775, 1998.

Frueh BC et al: Procedural and methodological issues in telepsychiatry research and program development, *Psychiatr Serv* 51:1522, 2000.

Geller JL et al: A national survey of "consumer empowerment" at the state level, *Psychiatr Serv* 49:498, 1998.

Griffiths KM, Christensen H: Quality of web-based information on treatment of depression: cross sectional survey, *Br Med J* 321:1511, 2000.

Jenkins RL, White P: Telehealth advancing nursing practice, *Nurs Outlook* 49:100, 2001.

Kevin J: An examination of telephone triage in a mental health context, *Issues Ment Health Nurs* 23:757, 2002.

Manderscheid RW, Henderson MJ, editors: *Mental health, United States, 2001,* Washington, DC, 2002, Department of Health and Human Services, Center for Mental Health Services.

Mechanic D: *Mental health and social policy: the emergence of managed care,* Needham Heights, Mass, 1999, Allyn and Bacon.

Murray CJL, Lopez AD: Evidence-based health policy—lessons from the Global Burden of Disease Study, *Science* 274:740, 1996.

New Freedom Commission on Mental Health (NFCMH): *Achieving the promise: transforming mental health care in America, final report,* DHHS Pub. No. SMA-03-3832, Rockville, Md, 2003, USDHHS.

Peck MC, Scheffler RM: An analysis of the definitions of mental illness used in state parity laws, *Psychiatr Serv* 53:1089, 2002.

Sing M et al: *The costs and effects of parity for mental health and substance abuse insurance benefits,* Rockville, Md, 1998, US Department of Health and Human Services.

Unutzer J et al: A web-based data management system to improve care for depression in a multicenter clinical trial, *Psychiatr Serv* 53:671, 2002.

US Department of Health and Human Services (USDHHS): *Mental health: a report of the surgeon general,* Rockville, Md, 1999, National Institute of Mental Health.

US Department of Health and Human Services (USDHHS): *Healthy People 2010,* Washington, DC, 2000, USDHHS.

Wolff N, Schlesinger M: Clinicians as advocates: an exploratory study of responses to managed care by mental health professionals, *J Behav Health Serv Res* 29:274, 2002.

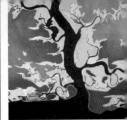

Pinel immediately led Couthon to the section for the deranged, where the sight of the cells made a painful impression on him. Couthon asked to interrogate all the patients. From most, he received only insults and obscene apostrophes. It was useless to prolong the interview. Turning to Pinel, Couthon said: "Now, citizen, are you mad yourself to seek to unchain such beasts?" Pinel replied calmly: "Citizen, I am convinced that these madmen are so intractable only because they have been deprived of air and liberty."

PHILIPPE PINEL, *TRAITE COMPLET DU REGIME SANITAIRE DES ALIENES* 56 (1836)

LEGAL AND ETHICAL CONTEXT OF PSYCHIATRIC NURSING CARE

10

Gail W. Stuart

LEARNING OBJECTIVES

After studying this chapter, the student should be able to:

1. Describe ethical standards, decision making, and dilemmas impacting psychiatric nursing practice (I).
2. Compare and contrast the two types of admission to a psychiatric hospital and the ethical issues raised by commitment (II).
3. Examine involuntary community treatment and its implications for improving the care received by psychiatric patients (III).
4. Analyze the common personal and civil rights retained by psychiatric patients and ethical issues related to them (IV).
5. Identify current legislative initiatives that affect the psychiatric care provided in the United States (V).
6. Discuss the insanity defense and the psychiatric criteria used in the United States to determine criminal responsibility (VI).
7. Evaluate the rights, responsibilities, and potential conflict of interest that arise from the three legal roles of the psychiatric nurse (VII).

TOPICAL OUTLINE

I. Ethical Standards
   A. Ethical Decision Making
   B. Ethical Dilemmas
II. Hospitalizing the Patient
   A. Voluntary Admission
   B. Involuntary Admission (Commitment)
   C. Commitment Dilemma
   D. Discharge
   E. Ethical Considerations
III. Involuntary Community Treatment
IV. Patients' Rights
   A. Right to Communicate With People Outside the Hospital
   B. Right to Keep Personal Effects
   C. Right to Enter Into Contractual Relationships
   D. Right to Education
   E. Right to Habeas Corpus
   F. Right to Privacy
   G. Right to Informed Consent
   H. Right to Treatment
   I. Right to Refuse Treatment
   J. Right to Treatment in the Least Restrictive Setting
   K. Role of Nursing
   L. Ethical Considerations
V. Legislative Initiatives
   A. Federal Budget Acts
   B. Protection and Advocacy Act
   C. Americans With Disabilities Act
   D. Advance Directives
   E. Mental Health Courts
VI. Psychiatry and Criminal Responsibility
   A. Disposition of Mentally Ill Offenders
VII. Legal Role of the Nurse
   A. Nurse As Provider
   B. Nurse As Employee
   C. Nurse As Citizen

evolve Visit Evolve for additional resources related to the content of this chapter.
http://evolve.elsevier.com/Stuart/principles/

The relationship between psychiatry and the law reflects the tension between individual rights and social needs. Both psychiatry and the law deal with human behavior and the relationships and responsibilities that exist among people. Both also play a role in controlling socially undesirable behavior, and together they analyze whether the care psychiatric patients receive is therapeutic, custodial, repressive, or punitive.

Differences also exist between psychiatry and the law. For example, psychiatry is concerned with the meaning of behavior and the life satisfaction of the individual. In contrast, the law addresses the outcome of behavior and the enforcement of a system of rules to encourage orderly functioning among groups of people.

The legal and ethical context of care is important for all psychiatric nurses because it focuses concern on the rights of patients and the quality of care they receive. In the past two decades civil, criminal, and consumer rights of patients have been established and expanded through the legal system. Many of the laws vary from state to state, and psychiatric nurses must become familiar with the laws of the state in which they practice. This knowledge enhances the freedom of both the nurse and the patient, informs their ethical decision making, and ultimately results in better care.

■ ETHICAL STANDARDS

Psychiatric nurses often encounter complex ethical situations in caring for patients and families suffering from mental illness. As professionals, they are held to the highest standards of ethical accountability in their clinical practice. A number of essential ethics skills or capacities have been identified for mental health providers (Box 10-1). They include the importance of recognition, knowledge, self-awareness, and focused activity. Possession of these skills will allow the nurse to provide care that is socially responsible and personally accountable.

An ethic is a standard of behavior or a belief valued by an individual or group. It describes what ought to be, rather than what is—a goal to which an individual aspires. These standards are learned through socialization, growth, and experience. As such, they are not static but evolve to reflect social change. Ethical standards, guidelines, and principles are not legally enforceable unless they have been incorporated into the law (Reid, 2002).

Ethical Decision Making

Ethical decision making involves trying to distinguish right from wrong in situations without clear guidelines. A decision-making model can help identify factors and principles that affect a decision. A model for critical ethical analysis that describes steps or factors that the nurse should consider in resolving an ethical dilemma is shown in Figure 10-1.

1. The first step is **gathering background information** to obtain a clear picture of the problem. This includes finding available information to clarify the underlying issues.
2. The next step is **identifying the ethical components** or the nature of the dilemma, such as freedom versus coercion or treating versus accepting the right to refuse treatment.
3. The third step is the **clarification of the rights and responsibilities of all ethical agents,** or those involved in the decision making. This can include the patient, the nurse, and possibly many others, including the patient's family, physician, health care institution, clergy, social worker, and perhaps even the courts. Those involved may not agree on how to handle the situation, but their rights and duties can be clarified.
4. **All possible options must then be explored** in light of everyone's responsibilities, as well as the purpose and potential result of each option. This step eliminates alternatives that violate rights or seem harmful.
5. The nurse then engages in the **application of principles,** which stem from the nurse's philosophy of life and nursing, scientific knowledge, and ethical theory. Ethical theories suggest ways to structure ethical dilemmas and judge potential solutions. Four possible approaches include the following:

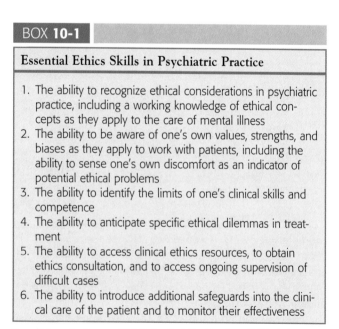

Essential Ethics Skills in Psychiatric Practice

1. The ability to recognize ethical considerations in psychiatric practice, including a working knowledge of ethical concepts as they apply to the care of mental illness
2. The ability to be aware of one's own values, strengths, and biases as they apply to work with patients, including the ability to sense one's own discomfort as an indicator of potential ethical problems
3. The ability to identify the limits of one's clinical skills and competence
4. The ability to anticipate specific ethical dilemmas in treatment
5. The ability to access clinical ethics resources, to obtain ethics consultation, and to access ongoing supervision of difficult cases
6. The ability to introduce additional safeguards into the clinical care of the patient and to monitor their effectiveness

From Roberts L, Geppert CM, Bailey R: *J Psychiatr Pract* 8:290, 2002.

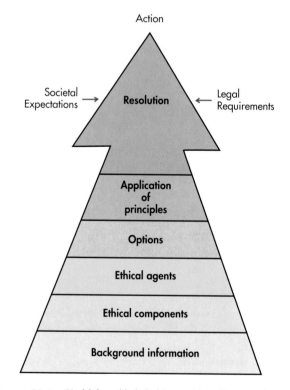

Figure 10-1 Model for ethical decision making. (From Curtin L: *Nurs Forum* 17:12, 1978.)

a. **Utilitarianism**, which focuses on the consequences of actions. It seeks the greatest amount of happiness or the least amount of harm for the greatest number, or "the greatest good for the greatest number."

b. **Egoism** is a position in which the individual seeks the solution that is best personally. The self is most important, and others are secondary.

c. **Formalism** considers the nature of the act itself and the principles involved. It involves the universal application of a basic rule, such as "do unto others as you would have them do unto you."

d. **Fairness** is based on the concept of justice, and benefit to the least advantaged in society becomes the norm for decision making.

6. The final step is **resolution into action**. Within the context of social expectations and legal requirements, the nurse decides on the goals and methods of implementation. Table 10-1 summarizes these steps and suggests questions nurses can ask themselves in making complex ethical choices in psychiatric nursing practice.

Think of an ethical problem you have encountered in caring for a psychiatric patient and family. Use the model for ethical decision making to decide on the best course of action. ■

Table 10-1	Steps and Questions in Ethical Decision Making
STEPS	**RELEVANT QUESTIONS**
Gathering background information	Does an ethical dilemma exist?
	What information is known?
	What information is needed?
	What is the context of the dilemma?
Identifying ethical components	What is the underlying issue?
	Who is affected by this dilemma?
Clarification of agents	What are the rights of each involved party?
	What are the obligations of each involved party?
	Who should be involved in the decision making?
	For whom is the decision being made?
	What degree of consent is needed by the patient?
Exploration of options	What alternatives exist?
	What is the purpose or intent of each alternative?
	What are the potential consequences of each alternative?
Application of principles	What criteria should be used?
	What ethical theories are subscribed to?
	What scientific facts are relevant?
	What is the nurse's philosophy of life and nursing?
Resolution into action	What are the social and legal constraints and ramifications?
	What is the goal of the nurse's decision?
	How can the resulting ethical choice be implemented?
	How can the resulting ethical choice be evaluated?

Ethical Dilemmas

An ethical dilemma exists when moral claims conflict with one another. It can be defined as:

- A difficult problem that seems to have no satisfactory solution.
- A choice between equally unsatisfactory alternatives.

Ethical dilemmas pose such questions as "What should I do?" and "What is the right thing to do?" They can occur both at the nurse-patient-family level of daily nursing care and at the policymaking level of institutions and communities. Although ethical dilemmas arise in all areas of nursing practice, some are unique to psychiatric and mental health nursing. Many of these dilemmas fall under the umbrella issue of **behavior control**.

At first glance, behavior control may seem a simple issue: Behavior is a personal choice, and any behavior that does not impose on the rights of others is acceptable. Unfortunately, this does not help to address complex situations. For example, a severely depressed person may choose suicide as an alternative to an intolerable existence. On one level, this is an individual choice not directly harming others, yet suicide is forbidden in American society. In many states it is a crime that can be prosecuted.

As another example, in some states it is illegal for consenting adults of the same sex to have sexual relations, although it is not illegal for a man to rape his wife. These examples raise difficult questions: When is it appropriate for society to regulate personal behavior? Who will make this decision? Is its goal personal adjustment, personal growth, or adaptation to social norms? And finally, how do we measure the costs and benefits of attempting to control personal freedom in a free society?

One of the most fundamental problems is the blurry line between science and ethics in the field of psychiatry. Theoretically, science and ethics are separate entities. Science is descriptive, deals with what is, and rests on validation; ethics is predictive, deals with what ought to be, and relies on judgment. However, psychiatry is neither purely scientific nor value-free.

Despite these ambiguities, nurses must identify their professional commitment. Are they committed to the happiness of the individual or the smooth functioning of society? Ideally, these values should not conflict, but in reality they sometimes do. The patient's rights to treatment, to refuse treatment, and to informed consent highlight this conflict-of-interest question. Nurses must consider whether they are forcing patients to be socially or politically acceptable at the expense of patients' personal happiness. Nurses may not be working for either the patient's best interests or their own; they may be acting as agents of society and not be aware of it.

All nurses participate in some therapeutic psychiatric regimens whose scientific and ethical bases are ambiguous. The American health care system continues to apply a medical model of wellness and illness to human behavior. Wellness is socially acceptable behavior, and illness is socially unacceptable. It becomes critically important for each nurse to analyze such ethical dilemmas as freedom of choice versus coercion, helping versus imposing values, and focusing on cure versus prevention. The nurse also must become active in defining adequate treatment and deciding important resource allocations.

■ HOSPITALIZING THE PATIENT

Hospitalization can be either traumatic or supportive for the patient, depending on the institution, attitude of family and friends, response of the staff, and type of admission. There are two major types of admission: voluntary and involuntary. Table 10-2 summarizes their distinguishing characteristics.

What were your impressions as you walked through the doors of a psychiatric hospital for the first time? How might you use your perceptions and responses to provide better nursing care for patients being admitted for inpatient treatment? ■

Voluntary Admission

Under voluntary admission any citizen of lawful age may apply in writing (usually on a standard admission form) for admission to a public or private psychiatric hospital. The person agrees to receive treatment and abide by hospital rules. People may seek help based on their personal decision or the advice of family or a health professional. If someone is too ill to apply but voluntarily seeks help, a parent or legal guardian may request admission. In most states children under the age of 16 years may be admitted if their parents sign the required application form.

Voluntary admission is preferred because it is similar to a medical hospitalization. It indicates that the patient acknowledges problems in living, seeks help in coping with them, and will probably actively participate in finding solutions. Most patients who enter private psychiatric units of general hospitals do so voluntarily.

When admitted in this way, the patient retains all civil rights, including the right to vote, hold a driver's license, buy and sell property, manage personal affairs, hold office, practice a profession, and engage in a business. It is a common misconception that all admissions to a mental hospital involve the loss of civil rights.

Although voluntary admission is the most desirable, it is not always possible. Sometimes a patient may be acutely disturbed, suicidal, or dangerous to self or others, yet rejects any therapeutic intervention. In these cases involuntary commitments are necessary.

Should a psychotic person be allowed to sign forms for voluntary admittance to the hospital? If not, should all voluntary patients be screened for competence before hospitalization? ■

Involuntary Admission (Commitment)

Involuntary admission or commitment is based on two legal theories. First, under its **police power**, the state has the authority to protect the community from the dangerous acts of the mentally ill. Second, under its **parens patriae powers**, the state can provide care for citizens who cannot care for themselves, such as some mentally ill people. The police power rationale for civil commitment has been emphasized over the parens patriae doctrine, using dangerousness as the standard for commitment.

Involuntary admission or commitment means that the patient did not request hospitalization and may have opposed it or was indecisive and did not resist it. Most laws permit commitment of the mentally ill on one or more of the following three grounds:

1. **Dangerous to self or others**
2. **Mentally ill and in need of treatment**
3. **Unable to provide for own basic needs**

The Commitment Process. State laws vary, but they try to protect the person who is not mentally ill from being detained in a psychiatric hospital against his or her will for political, economic, family, or other nonmedical reasons. Certain procedures are standard. The process begins with a sworn petition by a relative, friend, public official, physician, or any interested citizen stating that the person is mentally ill and needs treatment. Some states allow only specific people to file such a petition. One or two physicians must then examine the patient's mental status; some states require that at least one of the physicians be a psychiatrist.

The decision of whether to hospitalize the patient is made next. Precisely who makes this decision determines the nature of the commitment. **Medical certification** means that physicians make the decision. **Court** or **judicial commitment** is made by a judge or jury in a formal hearing. Most states recognize the patient's right to legal counsel, but only about half actually appoint a lawyer for patients if they do not have one. **Administrative commitment** is determined by a special tribunal of hearing officers.

If treatment is deemed necessary, the person is hospitalized. The length of hospital stay varies depending on the patient's needs. Figure 10-2 presents a clinical algorithm of the involuntary commitment process. It identifies three types of involuntary hospitalization: emergency, short term, and long term.

Table 10-2	Characteristics of the Two Types of Admission to Psychiatric Hospitals	
	VOLUNTARY ADMISSION	INVOLUNTARY ADMISSION
Admission	Written application by patient	Application did not originate with patient
Discharge	Initiated by patient	Initiated by hospital or court but not by patient
Civil rights	Retained fully by patient	Patient may retain none, some, or all, depending on state law
Justification	Voluntarily seeks help	Mentally ill and one or more of the following: Dangerous to self or others Need for treatment Unable to meet own basic needs

Most states specify that any physician, not necessarily a psychiatrist, can certify a person for involuntary commitment to a psychiatric hospital. Do you agree with this? What is required by law in your state? ■

Emergency Hospitalization. Almost all states permit emergency commitment for patients who are acutely ill. The goals are primarily intended to control an immediate threat to self or others. In states lacking such a law, police often jail the acutely ill person on a disorderly conduct charge, which is a criminal charge. Such a practice is inappropriate and often harmful to the patient's mental status. Most state laws limit the length of emergency commitment to 48 to 72 hours. Emergency hospitalization allows detainment in a psychiatric hospital only until proper legal steps are taken to provide for additional hospitalization.

Short-Term or Observational Hospitalization. This type of commitment is used primarily for diagnosis and short-term therapy and does not require an emergency situation. Again, the commitment is for a specified time that varies greatly from state to state. If at the end of the period the patient is still not ready for discharge, a petition can be filed for a long-term commitment.

Long-Term Hospitalization (Formal Commitment). A long-term commitment provides for hospitalization for an indefinite time or until the patient is ready for discharge. Patients in public or state hospitals have indefinite commitments more often than patients in private hospitals. Even when committed, these patients maintain their right to consult a lawyer at any time and to request a court hearing to de-

termine whether additional hospitalization is necessary. The hospital ultimately discharges the patient, however, and a court order is not needed for this action. Periodic reviews for long-term hospitalization may be made every 3, 6, or 12 months.

Do you agree with the criteria for committing patients to psychiatric hospitals? How would you assess whether a person met these criteria? ■

Commitment Dilemma

Because of the many people affected by involuntary commitment and the loss of personal rights that it can entail, it becomes a matter of great legal, ethical, social, and psychiatric significance. In general medicine there is no equivalent loss of individual rights, except for rare cases requiring quarantine for carriers of potentially epidemic diseases.

How ill does a person need to be to merit commitment? A person's dangerousness to self or others is a pertinent consideration. Certainly psychiatric professionals consider hospitalization in this instance to be a humanitarian gesture that protects both the individual and society. However, dangerousness is a vague term.

According to a survey commissioned by Parade *magazine, over 57% of Americans think mentally ill people are more likely to commit acts of violence than other people. How does this compare with the facts? How do the media contribute to this impression of the mentally ill?* ■

Dangerousness. Interestingly, courts guard the freedom of people who are mentally healthy but dangerous. For example, after a prison sentence is served, the person is automatically released and can no longer be retained. However, someone who is mentally ill and dangerous can be confined indefinitely. The idea of preventive detention does not exist in most areas of the law because the ability to predict an action does not confer the right to control it in advance. Only illegal acts result in prolonged confinement for most citizens, except the mentally ill.

Most mentally ill people are not dangerous to themselves or others. Studies show that the vast majority of people with serious mental illness are not inherently violent. Research does suggest, however, that a subgroup of people with mental illness may be more dangerous. Patients in this subgroup have a history of one or more of the following:

- **Violent behavior**
- **Psychosis**
- **Noncompliance with medications**
- **Current substance abuse**
- **Antisocial personality disorder**

These characteristics can serve as predictors of potential violence (McConnell and Catalano, 2001).

It is important that patients with severe psychiatric disorders be identified and appropriately treated. It also should be remembered that violent behavior by people with serious mental illness is only one aspect of a larger problem: the failure of public psychiatric services and the deinstitutionalization of the mentally ill without adequate community support.

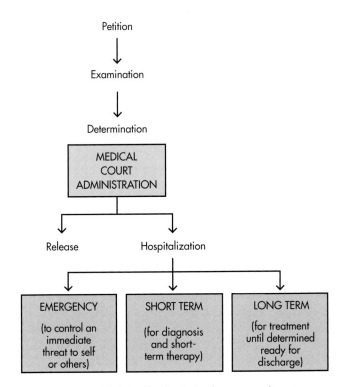

Figure 10-2   Clinical algorithm for the involuntary commitment process.

Other aspects of this problem include the large number of mentally ill among the homeless, the large number of mentally ill in jails and prisons, and the revolving door of psychiatric readmissions.

Another issue is that **no reliable indicators of dangerousness** have been identified. Even if some mentally ill people are thought to be potentially dangerous, psychiatrists cannot predict future violence. Psychiatrists often overpredict patients' potential for dangerous acts. This may result from their medical training, which cautions that underdiagnosis is more harmful than overdiagnosis. If psychiatrists underpredict a psychiatric illness and the patient later causes harm, they are held responsible. If they overpredict illness, however, a patient is subjected to treatment unwillingly. Therefore multidisciplinary teams should be involved in determining dangerousness (Haim et al, 2002). Input from those familiar with the patient's home setting and sociocultural background also might improve evaluations.

Some suggest that the underlying issue is nonconformity in ways that offend others. In this context, social role becomes important. For example, before the law all men and women are equal, but it is also true that most committed patients are members of the lower classes. This raises questions regarding the sociocultural context of psychiatric care (see Chapter 8) and the role of mental health professionals as enforcers of social rules and norms. Thus the behavioral standard of dangerousness can change the function of the psychiatric hospital from a place of therapy for mental illness to a place of confinement for offensive behavior.

How do you explain the fact that society condones certain kinds of dangerous behavior, such as race car driving, but objects to other kinds? ▪

Freedom of Choice. The legal and ethical question thus raised is freedom of choice. Some professionals believe that at certain times the individual cannot be self-responsible. To protect both the patient and society, it is necessary to confine the patient and make decisions for him or her. An example is the suicidal patient. In most states suicide is against the law, so law and psychiatry join to protect the person and help individuals resolve personal conflicts.

How does this compare with patients who have cancer or cardiac disease and decide to reject medical advice and the prescribed treatment? Should society, through law and medicine, attempt to cure these patients against their will? Some clinicians view civil commitment as basically a benevolent system that makes treatment available. They disagree with the assumption that mentally ill people are competent to exercise free will and make decisions in their own best interest, such as whether to take medications or remain outside a hospital. They contend that there are mentally ill people who may not be physically dangerous but still endanger their own prospects for a normal life. Because institutions can protect them and in many cases help them, they think it would be unethical to abolish involuntary civil commitment.

Others oppose commitment. They favor responsibility for self and the right to choose or reject treatment. If a person's actions violate criminal law, they suggest that the person be punished through the penal system. Currently a middle ground is being sought between meeting the needs of the severely mentally ill and preserving their legal rights and freedom of choice.

Who should decide what is in the patient's best interest if a patient is involuntarily committed? Should it be the patient, a family member, a health care professional, or the judicial system? ▪

Discharge

The patient who is voluntarily admitted to the hospital can leave at any time. The voluntarily admitted patient can be discharged by the staff when maximum benefit has been received from the treatment. Voluntary patients also may request discharge. Most states require written notice of patients' desire to leave and also require that patients sign a form that states they are leaving against medical advice (AMA). This form then becomes part of the patient's permanent record.

The issue of leaving AMA presents a particular ethical dilemma for the clinician who must weigh provider accountability for the patient's safety against the patient's right to refuse treatment. Two key factors in deciding to release a voluntary psychiatric patient are as follows:

- Assessment of the patient's competency
- Assessment of the patient's potential danger to self or others

Furthermore, documentation of AMA requests should include the following (McGihon, 1998):

- The mental status of the patient requesting to leave
- The patient's own description of why he or she wants to leave
- Content of discussions in which possible risks of leaving were described to the patient
- Instructions on medications and follow-up care
- Conversations with significant others who may have been present
- Destination of the patient and means of transportation

In some states, voluntarily admitted patients can be released immediately; in others they can be detained 24 to 72 hours after submitting a discharge request. This allows hospital staff time to confer with the patient and family members and decide whether additional inpatient treatment is indicated. If it is and the patient will not withdraw the request for discharge, the family may begin involuntary commitment proceedings, thereby changing the patient's status.

An involuntarily committed patient has lost the right to leave the hospital when he or she wishes. Short-term and emergency commitments specify the maximum length of detainment. Long-term commitments do not, although the patient's status should be reviewed periodically. The patient also may apply for another commitment hearing.

If a committed patient leaves before discharge, the staff has the legal obligation to notify the police and committing courts. Often these patients return home or visit family or friends and can be easily located. The legal authorities then return the patient to the hospital. Additional steps are not necessary because the original commitment is still in effect.

Ethical Considerations

Nurses must analyze their beliefs regarding the voluntary and involuntary hospitalization of psychiatric patients (Balevre, 2001). What should be done if the nonconformist does not wish to change behavior? Do nonconformists maintain freedom to choose even if their thinking appears to be irrational or abnormal? Is coercion fair? Can social interests be served by less restrictive methods such as outpatient therapy? Nurses are responsible for reviewing commitment procedures in their state and working for necessary clinical, ethical, and legal reforms.

The commitment dilemma exposes current practices and shines light on controversial issues, which will benefit from closer examination in the future. Studies show that more than half of the homeless population have psychiatric or substance abuse disorders. Homeless mentally ill people have a wider array of service needs than homeless people who use only social services. Many seriously mentally ill people cannot obtain or maintain access to community resources such as housing, a stable source of income, or treatment and rehabilitative services.

Homeless people lack supportive social networks and underuse psychiatric, medical, and welfare programs. Many avoid the mental health system entirely, often because they are too confused to respond to offers of help. As a consequence, they are often admitted into acute psychiatric hospitals or jailed because of their lack of shelter and other resources, even though such restrictive environments may not best address their psychiatric needs.

Unfortunately, local communities often deny the problem by resisting the establishment of halfway houses or sheltered homes in their neighborhoods. Third-party insurance seldom covers extended outpatient psychiatric care. In today's mobile society, family and friends are often unable to care for the newly discharged patient, who may end up in a boarding house with little to do but watch television.

These issues must be addressed by psychiatric nurses, patients, and citizens across the United States. The value of commitment, goals of hospitalization, quality of life, and rights of patients must be preserved through the judicial, legislative, and health care systems.

■ INVOLUNTARY COMMUNITY TREATMENT

Recently community initiatives have been developed to respond to the mandate to offer psychiatric patients treatment in the least restrictive setting. The most common of these is court-ordered treatment in the community or outpatient commitment.

Outpatient commitment is the process by which the courts can order patients committed to a course of outpatient treatment specified by their clinicians. This type of commitment is an alternative to inpatient treatment for people who meet the involuntary commitment criteria. Almost all states have laws permitting outpatient commitment, but its use varies greatly among states (Swartz and Monahan, 2001). Reasons for not using them include concerns about civil liberties, liability and financial costs, lack of information and interest, problems with enforcement and ways to deal with lack of compliance, and criteria that are too restrictive.

Guidelines to determine a patient's appropriateness for involuntary outpatient commitment are presented in Box 10-2. They are sequential in that a patient is not evaluated for appropriateness under a guideline unless the criteria for all preceding guidelines have been met. The guidelines also assume that the patient has a serious and persistent mental illness and a history of dangerous behavior toward self or others.

How might sociocultural factors influence a nurse's interpretation of the guidelines listed in Box 10-2? How might nurses guard against potential bias based on their personal worldview? ■

Like inpatient commitment, involuntary outpatient treatment is also the subject of controversy. Some believe that it is necessary to reach people who need help but do not realize it. These are people who lack insight because of their illness and subsequently refuse treatment and wind up homeless, in jails, or in hospitals. They point to research showing that patients in outpatient commitment had fewer hospital admis-

---

BOX 10-2

Guidelines for the Use of Outpatient Commitment

1. The patient must express an interest in living in the community.
2. The patient must have previously failed in the community.
3. The patient must have that degree of competency necessary to understand the stipulations of his or her involuntary community treatment.
4. The patient must have the capacity to comply with the involuntary community treatment plan.
5. The treatment or treatments being ordered must have demonstrated efficacy when used properly by the patient in question.
6. The ordered treatment or treatments must be such that they can be delivered by the outpatient system, are sufficient for the patient's needs, and are necessary to sustain community tenure.
7. The ordered treatment must be such that it can be monitored by outpatient treatment agencies.
8. The outpatient treatment system must be willing to deliver the ordered treatments to the patient and must be willing to participate in enforcing compliance with those treatments.
9. The public-sector inpatient support system must support the outpatient system's participation in the provision of involuntary community treatment.
10. The outpatient must not be dangerous when complying with the ordered treatment.

From Geller J: *Innovations Res* 2:23, 1993.

sions and hospital days after the court order requiring the outpatient treatment (Rohland, Rohrer, and Richards, 2000; Swartz et al 2001; Torrey and Zdanowicz, 2001), were less likely to be criminally victimized (Hiday et al, 2002), and had a decreased risk for homelessness (Compton et al, 2003).

Others disagree and say this law plays into the public's fear of the dangerous mentally ill. They believe that outpatient commitment may not improve public safety, may not be more effective than voluntary services, and may, in fact, drive consumers away from the mental health system (Allen and Smith, 2001). Questions also have been raised about the legality of limiting the rights of patients who are not incompetent and who would not qualify for inpatient commitment in a court of law (Hoge and Grottole, 2000).

The Bazelon Center for Mental Health Law opposes all involuntary outpatient commitment as an infringement of an individual's constitutional rights and believes that guidelines for commitment are based on speculation and are not legally permissible (Bazelon, 1999). Finally, it has been noted that the use of outpatient commitment is not a substitute for intensive treatment and that it requires a substantial allocation of treatment resources to be effective (Appelbaum, 2001).

■ PATIENTS' RIGHTS

In 1973 the American Hospital Association (AHA) issued a Patient's Bill of Rights that many hospitals and community-based settings throughout the United States have adopted. These rights were reaffirmed in 1990 (AHA, 1990). In 2003 this document evolved into "The Patient Care Partnership: Understanding Expectations, Rights, and Responsibilities" (AHA, 2003). This document is often given to patients on admission and read or explained to them.

The evolution of patients' rights has been uneven across the United States. Some states formally acknowledge very few rights, whereas other states guarantee certain categories of rights and ignore others. It is also unclear how well patients are actually informed about their rights, whether they understand the information given to them, how frequently patients exercise their rights, and what happens to them when they do so.

In your experience, are patients in general hospital settings granted their patient rights? How about patients in psychiatric inpatient units? What specific things could nurses do to see that these rights are honored in all hospitals? ■

Although the variation among states is great, psychiatric patients currently have the following rights:
- Right to communicate with people outside the hospital through correspondence, telephone, and personal visits
- Right to keep clothing and personal effects with them in the hospital
- Right to religious freedom
- Right to be employed if possible

- Right to manage and dispose of property
- Right to execute wills
- Right to enter into contractual relationships
- Right to make purchases
- Right to education
- Right to habeas corpus
- Right to independent psychiatric examination
- Right to civil service status
- Right to retain licenses, privileges, or permits established by law, such as a driver's or professional license
- Right to sue or be sued
- Right to marry and divorce
- Right not to be subject to unnecessary mechanical restraints
- Right to periodic review of status
- Right to legal representation
- Right to privacy
- Right to informed consent
- Right to treatment
- Right to refuse treatment
- Right to treatment in the least restrictive setting

Some of these rights deserve a more thorough discussion.

Did you know that many states still have laws on the books that restrict the right of some people with treatable psychiatric illnesses to vote? How do you think such laws perpetuate stigma, prejudice, and discrimination against people with mental illness? Does your state have such laws? ■

Right To Communicate With People Outside the Hospital

This right allows patients to visit and hold telephone conversations in privacy and send unopened letters to anyone of their choice, including judges, lawyers, families, and staff. Although the patient has the right to communicate in an uncensored manner, the staff may limit access to the telephone or visitors when it could harm the patient or be a source of harassment for the staff. The hospital also can limit the times when telephone calls are made and received and when visitors can enter the facility.

Right To Keep Personal Effects

The patient may bring clothing and personal items to the hospital, taking into consideration the amount of storage space available. The hospital is not responsible for their safety, and valuable items should be left at home. If the patient brings something of value to the hospital, the staff should place it in the hospital safe or otherwise provide for safekeeping. The hospital staff is also responsible for maintaining a safe environment and should take dangerous objects away from the patient if necessary.

 How are patients informed of their rights on your psychiatric unit? Talk to some of the patients and see whether they can recall any of the rights that were explained to them. ■

Right To Enter Into Contractual Relationships

The court considers contracts valid if the person understands the circumstances of the contract and its consequences. Once again, a psychiatric illness does not invalidate a contract, although the nature of the contract and degree of judgment needed to understand it are influencing factors.

Incompetency. Related to this right is the issue of mental incompetency. Every adult is assumed to be mentally competent, meaning mentally able to carry out personal affairs. To prove otherwise requires a special court hearing to declare an individual incompetent. Incompetence is a legal term without a precise medical meaning. **To prove incompetence in court, all of the following must be shown:**

- **The person has a mental disorder.**
- **This disorder causes a defect in judgment.**
- **This defect makes the person incapable of handling personal affairs.**

The psychiatric diagnosis of the person is not important. If a person is declared incompetent, the court will appoint a legal guardian to manage his or her affairs. This often is a family member, friend, or bank executive. Incompetency rulings are most often filed for people with senile dementia, cerebral arteriosclerosis, chronic schizophrenia, and mental retardation.

The legislative trend is to separate the concepts of incompetency and involuntary commitment because the reasons for each are different. Incompetency arises from society's desire to guard its citizens' assets from their inability to understand and transact business. Involuntary commitments are intended to protect patients from themselves, protect others from dangerous patients, and administer treatment. However, many states still consider the two to be the same.

If ruled incompetent, a person cannot vote, marry, drive, or make contracts. A release from the hospital does not necessarily restore competency. Another court hearing is required to reverse the previous ruling before the person can once again manage private affairs.

> *How is education provided for emotionally ill children living in your community? Are they mainstreamed in the school system, given special educational resources, or both?* ■

Right to Education

Many parents exercise the right to education on behalf of their emotionally ill or mentally retarded children. The U.S. Constitution guarantees this right to everyone, although many states have not provided adequate education to all citizens in the past and are now required to do so.

> *How is the right to education honored in a children's psychiatric inpatient setting? How does this compare with the education provided children in a pediatric hospital?* ■

Right to Habeas Corpus

Habeas corpus is an important constitutional right patients retain in all states even if they have been involuntarily hospitalized. It provides for the speedy release of any person who claims to be detained illegally. A committed patient may file a writ at any time on the grounds of being sane and eligible for release. The hearing takes place in court, where those who wish to restrain the patient must defend their actions. Patients are discharged if they are judged to be sane.

Right to Privacy

The right to privacy implies the person's right to keep some personal information completely secret or confidential. Confidentiality involves the nondisclosure of specific information about a person to someone else unless authorized by that person. **Every psychiatric professional is responsible for protecting a patient's right to confidentiality, including even the knowledge that a person is in treatment or in a hospital.** Revealing such information might result in damage to the patient. The protection of the law applies to all patients.

Clinicians are free from legal responsibility if they release information with the patient's written and signed request. Written consent makes clear to both parties that consent has been given, and if questions arise about the consent, a documentary record of it exists. Therefore it should be made a part of the patient's permanent chart. As a rule, it is best to reveal as little information as possible and discuss with the patient what will be released.

Confidentiality builds on the element of trust necessary in a patient-clinician relationship. Patients place themselves in the care of others and reveal vulnerable aspects of their personal life. In return they expect high-quality care and the protection of their interests. Thus the patient-clinician relationship is an intimate one that demands trust, loyalty, and privacy.

> *One of the adolescent girls on your unit runs away while going to the hospital cafeteria. When you speak to the girl's mother to let her know what has happened, the mother asks you to call the radio and television stations and have them announce it so that the girl can be found. How would you respond to this request?* ■

HIPAA. The issue of confidentiality is becoming increasingly important. Various agencies require information about a patient's history, diagnosis, treatment, and prognosis, and sophisticated methods for obtaining information through computer systems have been developed. These methods threaten the individual's right to privacy and, in part, contributed to the passage of the Health Insurance Portability and Accountability Act (HIPAA) that took effect April, 2003 (Appelbaum, 2002).

HIPAA provides patients with access to their medical records and more control over how their personal health information is used and disclosed. It is the first national, comprehensive privacy protection act. HIPAA guarantees patients four fundamental rights related to the release of information:

1. To be educated about HIPAA privacy protection
2. To have access to their own medical records
3. To request correction or amendment of their health information to which they object
4. To require their permission for disclosure of their own personal information.

The scope of HIPAA is extensive and applies to almost any institution or individual involved in health care. Specific patient protections included in the Act are listed in Box 10-3.

Most treatment facilities keep psychiatric records separately so that they are less accessible than medical records. The law and psychiatric professionals view them as more sensitive than medical records. If a patient requests access to his or her own records, the clinician should explore the reasons for the request, prepare the patient for the review, and be present with the patient to discuss any questions the patient might have. The clinician must not release material from any other sources and must not alter or destroy any part of the record.

It is important for the nurse to realize that the physical record itself is the property of the treatment facility or therapist, but the information contained in the record belongs to the patient. Thus the original record should never be given to the patient; only a copy of it should be provided. A patient's record or chart can be brought into court and its contents used in a lawsuit because privilege does not apply to records or charts.

Privileged Communication. The legal term **privilege** or, more accurately, testimonial privilege, applies only in court-related proceedings. It includes communications between husband and wife, attorney and client, and clergy and church member. The right to reveal information belongs to the person who spoke, and the listener cannot disclose the information unless the speaker gives permission. This right protects the patient, who could sue the listener for disclosing privileged information.

Testimonial privilege between health professionals and patients exists only if established by law. It varies greatly among professions, even within the same state. A minority of the states allow privilege between nurses and patients. Nurses also may be covered in states that have adopted privileges between psychotherapists and patients. The psychotherapist-patient privilege is usually limited. It applies only when a therapist-patient relationship exists, and only communications of a pro-

---

BOX 10-3

Patient Protections Provided by HIPAA

The new privacy regulations specified in the Health Insurance Portability and Accountability Act (HIPAA) ensure a nation-wide span of privacy protections for patients by limiting the ways that health plans, pharmacies, hospitals, and other covered entities can use patients' personal medical information. The regulations protect medical records and other individually identifiable health information, whether it is on paper, in computers, or communicated orally. Key provisions of these new standards include the following:

Access to Medical Records
Patients generally should be able to see and obtain copies of their medical records and request corrections if they identify errors and mistakes. Health plans, doctors, hospitals, clinics, nursing homes, and other covered entities generally should provide access to these records within 30 days and may charge patients for the cost of copying and sending the records.

Notice of Privacy Practices
Covered health plans, doctors, and other health care providers must provide a notice to their patients regarding how they may use personal medical information and their rights under the new privacy regulation.

Limits on Use of Personal Medical Information
The privacy rule sets limits on how health plans and covered providers may use individually identifiable health information. To promote the best quality care for patients, the rule does not restrict the ability of doctors, nurses, and other providers to share information needed to treat their patients. In other situations, though, personal health information generally may not be used for purposes not related to health care, and covered entities may use or share only the minimum amount of protected information needed for a particular purpose. In addition, patients would have to sign a specific authorization before a covered entity could release their medical information to a life insurer, a bank, a marketing firm, or another outside business for purposes not related to their health care.

Prohibition on Marketing
The privacy rule sets new restrictions and limits on the use of patient information for marketing purposes. Pharmacies, health plans, and other covered entities must first obtain an individual's specific authorization before disclosing their patient information for marketing purposes.

Confidential Communications
Under the privacy rule, patients can request that their doctors, health plans, and other covered entities take reasonable steps to ensure that their communications with the patient are confidential. For example, a patient could ask a doctor to call his or her office rather than home, and the doctor's office should comply with that request if it can be reasonably accommodated.

Complaints
Consumers may file a formal complaint regarding the privacy practices of a covered health plan or provider. Consumers can find out more information about filing a complaint at http://www.hhs.gov/ocr/hipaa or by calling (866) 627-7748.

From U.S. Department of Health and Human Services: *Fact sheet,* Monday, April 14, 2003.

fessional nature are protected. Third persons present during the communication between the therapist and the patient may be required to testify and are not included in privilege.

What is the law in your state regarding testimonial privilege between nurses and patients? How would you change the law if it does not include nurses? ■

Circle of Confidentiality. Figure 10-3 depicts a circle of confidentiality that is a useful model for the nurse. Within the circle, patient information may be shared. Those outside the circle require the patient's permission to receive information. Within the circle are treatment team members, staff supervisors, health care students and their faculty working with the patient, and consultants who actually see the patient. All of these people must be informed about the patient's clinical condition to be able to help. The patient is also inside the circle (an obvious point, but one that is often overlooked). The patient can reveal any aspect of his or her life, problems, treatments, and experiences, to anyone. This is an important point for the nurse to remember in situations where the requirements of confidentiality are uncertain.

Many people are outside the circle, and these relationships must be carefully considered by the nurse. For example, family members of adult patients are not automatically entitled to clinical information about the patient. Although nurses may wish to engage the family in a therapeutic alliance, it is equally important to remember that information about the patient belongs to the patient. It is essential, therefore, that the nurse first discuss with the patient the benefits of involving the family in the treatment process and obtain clear consent from the patient before doing so. A specific form for release of information to families indicating the types of information that may be released has been found useful (Bogart and Solomon, 1999). This may create uncomfortable situations for the nurse who is pressured by a family to reveal patient information, but it is a critical aspect of patient confidentiality and the nurse-patient relationship.

Legal representatives, outside or previous therapists, reimbursers or insurance companies, students, health care professionals and support staff not directly involved in the care of the patient, and the police or other law enforcement or regulatory agencies are outside the circle of patient confidentiality. A signed written consent from the patient is required to release information to any of these parties. However, in some situations breaching confidentiality and testimonial privilege is both ethical and legal. These exceptions are listed in Box 10-4.

The parents of one of your patients ask for information about their adult son. The patient has been very specific about not wanting to see his family and not wanting them to know anything about his treatment. How would you respond? ■

BOX 10-4

Exceptions Allowing the Release of Information Without the Patient's Consent

- Emergency situations when acting in the patient's best interests
- Court-ordered evaluations or reports
- If the patient is incompetent and consent is obtained from a guardian or is not available
- Commitment proceedings
- Criminal proceedings
- Acting to protect third parties
- Child custody disputes
- Reports required by state law (contagious diseases, gunshot wounds, child abuse)
- Patient-litigant exceptions
- Child abuse proceedings

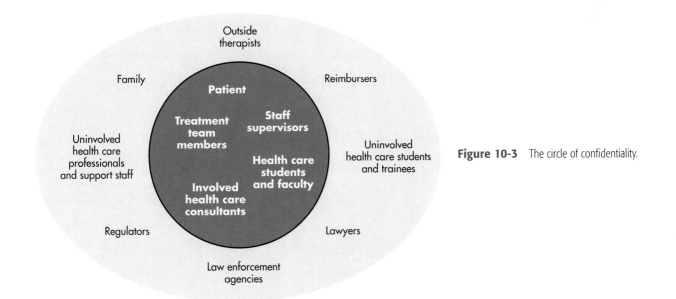

Figure 10-3 The circle of confidentiality.

Protecting a Third Party. Another aspect of confidentiality and privilege stems from the case of *Tarasoff v Regents of the University of California et al* (1974). In this case the psychotherapist did not warn Tatiana Tarasoff or her parents that his client had stated he intended to kill Tatiana when she returned from summer vacation. In the lawsuit that followed Tatiana Tarasoff's death, California's Supreme Court decided that the treating therapist had a duty to warn the intended victim of his patient's violence. When a therapist is reasonably certain that a patient is going to harm someone, the therapist has the responsibility to breach the confidentiality of the relationship and warn or protect the potential victim (Mason, 1998).

Most states now recognize some variation of the **duty to warn**. This duty obliges the clinician to do the following:
- **Assess the threat of violence to another**
- **Identify the person being threatened**
- **Implement some affirmative, preventive act**

A clinical algorithm to assist clinicians in making decisions regarding protective measures is presented in Figure 10-4. Four important questions for the clinician to consider are as follows (Felthous, 1999):

1. Is the patient dangerous to self or others?
2. Is the danger due to serious mental illness?
3. Is the danger imminent?
4. Is the danger targeted at an identifiable victim?

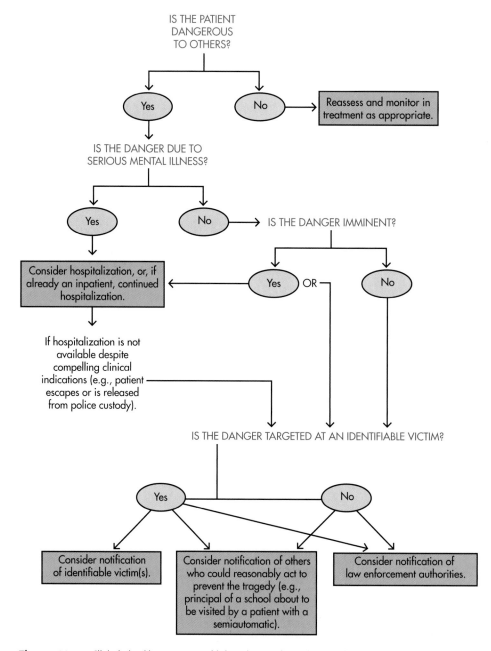

Figure 10-4 Clinical algorithm to protect third parties. (Redrawn from Felthous A: *Psychiatr Clin North Am* 22:52, 1999.)

More recently, courts have extended the Tarasoff duty to include mental health paraprofessionals and a duty to protect property, as well as persons. Current controversy exists about how long after treatment therapists can be held liable for the actions of their patients, and whether after issuing a Tarasoff warning, therapists can be called as prosecution witnesses in cases against patients arrested for serious violent crimes.

Right to Informed Consent

The goal of informed consent is to help patients make better decisions. Informed consent means that a clinician must give the patient a certain amount of information about the proposed treatment and must attain the patient's consent, which must be informed, competent, and voluntary.

The clinician should explain the treatment and possible complications and risks. The information to be disclosed in obtaining informed consent is listed in Box 10-5. The patient must be able to consent and not be a minor or judged legally incompetent (Reid, 2001). Even if a patient is psychotic, the clinician is not relieved from attempting to obtain informed consent for treatment. Psychosis does not necessarily mean that a person is unable to consent to treatment, and many psychotic patients are capable of giving informed consent. For patients not able to consent and for minors, informed consent should be obtained from a substitute decision maker.

The doctrine of informed consent is consistent with the provision of good clinical care. It allows patients and clinicians to become partners in the treatment process and re-spects patients' autonomy, needs, and values. Furthermore, informed consent should be viewed as a continuing educational process rather than a procedure done merely to comply with the law.

In obtaining informed consent the clinician should adhere to the principles listed in Box 10-5. Consent forms usually require the signature of the patient, a family member, and two witnesses. Nurses are often called on to be witnesses. The form then becomes part of the patient's permanent record.

Informed consent should be obtained for all psychiatric treatments, including medication, particularly antipsychotics; somatic therapies, such as electroconvulsive therapy (ECT); and experimental treatments. Whether consent should be obtained for psychotherapy is unclear at present (Beahrs and Gutheil, 2001), and other aspects related to obtaining informed consent remain controversial (see Critical Thinking About Contemporary Issues).

BOX **10-5**

Obtaining Informed Consent

Information to Disclose
Diagnosis
Description of the patient's problem
Treatment
Nature and purpose of the proposed treatment
Consequences
Risks and benefits of the proposed treatment including physical and psychological effects, costs, and potential resulting problems
Alternatives
Viable alternatives to the proposed treatment and their risks and benefits
Prognosis
Expected outcome with treatment, with alternative treatments, and without treatment

Principles of Informing
- **Assess** the patient's ability to give informed consent.
- **Simplify** the language so that a layperson can understand.
- **Offer** opportunities for the patient and family to ask questions.
- **Test** the patient's understanding after the explanation.
- **Reeducate** as often as needed.
- **Document** all relevant factors, including what was disclosed, the patient's understanding, competency, voluntary agreement to treatment, and the actual consent.

Critical Thinking *About* Contemporary Issues

Can Patients With Mental Disorders Give Informed Consent?

Informed consent is a critical variable in the self-determination of consumers receiving health and mental health services. Obtaining informed consent from psychiatric patients has received recent attention as questions have been raised regarding the capacity of these patients to understand the risks and benefits of consenting both to treatment and to participation in clinical research trials.

Empirical studies indicate that (Roberts, Warner, and Brody, 2000):
- Psychiatric symptoms significantly affect informed consent.
- Psychiatric patients may possess certain strengths with respect to research involvement.
- Proxy decision making is problematic.
- Informed consent is also difficult to attain with the medically ill and others.
- Patients are motivated to participate in research by the hope of personal benefit.
- Ethical aspects of research are poorly documented.
- Institutional review processes may not be adequate to protect vulnerable subjects.

The National Bioethics Advisory Commission (1998) has thus issued a series of recommendations designed to protect psychiatric patients who participate in medical research. Their 21 recommendations cover six areas: review bodies, research design, informed consent and capacity, categories of surrogate decision making, and education, research, and support.

Patient-focused studies have identified a clinical tool, the MacCAT-T that offers a flexible yet structured method to assess, rate, and report patients' capacities to make treatment decisions (Grisso, Appelbaum, and Hill-Fotoyh, 1997). Studies also show that patients with schizophrenia who were research subjects were able to understand and retain critical components of informed consent information when adequate procedures are followed (Carpenter et al, 2000; Moser et al, 2002, Stiles et al, 2001). Thus the real issue may not be related as much to a patient's capacity as it is to the procedures and process used to obtain informed consent by health care providers.

How is informed consent obtained in your psychiatric treatment setting? Ask to observe this process and evaluate it based on the criteria listed in Box 10-5. ■

Right to Treatment

Early court cases extended the right to treatment to all mentally ill and mentally retarded people who were involuntarily hospitalized. The courts defined three criteria for adequate treatment:

1. A humane psychological and physical environment
2. A qualified staff with a sufficient number of members to administer adequate treatment
3. Individualized treatment plans

Most important is the requirement for an individualized treatment plan. Failure to provide it means that the patient must be discharged unless he or she agrees to stay voluntarily.

The right to treatment is not a guarantee of treatment for all patients. It applies only to involuntary or committed patients. In addition, the right to treatment identifies minimal treatment standards, not optimal treatment; it does not guarantee that adequate treatment occurs and it does not require that a range of treatments be available (one treatment choice is adequate). Thus, although much has been gained through this legislation, much remains to be done.

Right To Refuse Treatment

The relationship between the right to treatment and the right to refuse treatment is complex. The right to refuse treatment includes the right to refuse involuntary hospitalization. It has been called the right to be left alone.

Some people believe that therapy can control a person's mind, regulate thoughts, and change personality, and the right to refuse treatment protects the patient. This argument states that involuntary therapy conflicts with two basic legal rights: freedom of thought and the right to control one's life and actions as long as they do not interfere with the rights of others.

Forcing Medications. Patients may refuse medication for many reasons. Symptoms such as delusions and denial may cause the refusal, and patients who refuse medication are often sicker than those who comply. Nurses should judge each situation on a case-by-case basis. Three criteria that may justify coerced treatment are as follows:

- The patient must be judged to be dangerous to self or others.
- It must be believed by those administering treatment that it has a reasonable chance of benefiting the patient.
- The patient must be judged to be incompetent to evaluate the necessity of the treatment.

Even if these three conditions are met, the patient should not be deceived but should be informed regarding what will be done, the reasons for it, and its probable effects.

Is the refusal of treatment the same as noncompliance? If not, how would you distinguish between them and what nursing intervention would be most appropriate for each? ■

Nurses are often on the front line in dealing with patients who refuse treatments and medications. It is clear that voluntary patients have the right to refuse any treatment and should not be forcibly medicated except in exceptional situations when the patient is actively violent to self or others and when all less restrictive means have been unsuccessful. The behavior of the patient should be clearly documented and all interventions recorded.

Nurses must know the guidelines identified by the courts and the legislature in the state in which they practice to administer medication properly to involuntarily committed patients. Some questions that can help guide the nurse's decision are as follows:

- Has the patient been given a psychiatric diagnosis?
- Is the treatment consistent with the diagnosis?
- Is there a set of defined target symptoms?
- Has the patient been informed about the treatment outcome and side effects?
- Have medical and nursing assessments been completed?
- Are therapeutic effects of treatment being monitored?
- Are side effects being monitored?
- Is the patient overmedicated or undermedicated?
- Is drug therapy being changed too quickly?
- Are pro re nata (prn, when required) and stat doses being used too often?
- Is drug therapy being prescribed for an indefinite period of time?

Finally, it is important for the nurse to remember that a therapeutic nurse-patient relationship is critical in working with a patient who refuses to take medication. A positive, caring relationship between the nurse and patient can play a vital role in reversing treatment refusal.

Imagine that your mother was admitted to a psychiatric hospital in need of treatment. Once there, however, she refused to take any medication. How would you feel if the staff forced medication on her? How would you feel if they honored her right to refuse treatment? What could you do to help your mother get the treatment she needed? ■

Right to Treatment in the Least Restrictive Setting

The right to treatment in the least restrictive setting is closely related to the right to adequate treatment. Its goal is evaluating the needs of each patient and maintaining the greatest amount of personal freedom, autonomy, dignity, and integrity in determining treatment. This right applies to both hospital-based and community programs. Another consideration in the right to the least restrictive alternative is that it applies not only to when a person should be hospitalized but also to how a person is cared for. It requires that a patient's progress be carefully monitored so that treatment plans are changed based on the patient's current condition.

Issues related to the use of **seclusion** and **restraints** are of particular concern. There must be adequate rationale for the use of these practices. Documentation should include a description of the event that led to seclusion or restraint, alternatives attempted or considered, the patient's behavior while

Hierarchy of Restrictiveness

1. Body movement, for example, four-point restraint (hands and feet)
2. Movement in space, for example, seclusion rooms, restriction to the unit
3. Decisions of daily life, for example, selection of food or a television program, the choice of when or where to smoke or with whom to socialize
4. Meaningful activities, for example, participation in treatment, access to work
5. Treatment choice, for example, court-mandated treatment, unwanted social interventions
6. Control of resources, for example, use of money
7. Emotional or verbal expression, for example, censorship, discouraging personal expression

From Olsen DP: *J Clin Ethics* 9:235, 1998.

secluded or restrained, nursing interventions, and ongoing evaluation of the patient. It is important to remember that seclusion and restraint must be therapeutically indicated and justified (see Chapter 30).

Restriction has two aspects: (1) the nature of the choices being restricted and (2) the method by which choices are restricted. Box 10-6 presents a hierarchy of restrictiveness that proceeds from the most restrictive to the least restrictive.

Which do you think is more restrictive—to be living in the community while being actively psychotic or to be involuntarily committed to a psychiatric hospital for treatment? ■

Role of Nursing

The National League for Nursing (1977) issued a statement on the nurse's role in patients' rights. It identified respect and concern for patients and competent care as basic rights, along with patients receiving the necessary information to be able to understand their illness and make decisions about their care. The League urged nurses to get involved in ensuring patients' human and legal rights.

The League identified many of the previously mentioned rights, plus the following:

- Right to health care that is accessible and meets professional standards, regardless of the setting
- Right to courteous and individualized health care that is equitable, humane, and given without discrimination based on race, color, creed, sex, national origin, source of payment, or ethical or political beliefs
- Right to information about their diagnosis, prognosis, and treatment, including alternatives to care and risks involved
- Right to information about the qualifications, names, and titles of health care personnel
- Right to refuse observation by those not directly involved in their care
- Right to coordination and continuity of health care

- Right to information on the charges for services, including the right to challenge these charges
- Above all, the right to be fully informed about all their rights in all health care settings

Perhaps the most important factors in ensuring patients' rights are the attitude, knowledge, and commitment of the mental health professional. Sensitivity to patients' rights cannot be imposed by the court, the legislature, administrative agencies, or professional groups. If nurses ignore them, implement them casually, or are outwardly hostile about honoring them, patients' rights are an empty legal concept. But if professionals are sensitive to patients' needs in all aspects of their relationships with them, they will secure these human and legal rights.

Ethical Considerations

Ensuring patients' rights is often complicated by ethical considerations. For example, consider the crucial element of power. In the psychiatric setting the nurse can function in many roles, from a custodial "keeper of the keys" to a skilled therapist. Each of these roles includes a certain amount of power because all nurses have the ability to influence the patient's treatment and serve as the major source of information regarding a patient's behavior. This is particularly true in inpatient settings, in which a nurse and patient spend more time together and the nursing staff is the only group to work a 24-hour day. Nurses also participate in team meetings, individual and group psychotherapy, and behavior modification programs. Finally, nurses can greatly influence decisions about patient medications, such as type, dosage, and frequency.

Many ethical dilemmas arise from health care professionals' paternalistic attitude toward patients (Breeze, 1998; Balevre, 2001). **Paternalism** can be defined as deciding what is best for another person without consideration of the person's thoughts, feelings, or preferences. It occurs when something is done "for the patient's own good" even though the patient may disagree with the action. This attitude reduces adult patients to the status of children and interferes with their freedom of action.

An example of this is seen in a study of patients' and staff members' attitudes about the rights of hospitalized psychiatric patients. The most consistent finding of the study was that staff were more likely to express the view that patients' rights should be compromised if they conflicted with what the staff perceived to be a clinical need (Roe et al, 2002).

The right to treatment also poses several ethical questions. One involves the appropriateness of treatment and whether confinement itself can be therapeutic. A second question deals with the untreatable patient. Should such a patient be released after a certain length of time? Another problem is the unwilling patient. Might a person refuse treatment and then seek release, claiming that the right to adequate treatment was denied?

Ethical dilemmas also arise in considering the right to refuse treatment. Does the right apply to all treatments, including medications, or only to those that are hazardous, intrusive, or severe? How can staff meet their obligation for the right to

CITING THE EVIDENCE ON

Ethics, Human Rights Issues, and Psychiatric Nurses

BACKGROUND: This study examined the ethics and human rights issues experienced by psychiatric–mental health and substance-abuse registered nurses in their daily work.

RESULTS: Of the nurses surveyed, 41% reported experiencing ethics and human rights issues daily or one to four times a week in their clinical practice. The issues most often experienced were (1) protecting patients' rights and human dignity; (2) providing care with possible risks to RN's health; (3) use/nonuse of physical and chemical restraints; (4) involvement in informed consent to treatment; (5) staffing patterns that limit patient access to nursing care; (6) conflicts in nurse/physician relationships; (7) allocating scarce resources; (8) working with unethical/incompetent/impaired colleagues; (9) caring for patients and families who lacked accurate information; and (10) implementing managed care policies that threaten quality of care.

IMPLICATIONS: The issues faced by psychiatric nurses on a daily basis are stressful and can negatively impact quality nursing care. The study findings suggest important areas for inservice education programs that can assist nurses in identifying relevant information and support services that are available to help them deal with these issues. Additional research is needed to identify what would help nurses practice ethically under difficult patient care situations, including those in which the nurse's own safety is at risk.

Grace P et al: *J Am Psychiatr Nurs Assoc* 9:17, 2003.

treatment when a patient refuses to be treated? How can refusal, resisting treatment, and noncompliance be differentiated, and does each of these require a different response?

Finally, the right to treatment in the least restrictive setting raises a number of difficult questions (Lin, 2003). How do mental health professionals balance human rights with the human needs of patients? Are sufficient funds available to provide adequate supportive care in the community? Can community centers provide better care than institutions? How can one deal with community resistance to local placement of mentally ill patients? And most important, given economic constraints, how can limited resources be used wisely to provide a full range of needed mental health services?

No easy solutions to these complex issues are known, but these issues are still of concern to nurses who are responsible for quality of care (see Citing the Evidence). It is clear that many challenges exist in the field.

■ LEGISLATIVE INITIATIVES

The connection between psychiatry and the law is becoming increasingly complex. Mental health professionals are concerned about the quantity and quality of psychiatric care. Legal reformers are indignant about perceived violations of patients' rights. Judges are angry that in the day-to-day implementation of the commitment law, their only option is

to prosecute the mentally ill defendant. Psychiatric hospitals are understaffed, underfunded, and attacked on all sides for their inability to care for and cure psychiatric patients. Community programs are few and poorly supported, often resulting in deinstitutionalized patients living without treatment in urban ghettos or being treated as criminals. The public is frightened at the thought of psychiatric patients in their neighborhoods. Concerned citizens demand that mental health programs exercise greater control over this population, whom they perceive as dangerous.

Clearly, mechanisms are needed by which patients, families, mental health professionals, attorneys, and concerned citizens can work together to advance mental health care and the rights of all patients. The mentally ill need protection not only of their legal rights but also of their clinical needs and general welfare. No one profession can fulfill all these needs, but increased cooperation among mental health advocates can achieve this goal.

Federal Budget Acts

Legislation has changed the nature of psychiatric care and service delivery in the United States. One major event was passage of the Omnibus Budget Reconciliation Act (OBRA) in 1981. It placed mental health service programs formerly administered by the federal government into alcohol and drug abuse and mental health service block grants to be administered by the states. Overall this had a negative impact on the quality of mental health services provided throughout the United States because each state was able to allocate resources to mental health based on its own priorities and political climate. Although some states made significant progress in developing community-based systems, in most state governments mental health funding was not given high priority.

In 1985 the Consolidated OBRA (COBRA) prohibited the transfer of indigent patients with acute medical conditions from general medical hospitals or emergency departments to public psychiatric hospitals that are ill equipped to provide medical care. The OBRA passed in 1987 established criteria for Medicaid- or Medicare-certified nursing homes to use in admitting or retaining mentally ill patients. The effect of this law was to reduce the use of antipsychotic medications and physical restraints in nursing homes (Snowden and Roy-Byrne, 1998).

The federal Balanced Budget Act of 1997 led to further restrictions in mental health services, especially for the severely mentally ill. Programs such as Medicare, as well as Medicaid and disability benefits, have been decreased or are being phased out.

Protection and Advocacy Act

Under the Protection and Advocacy for Mentally Ill Individuals Act of 1986, all states must designate an agency that is responsible for protecting the rights of the mentally ill. A primary mission of the agency is to investigate reported incidents of abuse, neglect, and civil rights violations of persons with mental illness who live in institutions (Hennessy, Green-

Hennessy, and Higgazi, 2002). The following three areas of advocacy help maximize the fulfillment of patients' rights:

1. Education of the mental health staff and implement policies and procedures that recognize and protect patients' rights
2. Establishment of an additional procedure to permit the speedy resolution of problems, questions, or disagreements that occur based on legal rights
3. Providing access to legal services when patients' rights have been denied

In addition to representing individuals, protection and advocacy programs agencies provide referral and information services, public education, outreach, training, and class-action representation. As mental health systems change and more patients are treated in outpatient settings, access to protection and advocacy services for people living in the community is becoming increasingly important, and psychiatric nurses have the opportunity to participate in these initiatives.

Americans With Disabilities Act

The Americans with Disabilities Act (ADA), passed in 1990, protects over 43 million Americans with physical or mental disabilities from discrimination in jobs, public services, and accommodations. It prohibits discrimination against people with physical and mental disabilities in hiring, firing, training, compensation, and advancement in employment. Employers are prohibited from asking job applicants whether they have a disability, and medical examinations and questions about disability may be required only if the concerns are job related and necessary.

Each of these prohibitions has major implications for people with psychiatric disabilities. However, because the disability is often not obvious, and because of widespread stigma and discrimination, or simply as a statement of self-sufficiency, many people choose not to identify themselves as disabled. If they do, they have concern that employers and co-workers will assume that any work or personal difficulties they have are related to the psychiatric disability. Thus discrimination and unintended negative consequences in psychiatric disability coverage has been one outcome of the ADA (Appelbaum, 1998).

Although the act has produced some encouraging advances in job placement, education, and training, the majority of people with psychiatric disabilities remain unemployed or continue to work in sheltered settings. Partly because of the ambiguity of the wording of the act, instructions were issued in 1995 to eliminate pregnancy, physical characteristics, common personality traits, cultural and economic disadvantages, a range of sexual disorders, and current illegal drug use. In 1999 the court issued three decisions that made it more difficult for individuals, including people with mental illness, to prove a disability under the ADA (Petrila, 2002).

Finally, although the ADA provides a cultural and legal mandate to include people with disabilities in the social and economic mainstream, it is not likely to totally eliminate the myths, fears, and discrimination faced by people with disabilities. However, it does contribute to the educational effort needed to combat widespread biases and misperceptions about people with disabilities, including mental illness.

Early in the semester, one of your friends shared with you that she has been diagnosed with bipolar disorder and has been successfully stabilized with treatment. One day she arrives in class very agitated and verbal. How might you interpret this behavior? Would your interpretation be different if she had not shared her psychiatric history with you? ■

Advance Directives

Advance directives came about as a result of the Patient Self-Determination Act (PSDA) of 1990. They are documents, written while a person is competent, that specify how decisions about treatment should be made if the person becomes incompetent. They can prevent unwanted treatment and identify preferred treatment. They allow mentally ill persons to exercise autonomous control over their care, even at times when they are in crisis. The Bazelon Center for Mental Health Law (1998) has sample forms or templates that can be used to prepare such a directive.

Use of psychiatric advance directives is particularly appropriate for people with mental illness who may alternate between periods of competence and incompetence. For example, they could formalize a patient's wishes about forced medication, treatment approach, treatment setting, methods for handling emergencies, persons who should be notified, and willingness to participate in research studies.

Federal regulations require all facilities that receive Medicare or Medicaid to inform patients, including psychiatric patients, at the time of admission about their rights under state law to sign advance directives. To date, advance directives have not had a major impact on psychiatric treatment, but that may change. Potential effects of mental health advance directives include enhanced consumer empowerment; improved functioning; better communication among consumers, family members, and providers; increased tolerance for consumer autonomy in community mental health agencies; and reduced use of hospital services and court proceedings.

Nurses and other mental health providers should be informed about the intended benefits and limitations of psychiatric advanced directives so that they can support the creation of these documents. In addition, a shift in values may be necessary to more consistently recognize and honor patients' treatment preferences as specified in the directives (Srebnik et al, 2003; Vuckovich, 2003).

Does your psychiatric setting comply with federal law that requires having patients sign advanced directives? If so, talk with some patients and ask them what this document means to them. ■

Mental Health Courts

Congress first authorized the federal Mental Health Courts program in 2000 to assist states and communities in creating innovative approaches to diverting offenders into treatment programs and easing the burden on the criminal justice and corrections systems. Mental Health Courts keep people who have severe and persistent mental illness and commit minor offenses from being incarcerated in jails and prisons and allow them to get into treatment instead.

Those courts that are federally funded must:

- Continue to supervise cases for up to 1 year after the individual's court date.
- Provide specialized training for law enforcement and judicial personnel to address the mental health needs of offenders.
- Provide inpatient and outpatient treatment that may result in the dismissal of charges or reduced sentences for the individual.
- Coordinate mental health treatment plans and social services for the individual, including housing, job placement, and relapse prevention.

The purpose of Mental Health Courts is to reduce recidivism among the mentally ill, decrease the use of jails to warehouse the mentally ill, and increase public safety. Given the number of mentally ill languishing in the criminal justice system, it is hoped that this newest federal program may be an idea whose time has come in providing more compassionate and appropriate care to the mentally ill (Haimowitz, 2002).

■ PSYCHIATRY AND CRIMINAL RESPONSIBILITY

The determination of criminal responsibility concerns the accused person's condition when the crime was committed. It has received much public attention as the "insanity defense." It proposes that a person who has committed an act usually considered criminal is not guilty by reason of "insanity."

It has been estimated that a successful insanity defense occurs in less than 1% of all criminal prosecutions (Moran, 2002). Proving the state of another person's mind is quite difficult. A clear example of this was the guilty verdict rendered in Texas in 2002 against Andrea Yates, who drowned all five of her children in a bathtub. Nurses should understand the law regarding this issue both as citizens and as psychiatric professionals.

This "insanity" defense is based on the humanitarian rationale that people should not be blamed for crimes if they did not know what they were doing or could not help themselves. A more recent change is the movement away from using the defense "not guilty by reason of insanity" (NGBI) to the more recent "guilty but mentally ill" (GBMI). In addition, five states—Montana, Idaho, Nevada, Utah, and Kansas—have abolished the insanity defense completely.

Three sets of criteria are used in the United States to determine the criminal responsibility of an offender who is mentally ill: the M'Naghten Rule, the Irresistible Impulse Test, and the American Law Institute's Test (Table 10-3). The M'Naghten Rule is used in 24 states; the American Law Institute's Test is used in 19 states. Texas used the M'Naghten Rule and Andrea Yates was found guilty and convicted because the jury believed that she knew that what she did was wrong.

In the 1994 case of Lorena Bobbitt, who was found not guilty by reason of insanity, the jury concluded that she could not resist the impulse to sever her husband's penis. Mrs. Bobbitt was committed to a psychiatric hospital for observation and was released when she was found not to be psychiatrically ill. Do you agree with the court's decision? Defend your position. ■

Table 10-3	Three Sets of Criteria Used To Determine the Criminal Responsibility of a Mentally Ill Offender
NAME OF TEST	**CRITERIA**
M'Naghten Rule	The person did not know the nature and quality of the act. The person did not know that the act was wrong.
Irresistible Impulse Test	A person is impulsively driven to commit the criminal act with lack of premeditation and a strong urge to do so. This test typically used with the M'Naughten test.
American Law Institute's Test	A person lacks the capacity to appreciate the wrongfulness of an act or to conform conduct to the requirements of the law.

Disposition of Mentally Ill Offenders

Those found not guilty by reason of insanity (NGBI) are rarely set free. In some states they may be committed at the court's discretion, and in almost a third of the states they are automatically hospitalized. Some offenders are treated in special hospitals, others are sent to state mental hospitals, and still others go to prison treatment facilities. Those found guilty but mentally ill (GBMI) are never freed. Because the insanity defense is used most often in capital offenses, it is usually better to send the offender to a place with good security, and penal institutions or maximum security forensic psychiatric hospitals are the best option.

After hospitalization and recovery, the patient may be discharged by the court that ordered the commitment. In other states the governor may discharge the patient. Still others allow the mental institution to make that decision. The major criteria for discharge are that the patient is not likely to repeat the offense and that it is safe to release the patient to the community.

Do you believe in the legal defenses of NGBI and GBMI? What are the pros and cons of each insanity defense? ■

■ LEGAL ROLE OF THE NURSE

Professional nursing practice is not determined by simply following patients' rights. Rather, it is an interplay between the rights of patients, the legal role of the nurse, and concern for quality psychiatric care. The psychiatric nurse as provider performs three roles while completing professional and personal responsibilities: provider of services, employee or contractor of services, and private citizen (Figure 10-5). These roles are fulfilled simultaneously, and each carries certain rights and responsibilities.

Nurse As Provider

Malpractice. All psychiatric professionals have legally defined duties of care and are responsible for their own work. If these duties are violated, malpractice exists. Malpractice involves the failure of professionals to provide the proper and competent care that is warranted by members of their profession, a failure that results in harm to the patient. Nurses are held to national standards of care.

Most malpractice claims are filed under the law of **negligent tort**. A tort is a civil wrong for which the injured party is entitled to compensation. Under the law, individuals are responsible for their own torts, so each nurse can be held responsible in malpractice claims. For this reason, all nurses should carry malpractice liability insurance. Under the law of negligent tort, the plaintiff must prove the following:

- **A legal duty of care existed.**
- **The nurse performed the duty negligently.**
- **Damages were suffered by the plaintiff as a result.**
- **The damages were substantial.**

When patients are admitted to a psychiatric hospital, the problems of litigation in connection with their care are many and varied (Wysoker, 2002).

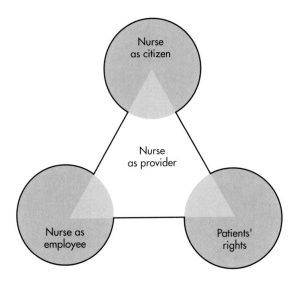

Figure 10-5   Legal influences on psychiatric nursing practice.

Litigation. Lawsuits alleging malpractice in psychiatric diagnosis or treatment are increasing. Some of the more common sources of malpractice suits are listed in Box 10-7. Lawsuits against nurses can occur when the nurse errs while acting either dependently or independently.

The most common causes of malpractice suits against psychiatric nurses are negligence in preventing a suicide and while assisting in ECT. Other causes for malpractice suits against nurses include patient falls; failing to follow physician orders or established protocols; medication errors; improper use of equipment; inadequate discharge planning, failure to remove foreign objects; failure to provide sufficient monitoring; and failure to communicate. Box 10-8 describes three cases involving psychiatric nurses.

Legal Responsibilities. The nurse is responsible for reporting pertinent information to co-workers involved in the pa-

---

BOX 10-7

Common Areas of Liability in Psychiatric Services

- Sexual contact with a patient
- Patient suicide
- Failure to diagnose
- Problems related to electroconvulsive therapy
- Misuse of psychoactive prescription drugs
- Breach of confidentiality
- Failure to refer a patient
- False imprisonment in civil commitment
- Failure to obtain informed consent
- Inadequate supervision of trainees and employees
- Failure to warn potential victims
- Failure to report abuse

BOX 10-8

Selected Litigation Involving Psychiatric Nurses

Case 1: Valentine v Strange (597 F. SUPP. 1316 VA.)
Problem: Nurses were sued when psychiatric patient set self on fire.
Facts: Despite two previous attempts to burn herself, the health care providers permitted the patient to keep her cigarettes and lighter. Patient subsequently set fire to her clothing and suffered third-degree burns.
Legal lesson: The failure of health care professionals to take precautions in the face of imminent danger to the life of an involuntarily committed patient constitutes a violation of liberty interests protected by the due process clause of the Fourteenth Amendment.

Case 2: Delicata v Bourlesses (404 N.E. 2ND 667-MASS.)
Problem: Nursing psychiatric assessment disagreed with the psychologist's assessment.
Facts: A nursing assessment indicated that a depressed patient should be closely supervised as being potentially suicidal. An evaluation by the staff psychologist advised that suicidal precautions were not necessary. The patient subsequently killed herself in a locked bathroom.

Legal lesson: Medical orders by a staff psychiatrist or an evaluation by a staff psychologist must be questioned when there is a change or deterioration in a patient's condition. Nursing assessments should include the evaluation of such changes in the patient's apparent physical and psychological condition. The responsibility of nursing assessment includes the necessity for making appropriate nursing judgments and implementing nursing actions based on these nursing assessments.

Case 3: Vattimo v Lower Bucks Hospital (428 A. 2ND 765-PA.)
Problem: Patient required restraint and supervision by psychiatric nurses.
Facts: A patient with a psychotic fascination with fire set fire to his hospital room, resulting in the death of the other occupant. The patient had been diagnosed as a paranoid schizophrenic, and staff had been warned of his preoccupation with fire.
Legal lesson: The hospital was required to exercise reasonable care under the circumstances, that is to restrain, supervise, and protect mentally deficient patients.

Characteristics of Good Nursing Records

- Accurate
- Clear
- Complete
- Concise
- Descriptive
- Factual
- Legible
- Objective
- Relevant
- Timely

tient's care. The degree of nursing care depends on the patient's condition, with the seriously ill demanding a higher degree of care to protect them from injury and self-destruction.

Reporting information includes written as well as oral communication, and accurate records are crucial. Box 10-9 lists characteristics of good nursing records. For example, notes that record specific suicidal precautions clarify the nurse's actions. The nurse also should record all patient and family education, such as explaining the food precautions needed when taking monoamine oxidase inhibitor (MAOI) medication. Such a note would provide a good defense against a possible lawsuit if the patient were to violate dietary restrictions and become ill.

Unlike patients' charts, some hospital records, such as incident reports, are not admissible in court to prove facts, but they can cast doubt on the credibility of the involved parties. Currently, many insurance companies are requiring hospitals to keep incident reports, and more state and federal agencies are demanding the right to review them. Because they can be seen and used by so many people, what a nurse writes on an incident report should be carefully considered, and unfounded statements, opinions, interpretations, and vague descriptions should be avoided.

In summary, a psychiatric nurse can follow the preventive measures listed below to avoid possible lawsuits:

- Implement nursing care that meets the *Scope and Standards of Psychiatric–Mental Health Nursing Practice* as described by the American Nurses Association (2000) (see Chapter 12).
- Know the pertinent laws of the specific state in which they practice, including the rights and duties of the nurse and the rights of the patients.
- Stay current with advances and new knowledge in the field.
- Keep accurate and concise nursing records.
- Maintain the confidentiality of patient information.
- Maintain current malpractice liability insurance coverage.
- Consult a lawyer if any questions arise.

Nurse As Employee

The role of the nurse as employee, or contractor of service, is less often studied but also very important. It involves the practitioner's rights and responsibilities in relation to employers, partners, consultants, and other professional colleagues. Professionals often do not know the rights and responsibilities of employees and contractors of service. However, these are the basis of the practitioner's economic security, professional future, and peer relationships.

As employees, nurses have the responsibility to supervise and evaluate those under their authority for the quality of care given. They also must observe their employer's rights and responsibilities to clients and other employees, fulfill the obligations of the contracted service, inform the employer of circumstances and conditions that impair the quality of care, and report negligent care by others. This includes the legal duty to communicate any concerns about other nurses and other mental health providers.

You have seen a colleague sexually touching a patient on the unit. What should you do based on your legal and professional obligations?

In return, nurses can expect certain rights from their employer. These include consideration for service, adequate working conditions, adequate and qualified assistance when necessary, documented grievance procedures, and the right to respect all of their other rights and responsibilities.

You arrive for work one morning and are told that you and an aide are the only staff assigned to work the day shift on a 25-bed closed acute psychiatric unit. Based on your legal roles, rights, and responsibilities, how should you respond?

Nurse As Citizen

The third role that the nurse plays is that of citizen. This role is significant because all other roles, rights, responsibilities, and privileges are based on the inherent rights of citizenship. The U.S. government grants these as inherent: civil rights, property rights, right to protection from harm, right to a good name, and right to due process. These form the foundation for the nurse's other legal relationships.

Unfortunately, the best interests of the patient, nurse, and employer do not always coincide. Conflict can occur when, for example, the nurse's right to live and work without threat to personal security is violated by a patient who harms the nurse, as is evident in the following clinical example.

CLINICAL EXAMPLE

A psychotic patient who has hallucinations that are adequately controlled with psychotropic medications but who refuses to take them was recently admitted to a locked psychiatric unit. Before intervening, the staff considered the following possibilities:

Failing to medicate may deny the patient's right to treatment.

Failing to medicate the patient could have harmful side effects, such as the unnecessary and possibly irreversible continuation of illness.

Failing to medicate the patient may lead to a psychotic episode and result in injury to self, other patients, or the staff.

Failing to medicate the patient may lead to a psychotic episode but no violence.

Medicating the patient in the absence of an emergency situation and without a clear threat of violence violates the patient's right to refuse treatment.

The staff decided not to medicate the patient. When the night nurse checked on the patient in his room that evening, he struck the nurse in the face, resulting in severe bruises and the loss of several teeth. This development leads to new questions:

Was the patient competent and legally liable for his actions?

What were the circumstances of the incident?

Was the nurse sufficiently aware of the potential hazard and, if so, was she responsible for assuming the risk?

Was staffing adequate to discourage, respond to, and control a potentially violent situation?

Was there a provision in the unit for potentially violent patients and, if so, why wasn't it used for this patient?

Was the nurse able to sue the patient for assault and battery? ■

Obviously, there are no simple or perhaps even equitable solutions to such clinical dilemmas, yet they are real and ever present. All mental health professionals must focus on prevention. This requires a knowledge of legislation, rights, responsibilities, and potential conflicts. In addition, professional nursing judgment requires examining the ethical context of nursing care, the possible consequences of nurses' actions, and practical alternatives. Only then do rights and responsibilities become meaningful.

CHAPTER **FOCUS POINTS**

- The legal and ethical context of care is important for all psychiatric nurses because it focuses concern on the rights of patients and the quality of care they receive.

- An ethic is a standard of behavior or a belief valued by an individual or group. An ethical dilemma exists when moral claims conflict with one another. Ethical dilemmas unique to psychiatric nursing often fall under the umbrella issue of behavior control.

- There are two types of admission to a psychiatric hospital: voluntary and involuntary commitment. Voluntary admission indicates that the patient acknowledges problems in living, seeks help in coping with them, and will probably actively participate in finding solutions.

- Involuntary admission or commitment means that the patient did not request hospitalization and may have opposed it or was indecisive and did not resist it. Most laws permit commitment of the mentally ill on the following three grounds: dangerous to self or others; mentally ill and in need of treatment; and unable to provide for own basic needs.

- Most mentally ill people are not dangerous to themselves or others. People with mental illness who may be more dangerous include those with a history of violent behavior, psychosis, noncompliance with medications, current substance abuse, and antisocial personality disorder.

- The patient who is voluntarily admitted to the hospital can leave at any time. An involuntarily committed patient has lost the right to leave the hospital when he or she wishes.

- Outpatient commitment is the process by which the courts can order patients committed to a course of outpatient treatment specified by their clinicians.

- Psychiatric patients have a wide variety of personal and civil rights. They should be informed of these rights, and hospitals must honor them.

- The right to communication allows patients to visit and hold telephone conversations in privacy and send unopened letters to anyone of their choice, including judges, lawyers, families, and staff.

- The patient may bring clothing and personal items to the hospital, taking into consideration the amount of storage space available. The hospital is not responsible for their safety, and valuable items should be left at home.

- Incompetence is a legal term without a precise medical meaning. To prove incompetence in court, it must be shown that the person has a mental disorder; this disorder causes a defect in judgment; and this defect makes the person incapable of handling personal affairs.

- All emotionally ill or mentally retarded children have the right to education.

- Habeas corpus is an important constitutional right patients retain in all states even if they have been involuntarily hospitalized. It provides for the speedy release of any person who claims to be detained illegally.

- Every psychiatric professional is responsible for protecting a patient's right to confidentiality, including even the knowledge that a person is in treatment or in a hospital.

- HIPAA provides patients with access to their medical records and more control over how their personal health information is used and disclosed. The physical record itself is the property of the treatment facility or therapist, but the information contained in the record belongs to the patient.

- Testimonial privilege between health professionals and patients exists only if established by law. It varies greatly among professions, even within the same state. A minority of the states allow privilege between nurses and patients.

- When a therapist is reasonably certain that a patient is going to harm someone, the therapist has the responsibility to breach the confidentiality of the relationship and warn or protect the potential victim.

- Informed consent means that a clinician must give the patient a certain amount of information about the proposed treatment and must attain the patient's consent, which must be informed, competent, and voluntary. It should be obtained for all psychiatric treatments, including medication, somatic therapies, and experimental treatments.

- In determining the right to treatment, the courts defined three criteria for adequate treatment: a humane psychological and physical environment, a qualified staff with a sufficient number of members to administer adequate treatment, and individualized treatment plans.

- The right to refuse treatment includes the right to refuse involuntary hospitalization.

- The goal of the right to treatment in the least restrictive setting is to evaluate the needs of each patient and maintain the greatest amount of personal freedom, autonomy, dignity, and integrity in determining treatment. This right applies to both hospital-based and community programs.

- The most important factors in ensuring patients' rights are the attitude, knowledge, and commitment of the mental health professional.

- Legislation has changed the nature of psychiatric care and service delivery in the United States. Advance directives are documents, written while a person is competent, that specify how decisions about treatment should be made if the person becomes incompetent.

- Mental Health Courts keep people who have severe and persistent mental illness and commit minor offenses from being incarcerated in jails and prisons and allow them to get into treatment instead.

- Three sets of criteria are used in the United States to determine the criminal responsibility of an offender who is mentally ill: the M'Naghten Test, the Irresistible Impulse Test, and the American Law Institute's Test.

- The psychiatric nurse has three roles in performing professional and personal duties: provider of services, employee or contractor of services, and private citizen.

- Malpractice involves the failure of professionals to provide the proper and competent care that is given by members of their profession, resulting in harm to the patient.

KEY TERMS

advance directives, 163
commitment, 150
confidentiality, 155
ethic, 148

ethical dilemma, 149
habeas corpus, 155
incompetence, 155
informed consent, 159

malpractice, 164
outpatient commitment, 153
testimonial privilege, 156

CHAPTER REVIEW QUESTIONS

1. **Indicate whether the following statements are true (T) or false (F).**

_____ A. Patients who are voluntarily admitted to a psychiatric hospital retain all civil rights.

_____ B. The parens patriae doctrine for civil commitment is currently emphasized over the police power rationale.

_____ C. Mental Health Courts were designed to decide which patients who are mentally ill would benefit from special therapeutic units in prisons.

_____ D. People with mental illness are more likely to commit acts of violence than other people.

_____ E. Involuntary community treatment is underused in the current mental health care system.

_____ F. Incompetent is a legal term without precise medical meaning.

_____ G. Police and lawyers are always entitled to information about committed psychiatric patients.

_____ H. Information can be released without a patient's consent when it is related to child custody disputes.

_____ I. Patients are allowed to keep their records when they are discharged from treatment.

_____ J. Fairness is the ethical theory that seeks the greatest good for the greatest number.

_____ K. None of the states in the United States have abolished the insanity defense.

2. **Fill in the blanks.**

A. Emergency commitment is usually limited to _____ hours.

B. Psychiatric patients who appear to be prone to violence dis

play a _____, _____,

_____ and _____.

C. _____ is the process by which courts can order patients committed to a course of outpatient treatment specified by their clinicians.

D. Informed consent must be _____,

_____, and _____.

E. The _____ Act mandates that all states designate an agency that is responsible for protecting the rights of the mentally ill.

F. Documents, written while a person is competent, that specify how decisions about treatment should be made if the person

becomes incompetent are called _____.

G. An _____ is a standard of behavior or a belief valued by an individual or group that describes what ought to be rather than what is.

3. **Provide short answers for the following questions.**

A. List the three grounds that permit commitment or involuntary hospitalization of the mentally ill. Do you believe these are justifiable? Defend your answer.

B. How is confidentiality different from privilege or testimonial privilege? If you were seeing a therapist, would the concept of privileged communication be important to you? Why or why not?

C. What is the duty to warn, and how might it affect you first as a nurse and then as a citizen?

D. Describe an ethical dilemma you have experienced in relation to your psychiatric nursing experience and the process you used to choose a course of action.

Visit Evolve for additional resources related to the content of this chapter.
http://evolve.elsevier.com/Stuart/principles/
• Topical Course Outline • Student Workbook Exercises • Critical Thinking Questions and Activities • Case Studies • Research Topics
• Monthly Content Updates • WebLinks

Student Study CD-ROM

Access the accompanying CD-ROM for animations, interactive exercises, review questions for the NCLEX examination, and an audio glossary.

REFERENCES

Allen M, Smith VF: Opening Pandora's box: the practical and legal dangers of involuntary outpatient commitment, *Psychiatr Serv* 52:342, 2001.

American Hospital Association (AHA): *A patient's bill of rights*, Chicago, 1990, The Association.

American Hospital Association (AHA): *The patient care partnership: understanding expectations, rights, and responsibilities*, Chicago, 2003, The Association.

American Nurses Association: *Scope and standards of psychiatric—mental health nursing practice*, Washington, DC, 2000, The Association.

Appelbaum PS: Discrimination in psychiatric disability coverage and the Americans with Disabilities Act. *Psychiatr Serv* 49:875, 1998.

Appelbaum PS: Thinking carefully about outpatient commitment, *Psychiatr Serv* 52:347, 2001.

Appelbaum PS: Privacy in psychiatric treatment: threats and responses, *Am J Psychiatry* 159:1809, 2002.

Balevre P: Is it legal to be crazy: an ethical dilemma, *Arch Psychiatr Nurs* 15:241, 2001.

Bazelon Center for Mental Health Law: *Psychiatric advance directive*, Washington, DC, 1998, Bazelon Center.

Bazelon Center for Mental Health Law: *Position statement on involuntary commitment*, Washington, DC, 1999, Bazelon Center.

Beahrs JO, Gutheil TG: Informed consent in psychotherapy, *Am J Psychiatry* 158:4, 2001.

Bogart T, Solomon P: Procedures to share treatment information among mental health providers, consumers, and families, *Psychiatr Serv* 50:1321, 1999.

Breeze J: Can paternalism be justified in mental health care? *J Adv Nurs* 28:260, 1998.

Carpenter WT et al: Decisional capacity for informed consent in schizophrenia research, *Arch Gen Psychiatry* 57:533, 2000.

Compton SN et al: Involuntary outpatient commitment and homelessness in persons with severe mental illness, *Ment Health Serv Res* 5:27, 2003.

Felthous AR: The clinician's duty to protect third parties, *Psychiatr Clin North Am* 22:49, 1999.

Grisso T, Appelbaum PS, Hill-Fotouhi C: The MacCAT-T: a clinical tool to assess patients' capacities to make treatment decisions, *Psychiatr Serv* 48:1415, 1997.

Haim R et al: Predictions made by psychiatrists and psychiatric nurses of violence by patients, *Psychiatr Serv* 53:622, 2002.

Haimowitz S: Can mental health courts end the criminalization of persons with mental illness? *Psychiatr Serv* 53:1226, 2002.

Hennessy KD, Green-Hennessy S, Hijjazi K: State variations in compliant rates to protection and advocacy systems, *Psychiatr Serv* 53:535, 2002.

Hiday VA et al: Impact of outpatient commitment on victimization of people with severe mental illness, *Am J Psychiatry* 159:1403, 2002.

Hoge MA, Grottole E: The case against outpatient commitment, *J Am Acad Psychiatry Law* 28:165, 2000.

Lin CY: Ethical exploration of the least restrictive alternative, *Psychiatr Serv* 54:866, 2003.

Mason T: Tarasoff liability: its impact for working with patients who threaten others, *Int J Nurs Stud* 35:109, 1998.

McConnell WA, Catalano R: A challenge for the field: the association between violence and mental illness, *Behav Healthc Tomorrow* 10:16, 2001.

McGihon NN: Discharges against medical advice: provider accountability and psychiatric patients' rights, *J Psychosoc Nurs Ment Health Serv* 36:22, 1998.

Moran M: Insanity standards may vary, but plea rarely succeeds, *Psychiatr News* 37:24, 2002.

Moser DT et al: Capacity to provide informed consent for participation in schizophrenia and HIV research, *Am J Psychiatry* 159:1201, 2002.

National Bioethics Advisory Commission: *Research involving persons with mental disorders that may affect decisionmaking capacity*, Washington, DC, 1998, The Commission.

National League for Nursing: *Nursing's role in patient's rights*, Pub No 11-1671, New York, 1977, The League.

Petrila J: The US Supreme Court narrows the definition of disability under the Americans with Disabilities Act, *Psychiatr Serv* 53:797, 2002.

Reid WH: Competence to consent, *J Psychiatr Pract* 7:276, 2001.

Reid WH: Ethics and forensic work, *J Psychiatr Pract* 8:380, 2002.

Roberts LW, Warner TD, Brody JL: Perspectives of patients with schizophrenia and psychiatrists regarding ethically important aspects of research participation, *Am J Psychiatry* 157:67, 2000.

Roe D et al: Patients' and staff members' attitudes about the rights of hospitalized psychiatric patients, *Psychiatr Serv* 53:87, 2002.

Rohland BM, Rohrer JE, Richards CC: The long-term effect of outpatient commitment on service use, *Adm Policy Ment Health* 27:383, 2000.

Snowden M, Roy-Byrne P: Mental illness and nursing home reform: OBRA-87 ten years later. Omnibus Budget Reconciliation Act, *Psychiatr Serv* 49:229, 1998.

Srebnik DS et al: Interest in psychiatric advance directives among high users of crisis services and hospitalization, *Psychiatr Serv* 54:981, 2003.

Stiles PG et al: Improving understanding of research consent disclosures among persons with mental illness, *Psychiatr Serv* 52:780, 2001.

Swartz MS et al: A randomized controlled trial of outpatient commitment in North Carolina, *Psychiatr Serv* 52:325, 2001.

Swartz MS, Monahan J: Special section on involuntary outpatient commitment, *Psychiatr Serv* 52:323, 2001.

Tarasoff v Regents of the University of California et al, 529 p 2d 553, 1974.

Torrey EF, Zdanowicz M: Outpatient commitment: what, why and for whom? *Psychiatr Serv* 52:337, 2001.

Vuckovich P: Psychiatric advance directives, *J Am Psychiatr Nurs Assoc* 9:55, 2003.

Wysoker A: Lawsuits: should psychiatric nurses be concerned? *J Am Psychiatr Nurs Assoc* 8:106, 2002.

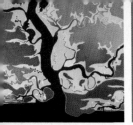

To multiply the harbors does not reduce the sea.

EMILY DICKINSON

11

FAMILIES AS RESOURCES, CAREGIVERS, AND COLLABORATORS

Victoria Conn ▪ Gail W. Stuart

LEARNING OBJECTIVES

After studying this chapter, the student should be able to:
1. Describe the components of family assessment (**I**).
2. Examine issues related to working with families of the mentally ill, including the competence paradigm and psychoeducation (**II**).
3. Examine the benefits and barriers to family involvement in the continuum of care (**III, IV**).
4. Discuss how family members of a relative with mental illness are a population at risk (**V**).
5. Analyze ways to collaborate with family advocacy organizations (**VI**).

TOPICAL OUTLINE

I. Family Assessment
   A. Characteristics of the Functional Family
   B. Family History
   C. Family APGAR
II. Working with Families
   A. Competence Paradigm
   B. Psychoeducational Programs
III. Benefits of Family Involvement
IV. Barriers to Family Involvement
V. Families as a Population at Risk
VI. Building Bridges

 Visit Evolve for additional resources related to the content of this chapter.
http://evolve.elsevier.com/Stuart/principles/

Ever since Florence Nightingale, nurses have involved family members in the care of patients with heart disease, cancer, diabetes, and similar disorders. In contrast, the families of patients with mental illnesses were for many years considered to be part of the problem, not part of the solution. However, during the 1990s professional perceptions of families changed dramatically.

Psychiatric nurses now work with families at all levels of functioning. Patients are or have been members of a "family" system. Thus past and present family relationships affect a patient's self-concept, behavior, expectations, values, and beliefs. Understanding principles of family dynamics and interventions is important; it helps the nurse make more acute observations of the individual patient as well as the family.

Competence in this area will enhance the nurse's assessment of the individual's and the family's needs and resources; it will enhance the ability to select interventions needed to promote adaptive functioning; and it will facilitate the use of positive coping strategies. Having skills in the area of family dynamics and interventions can help the nurse more readily identify problems and strengths displayed by an individual and a family, can help the nurse learn when and how to intervene appropriately, and can help the nurse in discerning when referral to other appropriate resources is necessary.

In loving memory of Victoria Conn, 2003.

This chapter is intended to encourage psychiatric nurses to partner with families as resources, caregivers, and collaborators in their clinical practice.

▪ FAMILY ASSESSMENT

The concept of "family" has evolved from the "two married heterosexual parents with several children of their own" household of several decades ago to a variety of extended and creative nontraditional "family" systems. Nurses thus encounter many different configurations of the family unit in their clinical work. Figure 11-1 presents an overview of four dimensions of parent status that can be used to describe families in contemporary society. These include biological ties, marital status, sexual orientation, and gender roles.

Although the definitions of family have become more fluid in recent decades, a family is usually defined in terms of kinship: individuals joined by marriage or its equivalent, or parenthood. A nuclear family refers to parents and their children, whereas an extended family includes other people related by blood or marriage. A household is a residence consisting of an individual living alone or a group of people sharing a common dwelling and cooking facilities (Puri and Tyrer, 1999). The many potential variations of family configurations provide challenges to the nurse's evaluation skills and perhaps to her or his own value system.

Biological Tie	**Marital Status**
•Both parents biologically related to the child

•One parent biologically related (artificial insemination, surrogate parenting, lesbian families, blended families)

•Neither parent biologically related (adoption)

•Biologically related grandparents fulfilling the parenting role | •Single parent
By choice: child product of heterosexual union or insemination, or due to adoption
Result of divorce

•Married parents
Both biological parents
One biological parent and one stepparent
Adoptive parents

•Cohabiting parents
Heterosexual
Gay or lesbian |

Sexual Orientation	**Gender Roles/ Employment Status**
•Heterosexual

•Gay or lesbian | •Traditional

•Nontraditional |

Figure 11-1 Parent status in the contemporary family.

Examine the potential problems a nontraditional family may encounter regarding values held by their health care providers, neighbors, employers, school system, church, and the legal system in your state. ∎

Families differ in ways other than just their configuration of members. Many families face special challenges because one member has experienced something out of the ordinary. This includes families with a mentally ill member, families who have a member with human immunodeficiency virus (HIV) or another significant health-related problem, families with genetically linked problems or birth anomalies, and families affected by violence or abuse from within or outside of the household, natural disasters, poverty, or stigma.

Characteristics of the Functional Family

A well-functioning family can shift roles, levels of responsibility, and patterns of interaction as it experiences stressful life changes. A well-functioning family may, under acute or prolonged stress or increased vulnerability, express maladaptive responses, but should be able to rebalance as a system over time.

A functional family can rebalance, even when faced with various life stressors, as the function of all members is restored and symptoms fade. Ultimately, family members remain focused on healthy patterns and established values, and family relationships remain intact. Characteristics of such a family include the following:

- It completes important life cycle tasks.
- It has the capacity to tolerate conflict and to adapt to adverse circumstances without long-term dysfunction or disintegration of family cohesion.

- Emotional contact is maintained across generations and between family members without blurring necessary levels of authority.
- Overcloseness or fusion is avoided, and distance is not used to solve problems.
- Each twosome is expected to resolve the problems between them. Bringing a third person in to settle disputes or to take sides is discouraged.
- Differences between family members are encouraged to promote personal growth and creativity.
- Children are expected to assume age-appropriate responsibility and to enjoy age-appropriate privileges negotiated with their parents.
- The preservation of a positive emotional climate is more highly valued than doing what "should" be done or what is "right."
- Within each adult there is a balance of affective expression, careful rational thought, relationship focus, and care taking; each adult can selectively function in the respective modes.
- There is open communication and interactions among family members.

These functional characteristics represent an ideal family that may be more fictional than real. Most families have some but not all of these elements and still operate with integrity and respect.

Culture. Nurses also have a professional responsibility to be aware of and be sensitive to aspects of family structures that are due to cultural and ethnic differences. Specifically, culture within a family determines the following:

- The definition of family
- The beliefs governing family relationships
- The conflict and tensions present in a family and the adaptive or maladaptive responses to them
- The norms of a family
- How outside events are perceived and interpreted
- When, how, and what type of family interventions are most effective

Describe the potential impact on family functioning you might observe among families related to their particular family configuration: families that include a single parent, an interracial marriage, a homosexual partnership, and a family with several members who have a severe mental illness. ∎

Family History

Family history information usually includes all family members across three generations. It is convenient to use a family genogram as the organizing structure for collecting this information. A three-generation family genogram is a structured method of gathering information and graphically depicting the factual and emotional relationship data in the initial interview and during subsequent family meetings (Jorde, 2003). A sample genogram is presented in Figure 11-2. Drawing a family genogram in full view of the family on large easel paper or a blackboard broadens the

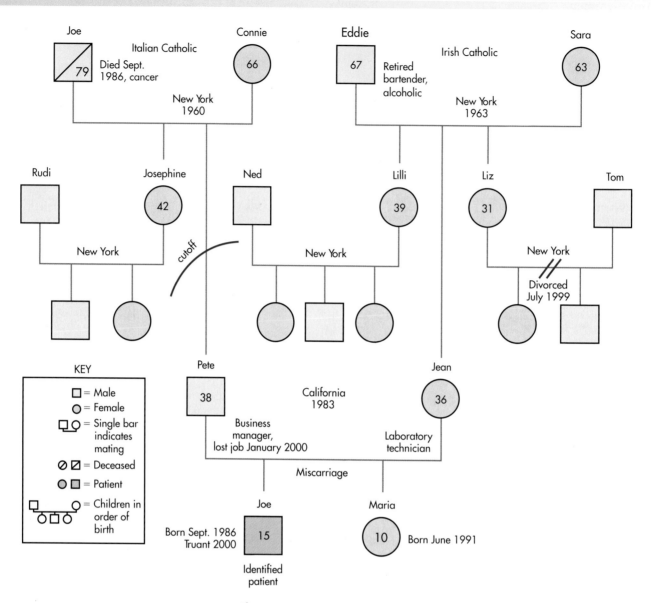

Figure 11-2   Example of a family genogram.

family's focus and facilitates an understanding of the family constellation.

The genogram is usually designed around the patient and all relatives are included. First-degree relatives include parents, siblings, and children of the patient. Second-degree relatives include grandparents, uncles, aunts, nephews, nieces, and grandchildren. All family members by marriage or partnership, adoption, and step-family members also are included.

The health status of each is noted, as are the current household configurations. Relationships between members also are recorded. The genogram provides an invaluable family map for discovering both individual and family insights and for generating discussions and can be updated by the family indefinitely.

Do a genogram of your own three-generational family. Ask family members to join you in this project. ■

Family APGAR

Once the family structure is clear, the nurse can explore roles and relationships to determine to whom the patient is attached and how the patient's family dynamics work. An evidence-based tool commonly used to assess the patient's satisfaction with relationships in the immediate family is the Family APGAR (Barkauskas et al, 2002). Functions measured by the Family APGAR include how the following are shared within the family:

- **Resources,** or the degree to which a member is satisfied with the assistance received when family resources are needed.
- **Decisions,** or the member's satisfaction with mutuality in family communication and problem solving.
- **Nurturing,** or the member's satisfaction with the freedom available within the family to change

roles and attain physical and emotional growth or maturation.

- **Emotional experiences,** or the member's satisfaction with the intimacy and emotional interaction that exist in the family.
- **Time, space,** and **money,** or the member's satisfaction with the time commitment that has been made to the family by its members.

■ WORKING WITH FAMILIES

Partnering with patients' families is an essential part of nursing care. Nurses have always made intuitive observations about family dynamics. Although many nurses have gained additional knowledge and received training in formal family therapy techniques, all nurses use various nonclinical techniques, such as psychoeducational programs developed from a competence paradigm, in order to more competently work with families in everyday nursing practice.

Competence Paradigm

The competence paradigm provides a significant shift in how family interventions are considered (Marsh, 2000). **Older conceptual models tended to focus on family pathological states and dysfunction whereas the competence model focuses on family strengths, resources, and competencies.**

The competency paradigm used in working with families values empowerment instead of a dependency-producing helper-helpee ideology and stresses the importance of treating people as collaborators who are the masters of their own fate and capable of making healthy changes (Table 11-1).

An empowerment model has been used increasingly as a framework for professional practice dealing with families who are coping with a member who is mentally ill. Its use is likely to increase the understanding of familial traits that are relevant to coping with mental illness. This empowerment model also is likely to facilitate the assessment of positive attributes among family members, offer a blueprint for designing effective interventions for patients and families, and advance efforts to evaluate the outcome of family-oriented services.

In addition, unlike pathology models that may stigmatize and alienate families, a competence paradigm attempts to foster positive alliances between families and health care providers and enhance the delivery of services. The competence paradigm emphasizes the following points:

- Focus is on growth-producing behaviors rather than on treatment of problems or prevention of negative outcomes
- Promotion and strengthening of individual and family functioning occurs by way of fostering prosocial, self-sustaining, and self-efficacious behaviors, and other adaptive behaviors as well
- Definition of the relationship between the help seeker and help giver embodies a cooperative partnership that assumes joint responsibility
- Encouragement of assistance that is in line with the family's culture and congruent with the family's appraisal of problems and needs
- Promotion of the family's use of natural support networks

In this framework it is expected that families will play a major role in deciding what is important to them, what options they will choose to achieve their goals, and whether they will accept help that is offered to them.

Watch a popular television show that depicts a family situation. Evaluate the family's level of functioning in terms of culture, competence, and dynamics. ■

Psychoeducational Programs

Psychoeducational programs for families are designed primarily for education and support. They are the result of the emergence of the family self-help movement in psychiatry. Due mainly to the efforts of the National Alliance for the Mentally Ill (NAMI) and other family groups, a variety of psychoeducational programs have been developed for families of the mentally ill. Although these programs vary, they share certain features.

Psychoeducational programs are educational and pragmatic in approach. Their aim is to improve the course of the family member's illness, reduce relapse rates, and improve

Table 11-1	Paradigms Used in Working With Families	
	PATHOLOGY PARADIGM	COMPETENCE PARADIGM
Nature of paradigm	Disease-based medical model	Health-based developmental model
View of families	Pathological, pathogenic, or dysfunctional	Basically or potentially competent
Emphasis	Weakness, liabilities, and illness	Strengths, resources, and wellness
Role of professionals	Practitioners who provide psychotherapy	Enabling agents who help families achieve their goals
Role of families	Clients or patients	Collaborators
Basis of assessment	Clinical typologies	Competencies and competence deficits
Goal of intervention	Treatment of family pathology or dysfunction	Empowerment of families in achieving mastery and control over their lives
Modus operandi	Provision of psychotherapy	Strengthening of the relevant competencies
Systemic perspective	Family systems framework	Ecological systems framework

From Marsh DT: *Serious mental illness and the family: the practitioners guide,* New York, 2000, John Wiley & Sons.

patient and family functioning. These goals are achieved through educating the family about the illness, teaching families techniques that will help them cope with symptomatic behavior, and reinforcing family strengths (McFarlane, 1995). Not all programs include the ill family member, but they do promote regular contact of the family with other affected families.

In general, a comprehensive program for working with families should include the following components (Marsh, 2000):

- A **didactic** component that provides information about mental illness and the mental health system
- A **skill** component that offers training in communication, conflict resolution, problem solving, assertiveness, behavioral management, and stress management
- An **emotional** component that provides opportunities for ventilation, sharing, and mobilizing resources
- A **family process** component that focuses on coping with mental illness and its sequelae for the family
- A **social** component that increases use of informal and formal support networks

Although no single program works equally well in all situations, it is possible to describe a general structure that can be modified to meet individual needs. The educational program outlined in Box 11-1 is time limited and didactic and is designed to primarily meet the cognitive and behavioral needs of families. However, it is important that psychoeducational programs for families meet a range of needs and that families have an opportunity to ask questions, express feelings, and socialize with each other and with mental health professionals.

■ BENEFITS OF FAMILY INVOLVEMENT

The benefits of involving family in the care of their loved ones with mental illness are well documented. Research confirms that family input in treatment decisions improves consumer outcomes, with maximum benefits occurring when the families are supported and educated for these partnership roles. Controlled clinical studies based on the belief that schizophrenia is a brain disorder responsive to the social and familial environment have shown a reduction in annual relapse rates for medicated, community-based consumers of as much as 60% (Falloon, 1999; Dixon et al, 2001).

Family interventions consisting of educational, supportive, cognitive, and behavioral strategies of at least 9 months' duration are considered to be evidence-based practice. They are called for in the national practice guidelines formulated by a number of organizations including the American Psy-

---

BOX 11-1

10-Week Educational Program for Families of the Mentally Ill

Nature and Purpose of Program
Introductions of family members and staff
Purpose and scope of program
Description of treatment program, policies, and procedures
Brief, written survey of specific family needs and requests

The Family Experience
Family burden and needs
The family system
Family subsystems
Life-span perspectives

Mental Illness I
Diagnosis
Etiology
Prognosis
Treatment

Mental Illness II
Symptoms
Medication
Diathesis-stress model
Recent research

Managing Symptoms and Problems
Bizarre behavior
Destructive and self-destructive behavior
Hygiene and appearance
Distressing symptoms

Stress, Coping, and Adaptation
The general model
The stressor of mental illness
The process of family adaptation
Increasing coping effectiveness

Enhancing Personal and Family Effectiveness I
Behavior management
Conflict resolution
Communication skills
Problem solving

Enhancing Personal and Family Effectiveness II
Stress management
Assertiveness training
Achieving a family balance
Meeting personal needs

Relationships Between Families and Professionals
Historical context
New modes of family-professional relationships
Barriers to collaboration
Breaking down barriers

Community Resources
The consumer-advocacy movement
Accessing the system
Legal issues
Appropriate referrals

chiatric Nurses' position paper on *Collaboration*; the American Psychiatric Association's treatment guidelines for schizophrenia and for bipolar disorder; the *Expert Consensus Guidelines* for schizophrenia and bipolar disorder; and the *Diagnostic and Statistical Manual of Mental Disorders (DSM)*. Furthermore, the provision of education for families is now a criterion for accreditation by the Joint Commission on Accreditation of Health Care Organizations (JCAHO).

So important is this aspect of care that it was identified as a goal in the report of the New Freedom Commission on Mental Health, *Achieving the Promise: Transforming Mental Health Care in America*, (2003): "Mental health care is consumer and family driven."

Unfortunately, the good intentions promoted at the policy level have not translated well into practice. According to the landmark Schizophrenia Patient Outcomes Research Team (PORT) Study, fewer than 1 in 10 families were receiving needed education and support services, and overall a significant gap exists between best practices and usual practices for families of persons with schizophrenia (Dixon et al, 1999). The same pessimistic conclusion was reached in the *Mental Health: a Report of the Surgeon General* (USDHHS,1999). This remains true currently despite worldwide advocacy for family involvement on the part of international family organizations under the leadership of the World Fellowship of Schizophrenia and Allied Disorders.

Is a family psychoeducation program offered at your clinical facility? If so, attend a session. If not, ask if they have considered starting one. ■

■ BARRIERS TO FAMILY INVOLVEMENT

The barriers to educating families for involvement in their loved one's treatment include the following:

- **Professional bias** against families based on exposure to family systems theories that suggest families cause or perpetuate the illness
- **Family attitudes** that equate all family interventions with past, unwelcome experiences with family therapy
- **Professional fears** that an alliance with the family will endanger confidentiality and threaten the therapeutic alliance with the patient
- **Administrative restraints** in a managed-cost environment, where services to families (as nonpatients) receive the lowest priority

These barriers are gradually disappearing, but only when the considerations of treatment and prevention are drawn around the family unit (as opposed to simply the individual) will they disappear completely.

As with a large stone skipping across water, the ripple effect of mental illness on the entire family is enormous (Wasow, 1995).

The meaning of mental illness to the family and the impact it can have on parents, children, siblings, or a spouse are presented in Box 11-2. To the extent that professional caregivers truly understand the impact of long-term mental ill-

ness on the family, the more they will work to involve family members as treatment resources, caregivers, and collaborators and provide them with preventive intervention strategies (see Citing the Evidence).

Everyone needs to understand that when a family member has a mental illness, you and your loved one are, like Alice in Wonderland, going to fall down the rabbit hole. The world you are entering is overwhelmed by the demand for services and ill equipped to meet your needs. You are up against centuries of bias against you, against the illnesses, against getting organized to do anything about them. What is important here is to recognize system failure and stigma as part of the reality we must deal with. It is also essential to realize how difficult this makes it for our ill relatives to get the help they deserve and to "rejoin" society. (Burland, 2002)

An extensive body of family literature is now available to help nurses understand the family experience of mental illness, often conceptualized as family burden (Muhlbauer, 2002; Saunders, 2003) (see Chapter 15). Nurses can read this literature, as well as attend NAMI meetings as members or guests in order to speak directly with NAMI families.

In response to learning about families in these ways, increasing numbers of nurse researchers are using theoretical models that help professionals empathize with family caregivers (Scharer, 2002). An example of this is symbolic interactionism, which suggests that nurses learn to "walk in the shoes" of family members by asking questions such as these (Saunders, 1997):

- What situations create stress in your family?
- How do you feel about your family member's dependency, social interactions, or response to treatment?
- How much support do you receive from mental health professionals, the community, or your extended family?

▌ CITING THE EVIDENCE ON
Stigma of Families of the Mentally Ill

BACKGROUND: Stigma affects not only people with mental illness but also their families. Understanding how stigma affects family members in terms of both their psychological responses to the ill person and their contacts with psychiatric services will improve interactions with the family. This study investigated factors of psychological significance related to stigma of relatives.

RESULTS: A majority of relatives experienced psychological factors of stigma by association; 18% of the relatives had at times thought that the patient would be better off dead, and 10% had themselves experienced suicidal thoughts. Stigma by association was greater in relatives experiencing mental health problems of their own and was unaffected by patient background characteristics.

IMPLICATIONS: Interventions are greatly needed to reduce the negative effects of psychological factors related to stigma by association in relatives of people with mental illness.

Ostman M, Kjellin L: *Br J Psych* 181:494, 2002.

BOX 11-2

The Meaning of Mental Illness to the Family

When a loved one is stricken with mental illness, every member of the family feels pain. Whether the patient is your mother, father, son, daughter, sister, brother, grandchild, or grandparent, you share in the suffering. But you also have other feelings that confuse and frighten you.

Before the doctors gave you a diagnosis, you probably went through a long period of uncertainty—trying to make sense of what was happening. You were stunned and bewildered. You hoped that the odd behavior and scary talk would stop, that soon things would be back to normal. Instead, maybe a crisis occurred.

In one way or another, your family member was brought in for treatment. Once the diagnosis was made, you began asking questions: "Will my loved one get better and lead a normal life again?" "What have I done wrong?" "Why did this happen to me, to us?"

Your questions and your feelings are quite natural. Your grief, shame, and anger, your sense of helplessness, your hours of anxiety: All are shared by others going through similar experiences. But depending on your relationship to the mentally ill family member, you also have feelings that are not shared by others.

Perhaps it is your child who has fallen ill. Suddenly a promising young person, on the threshold of becoming an adult, takes a sharp turn. Now there is a stranger in your midst. Your once happy and content son or daughter becomes withdrawn, unkempt, and unable to function. He argues, destroys possessions, says and does things that make no sense. You, like other parents, want to protect and nurture your child. When your desire is thwarted, you feel that you have failed. Perhaps you blame him. Such feelings are not unique to parents of mentally ill persons. Parents of children with severe physical illnesses such as cancer or heart disease also tend to blame themselves, to harbor feelings of resentment toward the victim. Because mental illness affects such intensely personal aspects of our being, it is not surprising that parents of mental patients do likewise. Professionals—often unwittingly—may augment your guilt by blaming you for the tragedy.

When it is your spouse who becomes mentally ill, you have special problems. This is, after all, the person you chose to marry: your mate, companion, and lover. Not only do once-shared responsibilities fall solely on you, but you also must try to find help for your spouse. Perhaps help is not welcomed. Without diminishing your partner's status, you must juggle the roles of mother, father, homemaker, and breadwinner all at once.

Other family members may escape the responsibilities that fall to a parent or spouse of the mentally ill person, but they share equally painful feelings. Brothers and sisters are bewildered, hurt, and sometimes ashamed and angry. Grandparents are perplexed and saddened. Adult children find it difficult to assume the role of caretaker when a parent becomes incompetent.

One out of four families has a close relative who is mentally ill. They, like you, typically go through a period of intense searching. Patients, family members, and doctors alike tend to place blame in an effort to identify an event or a person responsible for the breakdown. "Why me?" is an understandable cry.

In time, most families come to accept the illness. Somehow, they find resources to sustain themselves over the rocky period. Many become stronger in the process. When they look back over years of living with chronic mental illness, they almost invariably remember the earliest period as the hardest. They may have been surprised by the amount of energy, resourcefulness, and courage they were able to muster. They come to feel pride in their capacity to face tragedy and conquer defeat.

Although no cure is now known for the more severe, chronic mental illnesses, almost everyone can be helped to live worthwhile and meaningful lives. Caring relatives must continue to hope for improvement, set reasonable expectations, and maintain faith in the patient's recuperative and restorative powers. Realities change. What may have been impossible at one time may become quite possible. There will be regressions, plateaus when all anyone can expect to do is "hang on," without any forward movement.

A short time ago families who had known mental illness for a long time were asked how it had affected them. As might be expected, many reported the negative consequences. But many also saw positive changes in their lives. One mother said she no longer takes life for granted. "I've learned to appreciate the little things in life," she said. "I make it a point to find something to enjoy each day." Other family members reported that they were more compassionate, less judgmental, and more understanding of others. Most had made what they considered a more mature reevaluation of their lives, thereby achieving a truer vision of what really counts. They believed that their lives had become more significant, more basic, and more meaningful.

Most families, in short, found they had wellsprings of strength they never knew they had until they met the great challenge of mental illness.

From Hatfield A: *Coping with mental illness in the family: a family guide,* Arlington, Va, 1986, The National Alliance for the Mentally Ill.

Other nurse researchers, after examining international data sets about the family experience of mental illness, concluded that there is a moral imperative for family education to be part of every treatment plan. It has been proposed that nurses assume educator roles and suggested that curriculum content be tailored to the specific needs of spouses, siblings, parents, or children and be adapted for different cultural and geographical groups (Yamashita and Forsyth, 1998).

Find out if a NAMI group meets in your community. Attend a meeting and share your experience with your peers and instructor. ■

Nurses who take the time to talk with family caregivers about the history of the illness often learn that family members were the first to notice that something was not right. During the prodromal stages of the patient's illness, families are likely to notice changes in sleep and appetite patterns, loss of interest in favorite pastimes, or unexpected interest in religion or philosophy. However, without professional input, they rarely connect these changes with mental illness.

> We thought at first he was just having a difficult adolescence. Then we thought he might be into drugs. But mental illness? Not in our family!

> When our daughter started sending hundred dollar contributions to TV evangelists, we assumed she was just another born again Christian.

Usually as the result of a crisis, families are shocked into the realization that they are dealing with something very serious. At this point, if asked, they are often able to provide important diagnostic clues not otherwise available to the psychiatric team. Even further along in treatment, family members who see the patient on a daily basis are often more reliable informants than the patient.

> My brother who lives with us was seeing a therapist once a week, and we couldn't figure out why his only treatment was reading books the therapist recommended. He really wasn't reading them because he couldn't concentrate on account of the voices he was hearing most of the time. Finally, I called the therapist and told her what was going on. She was surprised, because my brother hadn't told her he was still hallucinating.

But families have roles other than that of informant, and other crucial needs. They may need to unwind by verbally replaying the events that led up to the crisis. They may need to be told they have done the right thing by bringing their loved one to a treatment setting, or by calling the police to do this, and they need to be kept informed about what is happening to him or her. These needs are superimposed on basic needs that may have gone unmet during the emergency, such as the need for rest, food, and drink.

> When I brought my husband to the emergency room for a psychiatric evaluation, the nurse allowed me to stay nearby, but out of his sight, because he was yelling at me to get out of there. She listened to my story, kept me informed, and brought me coffee. She helped me through the worst night in my life.

When the immediate crisis has settled down, nurses should complete their assessment of the mental and physical status of family members. At a minimum, families will need an explanation of the likely diagnosis, the proposed treatment, and a referral to a family support group. Some families may opt for a continuing program of family consultation, and family therapy also may be an option (see Chapter 33). In response to the need for continuing support and education, some hospitals have established a Family Resource Center staffed by volunteers and stocked with books, journal articles, videos, and access to mental health websites.

Of all the barriers to collaboration, confidentiality issues may well be the most problematic because of the perception that professionals are caught between the patient's right to a confidential therapeutic relationship and the family caregiver's right to information (see Chapter 10). However, professionals who believe in the value of collab-

oration can usually find ways to obtain the patient's permission to communicate with the family (Bogart and Solomon, 1999).

Failure to include family caregivers in treatment planning that directly involves them is not only unfair but may precipitate or perpetuate troubled family relationships, as was the case in the following scenario.

> The treatment plan for a 35-year-old single, pregnant woman who was suffering from depression and addiction to cocaine called for her and the future baby to live in the parents' home after her discharge from the hospital. When the father and mother came in to visit, they were stunned to learn that the discharge date had been moved up, and their daughter would be coming home the following day. They wondered aloud if their efforts to hide their resentment at being excluded from the discharge planning would be successful.

Even when a treatment objective involves increasing the patient's autonomy and separation from the family, there are advantages to family involvement. Such a plan is more likely to be carried out if the parents and other relatives understand the goal, agree with it, and contribute their ideas as to how it can be achieved. Conversely, to drive a wedge between the patient and family could rob a vulnerable person of a family resource that is likely to outlast any single professional resource.

Although not all patients with serious mental illness will have family members who are willing or able to provide care, the point is that family collaboration, support, and education must become the rule, not the exception.

> How would you respond to a colleague who says, "We have no time to work with families. They just slow us down, and we can't get reimbursed for the time we spend meeting with them"? ■

■ FAMILIES AS A POPULATION AT RISK

Following the terrorist attack on the World Trade Center in New York, nurses were deployed to minister to the victims' shocked and grieving families. The impact of mental illness is also a shattering, traumatic event in the life of a family and, as such, family members are ideal candidates for secondary prevention strategies (Burland, 1998).

Aging parents who expected to have an empty nest find themselves in their fifties, sixties, and seventies, sharing the nest with adult children who have a mental illness. Not only must their dreams for their young people be revised, but these parents must learn to live with loved ones whose moods and behaviors are often baffling and sometimes dangerous. The subjective and objective burden of living with a loved one for whom effective treatment has not been found has been called "mourning without end" (Cuijpers and Stam, 2000). At the same time, some families say their lives have been strengthened by such an experience.

> We have this terrible feeling of loss and grieve for the son we knew. We feel cheated out of watching him mature and

flower the way adolescents do as they grow into young adults. When I meet his former classmates who are now working, finishing graduate degrees, or are married, I am always aware that these things are not possible for him, just the same as someone would feel had their son died. Yet this mourning is strange, because our son is not dead at all. He is very much still with us, seemingly eternally 13 years old, needing care and attention.

In the dark soul of the night, I grieve for all of us—for the anguish of the past and the present, and the uncertainty of the future. Most of all, I grieve for my daughter, for her lost hopes and expectations. At the same time, we have emerged from this emotional holocaust as better, stronger, and more tolerant people.

It is not surprising when NAMI chapter newsletters report heart attacks or strokes suffered in apparent response to a loved one's relapse, suicide attempt, or encounter with the law. Less dramatic but also unfortunate are the reports of family members who suffer from depression, couples who separate or divorce, and those who become addicted to cigarettes, alcohol, or drugs.

Critical Thinking *About* Contemporary Issues

What Is the Future for Children With Mentally Ill Parents?

Living with a mentally ill parent does not necessarily mean that the child will develop the disorder, but it can make growing up more difficult. Although the mechanisms for transmitting psychiatric illness across generations are controversial, many studies support the fact that parental illness affects children. For example, it has been noted that coping with a mentally ill parent may be more difficult than coping with parental loss. These children also feel psychologically vulnerable and fear becoming ill themselves. The major research findings on this topic are as follows:

- Children of mentally ill parents are at greater risk for psychiatric and developmental disorders than are children of well parents.
- The risk to children is greater if the mother rather than the father is the ill parent.
- In studies of depressed versus nondepressed groups, differences in the mother-child interaction are evident as early as 3 months postpartum.
- Many children with emotionally disturbed parents do not become disordered themselves. The nature of the parent's illness, the child's genetic and constitutional make-up, the family's functional ability, and the availability of healthy attachment figures all play an important role in the mental health of the child.

The evidence suggests that psychiatric nurses need to focus more attention on the children of mentally ill parents. They should assess parenting problems whenever parents with children at home are hospitalized for psychiatric care. They also can implement psychoeducational, preventive nursing interventions that will enhance mental health in high-risk children and families (Butler et al., 2000).

Well siblings attracted the attention of early researchers primarily because they had escaped the illness. The question was, "How did the schizophrenic mother manage to raise well children?" Some theorized that the siblings were only superficially normal; others guessed that they escaped major pathology by detaching themselves from the family, or because they were neglected by their mothers.

Contemporary researchers have made similar observations, but have different interpretations about the status of siblings (see Critical Thinking About Contemporary Issues). Many surveys have revealed that siblings suffer problems in living (Friedrich et al, 1999). The reality is that when the emotional and financial resources are devoted disproportionately to the son or daughter with the illness, less is available for the siblings. They may be resentful but are unable to express their resentment because of survivor's guilt. Some siblings detach from the family. Others remain involved, often at the expense of career and marriage options. Many become members of helping professions.

Siblings and offspring are likely to have problems as adults because they had less parental attention than they needed as children and adolescents. It is ironic that professional caregivers who are very knowledgeable about the effects of childhood trauma in general terms are often unaware of the specific difficulties faced by children growing up in families preoccupied by mental illness.

Despite the known genetic risks for the offspring of parents with schizophrenia, and the even greater risk for those who have parents with bipolar disorder or major depression, these children are underserved in the mental health system. This lack of service results in part from the fact that women in treatment for serious mental illnesses often do not reveal that they have children, for fear that they will be removed from their care. Consequently, offspring and siblings may present for treatment years later, exhibiting problems with identity, self-esteem, and dependence on the approval of others. There may be difficulties with trust and intimacy, an excessive need for perfectionism and control, and developmental delays with respect to marriage and careers.

On the other hand, children raised in the shadow of mental illness can achieve success in life and even become prominent public figures. A case in point is the actress, Marilyn Monroe, whose mother suffered from schizophrenia and whose grandmother (also afflicted) tried to suffocate her with a pillow when she was 13 months old (Marshall, 1996).

In keeping with the theme that siblings and offspring gravitate toward the helping professions, a number of nurses and social workers contributed their personal accounts to the *Journal of the California Alliance for the Mentally Ill.*

I had to grow up fast as a child. I recognize that my mother's illness deprived me of having any sort of a carefree, normal childhood. Periodically, I have been angry at one or both of my parents for the atmosphere at home (Bruge, 1996).

As a child it was often difficult to know which of my mother's behaviors were normal and which were due to the illness (List, 1996).

Daddy always had to tell us, "Don't step off the curb" before we left for school. I was so used to it; it was such a part of my daily routine, that I never realized the absurdity of it (Poe, 1996).

The professor had just finished a compressed overview on what was known about schizophrenia. "Oh, my God!" I gasped, to myself. "That's what my father has" (Steinert, 1996).

The following have been suggested as ways in which professionals can help young people living in families with mental illness (Marsh and Johnson, 1997):

- Become informed about the family experience of mental illness.
- Strengthen and support the family system.
- Reach out as early as possible and assure them they are not to blame.
- Address the needs of young family members in an age-appropriate manner.
- Enlist the help of teachers, principals, guidance counselors, and school psychologists.
- Assure them that their needs matter and support their goals.
- Offer counseling for those who are experiencing particular difficulty.

What personal and social impact do you think stigma has on the siblings of those who are mentally ill? ■

■ BUILDING BRIDGES

In the late 1980s NAMI's Curriculum and Training Network offered a program to train two persons from each state affiliate as "family education specialists." Later, a 30-hour curriculum known as the NAMI Family-to-Family Education Program was written (Box 11-3). This peer-taught program has been presented free of charge to over 50,000 families across the nation. It is no coincidence that many of the family members trained to teach the course have a nursing background. To make this unique referral resource better known to mental health professionals, a Clinician's Guide to the NAMI Family-to-Family Education Program was written (Weiden, 1999).

In 1990 NAMI and the Human Interaction Research Institute of Los Angeles collaborated on a Center for Mental Health Services–funded project that identified seven competencies that professionals need in order to involve families as partners in treatment. Psychiatric nurses should assess the extent to which they practice these skills (Box 11-4).

The American Psychiatric Nurses Association (APNA) also has formed a working alliance with NAMI for the purpose of jointly promoting public policy pertaining to mental health/illness issues. APNA also testified before Congress on behalf of NAMI's policy on the limitations on restraints and seclusion (see Chapter 30). As a result, legislation protecting patients from the inappropriate use of seclusion and restraints has been enacted in several states. This is but one example of the potential impact that joint advocacy between nursing and family organizations can have on the field.

BOX 11-3

NAMI Family-to-Family Curriculum

Class 1. Introduction. Special features of the course, emotional reactions to the trauma of mental illness; your goals for your family member with mental illness

Class 2. Schizophrenia, Major Depression, Mania, Schizoaffective Disorder. Diagnostic criteria; characteristic features of psychotic illnesses; keeping a Crisis File

Class 3. Mood Disorders and Anxiety Disorders. Types and subtypes of depression and bipolar disorder; causes of mood disorders; diagnostic criteria for panic disorder and obsessive-compulsive disorder

Class 4. Basics About the Brain. Functions of key brain areas; research on functional and structural brain abnormalities; chemical messengers in the brain; genetic research; the biology of recovery; NAMI Science and Treatment Video

Class 5. Problem Solving Skills Workshop. How to define a problem; sharing our problem statements; solving the problem; setting limits

Class 6. Medication Review. How medications work; basic psychopharmacology of mood disorders, anxiety disorders, and schizophrenia; side effects; key treatment issues; stages of adherence to medications; early warning signs of relapse

Class 7. Inside Mental Illness. The subjective experience of coping with a brain disorder; maintaining self-esteem and positive identity; gaining empathy for your relative's psychological struggle to protect one's integrity despite mental illness

Class 8. Communication Skills Workshop. How illness interferes with the capacity to communicate; learning to be clear; how to respond when the topic is loaded; talking to the person behind the symptoms

Class 9. Self-Care. Learning about family burden; handling feelings of anger, entrapment, guilt, and grief; how to balance our lives

Class 10. The Vision and Potential of Recovery. Learning about key principles of rehabilitation and model programs of community support; a first hand account of recovery

Class 11. Advocacy. Challenging the power of stigma in our lives; learning how to change the system; the NAMI Campaign to End Discrimination; meet a NAMI advocate

Class 12. Review, Sharing, and Evaluation. Certification ceremony. Celebration!

BOX 11-4

Family Involvement Competencies for Mental Health Professionals

Developing a Collaboration With the Family
Make a positive first contact.
Identify family's needs.
Address confidentiality.

Offering Information on Mental Illness
Diagnosis, etiology, prognosis, treatments
Long-term course of serious mental illness
Educational sessions

Enhancing Family Communication and Problem Solving
Teach principles of effective communication.
Teach problem-solving strategies.

Helping With Service System Use
Help access entitlements, support, and rehabilitation.
Explain the roles of different mental health providers.
Establish needed linkages.
Translate the language of mental health services.
Help access crisis services.
Help access housing.

Helping Family Members Meet Own Needs
Help family members access support services.
Understand burden and grief.
Assess for stress-related disorders.
Offer services or referrals.
Encourage self-care.
Encourage advocacy.

Addressing Special Issues Concerning the Patient
Treatment is not working.
Illness is of recent onset.
Patient has multiple diagnoses.
Patient is in jail.
Patient refuses treatment.

Addressing Special Issues Concerning the Family
The family does not speak English.
The family is very important or of high status in the community.
The family belongs to an ethnic minority.
The family is missing.
The family is disinterested.

Modified from Glynn S et al: *Involving families in mental health services: competencies for mental health workers*, Los Angeles, 1997, Human Interaction Research Institute.

CHAPTER FOCUS POINTS

- Competence in working with families will enhance the nurse's assessment of the individual's and the family's needs and resources, enhance selection of interventions needed to promote adaptive functioning, and facilitate the use of positive coping strategies.
- A well-functioning family can shift roles, levels of responsibility, and patterns of interaction as it experiences stressful life changes. It may, under acute or prolonged stress or increased vulnerability, express maladaptive responses, but should be able to rebalance as a system over time.
- Nurses have a professional responsibility to be aware of and be sensitive to aspects of family structures that are due to cultural and ethnic differences.
- Information about family history generally includes all family members across three generations. It is convenient to use a family genogram as the organizing structure for collecting this information.
- The competency paradigm used in working with families values empowerment instead of a dependency-producing helper-helpee ideology and stresses the importance of treating people as collaborators who are the masters of their own fate and capable of making healthy changes.
- Psychoeducational programs are educational and pragmatic in approach, with the aim of improving the course of the family member's illness, reducing relapse rates, and improving patient and family functioning. These goals are achieved through educating the family about the illness, teaching families techniques that will help

them cope with symptomatic behavior, and reinforcing family strengths.
- Family interventions consisting of educational, supportive, cognitive, and behavioral strategies of at least 9 months' duration are considered evidence-based practice.
- Barriers to family involvement are gradually disappearing, but only when the considerations of treatment and prevention are drawn around the family unit (as opposed to simply the individual) will they disappear completely.
- Of all the barriers to collaboration, confidentiality issues may well be the most problematic because of the perception that professionals are caught between the patient's right to a confidential therapeutic relationship and the family caregiver's right to information.
- The impact of mental illness is a shattering, traumatic event in the life of a family, and as such, family members are ideal candidates for secondary prevention strategies.
- Despite the known genetic risks for the offspring of parents with schizophrenia, and the even greater risk for those who have parents with bipolar disorder or major depression, these children are underserved in the mental health system.
- Collaboration between psychiatric nurses and families (and psychiatric nursing organizations and family advocacy groups) can reap rich rewards in terms of advancing prevention, treatment, and recovery in the field.

KEY TERMS

extended family, 170
family, 170
genogram, 171

household, 170
nuclear family, 170

CHAPTER REVIEW QUESTIONS

1. Fill in the blanks.

A. Using the competency paradigm, a family's _____ are emphasized as compared to a pathology paradigm that emphasizes a family's _____.

B. Psychoeducational interventions with families are designed primarily to _____ and _____.

C. The largest self-help and consumer advocacy group in the United States is _____.

2. Read the following two interactions and answer the questions at the end.

Mr. Silverman, the father of a 30-year-old son diagnosed with schizophrenia enters the community mental health center office of the nurse who sees his son for blood work and a weekly assessment.

Dialogue 1

Nurse: Is Eric with you?

Mr. S.: No, he refused to come.

Nurse: Mr. Silverman, it's very important that Eric gets his blood work done. Why didn't you bring him? What's wrong?

Mr. S.: Eric threw a chair though the living room wall. That's what's wrong!

Nurse: (thinking) Hmmm. Mr. Silverman, what is going on at home?

Mr. S.: (baffled) I just told you. Eric got mad and threw a chair through the wall.

Nurse: I heard what you said, Mr. Silverman. But, I mean, have you and Mrs. Silverman been having any problems lately? Perhaps some arguments?

Mr. S.: (defensively) What's that got to do with anything? It's Eric we're talking about!

Dialogue 2

Nurse: Good morning, Mr. Silverman. Is Eric with you?

Mr. S.: No, he refused to come.

Nurse: Why? What's wrong?

M. S.: Eric threw a chair through the living room wall.

Nurse: That's terrible! You must be very upset.

Mr. S.: To tell the truth, I am. I just can't figure out what got into Eric.

Nurse: Maybe we can figure it out together. Tell me more about it.

Mr. S.: Well, for one thing, I suspect he hasn't been taking medicine the way he's supposed to. His mother keeps tabs on that, and she's been away since Friday.

Nurse: Where did she go?

Mr. S.: She went to Ohio to see her mother, and while she was there, her mother had a slight stroke.

Nurse: I am so sorry to hear that. Eric has mentioned his grandmother to me, and I know he's very fond of her. How did he take the news?

Mr. S.: You know that's a funny thing. Eric didn't seem bothered at all when his mother called about the stroke. He just went into his room for a real long time, and when he came out, that's when he threw the chair through the wall.

Nurse: Mr. Silverman, I can see you're having a rough time and a lot is going on just now. What can I do to help?

A. How do you think Mr. S. was feeling when he entered the office?

B. How did he feel as a result of the nurse's responses in Dialogue 1? Dialogue 2?

C. What was the nurse's hypothesis about what caused Eric's behavior in Dialogue 1?

D. What was accomplished when, in Dialogue 2, the nurse said, "Tell me more about it."

 Visit Evolve for additional resources related to the content of this chapter.
http://evolve.elsevier.com/Stuart/principles/
• Topical Course Outline • Student Workbook Exercises • Critical Thinking Questions and Activities • Case Studies • Research Topics
• Monthly Content Updates • WebLinks

 Student Study CD-ROM

Access the accompanying CD-ROM for animations, interactive exercises, review questions for the NCLEX examination, and an audio glossary.

REFERENCES

Barkauskas V et al: *Health and physical assessment*, ed 3, St Louis, 2002, Mosby.

Bogart T, Solomon P: Procedures to share treatment information among mental health providers, consumers, and families, *Psychiatr Serv* 50:1321, 1999.

Bruge D: Thoughts about my mother, *J Calif Alliance Mentally Ill* 7:15, 1996.

Burland J: Personal communication, 2002.

Burland J: Family-to-family: a trauma-and-recovery model of family education, *New Dir Ment Health Serv* 77:33, 1998.

Butler S et al: Risk reduction in children from families with parental depression: a videotape psychoeducation program, *Natl Acad Pract Forum* 2:267, 2000.

Cuijpers P, Stam H: Burnout among relatives of psychiatric patients attending psychoeducational support groups, *Psychiatr Serv* 51:375, 2000.

Dixon L et al: Services to families of adults with schizophrenia: from treatment recommendations to dissemination, *Psychiatr Serv* 50:233, 1999.

Dixon L et al: Evidence-based practices for services to families of people with psychiatric disabilities, *Psychiatr Serv* 52:903, 2001.

Falloon I: Newsletter of the World Fellowship of Schizophrenia and Allied Disorders, Toronto, Canada, 1999, World Fellowship of Schizophrenia and Allied Disorders.

Friedrich RW et al: Well siblings living with schizophrenia, *J Psychosoc Nurs Ment Health Serv* 37:11, 1999.

Jorde L: *Medical genetics*, ed 3, St Louis, 2003, Mosby.

List A: On becoming authentic: a daughter's story, *J Calif Alliance Mentally Ill* 7:37, 1996.

Marsh D, Johnson D: The family experience of mental illness: implications for interventions, *Professional Psychology: Res Pract* 28:232, 1997.

Marsh DT: *Serious mental illness and the family: the practitioners guide*, New York, 2000, John Wiley & Sons.

Marshall L: Marilyn Monroe: a child of mental illness, *J Calif Alliance Mentally Ill* 7:31, 1996.

McFarlane W: Multiple family groups and psychoeducation in the treatment of schizophrenia, *Arch Gen Psychiatr* 52:679, 1995.

Muhlbauer S: Experience of stigma by families with mentally ill members, *J Am Psychiatr Nurs Assoc* 8:76, 2002.

New Freedom Commission on Mental Health: *Achieving the promise: transforming mental health care in America, final report*, DHHS Pub. No. SMA-03-3832, Rockville, Maryland, 2003, USDHHS.

Poe S: Sailing similar seas, *J Calif Alliance Mentally Ill* 7:16, 1996.

Puri BK, Tyrer PJ: *Sciences basic to psychiatry*, ed 2, Edinburgh, 1999, Churchill Livingstone.

Saunders JC: Walking a mile in their shoes: symbolic interactionism for families living with severe mental illness, *J Psychosoc Nurs Ment Health Serv* 35:10, 1997.

Saunders JC: Families living with severe mental illness: a literature review, *Issues Ment Health Nurs* 24:175, 2003.

Scharer K: What parents of mentally ill children need and want from mental health professionals, *Issues Ment Health Nurs* 23:617, 2002.

Steinert P: Why didn't you tell me? *J Calif Alliance Mentally Ill* 7:22, 1996.

U.S. Department of Health and Human Services (USDHHS): *Mental health: a report of the Surgeon General*, Rockville, MD, 1999, USDHHS, SAMHSA, CMHS, NIH, NIMH.

Wasow M: *The skipping stone: ripple effects of mental illness in the family*, ed 2, Palo Alto, Calif, 1995, Science and Behavior Books.

Weiden P: The road back: working with those with severe mental illness, *J Pract Psychiatr Behav Health* 4:354, 1999.

Yamashita M, Forsyth D: Family coping with mental illness: an aggregate from two studies, Canada and United States, *J Am Psychiatr Nurs Assoc* 4:1, 1998.

> *The professional motive is the desire and perpetual effort to do the thing as well as it can be done, which exists just as much in the Nurse, as in the Astronomer in search of a new star, or in the Artist completing a picture.*
>
> FLORENCE NIGHTINGALE

IMPLEMENTING THE NURSING PROCESS: STANDARDS OF CARE AND PROFESSIONAL PERFORMANCE

12

Gail W. Stuart

evolve Visit Evolve for additional resources related to the content of this chapter.
http://evolve.elsevier.com/Stuart/principles/

The nurse-patient relationship is the vehicle for applying the nursing process. The goal of psychiatric nursing care is to **maximize the patient's positive interactions with the environment, promote a level of wellness,** and **enhance self-actualization**. By establishing a therapeutic nurse-patient relationship and using the nursing process, the nurse strives to promote and maintain patient behavior that contributes to integrated functioning. This is the essence of the nursing therapeutic process and the framework on which this text is based.

This chapter discusses the Standards of Care and the Professional Performance Standards as described in the *Scope and Standards of Psychiatric–Mental Health Nursing Practice* (ANA, 2000). The Standards of Care from the *Scope and Standards of Psychiatric–Mental Health Nursing Practice* describe what the psychiatric nurse does. The Standards of Professional Performance from the same document describe the context in which the psychiatric nurse performs these activities. Neither set of standards can be taken in isolation. Together they complete the picture of contemporary psychiatric nursing practice.

■ THE NURSING PROCESS

The nursing process is an interactive, problem-solving process and a systematic and individualized way to achieve the outcomes of nursing care. The nursing process respects the individual's autonomy and freedom to make decisions and be involved in nursing care. The nurse and patient emerge as partners in a relationship built on trust and directed toward maximizing the patient's strengths, maintaining integrity, and promoting adaptive responses to stress.

In dealing with psychiatric patients, the nursing process can present unique challenges. Mental health problems may be vague and elusive, not tangible or visible like many physiological illnesses. Mental health problems also can show different symptoms and arise from a number of causes. Many psychiatric patients are initially unable to describe their problems. They may be withdrawn, highly anxious, or out of touch with reality. Their ability to participate in the problem-solving process also may be limited if they see themselves as powerless victims or if their illness impairs them from fully engaging in the treatment process.

It is essential that the nurse and the patient become partners in the problem-solving process. Nurses may be tempted to exclude patients, particularly if they resist becoming involved, but this should be avoided for two reasons. First, learning is most effective when patients participate in the learning experience. Second, by including patients as active participants in the nursing process, the nurse helps restore their sense of control over life and their responsibility for action. They reinforce the message that patients, whether they have an acute crisis or a serious and persistent mental illness, can choose either adaptive or maladaptive coping responses.

■ STANDARDS OF CARE

The phases of the nursing process as described by Standards of Care in the *Scope and Standards of Psychiatric–Mental Health Nursing Practice* are assessment, diagnosis, outcome identification, planning, implementation, and evaluation. **Validation** is part of each step, and all phases may overlap or occur simultaneously. The nursing conditions and nursing behaviors related to each of these phases are shown in Figure 12-1. Each of these phases, as it applies to psychiatric nursing practice, is described here.

> *Some psychotic patients are discouraged and dispirited by their illness. As a result, it may be difficult to engage them in the treatment process. What strategies might you use to connect with these patients and develop a therapeutic alliance with them?* ■

■ ASSESSMENT

STANDARD I: ASSESSMENT
The psychiatric–mental health nurse collects patient health data.
■ **Rationale**
The assessment interview—which requires linguistically and culturally effective communication skills, interviewing, behavioral observation, record review, and comprehensive assessment of the patient and relevant systems—enables the psychiatric–mental health nurse to make sound clinical judgments and plan appropriate interventions with the patient.
■ **Nursing Conditions**
Self-awareness
Accurate observations
Therapeutic communication
Responsive dimensions of care
■ **Nursing Behaviors**
Establish nursing contract
Obtain information from patient and family
Validate data with patient
Organize data
■ **Key Elements**
Identify the patient's reason for seeking help
Assess for risk factors related to the patient's safety including potential for:
Suicide or self-harm
Assault or violence
Substance abuse withdrawal
Allergic reaction or adverse drug reaction
Seizure
Falls or accidents

Elopement (if hospitalized)
Physiological instability
Complete a biopsychosocial assessment of patient needs related to this treatment encounter including:
Patient and family appraisal of health and illness
Previous episodes of psychiatric care in self and family
Current medications
Physiological coping responses
Mental status coping responses
Coping resources, including motivation for treatment and functional supportive relationships
Adaptive and maladaptive coping mechanisms
Psychosocial and environmental problems
Global assessment of functioning
Knowledge, strengths, and deficits

In the assessment phase, information is obtained from the patient in a direct and structured manner through **observations, interviews**, and **examinations**. An assessment tool or nursing history form can provide a systematic format that becomes part of the patient's written record. It should include components of the mental status examination (see Chapter 7).

A standardized format enables the nurse to assess the patient's level of functioning and serves as a basis for diagnosis, outcome identification, planning, implementation, and evaluation of nursing care. Using a specified data collection format helps ensure that the necessary information is obtained. It also reduces repetition of the patient's medical history and provides a source of information available to all health care team members.

The nurse also should use the most appropriate **behavioral rating scales**. These can help define current pretreatment aspects of the patient's problems, increase the patient's involvement in treatment, document the patient's progress over time and the efficacy of the treatment plan, and compare the patient's responses to those of groups of people with the same illness (see Citing the Evidence). This information

■ CITING THE EVIDENCE ON
Usefulness of Behavioral Rating Scales

BACKGROUND: This study sought to determine whether psychiatric inpatients who completed a self-report symptom and problem rating scale on admission and reviewed the results with a clinician would perceive at discharge that they had been more involved in their treatment than patients who did not complete the scale.

RESULTS: Patients in the intervention group rated their involvement in decisions about their treatment significantly higher than patients in the comparison groups. They also more frequently reported that they were treated with respect and dignity by the staff. Treatment outcomes did not differ among the groups.

IMPLICATIONS: The results suggest that a behavioral rating scale can be a useful tool for engaging patients in the treatment process.

Eisen S et al: *Psychiatr Serv* 51:349, 2000.

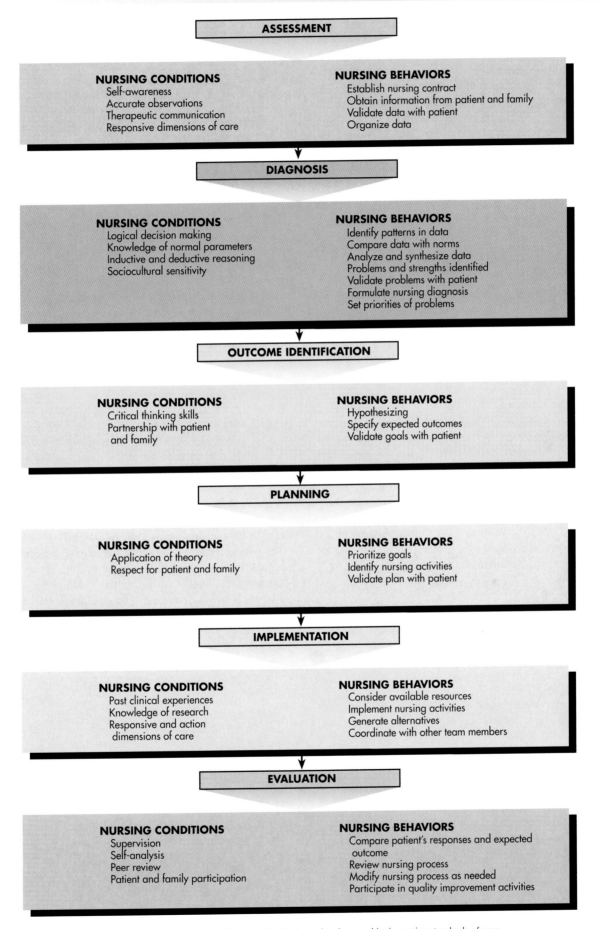

Figure 12-1   Nursing conditions and behaviors related to psychiatric nursing standards of care.

can help formulate diagnoses and treatment plans, as well as document clinical outcomes of care.

The patient data identified in Standard I relate to all of the components of the Stuart Stress Adaptation Model used in this text: predisposing factors, precipitating stressors, appraisal of stressor, coping resources, coping mechanisms, and coping responses as described in Chapter 4.

The baseline data should reflect both content and process, and the patient is the ideal source of validation. The nurse should select a private place, free from noise and distraction, in which to interview the patient. Interviewing is a goal-directed method of communication that is required in a formal admission procedure.

It should be focused but open ended, progressing from general to specific and allowing spontaneous patient self-expression. The nurse's role is to maintain the flow of the interview and to listen to the verbal and nonverbal messages conveyed by the patient. Nurses also must be aware of their responses to the patient.

Although the patient should be regarded as a source of validation, the nurse also should be prepared to consult with family members or other people knowledgeable about the patient. This is particularly important when the patient is unable to provide reliable information because of the symptoms of the psychiatric illness.

The nurse also might consider using a variety of other information sources, including the patient's health care record, nursing rounds, change-of-shift reports, nursing care plan, and evaluation by other health professionals such as psychologists, social workers, or psychiatrists. In using secondary sources, nurses should not simply accept the assessment of another health care team member. Rather, they should apply the information they obtain to their nursing framework for data collection and formulate their own impressions and diagnoses. This brings another perspective to the work of the health care team and an unbiased receptivity to patients and their problems.

◀ DIAGNOSIS

STANDARD II: DIAGNOSIS
The psychiatric–mental health nurse analyzes the assessment data in determining diagnoses.

■ Rationale
The basis for providing psychiatric–mental health nursing care is the recognition and identification of patterns of response to actual or potential psychiatric illnesses, mental health problems, and potential comorbid physical illnesses.

■ Nursing Conditions
Logical decision making
Knowledge of normal parameters
Inductive and deductive reasoning
Sociocultural sensitivity

■ Nursing Behaviors
Identify patterns in data
Compare data with norms
Analyze and synthesize data
Identify problems and strengths
Validate problems with patient

Formulate nursing diagnoses
Set priorities of problems

■ Key Elements
Diagnoses should reflect adaptive and maladaptive coping responses based on nursing frameworks such as those of the North American Nursing Diagnosis Association (NANDA).

Diagnoses should incorporate health problems or disease states such as those identified in the *Diagnostic and Statistical Manual of Mental Disorders* (*DSM-IV-TR*) (American Psychiatric Association, 2000) and the *International Classification of Diseases and Related Health Problems* (WHO, 1993).

Diagnoses should focus on the phenomena of concern to psychiatric–mental health nurses as described in Box 12-1.

After collecting all data, the nurse compares the information to documented norms of health and adaptation. Because standards of behavior are culturally determined, the nurse should allow for both the patient's individual characteristics and the characteristics of the larger social group to which the patient belongs.

The nurse then analyzes the data and derives a nursing diagnosis. A nursing diagnosis is a clinical judgment about individual, family, or community responses to actual or potential health problems/life processes. A nursing diagnosis provides the basis for selection of nursing interventions to achieve outcomes for which the nurse is accountable (NANDA, 2003). The subject of nursing diagnoses is the **patient's behavioral response to stress**. This response may lie anywhere on the coping continuum from adaptive to maladaptive.

According to NANDA, the components of a nursing diagnosis are the label or name of the diagnosis; its definition; the defining characteristics of the diagnosis; related factors; and risk factors. The defining characteristics are particularly helpful because they reflect the behaviors that are the target of nursing intervention. They also provide specific indicators for evaluating the outcomes of psychiatric nursing interventions. The actual or potential mental health problems focused on by psychiatric nurses are listed in Box 12-1.

NANDA diagnoses were first developed in 1973, whereas the DSM was first published in 1952. What impact do you think that this time difference has had on the use and acceptance of each classification system? ■

The relationship between medicine and nursing includes sharing information, ideas, and analyses and developing appropriate care plans for the patient. Interventions are based on the nursing assessment as well as the medical evaluation and ensure a thorough and coordinated plan of treatment. Therefore, while formulating nursing diagnoses and using the nursing process, nurses also should be familiar with medical diagnoses and treatment plans.

A medical diagnosis is the health problem or disease state of the patient. In the medical model of psychiatry, the health problems are mental disorders or mental illnesses. These are classified in the *DSM-IV-TR* (American Psychiatric Association, 2000), which comprehensively describes the symptoms

Psychiatric–Mental Health Nursing's Phenomena of Concern

Actual or Potential Mental Health Problems of Patients Pertaining to:

- The maintenance of optimal health and well-being and the prevention of psychobiological illness
- Self-care limitations or impaired functioning related to mental and emotional distress
- Deficits in the functioning of significant biological, emotional, and cognitive systems
- Emotional stress or crisis components of illness, pain, and disability
- Self-concept changes, developmental issues, and life process changes
- Problems related to emotions such as anxiety, anger, sadness, loneliness, and grief
- Physical symptoms that occur along with altered psychological functioning
- Psychological symptoms that occur along with altered physiological functioning
- Alterations in thinking, perceiving, symbolizing, communicating, and decision making
- Difficulties in relating to others
- Behaviors and mental states that indicate that the patient is a danger to self or others or has a severe disability
- Symptom management, side effects/toxicities associated with psychopharmacological intervention, and other aspects of the treatment regimen
- Interpersonal, systemic, sociocultural, spiritual, or environmental circumstances or events that affect the mental and emotional well-being of the individual, family, or community

From American Nurses Association: *Scope and standards of psychiatric–mental health nursing practice*, Washington, DC, 2000, The Association.

of mental disorders but does not attempt to discuss cause or how the disturbances come about. However, specific diagnostic criteria are provided for each mental disorder.

If nurses are to be familiar with DSM-IV-TR *medical diagnoses, should physicians be similarly knowledgeable about NANDA diagnoses?* ◼

OUTCOME IDENTIFICATION

STANDARD III: OUTCOME IDENTIFICATION
The psychiatric–mental health nurse identifies expected outcomes individualized to the patient.

◼ Rationale
Within the context of providing nursing care, the ultimate goal is to influence mental health outcomes and improve the patient's health status.

◼ Nursing Conditions
Critical thinking skills
Partnership with patient and family

◼ Nursing Behaviors
Hypothesizing
Specifying expected outcomes
Validating goals with patient

◼ Key Elements
Outcomes should be mutually identified with the patient.
Outcomes should be identified as clearly and objectively as possible.
Well-written outcomes help nurses determine the effectiveness and efficiency of their interventions.
Before defining expected outcomes, the nurse must realize that patients often seek treatment with goals of their own.

Patient outcomes may include relieving symptoms or improving functional ability. Sometimes a patient cannot identify specific goals or may describe them in general terms. Translating nonspecific concerns into specific goal statements is not easy. The nurse must understand the patient's coping responses and the factors that influence them.

The patient may view a personal problem as someone else's behavior. This may be the case of a father who brings his adolescent son in for counseling. The father may view the son as the problem, whereas the adolescent may feel his only problem is his father. One approach to this situation is to focus help on the person who brought the problem into treatment because he "owns" the problem at that moment. The nurse might suggest, "Let's talk about how I could help you deal with your son. A change in your response might lead to a change in his behavior also."

The patient may express a problem as a feeling, such as, "I'm lonely," or "I'm so unhappy." Besides trying to help the patient clarify the feeling, the nurse might ask, "What could you do to make yourself feel less alone and more loved by others?" This helps patients see the connection between actions and feelings and increase their sense of responsibility for themselves.

The patient's problem may be one of lacking a goal or an idea of exactly what is desired out of life. In this case it might be helpful for the nurse to point out that values and goals are not magically discovered but must be created by people for themselves. The patient can then actively explore ways to construct goals or adopt the objectives of a social, service, religious, or political group with whom the patient identifies.

The patient's goals may be inappropriate, undesirable, or unclear. However, the solution is not for the nurse to impose goals on the patient. Even if the patient's desires seem to be against self-interests, the most the nurse can do is reflect the patient's behavior and its consequences. If the patient then asks for help in setting new goals, the nurse can help.

The patient's problem may be a choice conflict. This is especially common if all the choices are unpleasant, unacceptable, or unrealistic. An example is a couple who wants to divorce but do not want to see their child hurt or suffer the financial hardship that would result. Although undesirable choices cannot be made desirable, the nurse can help patients use the problem-solving process to identify the full range of alternatives available to them.

The patient may have no real problem but may just want to talk. Nurses must then decide what role to play and carefully distinguish between a social and a therapeutic relationship.

Mutually identifying goals and expected outcomes is an essential step in the therapeutic process. In this process, a well-intentioned nurse sometimes overlooks the patient's goals and devises a treatment plan leading to an outcome that the nurse believes is better. However, this is a mistake because the experience of working cooperatively with the nurse to evolve mutually acceptable goals is extremely valuable. If the patient does not share one of the nurse's goals, it may be best to defer it until the patient agrees on its importance.

Once overall goals are agreed on, the nurse must state them explicitly. Box 12-2 lists qualities of well-written outcome criteria. Expected outcomes are derived from diagnoses, guide later nursing actions, and enhance the evaluation of care. Expected outcomes can be documented using standardized classification systems, such as the Nursing Outcomes Classification (NOC) (Moorhead, Johnson, and Maas, 2004).

Review some of the treatment plans in your clinical setting. Are the expected outcomes and long- and short-term goals well written given the qualities listed in Box 12-2? ■

Long- and short-term goals should contribute to the expected outcomes. Following is a sample expected outcome and long- and short-term goals:

Expected outcome: Patient will be socially engaged in the community.

Long-term goal:
• The patient will travel about the community independently within 2 months.

Short-term goals:
• At the end of 1 week the patient will sit on the front steps at home.
• At the end of 2 weeks the patient will walk to the corner and back home.
• At the end of 3 weeks the patient, accompanied by the nurse, will walk in the neighborhood.
• At the end of 4 weeks the patient will walk in the neighborhood alone.
• At the end of 6 weeks the patient will drive her car in the neighborhood.
• At the end of 8 weeks that patient will drive to the mall and meet a friend for dinner.

Each goal is stated in terms of an observable behavior and includes a period of time in which it is to be accomplished. It also includes any other relevant conditions, such as whether the patient is to be alone or accompanied by the nurse.

BOX **12-2**

Qualities of Well-Written Outcome Criteria

• Specific rather than general
• Measurable rather than subjective
• Attainable rather than unrealistic
• Current rather than outdated
• Adequate in number rather than too few or too many
• Mutual rather than one-sided

In writing goals, psychiatric nurses should remember that they can be classified into the "ABCs" or three domains of knowledge:
1. **A**ffective (feeling)
2. **B**ehavioral (psychomotor)
3. **C**ognitive (thinking)

Correctly identifying the domain of the expected outcome is very important in planning nursing interventions. Some psychiatric nurses assume that the only outcomes necessary are those related to learning new information (cognitive). They forget about the equally important needs of patients to acquire new values (affective) or master new skills (behavior).

For example, it would be of limited help to teach a patient about medication if the patient did not value taking medications based on a personal belief system or previous life experiences. It would be equally unsuccessful to engage in medication education if the patient did not know how to take public transportation to fill the prescription.

Finally, it is important to explore with the patient the cost/benefit effect of all identified goals, that is, what is being given up (cost) versus what is being gained (benefit) from attaining the goal. This can be thought of as exploring advantages, or positive effects, and disadvantages or negative effects. Patients are not likely to commit themselves to a goal or to work toward attaining a goal if the stakes are too high and the payoffs too low.

Exploring advantages and disadvantages helps the patient anticipate what price will be paid to achieve the goal and then decide if the change is worth the cost to oneself or significant others. Sometimes it is helpful to write these down in the form of two columns (advantages and disadvantages) that can be added to or changed at any time.

PLANNING

STANDARD IV: PLANNING
The psychiatric–mental health nurse develops a plan of care that is negotiated among the patient, nurse, family, and health care team and prescribes evidence-based interventions to attain expected patient outcomes.

■ **Rationale**
A plan of care is used to guide therapeutic interventions systematically, document progress, and achieve the expected patient outcomes.

■ **Nursing Conditions**
Application of theory
Respect for patient and family

■ **Nursing Behaviors**
Prioritize goals
Identify nursing activities
Validate plan with patient

■ **Key Elements**
The plan of nursing care must always be individualized for the patient.
Planned interventions should be based on current knowledge in the field and contemporary clinical psychiatric–mental health nursing practice.
Planning is done in collaboration with the patient, the family, and the health care team.
Documentation of the plan of care is an essential nursing activity.

One of the most important tasks facing the nurse and patient is to assign **priorities** to the goals. Often several goals can be pursued at the same time. Those related to protecting the patient from self-destructive impulses always receive top priority. When identifying expected outcomes and long- and short-term goals, the nurse must keep the proposed time sequence firmly in mind.

Because the nursing care plan is dynamic and should adapt to the patient's coping responses throughout contact with the health care system, priorities are constantly changing. If the focus is always on the patient's behavioral responses, priorities can be set and modified as the patient changes. This personalizes nursing care, and the patient participates in its planning and implementation.

Once the goals are chosen, the next task is to outline the plan for achieving them. The nursing care plan applies theory and research from nursing and related biological, behavioral, and social sciences to the unique responses of the individual patient. This assumes that as the nurse identifies patient needs, appropriate resources will be consulted. Skilled psychiatric nursing requires a commitment to the ongoing pursuit of knowledge that will enhance professional growth.

The patient's active involvement leads to a more successful care plan. After writing a tentative care plan, the nurse must validate this plan with the patient. This saves time and effort for them both as they continue to work together. It also communicates to the patient a sense of self-responsibility in getting well.

The patient can tell the nurse that a proposed plan is unrealistic regarding financial status, lifestyle, value system, culture or, perhaps, personal preference. Usually several approaches to a patient's problem are possible. Choosing the one most acceptable to the patient improves the chances for success.

If a goal answers the question of **what**, the plan of care answers the questions **how** and **why**. The plan chosen obviously depends on the nursing diagnosis, the nurse's theoretical orientation, the evidence supporting the intended intervention, and the nature of the outcomes pursued. Failure to reach a goal through one plan can lead to the decision to adopt a new approach or reevaluate the goal. These activities commonly occur in the working phase of the relationship.

The Joint Commission on Accreditation of Healthcare Organizations (JCAHO) standards specify that the nursing plan of care must contain the six elements listed in Box 12-3 and that the primary place to document the nursing process is in the patient's health care record.

Psychiatric nurses are beginning to use a variety of formats that often differ from the traditional nursing care plan. Many of these changes have been prompted by changes in the treatment settings and by the advanced computer technology available.

For example, computerized programs have been developed that can provide rapid entry of patient data, retrieve psychiatric treatment plans, and produce a finished document that is clinically useful and highly readable. Another advantage of a computerized information system is its ability to store clin-

---

BOX 12-3

Essential Elements of the Nursing Plan of Care

- Initial assessment and reassessment
- Nursing diagnoses or patient care needs
- Interventions identified to meet the patient's nursing care needs
- Nursing care provided
- Patient's response to and the outcomes of the nursing care provided
- Ability of the patient or significant other to manage continuing care needs after discharge

---

ical data that also can be used for outcome research, quality improvement activities, and resource management. In addition to computerized plans of care, psychiatric nurses use clinical practice guidelines, clinical protocols, flow sheets, clinical pathways, and treatment algorithms in their practice settings.

What are the potential problems in using computerized patient information systems in psychiatric health care facilities? ■

IMPLEMENTATION

STANDARD V: IMPLEMENTATION
The psychiatric–mental health nurse implements the interventions identified in the plan of care.

■ **Rationale**
In implementing the plan of care, psychiatric–mental health nurses use a wide range of interventions designed to prevent mental and physical illness and to promote, maintain, and restore mental and physical health. Psychiatric–mental health nurses select interventions according to their level of practice. At the basic level, nurses may select counseling, milieu therapy, promotion of self-care activities, intake screening and evaluation, psychobiological interventions, health teaching, case management, health promotion and health maintenance, crisis intervention, community-based care, psychiatric home health care, telehealth, and a variety of other approaches to meet the mental health needs of patients. In addition to the intervention options available to the basic-level psychiatric–mental health nurse, at the advanced level the Advanced Practice Registered Nurse in Psychiatric–Mental Health (APRN-PMH) may provide consultation, engage in psychotherapy, and prescribe pharmacological agents where permitted by state statutes or regulations.

■ **Nursing Conditions**
Past clinical experiences
Knowledge of research
Responsive and action dimensions of care

■ **Nursing Behaviors**
Consider available resources
Implement nursing activities
Generate alternatives
Coordinate with other team members

■ **Key Elements**
Nursing interventions should reflect a holistic, biopsychosocial approach to patient care.
Nursing interventions are implemented in a safe, efficient, and caring manner.

The level at which a nurse functions and the interventions implemented are based on the nursing practice acts in one's state, the nurse's qualifications (including education, experience, and certification), the caregiving setting, and the nurse's initiative.

STANDARD VA: COUNSELING

The psychiatric–mental health nurse uses counseling interventions to assist patients in improving or regaining their previous coping abilities, fostering mental health, and preventing mental illness and disability.

STANDARD VB: MILIEU THERAPY

The psychiatric–mental health nurse provides, structures, and maintains a therapeutic environment in collaboration with the patient and other health care clinicians.

STANDARD VC: PROMOTION OF SELF-CARE ACTIVITIES

The psychiatric–mental health nurse structures interventions around the patient's activities of daily living to foster self-care and mental and physical well-being.

STANDARD VD: PSYCHOBIOLOGICAL INTERVENTIONS

The psychiatric–mental health nurse uses knowledge of psychobiological interventions and applies clinical skills to restore the patient's health and prevent further disability.

STANDARD VE: HEALTH TEACHING

The psychiatric–mental health nurse, through health teaching, assists patients in achieving satisfying, productive, and healthy patterns of living.

STANDARD VF: CASE MANAGEMENT

The psychiatric–mental health nurse provides case management to coordinate comprehensive health services and ensure continuity of care.

STANDARD VG: HEALTH PROMOTION AND HEALTH MAINTENANCE

The psychiatric–mental health nurse employs strategies and interventions to promote and maintain health and prevent mental illness.

ADVANCED PRACTICE INTERVENTIONS Vh-Vj

The following interventions (Vh-Vj) may be performed only by the APRN-PMH.

STANDARD VH: PSYCHOTHERAPY

The APRN-PMH uses individual, group, and family psychotherapy, and other therapeutic treatments to assist patients in preventing mental illness and disability, treating mental health disorders, and in improving mental health status and functional abilities.

STANDARD VI: PRESCRIPTIVE AUTHORITY AND TREATMENT

The APRN-PMH uses prescriptive authority, procedures, and treatments in accordance with state and federal laws and regulations, to treat symptoms of psychiatric illness and improve functional health status.

STANDARD VJ: CONSULTATION

The APRN-PMH provides consultation to enhance the abilities of other clinicians to provide services for patients and effect change in the system.

Implementation is the actual delivery of nursing care to the patient and his or her response to that care. Nursing interventions should be based on existing evidence of the efficacy of the intended treatment. The use of a standardized classification system of interventions that nurses perform, such as the Nursing Interventions Classification (NIC) (Dochterman and Bulechek, 2004) is useful for clinical documentation, communication of care across settings, integration of data across systems, effectiveness research, productivity measurement, competency evaluation, and reimbursement (Aquilino and Keenan, 2000).

Good planning increases the chances of successful implementation. Such factors as available people, equipment, resources, time, and money must be considered as nursing actions are planned. It is helpful when planning care to identify alternative nursing actions that are also appropriate to the goal. If this is done, the nurse is not left floundering if the first approach fails. Considering several alternatives makes the implementation phase of the nursing process highly flexible.

In implementing psychotherapeutic interventions, the nurse helps the psychiatric patient do two things: **develop insight** and **change behavior**. These two areas for nursing intervention correspond with the responsive and action dimensions of the nurse-patient relationship described in Chapter 2. **Insight** is the patient's development of new emotional and cognitive understandings (Baier, Murray, and McSweeney, 1998). Often the patient becomes more anxious as defense mechanisms are broken down. This is the time when resistance commonly occurs.

But knowing something on an intellectual level does *not* inevitably lead to a **change in behavior.** Nurses who terminate their interventions at this point are not fully carrying out the therapeutic process to the patient's benefit. An additional step is needed. Patients must decide whether they will revert to maladaptive coping mechanisms, remain in a resisting, immobilized state, or adopt new, adaptive, and constructive approaches to life.

The first step in helping a patient translate insight into action is to build adequate incentives to abandon old patterns of behavior. The nurse should help the patient see the consequences of actions and that old patterns do more harm than good. The patient will not learn new patterns until the motivation to acquire them is greater than the motivation to retain old ones. The nurse should encourage the patient's desires for mental health, emotional growth, and freedom from suffering. The nurse also should continue to motivate and support patients as they test new behaviors and coping mechanisms.

Many of the patient's maladaptive patterns have built up over years; the nurse cannot expect the patient to change them in a matter of days or weeks. Finally, the nurse must help the patient evaluate these new patterns, integrate them into life experiences, and practice problem solving to prepare for future experiences.

The standards of care for implementation are detailed and explicit. The standards identify the range of activities psychiatric nurses use. Information related to each of these implementation standards appears in various chapters throughout this text.

Psychiatric nurses need to be skilled in biological, psychological, and sociocultural skills to implement these nursing interventions. The current psychiatric population has a higher level of acuity, increased mortality rates, and more complex problems than in the past. Specifically, 50% of people with mental illness are estimated to have a known co-

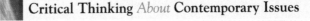

morbid medical disorder; another 35% are estimated to suffer from undiagnosed and untreated medical disorders; and on average, people with mental illness die 10 to 15 years earlier than the general population. Thus it is essential that psychiatric nurses stay current with their biomedical as well as psychosocial skills.

Graduating nursing students are sometimes advised to work in a medical-surgical setting before going into psychiatry so that they can learn "basic nursing skills." Why is this suggestion no longer valid given the treatment afforded contemporary psychiatric patients and the range of treatment settings? ■

A final issue for the psychiatric nurse to consider in the implementation process is that there are four possible treatment stages:

- Crisis
- Acute
- Maintenance
- Health promotion

These stages reflect the range of adaptive/maladaptive coping responses, and patients can move between these stages at any time. The goal, assessment, intervention, and expected outcome vary with each stage, as described in Chapter 4. It is critically important for psychiatric nurses to determine the patient's stage of treatment and then implement nursing activities that target the treatment goal in the most cost-effective and efficient manner.

EVALUATION

STANDARD VI: EVALUATION
The psychiatric–mental health nurse evaluates the patient's progress in attaining expected outcomes.
■ **Rationale**
Nursing care is a dynamic process involving change in the patient's health status over time, giving rise to the need for data, different diagnoses, and modifications in the plan of care. Therefore evaluation is a continuous process of appraising the effect of nursing and the treatment regimen on the patient's health status and expected outcomes.
■ **Nursing Conditions**
Supervision
Self-analysis
Peer review
Patient and family participation
■ **Nursing Behaviors**
Compare patient's responses and expected outcome
Review nursing process
Modify nursing process as needed
Participate in quality improvement activities
■ **Key Elements**
Evaluation is an ongoing process.
Patient and family participation in evaluation is essential.
Goal achievement should be documented and revisions in the plan of care should be implemented as appropriate.

When evaluating care, the nurse should review all previous phases of the nursing process and determine whether the

Critical Thinking *About* Contemporary Issues

Does Psychiatric Nursing Care Really Make a Difference?

Most nurses reading the question in the box title would automatically and emphatically say, "Yes, of course it does!" But does it really? More specifically, what evidence exists that the care provided by psychiatric nurses actually results in a decrease in patients' symptoms, improvement in patients' functional status, or improved quality of life? What evidence would you provide a hospital administrator who was proposing that all but one of the psychiatric nursing positions on the units be replaced with counselors? How would you convince the director of a community mental health program for the seriously mentally ill that, as a nurse, you should be hired to work with this population rather than the social worker who is also being interviewed?

In fact, very few well-designed psychiatric nursing studies have demonstrated the effectiveness of psychiatric nursing care. Of the hundreds of articles cited in recent reviews, very few psychiatric nursing studies are mentioned. It is clear that psychiatric nurses believe they make a valuable contribution to the health care of patients. However, providing the evidence of this contribution remains a challenge for the field.

expected outcomes for the patient have been met. Key words for the evaluation phase of the nursing process are **mutual, competent, accessible, effective, appropriate, efficient,** and **flexible.** Often, progress with psychiatric patients is slow and occurs in small steps rather than dramatic leaps. Realizing that progress has been made can produce growth and inspire new enthusiasm in both the patient and the nurse.

Above all, evaluation is a mutual process based on the patient's and family's previously identified goals and level of satisfaction. Patients, families, and psychiatric nurses often have different views of treatment and the effectiveness of care. It is therefore critical that psychiatric nurses have a systematic and objective way to learn from patients and families which aspects of the nursing care provided were helpful and what additional nursing actions may have further enhanced their well-being.

Finally, evaluation is a **continuous, active process** that begins early in the relationship and continues throughout. It is an activity that must be documented by psychiatric nurses so that they can demonstrate the value of psychiatric nursing services to consumers, administrators, reimbursers, and other health care providers (see Critical Thinking About Contemporary Issues). Perhaps more than any other phase of the nursing process, evaluation and outcome measurement will be the key aspects of psychiatric nursing activities in the decade to come.

■ ACCOUNTABILITY AND AUTONOMY

The Standards of Professional Performance apply to self-definition, self-regulation, accountability, and autonomy for practice by psychiatric nurses, both individually and as a group. As such, the standards of performance are critical.

Accountability means to be answerable to someone for something. It focuses responsibility on the individual nurse for personal actions, or perhaps lack of action. The preconditions of accountability include ability, responsibility, and authority. Accountability also includes formal review processes and an attitude of integrity and vigilance.

Autonomy implies self-determination, independence, and shared power. It is the condition that allows for definition of and control over one's work domain. For psychiatric nursing, attaining autonomy means being able to define the domain of nursing and being able to exercise control over psychiatric nursing practice.

This idea of shaping destiny, rather than letting outside forces be in control, views power as a positive force that allows nurses to attain goals. It involves a conscious decision to identify objectives, plan strategy, assume responsibility, exercise authority, and be held accountable. In contrast, burnout and emotional exhaustion are caused by a sense of failure in the psychiatric nurse's attempt to find meaning through work (Malach-Pines, 2000; Robinson, Clements, and Land, 2003)

Autonomy has two major interrelated components. The first is **control over nursing tasks**, which means:

- Having the opportunity for independent thought and action.
- Having use of time, skills, and ability by way of being able to eliminate, refuse, or delegate nonnursing tasks.
- Having the authority and responsibility for implementing goals related to the quality of care.
- Being able to initiate changes and innovations in practice.

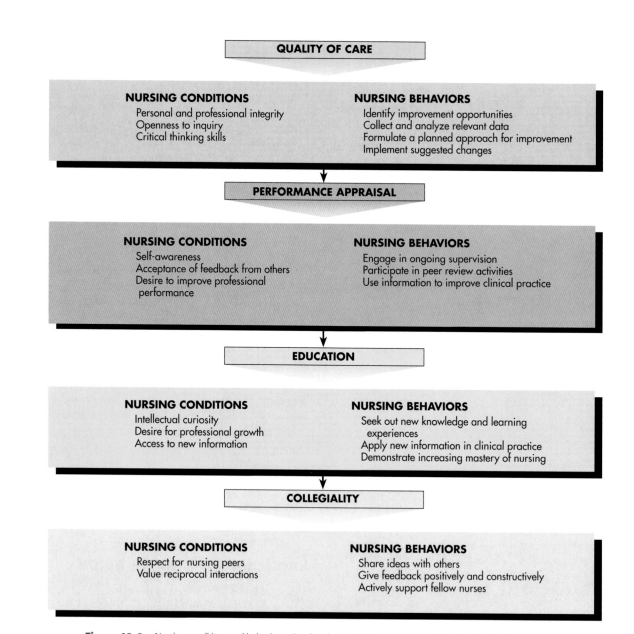

Figure 12-2 Nursing conditions and behaviors related to the psychiatric nursing standards of professional performance.

The second component of autonomy is **participation in decision making**. It requires the nurse's participation in the following:

- Determining and implementing quality standards
- Making decisions affecting each nurse's job context, including salary, staffing, and professional growth
- Setting institutional policies, procedures, and goals

The full realization of nursing's potential will be obtained through a negotiated process with other health professionals, consumers, and society at large. It requires increased access to resources, demonstration of expertise, and acknowledgment of the skills of nurses by other professionals. Psychiatric nursing is practiced largely in collaboration, coordination, and cooperation with a variety of other professionals working with and on behalf of the patient. As nurses see themselves

in a positive way, they will increase their ability to assert themselves, articulate the contributions they make, and function effectively.

The conditions and behaviors related to each standard of professional performance are shown in Figure 12-2. Each of these standards is discussed here.

■ PROFESSIONAL PERFORMANCE STANDARDS

QUALITY OF CARE

STANDARD I: QUALITY OF CARE
The psychiatric–mental health nurse systematically evaluates the quality of care and effectiveness of psychiatric–mental health nursing practice.

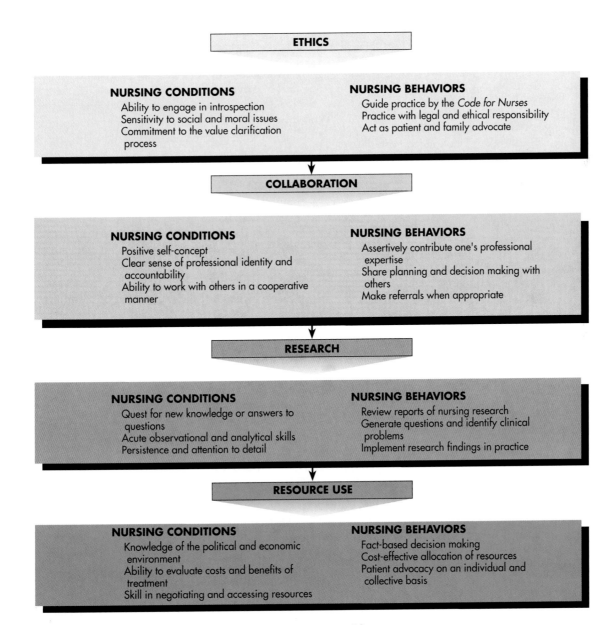

Figure 12-2, cont'd

■ **Rationale**

The dynamic nature of the mental health care environment and the growing body of psychiatric nursing knowledge and research provide both the impetus and the means for the psychiatric–mental health nurse to be competent in clinical practice, to continue to develop professionally, and to improve the quality of patient care.

■ **Nursing Conditions**

Personal and professional integrity
Openness to inquiry
Critical thinking skills

■ **Nursing Behaviors**

Identify improvement opportunities
Collect and analyze relevant data
Formulate a planned approach for improvement
Implement suggested changes

■ **Key Elements**

The nurse should be open to critically analyzing the caregiving process.
The patient and family should be partners with the nurse in the evaluation of care activities.
Improving the quality of care provided goes beyond discussion and analysis to actually implementing actions that will improve practice.

Psychiatric nurses actively participate in the formal organizational evaluation of overall patterns of care through a variety of **quality improvement** or **process improvement activities**. In these activities the focus is not on the nurse clinician but on the patient, the overall program of care, and health-related outcomes of care. The current commitment to critically reviewing health care stems from several sources: consumer demand for high-quality but reasonably priced health care, third-party payer demand for controlled health care costs, increased professional accountability, and regulatory and federal groups that monitor the quality of care.

The purpose of quality or process improvement programs is to design, implement, evaluate, guide, and modify a process for improving the performance of a health care organization and to initiate improvement activities. Specific objectives include the following:

- Continuous improvement of customer satisfaction
- Continuous improvement of patient outcomes
- Efficient use of resources
- Adherence to professional and regulatory standards

Psychiatric nurses play essential roles in identifying opportunities for improvement, collecting data for analysis of the current process, evaluating the effectiveness of the new processes, and representing nursing's perspective in the improvement team's deliberations.

Find out about a quality improvement project that is currently underway in your clinical facility. Does it relate to customer satisfaction, patient health outcomes, use of resources, or adherence to standards? ■

PERFORMANCE APPRAISAL

STANDARD II: PERFORMANCE APPRAISAL

The psychiatric–mental health nurse evaluates one's own psychiatric–mental health nursing practice in relation to professional practice standards and relevant statutes and regulations.

■ **Rationale**

The psychiatric–mental health nurse is accountable to the public for providing competent clinical care and has inherent responsibility as a professional to evaluate the role and performance of psychiatric–mental health nursing practice according to standards established by the profession.

■ **Nursing Conditions**

Self-awareness
Acceptance of feedback from others
Desire to improve professional performance

■ **Nursing Behaviors**

Engage in ongoing supervision
Participate in peer review activities
Use information to improve clinical practice

■ **Key Elements**

Supervision should be viewed as an essential and ongoing aspect of one's professional life.
The nurse should strive to grow and develop professional knowledge, skills, and expertise.

Performance appraisal for the psychiatric nurse is generally provided in two ways: administrative and clinical. **Administrative performance appraisal** involves the review, management, and regulation of competent psychiatric nursing practice. It involves a supervisory relationship in which a nurse's work performance is compared with role expectations in a formal way, such as in a nurse's annual performance evaluation. Administrative performance evaluations should identify areas of competency and areas for improvement. A method for recognizing quality performance also should be in place (see Critical Thinking About Contemporary Issues).

Many nursing departments have adopted clinical advancement programs or other formal mechanisms to recog-

Critical Thinking *About* Contemporary Issues

What Kind of Recognition Do Staff Nurses Value?

It is well known that recognition is central to nurses' morale. However, it is less clear what type of recognition is valued and why it is given. A survey asked 239 staff nurses about this issue. They found that verbal feedback was identified as the most meaningful type of recognition. This was followed by letters of praise for performance or achievement, organizational awards, honors, or public announcements of outstanding performance, promotion or a prestigious assignment with increased responsibility, being personally thanked and praised during an evaluation and, finally, monetary bonuses, salary increases, or gifts.

The main reasons given for receiving recognition included outstanding performance in patient care and positive attitude, followed by demonstrated expertise, willingness to assume extra work, involvement in professional activities, completion of a certification or degree program, and years of service in an organization. Recognition came most often from the head nurse, followed by the nurse administrator, patients and families, co-workers, physicians, and hospital administrators. Studies such as this help clarify meaningful aspects of administrative performance appraisals and ways to commend nurses for a job well done.

nize nursing excellence. Clinical advancement programs have been established to formally validate nurses for increasing mastery in practice. They allow the nurse to be promoted and economically rewarded for providing direct patient care. Such programs identify levels of professional development in nursing based on increased critical thinking and advanced application of nursing skills. These characteristics result in better care being provided by psychiatric nurses throughout their professional career.

One of your nursing colleagues tells you that she thinks nurses' pay should be based on their experience, not their education. After all, she argues, if two nurses do the same job, what does it matter if they have different educational degrees? How would you respond? ■

Clinical performance appraisal is guidance provided through a mentoring relationship and clinical supervision with a more experienced, skilled, and educated nurse. According to Lyth (2000), clinical supervision is a support mechanism for practicing professionals within which they can share clinical, organizational, developmental, and emotional experiences with another professional in a secure, confidential environment in order to enhance knowledge and skills. This process will lead to an increased awareness of other concepts including accountability and reflective practice.

The professional psychiatric nurse is aware of the need for ongoing mentorship to achieve increasing levels of mastery of psychiatric nursing practice. Clinical supervision not only reviews one's clinical care but also can serve as a support system for the nurse (Laskowski, 2001).

In many ways the process of supervision parallels the nurse-patient relationship. Both involve a learning process that takes place in the context of a meaningful relationship that facilitates positive change. Self-exploration is a critical element of both. The supervisor should provide the same responsive and action dimensions present in the nurse-patient relationship to help supervised nurses live effectively with themselves and others.

There are four common forms of supervision:

1. The **dyadic**, or one-on-one, relationship, in which the supervisor meets the one being supervised in a face-to-face encounter
2. The **triadic** relationship, in which a supervisor and two nurses of similar experience and training meet for supervision
3. **Group** supervision, in which several supervised nurses meet for a shared session with the supervisory nurse
4. **Peer review**, in which nurses meet without a supervisor to evaluate their clinical practice

All four forms have a similar purpose: exploring the problem areas and maximizing the strengths of the ones being supervised.

Despite its intensity, **supervision is not therapy**. The essential difference between the two is a difference of purpose. The aim of supervision is to teach psychotherapeutic skills, whereas the goal of therapy is to alter a person's characteristic patterns of coping to enable him or her to function more effectively in all areas of life.

The problems of the one being supervised in the supervisory and therapeutic relationships are dealt with only to the extent that they affect the nurse's ability to learn from the supervisor and be effective with patients. Therefore the problems are limited in scope and depth; they do not include all other aspects of the life of the one being supervised. With the resolution of the particular problem, the focus of supervision returns to the teaching of psychotherapeutic skills and their implementation by the nurse.

Supervision or consultation is necessary for the practicing psychiatric nurse. Although it is crucial for novices, it is equally important for experienced practitioners. Personal limitations create a need for assistance in remaining objective throughout the therapeutic process and the "normal" stresses it presents. Obviously, supervision is only as helpful as the skill of the supervisor, the openness of the supervised nurse, and the motivation of both to learn and grow.

EDUCATION

STANDARD III: EDUCATION
The psychiatric–mental health nurse acquires and maintains current knowledge in nursing practice.

■ **Rationale**
The rapid expansion of knowledge pertaining to basic and behavioral sciences, technology, information systems, and research requires a commitment to learning throughout the psychiatric–mental health nurse's professional career. Formal education, continuing education, independent learning activities, and experiential and other learning activities are some of the means the psychiatric–mental health nurse uses to enhance nursing expertise and advance the profession.

■ **Nursing Conditions**
Intellectual curiosity
Desire for professional growth
Access to new information

■ **Nursing Behaviors**
Seek out new knowledge and learning experiences
Apply new information in clinical practice
Demonstrate increasing mastery of nursing

■ **Key Elements**
Professional learning should be regarded as a lifelong process.
The nurse should pursue a variety of educational opportunities.
New knowledge should be translated into professional nursing practice.

The nature of psychiatric care, the mental health delivery system, and the boundaries of nursing are changing rapidly. In addition, the scientific basis for practice is expanding each day. Psychiatric nurses are expected to engage in a continuous learning process to keep up with this emerging knowledge. They may do this in the following ways:

- Formal educational programs
- Continuing education programs
- Independent learning activities
- Lectures, conferences, and workshops
- Credentialing
- Certification

Reading journals and textbooks and collaborating with colleagues are other important ways to remain current with

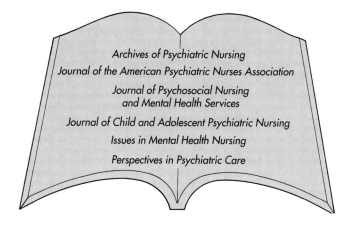

Archives of Psychiatric Nursing

Journal of the American Psychiatric Nurses Association

Journal of Psychosocial Nursing and Mental Health Services

Journal of Child and Adolescent Psychiatric Nursing

Issues in Mental Health Nursing

Perspectives in Psychiatric Care

Figure 12-3 Psychiatric nursing journals.

expanding areas of knowledge. Figure 12-3 lists journals that relate to psychiatric nursing practice and are good sources of new information.

One of the most exciting resources for psychiatric nurses is the Internet, which allows nurses access to information from around the globe. The Internet can help nurses communicate through e-mail and can help them network with other nurses through discussion groups or newsgroups found on-line.

The number of Web home pages is growing rapidly. These sites offer a wide range of information, from updates on current psychiatric medications, to information on various mental disorders, to resources on mental health organizations and delivery systems, to teaching modules for clinical training and continuing education. The amount of information available through this technology is revolutionizing the way in which psychiatric nurses acquire and maintain current knowledge in nursing practice.

With its access to the Evolve website, this textbook provides monthly updates on the latest findings in the field and facilitates the use of the Internet by providing WebLinks to home pages on the World Wide Web that are relevant to the content of each chapter. Nurses are encouraged to access these resources to further their knowledge and professional growth.

COLLEGIALITY

STANDARD IV: COLLEGIALITY

The psychiatric–mental health nurse interacts with and contributes to the professional development of peers, health care clinicians, and others, as colleagues.

■ **Rationale**

The psychiatric–mental health nurse is responsible for sharing knowledge, research, and clinical information with colleagues, through formal and informal teaching methods, to enhance professional growth.

■ **Nursing Conditions**

Respect for nursing peers

Value reciprocal interactions

■ **Nursing Behaviors**

Share ideas with others

Give feedback positively and constructively

Actively support fellow nurses

■ **Key Elements**

The nurse should regard other nurses as colleagues and partners in caregiving. Mentorship within nursing is important both to nurses as individuals and to the nursing profession as a whole.

Collegiality requires that nurses view their nurse peers as collaborators in the caregiving process who are valued and respected for their unique contributions, regardless of educational, experiential, or specialty background. It suggests that nurses view themselves as members of an organized professional group or unit and that nurses trust, remain loyal to, and demonstrate commitment to other nurses (DeMarco, Horowitz, and McLeod, 2000).

Many have observed that nursing, as a profession, has sometimes struggled with this concept. For example, nurses have voiced complaints about "ivory-tower" nurse educators, "nonsupportive" nurse administrators, "nonintellectual" nurse clinicians, and "irrelevant" nurse researchers in the past. Also, psychiatric nurses in various institutions or organizations have had difficulty joining forces and working together on a common psychiatric nursing agenda. However, this intradisciplinary conflict is not consistent with professional performance standards. It also has prevented the profession from acting as a unified group in pursuing health care initiatives at local, regional, and national levels.

Nurses need to work together as colleagues to blend their various skills and abilities in creating a better health care system and enhancing the quality and quantity of psychiatric nursing services provided. One specific way to do this is for psychiatric nurses to join a professional nursing organization. The largest psychiatric nursing organization that is open to nursing students and psychiatric nurses of all educational and experiential backgrounds is the American Psychiatric Nurses Association (APNA). The mission and goals of this organization are described in Box 12-4.

You approach a colleague about joining APNA, but she tells you that she does not have the money to join a nursing organization. You know that membership in APNA costs about $2 a week and it includes a subscription to the Journal of the American Psychiatric Nurses Association. *How would you respond?* ■

ETHICS

STANDARD V: ETHICS

The psychiatric–mental health nurse's assessments, actions, and recommendations on behalf of patients are determined and implemented in an ethical manner.

■ **Rationale**

The public's trust and its right to humane psychiatric–mental health care are upheld by professional nursing practice. Ethical standards describe a code of behaviors to guide professional practice. People with psychiatric–mental health needs are an especially vulnerable population. The foundation of psychiatric–mental health nursing practice is the development of a therapeutic relationship with the patient. Boundaries need to be established to safeguard the patient's well-being.

BOX 12-4

Overview of the American Psychiatric Nurses Association

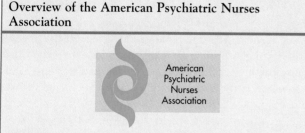
American Psychiatric Nurses Association

Mission

The American Psychiatric Nurses Association (APNA) provides leadership to promote psychiatric–mental health nursing, improve mental health care for culturally diverse individuals, families, groups, and communities, and shape health policy for the delivery of mental health services.

Goals

1. Practice: Drive psychiatric–mental health nursing practice
2. Education: Spearhead the professional development and certification of nurses who provide mental health care
3. Research: Maximize resources and opportunities to expand the science of psychiatric–mental health nursing
4. Mental health policy: Expand mental health public policy roles of APNA
5. Organizational development: Strengthen and expand the organization

Dues

Regular membership: $110
Student membership: $66
NSNA student member: $45

Internet

http://www.apna.org

- ■ **Nursing Conditions**
Ability to engage in introspection
Sensitivity to social and moral issues
Commitment to the values clarification process
- ■ **Nursing Behaviors**
Guide practice by the *Code for Nurses*
Practice with legal and ethical responsibility
Act as a patient and family advocate
- ■ **Key Elements**
Nurses should be sensitive to the social, moral, and ethical environment in which they practice.
Patient and family advocacy is a core aspect of nursing practice.
Ethical conduct is essential to the nurse-patient relationship.

Ethical considerations combine with legal and therapeutic issues to affect all aspects of psychiatric nursing practice. The legal and ethical context of psychiatric nursing care is discussed in Chapter 10. Boundary violations related to the nurse-patient relationship are described in Chapter 2.

Groups, such as professions, also can hold a code of ethics. Such a code guides the profession in serving and protecting consumers. It also provides a framework for decision making for members of the profession. Two major purposes for a code of ethics are structuring and sensitizing. **Structuring** is pre-

BOX 12-5

Code of Ethics for Nurses—Provisions, Approved as of June 30, 2001

1. The nurse, in all professional relationships, practices with compassion and respect for the inherent dignity, worth, and uniqueness of every individual, unrestricted by considerations of social or economic status, personal attributes, or the nature of health problems.
2. The nurse's primary commitment is to the patient, whether an individual, family, group, or community.
3. The nurse promotes, advocates for, and strives to protect the health, safety, and rights of the patient.
4. The nurse is responsible and accountable for individual nursing practice and determines the appropriate delegation of tasks consistent with the nurse's obligation to provide optimum patient care.
5. The nurse owes the same duties to self as to others, including the responsibility to preserve integrity and safety, to maintain competence, and to continue personal and professional growth.
6. The nurse participates in establishing, maintaining, and improving health care environments and conditions of employment conducive to the provision of quality health care and consistent with the values of the profession through individual and collective action.
7. The nurse participates in the advancement of the profession through contributions to practice, education, administration, and knowledge development.
8. The nurse collaborates with other health professionals and the public in promoting community, national, and international efforts to meet health needs.
9. The profession of nursing, as represented by associations and their members, is responsible for articulating nursing values, for maintaining the integrity of the profession and its practice, and for shaping social policy.

Reprinted with permission from the American Nurses Association: *Code of ethics for nurses with interpretive statements*, Washington, DC, 2001, American Nurses Publishing, American Nurses Foundation/American Nurses Association.

ventive and aims to restrain impulsive and unethical behavior. **Sensitizing** is educative, with the goal of raising members' ethical consciousness.

The American Nurses Association (2001) has revised their code of ethics for nurses (Box 12-5). It emphasizes that the nurse's primary commitment is to the patient and expands the ethical perspective of nurses to include the health care system and duties of the nurse to oneself (Daly, 2002).

COLLABORATION

STANDARD VI: COLLABORATION

The psychiatric–mental health nurse collaborates with the patient, significant others, and health care clinicians in providing care.

- ■ **Rationale**

Psychiatric–mental health nursing practice requires a coordinated, ongoing interaction between consumers and clinicians to deliver comprehensive services to the patient and the community. Through the collaborative process, different abilities of health care clinicians are used to identify problems, communicate, plan and implement interventions, and evaluate mental health services.

■ **Nursing Conditions**
Positive self-concept
Clear sense of professional identity and accountability
Ability to work with others in a cooperative manner
■ **Nursing Behaviors**
Assertively contribute one's professional expertise
Share planning and decision making with others
Make referrals when appropriate
■ **Key Elements**
Respect for others grows out of respect for self.
The nurse should be able to clearly articulate his or her professional abilities and areas of expertise to others.
Collaboration involves the ability to negotiate and formulate new solutions with others.

Collaboration is the shared planning, decision making, problem solving, goal setting, and assumption of responsibilities by individuals who work together cooperatively and with open communication. Three key ingredients are needed for collaboration:

1. Active and assertive contributions from each person
2. Receptivity and respect for each person's contribution
3. Negotiations that build on the contributions of each person to form a new way of conceptualizing the problem

Psychiatric nurses have many potential collaborators, including patients and families, interdisciplinary colleagues, and nursing peers (Figure 12-4). Each of these groups allows the psychiatric nurse an opportunity to solve problems in new ways and thus better plan and implement nursing care.

An essential part of contemporary practice is working with other health care providers (Akhavain et al, 1999). Nurses may be members of three different types of teams: uni-disciplinary, having all team members of the same discipline;

multidisciplinary, having members of different disciplines who provide specific services to the patient; and interdisciplinary, having members of different disciplines involved in a formal arrangement to provide patient services while maximizing educational interchange. Most organized mental health settings use an interdisciplinary team approach, which requires highly coordinated and often interdependent planning based on the separate and distinct roles of each team member (Table 12-1).

It has been said that nurses seek mutual collegiality, whereas physicians encourage teamwork with subordinates. How would these different views affect the process of collaboration? ■

Interdisciplinary collaboration does not always proceed smoothly. There are many barriers to interdisciplinary collaboration, including inappropriate education and training of mental health team members, traditional organizational structures, goal and role conflict, competitive and accommodating interpersonal interactions, power and status in-

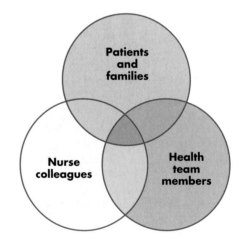

Figure 12-4   Collaborative relationships for psychiatric nurses.

Table 12-1	**Mental Health Personnel, Training, and Roles**	
PERSONNEL	**TRAINING**	**ROLE**
Psychiatric nurse	Registered nurse (RN) with specialized training in the care and treatment of psychiatric patients; may have an AD, BS, MS, or PhD degree	Accountable for the biopsychosocial nursing care of patients and their milieu
Psychiatrist	Medical doctor with internship and residency training in psychiatry	Accountable for the medical diagnosis and treatment of patients
Social worker	BS, MSW, or PhD degree with specialized training in mental health settings	Accountable for family casework and community placement of patients
Psychologist	PhD or PsyD degree with research and clinical training in mental health	Accountable for psychological assessments, testing, and treatments
Activity therapist	May have a BS degree with training in mental health settings	Accountable for recreational, occupational, and activity programs
Case worker	Varying degrees of training and usually works under supervision	Accountable for helping patients to be maintained in the community and receive needed services
Substance abuse counselor	Varying degrees of training in alcohol and substance use disorders	Accountable for evaluating and treating patients with substance use problems

equities, and personal qualities of individuals that do not promote shared problem solving.

If roles, functions, and channels of communication among the various team members are not clarified and agreed on, confusion, resentment, crossing of boundaries, and inappropriate use of psychiatric team members are likely to result. Steps that can be taken to facilitate the formation of interdisciplinary teams are listed in Box 12-6.

It is also important for nurses to maintain their professional integrity in the midst of interdisciplinary collaboration. Nurses must not abandon the nursing perspective when they participate in an interdisciplinary team (Lindeke and Block, 1998). Finally, psychiatric nurses must determine whether they as a group are ready to engage in collaborative practice. Questions that should be considered include the following:

- Can psychiatric nurses define, describe, and appropriately defend psychiatric nursing roles and functions?
- Is the psychiatric nursing leadership ready for collegial practice?
- Are psychiatric nursing roles and functions appropriate for nurses' education, experience, and expertise?
- Is nurse staffing appropriate in numbers, patterns, and ratios?
- Are the other disciplines prepared for and supportive of collaboration?
- Is the organizational climate conducive to collaboration?

With positive answers to these questions, psychiatric nurses should be able to move forward in implementing collaborative practice.

*Most people think that there are more **collaborative** interdisciplinary relationships in psychiatry than in other specialty areas because of the nature of the work. Others believe that there is more interdisciplinary **conflict** in psychiatry because roles overlap and boundaries are often unclear. What position would you take on this issue based on your observation of the mental health care team?* ■

BOX 12-6

Steps for Interdisciplinary Team Building

- Develop and agree on a team philosophy of care
- Understand and respect the contributions of each discipline
- Establish new professional interaction patterns
- Define disciplinary and individual roles and responsibilities
- Accept personal and professional changes in authority and status
- Specify lines of authority and decision making and conflict resolution procedures
- Accept shared authority and responsibility
- Communicate regularly, openly, and clearly
- Use multidisciplinary treatment plans and consolidated charting
- Strive for consistent leadership and low staff turnover
- Encourage constant review and exchange of ideas

RESEARCH

STANDARD VII: RESEARCH

The psychiatric–mental health nurse contributes to nursing and mental health through the use of research methods and findings.

■ **Rationale**

Nurses in psychiatric–mental health nursing are responsible for contributing to the further development of the field of mental health by participating in research. At the basic level of practice, the psychiatric–mental health nurse uses research findings to improve clinical care and identifies clinical problems for research study. At the advanced level, the psychiatric–mental health nurse engages and/or collaborates with others in the research process to discover, examine, and test knowledge, theories, and creative approaches to practice.

■ **Nursing Conditions**

Quest for new knowledge or answers to questions
Acute observational and analytical skills
Persistence and attention to detail

■ **Nursing Behaviors**

Review reports of nursing research
Generate questions and identify clinical problems
Implement research findings in practice

■ **Key Elements**

Research links nursing theory and practice and is essential to the development of a profession.
Outcome research helps to establish the value of nursing in an era of health care reform.

The progression of observing from practice, theorizing, testing in research, and subsequently modifying practice is an essential part of psychiatric nursing. The clinical problems are numerous, and as nurses gain the skills and experience to validate their work scientifically, they can make a significant contribution to psychiatric theory and practice through research. The nature and process of outcomes research and evidence-based practice are discussed in detail in Chapter 5.

It is important to encourage close collaboration between nurse researchers and nurse clinicians to ensure that the right questions are asked and the right variables are tested (Whittemore and Grey, 2002). It is also necessary to clearly define how nurses with different educational backgrounds can participate in research. Table 12-2 summarizes the research expectations for nurses based on educational preparation.

RESOURCE UTILIZATION

STANDARD VIII: RESOURCE UTILIZATION

The psychiatric–mental health nurse considers factors related to safety, effectiveness, and cost in planning and delivering patient care.

■ **Rationale**

The patient is entitled to psychiatric–mental health care that is safe, effective, and affordable. As the cost of health care increases, treatment decisions must be made in such a way as to maximize resources and maintain quality of care. The psychiatric–mental health nurse seeks to provide cost-effective, quality care by using the most appropriate resources and delegating care to the most appropriate, qualified health care clinician.

■ **Nursing Conditions**
Knowledge of the political and economic environment
Ability to evaluate costs and benefits of treatment
Skill in negotiating and accessing resources
■ **Nursing Behaviors**
Fact-based decision making
Cost-effective allocation of resources
Patient advocacy on an individual and collective basis
■ **Key Elements**
Nurses play a critical role in integrating and coordinating health
  care services.
Nurses should be fiscally accountable for the care they provide.
Resources should be allocated based on cost/benefit analyses and
  documented expected outcomes.

Resource use is one of the most important aspects of psychiatric nursing practice. Discussing the costs and benefits of treatment options with patients, families, providers, and re-imbursers is an essential part of the professional psychiatric nursing role.

To fulfill this performance standard, psychiatric nurses need to request and obtain both **cost** and **outcome information** related to tests, consultations, evaluations, therapies, and continuum of care alternatives. Nurses need to assume an active role in questioning, advising, and advocating for the most cost-effective use of resources.

One of the most critical resources in the mental health field is that of psychiatric labor. Because each team member has different competencies, a challenge for the mental health system is to use the best that each discipline has to offer and to develop an integrated set of clinical services that will offer the highest quality care (Stuart et al, 2000).

Psychiatric nurses must become increasingly cost and outcome conscious. Identify three commonly ordered tests for psychiatric patients. Find out how much they cost and analyze how helpful they are in planning treatment. ■

Table 12-2	Nursing Research Participation Based on Education
EDUCATIONAL PREPARATION	RESEARCH INVOLVEMENT
Associate degree in nursing	Help identify clinical problems in nursing practice, assist in data collection within a structured format, use research findings in practice with supervision
Baccalaureate degree in nursing	Identify clinical problems in need of research, help experienced investigators gain access to clinical sites, influence the selection of appropriate methods of data collection, participate in data collection and implementation of research findings
Master's degree in nursing	Collaborate in proposal development, data collection, data analysis, and interpretation; appraise the clinical relevance of research findings; provide leadership for integrating findings into practice
Doctoral education	Develop nursing knowledge through research and theory development, conduct funded independent research projects, develop and coordinate funded research projects, disseminate research findings to the scientific community

CASE STUDY

This case study describes the use of the nursing process with a psychiatric patient. It illustrates the interrelationship of the phases of the nurse-patient relationship, the therapeutic dimensions, and the various activities as the nurse works with the patient to foster adaptive coping behavior and more integrated functioning.

Assessment

Ms. G came to the psychiatric outpatient department of the local hospital requesting treatment with a female therapist. The psychiatric nurse specialist agreed to perform the initial screening and evaluation and consider serving as her primary therapist.

To collect the initial data, the nurse followed the admission format required by the department. A description of the presenting problem revealed that Ms. G was a 29-year-old single woman who was neat in appearance and markedly overweight. She reported feelings of "confusion and depression" and said that superficially she appeared "outgoing and friendly and played the role of a clown." In reality, however, she said she had few close friends, felt insecure about herself, felt unsuc-cessful in her job, and believed she "overanalyzed her problems." She said she had feelings of worthlessness and loss of pleasure in her daily activities on and off for the past 2 years.

Additional information was obtained in other significant areas of her life. Her psychosocial history revealed a disrupted family situation. Her mother died of tuberculosis when she was 11 years of age. Her father, age 73, was alive but had been an alcoholic for as long as Ms. G could remember. She had one sister, age 20, who married at age 16 and was now divorced. She also had one stepsister, age 45, who was married, had two adopted sons, and lived out of state. In giving this family information, Ms. G revealed that her stepsister was her natural mother, but she had continued to call her father's wife "mother." After her "mother" died, her stepsister took over the house. However, 2 years later this stepsister married and moved out of state. Ms. G reported feeling closest to this stepsister and felt abandoned when she left. Ms. G then took charge of the house until age 14, when her father placed her and her younger sister in a group home, where she had difficulty making friends.

CASE STUDY—cont'd

She completed high school and college. In college she had four good friends who were all married now. Her only close heterosexual relationship was in high school, and this boyfriend eventually married her best friend. Since that time she had never dated and stated she had no desire to marry.

After college she obtained a job as a "girl Friday" for a law firm and expressed much pleasure with it. She then saw the opportunity to make more money as a waitress and switched jobs. She currently worked at a restaurant, and her schedule involved day and night rotations as well as weekend shifts. She expressed dissatisfaction with many aspects of her job but was unable to identify alternatives. Her goal in life was to have a fulfilling career.

She lived alone. Her best friend was her immediate supervisor at work. She currently had no male friends and only two other female acquaintances.

Pertinent medical history revealed a major weight problem. She was 36 kg (80 pounds) overweight and extremely conscious of it. She viewed her body negatively and believed others were also "repulsed" by her weight. She also recently recovered from infectious hepatitis. She drank an occasional beer when out with friends (once or twice a month), denied any drug use, and smoked three fourths of a pack of cigarettes a day.

Diagnosis

After consultation the psychiatric nurse agreed to work with Ms. G as primary therapist. In the following session they established a contract for working together, and a fee was set. At this time they explored her expressed guilt over seeking help, the reason for her request for a female therapist, their mutual roles, and the confidential nature of the relationship. The nurse also shared with Ms. G the maladaptive coping responses she had noted and the inferences she had made. They discussed these areas, and the following nursing diagnoses were identified:

1. Chronic low self-esteem related to childhood rejection and unrealistic self-ideals, as evidenced by feelings of worthlessness
2. Social isolation related to ambivalence regarding male-female relationships and lack of socialization skills, as evidenced by lack of close friends
3. Ineffective role performance related to job dissatisfaction with working hours and nature of the work, as evidenced by feeling unsuccessful in her job
4. Disturbed body image related to weight control problem, as evidenced by negative feelings

Ms. G's DSM-IV-TR diagnosis was identified as dysthymia, a mood disorder.

Outcome Identification

They mutually agreed to work on her problem areas in weekly therapy sessions. After 3 months they would evaluate the achievement of the following expected outcomes: consistently positive self-esteem; substantial social involvement; substantially adequate role performance; and consistently positive body image. These expected outcomes would be met through the attainment of the following goals:

1. Ms. G will describe her expectations of the therapeutic process and her commitment to it.
2. Aspects of Ms. G's self-ideal will be identified and realistically evaluated.
3. Cognitive distortions influencing her self-concept and negative, stereotyped self-perceptions will be analyzed.
4. Interpersonal relationships will be examined to include her patterns of relating, her expectations of others, and specific areas of difficulty.
5. Alternative employment opportunities will be identified.
6. The advantages and disadvantages of a job change will be compared.

Planning

In discussing these areas they agreed that nursing diagnosis 1 was a central one and problems 2, 3, and 4 directly contributed to the low self-esteem. Her coping mechanisms included intellectualization and denial, and she compensated for her self-doubts by an outward appearance that was social, joking, and friendly, yet superficial. The strengths Ms. G brought to the therapy process included her introspective nature and ability to analyze events, her openness to new ideas, the resource people available to her in her immediate environment, and a genuine sense of humor.

Implementation

Because they were in the introductory phase of the relationship, many of the goals involved areas needing further assessment. During this phase of treatment, Ms. G displayed much anxiety, testing behavior, and ambivalence, and the nursing actions were focused on promoting respect, openness, and acceptance and minimizing her anxiety. Through the nurse's use of empathic understanding, Ms. G became less jovial and superficial and began to attain some intellectual insight into her behavior. With guidance she began to appraise her own abilities and became more open in expressing feelings.

She feared intimate personal involvement and could not tolerate physical closeness. The nurse incorporated this into nursing actions by initially minimizing confrontation, setting limits on anxiety-producing topics, and arranging the office seating to allow the patient to select her proximity to the nurse.

As they discussed the patient's relationships, the nurse confronted her with the dependent role Ms. G played and the unrealistic expectations she placed on others in the exclusiveness and amount of time she demanded from them. Her pattern of relating was also manipulative in that she elicited a sympathetic response and then used it to meet her own needs. She had great difficulty with mutuality and autonomy in relating to others. She was inexperienced in heterosexual relationships and missed many of the normal adolescent growth experiences in this area. Finally, she had much emotion and fear vested in her family of

Continued

CASE STUDY—cont'd

origin. The only trusting relationship Ms. G could recall was with her stepsister-mother. When this stepsister abruptly left home to marry, Ms. G perceived this as a personal rejection. She had since isolated herself from her family and continued to blame herself for her rejection by others, thus lowering her self-esteem and ability to trust others.

At the end of 2 months Ms. G was being considered for a promotion at work to hostess but, on the basis of an evaluation by her best friend and supervisor, was rejected for it. This precipitated a suicide attempt, which Ms. G revealed at her next regular session. At this point the issue of trust within the relationship became critical, as well as her inability to express anger because she feared rejection. The nurse now began more actively confronting Ms. G in her areas of ambivalence and inconsistency, setting limits on her self-destructive behavior, and suggesting alternatives. Ms. G then revealed that her relationship with her friend-supervisor was also a sexual one, and she expressed fears of homosexuality and loss of identity.

In later sessions Ms. G's relationship with this friend became a critical therapeutic issue because it reflected many of her conflicts. The therapy process presented a threat to the unhealthy parts of this relationship, and during the course of therapy Ms. G decided she needed to choose between maladaptive behaviors and more growth-producing options.

The nurse-patient relationship had now moved into the working phase, where focus was placed on specifics, and problem-solving activities began. After 3 months the nursing diagnoses were reevaluated to include the following:

1. Risk for self-directed violence related to perceived rejection by friend, as evidenced by suicide attempt
2. Disturbed personal identity related to childhood rejection and unrealistic self-ideals, as evidenced by self-statements
3. Social isolation related to inability to trust, lack of socialization skills, and feelings of inadequacy, as evidenced by relationship patterns
4. Powerlessness related to fear of rejection by others, as evidenced by perceived lack of control over life events
5. Ineffective role performance related to job dissatisfaction with working hours and nature of the work, as evidenced by feeling unsuccessful in her job

At this time the nurse sought consultation as she further evolved her plan of care. Neither medication nor hospitalization was indicated. These formulations were shared with Ms. G, who contracted for safety with the nurse, and together they collaborated about her future progress. They agreed to focus on changing Ms. G's maladaptive behavior by exploring past events and conflicts and helping her learn more productive patterns of living. Ms. G was now ready to commit herself to the work of therapy and interpersonal change, and she began to assume increased responsibility for this therapeutic work.

Because her self-ideal was unrealistically high, specific short-term goals became essential. The nurse's theoretical orientation incorporated the dynamics of Sullivan's and Peplau's interpersonal theories, Beck's cognitive framework, and Glasser's reality therapy. The relationship was focused on through the use of immediacy and became a model for examining many of her conflicts. This proved to be an excellent learning opportunity as Ms. G and the nurse dealt with resistance, transference, and countertransference reactions. During the next couple of months Ms. G made much progress, including the following changes:

1. She moved into an apartment with another girlfriend.
2. She left her previous job and resumed working in an office, where she received more personal satisfaction and a work schedule that allowed her to increase her social activities.
3. She began a diet regimen.
4. She participated in additional activities, such as a dancing class and a health spa.
5. She learned to verbalize her anger more freely with the nurse, friends, and others at work. This included discussing the many relationships in her past that were terminated without her agreement and in which she had internalized her anger.
6. She contacted her stepsister-mother and visited her. This was an important therapeutic goal because it allowed her to review her early experiences and provided her with actual feedback from those involved. Consequently, many of her misperceptions became evident and open to exploration in therapy.
7. She was able to admit her ambivalent feeling about her friend-supervisor and discuss the negative aspects of the relationship.
8. She stopped further sexual contact with the friend-supervisor because she felt exploited. Over time, the nature of this relationship changed, and it eventually became a casual acquaintance.
9. She learned about the variety of sexual feelings and responses and saw her needs in this area as appropriate developmental tasks. She became open to evaluating both heterosexual and homosexual expressions of her own sexual feelings.
10. Her perception of personal space changed, and her tolerance for physical closeness increased.
11. She developed new male and female friends and socialized frequently with them.

Evaluation

The terminating phase of the relationship began after about 6 months. At that time Ms. G was independently solving problems and, in therapy, the nurse primarily validated and supported her thinking. She was now receiving and accepting much positive feedback from others, had lost 15 kg (40 pounds), was

CASE STUDY—cont'd

continuing to diet, was planning future career goals, and had achieved more satisfactory interpersonal relationships with both men and women. The mutual goals for therapy had been met.

Terminating was difficult because of the close, trusting bond that had developed between them. The nurse had feelings of pleasure in Ms. G's growth, as well as personal satisfaction in her effectiveness as therapist. Ms. G openly described her feel- *ings about terminating and raised the question of a possible social relationship between them. Over the course of the sessions she came to realize that the premise of the relationship was therapy and changing individual perceptions or patterns of relating would not be feasible or desirable. Most important, she had control over terminating this relationship and the opportunity to work it through in a positive way.*

CHAPTER FOCUS POINTS

- The goal of psychiatric nursing care is to maximize the patient's positive interactions with the environment, promote a level of wellness, and enhance self-actualization.
- The Standards of Care describe what the psychiatric nurse does. The Standards of Professional Performance describe the context in which the psychiatric nurse performs these activities.
- In the assessment phase, information is obtained from the patient in a direct and structured manner through observations, interviews, and examinations. Patient data collected at this time relate to all of the components of the Stuart Stress Adaptation Model used in this textbook: predisposing factors, precipitating stressors, appraisal of stressor, coping resources, coping mechanisms, and coping responses.
- The subject of nursing diagnoses is the patient's behavioral response to stress. This response may lie anywhere on the coping continuum from adaptive to maladaptive.
- Mutually clarifying goals and identifying expected outcomes is an essential step in the therapeutic process.
- The nursing care plan applies theory and research from nursing and related biological, behavioral, and social sciences to the unique responses of the individual patient.
- In implementing psychotherapeutic interventions, the nurse helps the psychiatric patient do two things: develop insight and change behavior. It is important for psychiatric nurses to determine the patient's stage of treatment and then implement nursing activities that target the treatment goal in the most cost-effective and efficient manner.
- Key words for the evaluation phase of the nursing process are mutual, competent, accessible, effective, appropriate, efficient, and flexible. Evaluation is a continuous, active process that begins early in the relationship and continues throughout.

- The Standards of Professional Performance apply to self-definition, self-regulation, accountability, and autonomy for practice by psychiatric nurses, both individually and as a group.
- Psychiatric nurses actively participate in the formal organizational evaluation of overall patterns of care through a variety of quality improvement or process improvement activities.
- Performance appraisal for the psychiatric nurse is generally provided in two ways: administrative and clinical. Administrative performance appraisal involves the review, management, and regulation of competent psychiatric nursing practice. Clinical performance appraisal is guidance provided through a mentoring relationship and clinical supervision by a more experienced, skilled, and educated nurse.
- Psychiatric nurses are expected to engage in a continuous learning process to keep up with rapidly emerging knowledge in the field.
- Collegiality requires that nurses view their nurse peers as collaborators in the caregiving process who are valued and respected for their unique contributions, regardless of educational, experiential, or specialty background.
- Ethical considerations combine with legal and therapeutic issues to affect all aspects of psychiatric nursing practice.
- Collaboration is the shared planning, decision making, problem solving, goal setting, and assumption of responsibilities by individuals who work together cooperatively and with open communication.
- Clinical problems are numerous, and as nurses gain the skills and experience to validate their work scientifically, they can make a significant contribution to psychiatric theory and practice through research.
- Nurses need to assume an active role in questioning, advising, and advocating for the most cost-effective use of resources.

KEY TERMS

accountability, 192
autonomy, 192
clinical supervision, 195
collaboration, 198

collegiality, 196
interdisciplinary, 198
medical diagnosis, 186
multidisciplinary, 198

nursing diagnosis, 186
nursing process, 183
unidisciplinary, 198

CHAPTER REVIEW QUESTIONS

1. Match each of the phases of the nursing process identified in Column A with the appropriate nursing behavior in Column B.

Column A

_____ Data collection
_____ Evaluation
_____ Implementation
_____ Nursing
_____ Outcome
_____ Planning

Column B

A. Comparing responses and expected outcome, making modifications as needed
B. Considering available resources, generating alternatives, and coordinating with other team members
C. Establishing a contract and collecting, validating, and organizing data
D. Hypothesizing and validating goals with the patient diagnosis
E. Identifying patterns, analyzing, and synthesizing data identification
F. Prioritizing goals and identifying nursing activities

2. Fill in the blanks.

Well-written outcome criteria or goals are:

A. _____ rather than general.

B. _____ rather than subjective.

C. _____ rather than unrealistic.

D. _____ rather than outdated.

E. _____ rather than too few or too many.

F. _____ rather than one-sided.

G. The three advanced practice interventions for psychiatric

nurses are _____, _____,

and _____.

H. The four stages of psychiatric treatment are

_____, _____,

_____, and _____.

I. In implementing psychotherapeutic interventions, the nurse

helps the patient do two things: _____

and _____.

J. The _____ is the ideal source of validation of data.

K. It is important to explore with the patient the

_____ versus the _____

of all identified goals.

L. _____ focuses responsibility on the individual nurse for personal and professional actions.

M. The condition that allows for definition and control of a work domain and that implies self-determination, independence,

and shared power is _____.

N. The _____ is technology that allows nurses access to information from around the globe using a computer.

O. An _____ team is one in which members of different disciplines are involved in a formal arrangement to provide patient services while maximizing educational exchange.

3. Provide short answers for the following questions.

A. Why is it important for the psychiatric nurse to be knowledgeable about *DSM-IV-TR* diagnoses?

B. Discuss the special problems that can arise in establishing mutual goals when caring for psychiatric patients. How would you deal with them?

C. Discuss the differences between clinical supervision and therapy.

D. Do you think that the use of computers in health care dehumanizes it? Explain your position.

Visit Evolve for additional resources related to the content of this chapter.
http://evolve.elsevier.com/Stuart/principles/
• Topical Course Outline • Student Workbook Exercises • Critical Thinking Questions and Activities • Case Studies • Research Topics
• Monthly Content Updates • WebLinks

Student Study CD-ROM

Access the accompanying CD-ROM for animations, interactive exercises, review questions for the NCLEX examination, and an audio glossary.

REFERENCES

Akhavain P et al: Collaborative practice: a nursing perspective of the psychiatric interdisciplinary treatment team, *Holist Nurs Pract* 13:1, 1999.

American Nurses Association: *Code for nurses with interpretive statements*, Washington, DC, 2001, The Association.

American Nurses Association: *Scope and standards of psychiatric–mental health clinical nursing practice*, Washington, DC, 2000, The Association.

American Psychiatric Association: *Diagnostic and statistical manual of mental disorders*, ed 4, text revision, Washington, DC, 2000, American Psychiatric Association.

Aquilino ML, Keenan G: Having our say: nursing's standardized nomenclature, *Am J Nurs* 100:33, 2000.

Baier M, Murray RL, McSweeney M: Conceptualization and measurement of insight, *Arch Psychiatr Nurs* 12:32, 1998.

Daly BJ: Moving forward: a new code of ethics, *Nurs Outlook* 50:97, 2002.

DeMarco RF, Horowitz JA, McLeod D: A call to intraprofessional alliances, *Nurs Outlook* 48:172, 2000.

Dochterman JM, Bulechek GM: *Nursing interventions classifications (NIC)*, ed 4, St Louis, 2004, Mosby.

Laskowski C: The mental health clinical nurse specialist and the "difficult" patient: evolving meaning, *Issues Ment Health Nurs* 22:5, 2001.

Lindeke LL, Block DE: Maintaining professional integrity in the midst of interdisciplinary collaboration, *Nurs Outlook* 46:213, 1998.

Lyth GM: Clinical supervision: a concept analysis, *J Adv Nurs* 31:722, 2000.

Malach-Pines A: Nurses' burnout: an existential psychodynamic perspective, *J Psychosoc Nurs Ment Health Serv* 38:23, 2000.

Moorhead S, Johnson M, Maas ML: *Nursing outcomes classification (NOC)*, ed 3, St Louis, 2004, Mosby.

North American Nursing Diagnosis Association (NANDA): *Nursing diagnoses: definitions and classification 2003-2004*, Philadelphia, 2003, The Association.

Robinson JR, Clements K, Land C: Workplace stress among psychiatric nurses: prevalence, distribution, correlates, and predictors, *J Psychosoc Nurs Ment Health Serv* 41:32, 2003.

Stuart GW et al: Role utilization of nurses in public psychiatry, *Adm Policy Ment Health* 27(6):423, 2000.

Whittemore R, Grey M: The systematic development of nursing interventions, *J Nurs Scholarsh* 34:115, 2002.

World Health Organization (WHO): *International classification of diseases and related health problems*, ed 10, Geneva, 1992, The Organization.

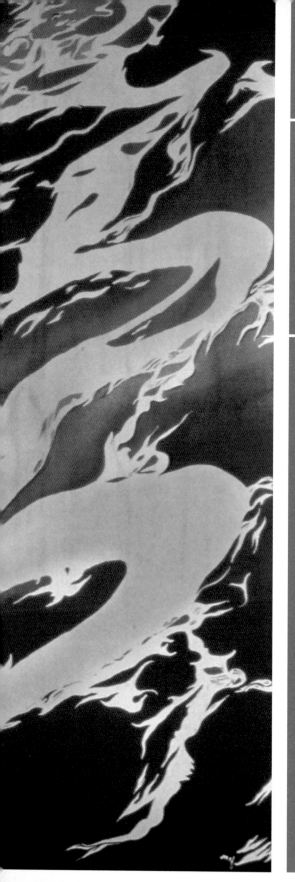

Unit Two

Curling River
144″ × 45″ batik on silk 1988

Artist's Note: When I was a vulnerable young mother, I made this batik of a river. Feeling the stress of living, this work is how I creatively moved through that period. It feels like a flaming dragon, but the calm misty blue river was where I strived to exist.

Continuum of Care

Continuum. What an interesting word. It means "a series of variations, or a sequence of things in regular order." As such, it is the perfect descriptor of the levels of contemporary psychiatric treatment. The continuum of psychiatric care allows nurses to use the full range of their skills and talents, often in new settings and innovative programs. Perhaps best of all, it provides patients, families, and communities with the healing ability to build competence, resilience, and health rather than merely to treat disability, illness, and disease. It therefore includes working with patients in crisis, acute, maintenance, and health promotion stages of treatment. Such is the brave new world of psychiatric and mental health nursing.

In this unit you will learn about intervening with primary, secondary, and tertiary prevention activities. All nurses, regardless of their specialty area, need to know how to promote mental health, intervene with patients and families in crisis, and build rehabilitative functioning in those who are ill. In the future you will use these skills more often than you might ever have imagined, and you will think back to this unit and the information it imparted with greater appreciation for the caregiving continuum.

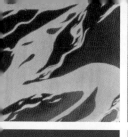

What is this thing called health? Simply a state in which the individual happens transiently to be perfectly adapted to his environment. Obviously, such states cannot be common, for the environment is in constant flux.

H. L. MENCKEN, *THE AMERICAN MERCURY*, MARCH 1930

13 MENTAL HEALTH PROMOTION AND ILLNESS PREVENTION

Gail W. Stuart

LEARNING OBJECTIVES

After studying this chapter, the student should be able to:
1. Define primary, secondary, and tertiary prevention (I).
2. Compare and contrast the public health, medical, and nursing models of primary prevention (I).
3. Assess the vulnerability of various groups to developing maladaptive coping responses (II).
4. Analyze the levels of intervention and activities related to the following primary prevention nursing interventions: health education, environmental change, social support, and stigma reduction (III).
5. Assess the importance of evaluation of the nursing process when applied to primary prevention (IV).

TOPICAL OUTLINE

I. Models of Primary Prevention
   A. Public Health Prevention Model
   B. Medical Prevention Model
   C. Nursing Prevention Model
II. Assessment
   A. Risk Factors and Protective Factors
   B. Target Populations
III. Planning and Implementation
   A. Health Education
   B. Environmental Change
   C. Social Support
   D. Stigma Reduction
IV. Evaluation

 Visit Evolve for additional resources related to the content of this chapter.
http://evolve.elsevier.com/Stuart/principles/

Mental health promotion and mental illness prevention are important parts of psychiatric care. The mere absence of mental illness does not mean that one has positive mental health or high quality of life. In the objectives of *Healthy People 2010* (USDHHS, 2000), mental health is defined in a positive way:

> Mental health is sometimes thought of as simply the absence of a mental illness but it is actually much broader. Mental health is a state of successful mental functioning, resulting in productive activities, fulfilling relationships, and the ability to adapt to change and cope with adversity. Mental health is indispensable to personal well-being, family and interpersonal relationships and one's contribution to society (p. 37).

So important is mental health that in the report of the New Freedom Commission on Mental Health, *Achieving the Promise: Transforming Mental Health Care in America,* (2003), the first goal and two recommendations were focused on it:

Goal 1: Americans understand that mental health is essential to overall health.

Recommendations: (1) Advance and implement a national campaign to reduce the stigma of seeking care and a national strategy for suicide prevention and (2) address mental health with the same urgency as physical health.

Thus a focus on mental health and mental illness prevention is long overdue.

■ MODELS OF PRIMARY PREVENTION

Primary prevention is often described with such slogans as "An ounce of prevention is worth a pound of cure" or "Curing is costly; prevention is priceless." However, the major emphasis in the United States has been on secondary prevention activities or the treatment of mental disorders. Only recently is primary prevention emerging as a substantial force in the mental health movement (Magyary, 2002; Papworth and Milne, 2001).

One of the reasons primary prevention is gaining momentum is because the health care system is beginning to provide some economic incentive for preventing illness rather than treating it. Another reason is that it has been found that good mental health improves the quality of life for people with serious physical illnesses and may contribute to longer life in general (NFCMH, 2003).

The idea of promoting mental health in general is attractive. Promotion sounds optimistic and positive. It is consistent with the idea of self-help and being self-responsible for health. It implies changing human behavior and draws on a holistic approach to health. Also, the ability to prevent the development of a psychiatric illness would be beneficial to individuals, families, communities, and society. Thus primary prevention activities in psychiatric care have two basic aims:

- **To help people avoid stressors or cope with them more adaptively**

- To change the resources, policies, or agents of the environment so that they no longer cause stress but rather enhance people's functioning

The terms **health promotion** *and* **illness prevention** *are often used interchangeably. In what ways do they overlap and how are they different?* ■

Health promotion and illness prevention activities are derived from a public health model of care. This model is intrinsic to nursing but distinct from the medical model. The differences emerge when comparing these two models.

Public Health Prevention Model

In the public health model, the "patient" is the **community** rather than the individual, and the focus is on the amount of mental health or illness in the community as a whole, including factors that promote or inhibit mental health. **The emphasis in this model is on reducing the risk of mental illness for an entire population by providing services to high-risk groups.** Use of the public health model requires that mental health professionals be familiar with such skills as community needs assessment, identifying and prioritizing target or high-risk groups, and intervening with treatment modalities such as consultation, education, and crisis intervention.

Do you believe it is possible to prevent mental illness in an individual or a community? ■

Community Needs Assessment. In the public health model services are developed and delivered based on a culturally sensitive assessment of community needs. Because it is not possible to interview each person in the community to determine mental health needs, four techniques are used to estimate service needs.

- **Social indicators** infer need for service from descriptive statistics found in public records and reports, especially statistics that are highly correlated with poor mental health outcomes. Examples of statistics most commonly used are income, race, marital status, population density, crime, and substance abuse.
- **Key informants** are people knowledgeable about the community's needs. Typical key informants are public officials, clergy, social service personnel, nurses, and primary care physicians.
- **Community forums** invite members of the community to a series of public meetings where they can express their ideas and beliefs about mental health needs in their community.
- **Epidemiological studies** examine the incidence and prevalence of mental disorders in a defined population. Incidence is the number of **new** cases of a disease or disorder in a population over a specified period of time. Prevalence is the number of **existing** cases of a disease or disorder in the total population at a specified point in time.

Identifying and Prioritizing High-Risk Groups. When the data from the various community needs assessments are analyzed, specific high-risk groups begin to emerge. For example, socioeconomic data might show that a large number of elderly widows live in the community. Community forums and surveys of key informants may find that there are few services and programs for the elderly, and epidemiological studies might suggest that elderly widows living alone are at high risk for depression. Therefore, elderly widows might become a target group for program development and intervention (Davis and Orb, 2001).

Demographic data also might show that a community has many preadolescent females, and socioeconomic indicators may suggest that many of these young women live in single-parent households and in poverty. Community forums and surveys of key informants may reveal few recreational and social services for children and adolescents. Finally, epidemiological studies may report high correlations among poverty, single-parent households, and adolescent pregnancy. Therefore community mental health providers might consider adolescents in this community to be at risk for mental health problems and target them for intervention.

Interventions. The public health model applies three levels of preventive intervention to mental illness and emotional disturbance (Caplan, 1964):

Primary prevention is lowering the incidence of a mental disorder by reducing the rate at which new cases of a disorder develop.

Secondary prevention involves decreasing the prevalence of a mental disorder by reducing the number of existing cases through early case finding, screening, and prompt effective treatment.

Tertiary prevention attempts to reduce the severity of a mental disorder and its associated disability through rehabilitative activities.

Each of these levels of intervention has implications for psychiatric nursing practice. **Primary prevention** is the focus of this chapter. **Secondary prevention** is addressed in Chapter 14, "Crisis Intervention." **Tertiary prevention** is described in Chapter 15, "Psychiatric Rehabilitation and Recovery."

Describe the characteristics of a group that was at high risk for developing mental illness in the community in which you grew up. ■

Medical Prevention Model

The medical prevention model focuses on biological and brain research to discover the specific causes of mental illness, with primary prevention activities focused on the prevention of illness in the **individual patient**. This model consists of the following steps:

1. Identify a **disease** that warrants the development of a preventive intervention program. Develop reliable methods for its **diagnosis** so that people can be divided into groups according to whether they do or do not have the disease.
2. By a series of epidemiological and laboratory studies, identify the most likely **cause** of the disease.

3. Launch and evaluate an experimental preventive intervention program based on the results of those studies.

This model has been effective for controlling a broad array of communicable diseases such as smallpox, typhus, malaria, diphtheria, tuberculosis, rubella, and polio and nutritional diseases such as scurvy, pellagra, rickets, kwashiorkor, and endemic goiter. It also has proved useful for preventing a variety of mental disorders caused by poisons, chemicals, licit or illicit drugs, electrolyte imbalances, and nutritional deficiencies. All of these diseases have one thing in common: a known necessary, but not always sufficient, causative factor.

Identify one psychiatric disorder that could be lessened or managed effectively by having the medical prevention model applied to it. ■

Nursing Prevention Model

The nursing prevention model stresses the importance of promoting mental health and preventing mental illness by focusing on risk factors, protective factors, vulnerability, and human responses. In the nursing prevention model, the "patient" may be an **individual, family, or community.** It is based on the understanding that mental disorders are multicausal in nature, requiring that mental illness prevention be thought of in a more behavioral way as the promotion of adaptive coping responses and the prevention of maladaptive responses to life stressors.

Stressors can include single-episode events, such as a divorce, or long-standing conditions, such as marital conflict. They can reflect either an acute health problem or a chronic health problem. For example, the following categories of maladaptive responses can arise from alcohol abuse:

- Acute health problems such as overdose or delirium tremens
- Chronic health problems such as cirrhosis of the liver
- Casualties, such as accidents on the road, in the home, or elsewhere, and suicide
- Violent crime and family abuse
- Problems of demeanor such as public drunkenness and use of alcohol by teenagers
- Default of major social roles (work or school and family roles)
- Problems of feeling state (demoralization and depression and experienced loss of control)

The nursing prevention model thus assumes that problems are multicausal, that everyone is vulnerable to stressful life events, and that any disability or problem may arise as a consequence. For example, four vulnerable people can face a stressful life event, such as the collapse of a marriage or the loss of a job. One person may become severely depressed, the second may be involved in an automobile accident, the third may head down the road to alcoholism, and the fourth may develop coronary artery disease.

The nursing prevention model does not search for a cause for each problem. Rather, it involves the following steps:

1. Identify a **stressor** that appears to result in a **maladaptive coping response** in a significant proportion of the population. Develop procedures for reliably identifying people who are **at risk** for the stressor and maladaptive response.
2. By epidemiological and laboratory methods, study the **consequences of that stressor** and develop hypotheses related to how its negative consequences might be reduced or eliminated.
3. Launch and evaluate an experimental preventive intervention program based on these hypotheses.

The nursing model also includes application of the nursing process, focusing on the primary prevention of maladaptive coping responses associated with an identified stressor. It thus incorporates the following aspects:

- **Assessment:** Identifying a stressor that precipitates maladaptive responses and a target or population group that is vulnerable or at risk for it
- **Planning:** Formulating specific prevention strategies and social institutions and situations through which the strategies may be applied
- **Implementation:** Applying selected nursing interventions aimed at decreasing maladaptive responses to the identified stressor and enhancing adaptation
- **Evaluation:** Determining the effectiveness of the nursing interventions with regard to short- and long-term outcomes, use of resources, and comparison with other prevention strategies

The nursing process can thus be used in a goal-directed way to decrease the incidence of mental illness and promote mental health.

Analyze the problem of child abuse from the nursing prevention perspective. ■

ASSESSMENT

Risk Factors and Protective Factors

The concepts of risk and protective factors are central to evidence-based prevention programs.

Risk factors are those predisposing characteristics that, if present for a person, make it more likely that he or she will develop a disorder. Some risk factors are fixed, such as gender and family history, whereas others can be changed, such as lack of social support and inability to read. Current research is focusing on the interplay between biological, psychosocial, and environmental risk factors and how they can be modified to eventually prevent a biological risk factor, such as the genes that may contribute to developing a mental illness, from being expressed (Dudley-Brown, 2002).

Protective factors are the coping resources and coping mechanisms that can improve a person's response to stress, resulting in adaptive behavior. These factors exist in the individual, family, and community. They can have a powerful effect on the influence of risk factors, and the potential for altering these factors is great.

Target Populations

Three types of preventive interventions based on target populations have been identified (Mrazek and Haggerty, 1994):

1. **Universal:** Targeted to the general population group without consideration of risk factors
2. **Selective:** Targeted to individuals or groups with a significantly higher risk of developing a particular disorder
3. **Indicated:** Targeted to high-risk individuals identified as having symptoms foreshadowing a specific mental disorder or biological markers indicating predisposition for the disorder

A knowledge of normal growth and development is essential for assessing a person's functioning and for being able to intervene with preventive nursing interventions. The nurse should be familiar with normative stages, tasks, and parameters; this will help the nurse understand what issues the person has faced in the past and what challenges lie ahead. In addition to understanding the person's development, the nurse must know about the family cycle because many nursing interventions are directed at the family, from mobilizing their support of a patient to modifying dysfunctional family patterns.

Assessment in primary prevention involves identifying individuals and groups of people who are vulnerable to developing mental disorders or who may display maladaptive coping responses to specific stressors or risk factors. To complete such an assessment, the nurse needs to draw on information generated from theory, research, and clinical practice.

It is also important for the nurse to realize that not all people in these groups are at equal risk. What these groups share is the experience of a life event, stressor, or risk factor that represents a loss of some kind or places an excessive demand on one's ability to cope. The more clearly the subgroup can be defined, the more specifically the prevention strategies can be researched, identified, and implemented.

Identify three groups of people vulnerable to the development of psychiatric illness, one based on biological factors, one based on psychological factors, and one based on sociocultural factors. ■

PLANNING AND IMPLEMENTATION

The Stuart Stress Adaptation Model presented in Chapter 4 is a useful tool for the nurse that can help in planning strategies for primary prevention. The overall nursing goal is to **promote constructive coping mechanisms and maximize adaptive coping responses.** Thus prevention strategies should be directed toward influencing predisposing factors, precipitating stressors, appraisal of stressors, coping resources, and coping mechanisms through the following interventions:

- Health education
- Environmental change
- Social support
- Stigma reduction

In each of these areas the nurse can focus on **decreasing risk factors or increasing protective factors.**

Furthermore, a single intervention can affect many parts of a person's life. For example, an environmental change, such as changing jobs, can affect an individual's predisposition to stress, decrease the amount of stress, change the appraisal of the threat, and perhaps increase financial or social coping resources. This interactive effect can thus justify the use of these prevention strategies for vulnerable groups.

Health Education

The health education strategy of primary prevention in mental health involves the strengthening of individuals and groups through competence building or resilience. It is based on the assumption that many maladaptive responses are the result of a lack of competence, that is, a lack of perceived control over one's own life and the lowered self-esteem that results.

Competence building is also referred to as resilience. The report of the New Freedom Commission on Mental Health, *Achieving the Promise: Transforming Mental Health Care in America,* (2003), offers a definition of resilience.

> Resilience means the personal and community qualities that enable us to rebound from adversity, trauma, tragedy, threats, or other stresses—and to go on with life with a sense of mastery, competence, and hope. We now understand from research that resilience is fostered by positive individual traits, such as optimism, good problem-solving skills, and treatments. Closely-knit communities and neighborhoods are also resilient, providing supports for their members (p. 5).

Thus competence building or resilience may be the single most important preventive strategy. A competent individual or community is aware of resources and alternatives, can make reasoned decisions about issues, and can cope adaptively with problems.

Self-Efficacy. Self-efficacy is a belief in one's personal capabilities. It is the notion that a person has control over the events in his or her life and that his or her actions will be effective. A high level of self-efficacy has been shown to positively affect one's thoughts, motivation, mood, and physical health (Bandura, 1997).

People with a low sense of efficacy tend to avoid difficult tasks. They have low aspirations and weak commitment to their goals. They turn inward on their self-doubts instead of thinking about how to perform successfully. When faced with stress, they dwell on obstacles and their personal deficiencies. They give up in the face of difficulty, recover slowly from setbacks, and easily fall victim to depression.

In contrast, people with high self-efficacy approach difficult tasks as challenges to be mastered rather than threats to be avoided. They are deeply interested in what they do, set high goals, and maintain strong commitments. This outlook sustains motivation, reduces stress, and lowers vulnerability to depression. Preventive interventions related to health education can equip people to take control of their lives and start a process of self-regulated change guided by a sense of resiliency and personal efficacy.

How is the concept of competency similar to the concept of positive mental health? ■

Types of Interventions. Health education related to competence building or increasing self-efficacy can include four types of interventions:

1. Increasing awareness of issues and events related to health and illness. Awareness of normal developmental tasks and potential problems is fundamental.
2. Increasing understanding of potential stressors, possible outcomes (both adaptive and maladaptive), and alternative coping responses.
3. Increasing knowledge of where and how to acquire the needed resources. Many health professionals assume that this is common knowledge, but for many people it is not.
4. Increasing the actual abilities of the individual or group. This means improving or maximizing coping skills such as problem solving, communication skills,

tolerance of stress and frustration, motivation, hope, anger management, and self-esteem.

Programs and Activities. Mental health education can take place in any setting, can have a formal or informal structure, can be directed toward individuals or groups, and can be related to predisposing factors or potential stressors (see Critical Thinking About Contemporary Issues). Health education activities identified by the Nursing Intervention Classification (NIC) system (Dochterman and Bulechek, 2004) are listed in Box 13-1.

Health education directed toward strengthening an individual's predisposition to stress can take various forms. Growth groups may be formed for parents that focus on parent-child relations, normal growth and development, or effective methods of child rearing (Gross and Grady, 2002). Groups of children or adolescents can discuss peer relationships, sexuality, or potential problem areas, such as drug abuse or promiscuity. Employee groups can discuss career burnout and related issues. A more activity-centered educational program also can be initiated, such as Outward Bound, which helps the individual discover that step-by-step competence can be expanded to master new, unexpected, and potentially stressful situations in an adaptive way.

Probably the most common type of health education program is one that helps the individual cope with a specific potential stressor (see Citing the Evidence). For example, families about to experience marital separation are vulnerable to emotional problems, physical complaints, and increased use of health care services. Such families may be offered educa-

---

Critical Thinking *About* Contemporary Issues

From Where Do Consumers Seek Health Information?

Questions still remain about how often consumers seek health information and where they go to obtain it. Contrary to the popular belief that Americans avidly seek health information, especially on the Internet, one study found that most Americans sought no information about a health concern (HSC, 2000-2001). And instead of surfing the Internet, the 38% of Americans who did obtain information relied more on traditional sources such as books, magazines, friends or relatives. People living with chronic conditions were more likely to seek information, yet more than half did not. Education was the key to explaining differences among people. Those with a college degree were twice as likely to seek health information as people without a high school diploma.

As consumers are confronted with more responsibility for making trade-offs among the cost, quality, and accessibility of care, credible and understandable information will need to be provided by nurses to empower consumers to take an active role in building competence, resilience, and self-efficacy.

Where Consumers Seek Health Information

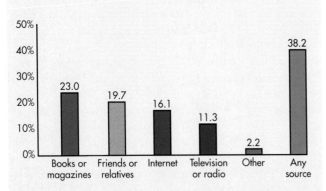

Note: Categories are not mutually exclusive; respondents could select multiple categories.
Source: HSC Community Tracking Study Household Survey, 2000–2001, Issue Brief, Health System Change 61:1, 2003.

CITING THE EVIDENCE ON
A Prevention Program for Married Women

BACKGROUND: The purpose of this study was to design an empirically-based, preventive intervention program for married women with school-age children. The daily hassles of 78 mostly white, middle-class, suburban, married women with children between 8 and 11 years old were explored.

RESULTS: The following hassles were reported in descending order of importance: not enough time; too many responsibilities; too many things to do; concerns about owing money; troubling thoughts about the future; concerns about weight; misplacing or losing things; health of a family member; overloaded with family responsibilities; and home maintenance. The results were then used to plan a three phase clinical intervention: hassle identification, hassle management, and integration of adaptive skills.

IMPLICATIONS: When conducting a prevention program, clinicians should first determine the specific stressor and coping responses of the at-risk population. This information can be used as the empirical foundation for directing the intervention. Behavioral rating scales should be incorporated into the program to assess its effectiveness.

McClowry S et al: *J Am Psychiatr Nurs Assoc* 6:107, 2000.

Health Education

Definition
Developing and providing instruction and learning experiences to facilitate voluntary adaptation of behavior conducive to health in individuals, families, groups, or communities

Activities
- Target high-risk groups and age ranges that would benefit most from health education.
- Target needs in *Healthy People 2000* or other local, state, and national needs.
- Identify internal or external factors that may enhance or reduce motivation for healthy behavior.
- Determine personal context and social-cultural history of individual, family, or community health behavior.
- Determine current health knowledge and lifestyle behaviors of individual, family, or target group.
- Assist individuals, families, and communities in clarifying health beliefs and values.
- Identify characteristics of target population that affect selection of learning strategies.
- Prioritize identified learner needs based on client preference, skills of nurse, resources available, and likelihood of successful goal attainment.
- Formulate objectives for health education program.
- Identify resources (e.g., personnel, space, equipment, money) needed to conduct program.
- Consider accessibility, consumer preference, and cost in program planning.
- Strategically place attractive advertising to capture attention of target audience.
- Avoid use of fear or scare techniques as strategy to motivate people to change health or lifestyle behaviors.
- Emphasize immediate or short-term positive health benefits to be received by positive lifestyle behaviors rather than long-term benefits or negative effects of noncompliance.
- Incorporate strategies to enhance the self-esteem of target audience.
- Develop educational materials written at a readability level appropriate to target audience.
- Teach strategies that can be used to resist unhealthy behavior or risk taking rather than give advice to avoid or change behavior.
- Keep presentation focused, short, and beginning and ending on main points.
- Use group presentations to provide support and lessen threat to learners experiencing similar problems or concerns as appropriate.
- Use peer leaders, teachers, and support groups in implementing programs to groups less likely to listen to health professionals or adults (e.g., adolescents) as appropriate.
- Use lectures to convey the maximum amount of information when appropriate.
- Use group discussions and role-playing to influence health benefits, attitudes, and values.
- Use demonstrations/return demonstrations, learner participation, and manipulation of materials when teaching psychomotor skills.
- Use computer-assisted instruction, television, interactive video, and other technologies to convey information.
- Use teleconferencing, telecommunications, and computer technologies for distance learning.
- Involve individuals, families, and groups in planning and implementing plans for lifestyle or health behavior modification.
- Determine family, peer, and community support for behavior conducive to health.
- Utilize social and family support systems to enhance effectiveness of lifestyle or health behavior modification.
- Emphasize importance of healthy patterns of eating, sleeping, exercising, and so on to individuals, families, and groups who model these values and behaviors to others, particularly children.
- Use variety of strategies and intervention points in educational program.
- Plan long-term follow-up to reinforce health behavior or lifestyle adaptations.
- Design and implement strategies to measure client outcomes at regular intervals during and after completion of program.
- Design and implement strategies to measure program and cost effectiveness of education, using these data to improve the effectiveness of subsequent programs.
- Influence development of policy that guarantees health education as an employee benefit.
- Encourage policy where insurance companies give consideration for premium reductions or benefits for healthful lifestyle practices.

From Dochterman JM, Bulechek GM: *Nursing interventions classifications (NIC)*, ed 4, St Louis, 2004, Mosby.

tional and supportive group intervention aimed at enhancing their ability to cope. Education groups can similarly be offered to those experiencing retirement, bereavement, or any other stress.

Parent education classes are a well-known example of anticipatory guidance that can be offered to high-risk groups. Although raising children is considered an important responsibility, relatively little attention has been directed to the belief that effective parenting is not an innate ability. Whether nurses subscribe to a specific set of beliefs and strategies for parenting or choose an eclectic approach, the opportunities for promoting mental health abound.

Possibly one of the most beneficial results of parent education is the acknowledgment that all parents become frustrated, angry, and ambivalent toward their children. Parent education goes beyond acknowledging feelings and includes learning and practicing alternative ways of interacting with children. During these classes, situations are anticipated, and discussions focus on identifying potential crisis situations and dealing with them through simulated encounters such as role playing. Education to promote mental health can thus address the needs of both children and parents as family roles shift and respond to societal change.

 Attend one of the self-help groups in your community. Describe the specific ways in which it promoted the mental health of those who attended. ■

Environmental Change

Activities in primary prevention involving environmental change have a social setting focus. They require the modification of an individual's or group's immediate environment or the modification of the larger social system. Such changes are particularly appropriate actions when the environment has become a source of new demands being made on the person, when it is not nurturing the person's developmental needs, and when it provides a diminished level of positive reinforcement.

Various environmental changes may promote mental health, including changes in **economic, work, housing,** or **family situations**. Economically, resources for financial aid or assistance in budgeting and money management may be obtained. Making changes in the work environment may be facilitated by vocational testing, guidance counseling, education, or retraining that can then result in a change in the work environment, even a completely different job. For an adolescent, a homemaker, or an older adult, this can entail starting a whole a new career. Changes in housing can involve moving to new quarters, which may mean leaving family and friends or returning to them, improvements in existing housing, or the addition or subtraction of coinhabitants, whether they are family, friends, or roommates. Environmental changes that may benefit the entire family include attaining child care facilities, enrolling in a nursery school, grade school, or camp, or gaining access to recreational, social, religious, or community facilities.

The potential benefit of all of these changes should not be minimized or overlooked by psychiatric nurses. They can promote mental health by increasing coping resources, modifying the nature of stressors, and increasing positive, rewarding, and self-enhancing experiences.

Organizations and Politics. Nurses also can effect environmental changes at a larger organizational and political level by influencing health care structures and procedures. Nurses might become involved in training community nonprofessional caregivers to increase the social supports available to vulnerable groups. Another approach would be to stimulate support for women's issues related to mental health, such as through studying the psychology of women; dispelling sex-role stereotypes; promoting feminist therapy; sponsoring programs, conferences, and workshops on women's issues; and recruiting more women into the mental health field.

Obviously, if nurses believe that their profession makes a valuable contribution to health promotion, they should document the cost-effectiveness and quality of nursing care, lobby for greater patient access by nurses, and seek adequate compensation and reimbursement for nursing services. Many of these goals can be obtained if nursing has greater participation in the decision-making structures of health care institutions, such as hospital boards, advisory groups, health system agencies, and legislative bodies.

Within organizations, environmental change can be achieved through program consultation. Such consultation with a large corporation, for example, may lead to the formulation of a preretirement counseling program or paternity leave for new fathers. Involvement in community planning and development can have an impact in many different areas. For instance, a community may be better able to meet the needs of the elderly in regard to educational opportunities, recreational programs, and access to social support networks by implementing telephone or transportation services. Also, the stress associated with environmental pollutants, such as chemicals and radiation, can be addressed at the community level.

Some environmental changes require involvement at the national level. For example, efforts to effect change may be directed toward modifying the media's portrayal of violence, enforcing laws on drunk driving, enacting gun control legislation, providing access to family planning services, and advocating changes in child-rearing practices, including the provision of day-care centers, flex time, and paternity leave by more businesses.

Of course, many aspects of the broader social system are in need of change, including racism, sexism, ageism, poverty, and inadequate housing and education. The dilemma is that global problems such as these are too broad, pervasive, and diffuse to be adequately addressed, let alone resolved. For any future prevention strategies to be successful, they will need to document three things: (1) the ways in which a particular group is vulnerable to a specific stressor, (2) how the proposed prevention program will be beneficial and cost-effective, and (3) to what degree the program can succeed.

 What legislation in your state is being considered that pertains to mental health care? What is your position on it and how can you influence its chances for passage? ■

Social Support

As a primary prevention strategy, supporting social systems means strengthening the social supports in place to enhance their protective factor and developing ways to buffer or cushion the effects of a potentially stressful event. Support system enhancement activities identified by the Nursing Intervention Classification (NIC) system (Dochterman and Bulechek, 2004) are listed in Box 13-2.

Social support systems can be helpful in emphasizing the strengths of individuals and families and in focusing on health rather than illness. This support is important for all levels of prevention—primary, secondary, and tertiary—and it influences all of the following:

- Encouraging health promotion behavior
- Helping people seek assistance earlier
- Improving the functioning of the immune system or other biological processes

BOX 13-2

Support System Enhancement

Definition
Facilitation of support to patient by family, friends, and community

Activities
- Assess psychological response to situation and availability of support system.
- Determine adequacy of existing social networks.
- Identify degree of family support.
- Identify degree of family financial support.
- Determine support systems currently used.
- Determine barriers to using support systems.
- Monitor current family situation.
- Encourage the patient to participate in social and community activities.
- Encourage relationships with persons who have common interests and goals.
- Refer to a self-help group as appropriate.
- Assess community resource adequacy to identify strengths and weaknesses.
- Refer to a community-based promotion/prevention/treatment/rehabilitation program as appropriate.
- Provide services in a caring and supportive manner.
- Involve family/significant others/friends in care and planning.
- Explain to concerned others how they can help.

From Dochterman JM, Bulechek GM: *Nursing interventions classifications (NIC)*, ed 4, St Louis, 2004, Mosby.

- Reducing the occurrence of potentially stressful events
- Fostering the ability to cope with stressful events
- Helping one to deal with chronic mental and physical illness

People with poor social support—whether it is defined by the number of social contacts, the satisfaction derived from them, or a combination of the two—have a higher risk of dying from all causes. The effects of isolation are even more dramatic in those with chronic illnesses. People with coronary artery disease who lack both a spouse and a confidant have a 50% death rate over a 5-year period. For those less isolated, the death rate is under 20% (Williams, 1999).

How can the goal of maximizing social support systems be achieved? First, the amount of social support needed by a high-risk group must be determined and compared with the amount of social support available. Although the question is straightforward, it is complicated by each element having many determinants.

The need for social support is influenced by predisposing factors, the nature of the stressors, and the availability of other coping resources such as economic assets, individual abilities and skills, and defensive techniques. The availability of social supports is also influenced by age, gender, socioeconomic status, the nature of the stressor, and the characteristics of the environment.

Acute episodic stressors tend to elicit more intense support, whereas support resources for chronic problems tend to fade away. Also, changes or stressors viewed in a positive way by the individual's social network, such as the birth of a baby or a promotion, may generate a great deal of support, whereas a negative event, such as a divorce, might stimulate little support. Finally, the quantity and type of social support that meets one need may not meet another.

Types of Interventions. Even though many variables related to social support need further study, social support can still be used to design and implement interventions in primary prevention. Four particular types of interventions are possible.

1. Social support patterns can be used to assess communities and neighborhoods to identify problem areas and high-risk groups. Not only will information about the quality of life be gained but also the social isolation of a particular group may become apparent, as may central individuals who can be enlisted to help develop community-based programs.

2. Links can be improved between community support systems and formal mental health services. Often mental health professionals are not aware of or comfortable with the existence or functioning of community support systems. They should be taught how to use and mobilize community resources and social support systems. All health care providers need to be able to recognize when patients are in need of social support and to provide them with access to appropriate community support systems.

3. Naturally existing caregiving networks can be strengthened. Health professionals can provide information and support to informal caregivers in the community, who serve a very important and somewhat different function than more formalized and organized support systems. Informal support systems provide:
   a. A natural training ground for the development of problem-solving skills
   b. A medium in which people grow and develop by learning to direct the process of change for themselves
   c. A supportive milieu that capitalizes on the strength of existing ties among people in communities, rather than fragmenting intact social units on the basis of diagnosed needs or specialized services.

4. Individuals and groups can be helped to develop, maintain, expand, and use their social networks. For example, network therapy involves bringing together all the important members of the family's kin and friendship network. The focus is then on tightening bonds within the network and breaking dysfunctional patterns. For families who are isolated and whose networks are depleted, too few network members may not be available for such a strategy to be feasible. In this case, arranging for the use of mutual support groups may be effective.

BOX **13-3**

Characteristics of Self-Help Groups

- Supportive and educational in nature rather than therapeutic
- Based on shared experiences and the premise that the individual is not alone
- Focused on a single life-disrupting event
- Purpose is to support personal responsibility and change
- Anonymous and confidential in nature
- Voluntary membership
- Members lead the group and implement principles of self-governance
- Nonprofit orientation

BOX **13-4**

Assessment Guidelines for Recommending Self-Help Groups

Questions for the Group
What is its purpose?
Who are the group members and leaders?
What are the beneficial aspects of the group?
For whom would the group not be suitable?
What problems are inherent in the group?
Is the group effective in preventing further emotional distress?

Questions for the Potential Member
How does the person feel about attending a self-help group?
How compatible is the group with the individual's approach to the problem?
How accessible is the group to the potential member?

Informal Support Groups. There are many informal support groups. They may include church groups, civic organizations, clubs, women's groups, or work and neighborhood support groups. Self-help groups are becoming more common as members organize themselves to solve their own problems. The members all share a common experience, work together toward a common goal, and use their strengths to gain control over their lives. Such groups are also forming on the Internet (Bacon, Condon, and Fernsler, 2000).

The processes involved in self-help groups are social affiliation, learning self-control, modeling methods to cope with stress, and acting to change the social environment. Characteristics of self-help groups are listed in Box 13-3.

Self-help groups such as Alcoholics Anonymous, Weight Watchers, Parents Without Partners, Recovery, and Parents Anonymous are familiar to the public. They have shown their ability to promote adaptive responses among people experiencing stress, such as the grief reactions of widows and of parents of children who died of sudden infant death syndrome.

Because self-help groups use a variety of stress coping methods and have differing membership criteria, each group should be assessed individually for its general effectiveness and appropriateness for particular individuals and families. Some areas for the nurse to assess before recommending involvement in a self-help group are presented in Box 13-4.

Working with naturally occurring, informal support systems should be done cautiously, however, to minimize undesirable consequences. The nurse should attempt to create the least amount of disruption possible and not suppress the natural repertoire of helping behaviors of informal caregivers.

Finally, although supporting social supports is an effective intervention, it is not limited to primary prevention activities. Rather, all nurses in all settings can use this strategy as a way of providing holistic care to maximize the health of individuals, families, and groups.

Stigma Reduction

An important aspect of mental health promotion involves activities related to dispelling myths and stereotypes associated with vulnerable groups, providing knowledge of normal parameters, increasing sensitivity to psychosocial factors affecting health and illness, and enhancing the ability to give sensitive, supportive, and humanistic health care.

Stigma is defined as a mark of disgrace or discredit that is used to identify and separate out people whom society sees as deviant, sinful, or dangerous. Misperceptions about vulnerable subgroups of the population must be corrected. In the report of the New Freedom Commission on Mental Health, *Achieving the Promise: Transforming Mental Health Care in America*, (2003), stigma is defined as "a cluster of negative attitudes and beliefs that motivate the general public to fear, reject, avoid, and discriminate against people with mental illness" (p. 4).

For the psychiatrically ill, stigma is a barrier that separates them from society and keeps them apart from others (Box 13-5). They are the result, in part, of the cultural stigma against mental illness that is prevalent in contemporary society.

The impact of this stigma is enormous. Nearly two thirds of people with diagnosable mental disorders do not seek treatment, and stigma related to mental illness is one of the major barriers that discourages people from seeking needed care. Another sign of stigma is evident in the public's reluctance to pay for mental health services and to provide the same coverage for physical and mental health care.

Patients and their families often report that the diagnosis of a mental illness is followed by increasing isolation and loneliness as family and friends withdraw (see Chapter 11). Patients feel rejected and feared by others, and their families are met by blame. Stigma against mental illness is a reflection of the cultural biases of contemporary society that are shared by consumers and health care providers alike (Box 13-6).

The stigma, misunderstanding, and fear surrounding mental illness are related to both the agencies providing mental health services and the people receiving these services, who are often elderly, poor, or members of social minority groups.

The Roots of Stigma

Stigma is ignorance. Stigma is fear. Stigma is guilt. Stigma is discrimination. Why is something so obviously wrong still so prevalent?

The roots of stigma in our society are stubborn, reaching back to the beginnings of human history. Anyone whose behavior was different was considered dangerous, and so those with mental diseases often became outcasts. With virtually no scientific data to enlighten people, ignorance of mental illness predominated for millennia. Medieval Christianity, for example, moralized about mental illness as an issue of good and evil. A person suffering from profound depression, for example, was assumed to be possessed by the devil and therefore in need of exorcism.

Fast forward to the twenty-first century. Though religious traditions endure through millennia, in our day, it's the police blotter that so often links mental illness to the evil of violence and other threatening behaviors. Reporters write stories from police reports often without real insights into mental illness. Thus we see the resultant newspaper accounts with headlines like:

"Schizo Son Smothers his Mom in Queens" (*New York Post*, 10/29/02).

The news media will always report on the sensational cases far out of proportion to the actual occurrences. The Andrea Yates story, serial murderers, random subway pushers, and the like get lots of ink compared to the millions of mental illness recovery stories that are not considered newsworthy.

Then we're exposed to TV shows and movies that entertain us by often linking mental illness to malevolence. Baby Jane, Norman Bates, and Hannibal Lecter are cultural icons. Cop shows on TV strive for realism, and yet they too can create distortions when their writers are inevitably influenced by newspaper stories generated by the police blotter.

What's the result of our society's steady diet of mass media fed by such cultural and religious beliefs, most of which associate mental illnesses with profound negativity? In a word, stigma.

From *Reintegration today*, Winter 2002, The Center for Reintegration.

Unlike physical illness, which tends to evoke sympathy and the desire to help, mental disorders tend to disturb and repel people.

Yet stigma must be overcome. Reducing stigma must involve programs of public advocacy, public education on mental health issues, and contact with persons with mental illness through schools and other social institutions. Another way to reduce stigma is to find causes and effective treatments for mental disorders (USDHHS, 1999; Jorm, 2000; NFCMH, 2003).

Finally, it must be understood that everyone encounters stress, and that all people are subject to maladaptive coping responses. Mental health professionals can educate the public and teach them that mental health is a continuum and mental illness is caused by a complex combination of factors. The public needs to realize that mental disorders are not the result of moral failings or limited will power, but rather they are legitimate medical illnesses that respond to specific treatments. Consumers need to understand that no one is immune to mental illness or emotional problems and that the fear, anxiety, and even anger we feel about people who suffer these problems may reflect some of our own deepest fears and anxieties.

Have you observed the stigma associated with psychiatric illness in your personal or professional life? If so, what steps have you taken or could you take to overcome it? ■

EVALUATION

When talking about primary prevention, there is a tendency to think in terms of the total elimination of mental illness and stress. Yet these are not realistic goals, and maintaining them can only discourage any possible action. Perhaps it is

Anti-Stigma: Do You Know the Facts?

- Do you know that an estimated 50 million Americans experience a mental disorder in any given year?
- Do you know that stigma is about disrespect and the use of negative labels to identify a person living with a mental illness?
- Do you know that many people would rather tell employers that they have committed a petty crime and were in jail than admit to being in a psychiatric hospital?
- Do you know that stigma results in inadequate insurance coverage for mental health services?
- Do you know that stigma results in fear, mistrust, and violence against people living with mental illness?
- Do you know that stigma results in families and friends turning their backs on people with mental illness?
- Do you know that stigma keeps people from getting needed mental health services?

From SAMHSA's Center for Mental Health Services, 1999, US Government Printing Office.

possible to set goals of reducing suffering and enhancing the capacity to cope, but even these may be unattainable, given that the environment is constantly changing and adaptation is an ongoing challenge. Rather, if the focus is directed toward specific problems of a vulnerable group in society, nursing activity becomes more concentrated and the chance of success increases.

Clearly a need exists for the evaluation of programs in primary prevention. In a world of shrinking resources, only programs with proven effectiveness are likely to be supported in the future. It must be demonstrated that the prevention strategy used has both short-term and long-term effects that will benefit the individual and society. Also, it is necessary to determine whether the specific strategy implemented was the most effective, appropriate, and efficient. Considering alternative approaches and comparing clinical and financial outcomes are essential aspects of the evaluation process.

Although preventing all illness is not possible, preventing some particular problems is. But a number of barriers exist that make expansion of primary prevention activities difficult. When faced with a choice, the needs of the ill consistently take precedence over promoting prevention. This holds true for nurses providing care as well as for the larger society. Yet by being more visionary, both groups could benefit greatly.

COMPETENT CARING

A Clinical Exemplar of a Psychiatric Nurse
PENELOPE CHASE, MSN, MEd, RN, CS

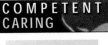

I was changing planes, having just left an inspiring psychiatric clinical nurse specialist conference in Florida, and was on my way to Boston to attend the reunion of my diploma nursing school. I was traveling alone and feeling safe from social interruptions. I was looking forward to some anonymity and a time to reflect and rest.

As I approached the check-in counter of the airport, I saw a young woman sitting nearby in the waiting area. The seats on either side of her were empty except for a soft knapsack on her left. She was wearing the loose-fitting cotton clothing and the nylon-strap sandals that college students often wear. She looked as if she were about to burst into tears or change her mind about being here and dash for the exit. I stopped in my tracks to observe her without being aware of deciding to do so. She turned her head with stiff, slightly jerky movements.

"Responding to internal stimuli," "seizure disorder," "hasn't taken her psychotropic medication" went through my professional mind, while "don't get involved" went through my personal mind, along with, "You're on vacation. Don't mess it up. Relax, you're not the only one who can help." So I went ahead and checked in. I chose to wait in a seat in the row behind the young woman. "She may not be able to ask for help. I should assess further," my professional self reasoned. "Maybe she's not alone. Maybe someone is traveling with her and will be back in a minute."

She compared her ticket information with the boarding announcement and sat back in her seat. A moment later, she shifted in her seat and put her hands over her face. It was then that I noticed that a man, somewhat older than she, seated two rows away and facing her was watching her intensely. My private self was afraid he might be a lonely traveler sizing up a vulnerable young woman that he could take advantage of. I intensified my vigil. I would be her advocate and protector.

I read a bit in my novel, keeping my peripheral vision and ears attuned in her direction. I had difficulty concentrating on my reading because I was constantly interrupted by imposing, opposing thoughts of "Do something" and "Let it be." At one point a uniformed airline employee passed near me on his way out the boarding door. I approached him and said, "I think there's a young lady in trouble here." "I'm a pilot," he replied. "The person you need to talk with is that gentleman at the counter." I wondered what I should do. If I were to say something, the young woman might be embarrassed, delayed, or asked to answer questions that might destroy whatever composure and dignity she was able to preserve. She had not indicated she needed any help . . . yet.

I was still deliberating when my flight was called. The young woman looked at her ticket, got up, and joined the line. I sat and waited until my row number was called. As the flight attendant checked the young woman's boarding pass, she looked carefully at the anguished face, then asked, "Are you okay?" The girl nodded. "Are you sure?" Another nod, but the flight attendant paused in her checking and turned briefly to watch as the girl began down the boarding ramp. It was then that I decided how to resolve my professional-helper's dilemma. I identified myself to the flight attendant as a psychiatric nurse and said that if there were an emergency, they could call on me. "Oh, you noticed her, too," the woman smiled. "Thank you."

I had just gotten settled in my seat when the flight attendant approached me. "I pulled her up in the computer. It's an emergency flight—a death in the family." "Oh," I ventured, the underlying cause of the scenario suddenly becoming clearer in my mind. "Loss and grief are one of my specialties. I'd be happy to sit with her if she'd like, but only if she says she'd like someone with her." I suddenly remembered traveling 450 miles, mostly alone, to my younger brother's funeral.

Within a few minutes the flight attendant returned saying, "She said she'd like that." So I took my purse and moved toward the back of the plane. As I approached her seat, the young woman looked up at me. I smiled, introduced myself by name, and said I was the person who would sit with her if that would be all right. She nodded assent, managed a wan smile, and said, "Thank you." I was trying to decide what my role would be. This was all happening rather quickly, yet somewhere in my gut or heart I knew it would be okay. I knew I wanted to stay in my role of a psychiatric nurse and a representative of my profession, and I was also aware that in a couple of hours our relationship would be ending. The time limit helped me focus on my goal of simply being available to her as a support.

Realizing that my seat partner was probably in the initial stage of shock in the grief process and thus lacked her usual coping skills, I decided to do a bit of framing for her. "The flight attendant told me you had a death in your family. I'm sorry," I said. "I'm a nurse who works with people who are going through losses. You could talk about it if you want to, or I could just sit here and read my book. It's up to you." I offered her two simple choices.

She sat silently, but with slightly changing facial expressions, and I thought she was getting ready to speak. I focused my attention softly on her and waited. "He wasn't supposed to die. He was going to have chemotherapy," she began. As her story unfolded, I listened, asked clarifying questions occasionally, and acknowledged her words and anguish. In between bits of content, I learned that she was being met by friends of the family and her sister at the airport with a subsequent 45-minute drive until she was in her

A Clinical Exemplar of a Psychiatric Nurse–cont'd
PENELOPE CHASE, MSN, MEd, RN, CS

hometown. At one point she said sadly, "Now he'll never see his grandchildren," and buried her head on my shoulder and sobbed for a little while. After a bit she said, "I think I need to sleep." That sounded like a good idea to me. As she slept, I evaluated what had unfolded and thought about where to go from here. I needed a plan for closure, for termination of the intervention.

I thought of how long she would have to stand in the aisle waiting to get off this big plane. I asked the flight attendant if there were some way the young woman could be one of the first passengers off the plane. We were moved to the first-class section near the door after she awoke. We talked briefly of how she wanted to depart. I let her know I was available to walk off the plane with her

if she wanted and that I thought she could manage "just fine" without me, as well. "I'll be all right," she said, giving me a hug as we stood up to disembark. "You don't know how much we appreciate this," the flight attendant said to me with sincere eye contact. I acknowledged her thanks. I motioned for my seat-mate to go ahead of me. As we approached the waiting area, I looked questioningly at her to see how she was managing. "I've got it," she said, and gave me the thumbs-up sign. I smiled and walked on. I was met by two classmates and felt clear, reflective, and exhilarated. I felt that my clinical skills had positively influenced the outcome. I felt I had acted in a professionally responsible and caring manner. I felt good about being a psychiatric nurse. ■

CHAPTER FOCUS POINTS

- Primary prevention activities in psychiatric care have two basic aims: (1) to help people avoid stressors or cope with them more adaptively and (2) to change the resources, policies, or agents of the environment so that they no longer cause stress but rather enhance people's functioning.
- In the public health model, the "patient" is the community rather than the individual; the focus is on the amount of mental health or illness in the community as a whole, including factors that promote or inhibit mental health; and emphasis is on reducing the risk of mental illness for an entire population by providing services to high-risk groups.
- Three levels of preventive intervention from the public health model include (1) primary prevention—the lowering of the incidence of a mental disorder or reducing the rate at which new cases of a disorder develop; (2) secondary prevention—decreasing the prevalence of a mental disorder by reducing the number of existing cases through early case finding, screening, and prompt effective treatment; and (3) tertiary prevention—reducing the severity of a mental disorder and associated disability through rehabilitative activities.
- The medical prevention model focuses on biological and brain research to discover the specific causes of mental illness, with primary prevention activities focused on the prevention of illness in the individual patient.
- The nursing prevention model stresses the importance of promoting mental health and preventing mental illness by focusing on risk factors, vulnerability, and human responses. In the nursing prevention model, the "patient" may be an individual, family, or community.
- Risk factors are those predisposing characteristics that, if present for a person, make it more likely that he or she will develop a disorder. Protective factors are the coping resources and coping mechanisms

that can improve a person's response to stress, resulting in adaptive behavior.
- Assessment in primary prevention involves identifying individuals and groups of people who are vulnerable to developing mental disorders or who may display maladaptive coping responses to specific stressors or risk factors.
- The overall goal of nursing care is to promote constructive coping mechanisms and maximize adaptive coping responses.
- The health education strategy of primary prevention in mental health involves the strengthening of individuals and groups through competence building or resilience. Preventive interventions related to health education can equip people to take control of their lives and start a process of self-regulated change guided by a sense of resiliency and personal efficacy.
- Various environmental changes may promote mental health, including changes in economic, work, housing, or family situations. Nurses also can effect environmental changes at a larger organizational and political level by influencing health care structures and procedures.
- Supporting social systems means strengthening the social supports in place to enhance their protective factor and developing ways to buffer or cushion the effects of a potentially stressful event.
- Mental health promotion includes activities related to reducing stigma by dispelling myths and stereotypes associated with vulnerable groups, providing knowledge of normal parameters, increasing sensitivity to psychosocial factors affecting health and illness, and enhancing the ability to give sensitive, supportive, and humanistic health care.
- It must be demonstrated that the prevention strategy used has both short-term and long-term effects that will benefit the individual and society. Also, it is necessary to determine whether the specific strategy implemented was the most effective, appropriate, and efficient.

KEY TERMS

incidence, 209
prevalence, 209
primary prevention, 209
protective factors, 210

resilience, 211
risk factors, 210
secondary prevention, 209
self-efficacy, 211

self-help groups, 216
stigma, 216
tertiary prevention, 209

CHAPTER REVIEW QUESTIONS

1. Match each term in Column A with its associated activity from Column B.

Column A

_____ Primary prevention

_____ Secondary prevention

_____ Tertiary prevention

Column B

A. Lowering incidence

B. Decreasing prevalence

C. Reducing severity

2. Fill in the blanks.

A. The two goals of primary prevention activities are to

_____ and _____.

B. The health education strategy of _____ is based on increasing perceived control over one's life, effective coping strategies, and self-esteem.

C. The model of prevention in which the "patient" is the community is called _____.

D. The term used to describe a mark of disgrace that separates out those people that society sees as deviant, sinful, or dangerous is called _____.

E. Becoming involved in health care organizations and political processes is a nursing intervention related to

_____.

F. Social support has important implications for

_____ levels of prevention.

3. Provide short answers for the following questions.

A. How do the medical and nursing prevention models differ?

B. Identify and describe three types of primary prevention interventions based on the assessment of targeted populations.

C. Describe the four aspects of health education and give an example of each.

D. Select one specific psychiatric disorder and research the impact of social support and stigma on its expression and resolution.

E. Relate one environmental change that would promote the mental health of people living in your community.

Visit Evolve for additional resources related to the content of this chapter.

http://evolve.elsevier.com/Stuart/principles/
• Topical Course Outline • Student Workbook Exercises • Critical Thinking Questions and Activities • Case Studies • Research Topics
• Monthly Content Updates • WebLinks

Student Study CD-ROM

Access the accompanying CD-ROM for animations, interactive exercises, review questions for the NCLEX examination, and an audio glossary.

REFERENCES

Bacon ES, Condon EH, Fernsler JI: Young widows' experience with an Internet self-help group, *J Psychosoc Nurs Ment Health Serv* 38:24, 2000.

Bandura A: *Self-efficacy: the exercise of control*, New York, 1997, Freeman.

Caplan G: *Principles of preventive psychiatry*, New York, 1964, Basic Books.

Davis PS, Orb A: The stratified-population-at-risk (SPAR) model for psychogeriatric nursing: a paradigm for the third millennium? *Arch Psychiatr Nurs* 15:62, 2001.

Dochterman JM, Bulechek GM: *Nursing interventions classifications (NIC)*, ed 4, St Louis, 2004, Mosby.

Dudley-Brown S: Prevention of psychological distress in persons with inflammatory bowel disease, *Issues Ment Health Nurs* 23:403, 2002.

Gross D, Grady J: Group-based parent training for preventing mental health disorders in children, *Issues Ment Health Nurs* 23:367, 2002.

Jorm AF: Mental health literacy: public knowledge and beliefs about mental disorders, *Br J Psychiatry* 177:396, 2000.

Magyary D: Positive mental health: a turn of the century perspective, *Issues Ment Health Nurs* 23:331, 2002.

Mrazek PJ, Haggerty RJ: *Reducing risks for mental disorders: frontiers for preventive intervention research*, Washington, DC, 1994, National Academy Press.

New Freedom Commission on Mental Health (NFCMH): *Achieving the promise: transforming mental health care in America, final report*, DHHS Pub. No. SMA-03-3832, Rockville, Md, 2003.

Papworth M, Milne D: Qualitative systematic review: an example from primary prevention in adult mental health, *J Community Appl Soc Psychol* 11:193, 2001.

US Department of Health and Human Services (USDHHS): *Mental health: a report of the surgeon general*, Rockville, Md, 1999, National Institute of Mental Health.

US Department of Health and Human Services (USDHHS): *Health People 2010*, Washington, DC, 2000, US Government Printing Office.

Williams R: Social ties and health, *Harvard Ment Health Lett* April 1999.

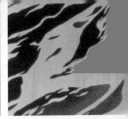

> *He knows not his own strength that hath not met adversity.*
>
> FRANCIS BACON, *OF FORTUNE*

CRISIS INTERVENTION 14

Sandra E. Benter

LEARNING OBJECTIVES

After studying this chapter, the student should be able to:

1. Describe a crisis and its characteristics, including crisis responses, types of crises, and crisis intervention (I).
2. Analyze aspects of the nursing assessment related to crisis responses (II).
3. Plan and implement nursing interventions for patients related to their crisis responses (III).
4. Develop a patient education plan to cope with crisis (III).
5. Evaluate nursing care for patients related to their crisis responses (IV).
6. Describe the settings in which crisis intervention may be practiced (V).
7. Discuss modalities of crisis intervention (VI).

TOPICAL OUTLINE

I. Crisis Characteristics
   A. Crisis Responses
   B. Types of Crises
   C. Crisis Intervention
II. Assessment
   A. Precipitating Event
   B. Perception of the Event
   C. Support Systems and Coping Resources
   D. Coping Mechanisms
III. Planning and Implementation
   A. Environmental Manipulation
   B. General Support
   C. Generic Approach
   D. Individual Approach
   E. Techniques
IV. Evaluation
V. Settings for Crisis Intervention
VI. Modalities of Crisis Intervention
   A. Mobile Crisis Programs
   B. Group Work
   C. Telephone Contacts
   D. Disaster Response
   E. Victim Outreach Programs
   F. Health Education

 Visit Evolve for additional resources related to the content of this chapter.
http://evolve.elsevier.com/Stuart/principles/

Stressful events, or crises, are a common part of life. They may be social, psychological, or biological in nature, and there is often little that a person can do to prevent them. As the largest group of health care providers, nurses are in an excellent position to help promote healthy outcomes for people in times of crisis.

Crisis intervention is a brief, focused, and time-limited treatment strategy that has been shown to be effective in helping people adaptively cope with stressful events. Knowledge of crisis intervention techniques is an important clinical skill of all nurses, regardless of clinical setting or practice specialty.

■ CRISIS CHARACTERISTICS

A crisis is a disturbance caused by a stressful event or a perceived threat. The person's usual way of coping becomes ineffective in dealing with the threat, causing anxiety. The threat, or precipitating event, usually can be identified. It may have occurred weeks or days before the crisis, and it may or may not be linked in the individual's mind to the crisis state he or she is experiencing. Precipitating events can be actual or perceived losses, threats of losses, or challenges.

Crisis Responses

After the precipitating event, the person's anxiety begins to rise, and four phases of a crisis response emerge. In the first phase, the anxiety activates the person's usual methods of coping. If these do not bring relief and support is inadequate, the person progresses to the second phase, which involves more anxiety because coping mechanisms have failed. In the third phase, new coping mechanisms are tried or the threat is redefined so that old ones can work. Resolution of the problem can occur in this phase. However, if resolution does not occur, the person goes on to the fourth phase, in which the continuation of severe or panic levels of anxiety may lead to psychological disorganization.

In describing the phases of a crisis, it is important to consider the balancing factors shown in Figure 14-1. These include the individual's **perception of the event, situational supports,** and **coping mechanisms.** Successful resolution of

the crisis is more likely if the person has a realistic view of the event, if situational supports are available to help solve the problem, and if effective coping mechanisms are present (Aguilera, 1998).

The phases of a crisis and the impact of balancing factors are similar to the components of the Stuart Stress Adaptation

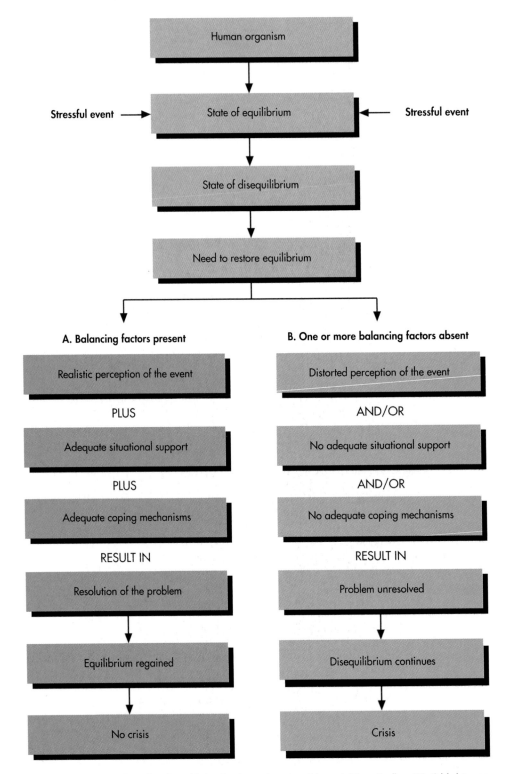

Figure 14-1 Paradigm: the effect of balancing factors in a stressful event. (From Aguilera DC: *Crisis intervention: theory and methodology,* ed 8, St Louis, 1998, Mosby.)

Model used in this textbook and described in Chapter 4. However, by definition, crises are self-limiting. People in crisis are too upset to function at such a high level of anxiety indefinitely. The time needed to resolve the crisis, whether it be a positive solution or a state of disorganization, may be **6 weeks or longer.**

It is also important to recognize that periods of intense conflict ultimately can result in increased growth. How the crisis is handled determines whether growth or disorganization will result. Growth comes from learning in new situations. People in crisis feel uncomfortable, often reach out for help, and accept help until they feel that their lives are back to normal. The fact that **crises can lead to personal growth** is important to remember when working with patients in crisis.

Think of a crisis you have experienced. Do you feel that the way you handled it made you a better person in some way? If so, how? ■

Types of Crises

There are two types of crises: maturational and situational. Sometimes these crises can occur simultaneously. For example, an adolescent who is having difficulty adjusting to a change in role and body image (maturational crisis) may at the same time undergo the stress related to the death of a parent (situational crisis).

Maturational Crises. Maturational crises are developmental events requiring role changes. For example, successfully moving from early childhood to middle childhood requires the child to become socially involved with people outside the family. With the move from adolescence to adulthood, financial responsibility is expected. Both social and biological pressures to change can precipitate a crisis.

The nature and extent of the maturational crisis can be influenced by role models, interpersonal resources, and the ease of others in accepting the new role. Positive role models show the person how to act in the new role. Interpersonal resources encourage the trying out of new behaviors to achieve role changes. Other people's acceptance of the new role is also important. The greater the resistance of others, the more stress the person faces in making the changes.

Transitional periods during adolescence, parenthood, marriage, midlife, and retirement are key times for the onset of maturational crises. Some conflicts related to maturational crises are seen in the clinical examples that follow.

■ ⌗ CLINICAL EXAMPLE

Ms. J was a 19-year-old black, single, unemployed woman who came to the mental health clinic a month after the birth of her first child. Ms. J complained of feeling depressed. Her symptoms included difficulty falling asleep, early morning awakening, crying spells, a poor appetite, and difficulty in caring for the baby because of fatigue and apathy. The patient lived with her parents and siblings and had never lived on her own. She had always depended on her mother to take care of her. Her mother worked, however, and the patient was totally responsible for her daughter's care each day. Also, Ms. J's mother was angry that she had a child and often refused to care for

the baby. The patient's boyfriend, who was the baby's father, had promised to marry her, but he had recently decided he was too young to handle the responsibility of a wife and child. In summary, the young woman who had unmet dependency needs of her own was now a parent and had to meet the dependency needs of her infant. This precipitated a crisis for her.

Selected Nursing Diagnoses

- Ineffective coping related to birth of a child, as evidenced by feelings of depression
- Interrupted family processes related to birth of a grandchild, as evidenced by lack of family support
- Impaired parenting related to being a single mother, as evidenced by difficulty caring for her baby ■

■ ⌗ CLINICAL EXAMPLE

Mr. R was a 67-year-old white, married pharmacist who came to the mental health clinic complaining of anxiety, depression, and insomnia. His symptoms had begun 2 weeks ago when his wife decided that they should move to a retirement community in Florida. He described his wife as a strong, willful woman who was also outgoing and charming and made friends easily. He considered himself a quiet, nervous person who was comfortable only with old friends and his two sons and their families. Mr. R, although at retirement age, had continued to work as a pharmacist, doing relief work for a drugstore chain when the regular pharmacists were absent. In moving to Florida, he would lose his pharmacist's license, which was valid only in his state of residence. He expressed difficulty in making the transition from work to retirement. He had fears of becoming directionless and useless. He was anxious about leaving his sons and his friends. The prospect of complete retirement and moving to another state precipitated his distress.

Selected Nursing Diagnoses

- Relocation stress syndrome related to pending retirement, as evidenced by feelings of anxiety
- Interrupted family processes related to conflict about lifestyle changes, as evidenced by inability to plan future ■

Situational Crises. Situational crises occur when a life event upsets an individual's or group's psychological equilibrium. Examples of situational crises include loss of a job, loss of a loved one, unwanted pregnancy, onset or worsening of a medical illness, divorce, school problems, and witnessing a crime.

The loss of a job can result in financial stress, feelings of inadequacy as a breadwinner, and marital conflict caused by a spouse's anger over the lost job. The loss of a loved one results in bereavement and also can cause financial stress, change in roles of family members, and loss of emotional support. Homelessness is another possible outcome of the loss of a job or a loved one. The onset or worsening of a medical illness causes anticipatory grief and fear of the loss of a loved one. Again, financial stress and change in roles of family members often occur.

Divorce is similar to the stress of losing a loved one, except that the crisis can recur with the stress of dealing with the ex-spouse. An unwanted pregnancy is stressful because it requires decisions to be made about whether to complete the pregnancy or to abort it, and whether to keep the baby or place it for adoption. If the pregnancy is aborted or adoption occurs, the mother may need to deal with feelings of grief or anger. If the baby is to be kept, changes in lifestyle are required. Finally, being the victim of or witnessing a crime can cause feelings of helplessness, distrust of others, fear, nightmares, and guilt about causing or not stopping the crime.

Situational crises can be accidental, uncommon, and unexpected events. For example, natural disasters, such as fires, tornadoes, earthquakes, hurricanes, or floods, which disrupt entire communities, are situational crises. Man-made disasters also can precipitate situational crises, events such as killings in the workplace or in schools, airplane crashes, suicide bombings, and acts of terrorism.

The terrorist attacks of September 11, 2001 in which airplanes were hijacked and flown into the World Trade Center in New York City presented unprecedented trauma and crisis to people throughout the United States (Haber et al, 2002). Entire communities, especially people living in New York City, experienced a sudden and unexpected violent act that resulted in multiple losses and extensive community disruption. In addition, the safety felt by all Americans across the country was affected. One study found that over half of the people who lived or worked in New York had some emotional sequelae 3 to 6 months after September 11; however, only a small portion of those with severe responses were seeking treatment (DeLisi et al, 2003).

Disaster-precipitated emotional problems can surface immediately, as well as weeks or even months after the disaster. The symptoms usually occur in roughly six phases, which are described in Table 14-1. Individuals and communities progress through these phases at different rates depending on the type of disaster and the degree and nature of disaster exposure. This progression may not be linear or sequential, because each person and community brings unique elements to the recovery process. Individual variables such as psychological resilience, social support, and financial resources influence a survivor's capacity to move through the phases.

The severe psychological stress resulting from situational crises is described in a study conducted among New York City school children in schools near the World Trade Center. Six months after the terrorist attack of September 11, 2001, children still experienced an increased incidence of separation anxiety, agoraphobia, conduct disorder, posttraumatic stress disorder, generalized anxiety, depression, and alcohol abuse (NY Board of Education, 2002).

Looking back on the Oklahoma City bombing, it is known that at least six people who survived or lost loved ones killed themselves in the months afterwards. Others lost marriages and custody rights as a result of new addictions (Ripley, 2001). Thus the impact of situational crises can be devastating in both the short term and the long term.

Table 14-1	**Phases of Disaster Response**
PHASE	**RESPONSE**
Warning or threat phase	Disasters vary in the amount of warning communities receive before they occur from little or no warning to hours or even days of warning. When no warning is given, survivors may feel more vulnerable, unsafe, and fearful of future unpredicted tragedies.
Impact phase	The impact period of a disaster can vary from the slow, low-threat buildup associated with some types of floods to the violent, dangerous, and destructive outcomes associated with tornadoes and explosions. The greater the scope, community destruction, and personal losses associated with the disaster, the greater the psychosocial effects.
Rescue or heroic phase	In the immediate aftermath, survival, rescuing others, and promoting safety are priorities. For some, post-impact disorientation gives way to adrenaline-induced rescue behavior to save lives and protect property. Although activity level may be high, actual productivity is often low. Altruism is prominent among both survivors and emergency responders.
Remedy or honeymoon phase	During the week to months following a disaster, formal governmental and volunteer assistance may be readily available. Community bonding occurs as a result of sharing the catastrophic experience and the giving and receiving of community support. Survivors may experience a short-lived sense of optimism that the help they will receive will make them whole again. When disaster mental health workers are visible and perceived as helpful during this phase, they are more readily accepted and have a foundation from which to provide assistance in the difficult phases ahead.
Inventory phase	Over time, survivors begin to recognize the limits of available disaster assistance. They become physically exhausted due to enormous multiple demands, financial pressures, and the stress of relocation or living in a damaged home. The unrealistic optimism initially experienced can give way to discouragement and fatigue.
Reconstruction or recovery phase	The reconstruction of physical property and recovery of emotional well-being may continue for years following the disaster. Survivors have realized that they will need to solve the problems of rebuilding their own homes, businesses, and lives largely by themselves and gradually assume the responsibility for doing so. Survivors are faced with the need to readjust to and integrate new surroundings as they continue to grieve losses. Emotional resources within the family may be exhausted and social support from friends and family may be worn thin.
	When people come to see meaning, personal growth, and opportunity from their disaster experience despite their losses and pain, they are well on the road to recovery. Although disasters may cause profound life-changing losses, they also bring the opportunity to recognize personal strengths and to reexamine life priorities.

From US Department of Health and Human Services: *Training manual for mental health and human service workers in major disasters*, ed 2, Washington, DC, 2000, Government Printing Office.

Some crises, such as obtaining a divorce, develop over time and are of longer duration. Other crises, such as an earthquake, are sudden and unexpected. How do you think the element of time affects the response to crisis? ■

Crisis Intervention

Crisis intervention is a short-term therapy focused on solving the immediate problem. It is usually limited to 6 weeks. **The goal of crisis intervention is for the individual to return to a precrisis level of functioning.** Often the person advances to a level of growth that is higher than the precrisis level because new ways of problem solving have been learned.

It is important for the nurse to remember that cultural attitudes strongly influence the communication and response style of the crisis worker. These attitudes are deeply ingrained in the processes of asking for, giving, and receiving help. They also affect the victimization experience, so it is essential to understand and respect the cultural values of the victims. Specific cultural factors to be considered in crisis intervention include the following:

- Migration and citizenship status
- Gender and family roles
- Religious belief systems
- Child-rearing practices
- Use of extended family and support systems

The age of the survivors is also important for the nurse to consider when providing crisis intervention. Responses to stressor events differ across the life span. Therefore age-appropriate interventions are most effective in helping survivors return to their previous level of functioning (Adams et al, 1999; Ball and Allen, 2000). For example, 4-year-old children may best express themselves through play, whereas adolescents may best work through crisis issues in peer group discussions.

Describe how sociocultural factors might affect a woman's decision to seek help after being raped. ■

ASSESSMENT

The first step of crisis intervention is assessment. At this time data about the nature of the crisis and its effect on the patient must be collected. From these data, an intervention plan will be developed.

People in crisis experience many symptoms, including those listed in Box 14-1. Sometimes these symptoms can cause further problems. For example, problems at work may lead to loss of a job, financial stress, and lowered self-esteem.

Crises also can be complicated by old conflicts that resurface as a result of the current problem, making crisis resolution more difficult. For example, a woman who was orphaned at an early age may have more difficulty resolving a crisis precipitated by the work injury of her husband than a woman who had not suffered an earlier loss.

Although the crisis situation is the focus of the assessment, more significant and long-standing problems may be identified by the nurse. It is important, therefore, to identify which ar-

BOX 14-1

Behaviors Commonly Exhibited After a Crisis

Anger	Irritability
Apathy	Lability
Backaches	Nightmares
Boredom	Numbness
Crying spells	Overeating or undereating
Diminished sexual drive	Poor concentration
Disbelief	Sadness
Fatigue	School problems
Fear	Self-doubt
Flashbacks	Shock
Forgetfulness	Social withdrawal
Headaches	Substance abuse
Helplessness	Suicidal thoughts
Hopelessness	Survivor guilt
Insomnia	Work difficulties
Intrusive thoughts	

eas can be helped by crisis intervention and which problems must be referred to other sources for further treatment.

During this phase the nurse begins to establish a positive working relationship with the patient. A number of balancing factors are important in the development and resolution of a crisis and should be assessed:

- Precipitating event or stressor
- Patient's perception of the event or stressor
- Nature and strength of the patient's support systems and coping resources
- Patient's previous strengths and coping mechanisms

Precipitating Event

To help identify the precipitating event, the nurse should explore the patient's needs, the events that threaten those needs, and the time at which symptoms appear. Four kinds of needs that have been identified are related to self-esteem, role mastery, dependency, and biological function.

1. **Self-esteem** is achieved when the person attains successful social role experience.
2. **Role mastery** is achieved when the person attains work, sexual, and family role successes.
3. **Dependency** is achieved when a satisfying interdependent relationship with others is attained.
4. **Biological function** is achieved when a person is safe and life is not threatened.

The nurse determines which needs are not being met by asking the patient to reflect on issues of self-image and self-esteem, the areas of life that are considered a success, one's relationships with others, and the degree of safety and security in life. The nurse looks for obstacles that might interfere with meeting the patient's needs. What recent experiences have been upsetting? What areas of life have had changes?

Coping patterns become ineffective and symptoms appear usually after the stressful incident. When did the patient begin to feel anxious? When did sleep disturbances begin? At what point in time did suicidal thoughts start? If symptoms began last Tuesday, ask what took place in the patient's life on Tuesday or Monday. As the patient connects life events with the breakdown in coping mechanisms, an understanding of the precipitating event can emerge.

Perception of the Event

The patient's perception or appraisal of the precipitating event is very important. What may seem trivial to the nurse may have great meaning to the patient. An overweight adolescent girl may have been the only girl in the class not invited to a dance. This may have threatened her self-esteem. A man with two unsuccessful marriages may have just been told by a girlfriend that she wants to end their relationship; this may have threatened his need for sexual role mastery. An emotionally isolated, friendless woman may have had car trouble and been unable to find someone to give her a ride to work. This may have threatened her dependency needs. A chronically ill man who has had a recent relapse of his illness may have had his need for biological function threatened.

Themes and surfacing memories of the patient give further clues to the precipitating event. Current issues of concern are often connected to past issues. For example, a female patient who talks about the death of her father, which occurred 3 years ago, may, on questioning, reveal a recent loss of a relationship with a male. A patient who talks about feelings of inadequacy he had as a child because of poor school performance may, on questioning, reveal a recent experience in which his feelings of adequacy on his job were threatened. Because most crises involve losses or threats of losses, the theme of loss is a common one. In assessment the nurse looks for a recent event that may be connected to an underlying theme.

Support Systems and Coping Resources

The patient's living situation and supports in the environment must be assessed. Does the patient live alone or with family or friends? With whom is the patient close, and who offers understanding and strength? Is there a supportive clergyman or friend? Assessing the patient's support system is important in determining who should come for the crisis therapy sessions. It may be decided that certain family members should come with the patient so that the family members' support can be strengthened. If the patient has few supports, participation in a crisis therapy group may be recommended.

Assessing the patient's coping resources is vital in determining whether hospitalization would be more appropriate than outpatient crisis therapy. If there is a high degree of suicidal or homicidal risk along with weak outside resources, hospitalization may be a safer and more effective treatment.

Identify people in your social system that you would turn to in a time of crisis. Compare your list with that of a friend. ■

Coping Mechanisms

Next, the nurse assesses the patient's strengths and previous coping mechanisms. How has the patient handled other crises? How were anxieties relieved? Did the patient talk out problems? Did the patient leave the usual surroundings for a period of time to think things through from another perspective? Was physical activity used to relieve tension? Did the patient find relief in crying? Besides exploring previous coping mechanisms, the nurse also should note the absence of other possible successful mechanisms.

▓ PLANNING AND IMPLEMENTATION

The next step of crisis intervention is planning; the previously collected data are analyzed and specific interventions are proposed. Dynamics underlying the present crisis are formulated from the information about the precipitating event. Alternative solutions to the problem are explored, and steps for achieving the solutions are identified. The nurse decides which environmental supports to engage or strengthen and how best to do this, as well as deciding which of the patient's coping mechanisms to develop and which to strengthen.

This process is outlined in the Patient Education Plan for coping with crisis in Table 14-2. The expected outcome of nursing care is that the patient will recover from the crisis event and return to a precrisis level of functioning. A more ambitious expected outcome would be for the patient to recover from the crisis event and attain a higher than precrisis level of functioning and improved quality of life.

Nursing interventions can take place on many levels using a variety of techniques. There are four levels of crisis intervention—environmental manipulation, general support, generic approach, and individual approach—that represent a hierarchy from the most basic to the most complex (Shields, 1975) (Figure 14-2). Each level includes the interventions of the previous level, and the progressive order indicates that the nurse needs additional knowledge and skill for implementing high-level interventions. It is often helpful to consult with others when deciding which approach to use.

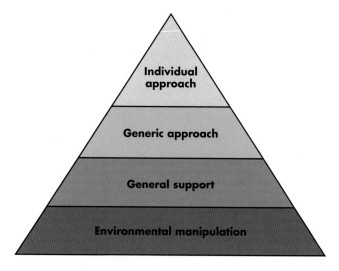

Figure 14-2 Levels of crisis intervention.

Table 14-2	PATIENT EDUCATION PLAN	Coping With Crisis
CONTENT	**INSTRUCTIONAL ACTIVITIES**	**EVALUATION**

Describe the crisis event.	Ask about the details of the crisis, including:
	   A timeline of the crisis
	   Who was affected
	   The events of the crisis
	   Any precipitating events
		Patient describes the crisis event in detail.

Explore feelings, thoughts, and behaviors related to the crisis event.	Determine precrisis level of functioning. Discuss patient's perception of the crisis event. Determine acute and long-term needs, threats, and challenges.	Patient discusses precrisis level of functioning and perceptions of the crisis event. Patient's needs are identified.
Identify coping mechanisms.	Ask how stressful events have been handled in the past. Analyze whether these are adaptive or maladaptive for the current crisis event. Suggest additional coping strategies.	Patient identifies adaptive coping mechanisms for the current crisis event.
Develop a plan for coping adaptively with the crisis event.	Reinforce adaptive coping mechanisms and healthy defenses. With the patient, construct a coping plan for the aftermath of the crisis event.	Patient develops a plan for coping with the crisis event.
Assign the patient activities from coping plan.	Review implementation of the coping plan. Help patient generalize coping strategies for use in future crisis events.	Patient reports satisfaction with coping abilities and level of functioning.

Environmental Manipulation

Environmental manipulation includes interventions that directly change the patient's physical or interpersonal situation. These interventions provide situational support or remove stress. Important elements of this intervention are mobilizing the patient's supporting social systems and serving as a liaison between the patient and social support agencies.

For example, a patient who is having trouble coping with her six children may temporarily send several of the children to their grandparents' house. In this situation some stress is reduced. Similarly, a patient having difficulty on his or her job may take a week of sick leave to be removed temporarily from that stress. A patient who lives alone may move in with his or her closest sibling for several days. Likewise, involving the patient in family or group crisis therapy provides environmental manipulation for the purpose of providing support.

General Support

General support includes interventions that convey the feeling that the nurse is on the patient's side and will be a helping person. The nurse uses warmth, acceptance, empathy, caring, and reassurance to provide this type of support.

Generic Approach

The generic approach is designed to reach high-risk individuals and large groups as quickly as possible. It applies a specific method to all people faced with a similar type of crisis. The expected course of the particular type of crisis is studied and mapped out. The intervention is then set up to ensure that the course of the crisis results in an adaptive response.

Grief is an example of a crisis with a known pattern that can be treated by the generic approach. Helping the patient to overcome ties to the deceased and find new patterns of rewarding interaction may effectively resolve the grief. Applying this intervention to people experiencing grief, especially with a high-risk group such as families of disaster victims, is an example of the generic approach.

Interventions following an acute stress are sometimes referred to as debriefing. Originally a military concept, debriefing is used as a therapeutic intervention to help people recall events and clarify traumatic experiences. Interventions consist of ventilation of feelings within a context of group support, normalization of responses, and education about psychological reactions to traumatic events. Although debriefing may be effective for some individuals, research findings about its effectiveness following extreme stress are inconclusive. Thus further research is needed before it can be endorsed as an evidence-based practice (Kaplan, Iancu, and Bodner, 2001).

Individual Approach

The individual approach is a type of crisis intervention similar to the diagnosis and treatment of a specific problem in a specific patient. The nurse must understand the specific patient characteristics that led to the present crisis and must use the intervention that is most likely to help the patient develop an adaptive response to the crisis.

This type of crisis intervention can be effective with all types of crises. It is particularly useful in combined situational and maturational crises. The individual approach is also helpful when symptoms include homicidal and suicidal risk. The individual approach also should be applied if the course of the patient's crisis cannot be determined and if resolution of the crisis has not been achieved using the generic approach.

Interventions are aimed at facilitating cognitive and emotional processing of the traumatic event and at improving coping. Five core interventions to assist survivors of acute stress are as follows (Osterman and Chemtob, 1999):

- Restore psychological safety
- Provide information
- Correct misattributions
- Restore and support effective coping
- Ensure social support

How might each level of crisis intervention be used in a high school after a star player of the football team commits suicide? ■

Techniques

The nurse should be creative and flexible, trying many different techniques. These should be active, focused, and explorative techniques that can facilitate achieving the targeted interventions. Some of these include catharsis, clarification, suggestion, reinforcement of behavior, support of defenses, raising self-esteem, and exploration of solutions.

The intervention must be aimed at achieving quick resolution. The nurse also must be active in guiding the crisis intervention through its various steps. A passive approach is not appropriate because of the time limitations of the crisis situation. A brief description of these techniques follows.

Catharsis is the release of feelings that takes place as the patient talks about emotionally charged areas. As feelings about the events are realized, tension is reduced. Catharsis is often used in crisis intervention. The nurse solicits the patient's feelings about the specific situation, recent events, and significant people involved in the particular crisis. The nurse asks open-ended questions and repeats the patient's words so that more feelings are expressed. The nurse does not discourage crying or angry outbursts but rather sees them as a positive release of feelings.

Only when feelings seem out of control, such as in cases of extreme rage or despondency, should the nurse discourage catharsis and help the patient concentrate on thinking rather than feeling. For example, if a patient angrily talks of wanting to kill a specific person, it is better to shift the focus to a discussion of the consequences of carrying out the act rather than to encourage free expression of the angry feelings.

Clarification is used when the nurse helps the patient identify the relationship between events, behaviors, and feelings. For example, helping a patient see that it was after being passed over for a promotion that he or she felt too sick to go to work is clarification. Clarification helps the patient gain a better understanding of feelings and how they lead to the development of a crisis.

Suggestion is influencing a person to accept an idea or belief. In crisis intervention the patient is influenced to see the nurse as a confident, calm, hopeful, empathic person who can

help. By believing the nurse can help, the patient may feel more optimistic and less anxious. It is a technique in which the nurse engages patients' emotions, wishes, or values to their benefit in the therapeutic process. Suggestion is a way of influencing the patient by pointing out alternatives or new ways of looking at things.

Reinforcement of behavior occurs when healthy, adaptive behavior of the patient is reinforced by the nurse, who strengthens positive responses made by the patient by agreeing with or positively acknowledging those responses. For example, when a patient who has passively allowed himself or herself to be criticized by the boss later reports asserting himself or herself in a discussion with the boss, the nurse can commend the patient on this assertiveness.

Support of defenses occurs when the nurse encourages the use of healthy defenses and discourages those that are maladaptive. Defense mechanisms are used to cope with stressful situations and to maintain self-esteem and ego integrity. When defenses deny, falsify, or distort reality to the point that the person cannot deal effectively with reality, they are maladaptive.

The nurse should encourage the patient to use adaptive defenses and discourage those that are maladaptive. For example, when a patient denies that her husband wants a separation despite the fact that he has told her so, the nurse can point out that she is not facing facts and dealing realistically with the problem. This is an example of discouraging the maladaptive use of the defense mechanism of denial. If a patient who is furious with his boss writes a letter to his boss's supervisor rather than assaulting his boss, the nurse should encourage the adaptive use of the defense mechanism of sublimation.

In crisis intervention, defenses are not attacked but rather are more gently encouraged or discouraged. When defenses are attacked, the patient cannot maintain self-esteem and ego integrity. Also the immediacy of crisis intervention does not allow enough time to replace the attacked defenses with new ones. Returning the patient to a prior level of functioning is the goal of crisis intervention, not the restructuring of defenses.

Raising self-esteem is a particularly important technique. The patient in a crisis feels helpless and may be overwhelmed with feelings of inadequacy. The fact that the patient has found it necessary to seek outside help may further increase feelings of inadequacy. The nurse should help the patient regain feelings of self-worth by communicating confidence that the patient can find solutions to problems. The nurse also should convey that the patient is a worthwhile person by listening to and accepting the patient's feelings, being respectful, and praising help-seeking efforts.

Exploration of solutions is essential because crisis intervention is geared toward solving the immediate crisis. The nurse and patient actively explore solutions to the crisis. Answers that the patient had not thought of before may become apparent during conversations with the nurse as anxiety decreases. For example, a patient who has lost her job and has not been able to find a new one may become aware of the fact that she knows many people in her field of work whom she could contact to get information regarding the job market and possible openings.

These crisis intervention techniques are summarized in Box 14-2. In addition to using these techniques, the crisis worker should have some other particular attitudes toward the care being given in order to be effective. The crisis worker should see this work as the treatment of choice for people in crisis rather than as a second-best treatment. Assessment of the present problem should be viewed as necessary for treatment, whereas a complete diagnostic assessment should be recognized as being unnecessary. The goal and time limitations of crisis intervention should be kept in mind constantly, and material unrelated to the crisis should not be explored. An active directive role must be taken by the crisis worker, and maintaining flexibility of approach is essential. If more complex problems are identified that are not suitable for crisis intervention, the patient should be referred for further treatment. Table 14-3 describes interventions for helping individuals and families cope with stress resulting from crisis.

EVALUATION

The last phase of crisis intervention is evaluation, when the nurse and patient evaluate whether the intervention resulted in a positive resolution of the crisis. Specific questions the nurse might ask include the following:

- Has the expected outcome been achieved, and has the patient returned to the precrisis level of functioning?
- Have the needs of the patient that were threatened by the event been met?
- Have the patient's symptoms decreased or been resolved?
- Does the patient have adequate support systems and coping resources on which to rely?

BOX 14-2

Techniques of Crisis Intervention

Technique: Catharsis
Definition: The release of feelings that takes place as the patient talks about emotionally charged areas
Example: "Tell me about how you have been feeling since you lost your job."

Technique: Clarification
Definition: Encouraging the patient to express more clearly the relationship between certain events
Example: "I've noticed that after you have an argument with your husband you become sick and can't leave your bed."

Technique: Suggestion
Definition: Influencing a person to accept an idea or belief, particularly the belief that the nurse can help and that the person will in time feel better
Example: "Many other people have found it helpful to talk about this and I think you will, too."

Technique: Reinforcement of behavior
Definition: Giving the patient positive responses to adaptive behavior
Example: "That's the first time you were able to defend yourself with your boss and it went very well. I'm so pleased that you were able to do it."

Technique: Support of defenses
Definition: Encouraging the use of healthy, adaptive defenses and discouraging those that are unhealthy or maladaptive
Example: "Going for a bicycle ride when you were so angry was very helpful because when you returned you and your wife were able to talk things through."

Technique: Raising self-esteem
Definition: Helping the patient regain feelings of self-worth
Example: "You are a very strong person to be able to manage the family all this time. I think you will be able to handle this situation, too."

Technique: Exploration of solutions
Definition: Examining alternative ways of solving the immediate problem
Example: "You seem to know many people in the computer field. Could you contact some of them to see whether they might know of available jobs?"

Table 14-3 Nursing Interventions for Crisis Events

TARGET AREAS	NURSING INTERVENTIONS
Basic Needs	Provide liaison to social agencies.
Physical Deficits	Attend to physical emergencies. Refer to other health care providers as necessary.
Psychological Effects	
Shock	Attentively listen to telling of the crisis details.
Confusion	Give nurturing support; permit regression.
Denial	Permit intermittent denial; identify patient's primary concern.
Anxiety	Provide structure, enact antianxiety interventions.
Lethargy/heroics	Encourage sublimation and constructive activity.
Protective Factors	
Coping	Encourage patient's favored, adaptive coping mechanisms; emphasize rationalization, humor, sublimation.
Self-efficacy	Support patient's previous successes and belief in own abilities, dilute irrational self-doubts, emphasize power of expectations to produce results.
Support	Add social supports to the patient's world, provide professional support, refer for counseling when necessary, help patient develop new coping strategies.

Modified from Hardin SB: Catastrophic stress. In McBride AB, Austin JK, editors: *Psychiatric–mental health nursing*, Philadelphia, 1996, WB Saunders.

Critical Thinking *About* Contemporary Issues

Should Medication Be Included As a Crisis Intervention Treatment for Acute Traumatic Stress?

Although people who are suffering from traumatic stress may experience a range of mental health symptoms in the acute phase of the trauma, it is unclear whether all problems share the same biological characteristics. It is also unclear in the initial phases of assessment which symptoms may quickly resolve with crisis intervention and which may last and ultimately meet criteria for a psychiatric disorder amenable to medication. Should psychopharmacological agents be offered to victims in the early stages of traumatic stress, which ones would be appropriate, and when in the process of crisis intervention would this be most helpful? Also, are there contraindications for biological interventions under some circumstances?

One might begin this decision-making process by assessing precrisis symptoms (and treatments, if any), history of substance use, family history of psychiatric disorders, and the person's belief system regarding psychiatric medications. Is the symptom already of long duration and, if so, how was it treated in the past? Does the person use substances such as alcohol that could complicate his or her reaction to the crisis or assessment of the crisis impact? If there is a family history of a psychiatric disorder, the person may be at greater risk for developing that or a similar disorder. Psychopharmacological interventions may be inappropri-

ate if many of the symptoms will be short-lived (given the fact that some medications take several weeks to work), if many of the symptoms are natural reactions to trauma rather than symptoms of psychiatric disorders, or if the medications will lead to adverse side effects and possibly stigmatize an already traumatized person.

Some may argue that medications might blunt a person's cognitive abilities at a time when concentration and problem solving are important, but an important question is whether withholding a treatment from a person who may benefit from it is an ethical decision. Could medication given immediately after exposure to a traumatic event avert a chronic posttraumatic illness? There are no clear-cut answers to these questions, but crisis clinicians are best guided by a few clinical principles:
- What bothers this person the most?
- Can this problem be controlled through psychotherapeutic, environmental, or psychopharmacological interventions?
- What treatment is most likely to make this person feel or function better?
- Is there a reason *not* to prescribe this treatment?

Answers will be governed by a careful assessment of each person's circumstances and a holistic view of care provided.

- Is the patient using constructive coping mechanisms?
- Is the patient demonstrating adaptive crisis responses?
- Does the patient need to be referred for additional treatment?

The nurse and patient also should review the changes that have occurred. The nurse should give patients credit for successful changes so that they can realize their effectiveness and understand that what they learned from a crisis may help in coping with future crises. If the goals have not been met, the patient and nurse can return to the first step, assessment, and progress through the phases again. At the end of the evaluation process, if the nurse and patient believe referral for additional professional help would be useful, the referral should be made as quickly as possible (see Critical Thinking About Contemporary Issues).

All of the phases of crisis intervention are presented in the Case Study on pp. 231 and 232.

Given that stress is experienced by all people, why aren't all nurses required to be competent in crisis intervention skills, just as they are in CPR skills? ■

■ SETTINGS FOR CRISIS INTERVENTION

Nurses work in many settings in which they see people in crisis. Hospitalizations are often stressful for patients and their families and are precipitating causes of crises. The patient who becomes demanding or withdrawn or the spouse who becomes bothersome to the nursing staff is a possible candidate for crisis intervention. The diagnosis of an illness, the limitations imposed on activities, and the changes in body image

because of surgery can all be viewed as losses or threats that may precipitate a situational crisis. Simply the stress of being dependent on nurses for care can precipitate a crisis for the hospitalized patient.

Nurses who work in obstetric, pediatric, geriatric, or adolescent settings often observe patients or family members undergoing maturational crises. The anxious new mother, the acting-out adolescent, and the newly retired depressed patient are all possible candidates for crisis therapy. If physical illness is an added stress during maturational turning points, the patient is at an even greater risk. Emergency room and critical care settings also are flooded with crisis cases. People who attempt suicide, psychosomatic patients, survivors of sudden cardiac arrest, and crime and accident victims are all possible candidates for crisis intervention. If the nurse is not in a position to work with the patient on an ongoing basis, a referral should be made.

Community and home health nurses work with patients in their own environments and can often spot and intervene in family crises. The child who refuses to go to school, the man who refuses to learn how to give himself an insulin injection, and the family with a member dying at home are possible candidates for crisis intervention. Community health nurses are also in an ideal position to evaluate high-risk families such as those with new babies, ill members, recent deaths, and a history of difficulty coping (Coombes, 2000).

Finally, nurses in community mental health centers, departments of psychiatry, managed care clinics, schools, occupational health centers, long-term care facilities, and home health agencies also may see patients in crisis, such as those experiencing depression, anxiety, marital conflict, suicidal

CASE STUDY

Assessment

Mr. A is a 39-year-old, medium-build, casually dressed black man who was referred to the mental health clinic by his primary care provider. The patient came to the center alone. The nurse working with Mr. A collected the following data.

The patient worked in a large naval shipyard that was recently scheduled for closing. It was laying off many workers and reassigning others. One month earlier Mr. A was assigned to an area where he had difficulty 2 years ago. The patient believed that the foreman was harassing him as he had had done previously. Two weeks ago the patient had become angry at the foreman and had thoughts of killing him. Instead of acting on these thoughts, Mr. A became dizzy, and his head ached. He requested medical attention but was refused. He then passed out and was taken by ambulance to the dispensary. Since that time Mr. A had had a comprehensive physical examination and was found to be in excellent health. He was prescribed diazepam (Valium) on an as-needed basis, which was only slightly helpful. He returned to work for 2 days this week but again felt sick.

Mr. A complained of being depressed, nervous, and tense. He was not sleeping well, was irritable with his wife and children, and was preoccupied with angry feelings toward his foreman. He denied suicidal thoughts but admitted that he felt like killing the foreman. He quickly added that he would really never do anything like that.

He appeared to have good comprehension, above-average intelligence, adequate memory, and some paranoid ideation related to the foreman at work. His thought processes were organized, and there was no evidence of a perceptual disorder. Ego boundary disturbance was evident in the patient's paranoid thoughts. It seemed that the foreman was a difficult man to get along with, but the description of personal harassment seemed distorted.

Mr. A was raised by his parents. His father beat him and his siblings often. His mother was quiet and always agreed with his father. The patient had a younger brother and sister and an older sister. The patient and his brother had always been close. The two of them had stopped their father's beatings by ganging up on him and "psyching him out." As a child, Mr. A hung around with a tough crowd and fought frequently. He believed that he could physically overpower others but tried to keep out of trouble by talking to people rather than fighting.

Mr. A had no psychiatric history. His physical health was excellent, and he was taking no medication other than the prescribed Valium. He had a tenth-grade education, and his work record up to this time was good. His interests included bowling and other sports. He had been married for 17 years and had three daughters, ages 16, 13, and 9. Mr. A stated that he had a good relationship with his wife and daughters and that both his wife and his brother were strong supports for him.

His usual means of coping were talking calmly with the threatening party and working hard on his job, at home, and in leisure activities. These coping mechanisms failed to work for him at this time but they had been successful in the past. He had

no arrest record and was able to think through his actions rather than act impulsively. Mr. A showed strong motivation for working on his problem. He was reaching out for help and was able to form a therapeutic relationship with the nurse. Although his wife and brother were supportive, he felt a need for outside support because his previous coping skills were not working.

Diagnosis

Mr. A was in a **situational crisis**. The threat or precipitating stress was his job transfer and supervision by a former boss, whom he felt was harassing him. The patient's need for role mastery was not being met because he was not feeling successful at his job. Soon after the transfer, Mr. A's usual means of coping became ineffective and he experienced increased anxiety.

His nursing diagnosis was ineffective coping related to changes at work, as evidenced by physical complaints of dizziness and tension. His DSM-IV-TR diagnosis was adjustment disorder with mixed anxiety and depressed mood.

Outcome Identification and Planning

The **expected outcome** of treatment was for Mr. A to return to his precrisis level of functioning. If possible, he could reach a higher level, having learned new methods of problem solving. The patient showed good potential for growth, and the nurse made a contract with him for crisis intervention. Mutually identified **short-term goals** included the following:

- Mr. A will explore his thoughts and feelings about recent work events.
- Mr. A will not harm his boss.
- Mr. A will describe coping mechanisms that have been successful for him in the past.
- Mr. A will identify three new ways of coping with work stress.
- Mr. A will implement two of the new coping strategies.
- Mr. A will be free of symptoms and function well at work.

Implementation

The level of intervention used by the nurse was the **individual approach**, which includes the generic approach, general support, and environmental manipulation.

Environmental manipulation involved having the patient remain home from work temporarily. Letters were written by the nurse to his employer explaining Mr. A's absence in general terms. Mr. A was encouraged to talk to his wife about his difficulties so that she could understand his anxiety and provide emotional support.

General support was given by the nurse, who provided an atmosphere of reassurance, nonjudgmental caring, warmth, empathy, and optimism. Mr. A was encouraged to talk freely about the problem, and the nurse assured him that his problem could be solved and that he would be feeling better soon.

The **generic approach** was used to decrease the patient's anxiety and guide him through the steps of problem solving.

Continued

CASE STUDY—cont'd

Levels of anxiety were assessed and ways of reducing anxiety and helping the patient tolerate moderate anxiety were identified. The patient was encouraged to use his anxiety constructively to solve his problem and develop new coping mechanisms.

The **individual approach** was used in assessing and treating the specific problems of Mr. A, who was strongly sensitive to mistreatment as a result of early childhood experiences. His emotional response was to strike out physically, as his father had struck out at him. Intellectually, Mr. A knew this would be disastrous, and his conflict was solved by becoming sick and passing out so that he could not assault his boss. Mr. A's intense anger was recognized, and a high priority was placed on channeling the anger in a positive direction. As a way of formalizing this intervention, Mr. A signed a safety contract with the nurse agreeing not to harm himself or others.

The first two meetings were used for data gathering and establishing a positive therapeutic relationship. Through the use of **catharsis** the patient vented angry feelings but did not concentrate on wanting to kill his boss. The nurse used **clarification** to help the patient begin to understand the precipitating event and its effect on him. **Suggestion** was used to allow the patient to see the nurse as one who could help. The nurse told the patient the problem could be worked out by the two of them and that he would soon be feeling better. Mr. A decided to contact several people at work to obtain information about transferring to another department and filing a formal complaint against the foreman. The patient and nurse therefore were **exploring solutions**. The nurse reinforced the patient's use of problem solving by telling him that his ideas about alternative solutions were good ones. Throughout these and other sessions the nurse **raised his self-esteem** by communicating her confidence that he could find solutions to his problems. She listened to and accepted his feelings and treated him with respect. By contacting others at work, the patient also found some supportive people.

During the third session the patient described an incident in which he became furious at a worker in an automobile repair shop. The repairs on the patient's car were repeatedly done incorrectly, and the patient had to keep returning the car. The patient shoved the worker but limited his physical assault to just that. He then felt nervous and jittery. The patient had previously expressed pride in his ability to control his angry feelings and not physically strike out at others. **Suggestion** was used by telling the patient that he showed control in stopping the assault before it had become a full-blown fight and he could continue to

do so. Mr. A's ability to honor the safety contract he made with the nurse was also reinforced. During this session the patient spoke of old, angry feelings toward his father. Some of this venting was allowed, but soon thereafter the focus was guided back to the present crisis.

In the fourth session the patient reported no episodes of uncontrollable anger. However, he still put much emphasis on being harassed by others. The nurse questioned the notion that others were out to intentionally harass the patient. Mr. A's defenses were not attacked, but his gross use of projection was discouraged. In the fifth session the patient reported that a car tried to run him off the road. At a red traffic light the patient spoke calmly to the offending driver and the driver apologized. The nurse **reinforced this behavior** and **supported his use of sublimation** as a defense. Discussion of termination of the therapy was begun.

In the sixth session Mr. A said that things were going well at work and that he would soon be going to a different department. He also talked about a course he had begun at a community college. He showed no evidence of anxiety, depression, or paranoia and thought he didn't need to come back to the mental health clinic.

Evaluation

The interventions resulted in an adaptive resolution of the crisis. The patient's need for role mastery was being met. He was once again comfortable and successful at work. His symptoms of anxiety, paranoia, dizziness, headaches, passing out, and homicidal thoughts had ended. He no longer felt harassed. His original coping mechanisms were again effective. He was talking calmly to people he was having difficulty with, and he was again working hard in a goal-oriented way (his college course). He had learned new methods of coping, which included talking about his feelings to significant others, following administrative or official avenues of protest, and seeking support. The patient and nurse discussed how Mr. A could use the methods of problem solving he had learned from the experience to help cope with future problems. The expected outcome, return to the precrisis level of functioning, had been attained.

It was also recommended to the patient that he engage in psychotherapy so that he could deal with the old angers that continued to interfere with his life. Mr. A refused the recommendation at that time and stated he would contact the clinic if he changed his mind.

---

thoughts, illicit drug use, and traumatic responses. Crisis intervention can be implemented in any setting and should be a competency skill of all nurses, regardless of specialty area.

■ MODALITIES OF CRISIS INTERVENTION

Crisis intervention modalities are based on the philosophy that the health care team must be aggressive and go out to the patients rather than wait for the patients to come to

them. Nurses working in these modalities intervene in a variety of community settings, ranging from patients' homes to street corners.

Mobile Crisis Programs

Mobile crisis teams provide front-line interdisciplinary crisis intervention to individuals, families, and communities. The nurse who is a member of a mobile crisis team may respond to a desperate person threatening to jump off a bridge in a suicide attempt, an angry person who is becoming violent toward family members at home, or a frightened person who has barricaded himself in an office building. By defusing the immediate crisis situation, lives can be saved, incarcerations and hospitalizations can be avoided, and people can be stabilized (Zealberg, Hardesty, and Tyson, 1998; Steadman et al, 2001; Gou et al, 2001).

Mobile crisis programs throughout the country vary in the services they provide and the procedures they use. However, they are usually able to provide on-site assessment, crisis management, treatment, referral, and educational services to patients, families, law enforcement officers, and the community at large. Studies of mobile crisis services show favorable outcomes for patients and families and lower hospitalization rates (see Citing the Evidence).

Ask if you can shadow a mobile crisis team in your community for a day. Observe the work they do and share your experience with your peers. ■

Group Work

Crisis groups follow the same steps that individual intervention follows. The nurse and group help the patient solve the problem and reinforce the patient's new problem-solving behavior. The nurse's role in the group is active, focal, and present oriented. The group follows the nurse's example and uses similar therapeutic techniques. The group acts as a support system for the patient and is therefore of particular benefit to socially isolated people.

Often the way the patient functions in the group suggests the faulty coping pattern that is responsible for the patient's current problem. For example, a patient's interaction with group members may show that he does not appear to listen to anything said by others. This same patient may be in a crisis because his girlfriend left him because she thought he did not care about her thoughts and feelings. The nurse can comment on the faulty coping behavior seen in the group and encourage group discussion about it.

Most crisis groups focus on people who have common traits or stressors. For example, groups have been established for children and parents to decrease traumatic distress after children had become victims of extrafamilial sexual abuse (Grosz, Kempe, and Kelly, 2000). Others who have evaluated the effects of bereavement groups for widowed survivors have found lower rates of depression, psychological distress, and grief, as well as a higher level of social adjustment (Constantino, Sekula, and Rubinstein, 2001). The common issue is that such groups provided the opportunity for members to express common concerns and experiences, foster hope, and build mutual support.

Nurses practicing on acute psychiatric units also can use crisis intervention in working with patients and families to prepare for discharge and prevent rehospitalization. With the shortened lengths of hospital stays, crisis intervention is often the treatment of choice. The hospitalization itself may be viewed as an environmental manipulation and part of the crisis intervention.

Telephone Contacts

Crisis intervention is sometimes practiced by telephone or Internet communication, rather than through face-to-face contacts. When individuals in crisis use the telephone or Internet, it is usually when they are at the peak of their distress. Nurses working for these types of hotlines or those who answer emergency telephone calls or electronic mail may find themselves practicing crisis intervention without having visual cues to rely on. Referrals for face-to-face contact should be made, but often, because of the patient's unwillingness or inability to cooperate, the telephone or Internet remain the only contact (Ottenstein, 2002). A variety of listening skills must therefore be emphasized in the nurse's role.

Most emergency telephone and Internet services have extensive training programs to teach this specialized type of crisis intervention. Manuals written for the crisis worker include content such as suicide-potential rating scales, community resources, drug information, guidelines for helping the caller or crisis worker discuss concerns, and advice on understanding the limitations of the crisis worker's role.

Disaster Response

As part of the community, nurses are called on when situational crises strike the community. Floods, earthquakes, airplane crashes, fires, nuclear accidents, and other natural and unnatural disasters precipitate large numbers of crises (Weaver et al, 2000). It is important that nurses in the immediate postdisaster period go to places where victims are likely to gather, such as morgues, hospitals, shelters, and areas surrounding the disaster site. This was a critically important part of nursing intervention in the aftermath of the Oklahoma City bombing (Flynn, 1995) and the World Trade Center and Pentagon attacks of September 11, 2001 (AJN News, 2002).

Rather than waiting for people to publicly identify themselves as being unable to cope with stress, it is suggested that nurses work with the American Red Cross, talk to people waiting in lines to apply for assistance, go door-to-door or, at a relocation site, ask people how they are managing their affairs and explore their reactions to stress.

Nurses are often called on to help out in times of disaster. What special needs might nurses have in situations where they are both victims and caregivers? ∎

Experts in the field of disaster response suggest that organized plans for crisis response be developed and practiced during nondisaster times. Disaster plans are needed for large and small communities so that multiple complex needs can be met. An epidemiological approach to evaluating and intervening in the effects of disasters is suggested. Specifically, disaster plans need to have a way of identifying those individuals who are at greatest risk for developing or worsening psychiatric illnesses (Norwood et al, 2002; Pandya and Weiden, 2001).

Common psychiatric responses to disaster should be considered when developing plans. These are listed in Box 14-3. Examples of agencies, organizations, and individuals to be included in disaster planning include hospitals, mental health programs, substance abuse agencies, departments of health, employee assistance programs, housing programs, university-affiliated nurses, and school district nurses (Drenkard et al, 2002; Franklin et al, 2000).

Nurses providing crisis therapy during large disasters use the generic approach to crisis intervention so that as many people as possible can receive help in a short amount of time. Tragedies such as workplace violence and school shootings may affect fewer people and may at times require the individual approach. The nurse may choose to work with families or groups rather than individuals during situational crises so that people can gain support from others in their family or community who are undergoing stresses similar to theirs.

Nurses and mental health professionals were active in providing crisis intervention to victims of the September 11th crisis. Although Red Cross and other official disaster plans were initiated, there were periods of disorganization due to the unexpected nature, magnitude, and violence of the event. Disaster planners are now using what was learned from that tragedy to design their plans and identify ways in which nurses and others can prioritize individuals in need of crisis intervention (Reid, 2001).

At the top of the list are those who have themselves been physically attacked or injured. This is followed by those who suffer immediate and direct loss, such as the families and neighbors of victims. Below that are people who have been less directly affected but have still experienced some significant changes in their lives, such as friends and co-workers of the injured person and rescue workers. Next are those who have not been directly affected but who are particularly sensitive to environmental uncertainty, such as physically and mentally ill patients. And finally, at the bottom, are the masses of people who have made some changes in their lives and feel fear as a result of the disaster.

Recently, attention has been focused on offering support and help to the helpers involved in disasters. Health and mental health professionals who are victims of disasters as well as providers of care during disasters often feel overwhelmed with stress (Badger, 2001). These care providers describe feelings of concern for both their patients and their own families, as well as themselves (French, Sole, and Byers, 2002). Crisis intervention strategies for the caregivers are essential.

For example, Stuart and Huggins (1990) described the actions that psychiatric nurse administrators used to care for their psychiatric nursing staff, and Stanley (1990) reported on a hospital-wide crisis stabilization program that provided large-group debriefing and small-group follow-up sessions for all nursing staff after Hurricane Hugo devastated South Carolina in 1989. Similarly, Tucker et al (1998) described debriefing services for firefighters, law enforcement officers, medical examiner personnel, and medical and mental health workers following the Oklahoma City bombing.

Victim Outreach Programs

Although crisis intervention is not considered the appropriate treatment for serious consequences of victimization, such as posttraumatic stress disorder (PTSD) or depression, it is very useful as a community support for victims in the immediate aftermath of crime and may provide an important link for referral to more comprehensive services when needed.

Violent crime has become a global issue, concerning people in every walk of life and in every country. Many victim outreach programs use crisis intervention techniques to identify the needs of victims and then to connect them with appropriate referrals and other resources. Patient concerns such as the personal meaning of the crime, who to tell, and the reaction of others should be discussed. A victim advocate can contact employers regarding the need for temporary time off, can mobilize community resources for food and shelter if necessary, and can arrange for grace periods with debtors to delay payment of bills without penalty until the victim recovers.

BOX 14-3

Common Psychiatric Responses to Disaster

Psychiatric Diagnoses
Organic mental disorders secondary to head injury, toxic exposure, illness, and dehydration
Acute stress disorder
Adjustment disorder
Substance use disorders
Major depression
Posttraumatic stress disorder
Generalized Anxiety Disorder
Psychological/Behavioral Responses
Grief reactions and other normal responses to an abnormal event
Family violence
Self-directed violence

Crisis intervention is successful in the immediate aftermath of rape. It uses an integrated framework of outreach, emergency care, and advocacy assistance. Nurses often work in rape crisis centers, where victims commonly are seen immediately after the rape. These victims need thorough evaluation, empathic support, information, and help with the legal system.

In this situation, the objectives of crisis intervention are to validate the crisis and criminal nature of the rape, carefully review the details of the rape, identify a supportive social network and self-enhancing ways of solving problems related to the rape and any subsequent events, and identify referral resources for follow-up care that may be needed to help the patient through the often prolonged aftermath (Osterman, Barbiaz, and Johnson, 2001; Resnick et al, 2000).

Another important issue is that of abusive relationships. Whether the victim is a spouse, a child, a date, an elderly person, or a caregiver, abusive relationships are experienced by people of both genders and of all racial, ethnic, economic, educational, and religious backgrounds. The widespread incidence and complex nature of abusive adult intimate relationships has been well documented. Nurses are often in ideal situations to identify and intervene with these people, most of whom are women. The nurse's validation of and response to people in abusive relationships is one component of a unified community-wide response that is headed by local domestic violence programs in many communities and is needed in all communities to prevent violence and abuse in the home. Chapter 39 presents more information regarding care of survivors of violence.

Health Education

Although health education can take place during the entire crisis intervention process, it is emphasized during the evaluation phase. At this time the patient's anxiety has decreased, so better use can be made of cognitive abilities. The nurse and patient summarize the course of the crisis, and the intervention is to teach the patient how to avoid other similar crises.

For example, the nurse helps the patient identify the feelings, thoughts, and behaviors experienced following the stressful event. The nurse explains that if these feelings, thoughts, and behaviors are again experienced, the patient should immediately become aware of being stressed and take steps to prevent the anxiety from increasing. The nurse then teaches the patient ways to use these newly learned coping mechanisms in future situations.

Nurses also are involved in identifying people who are at high risk for developing crises and in teaching coping strategies to help them avoid the development of the crises. For example, coping strategies that can be taught include how to request information, access resources, and obtain support.

The public also needs education so that they can identify those needing crisis services, be aware of available services, change their attitudes so that people will feel free to seek services, and obtain information about how others deal with potential crisis-producing problems. For example, a mother who learns about reactions to rape may identify her daughter as being a rape victim. She then may take her daughter to the nearest rape crisis center. The mother, in encouraging her daughter to go to the crisis center, tells her daughter that rape is not the fault of the victim, thus enabling her to change her attitude about the rape and feel positive about obtaining outside help. At the center the mother may be given a pamphlet that describes how to help rape victims, which she shares with friends so that they can cope quickly and effectively if their loved ones are raped.

Explain how conducting a group on stress management for critical care nurses is an example of health education as crisis intervention. ■

COMPETENT CARING

A Clinical Exemplar of a Psychiatric Nurse: Nurses Remember 9/11
MARIA GATTO, NYU DIVISION OF NURSING

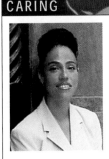

A Student's View

The doctor brought us to Firehouse 10, located at Greenwich and Liberty. I stood in amazement, taking in the environment that would be my home for the next few days. There was no front door or wall to the station house because it had been blown out. It was dark, dim and filthy with thick layers of dust, ash, and debris from the fallout. There were two small tables, one gurney, a coat rack that was fashioned into a makeshift IV pole, hung with a few bags of solution and tubing. There were also a few tanks of oxygen, a defibrillator, and an emergency crash box. Two other people, a retired lawyer turned EMT from Pennsylvania and a medical resident, walked into the station and joined us. We all sat down and looked out. For the first time that day, I really saw what no photograph, news report, or television footage could ever capture.

Ground Zero was a mountain of concrete, mangled steel, dirt, debris, and rubble . . . absolute devastation and destruction.

Silently we sat, exchanging a sober moment. There was nothing for us to do. Or was there?

Hundreds of people were working in a synchronized bucket brigade. A community banded together on their hands and knees trying to clear and unearth anything to bring home to the thousands waiting to celebrate or mourn. Our duty was right there in front of us. We joined the digging effort.

On our hands and knees, we dug with a purposeful rhythm. The ground underneath me was very hot, and the air was dense with choking fumes. I filled buckets with dirt and debris. Then signs of what was once a work force of thousands began to appear.

First it was the occasional business card, parts of a day planner with smeared notes, then pieces of a briefcase. This brought me closer to what I feared the most. A shoe—and then the foot.

I called out to a rescue worker, a towering man, rough and filthy with the day's events. He placed the remains carefully into a container and walked it down the mountain, cradling it like a baby. I said a silent prayer for this kind man who had just taught me one of the gravest lessons a nurse could learn:

In life we celebrate, in death we respect. ■

Continued

COMPETENT CARING

A Clinical Exemplar of a Psychiatric Nurse: Nurses Remember 9/11–cont'd
ANGELA APUZZO, NYU DIVISION OF NURSING

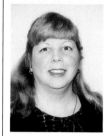

A Faculty's View

This is what I want to tell you about the profession of nursing. Nursing is not a nine-to-five job. It's a way of life that you have pledged yourselves to follow.

In school, professors cram your head with knowledge and nursing diagnoses. They help you develop critical thinking and try to show you how a nurse functions in clinical settings. They give you the tools you need to perform your professional duties. But we have to internalize this knowledge and make it our own.

We are nurses, members of a group that enjoys the highest level of trust of any profession. Patients believe nurses act as their advocates. In turn, we accept them as they are. We leave the security of our own selves and enter into the patients' worlds. When we are truly there, we can see their point of view and are able to help them to achieve healing and wellness.

Here's what I learned from September 11: *keep learning*, for nurses must function in unexpected settings and carry out a wide range of duties; *share yourself*, for it takes a brave heart to open yourself to pain and suffering; *always do your best*, for when you show that you care you are giving the best of clinical nursing. ■

The nurse educates the public by participating in programs in the media, by leading or participating in educational groups in the community, and by taking every opportunity to advertise crisis services. For instance, if a nurse is a member of a church group that has developed crisis services, the availability of these services should be shared with school staff members and parent-teacher associations. Nurses, as health care professionals, have a great opportunity to provide health education and crisis intervention, thus preventing mental illness and promoting mental health.

CHAPTER FOCUS POINTS

- A crisis is a disturbance caused by a stressful event or a perceived threat. The person's usual way of coping becomes ineffective in dealing with the threat, causing anxiety.
- Successful resolution of the crisis is more likely if the person has a realistic view of the event, if situational supports are available to help solve the problem, and if effective coping mechanisms are present.
- There are two types of crises: maturational and situational. Maturational crises are developmental events requiring role changes. Situational crises occur when a life event upsets an individual's or group's psychological equilibrium.
- Crisis intervention is a short-term therapy focused on solving the immediate problem, usually limited to 6 weeks. The goal of crisis intervention is for the individual to return to a precrisis level of functioning. Often the person advances to a level of growth that is higher than the precrisis level because new ways of problem solving have been learned.
- A number of balancing factors are important in the development and resolution of a crisis and should be assessed: precipitating event or stressor; patient's perception of the event or stressor; nature and strength of the patient's support systems and coping resources; and patient's previous strengths and coping mechanisms.
- To help identify the precipitating event, the nurse should explore the patient's needs, the events that threaten those needs, and the time at which symptoms appear. Four kinds of needs that have been identified are related to self-esteem, role mastery, dependency, and biological function.
- There are four levels of crisis intervention—environmental manipulation, general support, generic approach, and individual approach—that represent a hierarchy from the most basic to the most complex.
- Environmental manipulation includes interventions that directly change the patient's physical or interpersonal situation. These interventions provide situational support or remove stress.
- Important elements of this intervention are mobilizing the patient's supporting social systems and serving as a liaison between the patient and social support agencies.

- General support includes interventions that convey the feeling that the nurse is on the patient's side and will be a helping person. The nurse uses warmth, acceptance, empathy, caring, and reassurance to provide this type of support.
- The generic approach is designed to reach high-risk individuals and large groups as quickly as possible. It applies a specific method to all people faced with a similar type of crisis.
- The individual approach is a type of crisis intervention similar to the diagnosis and treatment of a specific problem in a specific patient. The nurse must understand the specific patient characteristics that led to the present crisis and must use the intervention that is most likely to help the patient develop an adaptive response to the crisis.
- The nurse should be creative and flexible, trying many different techniques. These should be active, focused, and explorative to carry out the interventions. Some of these include catharsis, clarification, suggestion, reinforcement of behavior, support of defenses, raising self-esteem, and exploration of solutions.
- The nurse should give patients credit for successful changes so that they can realize their effectiveness and understand that what they learned from a crisis may help in coping with future crises.
- Crisis intervention can be implemented in any setting and should be a competency skill of all nurses, regardless of specialty area.
- Crisis intervention modalities are based on the philosophy that the health care team must be aggressive and go out to the patients rather than wait for the patients to come to them. Nurses working in these modalities intervene in a variety of community settings, ranging from patients' homes to street corners.
- Mobile crisis programs throughout the country vary in the services they provide and the procedures they use. However, they are usually able to provide on-site assessment, crisis management, treatment, referral, and educational services to patients, families, law enforcement officers, and the community at large.
- Crisis groups follow the same steps that individual intervention follows. The nurse and group help the patient solve the problem and reinforce the patient's new problem-solving behavior.

CHAPTER **FOCUS POINTS**—cont'd

- Crisis intervention is sometimes practiced by telephone or Internet communication rather than through face-to-face contacts. When individuals in crisis use the telephone or Internet, it is usually when they are at the peak of their distress.
- As part of the community, nurses are called on when situational crises strike the community.
- Many victim outreach programs use crisis intervention techniques to identify the needs of victims and then to connect them with appropriate referrals and other resources.

- Although health education can take place during the entire crisis intervention process, it is emphasized during the evaluation phase. Nurses are involved in identifying people who are at high risk for developing crises and in teaching coping strategies to avoid the development of the crises. The public also needs education so that they can identify those needing crisis services, be aware of available services, change their attitudes so that people will feel free to seek services, and obtain information about how others deal with potential crisis-producing problems.

KEY TERMS

catharsis, 228
crisis, 221
crisis intervention, 225

debriefing, 227
maturational crises, 223
situational crises, 223

CHAPTER REVIEW QUESTIONS

1. Match each term in Column A with the correct definition in Column B.

Column A

_____ Catharsis
_____ Clarification between certain events
_____ Reinforcement of behavior
_____ Exploration of solutions
_____ Raising self-esteem
_____ Suggestion
_____ Support of defenses

Column B

A. Encourage the patient to express more clearly the relationship between certain events
B. Encourage the use of healthy, adaptive defenses and discourage those that are unhealthy or manipulative
C. Examining alternative ways of solving the immediate problem
D. Giving the patient positive responses to adaptive behavior
E. Helping the patient to regain feelings of self-worth
F. Influencing an individual to accept an idea or belief (for example, that the nurse can help and the patient will feel better)
G. The release of feelings that takes place as the patient talks about emotionally charged areas

2. Fill in the blanks.

A. A disturbance caused by a stressful event or perceived threat to self that challenges the individual's usual coping mechanisms is

a _____.

B. In crisis theory, perceived losses, threats of loss, or challenges that precede the stressor or threat are called

_____.

C. Crisis intervention is an active therapy, usually limited in time, with the goal of returning the patient to a

_____ level of functioning.

D. The first step of crisis intervention is _____.

E. When the nurse teaches the patient or the public principles of crisis intervention and healthy coping mechanisms in times of crisis, he or she is acting in the role of

_____.

3. Indicate whether the following statements are true (T) or false (F).

_____ A. When a person's usual way of coping becomes ineffective in dealing with a threat, the result is usually anxiety.

_____ B. A crisis, by definition, is a chronic, long-term event requiring 12 or more months of treatment.

_____ C. The fact that crises can lead to personal growth is important to remember when working with patients in crisis.

_____ D. The patient's perception or appraisal of the precipitating events of a crisis is a relatively unimportant factor in crisis intervention.

_____ E. The level of crisis intervention designed to reach high-risk individuals and large groups quickly, and that applies specific methods to similar types of crises, is the individual approach.

4. Provide short answers for the following questions.

A. List the two types of crisis and briefly describe each one.
B. Briefly describe cultural factors to be considered in crisis intervention.
C. Think of a crisis you have experienced in the past year. Identify which of the balancing factors of crisis intervention helped you cope positively with the event and which ones could have helped you even more.

Visit Evolve for additional resources related to the content of this chapter.

http://evolve.elsevier.com/Stuart/principles/
• Topical Course Outline • Student Workbook Exercises • Critical Thinking Questions and Activities • Case Studies • Research Topics
• Monthly Content Updates • WebLinks

Student Study CD-ROM

Access the accompanying CD-ROM for animations, interactive exercises, review questions for the NCLEX examination, and an audio glossary.

REFERENCES

Adams S et al: Mental health disaster response: nursing interventions across the life span, *J Psychosoc Nurs Ment Health Serv* 37:11, 1999.

Aguilera DC: *Crisis intervention: theory and methodology*, ed 8, St Louis, 1998, Mosby.

AJN News: September 11: health effects linger, *Am J Nurs* 102:18, 2002.

Badger JM: Understanding secondary traumatic stress, *Am J Nurs* 101:26, 2001.

Ball J, Allen K: Consensus recommendations for responding to children's emergencies in disasters, *Natl Acad Pract Forum* 2:253, 2000.

Constantino RE, Sekula LK, Rubinstein EN: Group intervention for widowed survivors of suicide, *Suicide Life Threat Behav* 31:428, 2001.

Coombes R: Home front, *Nurs Times* 96:54, 2000.

DeLisi L et al: A survey of New Yorkers after the Sept. 11, 2001, terrorist attacks, *Am J Psychiatry* 160:780, 2003.

Drenkard K et al: Healthcare system disaster preparedness, part 1: readiness planning, *J Nurs Adm* 32:461, 2002.

Flynn BW: Thoughts and reflections after the bombing of the Alfred P Murrah Federal Building in Oklahoma City, *J Am Psychiatr Nurs Assoc* 1:166, 1995.

Franklin J et al: Hurricane Floyd: response of the Pitt County Medical Community, *N C Med J* 61:384, 2000.

French ED, Sole ML, Byers JF: A comparison of nurses' needs/concerns and hospital disaster plans following Florida's Hurricane Floyd, *J Emerg Nurs* 28:111, 2002.

Gou S et al: Assessing the impact of community-based mobile crisis services on preventing hospitaltization, *Psychiatr Serv* 52:223, 2001.

Grosz CA, Kempe RS, Kelly M: Extrafamilial sexual abuse: treatment for child victims and their families, *Child Abuse Negl* 24:9, 2000.

Haber J et al: When trauma doesn't end…., *J Am Psychiatr Nurs Assoc* 8:174, 2002.

Kaplan Z, Iancu I, Bodner E: A review of psychological debriefing after extreme distress, *Psychiatr Serv* 52:824, 2001.

NY Board of Education, http://www.nycenet.edu/offices/spss/wtc_needs/firstep.pdf, 2002.

Norwood A et al: Disaster psychiatry: principles and practice, *Am Psychiatr Assoc Pract Psych*, www.psych.prg, 9/4/2002.

Osterman JE, Chemtob CM: Emergency intervention for acute traumatic stress, *Psychiatr Serv* 50:739, 1999.

Osterman JE, Barbiaz J, Johnson P: Emergency psychiatry: emergency interventions for rape victims, *Psychiatr Serv* 52:733, 2001.

Ottenstein RJ: Supporting remote and complicated critical incidents through e-mail support teams, *Int J Emerg Ment Health* 4:213, 2002.

Pandya A, Weiden P: Trauma and disaster in psychiatrically vulnerable populations, *J Psychiatr Pract* 7:426, 2001.

Reid W: Psychological aspects of terrorism, *J Psychiatr Pract* 7:422, 2001.

Resnick H et al: Emergency evaluation and intervention with female victims of rape and other violence, *Psychiatr Serv* 50:1317, 2000.

Ripley A: Grief lessons, *Time*, vol 96, October 29, 2001.

Shields L: Crisis intervention: implications for the nurse, *J Psychiatr Nurs* 13:37, 1975.

Stanley SR: When the disaster is over: helping the healers to mend, *J Psychosoc Nurs Ment Health Serv* 28:12, 1990.

Steadman H et al: A specialized crisis response site as a core element of police-based diversion programs, *Psychiatr Serv* 52:219, 2001.

Stuart G, Huggins E: Caring for the caretakers in times of disaster, *J Child Adolesc Psychiatr Nurs* 3:144, 1990.

Tucker P et al: Oklahoma City: disaster challenges mental health and medical administrators, *J Behav Health Serv Res* 25:93, 1998.

Weaver J et al: The American Red Cross disaster mental health services: development of a cooperative, single function, multidisciplinary service model, *J Behav Health Serv Res* 27:314, 2000.

Zealberg JJ, Hardesty SJ, Tyson SC: Mental health clinicians' role in responding to critical incidents in the community, *Psychiatr Serv* 49:301, 1998.

Of equality—as if it harm'd me giving others the same chances and rights as myself—as if it were not indispensable to my own rights that others possess the same.

WALT WHITMAN, *THOUGHT*

PSYCHIATRIC REHABILITATION AND RECOVERY

15

Sandra J. Sundeen

 Visit Evolve for additional resources related to the content of this chapter.
http://evolve.elsevier.com/Stuart/principles/

Any episode of illness may involve a lasting change in a person's level of functioning. A person who has been seriously ill is more likely to have problems living productively in the community. Hospitalization is especially disruptive, and it is often difficult to adjust after discharge. Nurses need to be aware of the total range of patient care needs both during and after hospitalization.

■ TERTIARY PREVENTION IN PSYCHIATRIC CARE

The goal of tertiary prevention is to limit the amount of disability and maladaptive functioning resulting from an illness. Although concepts of tertiary prevention can be applied to anyone who has experienced an episode of illness, they are particularly relevant to those with serious and persistent mental illnesses, sometimes called *chronic mental illness*. Because of the stigma associated with the term **chronic**, the term **serious mental illness** is used in this chapter.

It is estimated that 5.4% of adults in the United States have a serious mental illness. Nurses care for these people in a variety of settings: private and public psychiatric hospitals, psychiatric and medical-surgical units in general hospitals, emergency rooms, community-based treatment and rehabilitation programs, and patients' homes. As patients alternate between community-based and hospital-based care, nurses in all settings share responsibility for their care. Knowledge of the special needs and characteristics of this population is essential for all nurses.

Rehabilitation

Tertiary prevention is carried out through activities identified as rehabilitation, which is the process of helping the person return to the highest possible level of functioning. **Psychiatric rehabilitation is the range of social, educational, occupational, behavioral, and cognitive interventions used to increase the role performance of persons with serious and persistent mental illness and to enhance their recovery** (Barton, 1999).

Psychiatric rehabilitation grew out of a need to create opportunities for people diagnosed with severe mental illness to live, learn, and work in their own communities. It proposes that mental illness should be perceived as a disability. Like people with physical disabilities, people with psychiatric disabilities need a wide range of services, often for extended periods of time. Psychiatric rehabilitation uses a person-centered, people-to-people approach that differs from the traditional medical model of care (Table 15-1). It is supported by research findings related to people with long-term mental illness.

Table 15-1   **Comparison of Psychiatric Rehabilitation and Traditional Medical Models of Care**

ASPECT OF CARE	PSYCHIATRIC REHABILITATION	TRADITIONAL MEDICAL REHABILITATION
Focus	Focus on wellness and health, not symptoms	Focus on disease, illness, and symptoms
Basis	Based on person's abilities and functional behavior	Based on person's disabilities and intrapsychic functioning
Setting	Caregiving in natural setting	Treatment in institutional settings
Relationship	Adult-to-adult relationship	Expert-to-patient relationship
Medication	Medicate as appropriate and tolerate some illness symptoms	Medicate until symptoms are controlled
Decision making	Case management in partnership with patient	Physician makes decisions and prescribes treatment
Emphasis	Emphasis on strengths, self-help, and interdependence	Emphasis on dependence and compliance

---

BOX 15-1

Attributes of Effective Rehabilitation Treatment Teams

- Accessibility, preferably 24 hours a day and 7 days a week, as an entity or in league with other organizations or practitioners
- Consultation and coordination of services with agencies and practitioners external to the team, especially community support programs, such as housing agencies, employers, schools, residential care operators, Social Security offices, and state vocational agencies
- Priority given to persons with serious and disabling mental disorders
- Focus on improvement in symptoms, work and education, peer relationships, family relationships, community reintegration, personal hygiene, spiritual life, recreation, and housing
- Emphasis on community reintegration in normalized environments of work education, housing recreation, religious activities, and civic and political life
- Availability of personnel to meet the cultural and linguistic needs of consumers
- Maximization of clients' natural supports and self-help through encouraging their active participation in identifying personally relevant goals, selecting treatment plans, collaborating with the treatment team through problem solving, and advocating for their own needs with assistance from families and friends

- Flexible levels of intervention, from crisis services to long-term maintenance and reinforcement of stability and recovery, with an emphasis on clients' taking control of their own lives for community adaptation and reintegration
- Individualization of services so that evidence-based services are linked to phase, type, and severity of clients' disorders and adapted to enable clients to attain their own personally relevant goals in gradual steps
- Ongoing monitoring of clients' progress toward treatment and rehabilitation goals; with optimal remission of symptoms, recovery of psychosocial functioning, and improvements in quality of life, the primary aims of quality improvement in care plans
- Persistent effort with each client, linked with realistic optimism for gradual improvement in symptoms, functioning, and quality of life
- Accountability of the team to its administration and funding source; to team members; to clients, their families, and their natural supporters; and to all other stakeholders in the community
- Competencies available collectively to the team members that enable high-quality delivery of evidence-based services

From Liberman RP et al: *Psychiatr Serv* 52:1331, 2001.

Although research has reported that there are interventions that effectively assist people who have serious mental illnesses function productively in their communities, these have not been widely adopted by service providers, including nurses (Wang, Demler, and Kessler, 2002). This is reflected in the report of the New Freedom Commission on Mental Health, *Achieving the Promise: Transforming Mental Health Care in America* (2003), which endorses recovery as an essential goal of the mental health care system.

Following the publication of *Mental Health: Report of the Surgeon General* (USDHHS, 1999), the federal Substance Abuse and Mental Health Services Administration (SAMHSA) funded the development of a series of packages of training materials to disseminate evidence-based practices. This was the first phase of a "Science to Service" initiative intended to make approaches that are supported by research widely available to patients and their families.

The first group of evidence-based practices disseminated that support and enhance psychiatric rehabilitation included the following: assertive community treatment, supported employment, illness management and recovery, integrated treatment for co-occurring mental illness and substance abuse, family psychoeducation, and medication management. All of these practices except integrated treatment for co-occurring mental illness and substance abuse (see Chapter 24) and medication management (see Chapter 27) are addressed in this chapter.

Rehabilitative psychiatric nursing takes place in the context of a multidisciplinary treatment team. Other team members may include psychiatrists, psychologists, social workers, occupational therapists, rehabilitation counselors, case managers, consumer team members, family advocates, employment specialists, or job coaches (Liberman et al, 2001). The attributes of effective rehabilitation treatment teams are listed in Box 15-1.

Compare the principles of psychiatric rehabilitation with your knowledge of physical rehabilitation. How do the principles affect nursing intervention? ■

Rehabilitative psychiatric nursing also must be studied in the contexts of the patient and social system. This requires the nurse to focus on three elements: the individual, the family, and the community. The nursing care of people with serious mental illnesses is related to these three elements and the activities of assessment, planning and implementation, and evaluation.

Recovery

Traditionally, serious mental illness has been viewed as incurable, with a progressively deteriorating course. This assumption was discouraging to patients, families, and mental health professionals. It led to treatment focused mainly on maintenance of the person's existing level of functioning.

In the 1970s patients who were frustrated with the limited options that were available to them began to form consumer advocacy groups and brought forward the concept of recovery from serious mental illnesses. At the same time psychiatric care was moving from long-term hospitals to community settings, especially psychiatric rehabilitation programs. Traditional treatment had focused on deficits in functioning; psychiatric rehabilitation focuses on strengths and abilities. The rehabilitation philosophy is supportive of the goal of recovery.

Recovery is defined as the "process in which people are able to live, work, learn and participate fully in their communities. For some individuals, recovery is the ability to live a fulfilling and productive life despite a disability. For others, recovery implies the reduction or complete remission of symptoms. Science has shown that having hope plays an integral role in an individual's recovery" (NFCMH, 2003, p. 5).

The following are characteristics of recovery as described by persons recovering from serious mental illnesses themselves (Ralph, 2000):

- **Internal factors:** Factors that are within the consumer, such as awareness of the toll the illness has taken, recognition of the need to change, insight as to how this change can begin, and the determination it takes to recover
- **Self-managed care:** An extension of the internal factors in which consumers describe how they manage their own mental health and how they cope with the difficulties and barriers they face
- **External factors:** Include interconnectedness with others, the supports provided by family, friends, and professionals, and having people around them who believe that they can cope with, and recover from, their mental illness
- **Empowerment:** A combination of internal and external factors—where internal strengths are combined with interconnectedness to provide self-help, advocacy, and caring about what happens to oneself and to others

Another model proposes that recovery is related to the interaction between internal and external conditions (Jacobson and Greenley, 2001). These are presented in Box 15-2.

BOX 15-2

Internal and External Conditions That Influence Recovery

Internal Conditions
- **Hope:** The person's belief that recovery is possible
- **Healing:** Defining a self apart from illness and control
- **Empowerment:** Correction for feelings of lack of control, helplessness, and dependency
- **Connection:** Relating to others and finding one's roles in the world

External Conditions
- **Human rights:** Includes stigma and discrimination reduction and elimination; rights protection and promotion; equal opportunities for work, education, and housing; and access to needed resources
- **Positive culture of healing:** A service environment that demonstrates "tolerance, listening, empathy, compassion, respect, safety, trust, diversity, and cultural competence"
- **Recovery-oriented services:** Addressing consequences of serious mental illness by offering professional, consumer-to-consumer, and collaborative services that are based on a belief that recovery is possible

Adapted from Jacobson N, Greenley D: *Psychiatr Serv* 52:482, 2001.

ASSESSMENT

The Individual

Assessment of the need for rehabilitation and recovery begins with the initial contact between the nurse and the patient. A comprehensive psychiatric nursing assessment provides information that enables the nurse to help the patient achieve maximum possible functioning. In addition to identifying deficits, nurses are expected to identify and reinforce strengths as one means of helping the patient cope. This is basic to the concepts of rehabilitation and recovery. Thus good nursing care is really rehabilitative nursing care.

The Stuart Stress Adaptation Model can be applied within the context of rehabilitative nursing practice. It is important for the nurse to identify stressors that may interfere with the patient's adjustment to a health-promoting lifestyle. Nurses need to be aware of patients' perceptions of their experiences. It is also essential to validate each person's response to significant life changes.

When conducting an initial assessment, the nurse needs to assist the patient to plan for recovery by identifying strengths and discussing services available from the health care system and the person's social support network. In hospitals this process is provided through discharge planning. Nurses in community settings also should expect patients to progress to other levels of care as they recover. Although some people will need long-term outpatient care, others will be discharged from psychiatric care.

What changes does the recovery model require in the traditional attitudes and behaviors of psychiatric nurses? ■

Characteristics of Serious Mental Illness.

People who have serious mental illnesses are likely to have both primary and secondary symptoms. **Primary symptoms** are directly caused by the illness. For example, hallucinations and delusions are primary symptoms of schizophrenia, and elation and hyperactivity are primary symptoms of bipolar disorder. **Secondary symptoms** such as loneliness and social isolation are caused by the person's response to the illness or its treatment.

Behaviors related to primary symptoms may violate social norms and be considered deviant. Society then tries to protect itself from the person's norm violation. An example of this is community opposition to the establishment of group homes. As behavior problems become more serious, people increasingly identify themselves as mentally ill. They begin to relate to society in terms of this identity rather than others, such as wife, mother, husband, father, or worker.

The person's acceptance of mentally ill status and adjustment to society in terms of this role are accompanied by the secondary symptoms of serious mental illness. A nursing study of the perceptions of people with serious mental illness identified the following themes related to secondary symptoms (Vellenga and Christenson, 1994):

- **Stigmatization** or the sense of being discredited or shamed because of their illness
- **Alienation** caused by the outcome of being stigmatized and ostracized
- **Loss** of relationships and vocational opportunities
- **Distress** caused by the effects of the illness and one's related suffering
- **Acceptance** of oneself as having a mental illness and the need for acceptance by others

Behaviors Related to Serious Mental Illness.

People with serious mental illnesses are often unemployed, less likely to be involved in close relationships, and tend to have fewer financial resources than their peers. The exact causes of these characteristics have not been identified. Some could be related to primary and secondary symptoms or disabilities of the illness and others to society's reaction to the person with mental illness.

Attitudes that could contribute to this reaction are illustrated by the list of myths about people with mental illness (Box 15-3). None of these myths is true, but they are commonly believed and stigmatize people with mental illness (Dickerson et al, 2002). This often prevents people with mental illness from gaining access to needed services and opportunities.

Stigma experienced by those who are mentally ill also has been linked to low self-esteem. In a study of two aspects of stigma (devaluation-discrimination and social withdrawal because of perceived rejection), it was found that members of a psychiatric rehabilitation program who experienced higher amounts of stigma scored lower on measures of self-esteem (Link et al, 2001).

Copy the list of myths about mental illness and discuss them with a group of people who have little personal experience with mental illness.

Then discuss the list with a small group of people who have a serious mental illness. Compare the responses of the two groups. ■

Activities of daily living. Activities of daily living (ADLs) are the skills that are necessary to live independently, such as housekeeping, shopping, food preparation, money management, and personal hygiene. A major goal of psychosocial rehabilitation is to help the person develop independent living skills.

Interpersonal relations. People who have serious mental illnesses are often described as apathetic, withdrawn, and socially isolated. As more is learned about the nature of neurobiological disorders, it is becoming apparent that these difficulties are related to the primary symptoms of the illness. For instance, depression causes apathy and withdrawal, and schizophrenia leads to problems in perceiving and processing communications from others. These behaviors create serious problems in establishing close relationships. Nonetheless, formal and informal networks are needed by the seriously mentally ill (Pickens, 1999).

Low self-esteem. Self-esteem is the feeling of self-worth or regard for oneself. It is difficult to maintain high self-esteem when a person is aware of low achievement compared to cultural expectations. Lack of ability to maintain employment, live independently, marry, and have children contributes to low self-esteem. People who have serious mental illnesses often feel cheated of the life experiences they expected to enjoy before they became ill.

One mental health professional who also has a serious mental illness describes her experience of being diagnosed with schizophrenia during adolescence (Deegan, 1993):

> I was told I had a disease that was like diabetes, and if I continued to take neuroleptic medications for the rest of my life and avoided stress, I might be able to cope. I remember that as these words were spoken to me by my psychiatrist it felt as if my whole teenage world—in which I aspired to dreams of being a valued person in valued roles, of playing lacrosse for the U.S. Women's Team or maybe joining the Peace Corps—began to crumble and shatter. It felt as if these parts of my identity were being stripped from me. I was beginning to undergo that radically dehumanizing and devaluing transformation from being a person to being an illness; from being Pat Deegan to being a schizophrenic.

Motivation. For many people with serious mental illness, success and greater competence result in increased anxiety, causing regression, rather than in pride and continued progress. Patients attribute their uneasiness with success to fear that it will lead to higher expectations by others that they may not be able to attain. Fear of failure often results in reluctance to try new experiences. This may be perceived by others as lack of motivation. Apparent lack of motivation also may be caused by low energy. This can be related to the biological effect of the illness or to medication. In this case the person may want to be more active but is physically unable.

Strengths. Rehabilitation and recovery depend on the control of illness, as well as on the development of health po-

BOX **15-3**

Misconceptions About Mental Illness—Pervasive and Damaging

MYTH 1: Psychiatric disorders are not true medical illnesses like heart disease and diabetes. People who have a mental illness are just "crazy."

FACT: Brain disorders, like heart disease and diabetes, are legitimate medical illnesses. Research shows genetic and biological causes for psychiatric disorders, and they can be treated effectively.

MYTH 2: People with a severe mental illness, such as schizophrenia, are usually dangerous and violent.

FACT: Statistics show that the incidence of violence in people who have a brain disorder is not much higher than it is in the general population. Those suffering from a psychosis such as schizophrenia are more often frightened, confused, and despairing than violent.

MYTH 3: Mental illness is the result of bad parenting.

FACT: Most experts agree that a genetic susceptibility, combined with other risk factors, leads to a psychiatric disorder. In other words, mental illnesses have a physical cause.

MYTH 4: Depression results from a personality weakness or character flaw, and people who are depressed could just snap out of it if they tried hard enough.

FACT: Depression has nothing to do with being lazy or weak. It results from changes in brain chemistry or brain function, and medication and/or psychotherapy often help people recover.

MYTH 5: Schizophrenia means split personality, and there is no way to control it.

FACT: Schizophrenia is often confused with multiple personality disorder. Actually, schizophrenia is a brain disorder that robs people of their ability to think clearly and logically. The estimated 2.5 million Americans with schizophrenia have symptoms ranging from social withdrawal to hallucinations and delusions. Medication has helped many of these individuals to lead fulfilling, productive lives.

MYTH 6: Depression is a normal part of the aging process.

FACT: It is not normal for older adults to be depressed. Signs of depression in older people include a loss of interest in activities, sleep disturbances, and lethargy. Depression in the elderly is often undiagnosed, and it is important for seniors and their family members to recognize the problem and seek professional help.

MYTH 7: Depression and other illnesses, such as anxiety disorders, do not affect children or adolescents. Any problems they have are just a part of growing up.

FACT: Children and adolescents can develop severe mental illnesses. In the United States, 1 in 10 children and adolescents has a mental disorder severe enough to cause impairment. However, only about 20% of these children receive needed treatment. Left untreated, these problems get worse. Anyone talking about suicide should be taken very seriously.

MYTH 8: If you have a mental illness, you can will it away. Being treated for a psychiatric disorder means an individual has in some way "failed" or is weak.

FACT: A serious mental illness cannot be willed away. Ignoring the problem does not make it go away, either. It takes courage to seek professional help.

MYTH 9: Addiction is a lifestyle choice and shows lack of willpower. People with a substance abuse problem are morally weak or "bad."

FACT: Addiction is a disease that generally results from changes in brain chemistry. It has nothing to do with being a "bad" person.

MYTH 10: Electroconvulsive therapy (ECT), formerly known as "shock treatment" is painful and barbaric.

FACT: ECT has given a new lease on life to many people who suffer from severe and debilitating depression. It is used when other treatments such as psychotherapy or medication fail or cannot be used. Patients who receive ECT are asleep and under anesthesia, so they do not feel anything.

As printed in NARSAD's (National Alliance for Research on Schizophrenia and Depression) Research Newsletter, vol. 13, Issue 4, Winter 2001/2002.

tential by mobilizing strengths. A strength is an ability, skill, or interest that a person has used before. An emphasis on strengths provides hope that improved functioning is possible. Strengths may be related to recreational and leisure activities, work skills, educational accomplishments, self-care skills, special interests, talents and abilities, and positive interpersonal relationships. People with serious mental illness often need help in defining their skills, abilities, and interests as strengths. Low self-esteem may lead them to believe that they have only problems, not strengths.

Nonadherence. Failure to take medication is a common cause of rehospitalization. It is important to assess the reasons for nonadherence. There may be a denial of the illness or a lack of understanding of the reason for the treatment regimen. Sometimes the person wants to comply but needs help, such as transportation to a pharmacy or advice about obtaining a medical assistance card. Some patients do not like the side effects of their medication, but they may not be assertive enough to tell the prescriber about their discomfort.

The nurse can help patients by developing a therapeutic alliance with them, educating them about their illness and the beneficial effects of their treatment including medication, and engaging them in the treatment plan. Linking the benefits of medication to the achievement of personal goals is especially important. Teaching patients to write notes about their medicines and to keep lists of questions for the provider also may increase adherence.

Think about how medication adherence is influenced by all of the behaviors described above that are related to serious mental illness. How will this knowledge impact your work with patients in relation to their medication? ∎

Table 15-2	Potential Skilled Activities Needed To Achieve the Goal of Psychiatric Rehabilitation	
PHYSICAL	**EMOTIONAL**	**INTELLECTUAL**
Living Skills		
Personal hygiene	Human relations	Money
Physical fitness	Self-control	management
Use of public	Selective reward	Use of commu-
transportation	Stigma reduction	nity resources
Cooking	Problem solving	Goal setting
Shopping	Conversational skills	Problem
Cleaning		development
Sports participation		
Using recreational		
facilities		
Learning Skills		
Being quiet	Speech making	Reading
Paying attention	Question asking	Writing
Staying seated	Volunteering	Arithmetic
Observing	answers	Study skills
Punctuality	Following directions	Hobby activities
	Asking for directions	Typing
	Listening	
Working Skills		
Punctuality	Job interviewing	Job qualifying
Use of job tools	Job decision making	Job seeking
Job strength	Human relations	Specific job tasks
Job transportation	Self-control	
Specific job tasks	Job keeping	
	Specific job tasks	

From Anthony WA: *Principles of psychiatric rehabilitation*, Baltimore, 1999, University Park Press.

Living Skills Assessment. The nursing assessment of a patient who has a serious mental illness should include an analysis of the physical, emotional, and intellectual components of the skills needed for living, learning, and working in the community. Table 15-2 presents a matrix of the skills required for successful functioning in the community.

The nurse may use these examples in working with the patient to identify strengths, establish goals, and set priorities for skill development. Such a model provides a rational basis for assessing the patient's readiness to function productively in the community. It also provides objective information on quality of life that can be shared with other mental health care providers (Skinner et al, 1999).

The Family

The image of isolated people with serious mental illness who return to a community where they have no connections has been widely publicized. However, most people with mental illness are involved with their families and have frequent contact with family members while they are in the community. Approximately 65% of people who have mental illnesses live with their families. Therefore family resources must be assessed when a rehabilitation plan is being developed.

Families and other caregivers can be a major source of support for individuals who have serious mental illnesses. Family members can help by identifying potential problem areas and enhancing the patient's compliance with the treatment plan. Thus they should be viewed as resources, caregivers, and collaborators by psychiatric nurses (see Chapter 11).

Unfortunately they are often overlooked and not provided with education about mental illness. This is frustrating to the family and interferes with their ability to assist in the patient's recovery. Although issues of confidentiality and respect for the patient's wishes regarding disclosure of treatment information must always be primary, nurses should strive as much as possible to include family members as partners in the treatment process.

Components of Family Assessment. The nurse who assesses the family as part of a rehabilitation plan should consider the following aspects of family dynamics:

- Family structure, including developmental stage, roles, responsibilities, norms, and values
- Family attitudes toward the mentally ill member
- The emotional climate of the family (fearful, angry, depressed, anxious, calm)
- The social supports that are available to the family, including extended family, friends, financial support, religious involvement, and community contacts
- Past family experiences with mental health services
- The family's understanding of the patient's problem and the plan of care

Some of this information may be obtained from other members of the treatment team. However, it is the nurse's responsibility to be available to the family. This includes regular planned contacts with the family and inclusion of the family as part of the treatment team.

Family Burden. The mental illness of a family member affects the entire family (Saunders, 1999). This impact is often called family burden. A survey was conducted of behaviors that family members found most disturbing, broken out by diagnosis. The most disturbing behaviors associated with schizophrenia were poor grooming and personal care, suspiciousness, and talking to oneself. For bipolar illness the most disturbing behaviors were lack of consideration of others, excessive arguing, upsetting neighbors and friends, unusual religious beliefs, and inappropriate sexual behavior. Depressed people had more problematic eating and sleeping behaviors and suicide attempts. It is also important to note that on nine other behaviors, such as lack of motivation, poor handling of money, difficulty in completing tasks, and noncompliance with medication, there were no differences among diagnostic groups (Hatfield et al, 1994).

Burden may be objective or subjective. Objective burden is related to the patient's behavior, role performance, adverse effects on the family, need for support, and financial costs of the illness. Subjective burden is the person's own feeling of being burdened; it is individual and not consistently related to the elements of objective burden.

For instance, a patient may lack ambition and remain in a dependent role well into adulthood. Family members who value success and upward mobility would be likely to feel more subjective burden related to this situation than members who are comfortable with nurturing and supporting someone. One study found that aspects of objective burden including ability to cope with the ill family member's behavior, worrying about the patient, and a strained relationship with the patient were associated with higher levels of subjective burden (Cuijpers and Stam, 2003).

By assessing family burden the nurse can work with the family to identify concerns with which they would like help. Several responses are frequently noted in families who have members with serious mental illness. It is helpful to consider these when assessing subjective burden.

Grief is common and is related to the loss of the person they knew before the illness, as well as loss of the future that they expected to share with the ill family member. Because serious mental illness is usually cyclical, grief tends to be recurrent; it subsides during remissions and returns during exacerbations. This is especially difficult for families to handle. In addition, social support systems may not recognize or respond to their need because of discomfort with the situation or the related stigma.

Guilt is another emotion that families may experience in relation to their relative's illness. It is common for those who are close to a person with any serious illness to wonder whether they could have done something to prevent it. For instance, the wife of a heart attack victim may think she could have prevented it if she had not encouraged him to shovel snow. Similarly, parents of a depressed woman may believe that they could have prevented her depression if they had not shared their own worries with her.

In neither of these situations did relatives cause the illnesses, but they feel guilt because of their interpretation of the situation. Another source of guilt for relatives of people with mental illness is the need to set limits on the patient's behavior at times. For instance, the family of a patient who is physically agitated may need to arrange hospitalization to keep the patient safe.

Anger may be directed toward the patient, but it is more often felt toward other family members, mental health care providers, or the entire health care system. Anger within the family relates to differing perceptions of the patient and varied ideas about how to manage the illness. Prolonged stress results in irritability that is often taken out on those to whom one is closest. Anger at the system often is justified because it is related to deficiencies in the accessibility or acceptability of needed mental health services.

Powerlessness and **fear** often result from families' realization that they are dealing with a long-term recurrent illness. Most people believe that the health care system should cure illnesses. When this is impossible, they feel powerless and frustrated. This understanding also can result in fear about the future of the ill family member, as well as fear for themselves. Powerlessness and fear are especially troublesome for parents who are aging and worried about care arrangements for their mentally ill child when they can no longer provide care themselves. Some families also fear ill members who may become dangerous if they stop complying with their treatment.

Ask if you can speak with a family member of one of your patients about their experience with their mentally ill family member. Try not to talk much; listen closely to what they have to share with you. ■

Social Support Needs. Families who are providing care for members who have serious mental illnesses often feel isolated and alone in dealing with the challenges of caregiving. Previous sources of social support may be lost or limited because of the demands of attending to the mentally ill family member.

Caregivers may be embarrassed about the illness or fear that the person with mental illness will behave inappropriately in the presence of others. Sometimes a family member may decide to stop working outside the home so he or she can be more available for the ill person. All of the aspects of the subjective burden of the illness also may limit access to social support systems. These families will need assistance in rebuilding their social supports.

Support also may be found within the family. Even though a mental illness can be stressful for all family members, many families meet this challenge with a great deal of resilience. The person who has the mental illness can contribute to the family also, helping to ease the stress on other members.

Nurses can play an important role in offering family members opportunities to discuss their concerns and taking action to meet their needs whenever possible. Table 15-3 lists support needs expressed by family caregivers.

The Community

The community greatly influences the rehabilitation and recovery of its mentally ill members. Mental health professionals have a unique role in the community because they are community members and also advocates for people with mental illness and their families at the same time. Care providers, including nurses, should assume a leadership role in assessing the adequacy and effectiveness of community resources and in recommending changes to improve access and quality of mental health care.

Nurses in all settings must be familiar with the community agencies that provide services to people with mental illnesses. Most communities have a social and medical services directory that can be consulted for basic information such as location, type, and cost of the services provided. Most agencies serve people who come from a particular geographical area such as one part of a city or, in a rural area, one or several counties.

As nurses gain experience, they will become familiar with other agencies that provide services for the same people. Nurses should pay attention to patients' evaluations of the agencies from which they receive services. This information helps to identify agencies that are responsive and helpful as opposed to those that are difficult for patients to approach.

Table 15-3	Support Needs Expressed by Family Caregivers
NEED	**DESCRIPTION**

Emotional Support

Acceptance	Absence of stigmatization; acceptance of the caregiver despite his or her relationship to a mentally ill patient
Commitment	Demonstrating to the caregiver a commitment to the well-being of the patient, or sharing the burden of caregiving, if only through contact with the caregiver
Social involvement	Social contacts and companionship for the caregiver
Affective	Showing love and caring for the caregiver, including concern for his or her well-being (with qualities of sympathy, compassion, and occasionally true empathy)
Mutuality	Reciprocity in supportive exchanges

Feedback Support

Affirmation	Validation of the actions, feelings, and decisions associated with the caregiving role
Listening	Active listening by the support person, provision of a sounding board, and allowing for unburdening by the caregiver
Talking	The opportunity to talk with another person (without the quality of active listening, emotional presence, or the feeling of unburdening)

Informational or Cognitive Support

Illness information	Information about the patient's illness, care, or supervision
Behavior management	Information about behavior management strategies
Coping	Advice about personal coping strategies for the caregiver
Decision	Help in the decision-making process around caregiving issues and offering solutions
Perspective	Supportive interactions that give the caregiver a new perspective about caregiving or about the caregiving situation

Instrumental Support

Resources	Help in locating resources, negotiating systems, or advocating for needs
Respite	Provision of time off for the caregiver and support for the caregiver's own needs
Care help	Provision of help with the actual tasks of caregiving, including physical care assistance and monitoring activities (watching the patient and setting limits)
Backup	Help is available when needed, including financial help
Household	Help with such home activities as repairs, grocery shopping, and housecleaning

From Norbeck J et al: *Nurs Res* 40:208, 1991.

Personal contact with community agencies can be a very useful part of a community assessment. This may be done by making an appointment with an agency staff member. However, a more realistic picture of an agency's services can be obtained by going to the agency with someone who is requesting services. The nurse will see how the agency responds to the patient and how well the patient is able to handle personal affairs in the community. The nurse also can provide emotional support if the patient feels insecure in a new situation. Nurses should introduce themselves to the staff of the agency and explain that they, as well as the patient, would like to learn more about the services. Collaborative relationships between mental health care providers and community agencies are essential if rehabilitation is to succeed.

A wide range of community services must be available to patients. Those that are directed toward basic needs include provisions for shelter, food, and clothing; household management; income and financial support; meaningful activities; and mobility and transportation. Other services provide for special needs that may differ from one person to the next, such as general medical services, mental health services, habilitation and rehabilitation programs, vocational services, and social services. A third group of services coordinates the system. These include patient identifi-

cation and outreach, individual assessment and service planning, case management, advocacy and community organization, community information, and education and support (see Chapter 35).

You are approached by the parent of a hospitalized young adult patient who has a serious mental illness. The family is upset because the discharge plan is to refer the patient to a community program that has not been helpful in the past. What nursing interventions would you suggest in this case? ■

PLANNING AND IMPLEMENTATION

The Individual

Treatment planning and intervention in rehabilitative psychiatric nursing focus on fostering independence by maximizing the person's strengths. This is directly parallel to the nurse's role in physical rehabilitation. It differs from nursing care that is given to patients when they are acutely ill. During acute illness, people require nurturing. The nurse must provide for all of the basic life functions that the person is unable to manage. However, the relationship becomes less dependent as patients grow stronger and are able to care for themselves. Residual functional deficits may remain. The nurse and patient must work together to find ways for the patient to overcome any remaining impaired areas of functioning.

In promoting rehabilitation and recovery, the nurse helps the individual to:

- **Develop his or her strengths and potential**
- **Learn living skills**
- **Manage one's illness**
- **Access environmental supports**

The nursing treatment plan should be organized around very specific behavioral goals that are based on a comprehensive assessment of the person's living skills. These goals should build on those that are developed during the acute phase of the illness. This part of the nursing care plan may be called the discharge plan in an inpatient treatment setting. Discharge plans also should be developed in community care settings. This will remind the nurse and patient that the expected outcome of nursing care is independent functioning.

Patients who need long-term medication often can receive maintenance prescriptions from their primary care or family practitioner as part of their general health care program. This helps to put the mental illness into perspective as a chronic health problem that is not so different from other chronic problems the person might have.

The nurse and patient must decide together on the desired level of functioning. If the patient is unwilling to take on activities that the nurse thinks would be helpful, it is important to determine why. Sometimes nurses try to push a patient ahead too rapidly. Behavior that has developed gradually over time cannot be changed quickly. Learning new behavior patterns and giving up old ones is frightening and causes anxiety.

The nurse must be sure that the patient's coping skills are adequate to deal with the stress of growth. Feedback must be requested to be sure that the rehabilitation plan continues to address the patient's needs. It is a problem if the plan assumes greater importance than the patient. The nurse must prevent this from happening.

It has been noted that patient nonadherence to treatment is due to a failure of the patient-clinician alliance. In what ways is this true? ■

Developing Strengths and Potential.

The development of the patient's strengths and potential is critically important. Nursing interventions that develop strengths and potentials can help patients develop independent living skills, interpersonal relationships, and coping resources and thus help meet their special needs.

Ultimately, the expected outcome of such interventions is change in the patient's self-concept and an increase in self-esteem (see Chapter 18). The negative self-concept and low self-esteem that characterize people who have serious mental illnesses interfere with their ability to see themselves as individuals with strengths and potentials.

Nurses are especially capable of assisting patients who have schizophrenia with difficulties in social functioning such as limited performance of usual social roles; limited social integration and contacts; and limited intimacy and sexual functioning. Assisting individuals to improve their functioning in these areas has a positive impact on quality of life (McDonald and Badger, 2002).

Through experiences of adequacy, self-concept can be altered and self-esteem increased. One intervention that helps patients alter their negative self-perceptions is for nurses to describe their perception of patients' strengths. Nursing interventions in which patients become aware of their strengths fall into two categories: those that occur spontaneously and those that are planned. The following clinical example illustrates a nurse's use of spontaneously occurring situations to increase awareness of strengths.

CLINICAL EXAMPLE

Theresa, a woman in her fifties, had been in and out of psychiatric hospitals for 30 years and had been living in a supervised apartment in the community for 1 year. Theresa shared the apartment with two roommates. She was a talented musician and had her own baby grand piano. Despite her love for classical music, she played only the "oldies and goodies" her roommates preferred. She said that she didn't want to upset her roommates by practicing classical music. She was afraid that if she brought the issue out in the open she might get so upset she would hurt someone. She offered as evidence the numerous times she'd been placed in seclusion rooms for violent behavior. Clearly, keeping peace was her priority.

The nurse and Theresa discussed her strengths as a peacemaker, as well as ways in which she might calmly express her own needs to her roommates. The nurse offered to be with Theresa during the discussion. Declining the nurse's offer, Theresa said that even though she was somewhat anxious, she had a clearer understanding of the abilities she had to use in the situation, and she wanted to try to "pick up" for herself in a situation of interpersonal conflict. She carried out her plan and expressed surprise that her roommates accepted her need and quickly arranged 2 hours a day for her to practice. As she told of her success, Theresa smiled, saying she wondered what would have happened if she had tried expressing her needs many months earlier.

Cindy, in her early twenties, had recently moved into the supervised apartment with Theresa and one other roommate. Cindy arrived at the day treatment program crying because she had fainted while at her nursing home job the evening before. She felt that in addition to having been embarrassed, she had failed to live up to the trust invested in her by the director of the nursing home. She had decided to quit her job.

The nurse explored with Cindy the meaning of these events in terms of her many strengths in caring for others. Her sensitivity to anticipated criticism and rejection from the director was related to the same sensitivity that allowed her to respond creatively to others' needs. At this point, Cindy firmly stated that the job was important to her sense of being needed. The nurse encouraged her to call the nursing home, express both her embarrassment and sense of failure, yet state that she wanted to continue working there. Cindy made the phone call with the nurse present for support. Her pleasure at finding out the job was still hers, that she was not viewed unfavorably by the director of nursing, and her sense of personal achievement at having taken a risk and won were so visible and contagious that the other patients staged an impromptu celebration.

Selected Nursing Diagnoses

- Theresa: Impaired social interaction related to fear of aggressive impulses, as evidenced by social inhibition
- Cindy: Chronic low self-esteem related to fear of rejection, as evidenced by feelings of inadequacy ■

Learning Living Skills. Social skills training uses cognitive and behavioral techniques to help people gain the knowledge and skills they need to live in the community (see Chapter 31). The patient is taught a structured way of examining and modifying his or her own thoughts and behavior that can be continued with decreasing clinician involvement as the patient becomes more skillful at managing difficult situations. These include holding conversations, establishing and maintaining friendships, dating, managing medications, grooming, and the numerous other activities that are a part of leading a happy, successful life.

Persons participating in social skills training should be assisted to express their problems as positive goals (Liberman and Kopelowicz, 2002). For example instead of the negative "I'm tired of watching television all the time," encourage the positive "I am going to see at least one friend every week." Social skills training programs typically use videotapes, role-playing, practice, and homework assignments centered on practical problems.

Another important aspect of psychiatric rehabilitation and recovery relates to promoting the physical well-being of those with serious mental illness. Problems such as high tobacco use, low exercise level, poor oral health, high-risk sexual behavior, and limited contact with physicians and dentists are common among people who have serious mental illnesses. Thus psychiatric nurses need to intervene in a holistic way in all health care settings with patients who experience serious and long-term psychiatric illness (see Citing the Evidence).

Illness management. Illness management is an evidence-based practice that is focused on assisting the patient to assume control over the illness and function at the highest possible level of independence.

Four interventions that have been identified to support illness management in persons recovering from psychiatric illness are (Mueser et al, 2002):

1. **Psychoeducation**: An approach that supports the rehabilitation process by teaching the patient and family about the mental illness and the coping skills that will help with successful community living. It is defined as the process of imparting illness management information in a way that can be understood and carried out by the individual.
2. **Behavioral tailoring for medication**: Developing strategies with the patient that integrate medication regimens into the person's daily routine and simplifying the medication schedule.
3. **Training in relapse prevention**: Most people who have serious mental illnesses can learn to recognize signs and symptoms of an approaching relapse. This

CITING THE EVIDENCE ON

Providing Health Information

BACKGROUND: The purpose of this descriptive study was to identify the sources of health promotion information used by persons with serious mental illness, as well as their perceptions of the sources' reliability.

RESULTS: The most health information was provided by the following top five sources in order from most to least: nonpsychiatrist physicians, psychiatrists, nurses, pharmacists, and families. Each was regarded as a reliable source. Still, the most information provided by any of the sources was only rated as "some" rather than "a lot". In this study, nurses and pharmacists were seen as providing more, and media and print sources as providing less, information than in similar studies with non-mentally ill study subjects.

IMPLICATIONS: Health care professionals provide the greatest quantity of health promotion information and are regarded as the most reliable sources of this information for those who have a serious mental illness. Previous research has shown that with support and accurate information, these patients may readily try to stop smoking, engage in exercise, reduce weight, or attempt other health promoting lifestyle modifications. Mental health professionals can substantially contribute to improving and lengthening the lives of such individuals. Those with mental illness are equally deserving of good health and high quality of life.

MacHaffie S: *Arch Psychiatr Nurs* 16:263, 2002.

enables them to seek early intervention, thereby increasing the chance that the episode of illness will be less severe and treated in the community.
4. **Coping skills training**: Teaching the person techniques for coping with persistent symptoms of the mental illness. For instance, training a person who has auditory hallucinations to listen to music using headphones, thus alleviating the distraction of the voices.

Adult learners require an individualized approach to education that focuses on their self-identified needs and engages them as active participants in the teaching-learning process. Psychoeducational curricula and materials should be individualized based on the characteristics of the learner. Techniques vary but the information conveyed to the patient and family usually covers all aspects of the illness and its treatment, as shown in Box 15-4.

Behaviors related to the mental illness may affect the person's ability to learn. It is particularly important to assess memory and attention span when preparing to implement psychoeducation. Cognitive behavioral interventions such as a token economy approach may then be used to improve impaired functioning in these areas. This type of intervention is especially helpful for individuals who have a serious mental illness and difficulty learning from a social skills training curriculum.

Consumers expect health teaching to be a part of the health care services they receive. Nurses are well prepared to offer this important intervention to patients, families, and communities. A more general Patient Education Plan for coping with psychiatric illness is presented in Table 15-4.

Elements of a Psychoeducation Plan

- Signs and symptoms
- Natural course of the illness
- Possible etiologies
- Diagnostic tests and measures
- Indicated lifestyle changes
- Treatment options
- Expected treatment outcomes
- Medication effects and side effects
- Therapeutic strategies
- Adaptive coping responses
- Potential compliance problems
- Early warning signs of relapse
- Balancing needs and taking care of oneself

Accessing Environmental Supports. Supporting people who have serious mental illnesses in community settings requires the development of a wide array of community support programs. Some of these are rehabilitation centers, housing services, employment opportunities, education, crisis intervention and outreach, and case management. When these services are provided, it has been demonstrated that people who otherwise would have spent much of their time in the hospital can live successfully in the community.

Rehabilitation programs. Psychiatric rehabilitation programs (also called *psychosocial rehabilitation*) were developed in response to the plight of people who had been discharged from state mental hospitals lacking the skills and resources needed to live independently. Several models are presented here as an overview of some of the psychiatric rehabilitation approaches that have evidence supporting their effectiveness.

FOUNTAIN HOUSE. Fountain House, in New York City, was established in the late 1940s by a group of former state mental hospital patients. It began as a consumer-operated program, but a decade later employed a professional staff. Many of the current psychiatric rehabilitation programs are built on the Fountain House (1999) model.

Table 15-4 PATIENT EDUCATION PLAN   Coping With Psychiatric Illness

CONTENT	INSTRUCTIONAL ACTIVITIES	EVALUATION
Identify and describe the patient's diagnosis.	Provide handouts outlining behaviors. Discuss coping resources and behaviors. Assign homework from lay literature. Compare mental illness to physical illness.	Patient recognizes characteristics of the diagnosis. Patient distinguishes between cure and coping.
Describe the role of stress in contributing to psychiatric disorders.	Sensitize the patient to signs of increased stress. Define stress as a test of coping skills. Teach relaxation exercises.	Patient verbalizes level of stress. Patient performs relaxation exercises and describes a reduction in perceived stress.
Help to gain a sense of control by recognizing personal pattern of signs and symptoms and coping strategies.	Provide feedback when symptomatic behavior occurs Instruct patient to keep a diary of behavior to identify symptoms and coping strategies	Patient consistently identifies symptoms and uses an adaptive coping strategy.
Enhance social and living skills to enable full participation in vocational and recreational activities.	Role play social interaction in a variety of situations. Review vocational preparation and current level of functioning. Assess recreational activities and opportunities for future growth.	Patient participates in progressively more rewarding social and work activities.
Identify and describe community support systems.	Provide a list of community support programs, including self-help groups, mental health care agencies, and social agencies. Escort to first agency contact.	Patient selects community programs that offer needed resources. Patient becomes able to access agency independently.
Describe and discuss psychoactive medications.	Link the benefits of medication to the patient's personal goals. Instruct about actions, side effects, and contraindications. Distribute handouts describing the patient's medications. Suggest systems to help patient integrate the medication regimen into the personal routine and simplify the medication schedule if possible.	Patient states how medicine will help reach personal goals. Patient describes characteristics of prescribed medications. Patient reports effects of prescribed medications. Patient takes medication as prescribed.

Fountain House functions as a club in which patients are members. The usual hierarchical distinctions between staff (the healthy) and patients (the ill) do not exist. It is a place where members care about each other and pool their resources and abilities as they work toward increasing independence. Thus Fountain House combats loneliness and isolation while providing a variety of living and work situations that require differing levels of functional ability.

The first month at Fountain House is a residential phase, and members are taught skills necessary for apartment living. Fountain House owns and leases apartments that have staff on call, although not in residence. These supervised apartments allow people to make a gradual transition to independent living in the community.

Fountain House runs several businesses, providing a protected environment in which members can develop self-confidence and job skills. Progressing to a more complex work situation, Fountain House has creatively arranged for transitional employment placements (TEPs). Recognizing that job interviews are tremendously stressful, staff, rather than members, seek out and contract with businesses for jobs. The jobs are assigned to Fountain House rather than to individuals. Staff assign a member to a transitional employment position for as long as needed. The employer is promised that if members are unable to manage the job or do not show up, Fountain House staff will work in their place.

Fountain House members, who share responsibility for a job with staff, can assume increasing responsibility as they are able to handle it. A TEP can easily be transferred from a member who is ready for a more complex work experience to a member who needs a TEP. Furthermore, employers are satisfied because the quality of work is guaranteed.

Ronald Peterson speaks poignantly of the loneliness and isolation he felt when he left the state hospital to live alone in a small hotel room. Because he had no job, knew no one, and lived on welfare, it never occurred to him that things could be any different. He said, "You take what you can get. There is no choice." Eventually becoming a staff member of Fountain House, Peterson spoke for many people trying to adjust to community living when he described the wish for a place where one belongs and is needed.

> I think the greatest need is to have a place to go where you are expected each day, a place where you can be with people like yourself and do things that mean something to yourself and others . . . places to go and be with people who need us to contribute, to take part, to help, and who notice when we're not present and do something about it (Peterson, 1978).

ASSERTIVE COMMUNITY TREATMENT. Assertive community treatment (ACT) programs are an evidence-based psychiatric rehabilitation practice based on the Program of Assertive Community Treatment (PACT) that was developed in the 1970s by Stein and Test in Madison, Wisconsin. They are designed to provide intensive community supports to individuals who have serious mental illnesses. The goal is to prevent hospitalization and support the individual in achieving the highest possible level of functioning.

A multidisciplinary team is used, including nurses, social workers, case managers, employment counselors, addictions counselors, and a psychiatrist. Some programs also employ peer counselors, people who have mental illnesses. In one survey case managers ranked the presence of a full-time nurse as the most important ingredient of a successful ACT team (McGrew, Pescosolido, and Wright, 2003). These staff members are often effective in reaching individuals who are reluctant to participate in treatment, such as homeless people, and engaging them in treatment.

ACT is characterized by 24-hour, 7-days-a-week staff coverage; comprehensive treatment planning; ongoing responsibility; continuity of staff; and small caseloads. ACT and other community-based programs are discussed in Chapter 35.

CONSUMER-RUN SERVICES. Many of the consumers who founded Fountain House became dissatisfied with the program after it came under the control of professionals and left. There continues to be a strong feeling among some consumers that psychosocial rehabilitation programs are not truly responsive to their needs unless they are consumer run.

Leading consumer-advocates are also critical of the ACT/PACT model because it was designed to assist patients in the transition from long-term hospitalization to the community by replicating services provided by the hospital. This is not viewed as consistent with a recovery model of service (Ahern and Fisher, 2001).

The Empowerment Model of Recovery was developed by the National Empowerment Center, a research and training organization that is administered by ex-consumers of mental health services and explores issues related to recovery-oriented mental health services. These ex-consumers developed a training and education program called PACE (Personal Assistance in Community Existence) that is based on an empowerment model. The principles of PACE are presented in Box 15-5.

In recent years slow but steady growth of new consumer-run programs has occurred in many communities. Some of these are drop-in centers that provide peer support and a safe place to be, whereas others offer a full range of rehabilitative services. Successful consumer-run programs include specific elements. They should address needs identified by the members, and participation in all or part of the total program should be voluntary. Help is provided either by members or by others whom the member selects. Consumers are responsible for the administrative direction of the program, and they determine criteria for membership. Finally, the program is mainly accountable to the members and strict confidentiality is maintained.

One study of consumer-run services found that those who attended consumer-run programs had significantly more coping strategies and significantly higher social functioning scores than those who did not attend such programs (Yanos, Primavera, and Knight, 2001). A similar study found that program participants had increased personal empowerment and unchanged independent social functioning and needed less assisted social functioning (Segal and Silverman, 2002).

What is your response to the idea that consumers should run alternative treatment programs? Discuss positive and negative implications. ■

BOX 15-5

Principles of Personal Assistance in Community Existence (PACE)

- People fully recover from even the most severe forms of mental illness.
- Trust is the cornerstone of recovery.
- Control and coercion are emphasized in the absence of trust and interfere with recovery.
- People have to be able to follow their own dreams, not someone else's, to recover.
- Self-determination is vital to recovery.
- Human dignity and respect are vital to recovery.
- Understanding that mental illness is a label for severe emotional distress that interrupts a person's role in society helps in recovery.
- People who believe in people with mental illnesses help them recover.
- People with mental illnesses and those around them have to believe they will recover or they will not recover.
- There is always meaning, even in periods of severe emotional distress, and understanding that meaning helps in recovery.
- People can and do yearn to connect emotionally, especially when they are experiencing severe emotional distress.
- Feeling emotionally safe in relationships is vital to expressing feelings.
- Everything learned about the importance of human connections equally applies to people labeled with mental illnesses.

From Ahern L, Fisher D: *J Psychosoc Nurs Ment Health Serv* 39:22, 2001.

Critical Thinking *About* Contemporary Issues

Housing the Seriously Mentally Ill—Not In My Neighborhood?

One of the major problems of providing residential housing to the seriously mentally ill is the opposition some communities have raised under the cry of "not in my neighborhood." Neighbors often object to proposed group homes or other housing arrangements because of the presumed negative effect it will have on their neighborhood. They cite potential problems of resident safety, declining property values, changes in the residential character of the neighborhood, traffic problems, and noise (Cook, 1997). These concerns lead to neighborhood residents' opposition to the development of group homes through the use of restrictive local ordinances, bureaucratic obstacles, political pressure on elected officials, and occasional violence.

Neighbors' opposition to group homes has many negative effects. For example, as a result of such protests, group homes are often found in neighborhoods characterized by low socioeconomic status, high crime, low property values, and low voting frequency. Yet despite the opposition, many people are unaware that group homes even exist in their neighborhoods, and it has been noted that resistance tends to diminish over time. In addition, neighbors can and do provide significant support to group homes. Research in this area indicates that potential neighbors of group homes respond well to information, including letters, community meetings, video presentations, or visits to other group homes (Cook, 1998).

Nurses can be active in providing community members with opportunities to learn about programs that may be entering their neighborhood and in this way combat the "not in my neighborhood" phenomenon.

Residential services. Housing is consistently identified as a critical element of successful psychiatric rehabilitation services. Appropriate housing must be safe, affordable, and acceptable to the consumer. Early housing programs tended to focus on existing supervised living situations, such as foster care. More recently, an array of housing options has been developed under the leadership of consumers and psychiatric rehabilitation professionals.

Most recovering patients live at home with their families. For those who do not, group homes and supervised apartments are the predominant types of housing available. Most incorporate some form of rehabilitation program along with housing. Staff supervision ranges from intensive 24-hour awake staffing to telephone consultation, based on the consumer's level of need.

Most housing programs focus on providing a "normal" community living experience, but many fall short of this goal. Supervision needs may lead to organization of housing around levels of care, sometimes requiring consumers to move if their needs become more or less intensive. This can be very disruptive. Consumers rarely have a choice of housemates and they hardly ever lease or own the house in their own names. This type of housing program structure also leads to clustering of group homes or supervised apartments, rein-

forcing stigmatization and triggering community apprehension (see Critical Thinking About Contemporary Issues).

Some traditional residential programs are evolving into supported housing programs where housing is thought of as a basic service that should mirror the housing choices of others in the community. As such, it is permanent and under the control of the resident. Housing program staff helps consumers find affordable housing of their choice. If people decide to live together, it is also their choice. Staff may introduce consumers to each other, but they decide whether to establish a household. Mental health and rehabilitative services need to be flexible and designed to help the person live successfully in the community.

Some supported housing programs are part of comprehensive psychiatric rehabilitation programs and are an element of a broader supportive living approach. In this case, staff intervention is directed not only at maintaining the person in housing but also at assisting the consumer to become fully involved in community life. A personal future planning process helps the consumer identify goals, preferences, and the important people who can help in accomplishing these.

Although the supported housing approach works well for some consumers, it is still important to provide a choice of living arrangements. Many patients and families prefer a range of choices, from 24-hour supervised group residences to completely independent living (Friedrich et al, 1999).

Identify where supported housing for the mentally ill is in your community. Assess the location based on safety, convenience to stores and transportation, and access to recreational areas. ■

Vocational services. Psychiatric rehabilitation programs often provide vocational rehabilitation services. Prevocational training often begins within the program itself. Members may be organized into work teams around the activities needed to keep the program running, usually clerical, food service, and maintenance tasks. Aside from the development of marketable work skills, the goal of these programs is to foster good work habits.

Some members continue indefinitely in prevocational services. Others may move into temporary employment placements such as those developed at Fountain House and then into competitive employment. Some consumers use vocational services to achieve this goal (Donegan and Palmer-Erbs, 1998). Models of vocational rehabilitation services are presented in Box 15-6.

Supported employment has been identified as an evidence-based practice for psychiatric rehabilitation services. Supported employment programs assist participants in finding jobs in the community that are consistent with their own interests, pay at least minimum wage, and could be applied for by anyone (Bond et al., 2001). Job coaching is provided to assist the service recipient in mastering job skills and learning effective workplace behaviors. The employer is aware that the employee is participating in a vocational rehabilitation program, thereby avoiding the concern that many recovering patients have about disclosing their history of mental illness.

In a study that explored the critical components of supported employment programs that were correlated with positive participant outcomes, it was found that two components were most strongly correlated (Becker et al., 2001). The first was provision of services in the community, including participant engagement, job finding, and continuing supports. The second was the use of employment specialists who only provided vocational services rather than having this job responsibility added on to other assignments.

Although mental health service providers support the idea of vocational rehabilitation, they are reluctant and sometimes actively opposed to hiring consumers to work in mental health settings. If they do, it is often as a housekeeper, or groundskeeper. Consumers have begun to assert their unique qualifications as counselors and case managers. They have been successfully employed in this role and have achieved good outcomes for themselves and those to whom they provide services.

For example, an analysis was conducted on the benefits and limitations of a vocational program called Project WINS (Work Incentives and Needs Study) (Mowbray, Moxley, and Collins, 1998). This project employed consumers in the role of peer support specialists (PSSs). These staff members were

---

BOX 15-6

Models of Vocational Rehabilitation in Psychiatric Care

Supported Employment Programs (SEP)
This model is individualized and provides on-site, one-on-one support, and job-coaching services and occurs in competitive, "real work" settings; job-coach services are gradually removed.

Transitional Employment Programs (TEP)
This model offers a temporary work experience to individuals; it has the same supports and services as SEP. They must move on to competitive employment within an agreed-upon length of time. Staff often cover contract positions, working in the job for a day in cases of illness or with changes in participants' schedules.

Clubhouses
Programs are "member directed," with members defined as individuals with serious mental illness. Members have individual daily responsibilities and schedules to fulfill as preparation for entry or re-entry into the world of work.

Job Clubs
There are two main types: in-house clubs and postprogram graduate clubs. In-house clubs provide practical guidance in resume writing, work exploration, opportunities to practice interviewing skills and, in some cases, vocational assessment and interest identification. Postprogram graduate clubs provide essential offsite support services, such as working with new coworkers, adjusting to job requirements, handling issues of stigma and disclosure, and feelings of isolation.

Peer and Natural Supports
These circles of support are central to the continued success of individuals with serious psychiatric conditions who are attaining and maintaining employment. Circles include wider community links to religious organizations, recreational and activity groups, public libraries, volunteer activities, and peer support activities.

Modified from Donegan K, Palmer-Erbs VK: *J Psychosoc Nurs* 36:13, 1998.

---

responsible for such duties as helping consumers prepare resumes, open bank accounts, select clothing for interviews, work, or learn the bus system.

The PSSs were surveyed on the benefits and problems of the project from their perspective. Benefits to the PSS that were identified included earning money; satisfaction in having a job; skill development; having a work routine; learning interpersonal skills and ways to manage anger and frustration; feeling safe at work; positive attitudes from others; job security; positive feedback; finding a career direction; personal growth; and involvement with other PSSs.

Problems for the PSSs included dealing with difficult patients; personal stress related to disappointment with one's performance; lack of understanding about how to do the job; lack of administrative support; having too much responsibility; lack of a career path; and boundary issues.

In such programs it is very important to be aware of issues related to role change as experienced by the consumer-employees as well as by other staff in the program, especially if the consumer-employees have been members of the program. If these issues are not identified and discussed openly, they can interfere with the ability of the consumer-employees to be successful.

Educational services. Many people with serious mental illnesses have not completed formal education through high school or beyond because of the effects of the illness. Rehabilitation programs often offer remedial education related to vocational services. Education that is offered in a supportive environment can increase self-esteem, improve job qualifications, and encourage some consumers to pursue higher education. A study that examined the characteristics of people who were successful in supported education programs at the postsecondary level found that being married, involvement in a support network, dissatisfaction with doing housework, and lack of financial problems were related to success in educational programs (Collins, Mowbray, and Bybee, 2000).

Review a book intended for mental health consumers. Critique it in terms of accuracy, practical advice, reading level, and emotional tone. Ask a consumer or a family member of a consumer to review the book. Compare your critiques. ■

The Family

Family support is very important to the successful rehabilitation and recovery of a person with mental illness (see Chapter 11). The mental illness of a member is often a shock and a source of great stress to the family. One study found that many families that include members with serious mental illnesses do not receive adequate pertinent information about the illness or effective support from mental health professionals (Doornbos, 2001).

Nurses are in a favorable position to help families cope with the stress and adapt to changes in the family structure. Effective programs for families of people with serious mental illnesses include empowerment and education.

Empowerment. Several common trouble spots in family life can be anticipated. Learning ways to handle these troublesome areas empowers the family by giving them a sense of control over their lives. The problem areas include the following:
- Disrupted communications
- Mechanics of everyday life, including the need for privacy and control over personal space, keeping a regular schedule, television usage, money management, and grooming
- Responding to hallucinations, delusions, and odd behavior, particularly coping with violent or suicidal threats
- Alcohol and drug use
- Need for relatives to remember to take care of themselves

This last area of concern is often ignored by family members and professionals alike. However, it can be accomplished by the following:
- Accepting the fact that a family member has a mental illness
- Planning a self-care program
- Continuing to pursue personal activities and interests
- Getting involved with organizations such as self-help groups or churches
- Avoiding the advice and opinions of those who have not lived with a person with mental illness
- Remembering that happiness is possible
- Avoiding blaming oneself

Reviewing this list gives the nurse some understanding of the pain and stress experienced by the family of a person with mental illness.

The stigma associated with a member's mental illness is another challenge to a family's coping skills. Four areas of stigma management strategies that may be helpful to families include the following (Muhlbauer, 2002):
- Managing internalized feelings
- Learning how to disclose information
- Confronting direct, personal manifestations of stigma
- Dealing with institutionalized stigma

Families and mental health care providers sometimes become engaged in power struggles related to the care of the mentally ill family member. This interferes with their ability to work as a team. Nurses should strive to understand the family's fears and concerns and help members develop effective coping mechanisms.

Identifying feelings related to the illness is the first step toward coping. Sharing feelings with each other can be a great relief to people who feel isolated. When feelings are revealed, family members can be supportive of each other, including the ill person. Coping with feelings also allows the person to be receptive to information about the illness and mental health services. The combination of coping and education empowers the family and facilitates their involvement in the recovery process.

When working with aging families, it is particularly important to address issues related to the care of the mentally ill family member if the primary caregiver becomes disabled or dies. This is an uncomfortable subject that families often worry about but are reluctant to discuss (Smith, Hatfield, and Miller, 2000). Because nurses are usually viewed as supportive and helpful, they are in a good position to address the needs of families.

Describe the issues facing an aging parent of a young person with a serious and persistent mental illness. ■

Family Education. Family education has become a primary nursing intervention when providing rehabilitative services to relatives of people with serious mental illness is needed. Nurses have established workshops for family members that have been well received and have helped families cope with the challenges presented by the mental illness.

Programming for these workshops can include information and skill-building exercises (Wilson and Hobbs, 1999). The experiences of the more seasoned family members can be particularly helpful because they can share their successes and failures in using various coping strategies and provide needed social support.

Two major and complementary models of family education are widely accepted as being effective in assisting families to cope with mental illness. The Family-to-Family model is offered by chapters of the National Alliance for the Mentally Ill (NAMI) and is taught by family members who have been trained to present a standard curriculum as well as to assist group members to problem-solve situations related to the member's mental illness. The Family Psychoeducation model is an evidence-based practice that is designed to be led by mental health professionals and also includes educational and group supportive elements.

A study of the educational and support needs of family members of hospitalized patients found that 75% identified the following learning and support needs: advocacy in communicating with professionals, hospital treatment and rehabilitation, medication compliance, and side effects of medications (Gasque-Carter and Curlee, 1999). Family members also may find that the opportunity to meet one another for mutual support is especially important. These opportunities may be formal, such as in support groups or local chapters of NAMI, or informal, such as in family recreational gatherings.

If you were responsible for developing a nursing program for psychiatric rehabilitation, what would it be like? Describe the setting, the program, its goals, and the roles of staff and patients. ■

The Community

Nurses can intervene in the community to encourage the establishment of tertiary prevention programs in several ways. Among these are **health education**, **membership in advocacy groups**, **networking**, and **political action**. It has been noted that stigma decreases with increased familiarity and education (Corrigan et al, 2001).

Mental health education in the community can therefore have a real impact on the experience of patients in the community. Greater understanding of the behaviors and needs of people with mental illness could increase community acceptance, leading to the development of better services. Thus nurses should take advantage of opportunities to speak to community groups about mental health.

Psychiatric nurses also can perform a valuable service by educating their co-workers and professional colleagues about current research related to serious mental illnesses. Although they are seldom discussed, stigmatizing attitudes toward mental illness do exist among health care workers. These attitudes are transmitted to the general public. Professionals have even taken the lead in opposing the establishment of group homes in their neighborhoods. Well-informed nurses can make health care workers aware of their prejudices and assist them in changing their behavior.

Membership by nurses in community advocacy groups also can be helpful. Nurses can join forces with other professional and lay people who share concerns about the care of the mentally ill. The National Mental Health Association is the largest advocacy group that addresses mental health issues. Members of this organization have been influential in drawing attention to the needs of people with mental illness and in supporting positive legislation at the federal and state levels.

Nurses can promote working relationships among advocacy groups, professional organizations, self-help groups, and concerned citizens. With limited funding available and health care costs escalating, the formation of coalitions is essential if lobbying efforts focused on allocating needed resources to mental health care are to be successful. Psychiatric nurses have taken a leadership role in coalitions to influence reforms in the current health care system.

The activities of community-wide networks are often directed toward the political system. Aside from allocation of money and other resources, the nature of mental health care in a community is strongly influenced by the political structure of that community. Environmental, legal, and ethical issues have a great effect on mental health care delivery (see Chapters 9 and 10). Nurses need to be aware of and involved in the political process. They should communicate directly with legislators at all levels, sharing their interests and concerns. Politicians are well aware of the need to respond to the priorities of their constituents.

Finally, nurses can become more directly involved in the political system. They can run for office and support other nurses who are legislators. Nurses are often invaluable members of appointed boards and commissions on health care. Their knowledge can be shared with others who are planning community health care systems. These voluntary activities are time-consuming, but they can have great impact on the health care system.

Community-level policies can either inhibit or facilitate direct care efforts. Active involvement in professional organizations often leads to productive and rewarding community activities. A great sense of satisfaction is to be gained from selling a community on a new idea and seeing it become a reality.

Obtain a copy of a bill being considered by your state legislature that is relevant to psychiatric rehabilitation. Explain the effect this legislation would have on the mental health care system, including the potential effect on nursing. ■

EVALUATION

Evaluation of psychiatric rehabilitation services usually covers the impact on the patient and family and the effectiveness of the community service system.

Patient Evaluation

Evaluation of the services provided to patients and family members must focus on the achievement of the expected outcomes of the intervention. Most psychiatric rehabilitation evaluation programs rely on both objective and subjective measures of outcome. Objective measures are generally related to the following questions:

- Is the person living in housing of personal choice?
- Have days of hospitalization in the last year decreased?
- How many emergency room visits has the person made?
- How many days in the last year have been spent in a transitional employment placement? In competitive employment?
- How often does the person have contact with family members? Who are they?
- Can the person identify people to provide support in a crisis?
- Is the person involved in community activities?
- Is the person enrolled in an adult education course? In an academic education program?

The answers to such questions are compared with the individual rehabilitation plans, thereby providing a picture of the success of the services. They should be discussed with program participants and their families as a basis for further planning.

Subjective measures of effectiveness include periodic discussions with patients and families about the progress of rehabilitation. Staff members share their observations about the person's response to the program and invite feedback from the consumers. Many programs also conduct regular consumer satisfaction surveys. More recently, consumers have been employed as advocates to seek information about consumer dissatisfaction and present complaints to program administrators.

Program Evaluation

Program evaluation is conducted to inform administrators about the relevance and cost effectiveness of the services they offer. It is often required by funding, regulatory, and licensure agencies to confirm that public mental health dollars are being spent wisely. The Federal Substance Abuse and Mental Health Services Administration requires that states receiving Mental Health Block Grant funding conduct annual assessments of consumer satisfaction with public mental health services.

Program evaluation is evolving as program funders and the public demand greater accountability from service providers. Community advisory boards, legislators, and consumer advocates are all recognizing the importance of reviewing the effectiveness of individual programs and service systems. As comprehensive community-based service systems for people with serious mental illnesses continue to grow, evaluation approaches will provide direction.

COMPETENT CARING

A Clinical Exemplar of a Psychiatric Nurse
TANANARIEVE BROWN, BS, RN

It was a typical work day, and I was waiting outside the psychiatrist's office to consult with him about a patient. His door opened and the patient meeting with the psychiatrist emerged and headed for the receptionist's desk to check out. I went inside and, after finishing my consultation with him, came out of the office to find the patient who had just left still standing in the outer office. She asked if she could speak with me privately. We went into my office and shut the door. She began by thanking me for saving her life and the lives of her children. I honestly did not remember what I had done and I told her so. She reminded me that she had suffered from depression for many years beginning with the birth of the first of her three children.

She had come in 6 months ago to see me, and at that time was struggling with poor energy as well. She said that we talked about all the stress she was under and how she felt compelled to do for others but could never find time for herself. I remained confused as her complaints struck me as typical of a single mother of three young children. She went on to say that at our visit I asked her about her health and conducted a physical assessment. I found her blood pressure and pulse to be elevated and strongly recommended that she see her medical doctor as she had not had a recent physical examination.

She waited to see me this day to tell me that she did go to see her doctor. She was immediately admitted into the hospital when her doctor discovered she had been bleeding internally from a large uterine fibroid. He told her that any further delay would have cost her her life. Presently, she remains on antidepressants but her doses have been reduced and she is doing well. She is now working with vocational rehabilitation to find employment.

While I initially did not remember my actions, that patient reminded me that a psychiatric nurse is also a medical nurse who remains sensitive to how the mental and physical aspects of the patient profoundly affect one another. Often psychiatric patients present with complaints such as poor energy, sensory disturbances, and other symptoms that could be easily attributed to their psychiatric illness but may, in fact, have physical causes. This is especially pertinent when monitoring a patient's response to psychiatric medications as they can affect medical disorders such as hypertension and diabetes. All these issues must be considered even if the patient is hostile or psychotic.

Caring for the serious and persistently mentally ill and maintaining them in the community is both challenging and rewarding and often requires creativity. It demands a broad medical knowledge, emotional discipline, and keen psychiatric discretion, encompassed by sharp nursing intuition and skill. This is what I have learned in my practice as a psychiatric nurse. ■

CHAPTER **FOCUS POINTS**

- The goal of tertiary prevention is to limit the amount of disability and maladaptive functioning resulting from an illness.
- Psychiatric rehabilitation is the range of social, educational, occupational, behavioral, and cognitive interventions for increasing the role performance of persons with serious and persistent mental illness and enhancing their recovery.
- Evidence-based practices include assertive community treatment, supported employment, illness management and recovery, integrated treatment for co-occurring mental illness and substance abuse, family psychoeducation, and medication management.
- Recovery is the process in which people are able to live, work, learn, and participate fully in their communities. For some individuals, it is the ability to live a fulfilling and productive life despite a disability. For others, it implies the reduction or complete remission of symptoms. Hope plays an integral role in an individual's recovery.
- A comprehensive psychiatric nursing assessment provides information that enables the nurse to help the patient achieve maximum possible functioning. In addition to identifying deficits, nurses are expected to identify and reinforce strengths as one means of helping the patient cope.
- Primary symptoms of serious mental illness are directly caused by the illness, such as hallucinations and delusions. Secondary symptoms such as loneliness and social isolation are caused by the person's response to the illness or its treatment.
- The nursing assessment of a patient who has a serious mental illness should include an analysis of the physical, emotional, and intellectual components of the skills needed for living, learning, and working in the community.
- Families and other caregivers can be a major source of support for individuals who have serious mental illnesses. They can help by identifying potential problem areas and enhancing the patient's compliance with the treatment plan. The nurse should be available to the family through regular planned contacts and inclusion of the family as part of the treatment team.
- Care providers, including nurses, should assume a leadership role in assessing the adequacy and effectiveness of community resources and in recommending changes to improve access and quality of mental health care.
- A wide range of community services must be available to patients including provisions for shelter, food, and clothing; household man-

agement; income and financial support; meaningful activities; and mobility and transportation.
- In promoting psychiatric rehabilitation and recovery, the nurse helps the individual develop their strengths and potential; learn living skills; manage one's illness; and access environmental supports.
- Through experiences of adequacy, self-concept can be altered and self-esteem increased. Social skills training uses cognitive and behavioral techniques to help people gain the knowledge and skills they need to live in the community. Another important aspect of psychiatric rehabilitation and recovery relates to promoting the physical well-being of those with serious mental illness.
- Four interventions that have been identified to support illness management include psychoeducation, behavioral tailoring for medication, training in relapse prevention, and coping skills training.
- Supporting people who have serious mental illnesses in community settings requires the development of a wide array of community support programs including rehabilitation centers, housing services, employment opportunities, education, crisis intervention and outreach, and case management.
- Housing is consistently identified as a critical element of successful psychiatric rehabilitation services. Appropriate housing must be safe, affordable, and acceptable to the consumer.
- Supported employment programs assist participants in finding jobs in the community that are consistent with their own interests, pay at least minimum wage, and could be applied for by anyone.
- Education that is offered in a supportive environment can increase self-esteem, improve job qualifications, and encourage some consumers to pursue higher education.
- Effective programs for families of people with serious mental illnesses include empowerment and education.
- Nurses can intervene in the community to encourage the establishment of tertiary prevention programs in several ways. Among these are health education, membership in advocacy groups, networking, and political action.
- Evaluation of the services provided to patients and family members must focus on the achievement of the expected outcomes of the intervention. Program evaluation is conducted to inform administrators about the relevance and cost effectiveness of the services they offer.

KEY TERMS

assertive community treatment (ACT), 250
family burden, 244

recovery, 241
rehabilitation, 239
tertiary prevention, 239

CHAPTER REVIEW QUESTIONS

1. Indicate whether the following statements are true (T) or false (F).

_____ A. People who have serious mental illnesses and their families experience grief over the loss of potential life achievements.

_____ B. Serious mental illness prevents a person from being successful at work or school.

_____ C. Families of people with mental illness generally want and need to be involved with their ill family member.

_____ D. Consumers of mental health services should not be hired as providers of mental health services.

_____ E. Measures of skills and support, more than psychiatric diagnoses and symptom patterns, determine how well a person with a serious mental illness can function in the community.

2. Fill in the blanks.

A. Tertiary prevention is carried out by the performance of activities identified as _____.

B. The impact on the family of a member's mental illness is often called _____.

C. The rehabilitation philosophy is supportive of the goal of

patient _____.

D. _____ is the use of cognitive and behavioral techniques to help people gain the knowledge and skills they need to live in the community.

E. The approach that supports the rehabilitation process by teaching the patient and family about the mental illness and the coping skills that will help with successful community

living is called _____.

3. Provide short answers for the following questions.

A. Identify four common responses families have to the mental illness of a member.

B. Describe the four basic interventions used in psychiatric rehabilitation.

C. Think about someone you know who has a psychiatric illness. Relate three ways in which you, as a nurse, can help to empower this person and his or her family.

Visit Evolve for additional resources related to the content of this chapter.

http://evolve.elsevier.com/Stuart/principles/

• Topical Course Outline • Student Workbook Exercises • Critical Thinking Questions and Activities • Case Studies • Research Topics
• Monthly Content Updates • WebLinks

Student Study CD-ROM

Access the accompanying CD-ROM for animations, interactive exercises, review questions for the NCLEX examination, and an audio glossary.

REFERENCES

Ahern L, Fisher D: Recovery at your own PACE (Personal Assistance in Community Existence), *J Psychosoc Nurs Ment Health Serv* 39:22, 2001.

Barton R: Psychosocial rehabilitation services in community support systems: a review of outcomes and policy recommendations, *Psychiatr Serv* 50:525, 1999.

Becker DR et al: Fidelity of supported employment programs and employment outcomes, *Psychiatr Serv* 52:834, 2001.

Bond GR et al: Implementing supported employment as an evidence-based practice, *Psychiatr Serv* 52:313, 2001.

Collins ME, Mowbray CT, Bybee D.: Characteristics predicting successful outcomes of participants with severe mental illness in supported education, *Psychiatr Serv* 51:774, 2000.

Cook JR: Neighbors' perceptions of group homes, *Community Ment Health J* 33:287, 1997.

Cook JR: Interactions between group homes and neighbors: neighbor preferences, *J Behav Health Serv Res* 25:425, 1998.

Corrigan P et al: Familiarity with and social distance from people who have serious mental illness, *Psychiatr Serv* 52:953, 2001.

Cuijpers P, Stam H: Burnout among relatives of psychiatric patients attending psychoeducational support groups, *Psychiatr Serv* 51:375, 2003.

Deegan PE: Recovering our sense of value after being labeled mentally ill, *J Psychosoc Nurs Ment Health Serv* 31:7, 1993.

Dickerson FB et al: Experiences of stigma among outpatients with schizophrenia, *Schizophr Bull* 28:143, 2002.

Donegan KR, Palmer-Erbs VK: Promoting the importance of work for persons with psychiatric disabilities—the role of the psychiatric nurse, *J Psychosoc Nurs Ment Health Serv* 36:13, 1998.

Doornbos MM: Professional support for family caregivers of people with serious and persistent mental illnesses, *J Psychosoc Nurs Ment Health Serv* 39:38, 2001.

Fountain House: The wellspring of the clubhouse model for social and vocational adjustment of persons with serious mental illness, *Psychiatr Serv* 50:1473, 1999.

Friedrich R et al: Family and client perspectives on alternative residential settings for persons with severe mental illness, *Psychiatr Serv* 50:509, 1999.

Gasque-Carter KO, Curlee MB: The educational needs of families of mentally ill adults: the South Carolina experience, *Psychiatr Serv* 50:520, 1999.

Hatfield A et al: Family responses to behavior manifestations of mental illness, *Innovations Res* 3:41, 1994.

Jacobson N, Greenley D: What is recovery? A conceptual model and explication, *Psychiatr Serv* 52:482, 2001.

Liberman RP et al: Requirements for multidisciplinary teamwork in psychiatric rehabilitation, *Psychiatr Serv* 52:1331, 2001.

Liberman RP, Kopelowicz A: Teaching persons with severe mental disabilities to be their own case managers, *Psychiatr Serv* 53:1377, 2002.

Link BG et al: Stigma as a barrier to recovery: the consequences of stigma for the self-esteem of people with mental illnesses, *Psychiatr Serv* 52:1621, 2001.

McDonald J, Badger TA: Social function of persons with schizophrenia, *J Psychosoc Nurs Ment Health Serv* 40:42, 2002.

McGrew JH, Pescosolido B, Wright E: Case managers perspectives on critical ingredients of assertive community treatment and on its implementation, *Psychiatr Serv* 54:370, 2003.

Mowbray CT, Moxley DP, Collins ME: Consumers as mental health providers: first-person accounts of benefits and limitations, *J Behav Health Serv Res* 25:397, 1998.

Mueser KT et al: Illness management and recovery: a review of the research, *Psychiatr Serv* 53:1272, 2002.

Muhlbauer S: Experience of stigma by families with mentally ill members, *J Am Psychiatr Nurs Assoc* 8:76, 2002.

New Freedom Commission on Mental Health (NFCMH): *Achieving the promise: transforming mental health care in America, final report*, DHHS Pub. No. SMA-03-3832, Rockville, Md, 2003, USDHHS.

Peterson R: What are the needs of chronic mental patients? In Talbott JA, editor: *The chronic mental patient: problems, solutions, and recommendations for a public policy*, Washington, DC, 1978, The American Psychiatric Association.

Pickens JM: Social networks for women with serious mental illness, *J Psychosoc Nurs Ment Health Serv* 37:30, 1999.

Ralph RO: *Review of recovery literature: a synthesis of a sample of recovery literature 2000*, Alexandria, Va, 2000, National Technical Assistance Center for State Mental Health Planning.

Saunders JC: Family functioning in families providing care for a family member with schizophrenia, *Issues Ment Health Nurs* 20:95, 1999.

Segal SP, Silverman C: Determinants of client outcomes in self-help agencies, *Psychiatr Serv* 53:304, 2002.

Skinner E et al: Met and unmet needs for assistance and quality of life for people with severe and persistent mental disorders, *Ment Health Serv Res* 1:109, 1999.

Smith GC, Hatfield AB, Miller DC: Planning by older mothers for the future care of offspring with serious mental illness, *Psychiatr Serv* 51:1162, 2000.

US Department of Health and Human Services: *Mental health: a report of the Surgeon General*, Rockville, Md, 1999, USDHHS, SAMHSA, CMHS, NIH, NIMH.

Vellenga BA, Christenson J: Persistent and severely mentally ill clients' perceptions of their mental illness, *Issues Ment Health Nurs* 15:359, 1994.

Wang PS, Demler O, Kessler RC: Adequacy of treatment for serious mental illness in the United States, *Am J Public Health* 92:92, 2002.

Wilson JH, Hobbs H: The family educator: a professional resource for families, *J Psychosoc Nurs Ment Health Serv* 37:22, 1999.

Yanos PT, Primavera LH, Knight EL: Consumer-run service participation, recovery of social functioning and the mediating role of psychological factors, *Psychiatr Serv* 52:493, 2001.

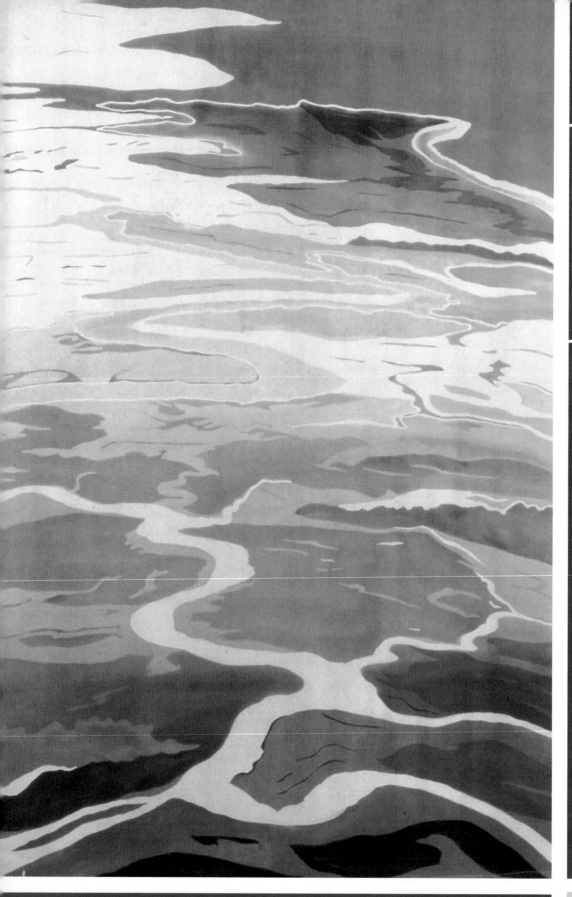

Unit Three

Coastal Flight
57″ × 36″ batik on silk, 2002

Artist's Note: Flying over the snaking tidal creeks near my home I am amazed at how orderly the earth is from the air. Our lives fluctuate from times of organization to pandemonium when we face illness or loss. Accepting this flow in its own time gives one the ability to confront pain and find acceptance.

Applying Principles in Nursing Practice

Have you thought that most people with psychiatric problems were suffering from schizophrenia? Did you ever suspect that one of your friends or family members had an emotional or psychiatric problem but dismissed the idea as impossible? Have you ever worried about the barometer of your own mental health but felt embarrassed to discuss it? If you have answered "yes" to any of these questions, you are in for an awakening. The fact is that almost half of all Americans experience some type of psychiatric problem in their lifetime. Most of these problems are not what nurses commonly think of as a psychiatric illness, but anxiety disorders, mood disorders, and substance use disorders are by far the most common psychiatric disorders, and they are experienced by people more often than many physical illnesses. They are disabling disorders that cause people significant distress, yet they are often underdiagnosed and undertreated. These facts are more than just interesting. They suggest that health care professionals need a wide variety of educational and treatment strategies to address these issues.

In this unit you will explore the adaptive and maladaptive coping responses used by people experiencing stress. Some of what you read will surprise you, some of it will concern you, and it is hoped that most of it will intrigue you. It is important that you understand, however, that these psychiatric problems are a common part of the human experience. As such, they merit careful study and consideration by nurses like yourself.

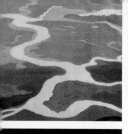

The fears we know are of not knowing. . . . It is getting late. Shall we ever be asked for? Are we simply not wanted at all?

WH AUDEN, *THE AGE OF ANXIETY*

16 ANXIETY RESPONSES AND ANXIETY DISORDERS

Gail W. Stuart

evolve   Visit Evolve for additional resources related to the content of this chapter.
http://evolve.elsevier.com/Stuart/principles/

Anxiety is a pervasive aspect of contemporary life. It has always existed and belongs to no particular era or culture. Anxiety derives from the Greek root meaning "to press tight." Anxious is related to the Latin word *angere*, which means "to strangle" and "to distress." It is also related to *anguish*, which is described as "acute pain, suffering, or distress." Anxiety disorders are the **most common psychiatric disorders** in America, affecting between 10% to 25% of the population. Anxiety involves one's body, perceptions of self, and relationships with others, making it a foundational concept in the study of psychiatric nursing and human behavior.

■ CONTINUUM OF ANXIETY RESPONSES

Anxiety is a diffuse apprehension that is vague in nature and associated with feelings of uncertainty and helplessness. Feelings of isolation, alienation, and insecurity are also present. The person perceives that the core of his or her personality is being threatened. Experiences provoking anxiety begin in infancy and continue throughout life. They end with the fear of the greatest unknown, death.

Defining Characteristics

Anxiety is an emotion and a subjective individual experience. It is an energy and cannot be observed directly. A nurse infers that a patient is anxious based on certain behaviors. The nurse needs to validate this inference with the patient.

Anxiety is an emotion without a specific object. It is provoked by the unknown and precedes all new experiences such as entering school, starting a new job, or giving birth to a child. This characteristic of anxiety differentiates it from fear. Fear has a specific source or object that the person can identify and describe. **Fear** involves the **intellectual appraisal** of a threatening stimulus; **anxiety** is the **emotional response** to that appraisal. A fear is caused by physical or psychological exposure to a threatening situation. Fear produces anxiety. These two emotions are differentiated in speech; we speak of **having** a fear but of **being** anxious.

Anxiety is communicated interpersonally. If a nurse is talking with a patient who is anxious, within a short time the nurse also will experience feelings of anxiety. Similarly, if a nurse is anxious in a particular situation, this anxiety will be communicated to the patient. The contagious nature of anxiety therefore can have positive and negative effects on the therapeutic relationship. The nurse must carefully monitor these effects. It is also important to remember that anxiety is part of everyday life. It is basic to the human condition and provides a valuable warning. In fact, the capacity to be anxious is necessary for survival.

The crux of anxiety is self-preservation. Anxiety occurs as a result of a threat to a person's selfhood, self-esteem, or identity. It results from a threat to something central to one's personality and essential to one's existence and security. It may be connected with the fear of punishment, disapproval, withdrawal of love, disruption of a relationship, isolation, or loss of body functioning.

Culture is related to anxiety because culture can influence the values one considers most important. Underlying every fear is the anxiety of losing one's own being. This anxiety is the frightening element, but a person can encompass the anxiety and grow from it to the extent that the person confronts, moves through, and overcomes anxiety-creating experiences.

Name two situations that provoke anxiety in you. Compare these to two situations that stimulate fear in you. ■

Levels of Anxiety

Peplau (1963) identified four levels of anxiety and described their effects:

1. **Mild anxiety is associated with the tension of day-to-day living.** During this stage the person is alert and the perceptual field is increased. The person sees, hears, and grasps more than before. This kind of anxiety can motivate learning and produce growth and creativity.
2. **Moderate anxiety, in which the person focuses only on immediate concerns, involves the narrowing of the perceptual field.** The person sees, hears, and grasps less. The person blocks selected areas but can attend to more if directed to do so.
3. **Severe anxiety is marked by a significant reduction in the perceptual field.** The person tends to focus on a specific detail and not think about anything else. All behavior is aimed at relieving anxiety, and much direction is needed to focus on another area.
4. **Panic is associated with awe, dread, and terror, and the person feeling it is unable to do things even with direction.** Panic involves the disorganization of the personality and can be life threatening. Increased motor activity, decreased ability to relate to others, distorted perceptions, and loss of rational thought are all symptoms of panic. Panic is a frightening and paralyzing experience. The panicked person is unable to communicate or function effectively. This level of anxiety cannot persist indefinitely because it is incompatible with life. A prolonged period of panic would result in exhaustion and death. It is a common and debilitating phenomenon, but can be safely and effectively treated.

The nurse needs to be able to identify which level of anxiety a patient is experiencing by the behaviors observed. Figure 16-1 shows the range of anxiety responses from the most adaptive response of anticipation to the most maladaptive response of panic. The patient's level of anxiety and its position on the continuum of coping responses is relevant to the nursing diagnosis and influences the type of intervention the nurse implements.

ASSESSMENT

Behaviors

Anxiety can be expressed directly through physiological and behavioral changes or indirectly through cognitive and affective responses, including the formation of symptoms or coping mechanisms developed as a defense against anxiety. The nature of the responses displayed depends on the level of anxiety, and the intensity of the response increases with increasing anxiety.

In describing anxiety's effects on **physiological responses**, mild and moderate anxiety heighten the person's capacities. Conversely, severe and panic levels paralyze or overwork capacities. The physiological responses associated with anxiety are modulated primarily by the brain through the **autonomic nervous system** (Figure 16-2). The body adjusts internally without a conscious or voluntary effort. Two types of autonomic responses exist:

1. **Parasympathetic** responses, which conserve body responses
2. **Sympathetic** responses, which activate body processes

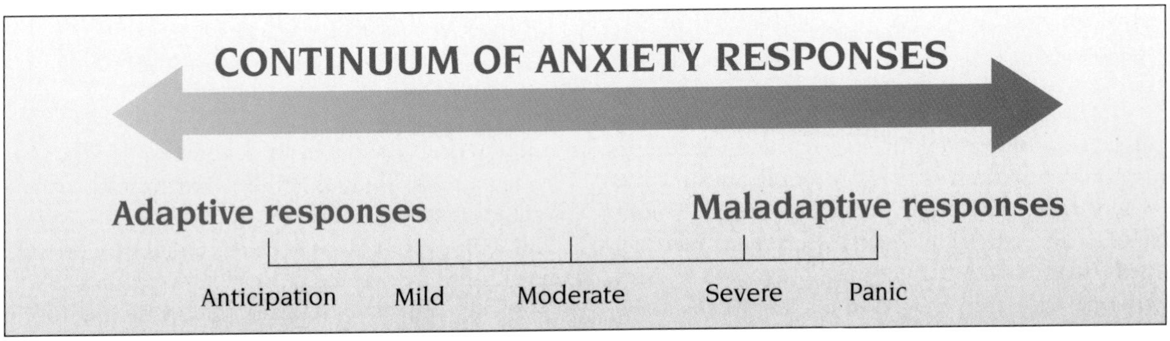

Figure 16-1   Continuum of anxiety responses.

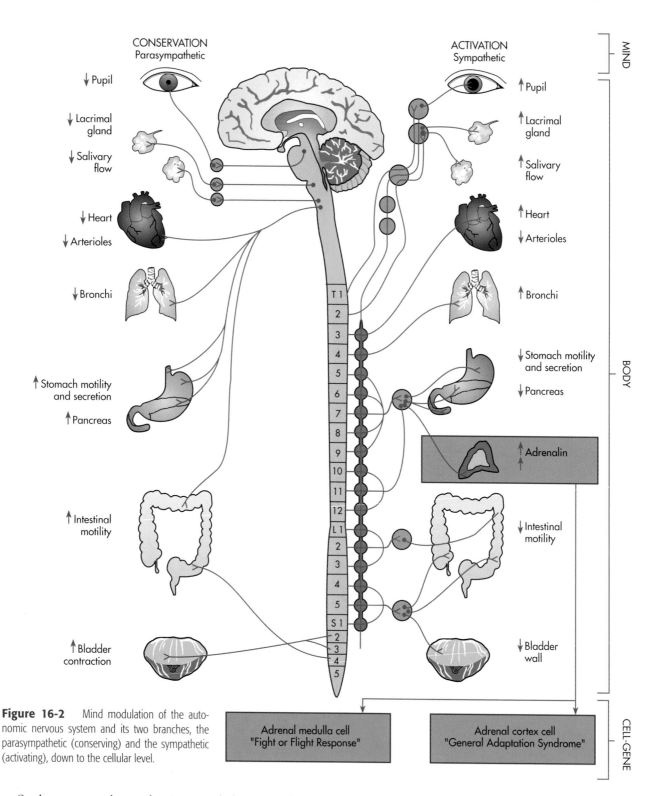

Figure 16-2 Mind modulation of the autonomic nervous system and its two branches, the parasympathetic (conserving) and the sympathetic (activating), down to the cellular level.

Studies support the **predominance of the sympathetic reaction** in anxiety responses. This reaction prepares the body to deal with an emergency situation by a *fight or flight* reaction. It can also trigger the *general adaptation syndrome*, as described by Selye (see Chapter 17). When the cortex of the brain perceives a threat, it sends a stimulus down the sympathetic branch of the autonomic nervous system to the adrenal glands. Because of a release of epinephrine, res-

piration deepens, the heart beats more rapidly, and arterial pressure rises. Blood is shifted away from the stomach and intestines to the heart, central nervous system, and muscles. Glycogenolysis is accelerated and the blood glucose level rises.

For some people, however, the parasympathetic reaction may coexist or predominate and produce opposite effects. Other physiological reactions also may be evident. The vari-

BOX 16-1

Physiological, Behavioral, Cognitive, and Affective Responses to Anxiety

Physiological
Cardiovascular
Palpitations
Racing heart
Increased blood
    pressure .
Faintness*
Actual fainting*
Decreased blood
    pressure*
Decreased pulse rate*
Respiratory
Rapid breathing
Shortness of breath
Pressure on chest
Shallow breathing
Lump in throat
Choking sensation
Gasping
Gastrointestinal
Loss of appetite
Revulsion toward food
Abdominal discomfort
Abdominal pain*
Nausea*
Heartburn*
Diarrhea*

Neuromuscular
Increased reflexes
Startle reaction
Eyelid twitching
Insomnia
Tremors
Rigidity
Fidgeting
Pacing
Strained face
Generalized
    weakness
Wobbly legs
Clumsy movement
Urinary tract
Pressure to urinate*
Frequent urination*
Skin
Flushed face
Localized sweating
    (e.g., palms)
Itching
Hot and cold
    spells
Pale face
Generalized
    sweating

Behavioral
Restlessness
Physical tension
Tremors
Startle reaction
Hypervigilance
Rapid speech
Lack of coordination
Accident proneness
Interpersonal withdrawal
Inhibition
Flight
Avoidance
Hyperventilation

Cognitive
Impaired attention
Poor concentration
Forgetfulness
Errors in judgment
Preoccupation
Blocking of thoughts
Decreased perceptual field
Reduced creativity
Diminished productivity
Confusion
Self-consciousness

Loss of objectivity
Fear of losing control
Frightening visual images
Fear of injury or death
Flashbacks
Nightmares

Affective
Edginess
Impatience
Uneasiness
Tension
Nervousness
Fear
Fright
Frustration
Helplessness
Alarm
Terror
Jitteriness
Jumpiness
Numbing
Guilt
Shame
Frustration
Helplessness

*Parasympathetic response.

ety of physiological responses to anxiety that the nurse may observe in patients is summarized in Box 16-1.

Psychomotor manifestations, or **behavioral responses**, also are observed in the anxious patient. Their effects have both personal and interpersonal aspects. High levels of anxiety affect coordination, involuntary movements, and responsiveness and also can disrupt human relationships. In an interpersonal situation, anxiety can warn a person to withdraw from a situation where discomfort is anticipated. The anxious patient typically withdraws and decreases interpersonal involvement. The possible behavioral responses the nurse might observe are presented in Box 16-1.

Mental or intellectual functioning also is affected by anxiety. **Cognitive responses** the patient might display when experiencing anxiety are described in Box 16-1.

Finally, the nurse can assess a patient's emotional reactions, or **affective responses,** to anxiety by the subjective description of the patient's personal experience. Often, patients describe themselves as tense, jittery, on edge, jumpy, worried, or restless. One patient described feelings in the following way: "I'm expecting something terribly bad to happen, but I don't know what. I'm afraid, but I don't know why. I guess you can call it a generalized bad feeling." All of these phrases are expressions of apprehension and overalertness. It seems clear that the person interprets his or her anxiety as a

kind of warning sign. Additional affective responses are listed in Box 16-1.

Anxiety is an unpleasant and uncomfortable experience that most people try to avoid. They often try to replace anxiety with a more tolerable feeling. Pure anxiety is rarely seen. Anxiety is usually observed in combination with other emotions. Patients might describe feelings of anger, boredom, contempt, depression, irritation, worthlessness, jealousy, self-depreciation, suspicion, sadness, or helplessness. This combination of emotions makes it difficult for the nurse to discriminate between anxiety and depression, for instance, because the patient's descriptions may be similar.

Close ties exist between anxiety, depression, guilt, and hostility. These emotions often function reciprocally; one feeling acts to generate and reinforce the others. The relationship between anxiety and hostility is particularly close. The pain experienced with anxiety often causes anger and resentment toward those thought to be responsible. These feelings of hostility in turn increase anxiety.

This cycle was evident in the case of a dependent and insecure wife who was very attached to her husband. She expressed numerous vague fears. In exploring her feelings, she also expressed great hostility toward him and their relationship. This hostility symbolized her helplessness and increased her feelings of weakness. Verbalizing these angry feelings further increased her anxiety and unresolved conflict. Thus anxiety is often expressed through anger, and a tense and anxious person is more likely to become angry.

Think of a patient you cared for recently who appeared to be angry or critical. Could this have been the patient's way of dealing with anxiety? If so, how would your nursing interventions have been different? ■

Predisposing Factors

Anxiety is a prime factor in the development of the personality and formation of individual character traits. Because of its importance, various theories of the origin of anxiety have been developed.

Psychoanalytic View. Freud (1969) identified two types of anxiety: primary and subsequent. Primary anxiety, the traumatic state, begins in the infant as a result of the sudden stimulation and trauma of birth. Anxiety continues with the possibility that hunger and thirst might not be satisfied. Primary anxiety therefore is a state of tension or a drive produced by external causes. The environment is capable of threatening as well as satisfying. This implicit threat predisposes the person to anxiety in later life.

With increased age and ego development, a new kind of anxiety arises. Freud viewed this subsequent anxiety as the emotional conflict between two elements of the personality: the id and the superego. The id represents instinctual drives and primitive impulses. The superego reflects conscience and culturally acquired restrictions. The ego, or I, tries to mediate the demands of these two clashing elements. Freud therefore suggested that one major function of anxiety was to warn the person that the ego was in danger of being overtaken.

Interpersonal View. Sullivan (1953) disagreed with Freud. He believed that anxiety could not arise until the organism had some awareness of its environment. He believed that anxiety is first conveyed by the mother to the infant. The infant responds as if he and his mother were one unit. As the child grows older, he sees this discomfort as a result of his own actions. He believes that his mother either approves or disapproves of his behavior. In addition, developmental traumas such as separations and losses can lead to specific vulnerabilities. Sullivan believed that anxiety in later life arises when a person perceives that he or she will be viewed unfavorably or will lose the love of a valued person.

A person's level of self-esteem is also an important factor related to anxiety. A person who is easily threatened or has a low level of self-esteem is more susceptible to anxiety. This is evident in students with test anxiety. Anxiety is high because they doubt they can succeed. This anxiety may have nothing to do with their actual abilities or how much they studied. The anxiety is caused only by their perception of their ability, which reflects their self-concept. They may be well prepared for the examination, but their severe level of anxiety reduces their perceptual field significantly. They may omit, misinterpret, or distort the meaning of the test items. They may even block out all their previous studying. The result

will be a poor grade, which reinforces their poor perception of self.

Behavioral View. Some behavioral theorists propose that anxiety is a product of frustration caused by anything that interferes with attaining a desired goal. An example of an external frustration might be the loss of a job. Many goals may thus be blocked, such as financial security, pride in work, and perception of self as family provider. An internal frustration is evidenced by young college graduates who set unrealistically high career goals and are frustrated by entry-level job offers. In this case their view of self is threatened by their unrealistic goals. They are likely to experience feelings of failure, insignificance, and mounting anxiety.

Other experimental psychologists believe that anxiety begins with the attachment of pain to a particular stimulus. If the reaction is strong enough, it may become generalized to similar objects and situations. Learning theorists believe that people who have been exposed in early life to intense fears are more likely to be anxious in later life. In this respect, parental influences are important. Children who see their parents respond with anxiety to every minor stress soon develop a similar pattern. Paradoxically, if parents are completely unmoved by potentially stressful situations, children feel alone and lack emotional support from their families. The appropriate emotional response of parents gives children security and helps them learn constructive coping methods.

Anxiety also may arise through conflict that occurs when the person experiences two competing drives and must choose between them. A reciprocal relationship exists between conflict and anxiety. Conflict produces anxiety, and anxiety increases the perception of conflict by producing feelings of helplessness. In this view, conflict derives from two tendencies: approach and avoidance. Approach is the tendency to do something or move toward something. Avoidance is the opposite tendency: not to do something or not to move toward something. There are four kinds of conflict:

1. **Approach-approach**, in which the person wants to pursue two equally desirable but incompatible goals. An example is having two very attractive job offers. This type of conflict seldom produces anxiety.
2. **Approach-avoidance**, in which the person wishes to both pursue and avoid the same goal. The patient who wants to express anger but feels great anxiety and fear in doing so experiences this type of conflict. Another example is the ambitious business executive who must compromise values of honesty and loyalty to be promoted.
3. **Avoidance-avoidance**, in which the person must choose between two undesirable goals. Because neither alternative seems beneficial, this is a difficult choice usually accompanied by much anxiety. An example is when a person observes a friend cheating and feels the need to report the act but worries about the loss of friends that might result from reporting the violation.

4. **Double approach-avoidance,** in which the person can see both desirable and undesirable aspects of both alternatives. An example of this is the conflict experienced by a person living with the pain of an unsatisfying social and emotional life, coupled with destructive coping patterns. The alternative is to seek psychiatric help and expose oneself to the threat and potential pain of the therapy process. Double approach-avoidance conflict feelings often are described as ambivalence.

Think of an example of each of the four kinds of conflict that you have experienced in your own life. ■

Family Studies. Epidemiological and family studies show that anxiety disorders run in families and that they are common and of different types (Hettema, Neale, and Kendler, 2001). Anxiety disorders can overlap, as do anxiety disorders and depression. People with one anxiety disorder are more likely to develop another or to experience a major depression within their lifetime. It has been estimated that only about a quarter of those with anxiety disorders receive treatment. However, these people are high users of health care facilities because they seek treatment for the various symptoms caused by anxiety, such as chest pain, palpitations, dizziness, and shortness of breath.

Biological Basis. The majority of studies point to a dysfunction in multiple systems rather than isolating one particular neurotransmitter in the development of an anxiety disorder. These systems include the following:

- **GABA system.** The regulation of anxiety is related to the activity of the neurotransmitter gamma-aminobutyric acid (GABA), which controls the activity, or firing rates, of neurons in the parts of the brain responsible for producing anxiety. GABA is the most common inhibitory neurotransmitter in the brain. When it crosses the synapse and attaches or binds to the GABA receptor on the postsynaptic membrane, the receptor channel opens, allowing for the exchange of ions. This exchange results in an inhibition or reduction of cell excitability, and thus a slowing of cell activity. The theory is that people who have an excess of anxiety have a problem with the efficiency of this neurotransmission process.

  When a person with anxiety takes a benzodiazepine (BZ) medication, which is from the antianxiety class of drugs, it binds to a place on the GABA receptor next to GABA. This makes the postsynaptic receptor more sensitive to the effects of GABA, enhancing neurotransmission and causing even more inhibition of cell activity (Figure 16-3). The effect of GABA and BZ at the GABA receptor in various parts of the brain is a reduced firing rate of cells in areas implicated in anxiety disorders. The clinical result is that the person becomes less anxious.

  The areas of the brain where GABA receptors are coupled to BZ receptors include the amygdala and hippocampus—both structures of the limbic system, which functions as the center of emotions (such as rage, arousal, and fear) and memory. Patients with anxiety disorders may have a decreased antianxiety ability of the GABA receptors in areas of the limbic system, making them more sensitive to anxiety and panic.

- **Norepinephrine system.** The norepinephrine (NE) system is thought to mediate the fight-or-flight response. The part of the brain that manufactures NE

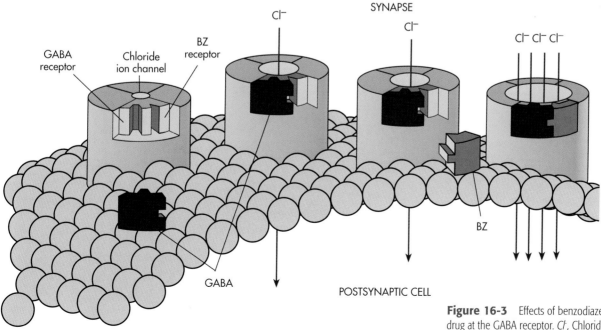

Figure 16-3   Effects of benzodiazepine (BZ) drug at the GABA receptor. *Cl*, Chloride ion.

is the locus ceruleus. It is connected by neurotransmitter pathways to other structures of the brain associated with anxiety, such as the amygdala, the hippocampus, and the cerebral cortex (the thinking, interpreting, and planning part of the brain). Medications that decrease the activity of the locus ceruleus (antidepressants such as the tricyclics) effectively treat some anxiety disorders. This suggests that anxiety may be caused in part by an inappropriate activation of the NE system in the locus ceruleus and an imbalance between NE and other neurotransmitter systems.

- **Serotonin system.** A dysregulation of serotonin (5-HT) neurotransmission may play a role in the etiology of anxiety, because patients experiencing these disorders may have hypersensitive 5-HT receptors. Drugs that regulate serotonin, such as the selective serotonin reuptake inhibitors (SSRIs), have been shown to be particularly effective in treating several of the anxiety disorders, suggesting a major role for 5-HT and its balance with other neurotransmitter systems in the etiology of anxiety disorders.

It also has been shown that a person's general health has a great effect on predisposition to anxiety. Anxiety may accompany some physical disorders such as those listed in Box 16-2. Coping mechanisms also may be impaired by toxic influences, dietary deficiencies, reduced blood supply, hormonal changes, and other physical causes. In addition, symptoms from some physical disorders may mimic or exacerbate anxiety.

Similarly, fatigue increases irritability and feelings of anxiety. It appears that fatigue caused by nervous factors predisposes the person to a greater degree of anxiety than does fatigue caused by purely physical causes. Thus fatigue may actually be an early symptom of anxiety. Patients complaining of nervous fatigue may already be suffering from moderate anxiety and be more susceptible to future stress situations.

Precipitating Stressors

Given these theories about the origin of anxiety, what kinds of events might precipitate feelings of anxiety? Clearly, experiencing or witnessing a source of trauma of any kind has been associated with a variety of anxiety disorders, particularly posttraumatic stress disorder (PTSD). Maturational and situational crises, as described in Chapter 14, can all precipitate a maladaptive anxiety response. Precipitating stressors can be grouped into two categories: threats to physical integrity and threats to self-system.

Threats to Physical Integrity. Threats to physical integrity suggest impending **physiological disability or decreased ability to perform the activities of daily living**. They may include both internal and external sources. External sources may include exposure to viral and bacterial infection, environmental pollutants, and safety hazards; lack of adequate housing, food, or clothing; and traumatic injury.

Internal sources may include the failure of physiological mechanisms such as the heart, immune system, or temperature regulation. The normal biological changes that can occur with pregnancy and failure to participate in preventive health practices are other internal sources. Pain is often the first indication that physical integrity is being threatened. It creates anxiety that often motivates the person to seek health care.

Threats to Self-System. Threats to one's self-system imply **harm to a person's identity, self-esteem,** and **integrated social functioning**. Again, both external and internal sources can threaten self-esteem. External sources may include the loss of a valued person through death, divorce, or relocation; a change in job status; an ethical dilemma; and other social or cultural group pressures.

Internal sources may include interpersonal difficulties at home or at work or when assuming a new role, such as parent, student, or employee. In addition, many threats to phys-

---

BOX **16-2**

Medical Disorders Associated With Anxiety

Cardiovascular/Respiratory Disorders
Asthma
Cardiac arrhythmias
Chronic obstructive pulmonary disease
Congestive heart failure
Coronary insufficiency
Hyperdynamic beta-adrenergic state
Hypertension
Hyperventilation syndrome
Hypoxia, embolus, infections

Endocrinological Disorders
Carcinoid
Cushing's syndrome
Hyperthyroidism

Hypoglycemia
Hypoparathyroidism
Hypothyroidism
Menopause
Pheochromocytoma
Premenstrual syndrome

Neurological Disorders
Collagen vascular disease
Epilepsy
Huntington's disease
Multiple sclerosis
Organic brain syndrome
Vestibular dysfunction
Wilson's disease

Substance-Related Disorders
Intoxications
Anticholinergic drugs
Aspirin
Caffeine
Cocaine
Hallucinogens including phencyclidine ("angel dust")
Steroids
Sympathomimetics
Withdrawal syndromes
Alcohol
Narcotics
Sedative-hypnotics

ical integrity also threaten self-esteem because the mind-body relationship is an overlapping one.

This distinction of categories is only theoretical. The person responds to all stressors, whatever their nature and origin, as an integrated whole. No specific event is equally stressful to all people or even to the same person at different times.

Appraisal of Stressors

A true understanding of anxiety requires integration of knowledge from all the various points of view. The Stuart Stress Adaptation Model integrates data from psychoanalytical, interpersonal, behavioral, genetic, and biological perspectives. It suggests a variety of causative factors and emphasizes the relationship among them in explaining present behavior as described in Box 16-3.

Coping Resources

The person can cope with stress and anxiety by mobilizing coping resources found internally and in the environment. Resources such as economic assets, problem-solving abilities, social supports, and cultural beliefs can help the person integrate stressful experiences into his or her being and learn to adopt successful coping strategies. They also can help the person extract meaning from stressful experiences and can foster the suggestion of alternative strategies for mediating stressful events.

How might a person's religious or spiritual belief system serve as a resource in coping with a moderate level of anxiety? ■

Coping Mechanisms

As anxiety increases to the severe and panic levels, the behaviors displayed by a person become more intense and potentially injurious, and quality of life decreases (see Citing the Evidence). People seek to avoid anxiety and the circumstances that produce it. When experiencing anxiety,

---

BOX 16-3

Causative Factors in Anxiety Disorders

- The body has a built-in neurobiological substance that prepares the person to cope with danger.
- Evolution has affected this substance in such a way that stimuli that threaten survival are selectively avoided.
- People may be born with a central nervous system that is overly sensitive to stimuli that are generally harmless.
- Childhood and adult learning experiences may determine the extent, severity, and nature of the situations that will evoke anxiety.
- Chronic inability to cope with dangerous situations adaptively could increase the tendency to respond with anxiety.
- Cognitive functions in some people might predispose them to continually focusing on anxiety reactions; so the mere anticipation of aversive stimuli would provoke anxiety.
- Such people might be more vulnerable to insecurities, especially if they are intelligent and introspective.

CITING THE EVIDENCE ON
Quality of Life

BACKGROUND: This was an integrated review of studies that have investigated quality of life in patients with panic disorder, social phobia, posttraumatic stress disorder, generalized anxiety disorder, and obsessive-compulsive disorder.

RESULTS: The studies show a uniform picture of anxiety disorders being illnesses that markedly compromise quality of life and psychosocial functioning. Effective pharmacological or psychotherapeutic treatment has been shown to improve the quality of life for these patients.

IMPLICATIONS: A more thorough understanding of the impact of quality of life may lead to increased public awareness of anxiety disorders as being serious mental illnesses worthy of further investment in research, prevention, and treatment.

Mendlowicz M, Stein M: *Am J Psychiatry* 157:669, 2000.

people use various coping mechanisms to try to relieve it (see A Patient Speaks).

The inability to cope with anxiety constructively is a primary cause of pathological behavior. To neutralize, deny, or counteract anxiety, the person develops patterns of coping. The pattern used to cope with mild anxiety dominates when anxiety becomes more intense. Anxiety plays a major role in the psychogenesis of emotional illness because many

---

A PATIENT SPEAKS

It's hard to describe what it feels like. You know something isn't right. Most people don't have to check their doors five or six times before they go to bed. Most people aren't afraid to be near children or feel like they have to count their money over and over again before they can put it back in their wallets. But that's the way my life has been ever since I was a little girl.

Of course I realized I needed help, so I saw a number of different professionals. With one psychologist we discussed every aspect of my childhood and my earliest memories of life. Unfortunately, I finished that therapy still counting everything around me. Next I went to a physician, but he told me that I was just nervous about getting married and things would get better with time. They didn't. Then my mother suggested I go to the university and see someone. That's where I met the psychiatric nurse who did a number of things I'll always remember. First she put me at ease and clearly told me that I wasn't crazy. Then she told me that what I had was called obsessive-compulsive disorder, and she gave me lots of great books and information to read. Finally, she told me that it was a treatable illness and together we devised a treatment plan. It included both medication and behavioral therapy and, wow, what a difference! I'm sure glad I was persistent, but I'm even more glad that there are caring professionals out there who can really help.

symptoms of illness develop as attempted defenses against anxiety.

The nurse needs to be familiar with the coping mechanisms people use when experiencing the various levels of anxiety. For mild anxiety, caused by the tension of day-to-day living, several coping mechanisms commonly used include crying, sleeping, eating, yawning, laughing, cursing, physical exercise, and daydreaming. Oral behavior, such as smoking and drinking, is another means of coping with mild anxiety. When dealing with other people, the individual copes with low levels of anxiety through superficiality, lack of eye contact, use of clichés, and limited self-disclosure. People also can protect themselves from anxiety by assuming comfortable roles and limiting close relationships to those with values similar to their own.

Moderate, severe, and panic levels of anxiety pose greater threats to the ego. They require more energy to cope with the threat. These coping mechanisms can be categorized as task-oriented and ego-oriented reactions.

Task-Oriented Reactions.
Task-oriented reactions are thoughtful, deliberate attempts to solve problems, resolve conflicts, and gratify needs. These reactions can include attack, withdrawal, and compromise. They are aimed at realistically meeting the demands of a stress situation that has been objectively appraised. They are consciously directed and action oriented.

In **attack behavior** a person attempts to remove or overcome obstacles to satisfy a need. There are many possible ways of attacking problems, and this type of reaction may be destructive or constructive. Destructive patterns are usually accompanied by great feelings of anger and hostility. These feelings may be expressed by negative or aggressive behavior that violates the rights, property, and well-being of others. Constructive patterns reflect a problem-solving approach. They are evident in self-assertive behaviors that respect the rights of others.

Withdrawal behavior may be expressed physically or psychologically. Physically, withdrawal involves removing oneself from the source of the threat. This reaction can apply to biological stressors, such as smoke-filled rooms, exposure to irradiation, or contact with contagious diseases. A person also can withdraw in various psychological ways, such as by admitting defeat, becoming apathetic, or lowering aspirations. As with attack, this type of reaction may be constructive or destructive. When it isolates the person from others and interferes with the ability to work, the reaction creates additional problems.

Compromise is necessary in situations that cannot be resolved through attack or withdrawal. This reaction involves changing usual ways of operating, substituting goals, or sacrificing aspects of personal needs. Compromise reactions are usually constructive and are often used in approach-approach and avoidance-avoidance situations. Occasionally, however, the person realizes with time that the compromise is not acceptable; a solution must then be renegotiated or a different coping mechanism adopted.

The capacity for task-oriented reactions and effective problem solving is influenced by the person's expectation of at least partial success. This prediction in turn depends on remembering past successes in similar situations. On this basis it is possible to go forward and deal with the current stressful situation. Perseverance in problem solving also depends on the person's expectation of a certain level of pain and discomfort and on the belief in one's being capable of tolerating the problem. Here lies the balance between courage and anxiety.

What coping mechanisms do you use when you are mildly, moderately, and severely anxious? How adaptive or maladaptive are they? ■

Ego-Oriented Reactions.
Ego-oriented reactions are used often to protect the self. These reactions, also called defense mechanisms, are the first line of psychic defense. Everyone uses defense mechanisms, and they often help people cope successfully with mild and moderate levels of anxiety. They protect the person from feelings of inadequacy and worthlessness and prevent awareness of anxiety. However, they can be used to such an extreme degree that they distort reality, interfere with interpersonal relationships, and limit the ability to work productively.

As coping mechanisms, they have certain drawbacks. First, ego-oriented reactions operate on unconscious levels. The person has little awareness of what is happening and little control over events. Second, they involve a degree of self-deception and reality distortion. Therefore, they usually do not help the person cope with the problem realistically. Table 16-1 lists some of the more common ego defense mechanisms, with an example of each.

The evaluation of whether the patient's use of certain defense mechanisms is adaptive or maladaptive involves four issues:

1. The accurate recognition of the patient's use of the defense mechanism by the nurse.
2. The degree to which the defense mechanism is used. Does it imply a high degree of personality disorganization? Is the person unresponsive to facts about his or her life situation?
3. The degree to which use of the defense mechanism interferes with the patient's functioning and his or her progress toward health.
4. The reason the patient used the ego defense mechanism.

The nurse will better understand the patient and plan more effective nursing care after considering these points.

Many coping mechanisms can be used to minimize anxiety. Some of them are essential for emotional stability. The exact nature and number of the defenses used strongly influence the personality pattern. When these defenses are overused or used unsuccessfully, they cause many physiological and psychological symptoms commonly associated with emotional illness.

◀ DIAGNOSIS

Nursing Diagnoses

The nurse who has adequately assessed a patient and uses the Stuart Stress Adaptation Model can formulate a nursing diagnosis based on the patient's position on the continuum of anxiety responses (Figure 16-4).

Table 16-1   Ego Defense Mechanisms

DEFENSE MECHANISM	EXAMPLE
Compensation: Process by which a person makes up for a perceived weakness by strongly emphasizing a feature that he or she considers more desirable.	A businessman perceives his small physical stature negatively. He tries to overcome this by being aggressive, forceful, and controlling in business dealings.
Denial: Avoidance of disagreeable realities by ignoring or refusing to recognize them; the simplest and most primitive of all defense mechanisms.	Mrs. P has just been told that her breast biopsy indicates a malignancy. When her husband visits her that evening, she tells him that no one has discussed the laboratory results with her.
Displacement: Shift of emotion from a person or object to another, usually neutral or less dangerous, person or object.	A 4-year-old boy is angry because he has just been punished by his mother for drawing on his bedroom walls. He begins to play war with his soldier toys and has them fight with each other.
Dissociation: The separation of a group of mental or behavioral processes from the rest of the person's consciousness or identity.	A man is brought to the emergency room by the police and is unable to explain who he is and where he lives or works.
Identification: Process by which a person tries to become like someone he or she admires by taking on thoughts, mannerisms, or tastes of that person.	Sally, 15 years old, has her hair styled like that of her young English teacher, whom she admires.
Intellectualization: Excessive reasoning or logic is used to avoid experiencing disturbing feelings.	A woman avoids dealing with her anxiety in shopping malls by explaining that shopping is a frivolous waste of time and money.
Introjection: Intense identification in which a person incorporates qualities or values of another person or group into his or her own ego structure. It is one of the earliest mechanisms of the child, important in formation of conscience.	Eight-year-old Jimmy tells his 3-year-old sister, "Don't scribble in your book of nursery rhymes. Just look at the pretty pictures," thus expressing his parents' values.
Isolation: Splitting off of emotional components of a thought, which may be temporary or long term.	A medical student dissects a cadaver for her anatomy course without being disturbed by thoughts of death.
Projection: Attributing one's thoughts or impulses to another person. Through this process one can attribute intolerable wishes, emotional feelings, or motivation to another person.	A young woman who denies she has sexual feelings about a co-worker accuses him without basis of trying to seduce her.
Rationalization: Offering a socially acceptable or apparently logical explanation to justify or make acceptable otherwise unacceptable impulses, feelings, behaviors, and motives.	John fails an examination and complains that the lectures were not well organized or clearly presented.
Reaction formation: Development of conscious attitudes and behavior patterns that are opposite to what one really feels or would like to do.	A married woman who feels attracted to one of her husband's friends treats him rudely.
Regression: Retreat to behavior characteristic of an earlier level of development.	Four-year-old Nicole, who has been toilet trained for over a year, begins to wet her pants again when her new baby brother is brought home from the hospital.
Repression: Involuntary exclusion of a painful or conflictual thought, impulse, or memory from awareness. It is the primary ego defense, and other mechanisms tend to reinforce it.	Mr. R does not recall hitting his wife when she is pregnant.
Splitting: Viewing people and situations as either all good or all bad. Failure to integrate the positive and negative qualities of oneself.	A friend tells you that you are the most wonderful person in the world one day, and how much she hates you the next day.
Sublimation: Acceptance of a socially approved substitute goal for a drive whose normal channel of expression is blocked.	Ed has an impulsive and physically aggressive nature. He tries out for the football team and becomes a star tackle.
Suppression: A process often listed as a defense mechanism, but really is a conscious counterpart of repression. It is intentional exclusion of material from consciousness. At times, it may lead to repression.	A young man at work finds he is thinking so much about his date that evening that it is interfering with his work. He decides to put it out of his mind until he leaves the office for the day.
Undoing: Act or communication that partially negates a previous one; a primitive defense mechanism.	Larry makes a passionate declaration of love to Sue on a date. At their next meeting he treats her formally and distantly.

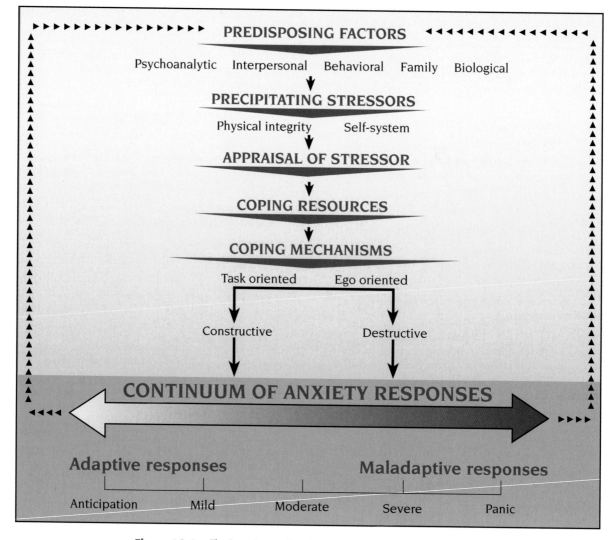

Figure 16-4   The Stuart Stress Adaptation Model as related to anxiety responses.

Initially the nurse needs to determine the quality and quantity of the anxiety experienced by the patient. In considering the quality of the anxiety, the nurse might question the appropriateness of the patient's response to the perceived threat. Is it adaptive or irrational? A problem may exist if the response is out of proportion to the threat. This disproportionate response would indicate that the patient's cognitive appraisal of the threat is unrealistic. The quantity of the reaction is the next consideration. When anxiety reaches the severe and panic levels, it indicates that the conflict is increasingly problematic for the patient.

The nurse also needs to explore how the patient is coping with the anxiety. Constructive coping mechanisms are protective responses that consciously confront the threat. Destructive coping mechanisms involve repression into the unconscious. They tend to be ineffective, inadequate, disorganized, inappropriate, and exaggerated. They may be evident in bizarre behavior or symptom formation.

Finally, the nurse needs to determine the overall effect of the anxiety. Is it stimulating growth? Or is it interfering with effective living and life satisfaction? Is it enhancing one's sense of self? Or is it depersonalizing? Whenever possible, the patient should be included in identifying problem areas. This involvement may not always be feasible, however, particularly if the patient's anxiety is at the severe or panic level.

There are four primary NANDA nursing diagnoses concerned with anxiety responses: **anxiety, ineffective coping, readiness for enhanced coping,** and **fear.** Many additional nursing problems may be identified from the way the patient's anxiety reciprocally influences interpersonal relationships, self-concept, cognitive functioning, physiological status, and other aspects of life.

Nursing diagnoses related to the range of possible maladaptive responses and related medical diagnoses are identified in the Medical and Nursing Diagnoses box (Box 16-4). The primary NANDA nursing diagnoses and examples of expanded nursing diagnoses are presented in the Detailed Diagnoses table (Table 16-2).

Table 16-2	*Detailed Diagnoses Related to* **Anxiety Responses**

NANDA DIAGNOSIS STEM	**EXAMPLES OF EXPANDED DIAGNOSIS**
Anxiety	Panic level of anxiety related to family rejection, as evidenced by confusion and impaired judgment
	Severe anxiety related to sexual conflict, as evidenced by repetitive hand washing and recurrent thoughts of dirt and germs
	Severe anxiety related to marital conflict, as evidenced by inability to leave the house
	Moderate anxiety related to financial pressures, as evidenced by recurring episodes of abdominal pain and heartburn
	Moderate anxiety related to assumption of motherhood role, as evidenced by inhibition and avoidance
	Moderate anxiety related to poor school performance, as evidenced by excessive use of denial and rationalization
Ineffective coping	Ineffective coping related to daughter's death, as evidenced by inability to recall events pertaining to the car accident
	Ineffective coping related to child's illness, as evidenced by limited ability to concentrate and psychomotor agitation
Readiness for enhanced coping	Readiness for enhanced coping related to adoption of grandchild because of death of the child's parents, as evidenced by engagement in family therapy and modification of living environment to promote the inclusion of a child in the home
Fear	Fear related to impending surgery, as evidenced by generalized hostility toward staff and restlessness

***DSM-IV-TR* DIAGNOSIS**	**ESSENTIAL FEATURES***
Panic disorder without agoraphobia	Recurrent unexpected panic attacks (Box 16-5), with at least one of the attacks followed by a month (or more) of persistent concern about having additional attacks, worry about the implications of the attack or its consequences, or a significant change in behavior related to the attacks. Also the absence of agoraphobia.
Panic disorder with agoraphobia	Meets the above criteria. In addition, includes the presence of agoraphobia, which is anxiety about being in places or situations from which escape might be difficult or embarrassing or in which help may not be available in the event of a panic attack. Agoraphobic fears typically involve characteristic clusters of situations that include being outside the home alone, being in a crowd or standing in a line, being on a bridge, and traveling in a bus, train, or car. Agoraphobic situations are avoided, or endured with marked distress or with anxiety about having a panic attack, or require the presence of a companion.
Agoraphobia without history of panic disorder	The presence of agoraphobia without meeting criteria for panic disorder.
Specific phobia	Marked and persistent fear that is excessive or unreasonable, cued by the presence or anticipation of a specific object or situation (such as flying, heights, animals, receiving an injection, or seeing blood). Exposure to the phobic stimulus almost invariably provokes an immediate anxiety response. The person recognizes the fear is excessive, and the distress or avoidance interferes with the person's normal routine.
Social phobia	A marked and persistent fear of social or performance situations in which the person is exposed to unfamiliar people or to possible scrutiny by others. The person fears that he or she will act in a way (or show anxiety symptoms) that will be humiliating or embarrassing. Exposure to the feared situation almost invariably provokes anxiety. The person recognizes the fear is excessive, and the distress or avoidance interferes with the person's normal routine.
Obsessive-compulsive disorder	Either obsessions or compulsions (Box 16-6) are recognized as excessive and interfere with the person's normal routine.
Posttraumatic stress disorder	The person has been exposed to a traumatic event in which both of the following were present: The person has experienced, witnessed, or been confronted with an event that involved actual or threatened death or serious injury, or a threat to the physical integrity of oneself or others. The person's response involved intense fear, helplessness, or horror. The traumatic event is reexperienced in the mind, and there is an avoidance of stimuli associated with the trauma and a numbing of general responsiveness.
Acute stress disorder	Meets the criteria for exposure to a traumatic event and person experiences three of the following symptoms: sense of detachment, reduced awareness of one's surroundings, derealization, depersonalization, and dissociated amnesia.
Generalized anxiety disorder	Excessive anxiety and worry, occurring more days than not for at least 6 months, about a number of events or activities. The person finds it difficult to control the worry and experiences at least three of the following symptoms: restlessness or feeling keyed up or on edge, fatigue, difficulty concentrating or mind going blank, irritability, muscle tension, sleep disturbance.

*From American Psychiatric Association: *Diagnostic and statistical manual of mental disorders*, ed 4, text revision, Washington, DC, 2000, American Psychiatric Association.

BOX 16-4 *Medical and Nursing Diagnoses Related to* Anxiety Responses

RELATED MEDICAL DIAGNOSES (*DSM-IV-TR*)*	RELATED NURSING DIAGNOSES (NANDA)†
Panic disorder without agoraphobia	Adjustment, Impaired
Panic disorder with agoraphobia	**Anxiety**‡
Agoraphobia without panic attacks	Breathing pattern, Ineffective
Specific phobia	Communication, Impaired verbal
Social phobia	Confusion, Acute
Obsessive-compulsive disorder	**Coping, Ineffective**‡
Posttraumatic stress disorder	**Coping, Readiness for enhanced**‡
Acute stress disorder	Denial, Ineffective
Generalized anxiety disorder	Diarrhea
	Fear‡
	Injury, Risk for
	Memory, Impaired
	Posttrauma syndrome
	Powerlessness
	Protection, Ineffective
	Role performance, Ineffective
	Self-esteem, Situational low
	Sensory perception, Disturbed
	Sleep pattern, Disturbed
	Social interaction, Impaired
	Thought processes, Disturbed
	Tissue perfusion, Ineffective

*From American Psychiatric Association: *Diagnostic and statistical manual of mental disorders*, ed 4, text revision, Washington, DC, 2000, American Psychiatric Association.
†From North American Nursing Diagnosis Association: *NANDA nursing diagnoses: definitions and classification 2003-2004*, Philadelphia, 2003, The Association.
‡**Primary nursing diagnosis for anxiety.**

BOX 16-5

Panic Attack Criteria

A panic attack is a discrete period of intense fear or discomfort in which at least four of the following symptoms develop abruptly and reach a peak within 10 minutes:
- Palpitations, pounding heart, or accelerated heart rate
- Sweating
- Trembling or shaking
- Sensations of shortness of breath or smothering
- Feeling of choking
- Chest pain or discomfort
- Nausea or abdominal distress
- Feeling dizzy, unsteady, lightheaded, or faint
- Derealization (feelings of unreality) or depersonalization (being detached from oneself)
- Fear of losing control or going crazy
- Fear of dying
- Paresthesias (numbness or tingling sensations)
- Chills or hot flushes

From American Psychiatric Association: *Diagnostic and statistical manual of mental disorders*, ed 4, text revision, Washington, DC, American Psychiatric Association, 2000.

Medical Diagnoses

Many patients with mild or moderate anxiety have no medically diagnosed health problem. However, patients with more severe levels of anxiety usually have neurotic disorders that fall under

the category of anxiety disorders in the *DSM-IV-TR* (American Psychiatric Association, 2000). These psychiatric disorders include **panic disorder with or without agoraphobia, agoraphobia, specific phobia, social phobia, obsessive-compulsive disorder, posttraumatic stress disorder, acute stress disorder,** and **generalized anxiety disorder.** The essential features of these medical diagnoses related to anxiety responses are presented in the Detailed Diagnoses table (see Table 16-2).

A neurosis is a mental disorder characterized by anxiety that involves no distortion of reality. Neurotic disorders are maladaptive anxiety responses associated with moderate and severe levels of anxiety. Psychosis is disintegrative and involves a significant distortion of reality. It can emerge with the panic level of anxiety. Psychotic people feel they are "breaking into pieces." They fear they are failing in the process of living and in the process of being (see Chapter 21).

The nurse also must discriminate between anxiety and other disorders. For example, a relationship has been established between anxiety disorders and alcohol use disorders (Kushner, Sher, and Erickson, 1999). So too, anxiety and depression often overlap because anxious patients are often depressed and depressed patients are often anxious. For example, both anxious and depressed patients share the following symptoms: sleep disturbances, appetite changes, nonspecific cardiopulmonary and gastrointestinal complaints, difficulty concentrating, irritability, and fatigue or lack of energy. Yet there are often discrete (if subtle) differences between the two groups. These are described in Box 16-7.

BOX **16-6**

Obsession and Compulsion Criteria

Obsession

Recurrent and persistent thoughts, impulses, or images are experienced during the disturbance as intrusive and inappropriate and cause marked anxiety or distress.

The thoughts, impulses, or images are not simply excessive worries about real-life problems.

The person attempts to ignore or suppress such thoughts or impulses or to neutralize them with some other thought or action.

The person recognizes that the obsessional thought, impulses, or images are a product of one's own mind.

Examples

Fear of dirt and germs

Fear of burglary or robbery

Worries about discarding something important

Concerns about contracting a serious illness

Worries that things must be symmetrical or matching

Compulsion

The person feels driven to perform repetitive behaviors or mental acts in response to an obsession or according to rules that one deems must be applied rigidly.

The behaviors or mental acts are aimed at preventing or reducing distress or preventing some dreaded event or situation; however, these behaviors or mental acts either are not connected in a realistic way with what they are designed to neutralize or prevent or are clearly excessive.

Examples

Excessive hand washing

Repeated checking of door and window locks

Counting and recounting of objects in everyday life

Hoarding of objects

Excessive straightening, ordering, or of arranging things

Repeating words or prayers silently

Modified from American Psychiatric Association: *Diagnostic and statistical manual of mental disorders*, ed 4, text revision, Washington, DC, 2000, American Psychiatric Association.

BOX **16-7**

Differences Between Anxiety and Depression

ANXIETY	DEPRESSION
Predominantly fear or apprehension	Predominantly sad or hopeless with feelings of despair
Difficulty falling asleep (initial insomnia)	Early morning awakening (late insomnia) or hypersomnia Diurnal variation (feels worse in the morning)
Phobic avoidance behavior	Slowed speech and thought processes
Rapid pulse and psychomotor hyperactivity Breathing disturbances Tremors and palpitations Sweating and hot or cold spells Faintness, lightheadedness, dizziness	Psychomotor retardation (agitation also may occur) Delayed response time
Depersonalization (feeling detached from one's body	Inability to experience pleasure
Derealization (feeling that one's environment is strange, unreal, or unfamiliar)	Loss of interest in usual activities
Selective and specific negative appraisals that do not include all areas of life	Negative appraisals are pervasive, global, and exclusive
Sees some prospects for the future	Thoughts of death or suicide Sees the future as blank and has given up all hope
Does not regard defects or mistakes as irrevocable	Regards mistakes as beyond redemption
Uncertain in negative evaluations	Absolute in negative evaluations
Predicts that only certain events may go badly	Global view that nothing will turn out right

Also, posttraumatic stress disorder (PTSD) is rarely a patient's only psychiatric diagnosis, and it is sometimes difficult to distinguish overlapping independent symptoms from effects of the trauma. Nearly half of all people with PTSD also suffer from major depression, and more than a third from phobias and alcoholism. Behavior that results from child abuse also may take the form of a personality disorder, and the symptoms of PTSD are occasionally mistaken for psychotic illness or an organic brain syndrome. PTSD is thus a highly prevalent and impairing condition (see Critical Thinking About Contemporary Issues).

Finally, about 25% or 1 of 4 people will experience an anxiety disorder sometime in their life. These are the most common psychiatric disorders in American society. Specifically, obsessive-compulsive disorder (OCD) affects about 2% of the

Critical Thinking *About* Contemporary Issues

Is Posttraumatic Stress Disorder the Disease of the New Millennium?

Posttraumatic stress disorder (PTSD) is a commonly occurring disorder that often has a duration of many years and is commonly associated with recurrences related to exposure to multiple traumas. PTSD describes a syndrome in which a trauma survivor is unable to get the event out of his or her mind. Scenes of the traumatic event return involuntarily as images, unwanted memories, nightmares, or flashbacks. Usually intense distress is associated with the reexperiencing of the event, and survivors report such unpleasant physical symptoms as palpitations, shortness of breath, and other panic symptoms. Often, in an attempt to cope with these memories, survivors develop a set of avoidance behaviors to restrict their exposure to persons, places, or things that will remind them of the event. Another type of avoidance behavior is to become emotionally numb, constricted, or unresponsive to the environment. Trauma survivors also have severe physiological disturbances, including trouble sleeping, irritability, impaired concentration, and hypervigilance to their environment.

It has long been known that stress response syndromes can result from exposure to war. For example, 30% of Viet Nam veterans developed PTSD within a few years of returning from the war. Although combat deaths in the Viet Nam war numbered 58,000, a greater number, between 60,000 and 70,000 Viet Nam veterans, committed suicide in the 20 years following because of PTSD. Recent evidence shows that PTSD can result from incidents of sex-

ual assault and other types of trauma as well. Specifically, it has been found that, in populations at risk, PTSD ranges from 18% in professional firefighters, 34% in adolescent survivors of motor vehicle accidents, and 48% in female rape victims to 67% in surviving prisoners of war (Lange, Lange, and Cabaltica, 2000). People with PTSD are 6 times more likely to attempt suicide, and as many as 80% of patients with PTSD have a comorbid psychiatric disorder such as depression, generalized anxiety disorder, substance abuse, or panic disorder. Potential links between PTSD, cognition, and behavioral problems in late life have been suggested (Cook, Ruzek, and Cassidy, 2003); and PTSD is also associated with a higher rate of general medical complaints, including anemia, arthritis, asthma, back pain, diabetes, eczema, and ulcers (Weisberg et al, 2002). Impairment resulting from PTSD can be considerable, including both failure to realize one's potential in terms of education, marriage, and employment and impairment even in day-to-day role functioning (Kessler, 2000).

Finally, the risk of PTSD is much greater after exposure to a trauma involving assaultive violence than to other forms of trauma. Given the prevalence of crime, terrorist acts, and political, racial, religious, and ethnic violence in contemporary society, it seems likely that PTSD will be a common illness in the years to come and that the processes of healing and recovery may have to be measured in terms of generations rather than years.

U.S. population; generalized anxiety disorder (GAD), about 3% to 6%; phobias, between 13% and 15%; panic disorder, about 1% to 3%; and posttraumatic stress disorder (PTSD), about 8% of the population.

Anxiety disorders occur twice as often in women as in men, and obsessive-compulsive disorder is about equally prevalent in women and men. No outstanding differences in the prevalence of anxiety disorders have been found on the basis of race, income, education, or rural versus urban dwelling.

OUTCOME IDENTIFICATION

Goals such as "decrease anxiety" and "minimize anxiety" lack specific behaviors and evaluation criteria. Therefore these goals are not particularly useful in guiding nursing care and evaluating its effectiveness. The expected outcome for patients with maladaptive anxiety responses is:

> *The patient will demonstrate adaptive ways of coping with stress.*

Short-term goals can break this expected outcome down into readily attainable steps. This identification of steps allows the patient and nurse to see progress even if the ultimate goal still appears distant.

When the nursing diagnosis describes the patient's anxiety at the severe or panic levels, the highest-priority short-term goals should address safety and lowering the anxiety level. Only after this decreased anxiety has been achieved can additional progress be made. The reduced level of anxiety should be evident in a reduction of behaviors associated with severe or panic levels.

When these goals are met, the nurse can assume that the patient's level of anxiety has been reduced. The nurse may

---

BOX **16-8**
NOC Outcome Indicators for Anxiety Self-Control

Monitors intensity of anxiety
Eliminates precursors of anxiety
Decreases environmental stimuli when anxious
Seeks information to reduce anxiety
Plans coping strategies for stressful situations
Uses effective coping strategies
Uses relaxation techniques to reduce anxiety
Monitors duration of episodes
Monitors length of time between episodes
Maintains role performance
Maintains social relationships
Maintains concentration
Monitors sensory perceptual distortions
Maintains adequate sleep
Monitors physical manifestations of anxiety
Monitors behavioral manifestations of anxiety
Controls anxiety response

From Moorhead S, Johnson M, Maas M, editors: *Nursing outcomes classification (NOC)*, ed 3, St Louis, 2004, Mosby.

---

then develop new short-term goals directed toward insight or relaxation therapy. In addition, since anxiety is a subjective response, a useful measure would be to ask the patient to rate his level of anxiety from 1 to 10. Obtaining a rating of 2 or 3 might be another expected outcome.

Outcome indicators related to "Anxiety Self-Control" from the Nursing Outcome Classification (NOC) project are presented in Box 16-8 (Moorhead, Johnson, and Maas, 2004).

PLANNING

The main goal of the nurse working with anxious patients is not to free them totally from anxiety. Patients need to develop the capacity to tolerate mild anxiety and to use it consciously and constructively. In this way the self will become stronger and more integrated. As they learn from these experiences, they will move on in their development.

Anxiety can be considered a war between the threat and the values people identify with their existence. Maladaptive behavior means that the struggle has been lost. The constructive approach to anxiety means that the struggle is won by the person's values. Thus a general nursing goal is to help patients develop sound values. This approach does not mean that patients assume the nurse's values. Rather, the nurse helps the patient sort out his or her own values.

Anxiety also can be an important factor in the patient's decision to seek treatment. Because anxiety is undesirable, the patient will seek ways to reduce it. If the patient's coping mechanism or symptom does not minimize anxiety, the motivation for treatment increases. Conversely, anxiety about the therapeutic process can delay or prevent the person from seeking treatment.

The patient should actively participate in planning treatment strategies. If the patient is actively involved in identifying relevant stressors and planning possible solutions, the success of the implementation phase will be maximized. A patient in extreme anxiety initially will not be able to participate in the problem-solving process. However, as soon as anxiety is reduced, the nurse should encourage patient involvement. This participation reinforces that patients are responsible for their own growth and personal development.

IMPLEMENTATION

Practice guidelines have been developed to treat a variety of anxiety disorders (American Psychiatric Association, 1998; Expert Consensus Guideline Series, 1999). **Empirically validated treatments** for some of the medical diagnoses related to anxiety disorders are summarized in Box 16-9 (Nathan and Gorman, 2002).

Severe and Panic Levels of Anxiety

Establishing a Trusting Relationship. To reduce the patient's level of anxiety, most nursing actions are purposely protective and supportive. Initially nurses need to establish an open, trusting relationship. Nurses should actively listen to patients and encourage them to discuss their feelings of anxiety, hostility, guilt, and frustration. Nurses should answer patients' questions directly and offer unconditional acceptance. Their verbal and nonverbal communications should convey awareness and acceptance of patients' feelings.

Nurses should remain available and respect the patient's personal space. A 6-foot distance in a small room may create the optimum condition for openness and discussion of fears. The more this distance is increased or decreased, the more anxious the patient may become.

Nurses' Self-Awareness. Nurses' feelings are particularly important in working with highly anxious patients. They may find themselves being unsympathetic, impatient, and frustrated.

These are common feelings of reciprocal anxiety. If nurses are alert to the development of anxiety in themselves, they can learn from it and use it therapeutically. Nurses should be alert to the signs of anxiety in themselves, accept them, and attempt to explore their cause. The nurse may ask the following questions:

- What is threatening me?
- Have I failed to live up to what I imagine to be the patient's ideal?
- Am I comparing myself to a peer or another health professional?
- Is the patient's area of conflict one that I have not resolved in myself?
- Is my anxiety related to something that will or may happen in the future? Is my patient's conflict really one of my own that I am projecting?

If nurses deny their own anxiety, it can have detrimental effects on the nurse-patient relationship. Because of their own anxiety, nurses may be unable to differentiate between levels of anxiety in others. They also may transfer their fears and frustrations to patients, thus compounding their problems.

Nurses who are anxious arouse defenses in patients and other staff that interfere with their therapeutic usefulness. Nurses should strive to accept their patients' anxiety without reciprocal anxiety by continually clarifying their own feelings and role, as indicated in the following clinical example.

CLINICAL EXAMPLE

Ms. R was a 35-year-old married woman and mother of three children, ages 4, 6, and 9. She was a full-time homemaker and mother. Her husband was a salesperson and spent about 2 nights each week out of town. She came to the clinic complaining of severe headaches that "come upon me very suddenly and are so terrible that I have to go to bed. The only thing that helps is for me to lie down in a dark and absolutely quiet room." She said that these headaches were becoming a real problem for everyone in the family, and her husband told her that she "just had to get over them and get things back to normal."

Mr. W, a psychiatric nurse, offered to see Ms. R in therapy once a week. After 3 weeks, he was asked to present his evaluation, treatment plans, and progress report to the clinic staff at their weekly team conference. Mr. W began his presentation by stating, "This case is really tough. I'll start with the progress report and say that there is none because I can't seem to get past all the complaining this patient does!" He then went on to discuss his evaluation and treatment plan in depth. It became obvious to the other members of the staff that Mr. W saw his patient as a woman who was not living up to her roles and responsibilities. He defended Ms. R's husband even though the husband refused to come to the sessions with his wife. When one of the team members asked about the possibility of a medication evaluation for Ms. R, the nurse replied, "Everyone gets headaches. I don't think we should reward or reinforce this woman's complaints."

In reviewing this case the staff noted that Mr. W appeared to have problems relating empathetically to his patient because of her particular set of problems and some of his own values and perceptions. Mr. W agreed with this and said he had thought of asking someone else to work with Ms. R. Mr. W's supervisor observed that the nurse had problems with this type of patient in the past, and a more constructive approach would be to increase his supervision on this case, focusing on the dynamics between the patient and nurse that were blocking learning and growth for both of them. Mr. W and his supervisor set a time when they could begin to meet for this purpose. ∎

What clinical situations or patient problems raise your level of anxiety? ■

Protecting the Patient. A major area of intervention is protecting and assuring the patient of his or her safety. One way to decrease anxiety is by allowing the patient to determine the amount of stress he or she can handle at the time. Nurses should not force severely anxious patients into situations they are not able to handle. Neither should they attack patients' coping mechanisms. Rather, nurses should attempt to protect patients' defenses.

The coping mechanism or symptom is attempting to deal with an unconscious conflict. Usually patients do not understand *why* the symptom has developed or *what* they are gaining from it. They know only that the symptom relieves some of the intolerable anxiety and tension. **Thus asking "why" questions of patients related to their behaviors or symptoms is not helpful.** If patients are unable to release this anxiety, their tension mounts to the panic level and they could lose control. It also is important to remember that the severely anxious patient has not worked through the area of

BOX **16-9**	SUMMARIZING THE EVIDENCE ON **Anxiety Disorders**
Disorder	Generalized anxiety disorder (GAD)
Treatment	◆ The most successful psychosocial treatments for GAD combine relaxation, exercise, and cognitive behavioral therapy in an effort to bring the worry process under the patient's control. ◆ Benzodiazepines, buspirone, tricyclic antidepressants, venlafaxine, and selective serotonin reuptake inhibitors (SSRIs) are all effective in reducing anxiety, although the first two medications are subject to abuse/dependence.
Disorder	Obsessive compulsive disorder (OCD)
Treatment	◆ Cognitive-behavioral therapy involving exposure and ritual prevention methods reduce or eliminate the obsessions and behavioral and mental rituals of OCD. ◆ Serotonin reuptake inhibitors (SRIs) reduce obsessions and compulsions in approximately 20% to 40% of cases.
Disorder	Panic disorder with or without agoraphobia
Treatment	◆ Situational in vivo exposure substantially reduces symptoms of panic disorder with agoraphobia. ◆ Cognitive-behavioral treatments that focus on education about the nature of anxiety and panic provide some form of exposure, and coping skills acquisition significantly reduces symptoms of panic disorder without agoraphobia. ◆ Tricyclic antidepressants and monoamine oxidase inhibitors reduce the number of panic attacks, anticipatory anxiety, and phobic avoidance. ◆ The benzodiazepines eliminate panic attacks in 55% to 75% of patients. ◆ SRIs and SSRIs reduce panic frequency, generalized anxiety, disability and phobic avoidance disorder with or without agoraphobia.
Disorder	Posttraumatic stress disorder (PTSD)
Treatment	◆ Monoamine oxidase inhibitors (MAOIs) reduce intrusive thoughts, improve sleep, and moderate anxiety and depression. ◆ Tricyclic antidepressants reduce intrusive thoughts and obsessions and moderate depression. ◆ SSRIs markedly reduce intrusive thoughts, avoidance, and sleep problems. ◆ Exposure therapies (systematic desensitization, flooding, prolonged exposure, and implosive therapy) and, to a lesser extent, anxiety management techniques (using cognitive-behavioral strategies) reduce PTSD symptoms, including anxiety and depression, and increase social functioning.
Disorder	Social phobia
Treatment	◆ Exposure-based procedures and cognitive-behavioral treatments reduce or eliminate the symptoms of the disorder. ◆ Social skills training and relaxation techniques are effective. ◆ MAOIs relieve the key symptoms of social phobia. ◆ Some of the SSRIs are helpful for some aspects of the disorder.
Disorder	Specific phobias
Treatment	◆ Exposure-based procedures, especially in vivo exposure, reduce or eliminate most aspects of specific phobic disorders. ◆ No pharmacological intervention has been shown to be effective for specific phobias.

From Nathan P, Gorman J: *A guide to treatments that work,* ed 2, New York, 2002, Oxford University Press.

conflict and therefore has no alternatives or substitutes for present coping mechanisms.

This principle also applies to severe levels of anxiety as seen in obsessive-compulsive reactions, phobias, and panic attacks. Nurses should not initially interfere with a patient's repetitive act or force patients to confront the avoided situation or phobic object. They should not ridicule the nature of the defense. Also, nurses should not attempt to argue with patients about it or reason them out of it. Patients need their coping mechanisms to keep anxiety within tolerable limits.

Neither should nurses reinforce the phobia, ritual, avoidance, or physical complaint by focusing attention on it and talking about it a great deal. With time, however, nurses can place some limits on patients' behavior and attempt to help them find satisfaction with other aspects of life.

Some nursing interventions can increase anxiety in severely anxious patients. These include pressuring the patient to change prematurely, being judgmental, verbally disapproving of the patient's behaviors, and asking the patient a direct question that brings on defensiveness. Focusing in a critical way on the patient's anxious feelings with others present, lacking awareness of one's own behaviors and feelings, and withdrawing from the patient also can be harmful.

Modifying the Environment.
The nurse can consult with others to identify anxiety-producing situations and attempt to reduce them. The nurse can set limits by assuming a quiet, calm manner and decreasing environmental stimulation. Limiting the patient's interaction with other patients will minimize the contagious aspects of anxiety. Supportive physical measures such as warm baths, massages, or whirlpool baths also may be helpful in decreasing a patient's anxiety.

Encouraging Activity.
The nurse needs to encourage the patient's interest in activities. This involvement limits the time available for destructive coping mechanisms and increases participation in and enjoyment of other aspects of life. The nurse might suggest physical activities such as walking, a sport, or an active hobby. This form of physical exercise helps to relieve anxiety because it provides an emotional release and directs the patient's attention outward. Family members should be involved in the planning because they can be very supportive in setting limits and stimulating outside activity (see A Family Speaks).

Medication.
Medications are very effective in treating anxiety disorders (Table 16-3). Because anxiety is a pervasive problem, large portions of the population take antianxiety drugs. Americans are now spending more than $500 million each year for drugs to relieve anxiety.

Table 16-3	Antianxiety Drugs
CHEMICAL CLASS **GENERIC NAME (TRADE NAME)**	**USUAL DOSAGE RANGE** **(MG/DAY)**
Antianxiety Drugs	
Benzodiazepines	
Alprazolam (Xanax)	1-4
Chlordiazepoxide (Librium)	10-40
Clonazepam (Klonopin)	0.5-10
Clorazepate (Tranxene)	10-40
Diazepam (Valium)	2-40
Halazepam (Paxipam)	60-160
Lorazepam (Ativan)	1-6
Oxazepam (Serax)	15-120
Prazepam (Centrax)	10-60
Antihistamines	
Diphenhydramine (Benadryl)	50
Hydroxyzine (Atarax)	100-300
Noradrenergic agents	
Clonidine (Catapres)	0.2-0.6
Propranolol (Inderal)	6-160
Anxiolytic	
Buspirone (BuSpar)	15-60
Antidepressant/Antianxiety Drugs	
Selective serotonin reuptake inhibitors	
Citalopram (Celexa)	20-40
Escitalopram (Lexapro)	20-40
Fluoxetine (Prozac)	20-60
Fluvoxamine (Luvox)	100-200
Paroxetine (Paxil)	20-50
Sertraline (Zoloft)	50-200
Other newer antidepressants	
Mirtazapine (Remeron)	15-45
Nefazodone (Serzone)	300-500
Trazodone (Desyrel)	150-300
Venlafaxine (Effexor)	75-375
Tricyclics	
Amitriptyline (Elavil)	50-300
Desipramine (Norpramin)	50-300
Clomipramine (Anafranil)	50-250
Imipramine (Tofranil)	50-300
Nortriptyline (Pamelor)	50-150
Monoamine oxidase inhibitor (MAOI)	
Phenelzine (Nardil)	45-90

A FAMILY SPEAKS

My daughter has obsessive-compulsive disorder (OCD). I didn't always know that, and I've spent many years of my life wondering what was wrong with her and if I were to blame. It's not easy living with someone who has an illness like that. At times it is just annoying. At other times it really makes you mad, and still other times you want to burst out laughing, but all that only makes it worse.

I think the one thing the family needs from the mental health care system is for health care professionals to talk with them. The nurse who sees my daughter told me that I can call her with questions, and she explained all about OCD to my husband and me in great detail. Families want to help and support their members who are suffering, but how can we help if we don't know what to do? I used to try to physically stop my daughter from checking things. Then I told her how ridiculous it was. I even tried ignoring it for a while. How was I supposed to know what to do? Things are different now. We've all learned about this illness and how we can best help our daughter. After all, that's all we ever really wanted.

Benzodiazepines are effective in the treatment of anxiety disorders. However, use of benzodiazepines in combination with alcohol may result in a serious or even fatal sedative reaction. Antidepressants have gained popularity in the treatment of anxiety disorders in light of studies documenting their effectiveness and the low side effect profile of some of them. Antipsychotic drugs are often prescribed for patients experiencing a panic level of anxiety of psychotic proportions.

Although some patients may need to take antianxiety drugs for extended periods, these drugs should always be used together with psychosocial treatments. Potential dangers of benzodiazepines include withdrawal syndrome side effects and addiction (see Chapter 24). It should be emphasized that medication is not a substitute for an ongoing therapeutic relationship, but it can enhance the therapeutic alliance. Chemical control of painful symptoms allows the patient to direct attention to the conflicts underlying the anxiety. More detailed information on medications is presented in Chapter 27.

The Nursing Treatment Plan Summary (Table 16-4) reviews interventions related to severe and panic levels of anxiety.

Moderate Level of Anxiety

The nursing interventions previously mentioned are supportive and directed toward the short-term goal of reducing severe- or panic-level anxiety. When the patient's anxiety is reduced to a moderate level, the nurse can begin helping with problem-solving efforts to cope with the stress. Long-term goals focus on helping the patient understand the cause of the anxiety and learn new ways of controlling it. Goals include recognition of anxiety, insight into the anxiety, and coping with the threat. They incorporate principles and techniques of cognitive behavioral therapy (see Chapter 31) and can be implemented in any setting: psychiatric, community, home, or general hospital.

Education. Education is an important aspect of promoting the patient's adaptive responses to anxiety. The nurse can identify the health teaching needs of each patient and then formulate a plan to meet those needs. Plans should be designed to increase patients' knowledge of their own predisposing and precipitating stressors, coping resources, and adaptive and maladaptive responses. Alternative coping strategies can

---

Table 16-4 NURSING TREATMENT PLAN SUMMARY Severe and Panic Anxiety Responses

Nursing Diagnosis: Severe/panic level anxiety
Expected Outcome: The patient will reduce anxiety to a moderate or mild level.

SHORT-TERM GOAL	INTERVENTION	RATIONALE
The patient will be protected from harm.	Initially accept and support, rather than attack, the patient's defenses. Do not ask the patient why the symptoms exist. Acknowledge the reality of the pain associated with the patient's present coping mechanisms. Do not focus on the phobia, ritual, or physical complaint itself. Give feedback to the patient about behavior, stressors, appraisal of stressors, and coping resources. Reinforce the idea that physical health is related to emotional health and that this is an area that will need exploration. In time, begin to place limits on the patient's maladaptive behavior in a supportive way.	Severe and panic levels of anxiety can be reduced by initially allowing the patient to determine the amount of stress that can be handled. If the patient is unable to release anxiety, tension may mount to the panic level and the patient may lose control. At this time the patient has no alternative coping mechanisms.
The patient will experience fewer anxiety-provoking situations.	Assume a calm manner with the patient. Decrease environmental stimulation. Limit the patient's interaction with other patients to minimize the contagious aspects of anxiety. Identify and modify anxiety-provoking situations for the patient. Administer supportive physical measures such as warm baths and massages.	The patient's behavior may be modified by altering the environment and the patient's interaction with it.
The patient will engage in a daily schedule of activities.	Initially share an activity with the patient to provide support and reinforce socially productive behavior. Provide for physical exercise of some type. Plan a schedule or list of activities that can be carried out daily. Involve family members and other support systems as much as possible.	By encouraging outside activities, the nurse limits the time the patient has available for destructive coping mechanisms while increasing participation in and enjoyment of other aspects of life.
The patient will experience relief from the symptoms of severe anxiety.	Administer medications that help reduce the patient's discomfort. Observe for medication side effects and initiate relevant health teaching.	The effect of a therapeutic relationship may be enhanced if the chemical control of symptoms allows the patient to direct attention to underlying conflicts.

be identified and explored. Health teaching also should address the beneficial aspects of mild levels of anxiety in motivating learning and producing growth and creativity.

Although further research is needed to clarify the mechanisms that cause anxiety disorders, the clinical significance of current findings can be reassuring to patients. Patients can be told, for example, that anxiety disorders are a dysregulation in the normal fight-or-flight response, which is important to survival. The way in which anxiety disorders present may be a combination of genetic vulnerability and a person's reactions to life's stressors. Perhaps most important, patients should be told that anxiety disorders can be successfully treated by a variety of evidence-based treatments. This information can give patients a sense of control over anxiety's seemingly uncontrollable and debilitating effects.

Recognition of Anxiety. After analyzing the patient's behaviors and determining the level of anxiety, the nurse helps the patient recognize anxiety by helping him or her explore underlying feelings with such questions as "Are you feeling anxious now?" or "Are you uncomfortable?"

It is also helpful for the nurse to identify the patient's behavior and link it to the feeling of anxiety (for example, "I noticed you have smoked three cigarettes since we started talking about your sister. Are you feeling anxious?"). In this way the nurse acknowledges the patient's feeling, attempts to label it, encourages the patient to describe it further, and relates it to a specific behavioral pattern. The nurse is also validating inferences and assumptions with the patient.

However, the patient's goal is often to avoid or deny anxiety, and he or she may use any of the resistive approaches described in Box 16-10. All of these approaches may create feelings of frustration, irritation, or reciprocal anxiety in the nurse, who must recognize personal feelings and identify the patient's behavior pattern that might be causing them.

At this time, a trusting relationship is very important. If nurses establish themselves as warm, responsive listeners, give patients adequate time to respond, and support the patient's self-expression, they will become less threatening. In helping patients recognize their anxiety, nurses should use open questions that move from nonthreatening topics to central issues of conflict. In time, supportive confrontation may be used to address a particularly resistive pattern. However, if the patient's level of anxiety begins to rise rapidly, the nurse might choose to refocus the discussion to another topic.

Insight Into the Anxiety. Once the patient is able to recognize anxiety, the nurse can help the patient gain insight by asking the patient to describe the situations and interactions that immediately precede the increase in anxiety. Together the nurse and patient make inferences about the precipitating causes or biopsychosocial stressors.

The nurse then helps the patient see which values are being threatened by linking the threat with underlying causes, analyzing how the conflict developed, and relating the patient's present experiences to past ones. It is also important to explore how the patient reduced anxiety in the past and what kinds of actions produced relief.

Coping With the Threat. If previous coping responses have been adaptive and constructive, the patient should be encouraged to use them. If not, the nurse can point out their maladaptive effects and help the patient see that the present way of life appears unsatisfactory and distressing. The patient needs to assume responsibility for actions and realize that limitations have been self-imposed. Other people must not be blamed.

In this phase of intervention, the nurse assumes an active role by interpreting, analyzing, confronting, and correlating cause-and-effect relationships. The nurse should proceed clearly so that the patient can follow while keeping anxiety within appropriate limits. If the patient's anxiety becomes too severe, the nurse may change topics temporarily.

The nurse can help the patient in problem-solving efforts in various cognitive and behavioral ways. Specifically,

---

BOX 16-10

Patient Resistances To Recognizing Anxiety

Screen symptoms. The patient focuses attention on minor physical ailments to avoid acknowledging anxiety and conflict areas.

Superior status position. The patient attempts to control the interview by questioning the nurse's abilities or asserting the superiority of the patient's knowledge or experiences. The nurse should not respond emotionally to this approach or accept the patient's challenge and compete because this would only further avoid the issue of anxiety.

Emotional seduction. The patient attempts to manipulate the nurse and elicit pity or sympathy.

Superficiality. The patient relates on a surface level and resists the nurse's attempts to explore underlying feelings or analyze issues.

Circumlocution. The patient gives the pretense of answering questions, but actually talks around the topic to avoid it.

Amnesia. This is a type of purposeful forgetting of an incident to avoid confronting and exploring it with the nurse.

Denial. The patient may use this approach only when discussing significant issues with the nurse or may generalize denial to all others, including self. The purpose is often to avoid humiliation.

Intellectualization. Patients who use this technique usually have some knowledge of psychology or medicine. They are able to express appropriate insights and analysis yet lack personal involvement in the problem they describe. They are not actually participating in the problem-solving process.

Hostility. The patient believes that offense is the best defense and therefore relates to others in an aggressive, defiant manner. The greatest danger in this situation is that the nurse will take this behavior personally and respond with anger. This reinforces the patient's avoidance of his or her anxiety.

Withdrawal. The patient may resist the nurse by replying in vague, diffuse, indefinite, and remote ways.

cognitive behavioral therapy has been shown to be very effective in treating many anxiety disorders across age-groups (Simpson and Kozak, 2000; Bryant et al, 1999; Wells, 1997; Valente, 2002a, 2002b). These treatments include a number of therapeutic strategies, which can be divided into three groups:

1. **Anxiety reduction**
2. **Cognitive restructuring**
3. **Learning new behavior**

The specific strategies for each group are listed in Box 16-11 and explained in detail in Chapter 31.

One way of helping the patient cope is to reevaluate the nature of the threat or stressor. Is it as bad as the patient perceives it? Is the cognitive appraisal realistic? Together the nurse and patient might discuss fears and feelings of inadequacy. Does the patient fear that others are as critical, perfectionistic, and rejecting as the patient is of others? Is the conflict based in reality, or is it the result of unvalidated, isolated, and distorted thinking? By sharing fears with family members, peers, and staff, the patient often gains insight into such misperceptions.

Another approach is to help the patient modify behavior and learn new ways of coping with stress. The nurse may act as a role model in this regard or engage the patient in role playing. This activity can decrease anxiety about new responses to problem situations. One nursing function therefore is to teach the patient how aspects of mild anxiety can be constructive and produce growth. Physical activity should be encouraged as a way to discharge anxiety. Interpersonal resources such as family members or close friends should be incorporated into the nursing plan of care to provide the patient with support.

Often the cause for anxiety arises from an interpersonal conflict. In this case, it is constructive to include the people involved when analyzing the situation with the patient. In this way, cause-and-effect relationships are more open to examination. Coping patterns can be examined in light of their effect on others, as well as on the patient.

Working through this problem-solving or reeducative process with the patient takes time because it has to be accepted both intellectually and emotionally. Breaking previous behavioral patterns can be difficult. Nurses need to be patient and consistent and continually reappraise their own anxiety.

Promote the Relaxation Response. In addition to problem solving, one also can cope with stress by regulating the emotional distress associated with it. Long-term goals directed toward helping the patient regulate emotional distress include promoting the relaxation response.

Relaxation can be taught individually, in small groups, or in large-group settings. A Patient Education Plan for teaching the relaxation response is presented in Table 16-5. It is within the scope of nursing practice, requires no special equipment, and does not need a physician's supervision.

As a group of interventions, relaxation can be implemented in various settings. A major benefit for patients is that after several training sessions, they can practice the techniques on their own. This puts the control in their hands and increases their self-reliance. Relaxation training is described in detail in Chapter 31. The Nursing Treatment Plan Summary for patients with moderate anxiety is presented in Table 16-6.

EVALUATION

Even before beginning to formulate the nursing diagnosis, the nurse should ask, "Did I critically observe my patient's physiological and psychomotor behaviors? Did I listen to my patient's subjective description of anxiety? Did I fail to see the relationships between my patient's expressed hostility or guilt and underlying anxiety? Did I assess intellectual and social functioning?"

After collecting the data, the nurse should analyze it: "Was I able to identify the precipitating stressor for the patient? What was the patient's perception of the threat? How was this influenced by physical health, past experiences, and present feelings and needs? Did I correctly identify the patient's level of anxiety and validate it?"

When using the criteria of adequacy, effectiveness, appropriateness, efficiency, and flexibility in evaluating the nursing goals and actions, the following questions can be raised:

- Were the planning, implementation, and evaluation mutual?
- Were goals and actions adequate in number and sufficiently specific to minimize the patient's level of anxiety?
- Were maladaptive responses reduced?
- Were new adaptive coping responses learned?
- Was the nurse accepting of the patient and able to monitor personal anxiety throughout the relationship?

The nurse also will identify personal strengths and limitations in working with the anxious patient. Plans may then be made for overcoming the areas of limitation and further improving nursing care.

BOX 16-11

Cognitive Behavioral Treatment Strategies for Anxiety Disorders

Anxiety Reduction	**Cognitive Restructuring**
Relaxation training	Monitoring thoughts and
Biofeedback	feelings
Systematic desensitization	Questioning the evidence
Interoceptive exposure	Examining alternatives
Flooding	Decatastrophizing
Vestibular desensitization	Reframing
training	Thought stopping
Response prevention	
Eye movement desensiti-	**Learning New Behavior**
zation and reprocessing	Modeling
(EMDR)	Shaping
	Token economy
	Role playing
	Social skills training
	Aversion therapy
	Contingency contracting

Table 16-5   PATIENT EDUCATION PLAN   The Relaxation Response

CONTENT	INSTRUCTIONAL ACTIVITIES	EVALUATION
Describe the characteristics and benefits of relaxation.	Discuss physiological changes associated with relaxation and contrast these with the behaviors of anxiety.	Patient identifies own responses to anxiety. Patient describes elements of a relaxed state.
Teach deep muscle relaxation through a sequence of tension-relaxation exercises.	Engage the patient in the progressive procedure of tensing and relaxing voluntary muscles until the body as a whole is relaxed.	Patient is able to tense and relax all muscle groups. Patient identifies muscles that become particularly tense.
Discuss the relaxation procedure of meditation and its components.	Describe the elements of meditation and help the patient use this technique.	Patient selects a word or scene with pleasant connotations and engages in relaxed meditation.
Help patient overcome anxiety-provoking situations through systematic desensitization.	With patient, construct a hierarchy of anxiety-provoking situations or scenes. Through imagination or reality, work through these scenes using relaxation techniques.	Patient identifies and ranks anxiety-provoking situations. Patient exposes self to these situations while remaining in a relaxed state.
Allow the rehearsing and practical use of relaxation in a safe environment.	Role play stressful situations with the nurse or other patients.	Patient becomes more comfortable with new behavior in a safe, supportive setting.
Encourage patient to use relaxation techniques in life.	Assign homework of using the relaxation response in everyday experiences.	Support success of patient. Patient uses relaxation response in life situations. Patient is able to regulate anxiety response through use of relaxation techniques.

Table 16-6   NURSING TREATMENT PLAN SUMMARY   Moderate Anxiety Responses

Nursing Diagnosis: Moderate level of anxiety
Expected Outcome: The patient will demonstrate adaptive ways of coping with stress.

SHORT-TERM GOAL	INTERVENTION	RATIONALE
The patient will identify and describe feelings of anxiety.	Help the patient identify and describe underlying feelings. Link the patient's behavior with such feelings. Validate all inferences and assumptions with the patient. Use open questions to move from nonthreatening topics to issues of conflict. In time, supportive confrontation may be used judiciously.	To adopt new coping responses, the patient first needs to be aware of feelings and to overcome conscious or unconscious denial and resistance.
The patient will identify antecedents of anxiety.	Help the patient describe the situations and interactions that immediately precede anxiety. Review the patient's appraisal of the stressor, values being threatened, and the way in which the conflict developed. Relate the patient's present experiences with relevant ones from the past.	Once feelings of anxiety are recognized, the patient needs to understand their development, including precipitating stressors, appraisal of the stressors, and available resources.
The patient will describe adaptive and maladaptive coping responses.	Explore how the patient reduced anxiety in the past and what kinds of actions produced relief. Point out the maladaptive and destructive effects of present coping responses. Encourage the patient to use adaptive coping responses that were effective in the past. Focus responsibility for change on the patient. Actively help the patient correlate cause-and-effect relationships while maintaining anxiety within appropriate limits. Help the patient reappraise the value, nature, and meaning of the stressor when appropriate.	New adaptive coping responses can be learned through analyzing coping mechanisms used in the past, reappraising the stressor, using available resources, and accepting responsibility for change.
The patient will implement two adaptive responses for coping with anxiety.	Help the patient identify ways to restructure thoughts, modify behavior, use resources, and test new coping responses. Encourage physical activity to discharge energy. Include significant others as resources and social supports in helping the patient learn new coping responses. Teach the patient relaxation exercises to increase control and self-reliance and reduce stress.	One also can cope with stress by regulating the emotional distress that accompanies it through the use of stress management techniques.

COMPETENT CARING

A Clinical Exemplar of a Psychiatric Nurse
MADELYN MYERS, MSN, RN, PMH-NP

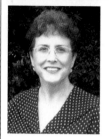

As the night shift charge nurse on an adult psychiatric unit, I learned that the graveyard shift was anything but routine. On return to the unit after my days off, I was told that Mr. B's behavior had deteriorated in the last few days. Mr. B was a 68-year-old man with a diagnosis of organic brain syndrome secondary to alcohol abuse. He was unable to stay in bed for more than a few minutes at a time, and he was at risk for falls because of his confusion and as a side effect of his tranquilizing medication. The previous nights the staff had found it necessary to contain Mr. B with soft restraints to keep him in bed and reduce the risk of his falling.

After shift report I made my nursing rounds, accounting for all patients and assessing the situation of the unit. Mr. B was obviously distraught and anxious. His first question to me was, "You're not going to rope me, are you?" I sat down to talk with Mr. B to reassure him and explain that it was time for him to get ready for bed. He refused to change his clothing, stating that he just needed to walk around a little longer. I asked the therapeutic assistants if they would walk him around a while longer to try calming him down. I went to the office to start verifying the day's orders, but found it impossible to get much done as Mr. B was calling me and coming to the nursing office to ask questions very frequently. The staff were also getting frustrated because he seemed very tired but would sit down for only a few minutes before he would jump up again.

After I did a few more tasks, I relieved the staff member sitting with Mr. B. I was able to get Mr. B to lie down on his bed only after he saw me take the posey off the bed and out of the room. I watched him as he lay down and he seemed to doze off to sleep almost immediately. Then again just as quickly he awoke and started out of bed. He said, "Something is very wrong with me—I'm afraid I might die." We discussed his anxiety, and I reassured him that one of the staff would sit with him if that would make him feel more secure. He nodded in affirmation. I sat by his bedside. He fell asleep immediately and again repeated his previous pattern of awakening with a start, but this time he just looked over, saw me, and returned to sleep.

A short while later, one of the other staff came to relieve me. I shared with her my concern that Mr. B had been quite anxious and that my plan was to sit at his bedside and gradually move the chair back until we were sitting just outside his room but still in his line of sight. This way, he would be reassured that staff were still close by, and we could observe him if he tried to get out of bed. That night he actually slept 4 hours with only two brief awakenings. The previous nights he had only dozed for minutes at a time.

The next morning I spoke with the nurse on his team about his fear of dying and of being "roped" with the posey. I shared with her the strategy we used of sitting with him and how he was able to sleep when we stayed nearby. The new plan of care was placed in his chart for all to follow. The next few nights we continued with our plan, and each night Mr. B slept a little longer. He would even change into his pajamas before bed. He no longer started to "escalate" at bedtime. As he was sleeping better, Mr. B was also feeling better physically, and his anxiety level decreased dramatically. He required less medication for his anxiety; thus he was much more stable on his feet and no longer at risk for falls. Mr. B's ability to perform his activities of daily living (ADLs) increased over the next week, and he was able to return to his previous living situation.

Many of his symptoms seemed to have been from sleep deprivation, high levels of anxiety, and the untoward effects of tranquilizers. This rewarding experience was not an isolated event on the night shift. It seems that many people sleep through the night and see only the shadows of the staff making rounds, but there are others for whom the care they receive during these darkened hours makes a critical difference. ■

CHAPTER FOCUS POINTS

- Anxiety disorders are the most common psychiatric disorders in America, affecting between 10% and 25% of the population. Anxiety is a diffuse apprehension that is vague in nature and associated with feelings of uncertainty and helplessness. It is an emotion without a specific object, a subjective individual experience, and an energy that cannot be observed directly. Anxiety is communicated interpersonally.

- The crux of anxiety is self-preservation. Anxiety occurs as a result of a threat to a person's selfhood, self-esteem, or identity.

- Mild and moderate levels of anxiety heighten the person's capacities, whereas severe and panic levels paralyze or overwork capacities. A panic level of anxiety can be life threatening.

- Anxiety can be expressed directly through physiological and behavioral changes or indirectly through cognitive and affective responses, including the formation of symptoms or coping mechanisms developed as a defense against anxiety.

- Behavioral changes with anxiety are most often the result of sympathetic reaction of the autonomic nervous system.

- Anxiety is a prime factor in the development of the personality and formation of individual character traits. Predisposing factors for anxiety responses can be explained by psychoanalytical, interpersonal, behavioral, family, and biological perspectives.

- Epidemiological and family studies show that anxiety disorders tend to run in families.

- The regulation of anxiety is related to the activity of the neurotransmitter gamma-aminobutyric acid (GABA), which controls the activity, or firing rates, of neurons in the parts of the brain responsible for producing anxiety. These are the limbic system, an area thought to be of central importance for emotional behavior; and the locus ceruleus, the primary manufacturing center of norepinephrine, which is an excitatory neurotransmitter.

- Both benzodiazepines and antidepressant drugs are effective, indicating that these disorders may involve additional alterations in synaptic functioning in the norepinephrine and serotonin pathways in the brain.

- A person's general health status also can be a predisposing factor for anxiety.

- Precipitating stressors include threats to physical integrity, such as impending physiological disability or decreased ability to perform the activities of daily living and threats to one's self-system that imply harm to one's identity, self-esteem, and integrated social functioning.

- Coping mechanisms can be task-oriented or ego-oriented reactions. Task-oriented reactions are thoughtful, deliberate attempts to solve problems, resolve conflicts, and gratify needs and include attack, withdrawal, and compromise. Ego-oriented reactions are defense mechanisms used to protect the self. They can be constructive or destructive in nature.

CHAPTER **FOCUS POINTS**—cont'd

- Initially the nurse needs to determine the quality and quantity of the anxiety experienced by the patient. The nurse also needs to explore how the patient is coping with the anxiety and then the overall effect of the anxiety.
- Primary NANDA diagnoses related to anxiety responses are anxiety, ineffective coping, readiness for enhanced coping, and fear.
- Primary *DSM-IV-TR* diagnoses are categorized as anxiety disorders. These psychiatric disorders include panic disorder with or without agoraphobia, agoraphobia, specific phobia, social phobia, obsessive-compulsive disorder, posttraumatic stress disorder, acute stress disorder, and generalized anxiety disorder.
- The expected outcome of nursing care for patients with maladaptive anxiety responses is that the patient will demonstrate adaptive ways of coping with stress.

- The main goal of the nurse working with anxious patients is not to free them totally from anxiety. Patients need to develop the capacity to tolerate mild anxiety and to use it consciously and constructively.
- Nursing interventions in severe and panic levels of anxiety include establishing a trusting relationship, self-awareness, protecting the patient, modifying the environment, encouraging activity, and medication.
- Nursing interventions in a moderate level of anxiety include education, recognizing anxiety, developing insight into the anxiety, learning new ways to cope, and promoting the relaxation response.
- The nurse should use the criteria of adequacy, effectiveness, appropriateness, efficiency, and flexibility in evaluating nursing care.

KEY TERMS

agoraphobia, 271
anxiety, 260
compensation, 269
compulsions, 271
defense mechanisms, 268
denial, 269
displacement, 269
dissociation, 269
identification, 269

intellectualization, 269
introjection, 269
isolation, 269
neurosis, 272
obsessions, 271
panic, 261
panic attacks, 271
projection, 269
psychosis, 272

rationalization, 269
reaction formation, 269
regression, 269
repression, 269
splitting, 269
sublimation, 269
suppression, 269
undoing, 269

CHAPTER REVIEW QUESTIONS

1. Match each term in Column A with the correct definition in Column B.

Column A
_____ Affective responses
_____ Anxiety
_____ Cognitive responses
_____ Ego-oriented reactions
_____ Fear
_____ Moderate anxiety
_____ Neurosis
_____ Panic
_____ Psychosis
_____ Task-oriented reactions

Column B
A. Diffuse, vague, subjective apprehension with feelings of uncertainty and helplessness
B. Attack behavior, withdrawal behavior, compromise
C. Forgetfulness, confusion, hypervigilance, fear of injury or death, poor concentration and judgment
D. Awe, dread, terror, loss of control, disorganization of the personality
E. A mental disorder characterized by anxiety that involves no distortion of reality
F. An individual ideation with a specific identifiable source
G. Edginess, impatience, uneasiness, tension, nervousness, fright, fear, alarm
H. A mental disorder that involves a disintegration of self, a fear of defeat in the process of being
I. Repression, splitting, denial, dissociation, projection, intellectualization, rationalization
J. Focus is only on immediate concerns, with a narrowing of the perceptual field

2. Fill in the blanks

A. Difficulty in falling asleep, psychomotor hyperactivity, and selective negative appraisals are characteristic of _____. Early morning wakening, psychomotor retardation or agitation, and absolute negative evaluations characterize _____.
B. Recurrent and persistent thoughts, impulses, or images that are intrusive and inappropriate, and cause marked anxiety or distress, are called _____.
C. The three major biological systems believed to be involved in the development of anxiety responses are the _____, _____ and _____.
D. Precipitating stressors that threaten the patient and cause anxiety fall into two categories: threats to _____ and _____.
E. The two main categories of medications to treat anxiety disorders are the _____ and _____.

3. Provide short answers for the following questions.

A. Explain the behavioral view that anxiety arises from conflict.
B. Consider the nursing intervention categories for working with the anxious patient. What are some principles you can follow to protect the patient with an anxiety disorder?
C. Describe the criterion of flexibility when evaluating nursing care. How could you have been more flexible last time you worked with an anxious patient?

Visit Evolve for additional resources related to the content of this chapter.
http://evolve.elsevier.com/Stuart/principles/
• Topical Course Outline • Student Workbook Exercises • Critical Thinking Questions and Activities • Case Studies • Research Topics
• Monthly Content Updates • WebLinks

Student Study CD-ROM

Access the accompanying CD-ROM for animations, interactive exercises, review questions for the NCLEX examination, and an audio glossary.

REFERENCES

American Psychiatric Association: *Diagnostic and statistical manual of mental disorders*, ed 4, text revision, Washington, DC, 2000, American Psychiatric Association.

American Psychiatric Association: Practice guideline for the treatment of patients with panic disorder, *Am J Psychiatry* 155:1, 1998.

Bryant RA et al: Treating acute stress disorder: an evaluation of cognitive behavior therapy and supportive counseling techniques, *Am J Psychiatry* 156:1780, 1999.

Cook JM, Ruzek JL, Cassidy E: Practical geriatrics: possible association of posttraumatic stress disorder with cognitive impairment among older adults, *Psychiatr Serv* 54:1223, 2003.

Expert consensus guideline series: treatment of posttraumatic stress disorder, The Expert Consensus Panels for PTSD, *J Clin Psychiatry* 60(suppl 16):3, 1999.

Freud S: *A general introduction to psychoanalysis*, New York, 1969, Pocket Books.

Hettema JM, Neale MC, Kendler KS: A review and meta-analysis of the genetic epidemiology of anxiety disorders, *Am J Psychiatry* 158:1568, 2001.

Kessler RC: Posttraumatic stress disorder: the burden to the individual and to society, *J Clin Psychiatry* 61 (suppl 5):4, 2000.

Kushner MG, Sher KJ, Erickson DJ: Prospective analysis of the relation between DSM-III anxiety disorders and alcohol use disorders, *Am J Psychiatry* 156:723, 1999.

Lange JT, Lange CL, Cabaltica RB: Primary care treatment of post-traumatic stress disorder, *Am Fam Physician* 62:1035, 2000.

Moorhead S, Johnson M, Maas M, editors: *Nursing outcomes classification (NOC)*, ed 3, St Louis, 2004, Mosby.

Nathan PE, Gorman JM: *A guide to treatments that work*, ed 2, New York, 2002, Oxford University Press.

Peplau H: A working definition of anxiety. In Burd S, Marshall M, editors: *Some clinical approaches to psychiatric nursing*, New York, 1963, Macmillan.

Simpson H, Kozak M: Cognitive-behavioral therapy for obsessive-compulsive disorder, *J Psychiatr Pract* 6:59, 2000.

Sullivan H: *The interpersonal theory of psychiatry*, New York, 1953, WW Norton.

Valente SM: Social phobia, *J Am Psychiatr Nurs Assoc* 8:67, 2002a.

Valente SM: Obsessive-compulsive disorder, *Perspect Psychiatr Care* 38:125, 2002b.

Weisberg RB et al: Nonpsychiatric illness among primary care patients with trauma histories and posttraumatic stress disorder, *Psychiatr Serv* 53:848, 2002.

Wells A: *Cognitive therapy of anxiety disorders: a practice manual and conceptual guide*, New York, 1997, John Wiley.

The cure of many diseases is unknown to the physicians of Hellas, because they disregard the whole, which ought to be studied also, for the part can never be well unless the whole is well.

PLATO

PSYCHOPHYSIOLOGICAL RESPONSES AND SOMATOFORM AND SLEEP DISORDERS

17

Gail W. Stuart

evolve Visit Evolve for additional resources related to the content of this chapter.
http://evolve.elsevier.com/Stuart/principles/

Throughout history, philosophers and scientists have debated the nature of the relationship between the mind (**psyche**) and body (**soma**). There is now a renewed interest in holistic health practices, based on the idea that mental processes influence physical well-being and vice versa. Research is identifying the links between thoughts, feelings, and body functioning. Many believe that all illness has a psychophysiological component: Physical disorders have a psychological component and mental disorders a physical one.

■ CONTINUUM OF PSYCHOPHYSIOLOGICAL RESPONSES

Current thinking about psychophysiological responses is related to an increased understanding of the role of stress in human life. Stress theory was significantly advanced when Hans Selye published *The Stress of Life* in 1956. Selye described the stress response in detail, creating a greater understanding of the effect of stressful experiences on physical functioning. He identified a three-stage process of response to

stress. This generalized response is called the **general adaptation syndrome (GAS)**. These levels of response are:

1. **The alarm reaction.** This reaction is the immediate response to a stressor in a localized area. Adrenocortical mechanisms respond, resulting in behaviors associated with the fight-or-flight response.
2. **Stage of resistance.** The body makes some effort to resist the stressor. The body adapts and functions at a lower than optimal level. This requires a greater than usual expenditure of energy for survival.
3. **Stage of exhaustion.** The adaptive mechanisms become worn out and then fail. The negative effect of the stressor spreads to the entire organism. If the stressor is not removed or counteracted, death will result.

Any experience believed by the individual to be stressful may stimulate a psychophysiological response. The stress does not have to be recognized consciously, and often it is not. If people recognize that they are under stress, they are often unable to connect the cognitive understanding of stress with the physical symptoms of the psychophysiological disor-

285

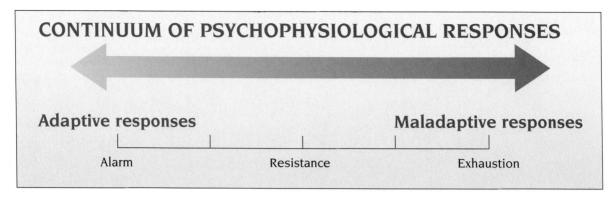

Figure 17-1   Continuum of psychophysiological responses.

der. Figure 17-1 illustrates the range of possible psychophysiological responses to stress, based on Selye's theory.

ASSESSMENT

Behaviors

Many behaviors are associated with psychophysiological disorders. Careful assessment is needed so that organic problems can be defined and treated. Such an illness should never be dismissed as being "only psychosomatic" or "all in one's head." Serious psychophysiological disorders can be fatal if not treated properly.

Physiological. The primary behaviors observed with psychophysiological responses are the physical symptoms. These symptoms lead the person to seek health care. Psychological factors affecting the physical condition may involve any body part. The most common organ systems involved are listed in Box 17-1. In addition, longer general hospital stays have

been reported to be associated with greater psychological comorbidity, particularly depression, anxiety, and organicity. Such research underscores the importance of linking physiological and psychological assessments.

People are often reluctant to believe that a physical problem may be related to psychological factors. In part, this is because being physically ill is more socially acceptable than having psychological problems. The situation is compounded because the patient does have real physical symptoms.

Denial of the psychological component of the illness may lead to "doctor shopping." The patient searches for someone who will find an organic cause for the illness. This tendency to experience and communicate psychological distress in the form of physical symptoms and to seek help for them in general medical settings is a widespread phenomenon. The following clinical example illustrates this problem.

CLINICAL EXAMPLE

Mr. R was a successful 42-year-old executive who had risen quickly to the top of his company. He worked long hours and had difficulty delegating any of his responsibilities. He set high standards for his employees and was believed to be insensitive to human concerns. He viewed himself as tough, but fair. However, he had little sympathy for a worker who requested extra time off for personal business.

Mr. R was married but saw little of his family. He expected his wife and children to do their part to maintain his standing in the community by associating with "the right people." He seldom interacted with his children except to reprimand them if they disturbed him while he was working. His wife reported that their sexual relationship was unsatisfying to her. Mr. R used it for physical release for himself but was not concerned about meeting her needs. She suspected that he was involved in an extramarital affair but did not want to endanger the marriage by confronting him.

Mr. R was expecting to be named to the board of directors of a prestigious philanthropic foundation. He expected that this would add to his social prominence in the community. Shortly before the announcement was to be made, his 14-year-old son was arrested in a drug raid in an undesirable part of town. Mr. R did not get the appointment to the board. He was furious with his son but dealt with his anger by withdrawing still more.

One day at work, he experienced an episode of dizziness, followed by a severe headache. He attributed it to tension, took some aspirin, and continued to work. However, after several similar episodes, he decided to consult

BOX **17-1**

Physical Conditions Affected by Psychological Factors

Cardiovascular	Colitis
Migraine	Obesity
Essential hypertension	
Angina	**Skin**
Tension headaches	Neurodermatitis
	Eczema
Musculoskeletal	Psoriasis
Rheumatoid arthritis	Pruritus
Low back pain (idiopathic)	
	Genitourinary
Respiratory	Impotence
Hyperventilation	Frigidity
Asthma	Premenstrual syndrome
Gastrointestinal	**Endocrinological**
Anorexia nervosa	Hyperthyroidism
Peptic ulcer	Diabetes
Irritable bowel syndrome	

his family doctor. The physician arrived at a diagnosis of essential hypertension. He tried to discuss work, family, and social behavior with Mr. R but received only superficial responses. Although concerned about Mr. R's condition and stress level, the doctor gave in to Mr. R's demand for medication to lower his blood pressure. He also advised Mr. R to exercise and to find a relaxing activity.

Selected Nursing Diagnoses

- Impaired adjustment related to family and work stress, as evidenced by denial and development of physical symptoms
- Interrupted family processes related to rigid role expectations, as evidenced by withdrawal and lack of communication ■

Mr. R is typical of many people with stress-related psychophysiological disorders. He is reluctant to admit to a lack of control over his mind and body. He expects a magical cure that will let him follow his usual lifestyle without interruption. He will probably stop taking his medication as soon as he feels better. Distance from the stressor may allow him to function for a while without noticeable symptoms of his hypertension. Sooner or later, however, new stressors will lead to another dizzy spell, headaches, or possibly myocardial infarction or cerebrovascular accident.

Psychological. Some people have physical symptoms without any organic impairment, and these are called somatoform disorders. They include the following:

- Somatization disorder, in which the person has many physical complaints
- Conversion disorder, in which a loss or alteration of physical functioning occurs
- Hypochondriasis, the fear of illness or belief that one has an illness
- Body dysmorphic disorder, in which a person with a normal appearance is concerned about having a physical defect
- Pain disorder, in which psychological factors play an important role in the onset, severity, or maintenance of the pain

The next clinical example is a case history of a person with a medical diagnosis of somatization disorder.

◢ CLINICAL EXAMPLE

Ms. P, a 28-year-old single woman, was admitted to the medical unit of a general hospital for a complete medical work-up. When asked about her main problem during the nursing assessment, she replied, "I've never been very well. Even when I was a child I was sick a lot." Ms. P listed multiple complaints during the physical assessment. These included palpitations, dizzy spells, menstrual irregularity, painful menses, blurred vision, dysphagia, backache, pain in her knees and feet, and a variety of gastrointestinal symptoms including stomach pain, nausea, vomiting, diarrhea, flatulence, and intolerance to seafood, vegetables of the cabbage family, carbonated beverages, and eggs. Except for the food intolerances, none of the symptoms was constant. They occurred at random, making her fearful of going out of her home.

The psychosocial assessment revealed that Ms. P lived with her parents. She was the youngest of three children. Her siblings were living away from the parental home. She had graduated from high school but had poor grades because of her frequent absences. She had tried to work as a clerk in a retail store but was fired because of absenteeism. She did not seem particularly bothered by the loss of her job. She had never tried to find other work, although she had been unemployed for 8 years. When asked how she spent her time, she said that she did some gardening and some housework when she felt well enough. However, she spent most of her time watching television.

Ms. P's parents visited her most of every day. Her mother asked whether she could spend the night in her daughter's room and was displeased when told no. The family had many complaints about the quality of the nursing care, mostly about failures to anticipate the patient's needs. Extensive diagnostic studies failed to reveal any organic basis for Ms. P's physical complaints. When informed that the problem was most likely psychological and advised to obtain psychotherapy, the family protested angrily and refused a referral to a psychiatric clinic. Ms. P was discharged and returned to her parents' home.

Selected Nursing Diagnoses

- Ineffective denial related to compromised physical and emotional health status, as evidenced by repeated medical care visits and refusal to obtain psychiatric treatment
- Interrupted family processes related to mother-daughter dependency issues, as evidenced by excessive caretaking by mother and passivity of daughter ■

Ms. P shows the dependent behavior that is typical of people with **somatization disorder**. Her many symptoms allowed her to be taken care of and to avoid the demands of adult responsibility. Her need to be cared for fit with her mother's need to nurture. Therefore, she had little incentive to give up her symptoms. A periodic hospital stay reinforced the seriousness of her problem.

Secondary gain related to the gratification of dependency needs is a powerful deterrent to change in many patients. Secondary gain is an indirect benefit, usually obtained through an illness or disability. Such benefits may include personal attention, release from unpleasant situations and responsibilities, or monetary and disability benefits.

Another type of somatoform disorder is **conversion disorder** in which symptoms of some physical illnesses appear without any underlying organic cause. The organic symptom reduces the patient's anxiety and usually gives a clue to the conflict. For example, a patient who has an impulse to harm his domineering father may develop paralysis of his arms and hands. The primary gain is that the patient is unable to carry out his impulses. He also may experience secondary gain in the form of attention, manipulation of others, freedom from responsibilities, and economic benefits. Conversion symptoms might include the following:

- Sensory symptoms such as numbness, blindness, or deafness
- Motor symptoms such as paralysis, tremors, or mutism
- Visceral symptoms such as urinary retention, headaches, or difficulty breathing

It is often difficult to diagnose this reaction. Other patient behaviors may be helpful in making the diagnosis. Patients often display little anxiety or concern about the conversion symptom and its resulting disability. The classic term for this lack of concern is **la belle indifference**. The patient also tends to seek attention in ways not limited to the actual symptom.

Hypochondriasis is another type of somatoform disorder. People with this disorder have an exaggerated concern with physical health that is not based on any real organic disorders. They fear presumed diseases and are not helped by reassurance. They also tend to seek out and use information about diseases to convince themselves that they are ill or about to become ill. Unlike the conversion reaction, no actual loss or distortion of function occurs. Patients appear worried and anxious about their symptoms. This concern may be based on physical sensations overlooked by most people or on symptoms of a minor physical illness that the patient magnifies. This is often a chronic behavior pattern accompanied by a history of visits to numerous practitioners (Barsky et al, 2001).

Hypochondriacal behavior is not related to a conscious decision. If a person decides to fake an illness, the behavior is called malingering. This behavior is usually done to avoid responsibilities the person views as burdensome. Many otherwise healthy people malinger at one time or another. For instance, a person involved in an automobile accident may feign neck pain to receive insurance money. Often, the person exaggerates symptoms, is evasive, and tells contradictory stories about the illness.

Pain. Pain is increasingly recognized as more than simply a sensory phenomenon, but as a complex sensory and emotional experience underlying potential disease. Pain is influenced by behavioral, cognitive, and motivational processes that require sophisticated assessments and multifaceted treatments for its control.

Acute pain is a reflex biological response to injury. By definition, chronic pain is pain of a minimum of 6 months' duration. Somatoform pain disorder is a preoccupation with pain in the absence of physical disease to account for its intensity. It does not follow a neuroanatomical distribution. A close correlation between stress and conflict and the initiation or exacerbation of the pain also may be a component of the disorder.

The experience, expression, and treatment of pain are subject to cultural norms and biases. For example, in Western cultures, being female is often a predictor of poor pain management because male expressions of pain are typically taken more seriously by health care practitioners. Also, members of minority groups who seek health care in culturally insensitive settings may have their requests for support in coping with pain misunderstood because support is culturally defined and varies across ethnic and racial groups.

Sleep. Sleep disorders are common in the general population and among people with psychiatric disorders. Sleep disturbances can influence the development and course of mental illnesses and addictive disorders and also can affect treatment and recovery.

Insomnia is the most prevalent sleep disorder. Up to 30% of the population have insomnia and seek help for it. Other sleep disturbances include excessive daytime drowsiness, difficulty sleeping during desired sleep time, and unusual nocturnal events such as nightmares and sleepwalking. Sleep disorders are more common in the elderly.

Sleep disorders are classified by the Association of Sleep Disorders Centers (ASDC) into four major groupings with considerable overlap (Lilie and Lahmeyer, 1991):

1. Disorders of initiating or maintaining sleep, also known as insomnia. Anxiety and depression are major causes of insomnia.
2. Disorders of excessive somnolence, also known as hypersomnia. This category includes narcolepsy, sleep apnea, and nocturnal movement disorders such as restless legs.
3. Disorders of the sleep-wake schedule, characterized by normal sleep occurring at the wrong time. These are transient disturbances associated with jet lag and work shift changes. They are usually self-limited and resolve as the body readjusts to a new sleep-wake schedule.
4. Disorders associated with sleep stages, also known as parasomnia. This category includes conditions such as sleepwalking, night terrors, nightmares, restless legs syndrome, and enuresis. These sleep problems are often experienced by children and can have a significant effect on functioning and well-being.

Approximately 40 million Americans suffer from chronic disorders of sleep and wakefulness, such as narcolepsy, sleep apnea, and the insomnias. The majority of those affected are undiagnosed and untreated. An additional 20 to 30 million people experience intermittent sleep-related problems. In addition, millions of other people get inadequate sleep because of demanding work schedules, school, and other lifestyle issues.

The consequences of sleep disorders, sleep deprivation, and sleepiness are significant and include reduced productivity, lowered cognitive performance, increased likelihood of accidents, higher morbidity and mortality risk, depression, and decreased quality of life. Furthermore, the consequences span all aspects of modern society, including health care, education, and family and social life (National Sleep Foundation, 2003).

The assessment of patients with sleep problems is multifaceted, involving a detailed history and medical and psychiatric examinations, extensive questionnaires, the use of sleep diaries or logs, and often psychological testing. Many patients are referred for formal sleep studies, which include all night polysomnography and physiological measures of daytime sleepiness. Many members of the health care team collaborate within sleep centers to deliver multidisciplinary care.

Have you ever had a problem sleeping? Which ASDC grouping would your problem have fit into, and what did you do to relieve it? ■

Predisposing Factors

A number of biopsychosocial factors influence psychophysiological responses to stress. Most of the relationships between physical and psychological processes are still not well described. Thus it is important for the nurse to consider all possibilities when assessing factors that might predispose the patient to a particular disorder.

Biological. Research has linked emotions to arousal of the neuroendocrine system through release of corticosteroids by the hypothalamic-pituitary-adrenal (HPA) axis, as well as to the actions of neurotransmitter systems, particularly norepinephrine and serotonin (Cohen, 2000). Neuroendocrine data provide evidence of insufficient glucocorticoid signaling in stress-related neuropsychiatric disorders. Impaired feedback regulation of relevant stress responses, especially immune activation and inflammation, may, in turn, contribute to stress-related pathology, including alterations in behavior, insulin sensitivity, bone metabolism, and acquired immune responses (Raison and Miller, 2003).

A biological tendency for particular psychophysiological responses may be inherited, underscoring the importance of genetic factors. For instance, epidemiological studies have shown that the lifetime prevalence for somatization disorder in the general population is 0.1% to 0.5% and is more common in women. However, in the mothers and sisters of affected patients, it increases to 10% to 20%. The rate in monozygotic (identical) twins is 29%, and in dizygotic (fraternal) twins, it is 10%. Thus an inherited tendency for this disorder clearly exists.

The genetic theory suggests that any prolonged stress can cause physiological changes, which result in a physical disorder. Each person has a "shock organ" that is genetically vulnerable to stress. Thus some patients may be prone to cardiac illness, whereas others may react with gastrointestinal distress or skin rashes. People who are chronically anxious or depressed are believed to have a greater vulnerability to psychophysiological illness.

Psychoneuroimmunology. Psychoneuroimmunology is the scientific field that explores the relationship between psychological states, the immune system, and health (see Chapter 6). This field is based on the mind-body connection that extends to the cellular level (Koenig and Cohen, 2002) (Figure 17-2).

For example, glial cells are found throughout the central nervous system. As numerous as neurons, they form an extensive defensive network in the brain, monitoring and even enhancing normal brain function, and migrating to trouble spots to ingest microbes, dying cells, and other debris. Research also has shown that these cells can begin to function

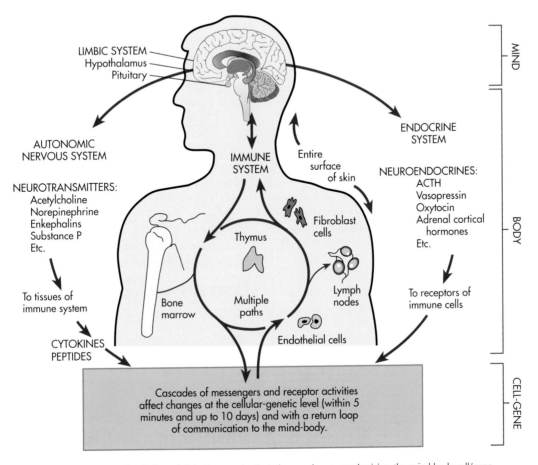

Figure 17-2   Updated view of Selye's general adaptation syndrome emphasizing the mind-body-cell/gene communication loop of the immune system. *ACTH,* Adrenocorticotropic hormone.

abnormally and then, in some people, exacerbate or even cause several disabling conditions such as stroke, Alzheimer's disease, multiple sclerosis, Parkinson's disease, dementia associated with HIV, and other neurodegenerative disorders.

The immune response can be modified by behavior modification techniques. Researchers are now investigating the possibility of modifying the immune response in the treatment of autoimmune illnesses such as rheumatoid arthritis, systemic lupus erythematosus, myasthenia gravis, and pernicious anemia. Other research is exploring the relationship between the immune system, stress, and cancer. It is suspected that high stress, especially if prolonged, can decrease the immune system's ability to destroy neoplastic growths.

Sleep. Scientists believe they may have identified the cause of the sleep disorder, narcolepsy. Studies show a dramatic reduction of up to 95% in the number of neurons containing a substance called hypocretin in the brains of people with narcolepsy as compared with normal controls. Hypocretin peptides are neurotransmitters that play an important role in regulating sleep and appetite. The researchers hypothesize that the pronounced loss of these neurons could be caused by either a neurodegenerative process or an autoimmune response.

The brains of those with narcolepsy also revealed signs of an inflammatory process called *gliosis*, which is linked to neuronal degeneration and may explain the loss of the hypocretin cells. These findings suggest that it may be possible to administer hypocretins to patients with narcolepsy as a potential treatment strategy (Stansberry, 2001).

Psychological. Philosophers and scientists have long speculated about the roles of personality and stress in the development of illness. In the 1930s and 1940s, personality profiles were developed of those prone to several diseases, including hypertension, coronary artery disease (CAD), cancer, ulcers, and rheumatoid arthritis.

Research suggests that a negative affective style marked by depression, anxiety, and hostility may be associated with the development or recovery from such diseases as asthma, headaches, ulcers, arthritis, and cancer (see Citing the Evidence). The clearest evidence to date relates to the negative effects of depression on cardiovascular disease (Ruo et al, 2003).

Type A behavior, which has been characterized by competitive drive, impatience, hostility, irritability, and aggressiveness, has been shown to predict both the physiological changes that are associated with CAD and the development of CAD itself. Type A people are also more likely to have accidents, to die as a result of accidents or violence, to have migraine headaches, to smoke more, and to have higher levels of serum cholesterol. Thus type A behavior appears to be a risk factor not only for cardiovascular disease but also for an array of other disorders.

Although such research suggests the possibility of a disease-prone personality, the exact nature of the relationship between personality and susceptibility is unknown. For example, a negative emotional state may:

CITING THE EVIDENCE ON
Survival in Breast Cancer

BACKGROUND: The psychological response to breast cancer has been suggested as a prognostic factor with an influence on survival. This study investigated the effect of psychological response on disease outcome in a large cohort of women with early-stage breast cancer.

RESULTS: A significantly increased risk of death from all causes by 5 years was found in women who scored high on the depression scales, and a significantly increased risk of relapse or death was noted for those who scored high on the helplessness and hopelessness scales. No significant results were found for the category of "fighting spirit."

IMPLICATIONS: The results reinforce the need to detect a response of helplessness or hopelessness and serious depression and to treat these responses vigorously to help women improve the quality of their lives and optimize their length of survival.

Watson M et al: *The Lancet* 354:1331, 1999.

- Produce pathological physiological changes.
- Lead people to practice high-risk behaviors for illness.
- Produce illness behavior but no underlying pathology.
- Be associated with illness through other unknown factors.

Complementing the research on negative emotional states and disease is the increasing focus on the protective role of positive emotional states. One idea regarding these traits is that of a self-healing personality, which is characterized by enthusiasm (Friedman, 1991). Self-healing, emotionally balanced people are believed to be alert, responsive, and energetic, although they also may be calm and conscientious. They are curious, secure, and constructive. Self-healing personalities also have a sense of continuous growth and **resilience** and an extra margin of emotional stability that they can call on when their capacities are challenged.

Two other positive traits are optimism and perceived control. Optimists appear to have fewer physical symptoms and may show faster recoveries from illness. Belief in personal control, or **self-efficacy**, affects the likelihood of developing illness by directly influencing the practice of health behaviors and by buffering people against the adverse effects of stress (Bandura, 1997).

Think of people you know who always seem to be ill. What personality characteristics do they share? How do they compare with people you know who are hardly ever ill? ■

Sociocultural. Health, illness, and suffering are patterned by culture and realized as personal worlds of experience (Donnelly and Long, 2003). Box 17-2 presents some unique somatoform syndromes of various cultures (American Psychiatric Association, 2000). In this view psychophysiological illness is derived from the relationships between body, psyche,

BOX 17-2

Somatoform Syndromes of Various Cultures

Ataque de nervios: Distress recognized by many Latin-American groups, with common symptoms of uncontrollable crying, trembling, heat in the chest rising to the head, fainting, and a sense of having lost control. These symptoms often occur after a stressful event affecting the individual or one's family.

Brain fag: A West-African term used to describe symptoms experienced by young people that is related to the stress of study, including difficulties in concentration, memory, and thinking.

Dhat: A folk term used by men in India relating to sexual dysfunction and signs of weakness and exhaustion.

Hwa-byung: A Korean folk syndrome attributed to the suppression of anger, with symptoms of insomnia, fatigue, indigestion, anorexia, and generalized aches and pains.

Shenjing shuairuo (neurasthenia): In China, a condition characterized by physical and mental fatigue, dizziness, headaches, concentration, and sleep difficulties.

Susto ("fright" or "soul loss"): A Latin-American folk illness that follows a frightening experience. Symptoms include appetite and sleep disturbance, lack of motivation, muscle pains, headaches, and abdominal pain and diarrhea.

Critical Thinking *About* Contemporary Issues

Is Chronic Fatigue Syndrome a Culturally Sanctioned Form of Illness Behavior?

Much interest has been shown in the recently defined chronic fatigue syndrome, which is characterized by exhaustion or fatigue and marked reduction in activity and correlated with a high prevalence of psychiatric disorders and psychophysiological symptoms secondary to stress. This interest results from reports of its growing frequency, substantial morbidity, and unclear pathogenesis. This interest is also fueled by debates about emotional factors related to the illness and questions as to whether it is a discrete disorder (Afari and Buchwald, 2003).

Currently the diagnosis of chronic fatigue syndrome is more common among women. It has been proposed that it is related to the struggle of American culture with the expanding role of women and the mismatch between women's ambitions and social possibilities. Today, illness and the sick role are the only socially legitimate excuses for abandoning work and the pursuit of achievement. Thus a diagnosis of chronic fatigue syndrome may provide a legitimate "medical" reason for a variety of psychophysiological responses, allowing the person to withdraw from situations that are intolerable. This example of the cultural shaping of illness and disease underscores society's greater understanding of physical illness and the continued stigmatization of psychiatric illness and emotional distress.

Compare this society's beliefs and expectations about the sick role for people with multiple sclerosis, alcoholism, lung cancer, and depression. Do they differ based on each diagnosis and, if so, how and why? ■

and society. Illness is not seen as simply the natural unfolding of an exclusively biological process. Rather, its course is also influenced by sociocultural factors (see Critical Thinking About Contemporary Issues).

The social course of illness has at least two meanings. The first is that the severity of the person's symptoms is influenced by aspects of the social environment. This means that subjectively experienced distress can be increased or decreased by the nature and number of problems in the person's world, changes in the emotional climate of that world, and by the ill person's social life.

In the second meaning, the symptoms shape and structure the person's social world, as the illness causes a series of changes in the person's environment. The resulting chain of illness-related interpersonal events thus becomes a part of the social course of the person's illness. This can be seen in the concept of the **sick role**, first described in the 1950s by Parsons. It proposes that being sick is a social role as well as a condition and that society places certain beliefs and expectations on the person who falls ill (Parsons, 1951). These include the following:

- The sick are allowed to be exempt from their usual social responsibilities.
- The sick are not seen as being responsible for being ill.
- The sick are expected to want to get well.
- The sick are expected to seek competent help and cooperate with the helper in trying to get well.

Although the premises of the sick role have been questioned, they do show the impact of sociocultural factors on the expression and resolution of psychophysiological responses.

Precipitating Stressors

Any experience that the person interprets as stressful may lead to a psychophysiological response. Some of these responses are mild and short-lived. Examples include diarrhea before an examination or a dry mouth when speaking before a large group of people. Sometimes the response is more serious and indicates a higher level of anxiety. For instance, a person might feel panicky and experience tachycardia when boarding an airplane. Because the psychophysiological disorder is an attempt to deal with anxiety, information on stressors related to anxiety (see Chapter 16) should be reviewed.

One type of stressor that has been shown to cause physical illness and even death is the loss of a significant interpersonal relationship. An increased mortality rate has been found among recently widowed people. Similar observations have been made about people admitted to institutions such as nursing homes, who are separated from significant others. Children who have been separated from their mothers, especially if placed in an impersonal environment, also show a decline in physical health. The effect of a loss may cause both physical and psychological symptoms for an extended period of time. Illnesses and deaths related to loss of a loved person seem to represent the exhaustion phase of the general adaptation syndrome.

Sometimes a psychophysiological problem is a response to an accumulation of rather small stressors. A patient may find it difficult to identify one specific stressor that preceded a particular problem. Careful assessment may reveal a pattern of overwork and overcommitment or a series of seemingly minor events that all required extra effort.

Most of the psychophysiological disorders come and go. This pattern of occurrence may be related to changes in the person's stress level. When the cumulative stress gets too high, the body "calls time out" by developing physical symptoms.

Appraisal of Stressors

The complex interaction between mind and body is perhaps most evident in psychophysiological responses to stress. These responses reinforce the need for an integrated approach to etiology and great sensitivity by the nurse to a person's appraisal of stress and its effects. Social and cultural factors play a particularly important role in the expression of adaptive and maladaptive behaviors. They also must be considered in planning effective, individualized treatment strategies (Servan-Schreiber, Kolb, Tabas, 2000a).

Coping Resources

One of the most important parts of promoting adaptive psychophysiological responses involves adopting positive health practices, because good health measures can prevent many illnesses. Patient Education Plans that include coping skills training, such as the one in Table 17-1, can increase a person's knowledge about the effect of stress, reduce anxiety, increase a person's feelings of purpose and meaning in life, reduce pain and suffering, and improve coping abilities.

Social support from family, friends, and caregivers also is an important resource for adaptive psychophysiological responses. It may lower the likelihood of developing maladaptive responses, speed the recovery from illness, and reduce the distress and suffering that accompany illness (see A Family Speaks). Social support groups are another coping resource that can satisfy needs that are unmet by family members and caregivers.

Coping Mechanisms

Psychophysiological disorders may be attempts to cope with the anxiety associated with overwhelming stress. Unconsciously the person links the anxiety to the physical illness. Secondary gain then adds to the psychological relief experienced.

Several of the defense mechanisms described in Chapter 16 may be seen in psychophysiological disorders. **Repression** of feelings, conflicts, and unacceptable impulses often leads to physical symptoms. The maintenance of repression over long periods of time requires a great deal of psychic energy. As the system approaches a state of exhaustion, physical symptoms occur. When a psychological basis for illness is suggested, the patient denies it. This denial indicates the inability to handle the anxiety that would otherwise be released if the person admitted the psychic conflicts being repressed. The need for this defense should be respected.

Some people respond to psychophysiological illness with **compensation**. They attempt to prove that they are actually healthy by being more active and exerting themselves physi-

A FAMILY SPEAKS

I worry about my husband. He drives himself so hard. I also feel guilty at times because I know he's doing it for me and the children. But I sure would like for him to slow down. Here's a good example of how things go in our house. Every year in the weeks before Christmas he works overtime to give us a little extra money. But then on Christmas Eve, without fail, his ulcer kicks up, and we wind up spending part of each holiday in the hospital visiting him.

I know every family has problems, and maybe ours aren't so bad. But then again, maybe they are. This last Christmas our doctor recommended that we see a family therapist to discuss the situation. I want to go, but my husband says it's silly. Maybe this year for Christmas I'll ask him to give me that as my present, and we'll finally have a really happy New Year.

Table 17-1	PATIENT EDUCATION PLAN	Coping With Stress
CONTENT	**INSTRUCTIONAL ACTIVITIES**	**EVALUATION**
Define and describe stress.	List feelings that indicate stress. Discuss behaviors associated with elevated stress.	Patient identifies general behaviors associated with stressful situations.
Recognize stressful situations.	Ask patient to describe situations personally experienced as stressful. Role play the situation (with videotape if possible). Discuss stress-related behaviors observed and feelings experienced.	Patient identifies stressful experiences. Patient describes own behaviors when stressed.
Review common life stressors.	Discuss common elements of stressful experiences.	Patient identifies stressful aspects of life.
Identify adaptive and maladaptive coping mechanisms.	Review the role-played stressful situations. Discuss alternative ways to cope with the stressors. Role play at least one adaptive coping mechanism.	Patient identifies and practices adaptive coping mechanisms.
Assign use of adaptive strategy to cope with stress.	Provide feedback about the effectiveness of the selected coping mechanism.	Patient selects an adaptive coping strategy when experiencing stress.

cally even if told to rest. This coping style is typical of type A people, who need desperately to prove that they are in control of their bodies, not controlled by them.

The opposite of this reaction is the person who uses **regression** as a coping mechanism. This person becomes dependent and embraces the sick role to avoid responsibility and conflict.

Common to each of these coping mechanisms is the need **not to confront the basic conflict** that is leading to stress and anxiety. This need is so strong that premature attempts to convince the person of psychological conflicts may result in the use of a less adaptive coping mechanism. In extreme cases, if the person is stripped of all efforts to cope and not provided with a substitute, death can result, either from worsening of the organic disorder or from suicide.

DIAGNOSIS

Nursing Diagnoses

The nursing diagnosis must reflect the complex biopsychosocial interaction that is the hallmark of psychophysiological disorders. The patient's effort to cope with stress-related anx-

iety may result in many somatic and emotional disorders. All possible disruptions must be considered when formulating a nursing diagnosis.

The Stuart Stress Adaptation Model (Figure 17-3) may help in the diagnostic process. A thorough interview will reveal many of the predisposing factors and precipitating stressors present. The nurse must use good communication skills during the interview to enable the patient to share his or her experience as completely as possible. Areas of resistance and gaps in information should be noted as possible indicators of a conflict. These may be explored more completely as trust is established in the nurse-patient relationship.

Questions related to lifestyle and activities may help identify precipitating stressors and coping behaviors. It is particularly important to elicit the patient's view of what is happening. This response will provide valuable information about the patient's awareness of the relationship between mind and body. Nonverbal behaviors also give clues about the patient's concerns. Apparent lack of concern may reveal the use of denial suggestive of a conversion disorder.

As the diagnosis is formulated, the nurse must consider the patient's coping in the context of the stress response. Is

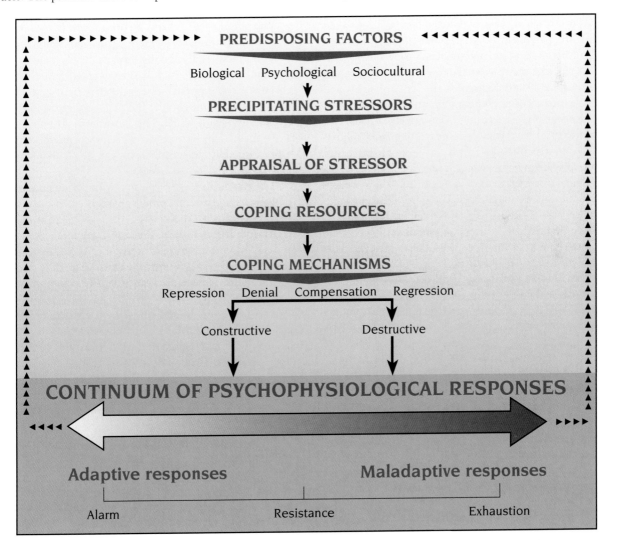

Figure 17-3 The Stuart Stress Adaptation Model as related to psychophysiological responses.

BOX 17-3 *Medical and Nursing Diagnoses Related to* **Psychophysiological Responses**

RELATED MEDICAL DIAGNOSES (*DSM-IV-TR*)*	RELATED NURSING DIAGNOSES (NANDA)†
Somatization disorder	**Adjustment, Impaired**‡
Conversion disorder	Anxiety
Hypochondriasis	Body image, Disturbed
Body dysmorphic disorder	Coping, Ineffective
Pain disorder	**Denial, Ineffective**‡
Primary insomnia	Family processes, Interrupted
Primary hypersomnia	Health maintenance, Ineffective
Narcolepsy	Hopelessness
Breathing-related sleep disorder	**Pain, Chronic**‡
Circadian rhythm sleep disorder	Powerlessness
Psychological factors affecting medical conditions	Self-esteem, Situational low
	Sleep pattern, Disturbed‡
	Spiritual distress

*From American Psychiatric Association: *Diagnostic and statistical manual of mental disorders*, ed 4, text revision, Washington, DC, 2000, American Psychiatric Association.
†From North American Nursing Diagnosis Association: *NANDA nursing diagnoses: definitions and classification 2003-2004*, Philadelphia, 2003, The Association.
‡**Primary nursing diagnosis for maladaptive psychophysiological responses.**

---

the patient in a stage of alarm with many coping resources at hand? Or is the patient in the stage of resistance, using coping mechanisms but depleting personal energy resources? Has the patient reached the stage of exhaustion, needing intensive intervention? Determination of the level of stress and coping being used influences the interventions chosen.

There are four primary nursing diagnoses for maladaptive psychophysiological responses. The first is **impaired adjustment**, a state in which the patient is unable to modify his or her lifestyle in order to improve health status. The second is **ineffective denial** in which disavowal is used to reduce anxiety but leads to the detriment of health. The third is **chronic pain**, a state that continues for more than 6 months. The fourth is **sleep pattern disturbance**, which is a disruption of sleep time that causes discomfort or interferes with desired lifestyle.

Nursing diagnoses related to the range of possible maladaptive responses and related medical diagnoses are identified in the Medical and Nursing Diagnoses box (Box 17-3). The primary NANDA diagnoses and examples of expanded nursing diagnoses are presented in the Detailed Diagnoses table (Table 17-2).

Medical Diagnoses

Medical disorders related to maladaptive psychophysiological responses are classified under the general categories of **somatoform disorders, sleep disorders**, and **psychological factors affecting medical condition** (American Psychiatric Association, 2000). The specific medical diagnoses and essential features in each of these diagnostic classes in the *DSM-IV-TR* are described in the Detailed Diagnoses table (see Table 17-2).

■ OUTCOME IDENTIFICATION

The expected outcome when working with a patient with maladaptive psychophysiological responses is:

The patient will express feelings verbally rather than through the development of physical symptoms.

This expectation is a long-term goal, and some may never reach it. However, an increased level of self-awareness is beneficial and should be achievable by all patients. An improved ability to deal with conflict will reduce the patient's need to use repression and denial. This in turn will decrease stress and allow the patient to function with fewer episodes of physical illness. In addition, specific goals can be set to address problems related to pain and sleep.

The establishment of goals with these patients is often a problem. The patient's primary goal is to ease the physical symptoms of the illness, often through medical or surgical treatment. Exploration of psychological conflicts is likely to be seen as unnecessary. This resistance is related to the need to maintain defenses against the extreme anxiety that has led to the illness. The nurse must identify common treatment goals.

The nurse also wants the patient to obtain relief from physical symptoms. Many patients undergo medical or surgical treatment and related nursing care. At the same time, the nurse should try to build a trusting relationship so that the patient can feel safe in exploring interpersonal conflicts and feelings.

Significant others also must be considered in developing the plan of care. It is important to explore their understanding of the patient's problem. They can be valuable allies in encouraging the patient to make a lifestyle change, if this is necessary.

At the same time, the nurse must recognize that a change in one family member requires a change in all the others. The family may be active participants in the patient's maladaptive behavioral style. In this case, goals should include addressing the family relationships with the patient.

Table 17-2	*Detailed Diagnoses Related to* **Psychophysiological Responses**

NANDA DIAGNOSIS STEM	EXAMPLES OF EXPANDED DIAGNOSIS
Impaired adjustment	Impaired adjustment related to fear of assuming adult responsibilities, as evidenced by multiple somatic complaints
	Impaired adjustment related to inability to express hostile and competitive feelings, as evidenced by labile hypertension
Ineffective denial	Ineffective denial related to doubts about self-worth, as evidenced by chronic, unresponsive respiratory symptoms limiting one's work
Chronic pain	Chronic pain related to marital conflict, as evidenced by back problems and protected gait
	Chronic pain related to work pressures, evidenced by reports of headaches and facial mask
Disturbed sleep pattern	Disturbed sleep pattern related to financial and familial concerns, as evidenced by difficulty falling asleep and frequent awakening during the night

DSM-IV-TR DIAGNOSIS	ESSENTIAL FEATURES*
Somatization disorder	A history of many physical complaints beginning before the age of 30, occurring over a period of several years, and resulting in treatment being sought or significant impairment in social or occupational functioning. The patient must display at least four pain symptoms, two gastrointestinal symptoms, one sexual symptom, and one symptom suggesting a neurological disorder.
Conversion disorder	One or more symptoms or deficits affecting voluntary motor or sensory function, suggesting a neurological or general medical condition. Psychological factors are judged to be associated with the symptom or deficit because the initiation or exacerbation of the symptom or deficit is preceded by conflicts or other stressors. The symptom or deficit cannot be fully explained by a neurological or general medical condition and is not a culturally sanctioned behavior or experience.
Hypochondriasis	Preoccupation with fears of having, or ideas that one has, a serious disease based on the person's misinterpretation of bodily symptoms. The preoccupation persists despite appropriate medical evaluation and reassurance and has existed for at least 6 months. It causes clinically significant distress or impairment in functioning.
Body dysmorphic disorder	Preoccupation with an imagined or exaggerated defect in appearance that causes clinically significant distress or impairment in functioning.
Pain disorder	Pain in one or more anatomical sites is the predominant focus of the clinical presentation. It is of sufficient severity to warrant clinical attention and causes clinically significant distress or impairment in functioning. Psychological factors are judged to have an important role in the onset, severity, exacerbation, or maintenance of the pain.
Primary insomnia	Difficulty initiating or maintaining sleep, or nonrestorative sleep, for at least 1 month that causes clinically significant distress or impairment in functioning.
Primary hypersomnia	Excessive sleepiness for at least 1 month, as evidenced by prolonged sleep episodes or daytime sleep episodes occurring almost daily that cause clinically significant distress or impairment in functioning.
Narcolepsy	Irresistible attacks of refreshing sleep occurring daily over at least 3 months with cataplexy (brief episodes of sudden bilateral loss of muscle tone) and hallucinations or sleep paralysis at the beginning or end of sleep episodes.
Breathing-related sleep disorder	Sleep disruption leading to excessive sleepiness or insomnia judged to be caused by sleep apnea or central alveolar hypoventilation syndrome.
Circadian rhythm sleep disorder	Persistent or recurrent pattern of sleep disruption leading to excessive sleepiness or insomnia that is caused by a mismatch between the sleep-wake schedule required by a person's environment and one's circadian sleep-wake pattern that causes clinically significant distress or impairment in functioning.
Psychological factors affecting medical condition	Presence of a medical condition in which psychological factors influence its cause, interfere with its treatment, constitute additional health risks, or elicit stress-related physiological responses that precipitate or exacerbate its symptoms.

* From American Psychiatric Association: *Diagnostic and statistical manual of mental disorders*, ed 4, text revision, Washington, DC, 2000, American Psychiatric Association.

PLANNING

Treatment plans for these patients may be lengthy. The nurse must attend to all of the patient's biopsychosocial needs. Most patients, while having needs in all areas, have their most urgent needs in a limited area of functioning. Physical disorders are usually disabling and may be life threatening.

Psychosocial problems will hinder recovery from the physical illness and must also be given immediate attention.

How would you plan care with a patient who denies that problems with his ulcerative colitis are related to work stress and marital conflict, as reported by his wife? ■

IMPLEMENTATION

Patients with psychophysiological illnesses are most often seen in general hospital and outpatient settings. They usually seek health care because of symptoms related to physiological functioning. Only after a thorough medical examination can the role of psychosocial stressors in the disorder be evaluated.

In some cases a pathophysiological disruption requires physical nursing intervention. **If the physical condition is life threatening, this intervention is given highest priority.** For instance, a person with a bleeding ulcer needs intensive care to maintain life. However, once the physical crisis is past, the nurse can help the patient avoid similar problems in the future.

Physical illnesses with psychosocial etiologies require psychiatric nursing care. **Skilled and compassionate nursing care directed to the patient's physical needs is the first step in establishing the trusting relationship.** A person who is in pain, bleeding, or covered with a rash is unable to discuss emotions or interpersonal relationships.

The most important principle for patients with psychophysical disorders is to **assess the patient's stress level and, whenever possible, act to reduce it.** Stress and anxiety are at the root of the patient's problem. The nurse must care for immediate needs before addressing less obvious ones.

Empirically validated treatments for some of the medical diagnoses related to psychophysiological responses are summarized in Box 17-4 (Nathan and Gorman, 2002).

Psychological Approaches

The psychophysiological symptom defends the person from overwhelming anxiety. It provides a way to receive help and nurturance without admitting the need for it. Others are protected from expressing frightening aggressive or sexual impulses. Recognizing the defensive nature of the symptom, the nurse should never try to convince the patient that the problem is entirely psychological. Likewise, the attitude that the patient needs only to get his or her life under control to get better is not therapeutic. The patient has not made a conscious choice to be hypertensive or to develop a conversion disorder.

The dilemma of these disorders is that the patient consciously would like nothing more than to be cured but is unconsciously unable to give up the symptom. Conscious recognition of the psychological role of the symptom defeats its purpose and is therefore vigorously resisted. An example of this resistance is illustrated in the following clinical example.

CLINICAL EXAMPLE

Ms. W was a 20-year-old woman admitted to the general hospital after the sudden onset of blindness. There was no evidence of any pathophysiological process affecting her eyes. Assessment revealed that she had witnessed her father's suicide by gunshot at the age of 5, although she claimed to have no memory of this. Her boyfriend had recently been expressing suicidal thoughts to her.

It appeared that the blindness was a conversion reaction. To confirm the diagnosis, the physician decided to interview Ms. W while she was sedated with amobarbital sodium. The interview was videotaped. During the interview, Ms. W was able to see. She read the day's menu and told the time by looking at a clock across the room. She also described her father's suicide. However, when the sedation wore off, Ms. W was again blind. The decision was made to play the videotape for her so that she would recognize the psychogenic nature of her blindness. As the tape was played, she regained the ability to see. However, when it reached the part in which she described her father's suicide, she became deaf.

Selected Nursing Diagnoses

- Ineffective denial related to early life events, as evidenced by symptoms affecting sight and hearing
- Impaired social interaction related to boyfriend's depressive thoughts, as evidenced by development of physical symptoms ■

BOX 17-4	SUMMARIZING THE EVIDENCE ON **Psychological Responses**
Disorder	Body dysmorphic disorder
Treatment	◆ Cognitive-behavior therapy can help patients identify and challenge distorted body perceptions and interrupt self-critical thoughts.
Disorder	Hypochondriasis
Treatment	◆ Cognitive-behavior therapy is helpful in reducing attention to the distressing bodily sensations, correcting misinformation and exaggerated beliefs, and addressing the cognitive processes that maintain disease fears.
Disorder	Pain disorder
Treatment	◆ Individual and group cognitive-behavior therapy reduces pain-related distress and disability. ◆ Antidepressants decrease pain intensity.
Disorder	Sleep disorders
Treatment	◆ Benzodiazepines, zolpidem, and zaleplon reduce sleep onset by 15 to 30 minutes, decrease the number of awakenings to an absolute level of 1 to 3 per night, and increase total sleep time by about 15 to 45 minutes. These pharmacological agents act more reliably than behavioral interventions in the short term. ◆ Over the long term, behavioral interventions, including stimulus control, sleep restriction, relaxation strategies and cognitive-behavioral therapy reduce time elapsed before sleep onset, decrease awakenings, and increase total sleep time. These behavioral interventions produce more sustained effects than pharmacological agents.

From Nathan P, Gorman J: *A guide to treatments that work,* ed 2, New York, 2002, Oxford University Press.

It is not unusual for a person with a conversion disorder to substitute another symptom if the original one is taken away. This substitution happens because the basic conflict remains. The ego still needs to be defended from experiencing repressed anxiety. The patient really needs assistance in dealing with the conflict. When this is resolved, the symptom will disappear because it is no longer needed.

Great skill is needed to intervene therapeutically with patients with maladaptive psychophysiological responses. Psychological approaches include supportive therapy, insight therapy, group therapy, cognitive behavioral strategies, stress reduction, and relaxation training (Dudley-Brown, 2002; Schuyler and Brownfield, 2002; Servan-Schreiber, Tabas, Kolb, 2000b). The nurse should be supportive and available to talk with the patient and provide physical care (see A Patient Speaks). Alternative and complementary therapies also can be helpful (see Chapter 29).

The process of insight-oriented therapy for patients with psychophysiological disorders requires that the patient's underlying feelings be recognized and confronted in a supportive manner. As the patient becomes aware of the anger, appropriate expression of it may be difficult. The nurse should accept the patient's attempts to express anger and provide feedback. Sometimes patients in this phase of treatment are labeled as hostile or demanding and then avoided by health care providers. This reaction only reinforces their conviction that angry feelings are unacceptable.

The next step in therapy is to identify and explore the patient's defenses, proceeding very carefully to help the patient discover and test new, more adaptive coping mechanisms as the dysfunctional ones are given up. The nurse should support the patient in using new behaviors. Spending time with the patient and appreciating the patient's positive qualities will help the patient build self-esteem and confidence.

The nurse should be alert to signs of increased anxiety. The physical disorder may worsen if the therapy moves too rapidly. The therapist may recommend changes in the environment to help the patient function more comfortably. If the patient must consider a job change or another lifestyle change, the nurse can offer time to talk about alternatives.

Patients also may need help in explaining lifestyle change or changes in themselves to significant others. The family is a system, and a change in one part of the system requires adjustment in the other parts. For instance, a man who was very involved in his job and out several nights a week agreed to limit himself to 8-hour work days. This change affected the rest of the family. Although his wife had protested for years that he spent too much time away from home, she had built her life around his schedule. She spent several evenings a week doing outside activities. If he were now to be at home every evening, she would have to reevaluate her activities and decide whether she should go out or be with him. These are not easy decisions for family members to make.

It is important that any underlying feelings of resentment be revealed and discussed to prevent indirect expression of them, which would create a new stressor for the patient. Family therapy may be necessary if family members have been supporting the patient's disorder. For instance, families sometimes become adjusted to having a dependent member and unwittingly sabotage efforts to foster independence.

Because social support systems may help patients cope with their illnesses, the nurse may need to look for alternatives when the family is not supportive. Self-help groups often provide the needed social support. Group interventions also are helpful in decreasing overuse of health care services by patients with somatoform disorders.

Nurses must be aware that **countertransference** often occurs with these patients (see Chapter 2). It is easy to become impatient with a demanding patient who is not acutely ill when sicker patients also need nursing care. Reacting to this behavior by avoidance or anger only adds to the patient's anxiety. Clinical supervision by an experienced psychiatric nurse is highly recommended for nurses who work with these difficult patients. Frequent nursing care conferences also are helpful. If possible, a limited number of staff members should be assigned to the care of these patients. This consistent care fosters the development of a trusting relationship.

Patient Education

Health education is important in caring for the patient with a psychophysiological disorder. These patients usually need instruction about medications, treatments, and lifestyle changes. The patient and family will need information about mental health promotion (see Chapter 13), follow-up care, and crisis management (see Chapter 14), and education about ways to cope with anxiety and stress (see Chapter 16). Group classes on stress management may be productive. They may enable patients to share experiences and make suggestions to each other about coping behaviors. Former patients who have made successful life adjustments also can be effective teachers of coping strategies.

Do you think that patients with maladaptive psychophysiological responses will be more or less likely to comply with their treatment plans? How might you enhance their adherence? ■

A PATIENT SPEAKS

All I want to do is to feel better. My husband tells me that I make up all these complaints, but who would want to be sick? It isn't any fun missing out on family and church events because you don't feel good. It isn't fun going to bed with a headache and waking up with back pain day after day after day. On the other hand, my doctors tell me that they can't find anything wrong. Where does that leave me?

Right now I'm working with a nurse who is helping me to learn new habits that may help my physical condition. She has taught me how I can relax myself when I am tense and in pain. She has suggested some activities that I can start doing right now and is also reviewing with me situations and events that seem to trigger my physical problems. Will it help? I don't know, because we're just starting out, but I do know that she is at least one person I can talk to who supports me in my fight to feel like my old self again.

Physiological Support

A variety of physiological treatments also can be implemented by the nurse. Relaxation training, described in Chapter 31, can be very helpful in promoting adaptive psychophysiological responses. Encouraging physical activity is also a positive way of promoting stress reduction. Ideally, it should be an activity that the patient enjoys and can share with others. Diet counseling may be helpful in building the person's resistance to stress and illness. Patients under stress should not overuse dietary stimulants such as caffeine. They may need education about the elements of a healthful diet and help in planning balanced meals. A patient who has been relying on alcohol or drugs to cope with stress should identify and use more adaptive coping mechanisms. Antidepressant medication is useful if the patient has a comorbid depression.

Finally, the effective treatment of sleep disorders requires that the underlying cause of the sleep problem be identified. Drugs and alcohol often produce fragmented sleep, as does caffeine. Poor sleep hygiene habits also may be a problem, and the patient can be encouraged to develop good sleep hygiene habits (Box 17-5).

Medications (Table 17-3) also can be used to help with sleep problems, but these drugs should be used for a limited time only. Melatonin may be helpful when insomnia is related to shift work and jet lag; however, studies evaluating its safety and efficacy have been inconclusive. The dose ranges from 2 to 5 mg (Larzelere and Wiseman, 2002).

Although prescription medications and sleep hygiene behavior therapy have similar short-term efficacy, behavioral interventions are recommended as the first-line treatment because of their greater safety and long-term efficacy (Edinger et al, 2001; Smith et al, 2002).

The Nursing Treatment Plan Summary for patients with maladaptive psychophysiological responses is presented in Table 17-4.

◼ EVALUATION

The evaluation of the nursing care of the patient with psychophysiological illness is based on the identified patient care goals. If goal achievement is not attained, the nurse must ask the following questions:

- Was the assessment complete enough to correctly identify the problem?
- Did the patient agree with the goal?
- Was enough time allowed for goal achievement?
- Was I skilled enough to carry out the desired intervention?
- Were there environmental constraints that affected goal accomplishment?
- Did additional stressors change the patient's ability to cope?

BOX **17-5**

Sleep Hygiene Behavior Strategies

- Maintain a regular bedtime and wake-up time 7 days a week.
- Exercise daily to aid sleep initiation and maintenance; however, vigorous exercise too close to bedtime may make falling asleep difficult.
- Schedule time to wind down and relax before bed.
- Try relaxation exercises before bedtime.
- Avoid worrying when trying to fall asleep.
- Guard against nighttime interruptions.
- Earplugs may help with a noisy partner.
- Bedroom should be dark, quiet, cool, and comfortable. Heavy window shades help to screen out light.
- Create a comfortable bed.
- A warm bath or warm drink before bed helps some people fall asleep.
- Excessive hunger or fullness may interfere with sleep. Avoid large meals before bed. If hungry, a light carbohydrate snack may be helpful.
- Avoid caffeine, excessive fluid intake, stimulating drugs, and excessive alcohol in the evening and before bed.
- Excessive napping may make it difficult for some people to fall asleep at night.
- Do not eat, read, work, or watch television in bed. The bed and bedroom should be used only for sleep and sex.
- Maintain a reasonable weight. Excessive weight may result in daytime fatigue and sleep apnea.
- Get out of bed and engage in other activities if not able to fall asleep.

Table 17-3	Medications for the Treatment of Insomnia		
CLASS	GENERIC NAME (TRADE NAME)	RANGE (MG)*	HALF-LIFE (HR)†
Benzodiazepine short-acting	Triazolam (Halcion)	0.125-0.5	3
Benzodiazepine intermediate	Lorazepam (Ativan)	1-6	14
	Temazepam (Restoril)	7.5-30	8
	Estazolam (Prosom)	1-4	16
Benzodiazepine long-acting	Flurazepam (Dalmane)	15-30	100‡
	Quazepam (Doral)	7.5-15	39
Non-benzodiazepine	Zaleplon (Sonata)	5-10	1-2.5
	Zolpidem (Ambien)	5-10	1-2.5
Antidepressant	Trazodone (Desyrel)	50-200	4
Antihistamine	Diphenhydramine (Benadryl)	50	unknown

Modified from Bezchilbnyk-Butler K, Jeffries J: *Clinical handbook of psychotropic drugs*, ed 12, Seattle, 2002, Hogrefe & Huber Publishers.
*Dose range for adults.
†Elimination half-life is not synonymous with duration of effect, which varies significantly from patient to patient; another reason for individualizing treatment.
‡Active metabolite.

Table 17-4	NURSING TREATMENT PLAN SUMMARY	Maladaptive Psychophysiological Responses

Nursing Diagnosis: Impaired adjustment
Expected Outcome: The patient will express feelings verbally rather than through the development of physical symptoms.

SHORT-TERM GOAL	INTERVENTION	RATIONALE
The patient will identify areas of stress and conflict and relate feelings, thoughts, and behaviors to them.	Assist patient in identifying stressful situations by reviewing events surrounding the development of physical symptoms. Facilitate the association among cognitions, feelings, and behaviors.	Inability to deal with intrapsychic conflict leads to anxiety and stress, resulting in physiological dysfunction.
The patient will describe present defenses and evaluate whether they are adaptive or maladaptive.	Proceed slowly in analyzing defenses. Explore alternative coping behaviors with the patient. Teach the patient stress management techniques such as relaxation and imagery.	Defenses should not be attacked; rather, the nurse should support positive exploration by the patient and suggest alternative responses.
The patient will adopt two new coping mechanisms to deal with stress.	Give patient positive feedback for new adaptive behaviors. Actively support patient in testing new coping mechanisms. Enlist the support of family and significant others to reinforce change.	Change requires time and positive reinforcement from others. Family members can be important in promoting adaptive responses.
The patient will display a decrease in physical symptoms and greater biological integrity.	Encourage physical activity to reduce stress. Counsel the patient on diet and nutrition needs. Review the patient's sleep habits and promote good sleep hygiene practices.	Wellness requires a balance between biological and psychosocial needs. Interventions focused on the patient's physiological needs can help the patient restore biological integrity.

- Was the goal achievable for this patient?
- What alternative approaches should be tried?

It is very important that neither the patient nor the nurse interpret the lack of goal achievement as a failure. The nurse should look at it as a challenge and convey that attitude to the patient. It is not helpful to add *failure to achieve a goal* to the patient's collection of stressors. The care of these patients is very complex. The nurse may need to modify the treatment plan several times before finding a successful approach. The most important thing is to keep trying and to encourage the patient to persist in the effort to find health.

COMPETENT CARING	**A Clinical Exemplar of a Psychiatric Nurse**
	AUDREY JOSEPH, MSN, RN

Often it is difficult for health care professionals to communicate with their patients about psychosomatic illness. Also, the patient's denial or rejection of this diagnosis does not make the communication process any easier. Psychiatric staff and family members can get caught in the middle when primary care physicians fail to tell their patients that they need a psychiatric evaluation to rule out a psychosomatic illness. I know this from an experience I had that taught me much about psychiatric care.

I was working the evening shift as a staff nurse on an inpatient unit when Mrs. O, an elderly woman, presented herself on the unit for voluntary admission. She was well dressed and quite cheerful. Her medical history revealed that she had visited her family doctor and the emergency room weekly for the last 2 months. She had many diagnostic studies, the results of which were all negative. Mrs. O reported that she was referred by her family doctor for a diagnostic work-up. A psychosocial assessment revealed that her husband had recently died and that she lived alone. The patient was allowed to become acclimated to the unit. Then, as the staff explained to her why she was admitted, she became angry and left against medical advice.

About 3 weeks later Mrs. O's son arranged for her to be readmitted because she was still constantly going to the emergency room and to her family doctor. She was angry with her son for having her admitted. To keep her in the hospital, he told her that he would have her committed if necessary. On this admission, Mrs. O was neatly dressed but looked tired. Her chief complaint was choking, and a general infection throughout her body that was causing a vaginal discharge. Her family doctor again had not told her that he could find nothing physically wrong with her. She was started on a regimen of antidepressant medication. During the 2 weeks she was in the hospital, she spent most of her time socializing with other patients. She was not interested in psychotherapy and did not develop a therapeutic alliance with the staff.

On her third admission, approximately 2 months later, Mrs. O's family doctor still had not told her that he thought she had a psychosomatic illness. At this time she was disheveled and looked physically ill. Mrs. O spent most of the day in bed. She constantly complained of choking and a vaginal discharge. She admitted that she stopped taking the antidepressant medication right after discharge from the hospital. At this point she was angry with all her children and thought they were all against her. She could not understand why they would not accept the fact that she was physically ill. After 3 weeks of treatment, Mrs. O was discharged home. Two years later I met Mrs. O in another psychiatric hospital, where she was again admitted for treatment.

Clearly this is not a success story. In fact, it taught me much about the problems of nonintegrated physical and psychiatric systems of care in which patients are treated as parts rather than wholes. I also realized that I shared responsibility for not providing better care for Mrs. O. To this day, she is often in my thoughts, and I now advocate for treating patients broadly within the context of their worldview rather than within the narrow realm our society defines as medical care. ■

CHAPTER **FOCUS POINTS**

■ Many believe that all illness has a psychophysiological component in that physical disorders have a psychological component and psychiatric disorders a physical one.

■ The continuum of possible psychophysiological responses to stress based on Selye's theory includes the stages of alarm, resistance, and exhaustion. Any experience believed by the individual to be stressful may stimulate a psychophysiological response.

■ The primary behaviors observed with psychophysiological responses are the physical symptoms. These symptoms lead the person to seek health care. People are often reluctant to believe that a physical problem may be related to psychological factors.

■ Some people have physical symptoms without any organic impairment, and these are called somatoform disorders. Secondary gain, an indirect benefit usually obtained through an illness or disability and related to the gratification of dependency needs, is a powerful deterrent to change in many patients.

■ Pain is increasingly recognized as more than simply a sensory phenomenon, but as a complex sensory and emotional experience underlying potential disease. The experience, expression, and treatment of pain are subject to cultural norms and biases.

■ Sleep disturbances can influence the development and course of mental illnesses and addictive disorders and also can affect treatment and recovery. The consequences of sleep disorders, sleep deprivation, and sleepiness are significant and include reduced productivity, lowered cognitive performance, increased likelihood of accidents, higher morbidity and mortality risk, depression, and decreased quality of life.

■ Research has linked emotions to arousal of the neuroendocrine system through release of corticosteroids by the hypothalamic-pituitary-adrenal (HPA) axis, as well as to the actions of neurotransmitter systems, particularly norepinephrine and serotonin.

■ A biological tendency for particular psychophysiological responses may be inherited, underscoring the importance of genetic factors. Psychoneuroimmunology is the scientific field that explores the relationship between psychological states, the immune system, and health.

■ Research suggests that a negative affective style marked by depression, anxiety, and hostility may be associated with the development or recovery from such diseases as asthma, headaches, ulcers, arthritis, and cancer. Complementing the research on negative emotional states and disease is the increasing focus on the protective role of positive emotional states and resilience.

■ Health, illness, and suffering are patterned by culture and realized as personal worlds of experience. The social course of illness has at least two meanings. The first is that the severity of the person's symptoms is influenced by aspects of the social environment. The second is that the symptoms shape and structure the person's social world, as the illness causes a series of changes in the person's environment.

■ Any experience that the person interprets as stressful may lead to a psychophysiological response. One type of stressor that has been shown to cause physical illness and even death is the loss of a significant interpersonal relationship. In contrast, a psychophysiological problem also can be a response to an accumulation of rather small stressors.

■ One of the most important parts of promoting adaptive psychophysiological responses involves adopting positive health practices, because good health measures can prevent many illnesses. Social support from family, friends, and caregivers is also an important resource for adaptive psychophysiological responses.

■ Psychophysiological disorders may be attempts to cope with the anxiety associated with overwhelming stress. A variety of coping mechanisms are used in psychophysiological response such as repression, denial, compensation, and regression. Common to each of these coping mechanisms is the need not to confront the basic conflict that is leading to stress and anxiety.

■ Primary NANDA nursing diagnoses for psychophysiological responses are impaired adjustment, ineffective denial, chronic pain, and sleep pattern disturbance.

■ Primary *DSM-IV-TR* diagnoses are categorized as somatoform disorders, sleep disorders, and psychological factors affecting medical condition.

■ The expected outcome of nursing care is that the patient will express feelings verbally rather than through the development of physical symptoms.

■ Only after a thorough medical examination can the role of psychosocial stressors in the disorder be evaluated. If the physical condition is life threatening, this intervention is given highest priority. The most important principle for patients with psychophysical disorders is to assess the patient's stress level and, whenever possible, act to reduce it.

■ The dilemma of these disorders is that the patient consciously would like nothing more than to be cured but is unconsciously unable to give up the symptom. The process of insight-oriented therapy for patients with psychophysiological disorders requires that the patient's underlying feelings be recognized and confronted in a supportive manner.

■ The next step in therapy is to identify and explore the patient's defenses, proceeding very carefully to help the patient discover and test new, more adaptive coping mechanisms as the dysfunctional ones are given up. Patients also may need help in explaining lifestyle change or changes in themselves to significant others. Nurses must be aware that countertransference often occurs with these patients.

■ These patients usually need instruction about medications, treatments, and lifestyle changes.

■ A variety of physiological treatments can be implemented by the nurse, including relaxation training, encouraging physical activity, and diet counseling. Patients should be advised not to use alcohol or drugs to cope with stress. Antidepressant medication also is helpful.

■ The effective treatment of sleep disorders requires that the underlying cause of the sleep problem be identified. The patient should be encouraged to develop good sleep hygiene habits. Although prescription medications and sleep hygiene behavior therapy have similar short-term efficacy, behavioral interventions are recommended as the first-line treatment because of their greater safety and long-term efficacy.

◢ KEY TERMS

body dysmorphic disorder, 287
conversion disorder, 287
hypersomnia, 288
hypochondriasis, 287
insomnia, 288

malingering, 288
pain disorder, 287
parasomnia, 288
psychoneuroimmunology, 289

secondary gain, 287
somatization disorder, 287
somatoform disorders, 287
somatoform pain disorder, 288

CHAPTER REVIEW QUESTIONS

1. Match each term in Column A with the correct definition in Column B.

Column A

_____ Body dysmorphic disorder

_____ Conversion disorder

_____ Hypersomnia

_____ Hypochondriasis

_____ Insomnia

_____ Pain disorder

_____ Parasomnia

_____ Sleep pattern disturbance

_____ Somatization disorder

_____ Somatoform disorders

Column B

A. Physical symptoms without organic impairment

B. A history of many physical complaints

C. Loss or alteration of voluntary motor or sensory function that cannot be explained by a medical condition

D. Preoccupation with fears of having a serious disease

E. An imagined or exaggerated defect in appearance

F. A disorder in which psychological factors have an important role in the onset, severity, exacerbation, or maintenance

G. Sleepwalking, night terrors, nightmares, enuresis

H. Narcolepsy, sleep apnea, nocturnal movement disorders

I. Disorders of initiating or maintaining sleep

J. Difficulty falling asleep and frequent awakening during the night

2. Fill in the blanks.

A. The continuum of possible psychophysiological responses to stress, based on Selye's theory, include the stages of

_____, _____,

and _____.

B. A variety of coping mechanisms are used in psychophysiological response, such as _____,

_____, _____,

and _____.

C. The expected outcome of nursing care is that the patient will express feelings _____ rather than through the development of _____ symptoms.

D. It is not unusual for a person with _____ to substitute another symptom if the original one is taken away without attention being given to the underlying stressor.

E. _____ is the scientific field that explores the relationship between psychological states and the immune response.

3. Provide short answers for the following questions.

A. Describe four psychological interventions the nurse might use in the treatment of the patient with a maladaptive psychophysiological response to stress.

B. Define secondary gain. Give several examples from your personal experience.

C. Research indicates that people with clinical depression who smoke are at higher risk for lung cancer than people without depression who smoke. Based on this information, how would you differ in your educational approach to patients with and without depression who smoke?

Visit Evolve for additional resources related to the content of this chapter.

http://evolve.elsevier.com/Stuart/principles/
• Topical Course Outline • Student Workbook Exercises • Critical Thinking Questions and Activities • Case Studies • Research Topics
• Monthly Content Updates • WebLinks

Student Study CD-ROM

Access the accompanying CD-ROM for animations, interactive exercises, review questions for the NCLEX examination, and an audio glossary.

REFERENCES

Afari N, Buchwald D: Chronic fatigue syndrome: a review, *Am J Psychiatry* 160:221, 2003.

American Psychiatric Association: *Diagnostic and statistical manual of mental disorders,* ed 4, text revision, Washington, DC, 2000, American Psychiatric Association.

Bandura A: *Self-efficacy: the exercise of control,* New York, 1997, WH Freeman.

Barsky AJ et al: Hypochondriacal patients' appraisal of health and physical risks, *Am J Psychiatry* 158:783, 2001.

Cohen JI: Stress and mental health: a biobehavioral perspective, *Issues Ment Health Nurs* 21:185, 2000.

Donnelly TT, Long BC: Stress discourse and Western biomedical ideology: rewriting stress, *Issues Ment Health Nurs* 24:397, 2003.

Dudley-Brown S: Prevention of psychological distress in persons with inflammatory bowel disease, *Issues Ment Health Nurs* 23:403, 2002.

Edinger JD et al: Cognitive behavioral therapy for treatment of chronic primary insomnia: a randomized controlled trial, *JAMA* 285:1856, 2001.

Friedman HS: *The self-healing personality: why some people achieve health while others succumb to illness,* New York, 1991, Holt.

Koenig HG, Cohen HJ: *The link between religion and health: psychoneuroimmunology and the faith factor,* New York, 2002, Oxford University Press.

Larzelere MM, Wiseman P: Anxiety, depression, and insomnia. *Prim Care* 29:339, 2002.

Lilie JK, Lahmeyer H: Psychiatric management of sleep disorders, *Psychiatr Med* 9:245, 1991.

Nathan PE, Gorman JM: *A guide to treatments that work*, ed 2, New York, 2002, Oxford University Press.

National Sleep Foundation (NSF): www.sleepfoundation.org, 2003.

Parsons T: *The social system*, New York, 1951, The Free Press.

Raison CL, Miller AH: When not enough is too much: the role of insufficient glucocorticoid signaling in the pathophysiology of stress-related disorders, *Am J Psychiatry* 160:1554, 2003.

Ruo B et al: Depressive symptoms and health-related quality of life: the Heart and Soul Study, *JAMA* 290:215, 2003.

Schuyler D, Brownfield E: Somatization: a disorder about "nothing," *J S C Med Assoc* 98:1, 2002.

Selye H: *The stress of life*, New York, 1956, McGraw-Hill.

Servan-Schreiber D, Kolb NR, Tabas G: Somatizing patients. Part I: practical diagnosis, *Am Fam Physician* 61:1073, 2000a.

Servan-Schreiber D, Tabas G, Kolb R: Somatizing patients. Part II: practical management, *Am Fam Physician* 61:1423, 2000b.

Smith MT et al: Comparative meta-analysis of pharmacotherapy and behavior therapy for persistent insomnia, *Am J Psychiatry* 159:5, 2002.

Stansberry T: Narcolepsy: unveiling a mystery, *Am J Nurs* 101:50, 2001.

> *To venture causes anxiety, but not to venture is to lose one's-self. And to venture in the highest sense is precisely to be conscious of one's self.*
>
> SØREN KIERKEGAARD

SELF-CONCEPT RESPONSES AND DISSOCIATIVE DISORDERS

18

Gail W. Stuart

LEARNING OBJECTIVES

After studying this chapter, the student should be able to:

1. Describe the continuum of adaptive and maladaptive self-concept responses (I).
2. Identify behaviors associated with self-concept responses (II).
3. Analyze predisposing factors, precipitating stressors, and appraisal of stressors related to self-concept responses (II).
4. Describe coping resources and coping mechanisms related to self-concept responses (II).
5. Formulate nursing diagnoses related to self-concept responses (III).
6. Examine the relationship between nursing diagnoses and medical diagnoses related to self-concept responses (III).
7. Identify expected outcomes and short-term nursing goals for patients related to self-concept responses (IV).
8. Develop a patient education plan to improve family relationships (V).
9. Analyze nursing interventions related to self-concept responses (VI).
10. Evaluate nursing care related to self-concept responses (VII).

TOPICAL OUTLINE

 Visit Evolve for additional resources related to the content of this chapter.
http://evolve.elsevier.com/Stuart/principles/

Of all human attributes, the *self* is the most complex and intangible. It is the frame of reference through which one perceives, conceives, and evaluates one's world. Self-concept is defined as all the notions, beliefs, and convictions that constitute a person's self-knowledge and that influence relationships with others. It includes one's perceptions of personal characteristics and abilities, interactions with other people and the environment, values associated with experiences and objects, and goals and ideals.

The self-concept is critical to the understanding of people and their behavior. No two people have identical self-concepts. The self-concept emerges or is learned through each person's internal experiences, relationships with other people, and interactions with the outer world. Because it is the frame of reference through which the person interacts with the world, it has a powerful influence on human behavior.

It is impossible to understand a person fully or to predict behavior accurately without understanding the person's internal frame of reference. This involves sharing the person's perceptual world and view of the self. Thus understanding a patient's self-concept is a necessary part of all nursing care.

■ CONTINUUM OF SELF-CONCEPT RESPONSES

Self-Concept

Developmental Influences. From birth the self develops gradually as the infant recognizes and distinguishes others and begins to gain a sense of differentiation from others. The boundaries of the self are defined as the result of

303

exploratory activity and experience with one's own body. At first self-differentiation is slow, but with the development of language it accelerates. Use of the child's own name helps with the identification and perception of individuality—of being someone special, unique, and independent. Human language allows clear distinctions to be made between the self and the rest of the world and the ability to symbolize and understand experiences.

The continued process of self-concept development is greatly aided by the following:

- Interpersonal and cultural experiences that generate positive feelings and a sense of worth
- Perceived competence in areas valued by the individual and society
- Self-actualization, or the implementation and realization of a person's true potential

Significant Others. The self-concept is learned in part through accumulated social contacts and experiences with other people. This has been called "learning about self from the mirror of other people" (Sullivan, 1963). What a person believes about himself is a function of his interpretation of how others see him, as inferred from their behavior toward him. His concept of self therefore rests partly on what he thinks others think of him.

For a young child the most significant others are his parents, who help him grow and react to his experiences. The family provides the person with his earliest experiences of:

- Feelings of adequacy or inadequacy.
- Feelings of acceptance or rejection.
- Opportunities for identification.
- Expectations concerning acceptable goals, values, and behaviors.

Research indicates that parental influence is strongest during early childhood and continues to have a significant impact through adolescence and young adulthood. Over time, however, the power and influence of friends and other adults increase, and they become significant others to the person. Culture and socialization practices also affect self-concept and personality development. General cultural patterns and cultural subdivisions, such as social class, have formative influences on one's view of self.

What sociocultural factors had an impact on your self-concept as you were growing up? Which ones currently influence your self-concept?

Self-Perceptions. Each person can observe his or her own behavior the same way that others do and thereby form opinions about oneself. One's perception of reality is selective, however, according to whether the experience is consistent with one's current concept of self. The way a person behaves is a result of how he or she perceives the situation, and it is not the event itself that elicits a specific response, but rather the individual's subjective experience of the event.

One's needs, values, and beliefs strongly influence perceptions. People are more likely to perceive what is meaningful and consistent with present needs and personal values. Similarly, people behave in a manner consistent with what they believe to be true. In this case a fact is not what is but what one believes to be true.

Once perceptions are acquired and incorporated into one's self-system, they can be difficult to change. However, ways do exist that can change perceptions, including modifying cognitive processes, taking drugs, undergoing sensory deprivation, and the generation of biochemical changes within the body.

A person with a weak or negative self-concept who is unsure of himself is likely to have narrowed or distorted perceptions. Because he feels easily threatened, his anxiety level will rise quickly, and then he will become preoccupied with defending himself. In contrast, a person with a strong or positive self-concept can explore his world openly and honestly because he has a background of acceptance and success to support him. Positive self-concepts result from positive experiences leading to perceived competence.

In conclusion, people with positive self-concepts function more effectively. Negative self-concept is correlated with personal and social maladjustment. Figure 18-1 describes the continuum of self-concept responses from the most adaptive state of self-actualization to the most maladaptive response of depersonalization.

To provide the best care, the nurse therefore needs an understanding of various components of the self, including body image, self-ideal, self-esteem, role, and identity, which are briefly discussed here.

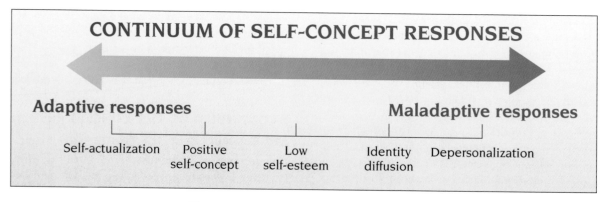

Figure 18-1   Continuum of self-concept responses.

Body Image

The concept of one's body is central to the concept of self. The body is the most material and visible part of the self, and although it does not account for one's entire sense of self, it remains a lifelong anchor for self-awareness. A person's attitude toward the body may mirror important aspects of identity. A person's feelings that his or her body is big or small, attractive or unattractive, or weak or strong also reveal something about the self-concept. Numerous research studies have documented the close positive relationship between self-concept and body image. This association appears to exist in all cultures.

Body image is the sum of the conscious and unconscious attitudes a person has toward one's own body. It includes present and past perceptions as well as feelings about size, function, appearance, and potential. Body image is dynamic because it is constantly changing as new perceptions and experiences are encountered in life. It is a target, or screen, on which the person projects significant personal feelings, anxieties, and values.

As one's body image develops, extensions of the body become important. Clothes become identified closely with the body, and in the same way toys, tools, money, and possessions serve as extensions of the body. Body image, appearance, and positive self-concept are related.

Studies indicate that the more a person accepts and likes his or her own body, the more secure and free from anxiety he or she feels. It also has been shown that people who accept their bodies are more likely to have high self-esteem than people who dislike their bodies. Problems related to body image are discussed in more detail in Chapter 25.

What does it mean when one says that "a child lives in his body but an adult lives in his mind"? ■

Self-Ideal

The self-ideal is the person's perception of how to behave, based on certain personal standards. The standard may be either a carefully constructed image of the type of person he or she would like to be or merely a number of aspirations, goals, or values that he or she would like to achieve. The self-ideal creates self-expectations based in part on society's norms, to which the person tries to conform.

Formation of the self-ideal begins in childhood and is influenced by significant others, who place certain demands or expectations on the child. With time the child internalizes these expectations, and they form the basis of the child's own self-ideal. New self-ideals are taken on during adolescence, formed from identification with parents, teachers, and peers. In old age additional adjustments must be made that reflect diminishing physical strength and changing roles and responsibilities.

Various factors influence self-ideal. First, a person tends to set goals within a range determined by personal abilities. A person does not ordinarily set a goal that is accomplished without any effort or that is entirely beyond his or her abilities. Self-ideals also are influenced by cultural factors as the person compares self-standards with those of peers. Other influencing factors include ambitions and the desire to excel and succeed, the need to be realistic, the desire to avoid failure, and feelings of anxiety and inferiority.

Based on these factors, one's self-ideal may be clear and realistic and thus facilitate personal growth and relations with others, or it may be vague, unrealistic, and demanding. The adequately functioning person demonstrates congruence between one's perception of self and self-ideal, that is, one sees oneself as being very similar to the person one wants to be.

In summary, self-ideals are important in maintaining mental health and balance. The self-ideal must be neither too high and demanding nor too vague and shadowy, yet it must be high enough and defined enough to provide continuous support to one's self-respect.

Self-Esteem

Self-esteem is a person's personal judgment of his or her own worth, based on how well behavior matches up with self-ideal. The frequency with which a person attains goals directly influences feelings of competency (high self-esteem) or inferiority (low self-esteem) (Figure 18-2). High self-esteem is a feeling based on unconditional acceptance of self, despite mistakes, defeats, and failures, as an innately worthy and important being. It involves accepting complete responsibility for one's own life.

Self-esteem comes from two primary sources: the self and others. It is first a function of being loved and gaining the respect of others. Self-esteem is lowered when love is lost and when one fails to receive approval from others. Conversely, it is raised when love is regained and when one is applauded and praised.

The origins of self-esteem can be traced to childhood and are based on acceptance, warmth, involvement, consistency, praise, and respect. The four best ways to promote a child's self-esteem are as follows (Coopersmith, 1967; Mruk, 1999):

1. Providing opportunities for success
2. Instilling ideals
3. Encouraging aspirations
4. Helping the child build defenses against attacks to his or her self-perceptions

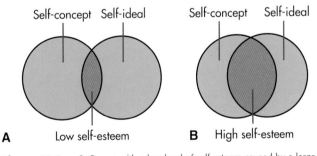

Figure 18-2   **A,** Person with a low level of self-esteem caused by a large discrepancy between self-concept and self-ideal. **B,** Person with a greater conformity of self-concept and self-ideal and therefore a high level of self-esteem. (From Sundeen SJ et al: *Nurse-client interaction: implementing the nursing process,* ed 6, St Louis, 1998, Mosby.)

These should provide the child with a feeling of significance or success in being accepted and approved of by others; a feeling of competence, or an ability to cope effectively with life; and a feeling of power, or control over one's own destiny.

Self-esteem increases with age and is most threatened during adolescence, when concepts of self are being changed and many self-decisions are made. The adolescent must choose an occupation and decide whether he or she is good enough to succeed in a given career. Adolescents also must decide whether they are able to participate or are accepted in various social activities.

With adulthood the self-concept stabilizes, and maturity provides a clearer picture of self. The adult tends to be more self-accepting and less idealistic than the adolescent. Adults have learned to cope with many self-deficiencies and to maximize self-strengths. Not all adults attain maturity; some continue to function as adolescents for many of their adult years.

In later life, self-esteem problems again arise because of the new challenges posed by retirement, loss of spouse, and physical disability. The impact of aging on self-esteem is also affected by the status of older people in American society. Being old in a society that values youth often leads to low status and prejudicial attitudes toward the aged. Negative stereotypes of the elderly and the stigmatization that results can decrease self-esteem. Two other potential negative factors are the decreased social interaction of the elderly and their loss of control over their environment, both of which can result in fewer opportunities to validate and confirm one's self-concept.

Research shows a clear relationship between self-reported physical health and self-esteem. The report of a health problem, regardless of its type or severity, is associated with significantly lower self-esteem than is the report of no health problem. In contrast, high self-esteem has been correlated with low anxiety, effective group functioning, and acceptance of others. It is a prerequisite to self-actualization; once self-esteem is achieved, the person is free to concentrate on achieving his or her potential.

Why do you think low self-esteem is associated with poor interpersonal relations and depressive states? ■

Role Performance

Roles are sets of socially expected behavior patterns associated with a person's functioning in different social groups. The person assumes various roles that he or she tries to integrate into one functional pattern. Because these roles overlap, an understanding of the person requires the nurse to see him or her in the context of the several roles occupied.

On the basis of one's perception of role adequacy in the most ego-involved roles, a person develops a level of self-esteem. High self-esteem results from roles that meet needs and are congruent with one's self-ideal. Factors that influence a person's adjustment to the role he or she occupies include the following:

- One's knowledge of specific role expectations
- The consistency of the response of significant others to one's role

- The compatibility and complementarity of various roles
- The congruency of cultural norms and one's own expectations for role behavior
- The separation of situations that would create incompatible role behaviors

Gender roles affect performance in other roles. They are particularly significant to family roles but permeate most others as well and are often the cause of role conflict. Another difficult problem faced in growing up is emancipation from one's parents and establishment of an independent life. This primarily occurs during adolescence and early adulthood, when great ambiguity in role definitions occurs. A final crisis is faced during old age, when role behavior must again be changed by aging parents. They rely on their children, yet strive to balance their lives with a sense of independence and a high level of self-esteem.

Role behavior is intimately related to self-concept and identity, and role disturbances often involve conflicts between independent and dependent functioning.

Personal Identity

The word *identity* is derived from the Latin root *idem*, meaning "the same." It is the organizing principle of the personality. Identity is the awareness of being oneself, as derived from self-observation and judgment. It is the synthesis of all self-representations into an organized whole. It is not associated with any one accomplishment, object, attribute, or role.

Identity is different from self-concept in that it is a feeling of distinctness from others. It implies consciousness of oneself as an individual with a definite place in the general scheme of things. The person with a sense of identity feels integrated, not diffuse. When a person acts in accordance with his or her self-concept, the sense of identity is reinforced; when he or she acts in ways contrary to the self-concept, he or she experiences anxiety and apprehension. The person with a strong sense of identity sees himself or herself as a unique individual.

Developmental Influences. The concept of ego identity was developed by Erikson (1963) and built within his formulation of the eight stages of human development. For each stage, Erikson describes a psychosocial crisis that must be resolved for further growth and personality development.

In adolescence the crisis of identity versus identity diffusion occurs. At no other phase of life are the promise of finding oneself and the threat of losing oneself so closely aligned. The adolescent's task is one of self-definition as one strives to integrate previous roles into a unique and reasonably consistent sense of self.

Important in achieving identity is the issue of sexuality, the image of oneself as a male or a female and what that implies. Society's ideals of masculinity and femininity are important standards for judging oneself as good, bad, superior, inferior, desirable, or undesirable. These ideals are passed down from generation to generation and become a part of the culture. If males are defined as superior, this idea becomes part of the self-image of both males and females. If passivity and obedience are feminine ideals in a society, most girls will be taught to be unassertive and obedient.

In addition, much of one's identity is expressed in relationships with others. How a person relates to other people is a central personality characteristic. This presents a paradox in that everyone is a part of humanity yet each person is also separate from all others. Achieving identity is a prerequisite for establishing an intimate relationship. Research has shown that only after a stable sense of identity has been established can one engage in genuinely intimate, mature, and successful relationships.

Healthy Personality

It is possible to describe the healthy personality according to developmental theory and the dynamics of the self (Clemens, 2002). This description may help give perspective to the many aspects of self. A person with a healthy personality would have the characteristics listed in Table 18-1 and be able to perceive both self and the world accurately. This insight would create a feeling of harmony and inner peace.

 How do you compare with the qualities of a healthy personality listed in Table 18-1? ■

■ ASSESSMENT

Behaviors

Assessing the various aspects of a patient's self-concept is a challenge to the nurse. Because self-concept is the cornerstone of the personality, it is intimately related to anxiety and depression, problems in relationships, acting out, and self-destructive behavior. All behavior is motivated by a desire to enhance, maintain, or defend the self, so the nurse has much information to evaluate. The nurse also must go beyond objective and observable behaviors to the patient's subjective and internal world. Only by exploring this area can the nurse understand the patient's actions.

The nurse can begin the assessment by observing the patient's appearance. Posture, cleanliness, makeup, and clothing provide data. The nurse might discuss the patient's appearance with him or her to determine what values are held related to body image. Observing or inquiring about eating, sleeping, and hygiene patterns gives clues to biological habits and self-care.

These initial observations should lead the nurse to ask: "What does my patient think about himself as a person?" The nurse might ask the patient to describe himself or how he feels about himself. What strengths does he think he has? What areas of weakness? What is his self-ideal? Does he conform to it? Does fulfillment of his self-ideal bring him satisfaction? Does he value his strengths? Does he view his weaknesses as important personality deficits, or are they unimportant to his self-concept? What are his priorities? Does he feel unified and self-directed or diffuse and other-directed?

The nurse can then compare the patient's responses to his behavior, looking for inconsistencies or contradictions. How does he relate to other people? How does he respond to compliments and criticisms? The nurse also can examine his or her own affective response to the patient. Is it one of hopelessness, despair, anger, or anxiety? The nurse's own response

Table 18-1	**Qualities of the Healthy Personality**	
CHARACTERISTIC	DEFINITION	DESCRIPTION
Positive and accurate body image	Body image is the sum of the conscious and unconscious attitudes one has toward one's body, function, appearance, and potential.	A healthy body awareness is based on self-observation and appropriate concern for one's physical well-being.
Realistic self-ideal	Self-ideal is one's perception of how one should behave or the standard by which behavior is appraised.	A person with a realistic self-ideal has attainable life goals that are valuable and worth striving for.
Positive self-concept	Self-concept consists of all the aspects of the person of which one is aware. It includes all self-perceptions that direct and influence behavior.	A positive self-concept implies that the person expects to be successful in life. It includes acceptance of the negative aspects of the self as part of one's personality. Such a person faces life openly and realistically.
High self-esteem	Self-esteem is one's personal judgment of one's own worth, which is obtained by analyzing how well one matches up to one's own standards and how well one's performance compares with others. It evolves through a comparison of the self-ideal and self-concept.	A person with high self-esteem feels worthy of respect and dignity, believes in his or her own self-worth, and approaches life with assertiveness and zest. The person with a healthy personality feels very similar to the person he or she wants to be.
Satisfying role performance	Roles are sets of socially expected behavior patterns associated with functioning in various social groups.	The healthy person can relate to others intimately, receive gratification from social and personal roles, trust others, and enter into mutual and interdependent relationships.
Clear sense of identity	Identity is the integration of inner and outer demands in one's discovery of who one is and what one can become. It is the realization of personal consistency.	The person with a clear sense of identity experiences a unity of personality and perceives herself or himself to be a unique person. This sense of self gives life direction and purpose.

to the patient is often a good indication of the quality and depth of the patient's pain.

Behaviors Associated With Low Self-Esteem.
Low self-esteem is a major problem for many people and can be expressed in moderate and severe levels of anxiety. It involves negative self-evaluations and is associated with feelings of being weak, helpless, hopeless, frightened, vulnerable, fragile, incomplete, worthless, and inadequate.

Low self-esteem is a major component of depression, which acts as a form of punishment and anesthesia. Low self-esteem indicates self-rejection and self-hate, which may be a conscious or unconscious process expressed in direct or indirect ways.

Direct behaviors. Direct expressions of low self-esteem may include any of the following areas.

SELF-CRITICISM. The patient has negative thinking and believes he or she is doomed to failure. Although the expressed purpose of the criticism may be self-improvement, no constructive value is found in it and the underlying goal is self-demoralization. The patient might describe himself as "stupid," "no good," or a "born loser." He views the normal stressors of life as impossible barriers and becomes preoccupied with self-pity.

SELF-DIMINUTION. Self-diminution involves minimizing one's ability by avoiding, neglecting, or refusing to recognize one's real assets and strengths.

GUILT AND WORRY. Guilt and worry are destructive activities by which the person punishes himself or herself. They may be expressed through nightmares, phobias, obsessions, or the reliving of painful memories and indiscretions. They indicate self-rejection.

PHYSICAL MANIFESTATIONS. These might include hypertension, psychosomatic illnesses, and the abuse of various substances, such as alcohol, drugs, tobacco, or food.

POSTPONING DECISIONS. A high level of ambivalence or procrastination produces an increased sense of insecurity.

DENYING ONESELF PLEASURE. The self-rejecting person feels the need to punish himself and expresses this by denying himself the things he finds desirable or pleasurable. This might be a career opportunity, a material object, or a desired relationship.

DISTURBED RELATIONSHIPS. The person may be cruel, demeaning, or exploitive with other people. This may be an overt or a passive-dependent pattern of relating, which indirectly exploits others. Another behavior included in this category is withdrawal or social isolation, which arises from feelings of worthlessness.

WITHDRAWAL FROM REALITY. When anxiety resulting from self-rejection reaches severe or panic levels, the person may dissociate and experience hallucinations, delusions, and feelings of suspicion, jealousy, or paranoia. Such withdrawal from reality may be a temporary coping mechanism or a long-term pattern indicating a profound problem of identity confusion.

SELF-DESTRUCTIVENESS. Self-hatred can be expressed through accident proneness or attempting dangerous feats. Extremely low levels of self-esteem can lead to suicide.

OTHER DESTRUCTIVENESS. People who have overwhelming consciences may choose to act out against society. This activity serves to paralyze their own self-hate and displaces or projects it onto victims.

Indirect behaviors. Indirect forms of self-hate complement and supplement the direct forms. They may be chronic patterns and difficult to change.

ILLUSIONS AND UNREALISTIC GOALS. Self-deception is the core element; the person refuses to accept a limited here and now. Illusions increase the possibility of disappointment and further self-hate. Examples of illusions are "If I were married, I would be happy" and "Money brings fulfillment." This indirect form of low self-esteem may make the person sensitive to criticism or overresponsive to flattery. It also may be evident in the defense mechanisms of blaming others for one's failures and becoming hypercritical to create the illusion of superiority.

EXAGGERATED SENSE OF SELF. The person also may attempt to compensate by expressing an exaggerated opinion of his ability. He may continually boast, brag of his exploits, or claim extraordinary talents. An extreme compensatory behavior for low self-esteem is grandiose thinking and related delusions. Another example is evident in the perfectionist. Such people strain toward impossible goals and measure their own worth entirely in terms of productivity and accomplishment.

BOREDOM. This involves the rejection of one's possibilities and capabilities. The person may neglect or reject aspects that have great potential for future growth.

POLARIZING VIEW OF LIFE. In this case the person has a simplistic view of life in which everything is worst or best, wrong or right. He tends to have a closed belief system that acts as a defense against a threatening world. Ultimately this view of life leads to confusion, disappointment, and alienation from others.

The behaviors associated with low self-esteem are described in the clinical example that follows and are summarized in Box 18-1.

◄ CLINICAL EXAMPLE

Mrs. G was a 66-year-old woman admitted to the psychiatric hospital because of a major depressive episode. She told the admitting nurse that "things have been building up for some time now" and that she had been seeing a private psychiatrist for the past 6 months who suggested that she enter the hospital. She had been employed in a community college as a librarian until 18 months earlier, when she was forced to retire.

Mrs. G said she had been married for 39 years and had two grown children who were married and lived out of state. Her husband had worked as an accountant but had retired a month before. She said that since her retirement she had felt "useless and lost" and "closed in by their apartment." She seldom left the apartment and had lost contact with many of her friends. She said she worried a great deal about their financial situation, especially now that her husband was also retired. He repeatedly reassured her that they had enough money, but she could not stop worrying about it.

Mrs. G said that she liked her old job very much and thought she was good at it. A younger woman took her place at the library, and Mrs. G was very bitter when talking about her. She said that, little by little, this woman took over duties Mrs. G was responsible for and one day even cleaned out

Mrs. G's desk and took it as her own. Since her retirement, she said, things had been "going downhill steadily." She said she was not a good housewife and disliked cooking. These tasks had become even more difficult since her husband retired because he was "always underfoot and criticizing" what she did. In the past couple of weeks, she had had great difficulty sleeping, a decreased appetite, fatigue, and little interest in her appearance. She said it seemed that all she had to do was "wait around to die."

Selected Nursing Diagnoses

- Situational low self-esteem related to developmental transition, as evidenced by self-criticism and lack of pleasure in life
- Ineffective role performance related to retirement, as evidenced by feeling useless and failing to complete routine activities
- Social isolation related to low self-worth, as evidenced by lack of contact with friends ■

In this clinical example, Mrs. G's perception of self was closely related to her ability to work. Her retirement created role changes difficult to adapt to. This example points out the close relationship between low self-esteem and role strain. The situation was further compounded by her husband's retirement. Mrs. G's feelings of low self-esteem were evident in her self-criticism, refusal to recognize her own strengths, worrying, physical complaints, and reduced social contacts. The diagnosis of major depressive episode was based on the severity of her feelings of self-deprecation, somatic problems, saddened emotional tone, history of losses, and absence of a manic episode.

Low self-esteem is also a major element of disturbed body image. The following clinical example illustrates the effect of the loss of a body part on a person's self-concept.

BOX **18-1**
Behaviors Associated With Low Self-Esteem
Criticism of self or others Decreased productivity Destructiveness Disruptions in relatedness Exaggerated sense of self-importance Feelings of inadequacy Guilt Irritability or excessive anger Negative feelings about one's body Perceived role strain Pessimistic view of life Physical complaints Polarizing view of life Rejection of personal capabilities Self-destructiveness Self-diminution Social withdrawal Substance abuse Withdrawal from reality Worrying

CLINICAL EXAMPLE

Mrs. M was an attractive 32-year-old married woman admitted to the general hospital for a total hysterectomy. Her history was presented in a nursing care conference because she was making many demands and the head nurse noticed that many of the staff were avoiding caring for her. Mrs. M had been married for 2 years and did not have any children. It was observed that Mr. M seldom visited his wife, although he did speak to her over the phone. Mrs. M complained that she was unable to sleep at night and often rang for the nurses with apparently minor requests. She appeared to have established a relationship with one of the evening nurses, who was able to describe some of Mrs. M's concerns.

Mrs. M appeared to have a severe level of anxiety about her hysterectomy. She feared the effect of the surgery on her sexual desires, attractiveness, and ability to have intercourse and respond to her husband. Without her reproductive organs she said she felt "inadequate and no longer like a woman." She said that she and her husband always planned on having children, and she wondered whether her husband might leave her in the future. She also feared that having the hysterectomy would cause her to lose her beauty and youth.

When the nursing staff became aware of Mrs. M's many fears and concerns, they were better able to understand her behavior and plan nursing care accordingly. They discussed with her the physiological implications of a hysterectomy and encouraged her to verbalize her feelings. Mr. M was not aware of his wife's concerns, and the nursing staff supported open discussions between them. As the staff were able to identify Mrs. M's concerns, they realized that some of their previous avoidance behavior resulted from their own fears and discomfort. The female nurses had identified with her, and the hysterectomy threatened their own concepts of self, body integrity, and sexual identity.

Selected Nursing Diagnoses

- Disturbed body image related to hysterectomy, as evidenced by expressed fears about her attractiveness and functioning as a woman
- Interrupted family processes related to lack of ability to bear children, as evidenced by limited communication with husband ■

Behaviors Associated With Identity Diffusion. Identity diffusion is the failure to integrate various childhood identifications into a harmonious adult psychosocial identity. Important behaviors that relate to identity diffusion include disruptions in relationships or problems of intimacy. The initial behavior may be withdrawal or distancing. If a person is experiencing an undefined identity, he may wish to ignore or destroy the people who threaten him. The problem is one of gaining intimacy, but it is reflected in isolation, denial, and withdrawal from others. Such patients lack empathy.

A contrasting behavior that may be evident is personality fusing. **Personality fusion** is a person's attempt to establish a sense of self by fusing with, attaching to, or belonging to someone else. Erikson has pointed out that true intimacy involves a sense of mutuality, which implies a firm self-delineation of the partners, not a diffused merger of two people. If a person is struggling to cope with a weak or undefined identity, however, he may try to establish his sense of self by fusing or belonging to someone else. This may occur in formal relationships, intense friendships, or brief affairs because each can be seen as a desperate attempt to outline one's own identity. However, personality fusion leads to a further loss of identity. Some of these behaviors are evident in this clinical example.

CLINICAL EXAMPLE

Mrs. P was seen by a psychiatric nurse in the psychiatric outpatient department of a general hospital. She was a well-dressed 24-year-old woman who had numerous somatic complaints, including decreased appetite, frequent headaches, fatigue, and difficulty falling asleep. She reported that she had no energy or interest in doing anything or being with people. She said she dreaded each day and felt abandoned and alone.

She was married at age 17 to the only boy she ever dated in high school. He was 19 at the time, and she "looked up to him tremendously." He established a successful career in the insurance business, and she stayed at home to care for the house. She described herself as centering her whole world around him. Three months earlier, he had told her that he wanted a separation and suggested she begin making a new life for herself. He said he intended to move out of the house at the end of the month, but Mrs. P said she hoped he would not do that when he saw how much she loved and needed him.

Mrs. P also described feelings of being unloved and unlovable. She said she felt empty inside and didn't really know who she was. She complained about her appearance and expressed much fear about living alone, finding a job, and getting along with people, especially men.

Selected Nursing Diagnoses

- Disturbed personal identity related to impending separation, as evidenced by feelings of loneliness and abandonment
- Situational low self-esteem related to doubts about self and her abilities, as evidenced by expressed fears of living alone, finding a job, and getting along with people ■

Many of Mrs. P's behaviors reflect the problem of identity diffusion. She married at an early age before defining her own sense of self as an autonomous individual. Her only experience in a close relationship was with her husband, and she attempted to establish her own identity by living through his. Within the security of the marriage, she managed to avoid any self-analysis, but the impending separation brought forth her fears and self-doubts. She displayed a low level of self-esteem and an unresolved conflict between dependence and independence.

Personality fusion and problems with identity also have serious implications for the larger family system. Dysfunctional families are often characterized by a fusion of ego mass that may be evident in severe symptomatology by one or more family members. This may be expressed in some form of family violence or abuse (see Chapter 39) or in the scapegoating of one family member, who becomes the "diagnosed" or "symptomatic" psychiatric patient.

People with identity diffusion may lack a historical-cultural basis of identity and thus display a peculiar lack of ethnicity. This is evident in their sense of history, cultural norms, group affiliations, lifestyle, and child-rearing practices. A related behavior is the absence of a moral code or any genuine inner value. The behaviors characteristic of identity diffusion are summarized in Box 18-2.

BOX **18-2**
Behaviors Associated With Identity Diffusion
Absence of moral code
Contradictory personality traits
Exploitive interpersonal relationships
Feelings of emptiness
Fluctuating feelings about self
Gender confusion
High degree of anxiety
Inability to empathize with others
Lack of authenticity
Problems of intimacy

Behaviors Associated With Depersonalization. A more maladaptive response to problems in identity involving withdrawal from reality occurs when the person experiences panic levels of anxiety. This panic state produces a blocking off of awareness, a collapse in reality testing, and feelings of depersonalization and dissociation. Depersonalization is a feeling of unreality in which one is unable to distinguish between inner and outer stimuli. In essence, it is a true alienation from oneself. The person has great difficulty distinguishing self from others, and his or her body has an unreal or strange quality.

Depersonalization is the subjective experience of the partial or total disruption of one's ego and the disintegration and disorganization of one's self-concept. Because of this, it is the most frightening human experience. It develops as an outcome of uncertainties in human relationships. The person feels unloved and, as a result of his failure to be loved, he fails to love himself.

Depersonalization serves as a defense, but it is destructive because it masks and immobilizes anxiety without diminishing its intensity. It can occur in a variety of clinical illnesses, including depression, schizophrenia, manic states, and organic brain syndromes, and it represents the advanced state of ego breakdown associated with multiple personality disorder and psychotic states.

Many behaviors are associated with depersonalization. Primarily, the patient feels estranged, as though he were hiding something from himself. He experiences a lack of inner continuity and sameness and feels as if life is happening to him rather than his living by his own initiative. The patient may say that the world appears queer, dreamlike, or frightening. He may experience a loss of identity and express confusion regarding his own sexuality. He may describe related feelings of insecurity, inferiority, frustration, fear, hate, shame, and a loss of self-respect and be unable to derive a sense of accomplishment from any activity.

In depersonalization a loss of impulse control and an absence of feeling and emotion may be present, which is shown in impersonality and stiffness in social situations. The person may become lifeless and lack spontaneity and animation. He

A FAMILY SPEAKS

My wife has multiple personality disorder, and it feels like I'm living with several different people. One moment everything is great, and the next thing I know, she is in a frenzy or a state of rage. There are other problems, too. For example, things keep appearing in our household, and no one knows where they came from, or I get calls at work from my wife telling me she is lost and doesn't know how she ended up there. At other times she tells me things and later denies she said them. Sometimes people come up to my wife and talk like they know her, but she says she's never seen them before. And then there are days when she dresses up and acts just like our teenage daughter.

What is it like to live with someone with this illness? Well, it's unreal and very upsetting. Most of all, it's like living in a world of doubt and uncertainty. Who is this woman I married 20 years ago? What is she all about? What is she capable of doing? These are the questions I ask myself each night as I fall asleep. They are the same ones that go unanswered in the early morning hours.

Behaviors Associated With Depersonalization

Affective
Feelings of loss of identity
Feelings of alienation from self
Feelings of insecurity, inferiority, fear, shame
Feelings of unreality
Heightened sense of isolation
Inability to derive pleasure or a sense of accomplishment
Lack of sense of inner continuity

Perceptual
Auditory and visual hallucinations
Confusion regarding one's sexuality
Difficulty distinguishing self from others
Disturbed body image
Dreamlike view of the world

Cognitive
Confusion
Distorted thinking
Disturbance of memory
Impaired judgment
Presence of separate personalities within the same person
Time disorientation

Behavioral
Blunted affect
Emotional passivity and nonresponsiveness
Incongruent or idiosyncratic communication
Lack of spontaneity and animation
Loss of impulse control
Loss of initiative and decision-making ability
Social withdrawal

may plod through each day in a state of numbness and may respond to situations ordinarily eliciting emotion without characteristic love, hate, anxiety, or guilt. The person may become increasingly passive, withdrawing from social contacts, failing to assert himself, losing interest in his surroundings, and allowing others to make decisions for him.

Another sign of depersonalization is a disturbance in perception of time, space, and memory (Guralnik, Schmeidler, and Simeon, 2000). The person may become disoriented and be unable to recognize events as pertaining to yesterday or tomorrow or unable to plan activities with reference to a schedule. A disturbance of memory may be characterized by aphasia, amnesia, or memory distortion. Thinking and judgment may be impaired and may reflect great confusion and distortion or focus on trivial details. Problems in information processing may be evident in visual hallucinations, and disturbed interpersonal relationships may be reflected in delusions, auditory hallucinations, and incongruent or idiosyncratic communication.

Another behavior associated with depersonalization is a confused or disturbed body image. The person may have a feeling of unreality about parts of the body. He may feel that his limbs are detached or that the size of his body parts is changed, or he is unable to tell where his body leaves off and the rest of the world begins. Some patients describe the feeling that they have stepped outside their bodies and are observing themselves as detached and foreign objects.

Finally, the person may exhibit behaviors related to dissociative identity disorder, formerly known as multiple personality disorder. In this case, distinct and separate personalities exist within the same person, each of which dominates the person's attitudes, behaviors, and self-view as though no other personality existed (see A Family Speaks). Because most patients with dissociative identity (multiple personality) disorder usually conceal their condition, the periods in their lives when they show overt symptoms are quite limited,

so diagnosing them is not easy. During these times the patients often show subtle dissociative signs in their affects, thoughts, memories, behaviors, object relations, and transferences. The many behaviors associated with depersonalization and dissociation are summarized in Box 18-3. The following clinical example may further clarify these behaviors.

CLINICAL EXAMPLE

Mr. S was a 40-year-old man with no history of psychiatric hospitalization. Two months before his present admission, he was severely burned while on the job in a steel-making plant. He sustained second- and third-degree burns over his face, hands, chest, and back and was treated in the burn center of a large university hospital. Three days before he was to be discharged from the burn unit, he experienced a psychotic episode. He reported hearing voices telling him to kill himself, and he was unable to recall any events surrounding the accident that produced his burns. He said he felt his arms were withering away and his eyes were falling into his skull. He was unable now to change the dressing on his burns even though he had done this before. When he looked at his arms or chest, his face remained impassive and he showed no emotion. He began to talk continuously about returning to work but was unable to identify how long he had been out on sick leave or the amount of time recommended by his physician for recovery.

With the onset of these symptoms, he was transferred from the burn unit to the psychiatric unit of the hospital. He remained socially isolated on the unit and refused to participate in ward meetings and group activities. At times he wandered into other patients' rooms and took pieces of their clothing. He was later seen wearing this clothing, and the staff intervened to return it to its owners.

Selected Nursing Diagnoses
- Panic level of anxiety related to severe burn injuries, as evidenced by confusion regarding identity, hearing voices, and reported body distortions
- Disturbed thought processes related to psychotic state, as evidenced by confusion and disorientation ∎

The various feelings and perceptions associated with depersonalization represent extreme defenses against threats to self that do not alleviate the anxiety and may add to it. The patient views his own behavior as foreign and sees himself as a strong, unknown, and unpredictable being whom he does not recognize. As both a participant and a spectator, he observes himself with great fear because he is unable to control his own impulses. He cannot completely escape the pain of self-awareness. He therefore disowns his behavior, feelings, thoughts, and body and becomes alienated from his true self.

Predisposing Factors

Factors Affecting Self-Esteem. Self-esteem is partly an inheritable trait, and genetic as well as environmental influences are very important in the development of self-esteem. Specifically, predisposing factors that begin in early childhood can contribute to problems with self-concept. Because the infant initially views himself as an extension of his parents, he is very responsive to both his parents' self-hate and any feelings of hatred toward himself. Parental rejection causes the child to be uncertain of himself and other human relationships. Because of his failure to be loved, the child fails to love himself and is unable to reach out with love to others.

As he grows older, the child may learn to feel inadequate because he is not encouraged to be independent, to think for himself, and to take responsibility for his own needs and actions. Overpossessiveness, overpermissiveness, or overcontrol, exercised by one or both parents, can create a feeling of unimportance and lack of self-esteem in the child. Harsh, demanding parents can set unreasonable standards, often raising them before the child has developed the ability to meet them.

Parents also may subject their children to unreasonable, harsh criticism and inconsistent punishment. These actions can cause early frustration, defeatism, and a destructive sense of inadequacy and inferiority. Another factor in creating such feelings may be the rivalry or unsuccessful imitation of an extremely bright sibling or a prominent parent, often creating a sense of hopelessness and inferiority. In addition, repeated defeats and failures can destroy self-worth. In this instance the failure in itself does not produce a sense of helplessness, but internalization of the failure as proof of personal incompetence does.

Unrealistic self-ideals. With age, other factors emerge that can cause feelings of low self-esteem. The person who lacks a sense of meaning and purpose in life also fails to accept responsibility for his own well-being and fails to develop his capabilities and potential. He denies himself the freedom of full expression, including the right to make mistakes and fail, and becomes impatient, harsh, and demanding with himself. He sets standards that cannot be met. Self-consciousness and observation turn to self-contempt and self-defeat. This results in a further loss of self-trust.

These self-ideals or goals are often silent assumptions, and the person may not be immediately aware of them. They reflect high expectations and are unrealistic. When the person judges his performance by these unreasonable and inflexible standards, he cannot live up to his ideals and, as a result, experiences guilt and low self-esteem. These inner dictates have been described as the "tyranny of the shoulds," and some of the common ones are identified in Box 18-4.

The person who overemphasizes these rules or ideals often makes a series of deductions such as the following: "Everyone should love me. If he or she doesn't love me, I have failed. I have lost the only thing that really matters. I am unlovable. There is no point in going on. I am worthless." This inner punishment results in feelings of depression and despair because no human being can fulfill the demands on self. Slavishly striving for these ideals interferes with other activities, such as living a healthy life and having satisfying relationships with other people. These predisposing factors lay the groundwork for feelings of low self-esteem.

Factors Affecting Role Performance

Gender roles. An important source of strain in contemporary society comes from values, beliefs, and behaviors about gender roles. Research demonstrates that society continues to have clearly defined gender-role stereotypes for men and women. Women are perceived as less competent, less independent, less objective, and less logical than men. Men are perceived as lacking interpersonal sensitivity, warmth, and expressiveness. Moreover, stereotyped masculine traits are more often perceived as desirable than are stereotyped feminine characteristics.

To the extent that these results reflect societal standards of gender-role behavior, both women and men are put in role

---

BOX **18-4**	
Unrealistic Self-Expectations: the Tyranny of the Shoulds	
I should have the utmost generosity, consideration, dignity, courage, and unselfishness.	
I should be the perfect lover, friend, parent, teacher, student, and spouse. Everyone should love me.	
I should be able to find a quick solution to every problem.	
I should never feel hurt; I should always be happy and serene.	
I should assert myself; I should never hurt anybody else.	
I should always be at peak efficiency. I should not be tired, get sick, or make mistakes.	

From Horney K: *Neurosis and human growth,* New York, 1950, WW Norton.

conflict by the difference in the standards. If a woman adopts behaviors desirable for a man, she risks criticism for her failure to be appropriately feminine; if she adopts behaviors seen as feminine, she is lacking in the values associated with masculinity. Likewise, if a man adopts the behaviors seen as desirable for a woman, his masculinity and sexuality may be questioned and his contributions may be devalued or ignored; if he adopts the behaviors associated with masculinity, he risks not being able to express warmth, tenderness, and responsiveness.

Thus when a woman steps out of her home, where her gender role has traditionally been defined and confined, and enters the outside world of work, she may experience heightened role strain. Similarly, the man who arrives home from work in the evening may feel uncertain or in conflict about how he should relate to his school-age son, infant daughter, or working wife.

Compare the value that two different cultures place on feminine and masculine roles and traits. ■

Work roles. Women are still in the minority in most high-status occupations and are clustered near the bottom in terms of professional status and income. In American society, women are socialized to seek an ideal that includes marriage, children, higher education, and satisfying work outside the home. They are increasingly expected to perform in both "feminine" and "masculine" spheres.

This situation has many negative aspects. First, it can be argued that it merely replaces the traditional woman's role with another equally confining one. As the new role is valued, the traditional roles of wife and mother become devalued. Second, although women are expected to assume more "masculine" qualities, there is only a small corresponding trend for men to assume more "feminine" behaviors. Third, the woman who seeks such an expanded role is faced with reconciling the often conflicting goals of work, marriage, homemaking, and parenting.

Despite social and economic changes, often little sharing of tasks occurs when men and women are both gainfully employed. Rather, most industrial societies have witnessed a gradual change in the obligations of women, who now perform a dual role: outside employment and continued responsibility for home and children.

The expectation exists that the woman will make the adjustments needed both at home and in her career, including housekeeping and managing; arranging meals, lessons, and appointments; entertaining; caring for the sick; and communicating with the family. The traditional expectation that the wife will be the primary caretaker of the children and will subsume other activities to this end are still prevalent as well.

Gender and work roles will continue as a source of stress until care of children, home, and career are viewed as equally valuable and important by both sexes and until gender is regarded as irrelevant to the abilities, personalities, and activities of the people involved.

Such a change in attitude should begin with nurses and other mental health clinicians, who indirectly increase role strain by accepting stereotyped views. The cause of mental health might be better served if psychiatric clinicians encourage both men and women to maximize individual potential rather than adjust to existing gender roles.

Factors Affecting Personal Identity. Constant parental intervention can interfere with adolescent choices. Parental distrust may lead a child to wonder whether his own choices are correct and to feel guilty if he goes against parental ideas. It also may devalue the child's opinions and lead to indecisiveness, impulsiveness, and acting out in an attempt to achieve some identity.

When the parent does not trust the child, the child ultimately loses respect for the parent. It has been found that parents and children do not disagree on significant issues, such as war, peace, race, or religion. Instead, personal and narrow concerns—dating, a party, use of the car, curfews, hairstyles, homework—create the conflict between parents and youth.

Peers also may create problems that inhibit identity development. The adolescent wants to belong, to feel needed and wanted. The peer group, with its rigid standards of behavior, gives him this feeling and provides a bridge between childhood and adulthood. The adolescent loses himself in the fads and the language of the group. However, the group is often a cruel testing ground that can hurt as much as it helps. Taught to be competitive, the young person competes with his friends, putting them down to bring himself up.

Membership in the peer group is bought at a high price; the adolescent must surrender much of his identity to belong. Often belonging to the group involves open destruction of self-esteem and insistence on conformity. Adolescents involved in sexual relationships introduce further uncertainty into their lives, which can interfere with developing a stable self-concept.

Discuss how belonging to a group affects an adolescent's identity. ■

Precipitating Stressors

Trauma. Specific problems with self-concept can be brought on by almost any difficult situation to which the person cannot adjust. Specifically, trauma such as physical, sexual, and psychological abuse in childhood has been reported by most patients with dissociative symptoms, depersonalization disorder, and dissociative identity disorder (Chu et al, 1999; Kluft, 1999). A small percentage of patients report no abuse but have experienced a trauma they perceived as life threatening to themselves or to someone else, such as a near drowning, witnessing a violent crime, or a terrorist act (Simeon et al, 2003). It is also believed that dissociation is more likely to be experienced by individuals who have experienced previous trauma (Morgan et al, 2001).

Role Strain. People who experience stress in fulfilling expected roles are said to experience role strain. Role strain is the frustration felt when the person is torn in opposite directions or feels inadequate or unsuited to enact certain roles. In the course of a lifetime, a person faces numerous role transitions. These transitions may require the incorporation of new knowledge and alterations in behavior. There are two categories of role transitions—developmental and health-illness. Each of these role transitions can precipitate a threat to one's self-concept.

Developmental transitions. Developmental transitions are normative changes associated with growth. Various developmental stages can precipitate threats to self-identity. Adolescence is perhaps the most critical because it is a time of upheaval, change, anxiety, and insecurity. A serious threat to identity in adulthood is cultural discontinuity. This occurs when a person moves from one cultural setting to another and experiences emotional upheaval. In addition, problems within the social structure, such as political upheavals, economic depression, and high unemployment, can pose threats to identity. In late maturity and old age, identity problems again arise. Menopause, retirement, and increasing physical disability are problems for which people must work out adaptive responses.

Health-illness transitions. Health-illness transitions involve moving from a well state to an illness state. Some stressors can cause disturbances in body image and related changes in self-concept. One threat is the loss of a major body part, such as an eye, breast, or leg. Disturbances also may result from a surgical procedure in which the relationship of body parts is disturbed. The results of the surgical intervention may be either visible, as with a colostomy or gastrostomy, or invisible, as with a hysterectomy or gallbladder removal.

Changes in body size, shape, and appearance can threaten the person's self-perceptions. Threats to body image can result from a pathological process that causes changes in the structure or function of the body, such as arthritis, multiple sclerosis, Parkinson's disease, cancer, pneumonia, and heart disease. The failure of a body part, as with paralysis, is particularly difficult to integrate into one's self-perceptions. The physical changes associated with normal growth and development also may pose problems, as may some medical or nursing procedures, such as enemas, catheterizations, suctioning, radiation therapy, dilation and curettage, and organ transplantation.

All these stressors can pose a threat to body image, with resultant changes in self-esteem and role perception. Factors that influence the degree of threat to body image are listed in Table 18-2.

Biological Stressors. Physiological (or biological) stressors also may disturb a person's sense of reality, interfere with an accurate perception of the world, and threaten ego boundaries and identity. Such stressors include oxygen deprivation, hyperventilation, biochemical imbalances, severe fatigue, and sensory and emotional isolation. Alcohol, drugs, and other toxic substances also may distort self-concept. Usually these stressors produce only temporary changes.

Appraisal of Stressors

Whether the problem in self-concept is precipitated by psychological, sociological, or physiological stressors, the critical element is the patient's perception of the threat. When assessing behaviors and formulating a nursing diagnosis, the nurse must continue to validate observations and inferences to establish a mutual, therapeutic relationship with the patient.

The incidence of breast cancer is rising in this country. What strategies are women using to promote adaptive self-concept responses? ■

Coping Resources

It is important that the nurse and patient review possible coping resources (see Citing the Evidence). **All people, no matter how disturbing their behavior, have some areas of personal strength.** These might include the following:

- Sports and outdoor activities
- Hobbies and crafts
- Expressive arts
- Health and self-care
- Education or training
- Vocation or position
- Special aptitudes
- Intelligence
- Imagination and creativity
- Interpersonal relationships

When the patient's positive aspects become evident, the nurse should share these observations with the patient to expand the patient's self-awareness and suggest possible areas for future intervention (Bjorklund, 2000).

Coping Mechanisms

Short-Term Defenses. An identity crisis may be resolved with either short-term or long-term coping mechanisms. These are used to ward off the anxiety and uncertainty of identity confusion. There are four categories of short-term defenses:

1. Activities that provide temporary escape from the identity crisis
2. Activities that provide temporary substitute identities
3. Activities that temporarily strengthen or heighten a diffuse sense of self

Table 18-2	Factors Influencing Self-Concept Based on Health-Illness Transitions
FACTOR	**QUESTION**
Meaning of the threat for the patient	Does it threaten the patient's ideal of youth or wholeness and decrease self-esteem?
Degree to which the patient's pattern of adaptation is interrupted	Does it jeopardize the patient's security and self-control?
Coping capacities and resources available	What is the response of significant others, and what help is offered?
Nature of the threat, extent of change, and rate at which it occurs	Is the change that of many small adjustments over time or a great and sudden adjustment?

4. Activities that represent short-term attempts to make an identity out of meaninglessness and identity diffusion—that try to assert that the meaning of life is meaningless itself

The first category of **temporary escape** includes activities that seem to provide intense immediate experiences. These experiences so overwhelm the senses that the issue of identity literally does not exist because the person's entire being is occupied with "right now" sensations. Examples include drug experiences, loud rock concerts, fast car and motorcycle riding, some forms of hard physical labor, exercise or sports, and even obsessive television watching.

The category of **temporary substitute identity** is derived from being a "joiner"; the identity of a club, group, team, movement, or gang may function as a basis for self-definition. The person temporarily adopts the group definition as his own identity in a type of devotion to the larger entity. Temporary substitute identities also can be obtained by playing a certain role within a group, such as clown, bully, or chauffeur, or by buying objects that are marketed with ready-made identities. Thus a certain type of cologne, make of car, or article of dress implies built-in personalities the person can adopt as his own.

The third category of defenses involves **confronting or challenging something** to feel more intensely alive. This is evident in risk taking for its own sake, which creates a feeling of bravado. Competitive activities, such as sports, academic achievement, and popularity contests, also fit into this category. The idea is that competition and comparison with an outsider more sharply define a sense of self. Another example is bigotry and prejudice. By adopting a bigoted stance toward some out group or scapegoat, the person can temporarily strengthen self-esteem or ego integrity.

The final category tries to devise an identity from the **meaninglessness of life**. It helps to explain why people indulge in fads with such fervor that seem so meaningless to others. The sheer force of commitment to fads is an attempt to transform them into something meaningful.

Long-Term Defenses. Any of the short-term defenses mentioned here may develop into a long-term one that will be evident in maladaptive behavior. Another type of long-term resolution has been identified as identity foreclosure. This occurs when people adopt the "ready-made" type of identity desired by others without really coming to terms with their own desires, aspirations, or potential. This is a less desirable long-term resolution, as is adopting a deviant or negative identity.

A negative identity is one that is at odds with the values of society. In this case the person tries to define the self in a nonprescribed or antisocial manner. The choice of a negative identity represents an attempt to retain some mastery in a situation in which a positive identity does not seem possible or desirable. The person may be saying, "I would rather be somebody bad than nobody at all." The following clinical example describes the negative identity assumed by an adolescent with a medical diagnosis of conduct disorder—undersocialized, aggressive.

CITING THE EVIDENCE ON

Enhancing Self-Esteem When Confronted With Catastrophic Illness

BACKGROUND: This qualitative study used grounded theory methods to determine how individuals were able to live with catastrophic illnesses and injuries.

RESULTS: Patients described using three principal strategies to cope—protecting, modifying, and boosting. Boosting consists of cognitive efforts to improve one's self-esteem and adjust to the emotional, social, and physical effects associated with their disability. Boosting efforts included comparing oneself to others, focusing on the positive, and building up courage. Patients compared themselves to others to enhance their feelings of well-being but needed to select their own comparison targets. They felt distressed and unsupported when health care professionals talked with them about other patients who were in worse situations.

IMPLICATIONS: This study points to the importance of social comparison as a coping strategy and offers an explanation as to why support groups are helpful to some people. However, patients need to select their own comparison groups. Nurses should be cautious before recommending that patients associate with individuals with worse situations because it can be threatening to see that one's own condition could deteriorate.

Dewar A: *J Psychosocial Nurs* 41:24, 2003.

CLINICAL EXAMPLE

Ken was a 17-year-old boy referred to the local community mental health center by his high school nurse. She made the referral after attending a team conference at school about Ken's repeated behavioral problems. He had a history of aggressive and destructive behavior, poor peer relationships, and low academic performance. The school had suspended him on three occasions, and the result of the team conference was to expel him for the remainder of the school year.

Mr. P, a psychiatric nurse at the mental health center, established a contract to work with Ken and his family. He noted that Ken was an obese young man (112.5 kg) who took little interest in his appearance. His dress was sloppy, his complexion unclean, and his hair oily. He sat slumped in the chair in a disinterested and slightly defiant posture.

As Ken talked about himself, he complained of many pressures he experienced in his part-time job at a local hardware store. He thought the work was too difficult and tiring and that he was qualified for better and more prestigious work. When asked for specifics, he could not identify another job in particular. He also expressed a great deal of harassment from his family. His mother and father had been married for 31 years, and he was the only child of the marriage. His mother worked part-time at a bakery, and his father was recently retired from his job as a supervisor at a local utility company, where he was highly regarded.

Ken said that his father "always had things for me to do." He described how his father signed him up for various team sports–baseball, basketball, football–without acknowledging how much Ken hated sports and how uncoordinated he was. His father also stressed good grades and the necessity of college for success in life. Ken described his mother as passive and polite and said he had little respect for her. He said his aggressive outbursts occurred both at home and at school—whenever he was frustrated. People reacted by staying out of his way. He said he never hurt anyone with his temper. He mostly destroyed property and objects.

Ken avoided the subject of peers but, when asked about friends, said he "hung out" with a couple of boys in the neighborhood. They were older than he was. Most had dropped out of high school and were employed in odd jobs. He denied drug use but said he drank heavily, especially on the weekends. He said he had no girlfriends and wasn't interested in complicating his life "with some broad."

Selected Nursing Diagnoses

- Disturbed personal identity related to fear of failure, as evidenced by aggressive and destructive behavior and poor school performance
- Interrupted family processes related to conflict with parents, as evidenced by avoidance and lack of communication ■

Ken displays many of the behaviors characteristic of a negative identity. The nurse working with Ken explored his underlying feelings and self-perceptions. Great anger with his father began to surface, and Ken was able to verbalize it. Because he was the only son, he believed he was competing with his father and had to live up to his father's ideals. Ken feared failing in trying to adopt a positive identity and resented the identity his father was trying to impose on him. He thought he had no part in defining it and that it did not represent his real self.

Ego Defense Mechanisms. Patients with alterations in self-concept may use a variety of ego-oriented mechanisms to protect themselves from confronting their own inadequacies. Typical ego defense mechanisms include **fantasy, dissociation, isolation, projection, displacement, splitting, turning anger against the self,** and **acting out.** These are described in Chapter 16.

Other, more damaging coping mechanisms also can be used to protect self-esteem. These may include the following:
- Obesity
- Anorexia
- Promiscuity
- Chronic overworking
- Suicide
- Delinquency
- Crime
- Drug use
- Family violence
- Incest

◀ DIAGNOSIS

Self-concept is a critical aspect of one's overall personality adjustment. Problems with self-concept are associated with feelings of anxiety, hostility, and guilt. These often create a circular, self-propagating process that ultimately results in maladaptive coping responses (Figure 18-3).

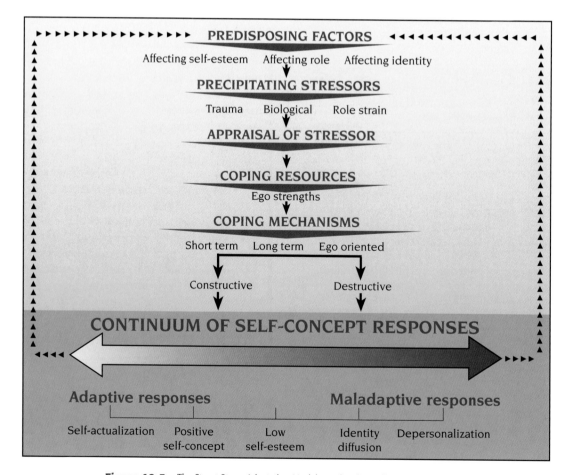

Figure 18-3   The Stuart Stress Adaptation Model as related to self-concept responses.

Nursing Diagnoses

Most people who express dissatisfaction with life, display deviant behavior, or have difficulty functioning in social or work situations have problems related to self-concept. The primary NANDA nursing diagnoses related to alterations in self-concept are **disturbed body image, readiness for enhanced self-concept, low self-esteem (chronic, situational, risk for situational), ineffective role performance,** and **disturbed personal identity**. Nursing diagnoses related to the range of possible maladaptive responses of the patient are identified in the Medical and Nursing Diagnoses box (Box 18-5).

Examples of expanded nursing diagnoses related to self-concept are presented in the Detailed Diagnoses table (Table 18-3). However, alterations in self-concept affect all aspects of a person's life. Therefore many additional problems may be identified by the nurse.

Medical Diagnoses

Maladaptive responses indicating alterations in self-concept can be seen in a variety of people experiencing threats to their physical integrity or self-system. These nursing diagnoses are not limited to the psychiatric setting and do not have a discrete category of medical diagnoses associated with them. Because they pertain to basic personality structure and feelings about oneself, they can emerge with many neurotic and psychotic disorders (see A Patient Speaks) and may be related to all the diagnostic categories identified in the *DSM-IV-TR* (American Psychiatric Association, 2000), because all of these disorders ultimately reflect on one's view of self.

Several specific medical diagnoses deserve particular attention, however, because their dominant features include alterations in self-concept. Related medical diagnoses include **identity problem, dissociative amnesia, dissociative fugue, dissociative identity disorder**, also known as *multiple personality disorder*, and **depersonalization disorder**. The essential features of these medical diagnoses related to alterations in self-concept are presented in the Detailed Diagnoses table (see Table 18-3).

OUTCOME IDENTIFICATION

The expected outcome when working with a patient with a maladaptive self-concept response is:

> *The patient will obtain the maximum level of self-actualization to realize his or her potential.*

Goals should be as clear and explicit as possible. They should identify realistic steps that the patient can accomplish. In this way the patient's self-confidence will increase, and this will build self-esteem. These goals should emphasize strengths instead of weaknesses. If they are mutually identified, they will motivate the patient and help the patient assume increased responsibility for his or her own behavior. Following are examples of goals related to role performance:

Long-term: Mrs. P will resolve role conflict by achieving greater congruency between work and family roles.

Short-term:

After 1 week:

- Mrs. P will describe her responsibilities in her work and home roles.
- She will identify aspects of these roles that provide her with satisfaction.
- She will identify areas of role incompatibility.

After 2 weeks:

- She will describe three alternative ways of increasing the complementarity of the roles.
- She will discuss the advantages and disadvantages of each alternative.

▪ BOX 18-5 *Medical and Nursing Diagnoses Related to* **Self-Concept Responses**

RELATED MEDICAL DIAGNOSES (*DSM-IV-TR*)*	RELATED NURSING DIAGNOSES (NANDA)†
Identity problem	Anxiety
Dissociative amnesia	**Body image, Disturbed‡**
Dissociative fugue	Communication, Impaired verbal
Dissociative identity disorder (multiple personality disorder)	Coping, Ineffective
Depersonalization disorder	Hopelessness
	Identity, Disturbed personal‡
	Powerlessness
	Role performance, Ineffective‡
	Self-concept, Readiness for enhanced‡
	Self-esteem, Chronic low, Situational low, Risk for situational low‡
	Sexuality pattern, Ineffective
	Social interaction, Impaired
	Spiritual distress
	Thought processes, Disturbed

*From American Psychiatric Association: *Diagnostic and statistical manual of mental disorders*, ed 4, text revision, Washington, DC, 2000, American Psychiatric Association.
†From North American Nursing Diagnosis Association: *NANDA nursing diagnoses: definitions and classification 2003-2004*, Philadelphia, 2003, The Association.
‡**Primary nursing diagnosis for alterations in self-concept.**

Table 18-3 *Detailed Diagnoses Related to* **Self-Concept Responses**

NANDA DIAGNOSIS STEM	EXAMPLES OF EXPANDED DIAGNOSIS
Disturbed body image	Disturbed body image related to fear of becoming obese, as evidenced by refusal to maintain body weight within normal limits
	Disturbed body image related to leukemia chemotherapy, as evidenced by negative feelings about one's body
	Disturbed body image related to cerebrovascular accident, as evidenced by lack of acceptance of body limitations
Readiness for enhanced self-concept	Readiness for enhanced self-concept related to birth of child, as evidenced by enrollment in parenting classes
Chronic or situational low self-esteem	Situational low self-esteem related to death of spouse, as evidenced by withdrawal from others and feelings of hopelessness
	Chronic low self-esteem related to overly high self-ideals, as evidenced by depressed mood and withdrawal from activities
Ineffective role performance	Ineffective role performance related to incompatibility of newly assumed work and family roles, as evidenced by feelings of frustration and criticism of others
	Ineffective role performance related to incongruence of cultural and self-role expectations about aging, as evidenced by feelings of frustration and criticism of others
Disturbed personal identity	Disturbed personal identity related to unrealistic parental expectations, as evidenced by running away from home
	Disturbed personal identity related to drug toxicity, as evidenced by confusion and loss of impulse control

DSM-IV-TR DIAGNOSIS	ESSENTIAL FEATURES*
Identity problem	Uncertainty about multiple issues relating to identity such as long-term goals, career choice, friendship patterns, sexual orientation and behavior, moral values, and group loyalties.
Dissociative amnesia	The predominant disturbance is episodes of inability to recall important personal information, usually of a traumatic or stressful nature, that is too extensive to be explained by ordinary forgetfulness.
Dissociative fugue	The predominant disturbance is sudden, unexpected travel away from home or one's customary place of work, with inability to recall one's past. Confusion about personal identity or assumption of a new identity.
Dissociative identity disorder (multiple personality disorder)	The presence of two or more distinct identities or personality states (each with its own enduring pattern of perceiving, relating to, and thinking about the environment and self). At least two of these identities or personality states recurrently take control of the person's behavior. Inability to recall important personal information that is too extensive to be explained by ordinary forgetfulness.
Depersonalization disorder	Persistent or recurrent experiences of feeling detached from, and as if one is an outside observer of, one's mental processes or body (for example, feeling as if one is in a dream). During the depersonalization experience, reality testing remains intact. The depersonalization causes clinically significant distress or impairment in functioning.

*From American Psychiatric Association: *Diagnostic and statistical manual of mental disorders*, ed 4, text revision, Washington, DC, 2000, American Psychiatric Association.

BOX **18-6**

NOC Outcome Indicators for Self-Esteem

Verbalizations of self-acceptance	Confidence level
Acceptance of self-limitations	Acceptance of compliments from others
Maintenance of erect posture	Expected response from others
Maintenance of eye contact	
Description of self	Acceptance of constructive criticism
Regard for others	
Open communication	Willingness to confront others
Fulfillment of personally significant roles	Description of success in work or school
Maintenance of grooming/hygiene	Description of success in social groups
Balance of participation and listening in groups	Description of pride in self
	Feelings about self-worth

From Moorhead S, Johnson M, Maas M, editors: *Nursing outcomes classification (NOC)*, ed 3, St. Louis, 2004, Mosby.

After 3 weeks:
- She will take the necessary measures to implement one of the identified alternatives.

Outcome indicators related to "Self-Esteem" from the *Nursing Outcome Classification (NOC)* project are presented in Box 18-6 (Moorhead, Johnson, and Maas, 2004).

PLANNING

The nurse's focus is to help the patient understand himself more fully and accurately so that he can direct his own life in a more satisfying way. This means helping him strive toward a clearer, deeper experience of his feelings, wishes, and beliefs; a greater ability to tap his resources and use them for constructive ends; and a clearer perception of his direction in life, assuming responsibility for himself, his decisions, and his actions.

Self-awareness is crucial in bringing about changes in self-concept, but people usually spend little time in introspection. However, certain conditions or events do stimulate self-

A PATIENT SPEAKS

It came to me—so clear that I could not deny it, the pain, the hurt, the anger—I am mentally ill. I've tried to pretend that I'd get better by putting the hurt away—gutting out the pain hoping it would eventually pass—yes, eventually pass. So I did therapy. I talked about what I had experienced. Perceptual disturbances, they said. I talked about the unrealness, the flatness—like cardboard. Depersonalization, they said. I talked about people making me nervous, about staying to myself. You must think rationally, do self-talk, change your behaviors. Take these drugs, they said, because I had heard a voice, or felt something they had not. I had psychotic symptoms—load her up on Mellaril, so what if she gets as fat as a pig—keep increasing the dosage. Too fat? Load her up on Haldol. But I'm not psychotic—oh, but you are schizo-affective; no—let's make that borderline; on second thought, maybe major depression with psychotic features? No, more like depersonalization disorder. Let's check for temporal lobe epilepsy; what the hell—it isn't our money; why are you complaining?

And the therapy goes on. I feel worse. The drugs don't work—you're resistant to treatment; take some more drugs—they will help you feel better. So I take the damn drugs—is one antidepressant any different from another? How much of the stuff can you take? It doesn't do any good. How many times do I have to say that? Why doesn't my doctor listen? Why does she keep writing prescriptions for more of the stuff? Who is taking this stuff—me, or her? I should know if it works.

I do therapy with the silicone people, they who make no mistakes, who are always clinically correct—always clean nice people—but inside I am not clean. I fear that I may be defective, that some loose part may come undone and all will be lost. I'm so scared and I work overtime to find something positive, something good to come out of all this chaos. When I talk to my therapist, I don't think he understands. I sometimes feel cheap and shallow because I've bought the time and I know he would not be talking to me if I hadn't.

I feel frustrated because I've been trapped in this sickness. How can they feel the humiliation—the stigma. The ones so well—that they can heal? Pain, hurt, and fear are subjectively private, but even for me the loneliness is too much. And so I ask the silicone people, have you ever been afraid? Yes, they say. But they don't feel the fear, and they don't connect with the fear. But I feel it, and I want the silicone folks to feel it, too. I do not want to hurt by myself; I want someone to also feel the hurt. So all you silicone therapists—hear me: to hurt when someone IS there but still is NOT is the worst kind of hurt of all—listen up.

Judy Hassam

From South Carolina Self-Help Association Regarding Emotions: *Share the News*, Spring 1993.

awareness. This may occur when stimuli from the body are intensified, as in states of pain, fatigue, or anger, or when stimuli from the environment are decreased, as in sensory deprivation or isolation.

Self-awareness may be triggered when something unexpected or extraordinary takes place, when the person has succeeded or failed, or when the person is confronted with himself by looking in a mirror, listening to his voice on a tape recorder, or reading an old letter. Special occasions, such as birthdays, anniversaries, New Year's Eve, or a death may stimulate introspection. It also may be initiated when others direct their attention to the person through conversation or touch.

Once the person begins to look at and analyze himself, changes in the self become possible. Often they are the result of feelings of failure, unhappiness, anxiety, inadequacy, doubt, or perceived discrepancies between one's concept of self and the demands of the environment or the expectations of others. Usually changes in the self occur only as a result of experiences and occur gradually. Occasionally, however, a change may take place suddenly. A traumatic experience may force a person to see that something drastic must be done. The nurse should take all these factors into consideration when planning nursing care.

Similarly, the family of origin is a source of many people's self-esteem. Adult contact with parents and siblings can correct misconceptions underlying low self-esteem and allow more positive beliefs. Learning to interact with family members with closeness, but without counterproductive forms of fusion and emotionality, can enable a more mature pattern to develop (see Chapter 11). Family relationships would therefore be an appropriate focus for patient education. A Patient Education Plan using family systems is presented in Table 18-4.

IMPLEMENTATION

The mutually identified goals can be reached by a problem-solving approach that focuses primarily on the present, removes much of the responsibility from the nurse, and actively engages the patient in working on personal difficulties. This approach requires that the patient first develop insight into one's problems and then take action to effect lasting behavioral changes. The outcome is an increase in the patient's self-confidence and self-esteem. The nurse thus must incorporate both the responsive dimensions (insight oriented) and the action dimensions (action oriented) of the therapeutic relationship described in Chapter 2.

The focus of this approach is on the patient's cognitive appraisal of life, which may contain faulty perceptions, beliefs, and convictions. Awareness of feelings and emotions is also important because they too may be subject to misconceptions. Only after examining the patient's cognitive appraisal of the situation and related feelings can one gain insight into the problem and bring about behavioral change.

These principles of nursing care for self-concept problems use a problem-solving approach in a progressive sequence.

Table 18-4	PATIENT EDUCATION PLAN	Improving Family Relationships
CONTENT	**INSTRUCTIONAL ACTIVITIES**	**EVALUATION**
Define the concept of self-differentiation within one's family of origin.	Discuss the differences between high and low levels of self-differentiation. Ask the patient to identify level of functioning among family members.	Patient identifies functioning level in family of origin.
Describe the characteristics of emotional fusion, emotional cutoff, and triangulation.	Analyze types and patterns of family relationships. Diagram family patterns.	Patient describes interactional patterns within family. Patient identifies own roles and behavior.
Discuss the role of symptom formation and symptom bearer in a family.	Sensitize the patient to family dynamics and manifestations of stress. Encourage communication with family of origin.	Patient recognizes family contribution to the stress of individual members. Patient contacts family members.
Describe a family genogram and show how it is constructed.	Use a blackboard to map out a family genogram. Assign family genogram as homework.	Patient obtains factual information about family. Patient constructs family genogram.
Analyze need for objectivity and responsibility for changing one's own behavior and not that of others.	Role-play interactions with various family members. Encourage testing out new ways of interacting with family members.	Patient demonstrates a higher level of differentiation in family of origin.

BOX 18-7	SUMMARIZING THE EVIDENCE ON **Self-Concept Responses**

Disorder	Dissociative disorders
Treatment	◆ Sodium pentobarbital, sodium amobarbital, and hypnosis are useful in facilitating the recovery of repressed and dissociated memories.
	◆ Psychotherapy helps patients work through and ultimately control access to traumatic memories.

From Nathan P, Gorman J: *A guide to treatments that work*, ed 2, New York, 2002, Oxford University Press.

They focus primarily on the level of the patient. However, they may be implemented with group or family interventions, and the nurse is expected to include the patient's family, significant others, and community supports whenever possible.

Empirically validated treatments for the medical diagnoses related to dissociative disorders are summarized in Box 18-7 (Nathan and Gorman, 2002).

Level 1: Expanded Self-Awareness

To avoid anxiety, most people resist change. In general, change in the self is easier when threat is absent. Threat forces a person to defend himself, perceptions are narrowed, and the person has difficulty forming new perceptions of himself (see Critical Thinking About Contemporary Issues).

To expand the patient's self-awareness and reduce the element of threat, the nurse should adopt an accepting attitude. Acceptance allows the patient the security and freedom to examine all aspects of oneself as a total human being with positive and negative qualities. The basis of a therapeutic relationship is established by listening to the patient with understanding, responding nonjudgmentally, expressing genuine interest, and conveying a sense of caring and sincerity.

Creating a climate of acceptance allows previously denied experiences to be examined. This broadens the patient's concept of self and helps the patient accept all aspects of one's personality. It also indicates that the patient is a valued person who is responsible for himself and is able to help himself. This is important because the nurse must work with whatever ego strength the patient possesses.

Most patients seen in clinics, the general hospital, and the community setting possess considerable ego strength. However, people who are hospitalized might have limited ego resources. Psychotic patients experiencing depersonalization and identity confusion often present difficult challenges for the nurse. They tend to isolate themselves and withdraw from reality, so little ego strength is available for problem solving.

For this type of patient, expanding self-awareness means first confirming the patient's identity. The nurse should attempt to provide supportive measures to decrease the panic level experienced by this patient. Additional interventions related to anxiety and psychotic states are described in Chapters 16 and 21.

The nurse can spend time with the patient in an undemanding way and approach the patient nonaggressively. Initially the nurse may accept the patient's need to remain nonverbal or attempt to clarify and understand the patient's verbal communication even though it may be distorted or lack apparent logic.

Critical Thinking *About* Contemporary Issues

When Do People Reach Out for Help?

We all write our own biographies, framing the narrative in ways that are congruent with the self we know and the one we want to be. It isn't that we lie to ourselves and to others, only that there are so many ways to interpret and assemble the facts of our lives.

So, for example, a woman who suffers some traumatic event like incest or rape can tell the story two ways. In one version it's the central fact of her life, the one she can never forget and never get past. It's a story of victimization that builds on itself until it defines who she is and what she can do. In another account it's a terrible event that marked her life but not her identity. It's a tale of transcendence in which the past isn't denied or forgotten; it simply doesn't form the core of the narrative she has constructed.

How we write the script depends on who we are and how we internalize the events of our world. Obviously, some stories are more psychologically functional than others. But every story changes with time, not just because memories grow dim but because we ourselves change, and the story we need to tell us where we've been and who we are now is different today that it was yesterday. It's when the tale remains fixed that therapy can be most effective by helping us to reframe the narrative to focus on change rather than stasis, on strength rather than weakness.

From Rubin L: *The man with the beautiful voice: and more stories from the other side of the couch*, Boston, 2003, Beacon Press.

Attempts should be made to prevent the patient from being isolated by establishing a simple routine for the patient. If the patient displays bizarre behavior, such as inappropriate laughing or mannerisms, the nurse can set limits on the behavior. It is important to orient the patient frequently to reality and reinforce appropriate behavior.

The patient should be helped to increase activities that provide positive experiences. This may involve the use of occupational therapy, recreational therapy, or activity groups because success at tasks and increased involvement with objects can increase self-esteem. Movement therapy or body ego technique is a goal-directed way to develop identity, body image, and ego structure. It is predominantly a nonverbal therapy because the emphasis is on movement, not on what the person says.

Depersonalization often leads to poor hygiene and an unkempt personal appearance. Nurses who are aware of their own value systems regarding cleanliness and grooming can help patients unable to care for themselves. They can use patience and repetition to establish health routines and can kindly but firmly encourage patients to care for themselves. Through verbal and nonverbal messages, nurses can encourage patients to take pride in their appearance and reinforce any progress made.

Another possible nursing intervention is photographic self-image confrontation. This involves taking photographs of patients and then discussing them. This intervention can provide a means for establishing a nurse-patient relationship and mutually exploring some aspects of the self.

Mutuality is often difficult to establish with a patient experiencing depersonalization. Initially the nurse will determine appropriate activities and incorporate the patient into them without asking for a response. Gradually, however, the nurse can expect greater participation and can involve the patient in decision making. Table 18-5 summarizes the nursing interventions appropriate to level 1.

Sometimes the nurse's attitudes or behaviors can block patients from expanding their own self-awareness. These behaviors can take the form of criticism, belittlement, condemnation, condescension, indifference, or insincerity. An impersonal attitude can decrease the patient's self-esteem. Excessive demands or direct challenges to self-concept can result in further withdrawal.

Nurses should not allow patients to remain alone or inactive, should not attempt to shame them into improving their habits, or not assume total care for them. If nurses refrain from these behaviors and instead strive to foster acceptance of the patients, they remove themselves as a source of threat and encourage patients to lower their defenses. Patients are then prepared to take the next step in problem solving (see A Patient Speaks on p. 319).

How do you think that the nurse's level of self-esteem affects nursing interventions in patients' self-concept responses? ■

Level 2: Self-Exploration

At this level of intervention nurses encourage patients to examine feelings, behavior, beliefs, and thoughts, particularly in relation to the current stressor. The cognitive behavioral strategies described in Chapter 31 are very useful at this time. Patients' feelings may be expressed verbally, nonverbally, symbolically, or directly. For example, structured writing activities, such as journaling, letters, poetry, and prose, can be used to facilitate self-examination (Dellasega, 2001).

Acceptance continues to be important because when nurses accept patients' feelings and thoughts, they are helping them accept themselves as well. Nurses should facilitate the expression of strong emotions, such as anger, sadness, and guilt. In a sense, patients' emotions or affects serve as clues to inner thoughts and current behavior.

As the patient focuses attention on the meaning that experiences have for him, he is clarifying his perceptions and concept of himself and his relationship to the people and events around him. The nurse can elicit his perception of strengths and weaknesses and have him describe his self-ideal. He can be made aware of his self-criticisms.

It is important for nurses to accept and deal with their own feelings before becoming involved in the self-exploration of others. Self-awareness limits the potential negative effects of countertransference in the relationship. It also allows nurses to demonstrate authentic behavior that, in turn, can be elicited and reinforced in the patient.

Table 18-5	Nursing Interventions in Alterations in Self-Concept at Level 1	
PRINCIPLE	**RATIONALE**	**NURSING INTERVENTIONS**
GOAL: Expand the patient's self-awareness		
Establish an open, trusting relationship.	Reduces the threat that the nurse poses to the patient and helps the patient to broaden and accept all aspects of one's personality.	Offer unconditional acceptance. Listen to the patient. Encourage discussion of thoughts and feelings. Respond nonjudgmentally. Convey to the patient that he is a valued person who is responsible for and able to help himself.
Work with whatever ego strength the patient has.	Some degree of ego strength, such as the capacity for reality testing, self-control, or a degree of ego integration, is needed as a foundation for later nursing care.	Identify the patient's ego strength. Guidelines for the patient with limited ego resources are as follows: 1. Begin by confirming his identity. 2. Provide support measures to reduce his level of anxiety. 3. Approach him in an undemanding way. 4. Accept and attempt to clarify any verbal or nonverbal communication. 5. Prevent him from isolating himself. 6. Establish a simple routine for him. 7. Set limits on inappropriate behavior. 8. Orient him to reality. 9. Reinforce appropriate behavior. 10. Gradually increase activities and tasks that provide positive experiences for him. 11. Help him in personal hygiene and grooming. 12. Encourage the patient to care for himself.
Maximize the patient's participation in the therapeutic relationship.	Mutuality is needed for the patient to assume responsibility for his own behavior and maladaptive coping responses.	Gradually increase the patient's participation in decisions that affect his care. Convey to the patient that he is a responsible person.

Often patients experience great difficulty in discussing or describing their feelings. This may be because society tends to discourage self-revelation or because some patients are honestly out of touch with their inner self. In these cases nurses can use themselves therapeutically through purposeful self-disclosure, such as in sharing feelings, verbalizing how they might feel in the situation, or mirroring their perception of patients' feelings. In this way nurses can help patients explore maladaptive thinking.

The nurse must be careful not to reinforce the patient's self-pity by responding with sympathy. Patients often deny any personal responsibility for their situation, and they fail to see how their own behavior precipitates the problem about which they complain. Examples include patients who seek treatment because of things that happened to them (his wife left him, her husband beat her, or his boss fired him, for example), and patients who seek help because of things that have not happened, such as not being happy or not having friends. These patients fail to see that they have a choice in life and that personal growth and satisfaction involve both risk and responsibility.

The nurse can clarify with the patient that he is not helpless or powerless. He is powerless when he sees himself as such and gives up control and responsibility for his behavior. The patient must accept responsibility for the logical consequences of the things he chooses to do or not to do. Only if a patient fully understands the implications of his actions and the scope of his choices can he set goals, explore alternatives, and effect change.

In stressing the importance of behavior, the nurse helps the patient see that he chooses to behave in certain ways. If the patient projects his problems onto the environment, the nurse can discuss with him the difficulty in changing other people and explore the possibilities of changing his own self. This means helping the patient realize that when he says, "I can't," he really means "I don't want to."

The nurse should not give the impression that she has the power to change a patient's life. That power lies with the patient alone. However, the nurse can help him maximize his strengths, use available resources, and see that life involves more than misery and pain.

Self-exploration need not take place solely within the one-to-one relationship. Family sessions and group meetings can help clarify how the patient appears to others. These meetings can supplement the individual sessions with the patient, and similar nursing interventions can be applied within family or group therapy.

Regardless of the setting, the nurse collects information on the patient's thoughts about himself, logical or illogical reasoning, and reported or observed reactions. Interventions at this level should facilitate the patient progressing from denying or attributing contradictory feelings to the external situation to recognizing a major conflict within himself. Table 18-6 summarizes the nursing interventions appropriate to level 2.

Do you believe contemporary society encourages or discourages personal responsibility for behavior? Defend your point of view. ■

Table 18-6	Nursing Interventions in Alterations in Self-Concept at Level 2	
PRINCIPLE	**RATIONALE**	**NURSING INTERVENTIONS**
GOAL: Encourage the patient's self-exploration		
Help the patient accept his own feelings and thoughts.	When nurses show interest in and accept the patient's feelings and thoughts, they are helping him to do so as well.	Attend to and encourage the patient's expression of his emotions, beliefs, behavior, and thoughts verbally, nonverbally, symbolically, or directly. Use therapeutic communication skills and empathic responses. Note his use of logical and illogical thinking and his reported and observed emotional responses.
Help the patient clarify his concept of self and his relationship to others through self-disclosure.	Self-disclosure and understanding one's self-perceptions are prerequisites for bringing about future change. This may, in itself, reduce anxiety.	Elicit his perception of self-strengths and weaknesses. Help him to describe his self-ideal. Identify his self-criticisms. Help him describe how he believes he relates to other people and events.
Be aware and have control of one's own feelings.	Self-awareness allows the nurse to model authentic behavior and limits the potential negative effects of counter-transference in the relationship.	Be open to and accept one's own positive and negative feelings. Practice therapeutic use of self by sharing your own feelings with the patient, verbalizing how another might have felt, or mirroring one's perception of the patient's feelings.
Respond empathically, not sympathetically, emphasizing that the power to change lies with the patient.	Sympathy can reinforce self-pity. The nurse should communicate that the patient's life situation is subject to his own control.	Use empathetic responses and monitor oneself for feelings of sympathy or pity. Reaffirm to the patient that he is not powerless in the face of his problems. Convey that the patient is responsible for his own behavior, including his choice of maladaptive or adaptive coping responses. Discuss the scope of his choices, his areas of ego strength, and coping resources that are available. Use the support systems of family and groups to facilitate the patient's self-exploration. Help the patient recognize the nature of his conflict and the maladaptive ways in which he tries to cope with it.

Level 3: Self-Evaluation

This level involves hard work for the patient as he critically examines his own behavior, accepts the consequences for it, and judges whether it is the best possible choice. At this point the problem should be clearly defined and the patient should be helped to understand that his beliefs influence his feelings and behavior. Only by actively and systematically challenging his faulty beliefs and perceptions can he hope for change. Previously identified misperceptions and distortions should be evaluated. Irrational beliefs and unrealistic self-ideals should be identified and analyzed.

The patient's hopelessness should be countered by exploring areas of realistic hope. It is important to point out the mature part of the patient's personality and contrast it to the immature part that causes problems. The behaviors that interfere with effective functioning should be put in perspective so that the patient can see that the maladaptive behavior is only a small part of his or her total personality.

Success and failure must be placed in perspective. Failures occur every moment of every day and are a natural consequence of human activity. As long as people strive to achieve, often they will not reach their goals. The only way to avoid failure is to do absolutely nothing. Failure may be caused by one's own mistakes, a lack of motivation, or circumstances beyond one's control.

Whatever the reason, failure is the unavoidable outcome of human effort. The problem arises when people are labeled or label themselves as failures. This is potentially destructive. As an inherent part of life, failure should be seen as either a neutral concept or a positive one for the learning experience it provides.

Unrealistic self-ideals, dependency patterns, and denial are all potential areas that can be analyzed. The patient can be helped to realize that all behavior and coping responses have positive and negative consequences. Contrasts can be drawn between behavior that is destructive, inhibitory, or sabotaging and behavior that is productive, enhancing, or growth producing.

The patient must see that he acts in self-defeating ways because some "payoff" or personal gain is in it for him. The patient is probably well aware of the drawbacks of his maladaptive coping responses. The payoffs, or secondary gains, may be more obscure and well repressed. Following are some common payoffs:

- Procrastination
- Avoiding risks
- Retreating from the present
- Evading responsibility for one's actions
- Avoiding working or having to change

Payoffs specific to the patient's problem should be identified. For example, possible **secondary gains** from being obese include having people feel sorry for you, having an excuse for not dating or being married, being the focus of dieting attention, or being easily recognized and noticed when with other people. Possible secondary gains for an adult remaining dependent on one's parents might include not having to make one's own decisions, having someone else to blame if things go wrong, being protected from risks and venturing out in the world, not establishing lasting intimate relationships, or not having to establish one's own identity, but rather adopting the values and goals of others.

The nurse becomes more active at this level of intervention by confronting, interpreting, persuading, and challenging. The goal is to increase the patient's objectivity in dealing with stressors. For example, the nurse can show the patient that the same person can nurture and gratify as well as anger and frustrate because both negative and positive qualities coexist in the same person.

Supportive confrontation may be particularly effective in pointing out inconsistencies in words and actions. The climate of acceptance established by the nurse in level 1 and the empathic communication developed in level 2 provide a basis for confrontation in level 3. This groundwork is necessary to prevent premature confrontation, which can be destructive.

The nurse may use various aspects of role theory during this level, including helping the patient in role clarification by identifying behaviors, clarifying expectations, and specifying goals related to the role. The nurse also can encourage the patient to participate in any activity in which he can observe his own behavior. Role playing may be particularly effective in providing the patient with feedback and increasing his insight. Through it, he may become more objective about the irrationality and self-destructiveness of his self-criticisms.

Another therapeutic intervention that is particularly useful in promoting the self-esteem and coping mechanisms of the elderly is the use of reminiscence. Reminiscence involves thinking about or relating past experiences, especially those that are personally significant. It has been used to help patients acquire a sense of integrity, enhance self-esteem, and stimulate thinking about oneself. As such, it provides nurses with an opportunity to focus, reflect, and reinforce their patients' uniqueness and enhance their sense of self-worth. Reminiscence is discussed in more detail in Chapter 38.

The nurse-patient relationship is a rich source of information for the patient. Within this relationship the patient is enacting and experiencing many problem areas, and the nurse can use this as a "study in miniature." The nurse can observe how the patient reacts in the one-to-one situation and share reactions with him to give him feedback on how he affects others.

The analysis and use of **transference** and **countertransference** reactions constitute the nurse's therapeutic use of self. When a block arises in the relationship or anxiety increases, the nurse should explore its meaning with the patient. The nurse should confront the problem and openly discuss it with him. This also can be done in family or group therapy sessions.

During this level of intervention, the patient and nurse critically evaluate the patient's behavior. Misperceptions, unrealistic goals, and distortions of reality are explored. This provides the patient with sufficient knowledge to progress to the next level of problem solving. Table 18-7 summarizes the nursing interventions appropriate to level 3.

Think of one of your less desirable habits. What payoff or personal gain does it provide you? ■

Table 18-7 **Nursing Interventions in Alterations in Self-Concept at Level 3**

PRINCIPLE	RATIONALE	NURSING INTERVENTIONS
GOAL: Assist the patient's self-evaluation		
Help the patient define the problem clearly.	Only after the problem is accurately defined can alternative choices be proposed.	Identify relevant stressors with the patient and his appraisal of them. Clarify that the patient's beliefs influence his feelings and behaviors. Mutually identify faulty beliefs, misperceptions, distortions, illusions, and unrealistic goals. Mutually identify areas of strength. Place the concepts of success and failure in the proper perspective. Explore the patient's use of coping resources.
Explore the patient's adaptive and maladaptive coping responses to the problem.	Examine the coping choices the patient has made and evaluate their positive and negative consequences.	Describe to the patient how all coping responses are freely chosen and have both positive and negative consequences. Contrast adaptive and maladaptive responses. Mutually identify the disadvantages of the patient's maladaptive coping responses. Mutually identify the advantages, or payoffs, of the patient's maladaptive coping responses. Discuss how these payoffs have perpetuated the maladaptive response. Use a variety of therapeutic skills (facilitative communication, supportive confrontation, role clarification, and the transference and countertransference reactions occurring in the one-to-one relationship).

Level 4: Realistic Planning

The nurse and patient are now ready to formulate possible solutions or alternatives. This begins by investigating what solutions were attempted in the past and evaluating their effectiveness.

When the patient holds inconsistent perceptions, he is faced with several choices. He can change his perceptions and beliefs to bring them closer to a reality that cannot be changed. Alternatively, he may seek to change his environment to bring it in line with what he believes. When his behavior is inconsistent with his self-concept, he can change his behavior, change the beliefs underlying his self-concept so that they include his behavior, or change his self-ideal while leaving his self-concept intact.

At this time, all possible alternatives and solutions should be openly discussed with the patient. Nurses must be careful not to use their influence to persuade the patient to do anything that represents their values rather than the patient's. The nurse should help the patient conceptualize goals. If they are within the patient's reach, his or her efforts can be supported. If the patient has conflicting goals, the nurse helps identify which are more realistic by discussing emotional and practical consequences.

The nurse can work with the patient in various ways. The patient may be encouraged to give up superhuman standards by which he judges his behavior. These standards may set him up for failure. The patient may need to lower his self-ideal and limit his goals. He should be encouraged to renew involvement with life and pursue new experiences for their growth potential.

Role rehearsal, role modeling, and role playing may be used. In **role rehearsal** the person imagines how a particular situation might take place and how his role might evolve. He mentally enacts his role and tries to anticipate the responses of significant others. Role rehearsal is important in anticipating and planning the course of future action. **Role modeling** occurs when the patient first watches someone else playing a certain role so that then he is able to understand and emulate those behaviors. The person he observes may be the nurse, a family member, a group member, or a peer. The nurse can help the patient in his role learning by modeling behavior such as expression of feelings, specific socialization skills, or realistic self-expectations. Proceeding one step further, the nurse and patient may **role play** certain situations to develop alternative solutions.

Visualization also can be used to enhance self-esteem through goal setting. Through the conscious programming of desired change with positive images, expectations are molded. Strong, positive expectations can then become self-fulfilling. To use visualization, the nurse should do the following:

1. Ask the patient to select a positive, specific goal, such as "I will call a friend and suggest we go out together."
2. Help the patient to relax, using a relaxation technique (see Chapter 31).
3. Have the patient repeat the goal phrase several times slowly.
4. Have the patient close his eyes and visualize the goal written on a piece of paper.
5. Have the patient, while relaxed, imagine accomplishing the goal.

The patient should then describe how he feels when the desired goal is reached and how other people respond to him. In this way the patient can gain positive control over his life.

Table 18-8 summarizes the nursing interventions appropriate to level 4. Ultimately the patient should choose a plan that includes a clear definition of the desired change. Converting a talking decision into an action decision is the final, but most important, step.

Level 5: Commitment to Action

The nurse helps the patient become committed to his decision and then achieve his goals. The patient's development of self-awareness, self-understanding, and insight is not the ultimate desired outcome of the nursing therapeutic process. Insight

Table 18-8	Nursing Interventions in Alterations in Self-Concept at Level 4	
PRINCIPLE	**RATIONALE**	**NURSING INTERVENTIONS**
GOAL: Help the patient formulate a realistic plan of action		
Help the patient identify alternative solutions.	Only when all possible alternatives have been evaluated can change be effected.	Help the patient understand that he can change only himself, not others. If the patient holds inconsistent perceptions, help him see that he can change his beliefs or ideals to bring them closer to reality, and change his environment to make it consistent with his beliefs. If his self-concept is not consistent with his behavior, he can change his behavior to confirm to his self-concept, change the beliefs underlying his self-concept to include his behavior, or change his self-ideal. Mutually review how coping resources may be better used by the patient.
Help the patient develop realistic goals.	Goal setting that includes a clear definition of the expected change is necessary.	Encourage the patient to formulate his own (not the nurse's) goals. Mutually discuss the emotional, practical, and reality-based consequences of each goal. Help the patient clearly define the concrete change to be made. Encourage the patient to pursue new experiences for growth potential. Use role rehearsal, role modeling, role playing, and visualization when appropriate.

alone does not make problems disappear or transform one's world in magical ways. Although a patient may have obtained a high level of insight, he may nevertheless continue to function at a minimum level. Such a patient may be able to discuss with great ease the nature of his problem and the contributing influences, but the problem continues to be unresolved.

Some patients actually use their insights to resist moving forward and avoid the hard work involved in making behavioral changes. The value of having the patient gain insight and increase his self-understanding is that he can gain perspective on why he behaves the way he does and what must be done to break maladaptive patterns.

Providing opportunity for the patient to experience success is essential at this time. To help him commit himself to his goal, the nurse can relate to the patient how she sees him, correcting his own poor self-image. In this mirroring technique the nurse can openly and honestly describe to the patient the healthy parts of his personality and how, by using these parts, he can achieve his goal. The nurse should reinforce his strengths or skills and provide him with opportunities to use them whenever possible.

Sometimes the lack of vocational or social skills is a causative factor for low self-esteem. If so, nursing intervention can be directed toward gaining vocational assistance for the patient. Group and family involvement may be helpful in raising self-esteem. The experience of being accepted by others, the sense of belonging and being important to others, and the opportunity to develop interpersonal competence all can enhance self-esteem.

At this point the patient needs much support and positive reinforcement in effecting and maintaining change. For many patients this means breaking chronic behavior patterns and exposing themselves to real risk. The patient must actively maintain the processes learned to avoid slipping back to the previous behavior. Doing this is difficult and requires that the patient build on the progress made in the other levels. Successful change is a continuing process of modifying not only one's behavior but also one's environment to help ensure that the change to new ways of behaving is permanent. Otherwise a relapse will occur.

The nurse serves as a transition between the pain of the past and the positive gratification of the future. **Both nurse**

Table 18-9	NURSING TREATMENT PLAN SUMMARY	Maladaptive Self-Concept Responses

Nursing Diagnosis: Chronic or situational low self-esteem
Expected Outcome: The patient will obtain the maximum level of self-actualization to realize his or her potential.

SHORT-TERM GOAL	INTERVENTION	RATIONALE
The patient will establish a therapeutic relationship with the nurse.	Confirm the patient's identity. Provide supportive measures to decrease level of anxiety. Set limits on inappropriate behavior. Work with whatever ego strengths the patient has. Reinforce adaptive behavior.	Mutuality is necessary for the patient to assume responsibility for his or her behavior.
The patient will express feelings, behaviors, and thoughts related to the present stressor.	Help the patient express and describe feelings and thoughts. Help the patient identify self-strengths and weaknesses, self-ideals, and self-criticisms. Respond empathetically, emphasizing that the power to change lies within the patient.	Self-disclosure and understanding are necessary to bring about future change. The use of sympathy is not therapeutic because it can reinforce the patient's self-pity. The nurse should communicate that the patient is in control.
The patient will evaluate the positive and negative consequences of his or her self-concept responses.	Identify relevant stressors and the patient's appraisal of them. Clarify faulty beliefs and cognitive distortions. Evaluate advantages and disadvantages of current coping responses.	Only after the problem is defined can alternative choices be examined. It is then necessary to evaluate the positive and negative consequences of current patterns.
The patient will identify one new goal and two adaptive coping responses.	Encourage the patient to formulate a new goal. Help the patient clearly define the change to be made. Use role rehearsal, role modeling, and visualization to practice the new behavior.	Only after alternatives have been explored can change be effected. Goal setting specifies the nature of the change and suggests possible new behavioral strategies.
The patient will implement the new adaptive self-concept responses.	Provide opportunity for the patient to experience success. Reinforce strengths, skills, and adaptive coping responses. Allow the patient sufficient time to change. Promote group and family involvement. Provide the appropriate amount of support and positive reinforcement for the patient to maintain progress and growth.	The ultimate goal in promoting the patient's insight is to have him or her replace the maladaptive coping responses with more adaptive ones.

and patient must allow sufficient time for change. A significant period may be required for patterns that developed over months or years to be broken and for new ones to be established.

The nurse's role now becomes less active and directive and more confirming of the value, potential, and accomplishments of the patient. A Nursing Treatment Plan Summary for maladaptive self-concept responses is presented in Table 18-9.

EVALUATION

Problems with self-concept are prominent in many psychological disorders. To evaluate the success or failure of the nursing care given, each phase of the nursing process should be reviewed and analyzed by the nurse and patient.

The nurse's assessment should include both the objective and the observable behaviors, as well as the subjective perceptions of the patient.

- Did the nurse explore the patient's strengths and weaknesses and elicit his self-ideal?
- Was information obtained on his body image, feelings of self-esteem, role satisfaction, and sense of identity?
- Did the nurse compare responses to his behavior, and were any inconsistencies or contradictions identified?
- Was the nurse aware of any personal affective response to the patient, and how did this affect the ability to be therapeutic?

The nurse should have adopted a problem-solving approach that placed responsibility for growth on the patient. The most fundamental nursing action should have been to create a climate of acceptance that confirmed the patient's identity and conveyed a sense of value or worth. In expanding the patient's self-awareness, the following should be evaluated:

- How effective was the nurse in promoting full and pertinent self-disclosure?
- Was the nurse able to show authentic behavior in the relationship and share thoughts and reactions?
- What interventions were used, and which ones were helpful (validation, reflection, confrontation, suggestion, role clarification, role playing)?
- Did the nurse progress on the basis of the patient's readiness and motivation?
- Was the patient able to transfer his new perceptions into possible solutions or alternative behavior?
- Did they both allow sufficient time for changes to occur?

The degree of overall success achieved through nursing care can be determined by eliciting the patient's perception of his own growth and comparing his behavior to the healthy personality described in this chapter. Not everyone will achieve all these characteristics, but success has been achieved if the patient's potential has been maximized.

COMPETENT CARING

A Clinical Exemplar of a Psychiatric Nurse
MONICA MOLLOY, MSN, RN, CS

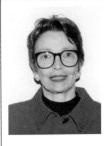

Last week one of my patients died. I have been a nurse for 20 years. I have experienced patients' deaths—many different kinds of deaths, some of them seemingly senseless. I think particularly of young patients with head injuries from motorcycle or automobile accidents. But I understood those deaths. I understood the concept of an accident. What I don't understand is the concept of murder.

In November, a woman was sitting apart from most of the members of a therapy group I lead with a graduate nursing student. I asked her why she didn't join the circle. She replied she was afraid the group didn't want her near them; she thought the odor of her cancer would offend them. When the women in the group responded that they hadn't noticed any odor, she seemed to accept the reassurance offered, but she continued to sit apart. Last week that woman was murdered.

She was a homeless woman, one of the women who embarrass us as a society. She lived in the Family Center of the homeless shelter. I'll call her C. I first met her 2 years ago, when the group began. I remember one group session in particular when she and another shelter guest talked about trust issues in the homeless community. Then she moved away. This past fall she returned to the shelter. In addition to neurofibromatosis, she now had cancer. She looked different; she had lost nearly 40 pounds. She had been discharged from a local hospital to the shelter. Despite her willingness to take a risk and to disclose her

fears about the odor she thought she had, she essentially remained alone and apart.

C's death has given me one more opportunity to examine what it is to practice psychiatric nursing in the community. When nurses practice in inpatient environments, one of our fundamental responsibilities is to ensure patient safety. Sometimes that safety is interpersonal, sometimes it is environmental. Among the homeless population, environmental safety is tenuous at best. One goal for the group intervention in the shelter community is to enable the women to use themselves and each other as resources to create their own safety zone. Somehow that didn't work with C. The day after her death, the graduate nursing student and I spent some time with the women in the Family Center community. We went there to be with the women to provide support. We also went there to grieve. And perhaps most of all, we went there to try to answer some questions for ourselves, the same questions all clinicians ask when a patient dies: Did we miss some signs? Could we have done something different?

C's death is mentioned in the group weekly now. New guests use her death to reify their fears about being homeless, as a metaphor for their own alienation experience. Through her death C has left a mark on that group and that community. I don't understand the concept of murder any better. I do understand more about the concept of alienation. Acknowledging alienation is a first step to creating a sense of personal safety. It is fundamental to the practice of psychiatric nursing in the community. I learned that from C, and for that I will always be grateful. ∎

CHAPTER **FOCUS POINTS**

- Self-concept is defined as all the notions, beliefs, and convictions that constitute a person's self-knowledge and that influence relationships with others. The self-concept emerges or is learned through each person's internal experiences, relationships with other people, and interactions with the outer world.

- Research indicates that parental influence is strongest during early childhood and continues to have a significant impact through adolescence and young adulthood. Over time, however, the power and influence of friends and other adults increase, and they become significant others to the person.

- One's needs, values, and beliefs strongly influence perceptions. People with positive self-concepts function more effectively. Negative self-concept is correlated with personal and social maladjustment.

- Body image is the sum of the conscious and unconscious attitudes a person has toward one's own body.

- The self-ideal is the person's perception of how to behave, based on certain personal standards. It must neither be too high and demanding nor too vague and shadowy, yet it must be high enough and defined enough to give continuous support to self-respect.

- Self-esteem is a person's personal judgment of his or her own worth, based on how well behavior matches up with self-ideal. Self-esteem increases with age and is most threatened during adolescence, when concepts of self are being changed and many self-decisions are made.

- Roles are sets of socially expected behavior patterns associated with a person's functioning in different social groups. On the basis of one's perception of role adequacy in the most ego-involved roles, a person develops a level of self-esteem.

- Identity is the awareness of being oneself, as derived from self-observation and judgment. It is the synthesis of all self-representations into an organized whole. The person with a strong sense of identity sees himself or herself as a unique individual. In adolescence the crisis of identity versus identity diffusion occurs. Achieving identity is a prerequisite for establishing an intimate relationship.

- All behavior is motivated by a desire to enhance, maintain, or defend the self, so the nurse has much information to evaluate. The nurse also must go beyond objective and observable behaviors to the patient's subjective and internal world.

- Low self-esteem indicates self-rejection and self-hate, which may be a conscious or unconscious process expressed in direct or indirect ways.

- Identity diffusion is the failure to integrate various childhood identifications into a harmonious adult psychosocial identity. Personality fusion is a person's attempt to establish a sense of self by fusing with, attaching to, or belonging to someone else.

- Depersonalization is the subjective experience of the partial or total disruption of one's ego and the disintegration and disorganization of one's self-concept. It can occur in depression, schizophrenia, manic states, and organic brain syndromes, and it represents the advanced state of ego breakdown associated with multiple personality disorder and psychotic states.

- Self-esteem is partly an inheritable trait, and genetic as well as environmental influences are very important.

- Gender and work roles will continue as a source of stress until care of children, home, and career are viewed as equally valu-

able and important by both sexes and until gender is regarded as irrelevant to the abilities, personalities, and activities of the people involved.

- Specific problems with self-concept can be brought on by almost any difficult situation to which the person cannot adjust. Role strain is the frustration felt when the person is torn in opposite directions or feels inadequate or unsuited to enact certain roles. There are two categories of role transitions—developmental and health-illness.

- All people, no matter how disturbing their behavior, have some areas of personal strength.

- An identity crisis may be resolved with either short-term or long-term coping mechanisms. These are used to ward off the anxiety and uncertainty of identity confusion.

- Typical ego defense mechanisms include fantasy, dissociation, isolation, projection, displacement, splitting, turning anger against the self, and acting out.

- Most people who express dissatisfaction with life, display deviant behavior, or have difficulty functioning in social or work situations have problems related to self-concept.

- Primary NANDA nursing diagnoses related to alterations in self-concept are disturbed body image, readiness for enhanced self-concept, low self-esteem (chronic, situational, risk for situational), ineffective role performance, and disturbed personal identity. These nursing diagnoses are not limited to the psychiatric setting and do not have a discrete category of medical diagnoses associated with them.

- Primary *DSM-IV-TR* diagnoses include identity problem, dissociative amnesia, dissociative fugue, dissociative identity disorder, also known as *multiple personality disorder*, and depersonalization disorder.

- The expected outcome of nursing care is that the patient will obtain the maximum level of self-actualization to realize his or her potential.

- The nurse's focus is to help the patient understand himself more fully and accurately so that he can direct his own life in a more satisfying way.

- The mutually identified goals can be reached by a problem-solving approach that focuses primarily on the present, removes much of the responsibility from the nurse, and actively engages the patient in working on personal difficulties. This approach requires that the patient first develop insight into one's problems and then take action to effect lasting behavioral changes.

- The focus of this approach is on the patient's cognitive appraisal of life, which may contain faulty perceptions, beliefs, and convictions. Awareness of feelings and emotions is also important because they too may be subject to misconceptions. Only after examining the patient's cognitive appraisal of the situation and related feelings can one gain insight into the problem and bring about behavioral change.

- Interventions include helping the patient expand self-awareness and engage in self-exploration, self-evaluation, realistic planning, and commitment to action.

- The degree of success achieved through nursing care can be determined by eliciting the patient's perception of his or her own growth and comparing his or her behavior to characteristics of a healthy personality.

KEY TERMS

body image, 305
depersonalization, 310
identity, 306
identity diffusion, 309
identity foreclosure, 315

multiple personality disorder, 311
negative identity, 315
reminiscence, 324
role strain, 313
roles, 306

self-concept, 303
self-esteem, 305
self-ideal, 305
visualization, 325

CHAPTER REVIEW QUESTIONS

1. Indicate whether the following statements are true (T) or false (F).

____ A. People behave in a manner consistent with what they believe to be true.

____ B. There is no evidence that genetics plays a role in the inheritance of self-esteem.

____ C. Most people who express dissatisfaction with life, display deviant behavior, or have difficulty functioning in social or work situations have problems related to self-concept.

____ D. The optimum outcome desired for a patient with alterations in self-concept is enhanced insight into self-concept and its influence on behavior.

____ E. Responding with sympathy is an appropriate nursing intervention to help a patient with self-exploration.

2. Fill in the blanks.

A. _____ is a person's perception of how one should behave based on certain personal standards.

B. A person's judgment of his or her own worth obtained by analyzing how well the person's behavior conforms to his or her self-ideal is called _____.

C. _____ are sets of socially expected behavior patterns associated with a person's functioning in various social groups.

D. The organizing principle of the personality is called

_____ .

E. _____ is the feeling of unreality in which one is unable to distinguish between inner and outer stimuli.

F. It is believed that _____ is a precipitating stressor for dissociative disorder and multiple personality disorder.

G. Thinking about or relating past experiences, especially those that are personally significant, is called _____.

3. Provide short answers for the following questions.

A. Describe the four best ways to promote a child's self-esteem.

B. Briefly describe the developmental crisis of adolescence.

C. List six qualities of the healthy personality. Think about someone you admire and evaluate him or her based on each of these qualities.

D. Describe your own body-image, self-ideal, and level of self-esteem. What changes would you like to make in each area?

Visit Evolve for additional resources related to the content of this chapter.

evolve   **http://evolve.elsevier.com/Stuart/principles/**
• Topical Course Outline • Student Workbook Exercises • Critical Thinking Questions and Activities • Case Studies • Research Topics
• Monthly Content Updates • WebLinks

Student Study CD-ROM

Access the accompanying CD-ROM for animations, interactive exercises, review questions for the NCLEX examination, and an audio glossary.

REFERENCES

American Psychiatric Association: *Diagnostic and statistical manual of mental disorders*, ed 4, text revision, Washington, DC, 2000, American Psychiatric Association.

Bjorklund P: Assessing ego strength: spinning straw into gold, *Perspect Psychiatr Care* 36:14, 2000.

Chu J et al: Memories of childhood abuse: dissociation, amnesia, and corroboration, *Am J Psychiatry* 156:749, 1999.

Clemens N: Subtleties of self, *J Psychiatr Pract* 8:377, 2002.

Coopersmith S: *The antecedents of self-esteem*, San Francisco, 1967, WH Freeman.

Dellasega CA: Using structured writing experiences to promote mental health, *J Psychosoc Nurs Ment Health Serv* 39:14, 2001.

Erikson EH: *Childhood and society*, New York, 1963, WW Norton.

Guralnik O, Schmeidler J, Simeon D: Feeling unreal: cognitive processes in depersonalization, *Am J Psychiatry* 157:103, 2000.

Kluft R: Current issues in dissociative identity disorder, *J Pract Psychiatr Behav Health* 5:3, 1999.

Moorhead S, Johnson M, Maas M, editors: *Nursing outcomes classification (NOC)*, ed 3, St Louis, 2004, Mosby.

Morgan C et al: Symptoms of dissociation in humans experiencing acute, uncontrollable stress: a prospective investigation, *Am J Psychiatry* 158:1239, 2001.

Mruk C: *Self-esteem: research, theory and practice*, ed 2, New York, 1999, Springer.

Nathan PE, Gorman JM: *A guide to treatments that work*, ed 2, New York, 2002, Oxford University Press.

Simeon D et al: Peritraumatic reactions associated with the world trade center disaster, *Am J Psychiatry* 160:1702, 2003.

Sullivan HS: *The interpersonal theory of psychiatry*, New York, 1963, WW Norton.

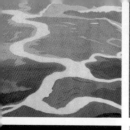

> Lying awake, calculating the future,
> Trying to unweave, unwind, unravel
> And piece together the past and the future,
>
> Between midnight and dawn, when the past is all
> deception,
> The future futureless . . .
>
> T.S. ELIOT

19 EMOTIONAL RESPONSES AND MOOD DISORDERS

Gail W. Stuart

LEARNING OBJECTIVES

After studying this chapter, the student should be able to:

1. Describe the continuum of adaptive and maladaptive emotional responses (I).
2. Identify behaviors associated with emotional responses (II).
3. Analyze predisposing factors, precipitating stressors, and appraisal of stressors related to emotional responses (II).
4. Describe coping resources and coping mechanisms related to emotional responses (II).
5. Formulate nursing diagnoses related to emotional responses (III).
6. Examine the relationship between nursing diagnoses and medical diagnoses related to emotional responses (III).
7. Identify expected outcomes and short-term nursing goals related to emotional responses (IV).
8. Develop a patient education plan to enhance social skills (V).
9. Analyze nursing interventions related to emotional responses (VI).
10. Evaluate nursing care related to emotional responses (VII).

TOPICAL OUTLINE

I. Continuum of Emotional Responses
   A. Grief Reactions
   B. Depression
   C. Mania
II. Assessment
   A. Behaviors
   B. Predisposing Factors
   C. Precipitating Stressors
   D. Appraisal of Stressors
   E. Coping Resources
   F. Coping Mechanisms
III. Diagnosis
   A. Nursing Diagnoses
   B. Medical Diagnoses
IV. Outcome Identification
V. Planning
   A. Acute Treatment Phase
   B. Continuation Treatment Phase
   C. Maintenance Treatment Phase
VI. Implementation
   A. Environmental Interventions
   B. Nurse-Patient Relationship
   C. Physiological Treatments
   D. Expressing Feelings
   E. Cognitive Strategies
   F. Behavioral Change
   G. Social Skills
   F. Mental Health Education
VII. Evaluation

 Visit Evolve for additional resources related to the content of this chapter.
http://evolve.elsevier.com/Stuart/principles/

Variations in mood are a natural part of life. They indicate that a person is perceiving the world and responding to it. Extremes in mood also are linked with extremes in human experience, such as creativity, madness, despair, ecstasy, romanticism, personal charisma, and interpersonal destructiveness.

Mood is a prolonged emotional state that influences the person's whole personality and life functioning. It pertains to prevailing and pervading emotion and is synonymous with the terms *feeling state* and *emotion*. Like other aspects of the personality, emotions or moods serve an adaptive role. The four adaptive functions of emotions are **social communica-**tion, physiological arousal, subjective awareness, and **psychodynamic defense**.

■ CONTINUUM OF EMOTIONAL RESPONSES

Emotions such as fear, joy, anxiety, love, anger, sadness, and surprise are all normal parts of the human condition. The problem arises in trying to evaluate when a person's mood or emotional state is maladaptive, abnormal, or unhealthy. Grief, for example, is a healthy, adaptive, separating process that attempts to overcome the stress of a loss. Grief work, or mourning, is not a pathological process; it is an adaptive response to a real stressor. The absence of grieving in the face of a loss suggests maladaptation.

The continuum of emotional responses is represented in Figure 19-1. At the adaptive end is **emotional responsiveness**. This involves the person being affected by and being an active participant in the internal and external worlds. It implies an openness to and awareness of feelings. If used in such a way, feelings provide us with valuable learning experiences. They are barometers that give us feedback about ourselves and our relationships, and they help us function more effectively. Also adaptive in the face of stress is an **uncomplicated grief reaction**. Such a reaction implies that the person is facing the reality of the loss and is immersed in the work of grieving.

A maladaptive response is the **suppression of emotions**. This may be a denial of one's feelings or a detachment from them. A transient suppression of feelings may at times be necessary to cope, as in an initial response to a death or tragedy. However, prolonged suppression of emotion, as in **delayed grief reaction**, will ultimately interfere with effective functioning.

The most maladaptive emotional responses or severe mood disturbances are recognized by their intensity, pervasiveness, persistence, and interference with social and physiological functioning. These characteristics apply to the clinical states of **depression** and **mania**, which complete the maladaptive end of the continuum of emotional responses.

Grief Reactions

Grief is the subjective state that follows loss. It is one of the most powerful emotional states and affects all aspects of a person's life. It forces the person to stop normal activities and focus on present feelings and needs. Most often, it is the response to the loss of a loved person through death or separation, but it also occurs following the loss of something tangible or intangible that is highly regarded. It may be a valued object, a cherished possession, an ideal, a job, or status.

As a response to the loss of a loved one, grief is a universal reaction. As a person's dependence on others grows, the chance increases that he or she will at some point face loss, separation, and death, which elicit intense feelings of grief. The capacity to form warm, satisfying relationships with others makes a person vulnerable to sadness, despair, and grief when those relationships are terminated.

As a natural reaction to a life experience, grief is universal; however, the way it is expressed is culturally determined (Clements et al, 2003). It involves stress, pain, and suffering, and an impairment of function that can last for days, weeks, or months. Thus understanding the stages of grief and its symptoms is of great importance because of grief's effect on both physical and emotional health (Egan and Arnold, 2003).

The ability to experience grief is gradually formed in the course of normal development and is closely related to the capacity for developing meaningful relationships. Grief responses may be either uncomplicated and adaptive or morbid and pathological. Uncomplicated grief runs a consistent course that is modified by the abruptness of the loss, the person's preparation for the event, and the significance of the lost object. It is a self-limited process of realization; it makes real the fact of the loss.

A maladaptive response to loss implies that something has prevented it from running its normal course (Piper et al, 2001). There are two types of pathological grief reactions: the **delayed grief reaction** and the **distorted grief reaction**. Persistent absence of any emotion may signal an undue delay in the work of mourning or a delayed grief reaction. The delay may occur in the beginning of the mourning process or slow the process once it has begun, or both. The delay and rejection of grief may occasionally last for many years. The emotions associated with the loss may be triggered by a deliberate recall of circumstances surrounding the loss or by a spontaneous occurrence in the patient's life. A classic example of this is the anniversary reaction, in which the person experiences incomplete or abnormal mourning at the time of the loss, only to have the grieving response recur at anniversaries of the original loss.

Depression is a type of distorted grief reaction. The person who does not mourn can experience the pathological grief reaction known as depression, or melancholia. It is an abnormal extension or overelaboration of sadness and grief.

Depression

Depression is the oldest and most common psychiatric illness. It was described as early as 1500 BC, and it is as familiar as it is mysterious. The word depression is used in a variety of ways. It can refer to a sign, symptom, syndrome, emotional state, reaction, disease, or clinical entity. In this chapter de-

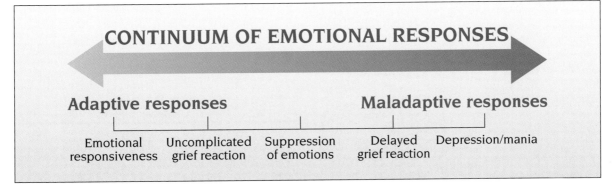

Figure 19-1   Continuum of emotional responses.

pression is viewed as a clinical illness that is severe, maladaptive, and incapacitating.

Depression may range from mild and moderate states to severe states with or without psychotic features. Psychotic depression is uncommon, however, accounting for less than 10% of all depressions. Major depression can begin at any age, although it usually begins in the mid-twenties and thirties. Symptoms develop over days to weeks. Approximately one of eight adults may experience major depression in his or her lifetime, and it affects 14 million people each year, 70% of whom are women. Other complications include significant marital, parental, social, and vocational difficulties (Wells et al, 2002). Finally, it has been estimated that depression costs the American economy $43.7 billion in worker absenteeism, lost productivity, and health care.

The lifetime risk for major depression is 7% to 12% for men and 20% to 30% for women. Among women, rates peak between adolescence and early adulthood. This difference holds true across cultures and continents (see Critical Thinking About Contemporary Issues). Other risk factors include a history of depressive illness in first-degree relatives and a history of major depression.

Most untreated episodes of major depression last 6 to 24 months. Although some people have only a single episode of major depression and return to presymptomatic functioning, it is estimated that over 50% of those who have such an episode will eventually have another, and **25% of patients will have chronic, recurrent depression.**

Depression often occurs along with other psychiatric illnesses (Table 19-1). Up to 40% of patients with major depressive disorders have histories of one or more nonmood psychiatric disorders. These statistics underscore the importance of this health problem and suggest the need for timely diagnosis and treatment. **Unfortunately, only one third of all people with depression seek help, are accurately diagnosed, and obtain appropriate treatment** (Kessler et al, 2003).

A high incidence of depression is found among all patients hospitalized for medical illnesses, although its intensity and frequency is higher in more severely ill patients (von Ammon Cavanaugh et al, 2001). These depressions are largely unrecognized and thus are often untreated by health care personnel. Studies suggest that about one third of medical inpatients report mild or moderate symptoms of depression and up to one fourth may have a depressive illness.

Certain medical conditions are often associated with depression, especially diabetes, cancer, stroke, epilepsy, multiple sclerosis, Parkinson's disease, cardiac disease, and a variety of endocrine disorders. Thus depression is a common accompaniment of many major medical illnesses.

Depressive conditions are also highly prevalent in primary care settings. One of every five patients seeing a primary care practitioner has significant symptoms of depression. Yet only about one in 100 patients cites depression as a reason for the most recent visit, and health care providers fail to diagnose major depression in their patients up to 50% of the time. Given the prevalence and disability associated with depression, the U.S. Preventive Services Task Force (Berg, 2002) recommends screening adults for depression in primary care settings that have systems in place to assure accurate diagnosis, effective treatment, and responsive follow-up.

Critical Thinking *About* Contemporary Issues

Does Culture Impact the Expression and Resolution of Depression?

As a psychiatric illness, depression exists in all countries across the globe. The World Health Organization has identified depression as the number one psychiatric cause of disability in the world and projected that it would rank second in the world as a cause of disability by 2020. Nonetheless, evidence suggests that culture impacts the symptomatic expression, clinical presentation, and effective resolution of depression.

Although depression has been linked to the loss of significant others, the way in which one expresses these feelings arises in a social and cultural context. Specifically, culture has an effect on the neural systems, psychological states, and interpersonal patterns that exist throughout one's life, and cultural variations in the composition of the family and child-rearing practices shape one's view of the world. Culture provides a release for one's emotional expression and also can influence one's source of distress, the form of illness experienced, modes of coping with distress, help-seeking behavior, and social response (Kirmayer, 2001).

In some cultures, disturbances of mood are viewed as moral problems, whereas in others they are repressed or seen as a sign of personal failure or lack of personal strength. This can lead some cultures to deny or minimize this aspect of their personal distress. In the United States, ethnic minorities have similar rates of mood disorders as do white Americans, but they are much less likely to receive appropriate care. Barriers to care include lack of insurance, scarcity of minority providers, and distrust of care providers (Miranda et al, 2002a). Clearly, clinicians need to work collaboratively with their patients, as well as with culture-brokers and colleagues from other cultural communities, to not only better understand and identify their patients' problems and eliminate disparities in care but also to uncover cultural resources that can complement and perhaps supplant conventional treatment.

A patient who just underwent cardiac surgery comes for a follow-up visit and tells the physician he is feeling depressed. He is told that depression is a normal response to cardiac illness and he will get over it in time. Do you agree? If not, what nursing actions are indicated? ■

Table 19-1	Comorbidity of Depression and Other Psychiatric Illness		
	MAJOR DEPRESSIVE DISORDER (%)	DYSTHYMIC DISORDER (%)	DEPRESSION NOS (%)
Alcohol abuse	10	30	67
Drug abuse	19	30	26
Panic disorder	19	7	21
Obsessive-compulsive disorder	35	15	40

Mania

In addition to severe depression, manic episodes may occur. These episodes, like those of depression, can vary in intensity and the accompanying level of anxiety from moderate manic states to severe and panic states with psychotic features. Mania is characterized by an elevated, expansive, or irritable mood. Hypomania is a clinical syndrome similar to but not as severe as mania.

In the *DSM-IV-TR* (American Psychiatric Association, 2000a), the major affective disorders are separated into two subgroups—bipolar and depressive disorders—based on whether manic and depressive episodes are involved over time. In this classification, major depression may involve a single episode or a recurrent depressive illness but does not include manic episodes. **When a person has experienced one or more manic episodes, with or without a major depressive episode, the category of bipolar disorder is used.**

Thus a depressive episode with no manic episodes would be classified as a depressive disorder. A depressive episode with previous or current manic episodes would be classified as a bipolar disorder or manic-depressive illness because the patient experiences both mania and depression. Although bipolar affective disorders are less common than depressive disorders, it is estimated that 1% of the adult population have bipolar disorder. Risk factors are being female and having a family history of bipolar disorder. The data suggest that people under age 50 years are at higher risk of a first attack, whereas those who already have the disorder face increased risk of a recurrent manic or depressive episode as they grow older.

Community-based studies indicate that 60% to 70% of individuals with bipolar disorder meet diagnostic criteria for a lifetime history of substance abuse or dependence. Thus the risk for alcohol or drug abuse is 6 to 7 times greater than would be expected by chance alone among people with bipolar disorder (Goldberg, 2001). Additional facts about depressive and bipolar disorders are presented in Box 19-1.

ASSESSMENT

Behaviors

Delayed Grief Reaction. Delayed grief reactions may be expressed by excessive hostility and grief, prolonged feelings of emptiness and numbness, an inability to weep or express emotions, low self-esteem, use of present tense instead of past when speaking of the loss, persistent dreams about the loss, retention of clothing of the deceased, an inability to visit the grave of the deceased, and the projection of living memories onto an object held in place of the lost one. The following clinical example illustrates some of the behaviors associated with a delayed grief reaction.

CLINICAL EXAMPLE

Mrs. G was a 38-year-old married woman with no history of depression. She came to the local community mental health center complaining of severe throbbing headaches, difficulty falling asleep, fitful and disturbing dreams when asleep, and poor appetite. She said she felt "disgusted" with herself and "useless" to her family. She was living only with her husband.

Her family history revealed that she had three children: two boys and a girl. Her eldest son, age 20, was attending college out of state, and her daughter, age 19, was living with a girlfriend in the same city. Her youngest son was killed in an automobile accident 2 years before at age 15. She described him as her "baby" and expressed much guilt for contributing to his death. She scolded herself for allowing him to drive to the seashore for the weekend with friends, and said she now worries a great deal about her other two children. She said she was trying to protect them from the dangers of the world, but they resented her advice and concern. On questioning by the nurse, Mrs. G reported that these feelings of sadness and guilt had emerged in the last month and seemed to be triggered by the graduation of her son's high school class.

Selected Nursing Diagnosis
*   Dysfunctional grieving related to son's death, as evidenced by somatic complaints and feelings of sadness and guilt ■

In this example Mrs. G was experiencing a delayed grief reaction precipitated by the event of her deceased son's would-be graduation. She had failed to progress through mourning after her son's death and was just now beginning grief work.

Depression. The behaviors associated with depression vary. Sadness and slowness may predominate, or agitation may occur. **The key element of a behavioral assessment is change:** Depressed people change their usual patterns and responses. Research indicates that people working through normal mourning respond to their loss with psychological symptoms often indistinguishable from depression, but these symptoms are accepted by them and by those around them as normal. In contrast, patients with depression experience their condition as a change from their usual selves, which often leads them to seek help.

Many behaviors are associated with depression. These can be divided into affective, physiological, cognitive, and behavioral (Box 19-2). The lists describe the spectrum of possible behaviors, and not all patients experience all of these behaviors.

The most common and **central behavior is that of depressive mood.** This is not necessarily described by the patient as depression but rather as feeling sad, blue, down in the dumps, unhappy, or unable to enjoy life. Crying often occurs. On the other hand, some depressed people do not cry and describe themselves as "beyond tears." The mood disturbance of the depressed patient resembles that of normal unhappiness multiplied in intensity and pervasiveness.

Another mood that often accompanies depression is **anxiety:** a sense of fear and intense worry. Both depression and anxiety may show diurnal variation, that is, a pattern whereby certain times of the day, such as morning or evening, are consistently worse or better.

Some patients may initially deny their anxious or depressed moods but do identify a variety of **somatic complaints.** These might include gastrointestinal distress, chronic or intermittent pain, irritability, palpitations, dizziness, appetite change, lack of energy, change in sex drive, or sleep disturbances. The person often focuses on these symptoms because they are more socially acceptable than the profound feeling of sadness, inability to concentrate, or loss of pleasure in usual activities. In addition, the physical symptoms may help the person with depression explain why nothing is fun anymore. When patients have a range of somatic symptoms, the nurse should carefully evaluate these complaints but also return to the issues of mood and interest, thus considering the possible diagnosis of depression.

It also may be helpful for the nurse to be familiar with the subgroups of major depressive disorder. The common subgroups and clinical relevance of each are presented in Table 19-2. These subgroups are not all-inclusive and may be varying clinical expressions of the same illness over time, in different age groups, or in relation to specific precipitating stressors. Two of these subgroups merit special attention.

Postpartum onset. Postpartum mood symptoms are divided into three categories based on severity: blues, depression, and psychosis.

1. **Postpartum blues** are brief episodes, lasting 1 to 4 days, of labile mood and tearfulness that occur in about 50% to 80% of women within 1 to 5 days of delivery. Treatment consists of reassurance and time to resolve this normal response.

2. **Postpartum depression** may occur from 2 weeks to 12 months after delivery, but usually occurs within 6 months. The risk of postpartum depression is 10% to

15%, but the rate is higher for people with a history of psychiatric disorders (Beck, 2001; Edler, 2000).

3. **Postpartum psychosis** can be divided into depressed and manic types. The incidence of postpartum psychosis is low, and the symptoms typically begin 2 to 3 days after delivery. The period of risk for postpartum psychosis is within the first month after delivery. The prognosis is good for acute postpartum psychosis. However, many patients subsequently develop a bipolar disorder. The recurrence rate is 33% to 51%.

Seasonal pattern. Seasonal affective disorder (SAD) is depression that comes with shortened daylight in winter and fall and disappears during spring and summer. It is characterized by hypersomnia, lethargy and fatigue, increased anxiety, irritability, increased appetite with carbohydrate craving, and often weight gain. It is believed to be related to abnormal melatonin metabolism. It also has been noted that two to three times as many people experience the winter recurrence

---

BOX 19-2

Behaviors Associated With Depression

Affective
Anger
Anxiety
Apathy
Bitterness
Dejection
Denial of feelings
Despondency
Guilt
Helplessness
Hopelessness
Loneliness
Low self-esteem
Sadness
Sense of personal
  worthlessness

Physiological
Abdominal pain
Anorexia
Backache
Chest pain
Constipation
Dizziness
Fatigue
Headache
Impotence
Indigestion
Insomnia
Lassitude
Menstrual changes
Nausea
Overeating
Sexual nonresponsiveness
Sleep disturbances
Vomiting
Weight change

Cognitive
Ambivalence
Confusion
Inability to concentrate
Indecisiveness
Loss of interest and
  motivation
Pessimism
Self-blame
Self-deprecation
Self-destructive thoughts
Uncertainty

Behavioral
Aggressiveness
Agitation
Alcoholism
Altered activity level
Drug addiction
Intolerance
Irritability
Lack of spontaneity
Overdependency
Poor personal hygiene
Psychomotor retardation
Social isolation
Tearfulness
Underachievement
Withdrawal

Table 19-2	Major Depressive Disorder Subgroups			
SUBGROUP	**ESSENTIAL FEATURES**	**DIAGNOSTIC IMPLICATIONS**	**TREATMENT IMPLICATIONS**	**PROGNOSTIC IMPLICATIONS**
Psychotic	Hallucinations Delusions	More likely to become bipolar than non-psychotic types May be misdiagnosed as schizophrenia	Antidepressant medication plus a neuroleptic is more effective than are antidepressants alone ECT is very effective	Usually a recurrent illness Subsequent episodes are usually psychotic Psychotic subtypes run in families Mood—incongruent features have a poorer prognosis
Melancholic	Anhedonia Unreactive mood Severe vegetative symptoms	May be misdiagnosed as dementia More likely in older patients	Antidepressant medication is essential ECT is 90% effective	If recurrent, consider maintenance medication
Atypical	Reactive mood Overeating/weight gain Oversleeping Rejection sensitivity Heavy limb sensation Fewer episodes	Common in younger patients May be misdiagnosed as personality disorder	TCAs may be less effective; MAOIs are preferred SSRIs preferred	Unclear
Seasonal	Onset, fall Offset, spring Recurrent	More common in nonequatorial latitudes Pattern occurs in major depressive and bipolar disorders	Medications have questionable efficacy Psychotherapy has questionable efficacy Phototherapy is an option	Recurs
Postpartum psychosis/ depression	Acute onset (<30 days) in postpartum period Severe, labile mood symptoms 1/1000 in psychotic form	Often heralds a bipolar disorder	Hospitalize Treat medically Antidepressants, antipsychotics are effective	50% chance of recurring in the next postpartum period

From Depression Guideline Panel: *Depression in primary care*, vol 1, *Detection and diagnosis, clinical practice guideline no 5*, pub no 93-0550, Rockville, Md, 1993, US Department of Health and Human Services, Public Health Service, Agency for Health Care Policy and Research.
ECT, Electroconvulsive therapy; *TCA*, tricyclic antidepressant, *MAOIs*, monoamine oxidase inhibitors; *SSRIs*, selective serotonin reuptake inhibitors.

of seasonal mood symptoms as those who actually exhibit behaviors severe enough to merit clinical diagnosis.

Conditions of light and darkness have often been noted to affect mood. Evaluate your own environment for exposure to light. Compare it with a hospital environment. ■

Suicide. Finally, the potential for suicide should always be assessed in those with severe mood disturbances. Approximately 15% of severely depressed patients commit suicide, and between 25% and 50% of patients with bipolar disorder attempt suicide at least once (Jamison, 2000). Suicide and other self-destructive behaviors are discussed in detail in Chapter 20. The intensity of anger, guilt, and worthlessness may precipitate suicidal thoughts, feelings, or gestures, as illustrated in the following clinical example.

CLINICAL EXAMPLE

Mr. W was a 60-year-old man who lived alone. His son and daughter were married and lived in the same state as Mr. W. His wife had died 2 years before, and since that time his children had often asked him to move in with either of them. He consistently refused to do this, believing that he and his children needed privacy in their lives. Six months before, he was diagnosed as having advanced prostatic cancer with metastasis. After the diagnosis and because of increasing disability, he left his job and began to receive disability compensation. He visited his children and their families about twice a month and kept his regularly scheduled visits with the medical clinic.

The nurses and physicians at the clinic noted that he was "despondent and withdrawn" but viewed this as a normal reaction to his diagnosis and family history. No interventions were implemented based on his emotional needs. A week after attending the clinic for a routine follow-up visit, he went to the cemetery where his wife was buried and at her gravestone shot himself in the head. A groundskeeper of the cemetery heard the shot, discovered what had happened, and called an ambulance. Mr. W was taken to the emergency room of the nearest hospital and, with prompt medical care, survived the suicide attempt.

Selected Nursing Diagnoses

- Risk for suicide related to feelings of depression, as evidenced by gunshot to the head
- Hopelessness related to medical diagnosis of metastatic cancer, as evidenced by withdrawal and despondency ■

This example dramatically makes three important points. First, medical illness often involves a loss of function, body part, or appearance. Therefore all patients should be assessed for depression. Second, all people experiencing depression and despair have the potential for suicide. Third, nurses can intervene to support the grieving and mourning process, whether it is uncomplicated or pathological. Nursing actions can be preventive, curative, or rehabilitative, based on the nursing assessment and diagnosis.

Mania.   The essential feature of mania is a distinct period of intense **psychophysiological activation**. Some of the behaviors of mania are listed in Box 19-3. The predominant mood is **elevated** or **irritable**, accompanied by one or more of the following symptoms: hyperactivity, the undertaking of too many activities, lack of judgment in anticipating consequences, pressured speech, flight of ideas, distractibility, inflated self-esteem, and hypersexuality.

If the mood is elevated or euphoric, it is often infectious. Patients report feeling happy, unconcerned, carefree, and devoid of problems. Although such experiences seem enviable, the person also has no concern for reality or the feelings of others. The mood is often expansive, and some patients have extraordinary delusions about their power and importance. They characteristically involve themselves in seemingly senseless and risky enterprises.

Alternatively, the mood may be irritable, especially when plans are blocked. Patients can be argumentative and provoked by seemingly harmless remarks. Self-esteem is inflated during a manic episode, and as activity level increases, feelings about the self become increasingly disturbed. Delusional grandiose symptoms are evident, and the patient is willing to undertake any project possible.

In contrast to depressed patients, manic patients are extremely self-confident, with an ego that knows no bounds; they are "on top of the world." Accompanying this magical omnipotence and supreme self-esteem is an equally inordinate lack of guilt and shame. Often they deny realistic danger. The patient's boundless energy, cunning, planning, scheming, and inability to anticipate consequences often lead to irresponsible activities and excessive spending, as well as problems of a sexual, aggressive, or possessive nature.

In contrast to depressed patients, manic patients have abundant energy and heightened sexual appetite. Characteristic physical changes are caused by inadequate nutrition, partly because manic patients have no time to eat; serious weight loss is also related to their insomnia and overactivity. Extremely manic patients may become dehydrated and require prompt attention.

In addition to mood alterations, the person with mania may exhibit disturbed speech patterns. As mania intensifies, formal and logical speech is replaced by loud, rapid, and confusing language. This is often referred to as *pressured speech.* As the activated state increases, speech becomes laced with numerous plays on words and irrelevancies that can escalate to *loose associations* and *flight of ideas* (see Chapter 7). Some of these behaviors are evident in the next clinical example.

CLINICAL EXAMPLE

Mr. B was a 30-year-old single man who was admitted to the psychiatric unit of the local community hospital. He had been hospitalized 2 years before for problems related to alcoholism. He was accompanied to the hospital by a friend who lived with him. His friend said that for the past 2 months Mr. B had been "running on 10 cylinders instead of four." He slept and ate little and talked constantly, sometimes so fast that no one could understand what he was trying to say. He had redecorated his bedroom in the apartment twice and had gone into debt buying a new wardrobe. His friend brought him in because his behavior was becoming more erratic and his physical condition was failing.

The nurse who admitted Mr. B asked about his social relationships. He revealed that his girlfriend of 7 years had left him 6 months before for another man. He said that initially he thought she would "see the light," but she had refused to see him since then. Mr. B said this "upset" him a little at the time, but he was sure it was for the best and there were plenty other women waiting for him.

Selected Nursing Diagnosis
- Risk for self-directed violence related to interpersonal rejection, as evidenced by agitated behavior and lack of self-care ■

Other behaviors found in those with mania include *lability of mood* with rapid shifts to brief depression. Such behavior accounts for patients who alternately laugh and cry. In addition, *hallucinations, ideas of reference,* and *delusions* (see Chapter 7) may be present, along with predominant feelings of guilt and thoughts of suicide.

Manic episodes are very likely to recur. **About 75% of manic patients have more than one episode,** and almost all

---

BOX 19-3

Behaviors Associated With Mania

Affective
- Elation or euphoria
- Expansiveness
- Humorousness
- Inflated self-esteem
- Intolerance of criticism
- Lack of shame or guilt

Physiological
- Dehydration
- Inadequate nutrition
- Little need of sleep
- Weight loss

Cognitive
- Ambitiousness
- Denial of realistic danger
- Easily distracted
- Has flight of ideas

- Thoughts of grandiosity
- Has illusions
- Lack of judgment
- Loose associations

Behavioral
- Aggressiveness
- Excessive spending
- Grandiose acts
- Hyperactivity
- Increased motor activity
- Irresponsibility
- Irritability or argumentativeness
- Poor personal grooming
- Provocativeness
- Sexual overactivity
- Increased social activity
- Verbosity

those with manic episodes also have depressive episodes. However, the duration and severity of the manic episodes vary among patients, as do the intervals between relapses and recurrences.

Finally, disturbances of mood are interrelated with self-esteem problems and disrupted relationships. Multiple aspects of the patient's life are affected, including that of physical health. Hypertensive crises, irritable bowel syndrome, coronary occlusions, rheumatoid arthritis, migraine headaches, and various dermatological conditions can occur with severe mood disturbances.

Predisposing Factors

Genetics. It is widely agreed that both heredity and environment play an important role in severe mood disturbances. Major depression and bipolar disorder are familial disorders, and their familiarity primarily results from genetic influences (Merikangas et al, 2002; Sullivan, Neale, and Kendler, 2000). The lifetime risk for mood disorders in the general population is 6%. Family, twin, and adoption studies show that the lifetime risk is 20% for relatives of people with depression and 24% for relatives of people with mania. A person with an identical twin (monozygotic, or MZ) with an affective disorder is two to four times more at risk for the disorder than are fraternal twins (dizygotic, or DZ) or siblings. Thus good evidence exists for the role of genetic factors in mood disorders.

Aggression-Turned-Inward Theory. The aggression-turned-inward theory of Freud views depression as the inward turning of the aggressive instinct, which for some reason is not directed at the appropriate object and accompanied by feelings of guilt. The process is initiated by the loss of an ambivalently loved object. The person feels angry and loving at the same time and is unable to express anger because it is considered inappropriate or irrational. Also, the person may have developed a pattern throughout life of containing feelings, especially those that are viewed negatively. Angry feelings are then directed inward. Freud believed that if a person went so far as to commit suicide, the act was a strike against the hated and loved object as well as against the self.

In fact, little evidence supports this theory. Furthermore, the redirection of hostility at outside objects has not been consistently correlated with clinical improvement. In some instances it actually may have negative effects on the patient's view of self and problem resolution.

Object Loss Theory. The object loss theory of depression refers to traumatic separation of the person from significant objects of attachment. Two issues are important to this theory: loss during childhood as a predisposing factor for adult depressions and separation in adult life as a precipitating stress. The first issue proposes that a child has ordinarily formed a tie to a mother figure by 6 months of age, and once that tie is ruptured, the child experiences separation anxiety, grief, and mourning. Furthermore, this mourning in the early years often affects personality development and predisposes the child to psychiatric illness.

From a research point of view, the connection between early object loss and adult depression is complex. Some cast doubt on the universality of the responses described and suggest that appropriate mothering during the separation period can prevent their occurrence. Other studies indicate that depressed patients seem to experience more parental loss from death, separation, and other causes than do normal and other diagnostic groups. However, that factor alone does not seem to account for all forms of depression. Some discussion suggests that successfully coping with an early loss can be beneficial or have immunizing effects in the development of resilience.

Another perspective on this theory focuses on the negative impact of maternal depression on infants and children. This is expressed by the infant as flat affect, lower activity, disengagement, and difficulty in being consoled. Among older children it is seen as sadness, submissive helplessness, and social withdrawal. Older children of depressed parents also have a three to four times higher than average rate of adjustment problems, including a range of emotional disorders (Biederman et al, 2001). These observations lend a different but related view to the object loss theory. They suggest that emotional unavailability may be more stressful to children than physical separation. They also underscore the need for early and aggressive intervention by nurses for parents suffering from depression and for their children.

Personality Organization Theory. The personality organization view of depression focuses on the major psychosocial variable of low self-esteem. The patient's self-concept is an underlying issue, whether expressed as dejection and depression or as overcompensation with supreme competence, as displayed in manic and hypomanic episodes. Threats to self-esteem arise from poor role performance, perceived low-level everyday functioning, and the absence of a clear self-identity.

Three forms of personality organization that could lead to depression have been identified (Arieti and Bemporad, 1980). One, based on the "dominant other," occurs because the patient has relied on another for self-esteem. Satisfaction is experienced only through an intermediary. Clinging, passivity, manipulativeness, and avoidance of anger characterize the person with this type of depression. A lack of personal goals and a predominant focus on problems is noticeable.

Another form of personality disorder results when a person realizes that a desired but unrealistic goal may never be accomplished. This is the "dominant goal" type of depression. This person is usually reclusive, arrogant, and often obsessive. The person sets unrealistic goals and evaluates them with an all-or-nothing standard. An inordinate amount of time is spent in wishful thinking and introverted searches for meaning.

The third type of depression is seen as a constant mode of feeling. These patients inhibit any form of gratification because of strongly held taboos. They experience emptiness, hypochondriasis, pettiness in interpersonal relationships, and a harsh critical attitude toward themselves and others.

This view of depression looks at patients' belief systems in relation to their experiences. Even in the absence of an apparent precipitating stressor, their depression appears to be preceded by a severe blow to their self-esteem. It emphasizes the crucial position of self-concept in adaptation or maladaptation and the importance of patients' appraisal of their life situations.

Cognitive Model. The cognitive model proposes that people experience depression because their thinking is disturbed (Beck et al, 1979). Depression is seen as a cognitive problem dominated by a person's negative evaluation of self, the world, and the future. It suggests that in the course of development certain experiences sensitize people and make them vulnerable to depression. Such people also acquire a tendency to make extreme, absolute judgments.

The depression-prone person, according to this theory, is likely to explain an adverse event as a personal shortcoming. For example, the deserted husband believes "she left me because I'm unlovable," instead of considering other possible alternatives, such as personality incompatibility, the wife's own problems, or her change of feelings toward him. As he focuses on his personal deficiencies, they expand to the point where they completely dominate his self-concept. He can think of himself only in a negative way and is unable to acknowledge his other abilities, achievements, and attributes. This negative set is reinforced when he interprets ambiguous or neutral experiences as additional proof of his deficiencies. Comparisons with other people further lower his self-esteem, and thus every encounter with others becomes a negative experience. His self-criticisms increase as he views himself as deserving of blame.

Depressed patients become dominated by pessimism. Their predictions tend to be overgeneralized and extreme. Because they see the future as an extension of the present, they expect their failure to continue permanently. Thus pessimism dominates their activities, wishes, and expectations.

Depressed people are capable of logical self-evaluation when not in a depressed mood or when only mildly depressed. When depression does occur, after some precipitating life stressors, the negative cognitive set makes its appearance. As depression develops and increases, the negative thinking increasingly replaces objective thinking.

Although the onset of the depression may appear sudden, it develops over weeks, months, or even years as each life experience is interpreted as further evidence of failure. As a result of this tunnel vision, depressed people become hypersensitive to experiences of loss and defeat and become oblivious to experiences of success and pleasure. They have difficulty acknowledging anger because they think they are responsible for, and deserving of, insults from others and problems encountered in living. Along with low self-esteem, they experience apathy and indifference. They are drawn to a state of inactivity and withdraw from life. They lack all spontaneous desire and wish only to remain passive. Because they expect failure, they lack the ordinary energy to even make an effort.

Suicidal wishes can be viewed as an extreme expression of the desire to escape. Suicidal patients see their life as filled with suffering, with no chance of improvement. Given this negative set, suicide seems a rational solution. It promises to end their misery and relieve their families of a burden, and they begin to believe that everyone would be better off if they were dead. The more they consider the alternative of suicide, the more desirable it may seem, and as their life becomes more hopeless and painful, the desire to end it becomes stronger.

Naturalistic, clinical, and experimental studies have provided substantial support for this cognitive model of depression. Strong evidence of the efficacy of cognitive therapy as a treatment strategy for depressed patients also exists (Jarret et al, 2001).

Relate the cognitive model of depression to the adage "mind over matter." ■

Learned Helplessness-Hopelessness Model. Helplessness is a "belief that no one will do anything to aid you" and hopelessness is a belief that neither "you nor anyone else can do anything." This theory proposes that it is not trauma per se that produces depression, but the belief that one has no control over the important outcomes in life and therefore refrains from adaptive responses (Seligman, 1975). Learned helplessness is both a behavioral state and a personality trait of one who believes that control over the reinforcers in the environment has been lost. These negative expectations lead to hopelessness, passivity, and an inability to assert oneself.

People resistant to depression have high self-efficacy and have experienced mastery in life. Their childhood experiences proved to them that their actions were effective in producing gratification and removing annoyances. In contrast, those susceptible to depression have low self-efficacy and have had lives devoid of mastery. Their experiences caused them to believe that they were helpless and incapable of influencing their sources of suffering and they developed no coping responses against failure.

This model has been revised to include the hopelessness theory of depression (Abramson et al, 1989). It suggests that inferred negative consequences and negative characteristics about the self contribute to the formation of hopelessness and, in turn, the symptoms of hopelessness contribute to depression. Hopelessness theory thus is very similar to the cognitive model of depression.

Behavioral Model. The behavioral model views people as being capable of exercising control over their own behavior (Lewinsohn et al, 1979). They do not merely react to external influences. They select, organize, and transform incoming stimuli. Thus people are not viewed as powerless objects controlled by their environments; nor are they absolutely free to do whatever they choose. Rather, people and their environment affect each other.

The concept of reinforcement is crucial to this view of depression. Person-environment interactions with positive outcomes provide positive reinforcement. Such interactions strengthen the person's behavior. Little or no rewarding interaction with the environment causes the person to feel sad.

Thus the key assumption in this model is that a low rate of positive reinforcement is the antecedent of depressive behaviors.

Two elements of this model are important. One is that the person may fail to produce appropriate responses that will initiate positive reinforcement. The other is that the environment may fail to provide reinforcement and thus worsen the patient's condition. This occurs because depressed patients are often deficient in the social skills needed to interact with others effectively. In turn, other people find the behavior of depressed people distancing, negative, or offensive and therefore often avoid them as much as possible.

Depression is likely to occur if certain positively reinforcing events are absent, particularly those that fall into the following categories:

- Competence experiences
- Rewarding social interaction
- Enjoyable outdoor activities
- Solitude
- Positive sexual experiences

These may be described as "being with friends," "being relaxed," "doing my job well," "being sexually attractive," and "doing things my own way." Depression also occurs in the presence of certain punishing events, particularly those that fall into three categories:

1. Marital or interpersonal discord
2. Work or school hassles
3. Negative reactions from others

The behavioral model of depression emphasizes an active approach to the person and relies heavily on an interactional view of personality. Treatment is aimed at helping the person increase the quantity and quality of positively reinforcing interactions and decrease aversive interactions.

How many positive reinforcing events have you experienced this month? How many punishing events? Relate these to your overall mood. ◼

Biological Model. The biological model explores chemical changes in the body during depressed states. Whether these chemical changes cause depression or are a result of depression is not yet understood. However, significant abnormalities can be seen in many body systems during a depressive illness, including electrolyte disturbances, especially of sodium and potassium; neurophysiological alterations; dysfunction and faulty regulation of autonomic nervous system activity; adrenocortical, thyroid, and gonadal changes; and neurochemical alterations in the neurotransmitters, especially in the biogenic amines, which act as central nervous system and peripheral neurotransmitters. The biogenic amines include three catecholamines—dopamine, norepinephrine, and epinephrine—as well as serotonin and acetylcholine. Most researchers agree that no single biochemical model adequately explains the affective disorders.

Endocrine system. The possibility of hormonal causes of depression has been considered for many years. Some symptoms of depression that suggest endocrine changes are decreased appetite, weight loss, insomnia, diminished sex drive, gastrointestinal disorders, and variations of mood. New assay techniques have recently detected alterations of hormone activity concurrent with depression. Mood changes also have been observed with a variety of endocrine disorders, including Cushing's disease, hyperthyroidism, and estrogen therapy. Further support for this theory is evident in the high incidence of depression during the postpartum period, when hormonal levels change.

Current study of neuroendocrine factors in affective disorders emphasizes the disinhibition of the hypothalamic-pituitary-adrenal (HPA) axis and the hypothalamic-pituitary-thyroid (HPT) axis. Two tests based on the neuroendocrine theory and performed clinically may prove to be useful in diagnosing affective illnesses. The first is the corticotropin-releasing factor stimulation test, which evaluates the pituitary's ability to respond to corticotropin-releasing hormone (CRH) and secrete sufficient amounts of adrenal corticotropin hormone (ACTH) to induce normal adrenal activity. The second test is the thyroid-releasing hormone (TRH) infusion test, which differs from CRH infusion by assessing the pituitary's ability to secrete sufficient amounts of thyroid-stimulating hormones (TSH) to produce normal thyroid activity. These tests may be helpful in differentiating unipolar from bipolar depression and mania from schizophrenic psychosis.

Cortisol. Many depressed patients exhibit hypersecretion of cortisol. This has been used in the dexamethasone suppression test (DST) (dexamethasone is an exogenous steroid that suppresses the blood level of cortisol). The DST is based on the observation that, in patients with biological depression, late afternoon cortisol levels are not suppressed after a single dose of dexamethasone. However, many physical illnesses and some medications can interfere with the test results.

Neurotransmission. One of the dominant theories in the neurobiology of mood disorders is the **dysregulation hypothesis**, which proposes that a problem exists in several of the neurotransmitter systems. Specifically, there is substantial evidence for the abnormal regulation of the **serotonin (5-HT)** neurotransmitter system (Figure 19-2). This dysregulation is in either the amount or the availability of 5-HT, in the sensitivity of its receptors in relevant regions of the brain and in its balance with other neurotransmitters and brain chemicals. Several areas of research support a role for serotonin in depression.

BEHAVIOR. 5-HT has an important role in brain functions such as aggression, mood, anxiety, psychomotor activity, irritability, appetite, sexual activity, sleep/wakefulness, circadian and seasonal rhythms, neuroendocrine function, body temperature, cognitive function, and pain perception, processes that are abnormal in people with depression.

BIOCHEMISTRY. Research has shown that there is decreased 5-HT availability in patients with depression—too little 5-HT, its precursor (tryptophan), or its major metabolite (5-HIAA) in the cerebrospinal fluid or blood of people with depression and in the postmortem brains of depressed people who died of other causes and in people who committed suicide.

NEUROENDOCRINE. 5-HT has an important role in the secretion of growth hormone, prolactin, and cortisol, all of which are found to be abnormal in people with depression.

TREATMENT. Most clinically effective biological antidepressant agents, such as drugs and electroconvulsive therapy (ECT), have been found to enhance the neurotransmission of 5-HT, although the mechanisms of actions differ from each other.

BRAIN IMAGING. Computed tomography (CT) and magnetic resonance imaging (MRI) studies find various abnormalities in the structure of brains in people with mood disorders. MRI studies of depressed patients show a decrease in the size of the hippocampus, supporting the hypothesis that increased levels of stress hormones are associated with damage to the hippocampus (a limbic structure involved in learning and memory). MRI studies also show that brain structures responsible for human mood are larger in bipolar patients compared with controls. Specifically, the amygdala (the limbic structure responsible for modulating feelings of aggression, anger, love, and shyness) is especially large, perhaps accounting for some of the heightened emotionality and problematic behaviors seen in manic patients.

Positron emission tomography (PET) studies of mood disorders consistently show decreased frontal lobe brain metabolism (hypometabolism), which is generally more pronounced on the left hemisphere in depression and on the right hemisphere in mania. This means that the frontal lobes, which have an important role in intellectual and emotional activities, are not using as much glucose as they should (Figure 19-3). Prefrontal cortex hypometabolism affects the function of many of the brain structures connected with it by way of the 5-HT system. It is hypothesized that these interconnections facilitate the varied symptoms of depression (Table 19-3).

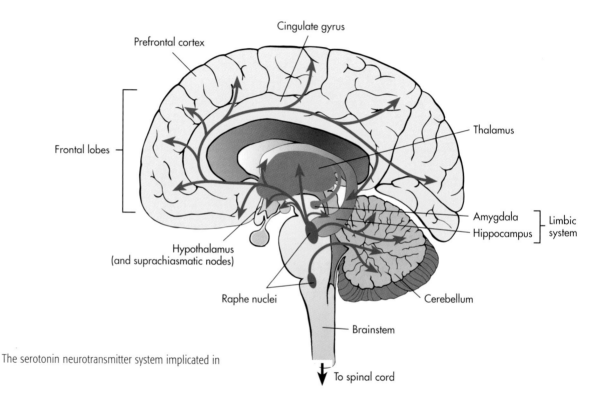

Figure 19-2 The serotonin neurotransmitter system implicated in depression.

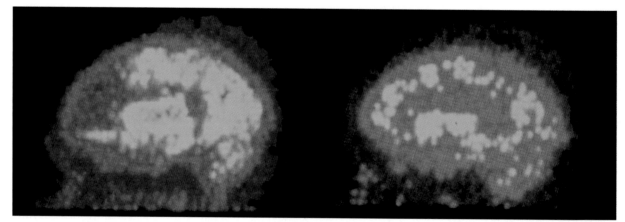

Figure 19-3 PET scan of glucose use in depressed subject *(figure on left)* showing frontal hypometabolism (left side of figure). This improves after treatment with antidepressant medication *(figure on right);* note increased glucose metabolism in frontal lobe (left side of figure).

Also, the amygdala shows increased blood flow, which is associated with intrusive ruminations in people with severe recurrent depression and a family history of mood disorders.

Several important implications of viewing depression as a brain-based illness of the prefrontal cortex are noted:

- Cognitive and interpersonal therapies may be viewed as prefrontal rehabilitation because they substitute for, then gradually bring back on line, some of the behaviors and cognitions compromised by prefrontal cortex (PFC) hypoactivity.
- Viewing depression as a disease with identified regional brain dysfunction helps destigmatize depression and reintegrate mood disorders into modern health care.
- Changes in brain metabolism identified by neuroimaging studies may help with the understanding of how psychosocial stressors such as grief (a hyperactivity in the PFC) may evolve into the clinical syndrome of depression (a hypoactivity in the PFC).

Biological rhythms. Mood disorders are also typified by periodic variations in physiological and psychological functions. Affective illnesses are usually recurrent, with episodes often occurring and remitting spontaneously. Two subtypes of mood disorders are specifically cyclical in nature: rapid cycling bipolar disorder and depressive disorder with seasonal patterns. In the first, cycles may endure for days, weeks, months, or years. In seasonal affective disorder (SAD), cycles occur annually in the same season each year, as people react to changes in environmental factors such as climate, latitude, or light.

People who are depressed or manic have certain characteristic changes in biological rhythms and related physiology. For instance, body temperature and certain hormones reach their peak earlier than normal; some depressed patients are more sensitive to the absence of sunlight than nondepressed people; and many depressed people experience circadian rhythm disturbances such as diurnal variation and early morning awakening.

The neurotransmitter **melatonin (a synthesis of serotonin in the pineal gland),** which is secreted with darkness and suppressed with bright light, is believed to regulate hypothalamic hormones involved in the generation of circadian rhythms and the synchronization of such rhythms to variations in environmental light. The human sleep cycle appears to be linked to the timing of human circadian rhythms and to malfunctions in the brain's ability to follow environmental cues such as light and darkness; to unusual environmental situations such as long, dark winters in northern latitudes; or to disturbances in the intensity of the circadian rhythm, such as those caused by sleep problems, body temperature changes, mood cycling, and endocrine system (hormones such as cortisol and thyrotrophin) abnormalities.

Sleep problems associated with depression have to do with the timing of rapid eye movement (REM) sleep. Sleep electroencephalograph (EEG) studies are abnormal in 90% of depressed patients. Normally on falling asleep, the brain cycles through each stage of sleep for 60 to 90 minutes before it reaches stage 5, or REM (dream sleep). The time between the initiation of sleep and the occurrence of the first REM period is called REM latency. Depressed patients reach REM too early in the night (in just 5 to 30 minutes); spend less time in the more refreshing slow wave stages of sleep (stages 3 and 4); spend too much time in REM sleep (up to twice as long as the first REM period in nondepressed people); and have increased periods of either very light sleep or awakenings during the night (Figure 19-4). This explains why depressed patients complain of feeling tired and unrefreshed after a night's sleep. They experience a decrease in total sleep time, an

Table 19-3	Prefrontal Cortex and Serotonin Interconnections: Implications in Depression	
INTERCONNECTED BRAIN STRUCTURES	**HYPOTHESIZED ROLE OF THESE INTERCONNECTIONS IN DEPRESSION**	
Prefrontal cortex	Covering the frontal lobes, it is unique within the CNS for its strong interconnections with all other areas of the brain; it receives information that has already been processed by other sensory areas and then merges this information with other emotional, historical, or relevant information, thus attending to both feelings and intellect.	
Limbic system structures	The prefrontal cortex modulates limbic system activities (emotional and instinctive) by way of these three structures:	
	Hippocampus	Major importance in cognitive function, including memory.
	Amygdala	Major importance in modulating feelings such as aggression, anger, love, and shyness.
	Cingulate gyrus	Involved in motivation and interest.
Brainstem	Responsible for regulating the general state of arousal and tone of brain function; also the location of structures that manufacture various neurotransmitters, such as serotonin (5-HT), norepinephrine (NE), and dopamine (DA).	
Raphe nuclei	Located in the brainstem, they manufacture 5-HT; they also modulate excessive stimuli, and the organization and coordination of appropriate responses to these stimuli.	
Hypothalamus	This interconnection allows for direct prefrontal input into neuroendocrine function via the hypothalamic-pituitary axes.	
Suprachiasmatic nucleus	Located in the hypothalamus, it regulates circadian (24-hour) rhythms and circannual rhythms; thus it is also implicated in seasonal affective disorder.	

CNS, Central nervous system.

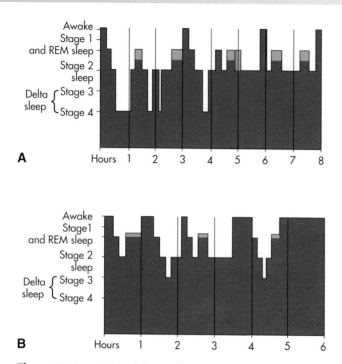

Figure 19-4 **A,** Normal sleep architecture. **B,** Depressed sleep architecture. Green areas indicate REM sleep.

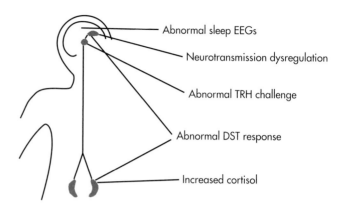

Figure 19-5 Biological factors related to depression. *EEGs,* Electroencephalograms, *TRH,* thyroid-releasing hormone, *DST,* dexamethasone suppression test.

increase in the percentage of dream time, difficulty in falling asleep, and an increased number of spontaneous awakenings.

Kindling. When an animal's brain is given intermittent and repeated stimulation by low-level electrical impulses or low-dose chemicals such as cocaine, the result is an increased responsiveness to stable, low doses of the stimulation over time, resulting eventually in seizures. A similar response can be elicited by environmental stimulation. **This sensitizing phenomenon is known as** kindling**.** Ultimately the animal becomes so sensitive that seizures continue to occur spontaneously after the stimulation is discontinued, demonstrating "behavioral sensitization." It is theorized that kindling underlies the addictive disorders and the cycling and recurrent psychiatric disorders.

Theoretically, early episodes of mania and depression in humans may be precipitated by psychosocial stressors in genetically vulnerable individuals, but later episodes can occur in the absence of any apparent external stimulus and with greater frequency and intensity over time. Additional evidence of a role for kindling in mood disorders is that many of the neurotransmitters implicated in the mood disorders inhibit kindling. Drugs used to treat bipolar disorder also affect kindling: lithium blocks behavioral sensitization and the anticonvulsants block kindling itself. Thus the effect of the environment on a vulnerable brain is the focus of ongoing research on these disorders.

The puzzle of the biology of mood disorders has many different pieces; as yet an all-inclusive hypothesis has not been formulated. It is likely, however, that mood disorders occur because integrated control systems are disrupted, as evidenced

by dysregulation in neurotransmitter systems and by the fact that the brain mechanisms that control hormonal balance and biological rhythms are implicated in mood disorders.

What is clear is that the etiologies are diverse, so the treatments must be both diverse and specific to the biopsychosocial context of the individual patient. Kindling and behavioral sensitization research suggest that early detection, aggressive treatment of acute episodes, and adequate long-term prophylactic treatment might inhibit or even prevent a progressively deteriorating course of illness. Some of the biological bases of depression are shown in Figure 19-5.

A pastor preaches about how depression results from "poor moral character" and "personal weakness." How would you respond? ■

Precipitating Stressors

Disturbances of mood are a specific response to stress. There are two major types of stress. The first is the stress of **major life events** that is evident to other people. The second type, the minor stress or **irritations of daily life** that a person may feel, may not be obvious to others. These are the small disappointments, frustrations, criticisms, and arguments that, when accumulated over time and in the absence of compensating positive events, have a major and chronic negative impact. Stressors that may produce disturbances of mood include loss of attachment, major life events, roles, and physiological changes.

Loss of Attachment. Loss in adult life can precipitate depression. The loss may be real or imagined and may include the loss of love, a person, physical functioning, status, or self-esteem. Many losses take on importance because of their symbolic meaning, which makes the reactions to them appear out of proportion to reality. In this sense, even an apparently pleasurable event, such as moving to a new home, may involve the loss of old friends, warm memories, and neighborhood associations. Loss of hope is another significant stressor often overlooked. Because of the actual and symbolic issues involved in loss, the patient's perception is of primary importance.

Factors That Influence the Mourning Process

- Childhood experiences, especially the loss of significant others
- Losses experienced later in life
- History of psychiatric illness, especially depression
- Occurrence of life crises before the loss
- Nature of the relationship with the lost person or object, including kinship, strength of attachment, security of attachment, dependency bonds, and intensity of ambivalence
- Process of dying (when applicable), including age of deceased, timeliness, previous warnings, preparation for bereavement, expression of feelings, and preventability of the loss
- Social support systems
- Secondary stresses
- Emergent life opportunities

The intensity of grief becomes meaningful only when the person understands earlier losses and separations. People reacting to a recent loss often behave as they did in previous separations. The intensity of the present reaction therefore becomes more understandable with the realization that the reaction is to earlier losses as well. By definition loss is negative, a deprivation. The ability to sustain, integrate, and recover from loss is a sign of personal maturity and growth.

An uncomplicated grief reaction is the process of normal mourning or simple bereavement. Mourning includes a complex sequence of psychological processes. It is accompanied by anxiety, anger, pain, despair, and hope. The sequence is not a smooth, unvarying course. It is filled with turmoil, regressions, and potential problems. Certain factors have been identified that influence the outcome of mourning (Box 19-4).

These factors should be assessed by the nurse for each person experiencing a loss. Two of the factors—the nature of the relationship with the lost person or object and the mourner's perception of the preventability of the loss—have been identified as prime predictors of the intensity and duration of the bereavement. Concurrent crises, the circumstances of the loss, and a pathological relationship with the lost person or object are other factors that contribute to a failure to resolve grief.

Inhibiting factors. Loss of a loved one is a major stressor that precipitates grief reactions. Most people resolve this loss through simple bereavement and do not experience pathological grief or depression. However, various external and internal factors can inhibit mourning. An external factor may be the immersion of the mourner in practical, necessary tasks that accompany the loss but are not directly connected to the emotional fact of the loss. These tasks may include funeral arrangements, unfinished business of the deceased, or a search for immediate employment. All of these tasks foster denial of the loss. Denial also may be encouraged by cultural norms that minimize or negate the finality of the loss. The American norm of "courage in the face of adversity" can prevent an open display of grief.

Mourning also may be inhibited when the bereaved lack support from their social network. Nonsupportiveness suppresses grieving when significant others inhibit mourners' expression of sadness, anger, and guilt, block their review of the lost relationship, and attempt to orient them too quickly to the future. Finally, the widespread use of tranquilizers and antidepressant medications may suppress normal grief and encourage pathological reactions.

Internal factors that inhibit mourning are often fostered by a society that encourages the control and concealment of feelings. Crying, for example, may be seen as weakness, especially in men. Grief and anger are particularly repressed in our society, and this repression may create many emotional problems. Another inhibitor is the belief that the quantity and quality of emotion are unique and cannot be communicated.

Finally, some studies have failed to demonstrate a relationship between loss and depression. Other studies support the relationship but suggest that depression may be the cause of alienation and object loss, and not vice versa. Thus the following conclusions may be proposed:

- Loss and separation events are possible precipitating stressors of depression.
- Loss and separation are not present in all depressions.
- Not all people who experience loss and separation develop depressions.
- Loss and separation are not specific to depression but may act as precipitating events for a variety of psychiatric and medical illnesses.
- Loss and separation may result *from* depression.

Life Events. Adverse life events are a potent factor in precipitating depression (Mazure et al, 2000). Such events include loss of self-esteem, interpersonal discord, socially undesirable occurrences, and major disruptions of life patterns. Events perceived as undesirable are most often the precipitants of depression. Exit events (separations and losses) more often than entrance events (additions and introductions) are followed by worsening of psychiatric symptoms, physical health changes, impairment of social role performance, and depressive illnesses. The concept of exit events overlaps with the psychiatric concept of loss.

Certain types of events also may prove to be more important than others. For example, childhood physical and sexual abuse has been found to be associated with high depressive symptoms in women. In addition, the presence of multiple family disadvantages, such as marital or family disruption, parental physical illness, poor physical care of child and home, social dependence, family overcrowding, and poor mothering in early life have been found to be associated with depression in adulthood. Research also suggests that although stressful life events do have a causal relationship with the onset of major depression, some of this effect may result because individuals who are predisposed to depression have chosen to live in high-risk environments.

Thus any conclusions about life events should be made with caution. All people experience stressful life events, but

Table 19-4	Physical Illness and Medications Associated With Depressive and Manic States	
	DEPRESSION	MANIA
Physical Illness		
Infectious	Influenza	Influenza
	Viral hepatitis	St. Louis encephalitis
	Infectious mononucleosis	Q fever
	General paresis (tertiary syphilis)	General paresis (tertiary syphilis)
	Tuberculosis	
Endocrine	Myxedema	Hyperthyroidism
	Hypothyroidism	
	Cushing's disease	
	Addison's disease	
	Diabetes mellitus	
Neoplastic	Occult abdominal malignancies (such as carcinoma of head of pancreas)	
	Carcinoid	
	Oat cell carcinoma	
Rheumatologic	Systemic lupus erythematosus	Systemic lupus erythematosus
	Chronic fatigue syndrome	Rheumatic chorea
	Fibromyalgia	Multiple sclerosis
	Rheumatoid arthritis	Diencephalic and third-ventricular tumors
Neurological	Multiple sclerosis	
	Cerebral tumors	
	Sleep apnea	
	Dementia	
	Parkinson's disease	
	Nondominant temporal lobe lesions	
Cardiovascular	Stroke	
	Coronary artery disease	
Nutritional	Pellagra	
	Pernicious anemia	
Metabolic	Electrolyte disturbance	
	Renal failure	
Gastrointestinal	Irritable bowel syndrome	
	Cirrhosis	
	Hepatic encephalopathy	
Medications		
	Alcohol	Amphetamines
	Alpha-methyldopa	Cocaine
	Amphetamine withdrawal	Levodopa
	Benzodiazepines	Methylphenidate
	Cycloserine	Monoamine oxidase inhibitors
	Glucocorticoids	Steroids
	Levodopa	Thyroid hormones
	Neuroleptics	Tricyclic antidepressants
	Physostigmine	
	Propranolol	
	Reserpine	
	Sedative-hypnotics	
	Steroidal contraceptives	

not all people become depressed. This suggests that specific events can contribute only partially to the development of depression.

Role Strain. In analyzing social role stressors, much of the literature focuses on women. This reflects the predominance of depression among women and the increasing interest in gender socialization processes and women's changing roles (Miranda et al, 2002b). Role strain in marriage emerges as a major stressor related to depression for both men and women. Research also suggests that being married has a protective effect for males but a detrimental effect for females.

Another role-related risk factor for women is exposure to chronic stressors such as those experienced in their classic role as caregivers. These present specific psychosocial and biological challenges, including the following:

- The perinatal period, with its subsequent sleep-disrupting infant care demands, which comes immediately after hormonal, biochemical, and social disruptions associated with pregnancy
- The predominantly female caretaking role for spouses and parents with age- or Alzheimer's-related dementias, which can cause the same sleep disruption experienced by mothers of infants
- Achievement-motivated women who take needed time from sleep in order to juggle full-time family and social roles in addition to work and educational commitments
- Shift work that does not follow a forward rotation (days to evenings to nights) with adequate adjustment for each shift change

If these special stressors for women are combined with other rhythm-disrupting processes, such as seasonal light changes, and other risk factors for depression, such as family history and inadequate support systems and primary relationships, a woman has a gender- and role-based risk for depression.

Describe how the early socialization of young girls in contemporary society might affect their cognitive and emotional coping responses. Compare this to the experiences of young boys. ■

Physiological Changes. Mood states are affected by a wide variety of physical illnesses and medications (Table 19-4). Drug-induced depressions can follow treatment with antihypertensive drugs, particularly reserpine, and the abuse of addictive substances such as amphetamines, barbiturates, cocaine, and alcohol. Depression also may occur secondary to medical illnesses, such as viral infections, nutritional deficiencies, endocrine disorders, anemias, and central nervous system disorders such as multiple sclerosis, tumors, and cerebrovascular disease. Most chronic debilitating illnesses, whether physical or psychiatric, are accompanied by depression.

The depressions of the elderly are particularly complex because the differential diagnosis often involves organic brain damage and clinical depression. Diagnostic differentiation is complicated (Alexopoulos et al, 2002; Ranga, 2002). People with early signs of senile brain changes, vascular disease, or other neurological diseases of aging may be more at risk for depression than the general population. In the United States there has been a tendency to overdiagnose arteriosclerosis and senility in people over age 65, without recognizing that depression may manifest itself by a slowing of psychomotor activity. Lowered intellectual function and a loss of interest in sex, hobbies, and activities may be taken as signs of brain disease.

Mania also can be a secondary reaction to taking drugs, particularly steroids, amphetamines, and tricyclic antidepressants. It can be triggered by infections, neoplasms, and metabolic disturbances. The evidence that mania can result from pharmacological, structural, and metabolic disturbances suggests that mania, like depression, is a clinical syndrome with multiple causes. The diversity of causes probably involves more than one pathophysiological pathway and challenges any one model of causation, whether biochemical, psychological, genetic, or structural.

Appraisal of Stressors

Debate continues over the nature of depression, that is, whether depression is a single illness with different signs and symptoms or whether several different forms of the disease exist. It is clear, however, that there is an interactive effect among predisposing and precipitating factors that are biological and psychosocial in origin. This underscores the importance of one's appraisal of one's life situation and related stressors. Table 19-5 summarizes these major theories of causation.

Coping Resources

Personal resources include one's socioeconomic status (income, occupation, social position, education), family (nuclear, extended), social support networks, and secondary organizations provided by the broader social environment (see

Table 19-5	Summary of Models of Causation of Severe Mood Disturbances
MODEL	MECHANISM
Genetic	Transmission through heredity and family history
Aggression turned inward	Turning angry feelings against oneself
Object loss	Separation from loved one and disruption of attachment bond
Personality organization	Negative self-concept and low self-esteem influence belief system and appraisal of stressors
Cognitive	Hopelessness experienced because of negative cognitive set
Learned helplessness-hopelessness	Belief that responses are ineffectual and that reinforcers in the environment cannot be controlled
Behavioral	Loss of positive reinforcement in life
Biological	Impaired monoaminergic neurotransmission
Life stressors	Response to life stress from four possible sources: loss of attachment, life events, role strain, and physiological changes
Integrative	Interaction of biopsychosocial predisposing and precipitating factors

A Family Speaks). The far-ranging effects of poverty, discrimination, inadequate housing, and social isolation cannot be ignored or taken lightly. Thus nursing interventions that foster the person's ability to develop capacities for coping with life's disruptions are very important. The **risk factors for depression** are listed in Box 19-5.

Coping Mechanisms

Uncomplicated grief reactions can be normal mourning or simple bereavement. Mourning includes all of the psychological processes set in motion by the loss. Mourning begins with the **introjection** of the lost object. In grieving the person's feelings are directed toward a mental image of the loved one. Thus the mechanism of introjection serves as a buffering mechanism. Through reality testing the person realizes that the loved person or object no longer exists, and then the

A FAMILY SPEAKS

It's hard for me to imagine how life could be so bad that my beautiful and loving 22-year-old daughter couldn't get out of bed in the morning and cried most of the day. It all started when she quit college and returned home and told us about the biggest mistake she had made in her life. While at school, she accidentally got pregnant and then had an abortion. Since that event, she said she had felt worthless, immoral, and extremely guilty.

We talked about it, and I suggested that she get help. She saw two different mental health professionals but dropped out of therapy with each one after only a couple of visits. Then one of my friends recommended a nurse who specialized in working with women with depression. My daughter saw her twice a week initially, then once a week, and finally monthly. My daughter was able to open up to this nurse and together they worked at changing my daughter's negative thoughts, feelings, and behaviors. She kept a diary and began to call friends and socialize once again.

Today, 8 months later, my daughter has a job and is going to college part-time in the evenings. Sometimes when I look at her, she seems like a different person to me—so much more grown up and mature. I'm sorry for her pain, but I know that now she is a stronger and wiser person for having endured it.

BOX 19-5

Risk Factors for Depression

- Prior episodes of depression
- Family history of depression
- Prior suicide attempts
- Female gender
- Age at onset less than 40 years
- Postpartum period
- Medical comorbidity
- Lack of social support
- Stressful life events
- Personal history of sexual abuse
- Current substance abuse

emotional investment is withdrawn from it. The ultimate outcome is that reality wins out, but this is accomplished slowly over time. When the mourning work is completed, the ego becomes free to invest in new objects.

A delayed grief reaction uses the defense mechanisms of denial and suppression in an attempt to avoid intense distress. Specific defenses used to block mourning are **repression, suppression, denial,** and **dissociation.** Denial of the loss in depression results in profound feelings of guilt, anger, and despair that focus on the person's own unworthiness. Manic and hypomanic episodes are more rare than depressive states. Some believe that mania is a mirror image of depression and that, even though the behaviors are dissimilar, the dynamics and coping mechanisms are related. According to this view, manic behavior is a defense against depression because the person attempts to deny feelings of worthlessness and helplessness.

DIAGNOSIS

The diagnosis of mood disturbances depends on an understanding of many interrelated concepts, including anxiety and self-concept. One task of the nurse in formulating a diagnosis is to determine whether the patient is experiencing primarily a state of anxiety or depression. It is often difficult to distinguish between the two because they may co-exist in one patient and are manifested by similar behaviors. The differences between anxiety and depression are presented in Chapter 16 (see Box 16-7).

Figure 19-6 presents the Stuart Stress Adaptation Model with the continuum of emotional responses. The maladaptive responses are a result of anxiety, hostility, self-devaluation, and guilt. This model suggests that nursing care should be centered around increasing self-esteem and encouraging expression of emotions.

Nursing Diagnoses

The primary NANDA nursing diagnoses related to maladaptive emotional responses are **dysfunctional grieving, hopelessness, powerlessness, spiritual distress, risk for suicide** and **risk for self-directed violence.** Nursing diagnoses related to the range of possible maladaptive responses are identified in the Medical and Nursing Diagnoses box (Box 19-6). Examples of expanded nursing diagnoses are presented in the Detailed Diagnoses table (Table 19-6).

How do you think "spiritual distress" relates to mood disorders? ■

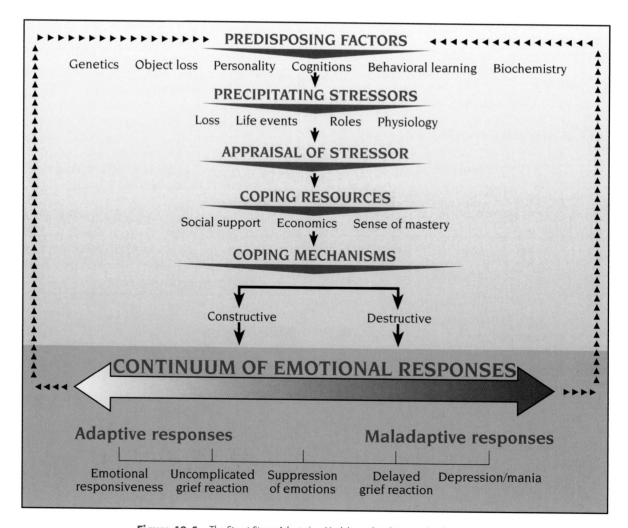

Figure 19-6   The Stuart Stress Adaptation Model as related to emotional responses.

■ ▦ **BOX 19-6** *Medical and Nursing Diagnoses Related to* **Emotional Responses**

RELATED MEDICAL DIAGNOSES (*DSM-IV-TR*)*	RELATED NURSING DIAGNOSES (NANDA)†
Bipolar I disorder	Anxiety
Bipolar II disorder	Communication, Impaired verbal
Cyclothymic disorder	Coping, Ineffective
Major depressive disorder	Grieving, Anticipatory
Dysthymic disorder	**Grieving, Dysfunctional‡**
	Hopelessness‡
	Powerlessness‡
	Self-esteem, Chronic low or Situational low
	Sexual dysfunction
	Sleep pattern, Disturbed
	Social isolation
	Spiritual distress‡
	Suicide, Risk for‡
	Violence, Risk for self-directed‡

*From American Psychiatric Association: *Diagnostic and statistical manual of mental disorders*, ed 4, text revision, Washington, DC, 2000, American Psychiatric Association.
†From North American Nursing Diagnosis Association: *NANDA nursing diagnoses: definitions and classification 2003-2004*, Philadelphia, 2003, The Association.
‡**Primary nursing diagnoses for disturbances in mood.**

Table 19-6   *Detailed Diagnoses Related to* **Emotional Responses**   ▦ ■

NANDA DIAGNOSIS STEM	EXAMPLES OF EXPANDED DIAGNOSIS
Dysfunctional grieving	Dysfunctional grieving related to death of sister, as evidenced by self-devaluation, sleep disturbance, and dejected mood
Hopelessness	Hopelessness related to loss of job, as evidenced by feelings of despair and development of ulcerative colitis
Powerlessness	Powerlessness related to new role as parent, as evidenced by apathy, uncertainty, and overdependency
Spiritual distress	Spiritual distress related to loss of child in utero, as evidenced by self-blame, somatic complaints, and pessimism about the future
Risk for self-directed violence	Risk for self-directed violence related to rejection by boyfriend, as evidenced by self-destructive acts
Risk for suicide	Risk for suicide related to impending divorce, as evidenced by giving away personal possessions and purchasing a handgun

DSM-IV-TR DIAGNOSIS	ESSENTIAL FEATURES*
Bipolar I disorder	Current or past experience of a manic episode, lasting at least 1 week, when one's mood was abnormally and persistently elevated, expansive, or irritable. The episode is severe enough to cause extreme impairment in social or occupational functioning. Bipolar disorders may be classified as manic (limited to manic episodes), depressed (a history of manic episodes with a current depressive episode), or mixed (presentation of both manic and depressive episodes).
Bipolar II disorder	Presence or history of one or more major depressive episodes and at least one hypomanic episode. No manic episode has developed.
Cyclothymic disorder	A history of 2 years of hypomania in which the person experienced numerous periods with abnormally elevated, expansive, or irritable moods. These moods did not meet the criteria for a manic episode, and many periods of depressed mood did not meet the criteria of a major depressive disorder.
Major depressive disorder	Presence of at least five symptoms during the same 2-week period, with one being either depressed mood or loss of interest or pleasure. Other symptoms might include weight loss, insomnia, psychomotor agitation or retardation, fatigue, feelings of worthlessness, diminished ability to think, and recurrent thoughts of death. Major depression may be classified as single episode or recurrent.
Dysthymic disorder	At least 2 years of a usually depressed mood and at least one of the symptoms mentioned for major depression without meeting the criteria for a major depressive episode.

*From American Psychiatric Association: *Diagnostic and statistical manual of mental disorders*, ed 4, text revision, Washington, DC, 2000, American Psychiatric Association.

Medical Diagnoses

A distinction has been made between primary and secondary affective disorders. **Primary affective disorders** occur in patients who have been well or whose only previous episodes of psychiatric disease were mania or depression. **Secondary affective disorders** include feelings of sadness, inadequacy, and hopelessness that occur with another preexisting psychiatric disorder, such as anxiety reactions. They also include symptoms secondary to medical illnesses.

Two major categories of mood or affective disorders are identified in the *DSM-IV-TR*: **bipolar disorders** and **depressive disorders**. Primary *DSM-IV-TR* diagnoses include **bipolar I and II disorders, cyclothymic disorder, major depressive disorder,** and **dysthymic disorder** (American Psychiatric Association, 2000a). Cyclothymia is a disorder resembling bipolar disorder with less severe symptoms, characterized by repeated periods of nonpsychotic depression and hypomania for at least 2 years. Dysthymia is a milder form of depression lasting 2 or more years. As such, it is a chronic condition, and almost all patients with dysthymia eventually develop major depressive episodes (Klein et al, 2000).

The specific disorders are described in the Detailed Diagnoses table (see Table 19-6). Diagnostic criteria for a major depressive episode and a manic episode are listed in Box 19-7.

BOX 19-7

Diagnostic Criteria for Major Depressive and Manic Episodes

Major Depressive Episode
At least five of the following (including one of the first two) must be present most of the day, nearly daily, for at least 2 weeks:
Depressed mood
Loss of interest or pleasure
Weight loss or gain
Insomnia or hypersomnia
Psychomotor agitation or retardation
Fatigue or loss of energy
Feelings of worthlessness
Impaired concentration
Thoughts of death or suicide

Manic Episode
At least three of the following must be present to a significant degree for at least 1 week:
Grandiosity
Decreased need for sleep
Pressured speech
Flight of ideas
Distractibility
Psychomotor agitation
Excessive involvement in pleasurable activities without regard for negative consequences

Modified from American Psychiatric Association: *Diagnostic and statistical manual of mental disorders*, ed 4, text revision, Washington, DC, 2000, American Psychiatric Association.

OUTCOME IDENTIFICATION

The expected outcome when working with a patient with a maladaptive emotional response is:
The patient will be emotionally responsive and return to a pre-illness level of functioning.

Goals of nursing care for patients with severe mood disturbance have the following aims:
- To allow recognition and continuous expression of feelings, including denial, hopelessness, anger, guilt, blame, helplessness, regret, hope, and relief, within a supportive therapeutic atmosphere
- To allow for gradual analysis of stressors while strengthening the patient's self-esteem
- To increase the patient's sense of identity, control, awareness of choices, and responsibility for behavior
- To encourage healthy interpersonal ties with others
- To promote understanding of maladaptive emotions and to acquire adaptive coping responses to stressors

Specific short-term goals should be generated in relation to behaviors of the patient, present areas of difficulty, and relevant stressors. Goal setting should involve a holistic view of the patient and the patient's world. Goals will most likely need to be developed regarding the patient's self-concept, physical status, behavioral performance, expression of emotions, and relationships. All of these areas can directly relate to the mood disturbance. The patient's participation in setting these goals can be a significant first step in regaining mastery over his or her life.

Outcome indicators related to "Grief Resolution" from the Nursing Outcome Classification (NOC) project are presented in Box 19-8 (Moorhead, Johnson, and Maas, 2004).

BOX 19-8

NOC Outcome Indicators for Grief Resolution

Resolves feelings about loss
Expresses spiritual beliefs about death
Verbalizes reality of loss
Verbalizes acceptance of loss
Describes meaning of the loss or death
Participates in planning funeral
Discusses unresolved conflict(s)
Reports absence of somatic distress
Reports decreased preoccupation with loss
Maintains living environment
Maintains grooming and hygiene
Reports absence of sleep disturbance
Reports adequate nutritional intake
Reports normal sexual desire
Seeks social support
Shares loss with significant others
Reports involvement in social activities
Progresses through stages of grief
Expresses positive expectations about the future

From Moorhead S, Johnson M, Maas M, editors: *Nursing outcomes classification (NOC)*, ed 3, St Louis, 2004, Mosby.

PLANNING

In planning care the nurse's priorities are the reduction and ultimate removal of the patient's maladaptive emotional responses, restoration of the patient's occupational and psychosocial functioning, improvement in the patient's quality of life, and minimization of the likelihood of relapse and recurrence (Keller, 2003). Treatment consists of three phases: acute, continuation, and maintenance (Figure 19-7).

Acute Treatment Phase

The goal of acute treatment is to eliminate the symptoms. If patients improve with treatment, they are said to have had a therapeutic response. A successful acute treatment brings patients back to an essentially symptom-free state and to a level of functioning comparable to that before the illness. This phase usually lasts 6 to 12 weeks, and if patients are symptom-free at the end of that time, they are then in remission.

Continuation Treatment Phase

The goal of continuation treatment is to prevent relapse, which is the return of symptoms, and to promote recovery. The risk of relapse is very high in the first 4 to 6 months after remission, and one of the greatest mistakes in the treatment of mood disorders is the failure to continue a successful treatment for a long enough time. This phase usually lasts 4 to 9 months.

Maintenance Treatment Phase

The goal of maintenance treatment is to prevent recurrence, or a new episode of illness. This concept is commonly accepted for bipolar illness, but it is now seen as important for major depressive disorder as well. Studies point out the effectiveness of both pharmacological and cognitive behavioral maintenance therapy in preventing new episodes or lengthening the interval between them. In the maintenance phase, patients may be on medication indefinitely.

Understanding the phases of treatment for mood disorders is critically important. The nurse should discuss them with the patient and family so that they may join in the therapeutic alliance and have clear expectations about the goals and course of treatment.

Your patient tells you she stopped taking her medicine after 2 months because she was feeling better. What would you tell her, based on your understanding of the treatment phases of depression? ■

IMPLEMENTATION

Maladaptive emotional responses may emerge at unpredicted moments, can vary in intensity from mild to severe, and can be transitory, recurrent, or stable conditions. Episodes of depression and mania can occur in any setting and can arise in conjunction with existing medical problems. Also, the treatment of mood disturbances can take place in various settings: at home, at an outpatient facility, or in a hospital.

The best treatment setting for the patient depends on the severity of the illness, available support systems, and resources of the treatment center. In timing intervention, remember that help given when maladaptive patterns are developing is likely to be more acceptable and effective than help given after these patterns have been established. Thus early diagnosis and treatment are associated with more positive outcomes.

A number of practice guidelines have been developed for the treatment of mood disorders (American Psychiatric Association, 2000b and 2002; Altshuler et al, 2001; Kahn et al, 2000). **Empirically validated treatments** for major depressive disorder and bipolar disorder are summarized in Box 19-9 (Nathan and Gorman, 2002). Research also has found that the nature of the therapeutic alliance is an important factor and has a significant impact on the treatment outcome in depression (Meredith et al, 2001; Zuroff et al, 2000).

The nursing interventions described for severe mood disturbances are based on a multicausal, integrative model of affective disorders. Such a model dismisses the notion of one cause or one cure. Rather, it proposes that affective problems have many causes and dimensions that affect all aspects of a person's life. Thus a single approach to nursing care would be inadequate.

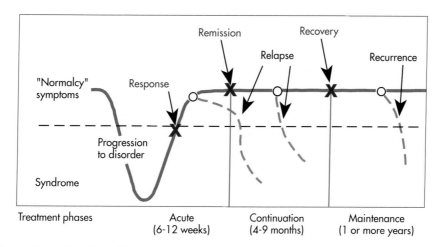

Figure 19-7   The phases of treatment for mood disorders. (From Kupfer DJ: *J Clin Psychiatry* 53[suppl]:28, 1991.)

BOX **19-9**	SUMMARIZING THE EVIDENCE ON **Mood Disorders**

Disorder	Major depressive disorder (MDD)
Treatment	◆ Interventions using behavior therapy, cognitive-behavior therapy, and interpersonal therapy are all effective treatments.
	◆ Because of their narrow safety margin and significant drug-induced adverse side effects, tricyclic antidepressants (TCAs) have now been largely replaced for the treatment of depression by selective serotonin reuptake inhibitors (SSRIs), including fluoxetine, sertraline, paroxetine, and citalopram, along with newer compounds such as venlafaxine, mirtazapine, buproprion, and nefazodone.
	◆ One large study supports the superior effectiveness of combined psychosocial and pharmacological treatment.
	◆ Because of adverse side effects, monoamine oxidase inhibitors (MAOIs) are generally reserved for treatment-refractory MDD patients.
Disorder	Bipolar disorder
Treatment	◆ Lithium, divalproex, and olanzapine are all effective in reducing the symptoms of acute bipolar manic episodes.
	◆ Carbamazepine; typical antipsychotics, risperidone and ziprasidone, are effective in the treatment of acute mania.
	◆ Although understudied, the pharmacological treatment of acute bipolar depression suggests that lithium, most antidepressants, and lamotrigine are effective antidepressants.
	◆ Lithium is effective with many patients in preventing or reducing the frequency of recurrent affective episodes, although side effects have been a problem with drug adherence.
	◆ Divalproex and carbamazepine are effective preventive treatments.
	◆ Although pharmacological interventions are treatments of choice, psychosocial treatments, including psychoeducation, cognitive-behavioral therapy, interpersonal therapy, and marital/family therapy help to increase medication adherence, improve quality of life, and enhance coping mechanisms of patients with bipolar disorder.

From Nathan P, Gorman J: *A guide to treatments that work*, ed 2, New York, 2002, Oxford University Press.

Nursing interventions must reflect the complex multicausal nature of the model and address all maladaptive aspects of a person's life. Intervening in as many areas as possible should have the maximum effect in modifying maladaptive responses and alleviating severe mood disturbances. The ultimate aim of these nursing interventions is to teach the patient coping responses and increase the satisfaction gained from interaction with the world.

Environmental Interventions

Environmental interventions are useful when the patient's environment is highly dangerous, impoverished, aversive, or lacking in personal resources. In caring for the patient with a severe mood disorder, **highest priority should be given to the potential for suicide**. Hospitalization is definitely indicated when suicide is deemed to be a risk. In the presence of rapidly progressing symptoms and in the absence of support systems, hospitalization is strongly indicated. Nursing care in this case means protecting patients and assuring them that they will not be allowed to harm themselves. Specific interventions for suicidal patients are described in Chapter 20.

Depressed patients must always be assessed for possible suicide. **They are at particular risk when they appear to be coming out of their depression** because they may then have the energy and opportunity to kill themselves. Acute manic states are also life threatening. These patients show poor judgment, excessive risk taking, and an inability to evaluate realistic danger and the consequences of their actions. In an acute manic episode, immediate measures must be instituted to prevent death.

Another environmental intervention involves changing the physical or social setting by helping the patient move to a new environment. Sometimes a change in the general pattern of living is indicated, such as taking a leave of absence from work, working at a different job, socializing with a new peer group, or leaving a family setting. Changes such as these decrease the immediate stress and mobilize additional support.

Nurse-Patient Relationship

Depressed Patients. Depressed patients resist involvement through withdrawal and nonresponsiveness. Because of their negative views, they tend to remain isolated, verbalize little, think that they are unworthy of help, and form dependent attachments.

In working with depressed patients, the nurse's approach should be quiet, warm, and accepting. The nurse should demonstrate honesty, empathy, and compassion. Admittedly, it is not always easy to give warm, personal care to a person who is unresponsive and detached. The nurse may feel angry, resent the patient's helplessness, or fear rejection. Patience and a belief in the potential of each person to grow and change are needed. If this is calmly communicated, both verbally and nonverbally, in time the patient may begin to respond.

Nurses should avoid assuming an overaggressive or lighthearted approach with the depressed person. Comments such as "You have so much to live for," "Cheer up—things are sure to get better," or "You shouldn't feel so depressed" convey little understanding of and respect for the patient's feelings.

They will create more distance and block the formation of a relationship. Also, nurses should not sympathize with the patient. Subjective overidentification by nurses can cause them to experience similar feelings of hopelessness and helplessness and can seriously limit their ability to provide therapy.

Rapport is best established with the depressed patient through shared time, even if the patient talks little, and through supportive companionship. The very presence of the nurse indicates belief that the patient is a valuable person. The nurse should adjust to the depressed patient's pace by speaking more slowly and allowing more time to respond. The patient should be addressed by name, talked with, and listened to. By studying the patient's life and interests, the nurse might select topics that lay the foundation for more meaningful discussions.

Manic Patients.
In contrast, elated patients may be very talkative and need simple explanations and concise, truthful answers to questions. Although manic patients may appear willing to talk, they resist involvement through manipulation, testing limits, and superficiality. Their hyperactivity, short attention span, flight of ideas, poor judgment, lack of insight, and rapid mood swings all present special problems to the nursing staff.

Manic patients can be very disruptive to a hospital unit and resist engagement in therapy. They may dominate group meetings or therapy sessions by their excessive talking and manipulate staff or patient groups. By identifying a vulnerable area in another person or a group's area of conflict, manic patients are able to exploit others. This provokes defensive and angry responses. Nurses are particularly susceptible to these feelings because they often have the most contact with patients and the responsibility for maintaining the psychiatric unit. When anger is generated, therapeutic care breaks down. Thus the maneuvers of manic patients act as diversionary tactics. By alienating themselves, patients can avoid exploring their own problems.

It is important for nurses to understand how manic patients are able to manipulate others and their reasons for doing so. The treatment plan for these patients should be thorough, well coordinated, and consistently implemented. **Constructive limit setting** on manic patients' behavior is an essential part of the plan. The entire treatment team must be consistent in their expectations of these patients, and progressive limits must be set as situations arise. Other patients also may be encouraged to carry out the agreed limits. Pressure applied by peers can sometimes be more effective than pressure applied by the staff. Frequent staff meetings are recommended to improve communication, share in understanding the manic patient's behavior, and ensure steady progress.

One goal of nursing care is to increase the patient's self-control, and this should be kept in mind when setting limits. Patients need to see that they can monitor their own behavior and that the staff is there to help them. Also, the nurse should point out the many positive aspects of their behavior. The ability to be outgoing, expressive, and energetic is a coping strength that can be maximized.

Physiological Treatments

Physiological treatments include **physical care, psychopharmacology,** and **somatic therapies.** They begin with a thorough physical examination and health history to identify health problems and current treatments or medications that may be affecting the patient's mood. The indications for physiological treatment include symptoms that will respond to physiological measures, greater severity of illness, suicidal potential, and need for speed in recovery.

Depressed Patients.
When depressed, the patient may forget to attend to physical well-being or may not be capable of self-care. The more severe the depression, the more important is the physical care. For example, the nurse may need to monitor the diet of a patient who has no appetite and consequently has lost weight. Staying with the patient during meals, arranging for preferred foods, and encouraging frequent small meals may be helpful. Recording intake and output and weighing the patient daily will help evaluate this need.

Sleep disturbances typically occur. It is best to plan activities according to each patient's energy levels; some feel best in the morning and others in the evening. A scheduled rest period may be helpful, but patients should not be encouraged to take frequent naps or remain in bed all day. Patients with depression experience less stage III and IV sleep, and because these stages depend on the period of wakefulness, napping may worsen sleep disturbances. For many patients, eating regularly, staying active during waking hours, and cutting back on caffeine (especially late in the day) may promote more normal sleep patterns.

The patient's physical appearance may be neglected and all movements may be slowed. Nurses may have to help with bathing or dressing. They should do this matter-of-factly, explaining that help is being offered because the patient is unable to do it independently right now. Cleanliness and interest in appearance can be noticed and praised. Nurses must allow patients to help themselves whenever possible. Often nurses might rush the patient or do a task themselves to save time, but this does not facilitate the patient's recovery and should be avoided.

Psychopharmacology. Antidepressant medications are often administered to elevate the mood of the depressed patient. They are particularly indicated in severe and recurrent depression. Many antidepressant medications are available on the market (Table 19-7) and new ones can be expected to be released each year. Antidepressant medications are equally effective in treating depression, and their overall success rate is 60% to 80%.

Despite the treatment success achieved with these drugs, antidepressant drugs have limitations. **Their therapeutic effects usually begin only after 2 to 6 weeks.** They also have side effects that can deter some patients from maintenance. Thus patient education is essential. Another major problem with some antidepressant medications is their toxicity. **Tricyclic antidepressants are lethal at high doses,** which makes them particularly dangerous for people most in need of them: suicidal patients. In contrast, the newer selective serotonin reuptake inhibitors (SSRI) antidepressants are safer in the event of an overdose. In addition, antidepressant medications do not help everyone, and it is difficult to predict who will respond to which drug. Fortunately, those who do not benefit from one drug often do well when switched to another. Antidepressant medications are discussed in detail in Chapter 27.

What would you say to a patient who tells you that she doesn't want to take medicines for her depression because they are addictive? ■

Somatic therapies. Electroconvulsive therapy (ECT) is also used with depressed patients, particularly those with recurrent depressions and those resistant to drug therapy. ECT is regarded by many as a specific therapy for patients with severe depressions characterized by somatic delusions and delusional guilt, accompanied by a lack of interest in the world, suicidal ideation, and weight loss.

Sleep deprivation therapy also may be effective in treating depression. Research indicates that depriving some depressed patients of a night's sleep will improve their clinical condition. How sleep deprivation works is not known, and the duration of improvement varies.

Another physiological treatment is that of phototherapy, or **light therapy,** in which patients are exposed to bright artificial light for a specified amount of time each day. Phototherapy appears to be effective in the short-term treatment of patients with mild to moderate seasonal affective disorder (SAD). Finally, two new treatments still being researched are **transcranial magnetic stimulation** (TMS) and **vagal nerve stimulation** (VNS). These somatic therapies are described in detail in Chapter 28.

Manic Patients. Manic patients primarily need protection from themselves. They may be too busy to eat or take care of themselves. Eating problems can be handled in the same way as with depressed patients. Manic patients may sleep very little, so rest periods should be encouraged, along with baths, soft music, and whirlpools. These patients also may need help in selecting clothes and maintaining hygiene. Setting limits and using firm actions are effective in physical care.

Psychopharmacology. For many years **lithium** was considered the drug of choice in the treatment of mania. Care must be taken regarding the narrow therapeutic index of this drug, which requires frequent blood levels and careful patient monitoring. The **anticonvulsants** divalproex and carbamazepine and **atypical antipsychotic** medications, including olanzapine, risperidone, and ziprasidone have added to the treatment alternatives for acute manic episodes in bipolar disorder (Table 19-8). **Caution must be used when prescribing antidepressants to patients with bipolar disorder because they may be switched into mania by these drugs.** Other drugs to treat this illness are

Table 19-7 **Antidepressant Drugs**

Drug Class Generic Name (Trade Name)	Usual Adult Daily Dose (mg/day)	Preparations
Selective Serotonin Reuptake Inhibitors (SSRIs)		
Citalopram (Celexa)	20-40	PO, L
Escitalopram (Lexapro)	20-40	PO
Fluoxetine (Prozac)	20-60	PO, L
Fluvoxamine (Luvox)	100-200	PO
Paroxetine (Paxil)	20-50	PO, CR
Sertraline (Zoloft)	50-200	PO, L
Other New Antidepressant Drugs		
Amoxapine (Asendin)	200-300	PO
Bupropion (Wellbutrin)	150-450*	PO, SR
Maprotiline (Ludiomil)	50-200*	PO
Mirtazapine (Remeron)	15-45	PO
Serotonin antagonist and reuptake inhibitors (SARIs)		
Nefazodone (Serzone)	300-500	PO
Trazodone (Desyrel)	150-300	PO
Serotonin-norepinephrine reuptake inhibitor (SNRI)		
Venlafaxine (Effexor)	75-375	PO, XR
Tricyclic Antidepressant Drugs (TCAs)		
Tertiary (parent)		
Amitriptyline (Elavil)	150-300	PO, IM
Clomipramine (Anafranil)	100-250	PO
Doxepin (Sinequan)	150-300	PO, L
Imipramine (Tofranil)	150-300	PO
Trimipramine (Surmontil)	150-300	PO
Secondary (metabolite)		
Desipramine (Norpramin)	150-300	PO, L
Nortriptyline (Pamelor)	50-150	PO, L
Protriptyline (Vivactil)	15-60	PO
Tetracyclics		
Amoxapine (Asendin)	150-400	PO
Maprotiline (Ludiomil)	150-225	PO
Monoamine Oxidase Inhibitors (MAOIs)		
Isocarboxazid (Marplan)	20-60	PO
Phenelzine (Nardil)	45-90	PO
Selegiline (Eldepryl, Emsam)	20-50	PO, TS
Tranylcypromine (Parnate)	20-60	PO

*Antidepressants with a ceiling dose due to dose-related seizures.
IM, Intramuscular; *L,* oral liquid; *PO,* tablet/capsule; *CR,* controlled release; *SR,* sustained release; *XR,* extended release; *TS,* transdermal system patch.

Table 19-8 **Mood-Stabilizing Drugs**

Drug Class Generic Name (Trade Name)	Usual Adult Dose (mg/day)	Preparations
Antimania		
Lithium (Eskalith, Lithobid)	600-2400	PO, CR, SR
Lithium citrate	600-2400	L/S
Anticonvulsants		
Valproic acid (Depakene), valproate (Depacon), divalproex (Depakote)	15-60 mg/kg/day	PO, L/S, ER, IM
Lamotrigine (Lamictal)	300-500	PO, Ch
Carbamazepine (Tegretol)	200-1600	PO, Ch
Gabapentin (Neurontin)	900-3600+	PO
Oxcarbazepine (Trileptal)	600-2400	PO, S
Topiramate (Topamax)	200-400	PO
Tiagabine (Gabatril)	4-32	PO

PO, Capsule/tablet by mouth; *CR,* controlled release; *SR,* sustained release; *L/S,* liquid/syrup; *ER,* extended release; *IM,* intramuscular; *Ch,* chewable tablets; *S,* suspension.

being investigated, including substance P blockers that show potential promise in regulating mood. A detailed discussion of mood stabilizing medications is presented in Chapter 27.

 Your patient with bipolar disorder tells you that she has stopped taking her medication because she misses the highs that she used to feel and the extra energy she used to have. What would your educational approach be to help her comply with treatment? ■

Expressing Feelings

Affective interventions are necessary because patients with mood disturbances have difficulty identifying, expressing, and modulating feelings. Feelings that are particularly problematic are hopelessness, sadness, anger, guilt, and anxiety. A range of interventions is available to the nurse in meeting patient needs in this area. Box 19-10 identifies nursing interventions used to facilitate grief work; these are taken from the Nursing Interventions Classification (NIC) project (Dochterman and Bulechek, 2004).

Intervening to guide patients in managing their emotions requires self-understanding by the nurse. Whether the interventions will be therapeutic depends greatly on the nurse's values regarding the various emotions, the nurse's emotional responsiveness, and the nurse's ability to offer genuine respect and nonjudgmental acceptance. Nurses must be able to experience feelings and express them if they expect to help patients.

Depressed Patients. Initially the nurse must express **hope** for depressed patients. Demoralization is a component of depression (Rickelman, 2002). They thus have a genuine need for believing that things can get better. The nurse should reinforce that depression is a self-limiting disorder and that the future will be better. This can be expressed calmly and simply. The intent is not to cheer the patient but to offer hope that, although recovery is a slow process involving weeks or months, the patient will feel progressively better. The nurse may acknowledge the patient's inability to take comfort from this reassurance. For the depressed, only the depression is real; past or future happiness is an illusion (see A Patient Speaks). By affirming belief in recovery, however, the nurse may make the patient's existence more tolerable.

A PATIENT SPEAKS

When in depression, this faith in deliverance, in ultimate restoration, is absent. The pain is unrelenting, and what makes the condition intolerable is the foreknowledge that no remedy will come—not in a day, an hour, a month, or a minute. If there is mild relief, one knows that it is only temporary; more pain will follow. It is hopelessness even more than pain that crushes the soul. So the decision making of daily life involves not, as in normal affairs, shifting from one annoying situation to another less annoying—or from discomfort to relative comfort, or from boredom to activity—but moving from pain to pain. One does not abandon, even briefly, one's bed of nails, but is attached to it wherever one goes. And this results in a striking experience—one which I have called, borrowing military terminology, the situation of the walking wounded. For in virtually any other serious sickness, a patient who felt similar devastation would be lying flat in bed, possibly sedated and hooked up to the tubes and wires of life-support systems, but at the very least in a posture of repose and in an isolated setting. His invalidism would be necessary, unquestioned, and honorably attained. However, the one suffering from depression has no such option and therefore finds himself, like a walking casualty of war, thrust into the most intolerable social and family situations. There he must, despite the anguish devouring his brain, present a face approximating the one that is associated with ordinary events and companionship. He must try to utter small talk, and be responsive to questions, and knowingly nod and frown and, God help him, even smile. But it is a fierce trial just attempting to speak a few simple words.

From Styron W: *Darkness visible*, New York, 1992, Vintage Books.

This initial reassurance is a way of acknowledging the patient's pain and despair while also conveying a sense of hope in recovery. It is not the premature reassurance of "Don't worry, everything's going to be just fine." It is an openness to the patient's feelings and acknowledgment of them. This is a very important first step. It lets the patient see that the present state is not permanent. For the depressed patient who lacks time perspective, it directs thoughts beyond the present with genuine hope for tomorrow.

Nursing actions in this area should convey that expressing feelings is normal and necessary. Blocking or repressing emotions is partly responsible for the patient's present pain. Nurses can help patients realize that their overwhelming feelings of dejection and worthlessness are defenses that prevent them from dealing with their problems. Encouraging a patient to express unpleasant or painful emotions can reduce their intensity and make the patient feel more alive and masterful. Thus nursing care should be directed toward helping the patient experience feelings and express them. These actions are a prerequisite to interventions in the cognitive, behavioral, or social areas.

Manic Patients. Manic patients may have the opposite problem of patients with depression in that they are often too expressive of their feelings. These patients are often hyperverbal and need help from the nurse in pacing and modulating their expression. The nurse must be careful to not criticize or negate the feelings expressed.

Helping patients speak more slowly and follow one line of thought are important areas for nursing intervention. Manic patients need feedback on the intensity of their self-expressions, as well as the impact of their behavior on other people. Social skills modeling and reinforcement are nursing care activities that can be incorporated into the daily routine. Setting limits, giving simple directions, and keeping focused are other useful nursing interventions.

When the nurse accepts without criticism the anger, despair, or anxiety expressed by the patient, the patient sees that expressing feelings is not always destructive or a sign of weakness. Sometimes, however, patients' expression of anger changes their cognitive set from self-blaming to blaming others. It may allow them to see themselves as more effective because it connotes power, superiority, and mastery. How this anger is expressed is important because aggressive behavior can be destructive and can further isolate them. Many patients experiencing both depressive and manic emotional states have problems with expressing anger and need to learn assertive behavior and anger management techniques. This important area of nursing intervention is explored in Chapter 30.

Relaxation techniques also may help both manic and depressed patients deal with their anxiety and tension and obtain more pleasure from life. Reducing anxiety to tolerable levels broadens one's perceptual field and allows the nurse to intervene in the cognitive and behavioral areas. Nursing actions used to reduce anxiety are described in Chapters 16 and 31.

To successfully implement any of these nursing actions related to the patient's affective needs, the nurse must use a variety of communication skills (see Chapter 2). Particularly important are empathy skills, reflection of feeling, open-ended feeling-oriented questions, validation, self-disclosure, and confrontation. The patient with a severe mood disturbance will challenge the nurse's therapeutic skills and stringently test the nurse's caring and commitment.

Cognitive Strategies

When intervening in the cognitive area, nurses have three major aims, which require that they begin with the patient's conceptualization of the problem:

- **To increase the patient's sense of control over goals and behavior**
- **To increase the patient's self-esteem**
- **To help the patient modify dysfunctional thinking patterns**

Depressed Patients. Depressed patients often see themselves as victims of their moods and environment. They do not see their behavior and their interpretation of events as possible causes of depression. They assume a passive stance and wait for someone or something to lift their mood. One task of the nurse, therefore, is to move patients beyond their limiting preoccupation to other aspects of their world that are related to it. To do this, the nurse must progress gradually.

The first step is to help patients explore their feelings. This is followed by eliciting their view of the problem. In so doing the nurse accepts the patient's perceptions but need not accept the patient's conclusions. Together they define the problem to give the patient a sense of control, a feeling of hope, and a realization that change may indeed be possible.

Nursing actions should then focus on modifying the patient's thinking. Depressed patients are dominated by negative thoughts (see Citing the Evidence). Often, despite a successful performance, the patient will view it negatively. Cognitive changes may be brought about in a variety of ways, as described in Chapter 31.

Often, negative thinking is an automatic process of which the patient is not even aware. The nurse can help patients identify their negative thoughts and decrease them through thought stopping or substitution. Concurrently, the patient can be encouraged to increase positive thinking by reviewing personal assets, strengths, accomplishments, and opportunities. Next, the patient can be helped to examine the accuracy of perceptions, logic, and conclusions. Misperceptions, distortions, and irrational beliefs become evident. The patient also should be helped to move from unrealistic to realistic goals and to decrease the importance of unattainable goals. All of these actions enhance the patient's self-understanding and increase self-esteem. More detailed interventions related to alterations in self-concept, which are inherent in disturbances of mood, are explored in Chapter 18.

Also, because the depressed patient tends to be overwhelmed by despair, it is important to limit the amount of negative evaluation in which he or she engages. One way is

CITING THE EVIDENCE ON
Reducing Negative Thinking in Depression

BACKGROUND: Although cognitive-behavioral interventions have been used successfully in treating depression, few studies focus on reducing negative thinking via group intervention as a means of preventing depression in high-risk groups. The purpose of this randomized controlled clinical trial was to test the effectiveness of a cognitive-behavioral group intervention in reducing depressive symptoms, decreasing negative thinking, and enhancing self-esteem in young women at-risk for depression.

RESULTS: Compared to those in the control group, women who received the intervention had a greater decrease in depressive symptoms and negative thinking and a greater increase in self-esteem, and these beneficial effects were maintained over 6 months.

IMPLICATIONS: The findings show the effectiveness of this cognitive-behavioral group intervention and indicate empirical support for the beneficial effects of reducing negative thinking by the use of affirmation and thought-stopping techniques on women's mental health. This represents a fertile area for focused nursing intervention.

Peden A et al: *J Nurs Scholarsh* 32:145, 2000.

to involve the patient in productive tasks or activities; another way is to increase the level of socialization. These benefit the patient in two complementary ways: They limit the time spent on brooding and self-criticism and they provide positive reinforcement.

Manic Patients. Manic patients also need to gain control over their thoughts and behaviors. Here, however, the challenge is to bring together a patient's scattered thoughts and ideas to help him or her engage in adaptive, goal-directed behavior. The communication skills of focusing, clarifying, and confrontation are useful in redirecting a patient's self-expressions. Once this is accomplished, the nurse can begin to help the patient modify dysfunctional thinking. Manic patients often have problems of grandiose thoughts, overestimation of self, and unrealistic pursuits. As in depression, cognitive interventions can help the patient evaluate these thought problems and identify more realistic and ego-supportive goals.

It is also important for the nurse to realize the meaning, nature, and value the manic patient places on behavior and mood change. For example, research has shown that patients with bipolar disorder receive pronounced short- and long-term positive effects from their illness. These include increases in productivity, creativity, sensitivity to surroundings, social friendliness, and sexual intensity. These effects can provide a great deal of secondary benefit from the illness and can be powerful reinforcers of maladaptive responses, thus making change more difficult. For some patients, at some times the perceived positive consequences of the illness may outweigh their perception of the negative consequences.

BOX 19-11

List of Possible Positive Activities

- Planning something you will enjoy
- Going on an outing (such as a walk, a shopping trip downtown, or a picnic)
- Going out for entertainment
- Going on a trip
- Going to meetings, lectures, or classes
- Attending a social gathering
- Playing a sport or game
- Spending time on a hobby or project
- Entertaining yourself at home (for example, reading, listening to music, or watching television)
- Doing something just for yourself (such as buying something, cooking something, or dressing comfortably)
- Spending time just relaxing (for example, thinking, sitting, napping, or daydreaming)
- Caring for yourself or making yourself attractive
- Persisting at a difficult task
- Completing a routine task or unpleasant task
- Doing a job well
- Cooperating with someone else on a common task
- Doing something special for someone else, being generous, going out of your way
- Seeking out people (for example, calling, stopping by, making a date or appointment, or going to a meeting)
- Initiating conversation (for example, at a store, party, or class)
- Discussing an interesting or amusing topic
- Expressing yourself openly, clearly, or frankly (expressing opinion, criticism, or anger)
- Playing with children or animals
- Complimenting or praising someone
- Physically showing affection or love
- Receiving praise, compliments, or attention

Behavioral Change

The ability to accomplish tasks and be productive depends on various factors that apply to both depressed and manic patients. First, expectations and goals should be small enough to ensure successful performance, relevant to their needs, and focused on positive activities. Box 19-11 presents a list of rewarding or potentially rewarding activities. Next, attention should be focused on the task at hand, not what has yet to be done or was done incorrectly in the past. Finally, positive reinforcement should be based on actual performance. If such an approach is used consistently over time, the nurse can expect the patient to demonstrate increasingly productive behavior.

Occupational and recreational tasks are usually easily identified by the nurse. These can be most valuable and are well represented in the positive activities list. Another source of accomplishment is movement and physical exercise. Jogging, walking, swimming, bicycling, and aerobics are popular forms of exercise that may be incorporated in a regular program of activity. They are beneficial because they improve the patient's physical condition, release emotions and tensions, and can have an antidepressant effect.

Successful behavior is a powerful reinforcer or antidepressant. However, this idea seldom occurs to depressed patients, who use their despondent mood as a rationalization for inactivity. They instead believe that once their mood lifts, they will be productive again. Such an idea is consistent with a negative cognitive set and a sense of helplessness. However, inactivity prevents satisfaction and social recognition. Thus it reinforces a depressive state. Likewise, overactivity or uncompleted activity lowers the self-evaluation of manic patients.

Therefore nursing interventions should focus on activating the patient in a realistic, goal-directed way. Directed activities, strategies, or homework assignments mutually determined by the nurse and patient can reveal alternative coping responses. Many depressed patients benefit from nursing actions that encourage them to redirect their self-preoccupation to interests in the outside world. The timing of these interventions is crucial. Patients should not be forced into activities initially. Also, they will not benefit from coming into contact with too many people too soon. Rather, the nurse should encourage activities gradually and suggest more involvement on the basis of patients' energy.

For severely depressed hospitalized patients, a structured daily program of activities can be beneficial. Because these patients lack motivation and direction, they are slow to initiate actions. The nurse should take into consideration the patient's tolerance to stress and probability of succeeding. The particular task should be neither too difficult nor too time consuming. Success tends to increase expectations of success, and failure tends to increase hopelessness.

Elated patients usually need little encouragement to become involved with others. Because of their short attention span and restless energy, however, they cannot deal with complicated projects. They need tasks that are simple and can be completed quickly. They need room to move about and furnishings that do not overstimulate them.

What physiological changes occur as a result of exercise? Relate these to what is currently known about the biology of depression. ■

Social Skills

Social factors play a major role in the causation, maintenance, and resolution of affective disorders. Socialization moderates depression by providing an experience incompatible with depressive withdrawal. It also provides increased self-esteem through the social reinforcers of approval, acceptance, recognition, and support.

A major problem is that patients with maladaptive emotional responses are less accomplished in social interaction. In addition, others may avoid them because of their self-absorption, pessimism, or elation. One nursing action that can be used to counteract this problem is to help patients improve their social skills. A Patient Education Plan for enhancing social skills is presented in Table 19-9. It applies to patients with either depression or mania.

Involvement with others often is a result of shared activities. The nurse can work with the patient to identify recreational, career, cultural, religious, and personal interests and how to pursue these interests through community groups, organizations, and clubs. Women's groups, single-parent groups, jogging clubs, church groups, and neighborhood associations are all opportunities. Although this may appear to be a simple nursing intervention, it often challenges the nurse's creativity and knowledge of resources.

Family and Group Treatment. In addition to a one-to-one relationship, patients with maladaptive emotional responses can benefit from family and group work. Behaviors associated with depression and mania may be contributed to and supported by other family members. The patient's problems in human relationships are examined in light of family patterns, and all members are expected to take responsibility for their share of the continuing pattern. The theory that friends and partners often reinforce and support the patient's maladaptive behavior has been well documented. Much attention and secondary gain are usually received from others, who respond by being helpful, nurturing, or annoyed. When the patient acts in a more adaptive way, however, attention given is

| Table 19-9 | **PATIENT EDUCATION PLAN** | Enhancing Social Skills |
CONTENT	INSTRUCTIONAL ACTIVITIES	EVALUATION
Describe behaviors interfering with social interaction.	Instruct the patient on corrective behaviors.	Patient identifies problematic and more facilitative behaviors.
Discuss positive social skills that could be used by the patient.	Model effective interpersonal skills for the patient.	Patient describes specific skills that could be acquired.
Analyze the way in which the patient could incorporate these specific skills.	Use role play and guided practice to allow patient to test these new behaviors.	Patient shows beginning skill in assumed social behaviors.
Encourage patient to test new skills in other situations.	Give the patient homework assignments to do in his or her natural environment.	Patient discusses ability to complete the assigned tasks.
Discuss generalization of new skills to other aspects of the patient's life and functioning.	Give feedback, encouragement, and praise for newly acquired social skills and their generalization.	Patient is able to integrate the new social behaviors in social interactions with others.

minimal. Therefore one goal of family therapy is to have the family reinforce adaptive behavior and ignore maladaptive mood responses.

Group therapy also can provide multiple benefits. For example, a format for group treatment of patients with depression or mania can have as its overall aim that of increasing self-worth and self-esteem through identification with the group and awareness of personal strengths. Specifically, group members can do the following:

- Learn more about their own behavior and relationships with others based on feedback from the group
- Increase social support through group relatedness
- Gain a heightened sense of identity, self-understanding, and control over their own lives
- Realize that other people have problems similar to their own, which helps reduce their sense of loneliness and isolation, thereby also decreasing feelings of hopelessness, helplessness, and powerlessness
- Learn new ways to cope with stress from others in the group
- More realistically modify their perceptions and expectations of self and others

- Allow for the expression of feelings of hopelessness and frustration within the supportive context of the group

Mental Health Education

A final but important aspect of nursing care related to maladaptive emotional responses is mental health education about the nature, extent, and treatments available for mood disorders (Box 19-12). Despite its prevalence, most people with depressive illnesses do not seek treatment because they do not know that they have a treatable disease or because they perceive stigma surrounding psychiatric illnesses (Raingruber, 2002). Outreach targeted to ethnic and racial minority communities is a particular need.

Nursing care also must address the specific needs of patients and families for education concerning mood disorders. A psychoeducational model can be used with families, who are a valuable resource in helping patients deal with their illness. The overall goal of such a program is to improve patient and family functioning and decrease symptomatology by increasing a sense of self-worth and control for both patients and families. Specific information about the reciprocal im-

---

BOX 19-12

Outline of Topics for Patient-Family Psychoeducational Sessions on Depression

I. Defining depression
  A. Definitions and descriptions of depression and mania
  B. How depression differs from "the blues" we all experience (duration, impact on mood, functioning, self-esteem, responsiveness to the environment)
  C. Possible causes: the Stuart Stress Adaptation Model
II. Depression and the interpersonal environment
  A. What depression looks like: interpersonal difficulties
    1. Oversensitivity and self-preoccupation
    2. Unresponsiveness (to reassurance, support, feedback, sympathy)
    3. Behaviors that appear willful
    4. Apparent lack of caring for others, unrealistic expectations
    5. Apparent increased need to control relationships
    6. Inability to function in normal roles, tasks
  B. Negative interactional sequences
    1. Family attempts to coax, reassure, protect (potential for overinvolvement)
    2. Patient is unresponsive, family escalates attempts to help or withdraws
    3. Patient feels alienated, family becomes withdrawn, angry, or both
    4. Family feels guilty and returns to overprotective stance
    5. Patient feels unworthy, hopeless, infantilized
    6. Families burn out over time but remain caught in guilt/anger dilemma
    7. Alienation or overprotection

III. Treatments
  A. Psychotropic medication
  B. Psychotherapies
  C. Other treatments
IV. Coping with depression
  A. What to avoid
    1. Too rapid reassurance
    2. Taking comments literally
    3. Attempting to be constantly available and positive
    4. Allowing the disorder to dominate family life
  B. Creating a balance (neither overresponsive nor underresponsive)
    1. Recognition of multiple realities
    2. Distinguishing between the patient and the disorder
    3. Decreasing expectations temporarily
    4. Providing realistic support and reinforcement
    5. Avoiding unnecessary criticism (but providing feedback when necessary)
    6. Communicating clearly and simply (proverbially)
    7. Providing activity, structure
  C. Taking care of self and family members other than the patient; skills for self-preservation
    1. Time out (away from patient)
    2. Avoiding martyrdom
    3. Accepting own negative feelings
    4. Minimizing the impact of the disorder
  D. Coping with special problems
    1. Suicide threats and attempts
    2. Medication
    3. Hospitalization
    4. Atypical responses

Modified from Anderson et al: *Fam Process* 25:185, 1986.

| Table 19-10 | NURSING TREATMENT PLAN SUMMARY | Maladaptive Emotional Responses |

Nursing Diagnosis: Hopelessness
Expected Outcome: The patient will be emotionally responsive and return to pre-illness level of functioning.

SHORT-TERM GOAL	INTERVENTION	RATIONALE
The patient's environment will be safe and protective.	Continually evaluate the patient's potential for suicide. Hospitalize the patient when there is a suicidal risk. Help the patient move to a new environment when appropriate (new job, peer group, family setting).	All patients with severe mood disturbances are at risk for suicide; environmental changes can protect the patient, decrease the immediate stress, and mobilize additional resources.
The patient will establish a therapeutic relationship with the nurse.	Use a warm, accepting empathetic approach. Be aware of and in control of your own feelings and reactions (anger, frustration, sympathy). *With the depressed patient:* Establish rapport through shared time and supportive companionship. Give the patient time to respond. Personalize care as a way of indicating the patient's value as a human being. *With the manic patient:* Give simple, truthful responses. Be alert to possible manipulation. Set constructive limits on negative behavior. Use a consistent approach by all health-team members. Maintain open communication and sharing of perceptions among team members. Reinforce the patient's self-control and positive aspects of patient behavior.	Both depressed and manic patients resist becoming involved in a therapeutic alliance; acceptance, persistence, and limit setting are necessary.
The patient will be physiologically stable and able to meet self-care needs.	Help the patient meet self-care needs, particularly in the areas of nutrition, sleep, and personal hygiene. Encourage the patient's independence whenever possible. Administer prescribed medications and somatic treatments.	Physiological changes occur in disturbances of mood; physical care and somatic therapies are required to overcome problems in this area.
The patient will be able to recognize and express emotions related to daily events.	Respond empathetically, with a focus on feelings rather than facts. Acknowledge the patient's pain and convey a sense of hope in recovery. Help the patient experience feelings and express them appropriately. Help the patient in the adaptive expression of anger.	Patients with severe mood disturbances have difficulty identifying, expressing, and modulating feelings.

pact of depression and family life can be outlined, along with suggestions and strategies designed to help family members cope more effectively with mood disorders.

In summary, the most important ideas that the nurse should try to communicate through mental health education include the following:

- **Mood disorders are a medical illness, not a character defect or weakness.**
- **Recovery is the rule, not the exception.**
- **Mood disorders are treatable illnesses, and an effective treatment can be found for almost all patients.**
- **The goal of intervention is not just to get better, but also to get and stay completely well.**

A Nursing Treatment Plan Summary for patients with maladaptive emotional responses is presented in Table 19-10.

EVALUATION

The effectiveness of nursing care is determined by changes in the patient's maladaptive emotional responses and the effect they have on functioning. Problems related to self-concept and interpersonal relationships merge and overlap. Because all people experience life stress and related losses, the nurse can ask a fundamental question related to evaluation: "Did I assess the patient for problems in this area?"

Supervision and peer support groups can be helpful to the nurse working with patients with mood disorders. Of particular significance are the many special aspects of transference and countertransference that may occur. The patient's heightened attachment and dependency behaviors and lowered defensiveness can lead to intense **transference reactions** that should be worked through. Themes

| Table 19-10 | NURSING TREATMENT PLAN SUMMARY | Maladaptive Emotional Responses—cont'd |

Nursing Diagnosis: Hopelessness
Expected Outcome: The patient will be emotionally responsive and return to pre-illness level of functioning.

SHORT-TERM GOAL	INTERVENTION	RATIONALE
The patient will evaluate thinking and correct faulty or negative thoughts.	Review the patient's conceptualization of the problem but do not necessarily accept conclusions. Identify the patient's negative thoughts and help to decrease them. Help increase positive thinking. Examine the accuracy of perceptions, logic, and conclusions. Identify misperceptions, distortions, and irrational beliefs. Help the patient move from unrealistic to realistic goals. Decrease the importance of unattainable goals. Limit the amount of negative personal evaluations the patient engages in.	This will help increase sense of control over goals and behaviors, enhance self-esteem, and modify negative expectations.
The patient will implement two new behavioral coping strategies.	Assign appropriate action-oriented therapeutic tasks. Encourage activities gradually, escalating them as the patient's energy is mobilized. Provide a tangible, structured program when appropriate. Set goals that are realistic, relevant to the patient's needs and interests, and focused on positive activities. Focus on present activities, not past or future activities. Positively reinforce successful performance. Incorporate physical exercise in the patient's care plan.	Successful behavioral performance counteracts feelings of helplessness and hopelessness.
The patient will describe rewarding social interactions.	Assess the patient's social skills, supports, and interests. Review existing and potential social resources. Instruct and model effective social skills. Use role playing and rehearsal of social interactions. Give feedback and positive reinforcement of effective interpersonal skills. Intervene with families to have them reinforce the patient's adaptive emotional responses. Support or engage in family and group therapy when appropriate.	Socialization is an experience incompatible with withdrawal and increases self-esteem through the social reinforcers of approval, acceptance, recognition, and support.

of loss and fear of loss, control of emotions and lack of control, and ambivalence predominate. Termination of the nurse-patient relationship may be difficult because the patient experiences it as another loss that requires mourning and integration.

Countertransference can be related to the nurse's own bereavements, attitudes about anger, guilt, sadness, and despair, the ability to confront these emotions openly and objectively, and most importantly, conflicts about death and loss. Difficulties with any of these issues can be evident in avoidance behavior, preoccupation with fantasies, blocking of feelings, or shortening of sessions. Nursing care will be more appropriate and effective if the nurse is aware of these issues and sensitive to personal feelings and conflicts regarding loss. Supervision and peer support groups can be of great help in this area.

COMPETENT CARING

A Clinical Exemplar of a Psychiatric Nurse
VIRGINIA A. REUGER, MSN, RN, C

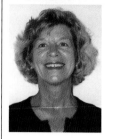

Sure, you read about therapeutic interactions in your nursing textbooks, but every person is not the same, so the only way you learn is by doing, by experiencing. Rarely in school do we have the time to become overly involved with our patients. We are taught on our psychiatric rotation not to let the boundaries between self and others become blurred. Yet the dynamics of a therapeutic relationship are not real until we come face to face with the situation.

It happened to me, subtly, soon after I started working in a private psychiatric hospital. I was working as a staff nurse on the intensive care unit. I was assigned to the next admission. From the intake sheet, I could see it was another depressed, suicidal patient. But when R and her husband walked onto the unit, I was immediately drawn to her with an empathic feeling. She was tiny, frail looking; her face was thin and drawn. Her long, dark hair partially hid her face. She ignored introductions and stared at the floor. My initial challenge was to establish trust to open channels of communication, assess her suicide potential, and provide a secure environment. Her potential for self-harm was quite high. She was put on strict suicidal precautions.

Initially, as I worked with R it required observations of her appearance, gestures, and interests, as well as nonverbal communication. I often had to make inferences, and I shared these with her. I felt like she was testing the waters of trust. R would often wrap herself up in her pink blanket and rock back and forth during our interactions. I found myself wondering what she was thinking.

One day during our time together I asked her about how it felt to be depressed. For her, it was the beginning of self-disclosure. She was able to acknowledge her fear and pain and unmet needs. She talked about what it was like growing up in New York City, living in rat-infested row houses. Her father worked at a bakery and sometimes their only food was the bread he brought home. She had two brothers and two sisters. Eventually she told me her uncle and grandfather lived with them, too. As she learned to trust me, she disclosed sexual abuse from her uncle and grandfather. At times the details became so vivid she trembled as she cried. It is hard to express, but there was a sense that we were making contact.

We talked about her present life, her frigidity, her 6-year-old daughter, and the nightmares. She often remarked that her husband and daughter would be better off without her. She believed she could not have a "normal life." R was very bright and talented. She had many hobbies. We started concentrating on these things. I knew her self-esteem was low, and this was the start of some good work. But being her primary nurse and assigned to her one-to-one daily made me realize I was becoming enmeshed in the situation. I went to my nurse manager for supervision. We discussed several options. I questioned whether I was helping her. I think sometimes nurses want to feel like omnipotent rescuers. I was not sure whether I was fostering independence or dependence. It was important to acknowledge my feelings to someone else openly, to discuss them, and then to move on.

Even though I felt a bond, I had to help R find strength on her own. We discussed her upcoming discharge date; we talked about priorities and decisions she had made. We talked about good choices, bad choices, and no choices. She had suffered many setbacks, but she was making plans.

I remember staying late the day of her discharge to say goodbye. R sent me cards at the hospital, dropped gifts off at the admissions office for me, and once tried to reach me at home. It was difficult to not acknowledge these things; I wanted so much to talk to her. But I knew the boundaries of a therapeutic relationship, and I knew she would be fine. I did talk to her outpatient therapist, and he told me she had completed a course in sign language (during her stay R befriended a deaf elderly woman), and she also was attending clown school, something she had always wanted to do—to make people laugh and feel good.

In psychiatric nursing it is important to remember that the art is to offer what you can without dictating the results while recognizing that you are not the only one to contribute to a person's health and happiness. I learned this important lesson from R. ■

CHAPTER **FOCUS POINTS**

- Mood is a prolonged emotional state that influences the person's whole personality and life functioning.
- The four adaptive functions of emotions are social communication, physiological arousal, subjective awareness, and psychodynamic defense.
- The continuum of emotional responses ranges from the most adaptive state of emotional responsiveness to the more maladaptive states of delayed grief reaction, depression, and mania.
- Grief is the subjective state that follows loss. As a natural reaction to a life experience, grief is universal; however, the way it is expressed is culturally determined. There are two types of pathological grief reactions: the delayed reaction and the distorted reaction.
- Depression may range from mild and moderate states to severe states with or without psychotic features. Psychotic depression accounts for less than 10% of all depressions.
- The lifetime risk for major depression is 7% to 12% for men and 20% to 30% for women.

- Most untreated episodes of major depression last 6 to 24 months.
- Over 50% of those who have had an episode of depression will eventually have another, and 25% of patients will have chronic, recurrent depression.
- Depression is a common accompaniment of many major medical illnesses. One of every five patients seeing a primary care practitioner has significant symptoms of depression. However, only one third of all people with depression seek help, are accurately diagnosed, and obtain appropriate treatment. The U.S .Preventive Services Task Force recommends screening adults for depression in primary care settings that have systems in place to assure accurate diagnosis, effective treatment, and responsive follow-up.
- Mania is characterized by an elevated, expansive, or irritable mood. Hypomania is a clinical syndrome similar to but not as severe as mania.
- A depressive episode with no manic episodes would be classified as a depressive disorder. A depressive episode with previous or cur-

CHAPTER **FOCUS POINTS**—cont'd

- rent manic episodes would be classified as a bipolar disorder or manic depressive illness because the patient experiences both mania and depression.
- The key element of a behavioral assessment is change: Depressed people change their usual patterns and responses. The most common and central behavior is that of the depressive mood. Some patients may initially deny their anxious or depressed moods but identify a variety of somatic complaints.
- Postpartum blues are brief episodes, lasting 1 to 4 days, of labile mood and tearfulness that occur in about 50% to 80% of women within 1 to 5 days of delivery. The incidence of postpartum psychosis is low, and the symptoms typically begin 2 to 3 days after delivery. The period of risk for postpartum psychosis is within the first month after delivery. Postpartum depression may occur from 2 weeks to 12 months after delivery, but usually occurs within 6 months.
- Seasonal affective disorder (SAD) is depression that comes with shortened hours of daylight in winter and fall and disappears during spring and summer.
- The potential for suicide always should be assessed in severe mood disturbances. About 15% of severely depressed patients commit suicide, and between 25% and 50% of patients with bipolar disorder attempt suicide at least once.
- The essential feature of mania is a distinct period of intense psychophysiological activation. Other behaviors found in mania include lability of mood with rapid shifts to brief depression. About 75% of manic patients have more than one episode, and almost all those with manic episodes also have depressive episodes.
- Current evidence suggests a significant genetic role in the cause of recurrent depression and bipolar disorder. Other predisposing factors affecting emotional responses include the aggression turned inward theory, object loss theory, personality organization theory, cognitive model, learned helplessness-hopelessness model, and behavioral model.
- Mood disorders occur because integrated biological control systems are disrupted, as evidenced by dysregulation in neurotransmitter systems, particularly serotonin, and by the fact that the brain mechanisms that control hormonal balance and biological rhythms are implicated in mood disorders.
- Precipitating stressors include loss of attachment, life events, role strain, and physiological changes. Mood states are affected by a wide variety of medications and physical illnesses. Most chronic debilitating illnesses, whether physical or psychiatric, are accompanied by depression.

- Uncomplicated grief reactions can be normal mourning or simple bereavement. A delayed grief reaction uses the defense mechanisms of denial and suppression in an attempt to avoid intense distress. Specific defenses used to block mourning are repression, suppression, denial, and dissociation.
- Primary NANDA nursing diagnoses related to maladaptive emotional responses are dysfunctional grieving, hopelessness, powerlessness, spiritual distress, risk for suicide, and risk for self-directed violence.
- Primary *DSM-IV-TR* diagnoses include bipolar I and II disorders, cyclothymic disorder, major depressive disorder, and dysthymic disorder. Cyclothymia is a disorder resembling bipolar disorder but with less severe symptoms, characterized by repeated periods of nonpsychotic depression and hypomania for at least 2 years. Dysthymia is a milder form of depression lasting 2 or more years.
- The expected outcome of nursing care is that the patient will be emotionally responsive and return to a pre-illness level of functioning.
- In planning care the nurse's priorities are the reduction and ultimate removal of the patient's maladaptive emotional responses, restoration of the patient's occupational and psychosocial functioning, improvement in the patient's quality of life, and minimization of the likelihood of relapse and recurrence.
- Treatment consists of three phases: acute, continuation, and maintenance. The goal of acute treatment is to eliminate the symptoms. The goal of continuation treatment is to prevent relapse, which is the return of symptoms, and to promote recovery. The goal of maintenance treatment is to prevent recurrence, or a new episode of illness.
- Early diagnosis and treatment are associated with more positive outcomes.
- Nursing interventions must reflect the complex multicausal nature of the model and address all maladaptive aspects of a person's life.
- In caring for patients with a severe mood disorder, highest priority should be given to the potential for suicide. They are at particular risk when they appear to be coming out of their depression because they may then have the energy and opportunity to kill themselves. Acute manic states are also life threatening.
- Nursing interventions address environmental issues, nurse-patient relationships, physiological treatments, expressing feelings, cognitive strategies, behavioral change, social skills, and mental health education.
- Supervision and peer support groups can be helpful to the nurse working with patients with mood disorders. Of particular significance are the many special aspects of transference and countertransference that may occur.

KEY TERMS

CHAPTER REVIEW QUESTIONS

1. Match each term in Column A with the correct examples in Column B.

Column A

_____ Behaviors related to emotional responses

_____ Coping mechanisms

_____ *DSM-IV-TR* diagnoses

_____ Precipitating stressors

_____ Predisposing factors

_____ Seasonal affective disorder

Column B

A. Introjection, denial, suppression
B. Loss, life events, role strain
C. Delayed grief reaction, depression/mania
D. Bipolar, cyclothymia, depression
E. Genetics, early childhood loss, turning anger inward
F. Depression that comes with shortened daylight

2. Fill in the blanks.

A. The somatic therapy of _____ is often used for patients with severe depression with somatic delusions and delusional guilt, suicidal ideation, and weight loss.

B. Substantial evidence exists for abnormal regulation of the _____ neurotransmitter system in depression.

C. Depressed patients with a history of manic episodes are said to have _____ disorder. Depressed patients who have had only episodes of depression are said to have _____ depression.

D. Prior episodes, family history, prior suicide attempts, female gender, and lack of social support are all _____ factors for depression.

E. The brain structure that is currently the focus of much research for its role in depression is the _____.

F. Two other psychiatric illnesses that often occur with depression are _____ disorders and _____ disorders.

G. When both medications and psychotherapy are used to treat depression and mania, the success rate of treatment is _____% to _____%.

H. The goal of the acute phase of treatment for depression is to eliminate symptoms and produce a therapeutic _____. This phase usually lasts _____ to _____ weeks. If patients are symptom free at the end of that time they are said to be in _____.

I. The goal of the continuation phase of treatment for depression is to promote _____ and prevent _____. This phase usually lasts _____ to _____ months.

J. The goal of the maintenance phase of treatment for depression is to prevent _____. This phase may last _____.

3. Provide short answers for the following questions.

A. List the responses on the continuum of emotional responses and give a brief definition of each one.

B. What are the three major aims when intervening in the cognitive area with a depressed patient?

C. You are asked to join a peer support group made up of nurses who work with patients with depression. How can such a group be helpful to you? What can you contribute to the group?

D. Design an intervention program for mothers who are depressed and their young children.

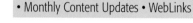

Visit Evolve for additional resources related to the content of this chapter.

 http://evolve.elsevier.com/Stuart/principles/
• Topical Course Outline • Student Workbook Exercises • Critical Thinking Questions and Activities • Case Studies • Research Topics
• Monthly Content Updates • WebLinks

Student Study CD-ROM

Access the accompanying CD-ROM for animations, interactive exercises, review questions for the NCLEX examination, and an audio glossary.

REFERENCES

Abramson L et al: Hopelessness depression: a theory-based subtype of depression, *Psychol Rev* 96:358, 1989.

Alexopoulos G et al: Comorbidity of late life depression: an opportunity for research on mechanisms and treatment, *Biol Psychiatry* 52:543, 2002.

Altshuler LL et al: Treatment of depression in women: a summary of the expert consensus guidelines, *J Psychiatr Pract* 7:185, 2001.

American Psychiatric Association: *Diagnostic and statistical manual of mental disorders*, ed 4, text revision, Washington, DC, 2000a, American Psychiatric Association.

American Psychiatric Association: Practice guideline for the treatment of patients with major depressive disorder (revision), *Am J Psychiatry* 157:1, 2000b.

American Psychiatric Association: Practice guideline for the treatment of patients with bipolar disorder (revision), *Am J Psychiatry* 159:1, 2002.

Arieti S, Bemporad JR: The psychological organization of depression, *Am J Psychiatry* 137:1360, 1980.

Beck A et al: *Cognitive therapy of depression*, New York, 1979, The Guilford Press.

Beck CT: Predictors of postpartum depression: an update, *Nurs Res* 50:275, 2001.

Berg AO: Screening for depression: recommendations and rationale, *Am J Nurs* 102:77, 2002.

Biederman J et al: Patterns of psychopathology and dysfunction in high-risk children of parents with panic disorder and major depression, *Am J Psychiatry* 158:49, 2001.

Clements PT et al: Cultural perspectives of death, grief and bereavement, *J Psychosoc Nurs Ment Health Serv* 41:18, 2003.

Dochterman JM, Bulechek GM, editors: *Nursing interventions classification (NIC)*, ed 4, St Louis, 2004, Mosby.

Edler CR: Beyond the baby blues: postpartum depression, *Nurs Spectrum*, October: 26, 2000.

Egan KA, Arnold RL: Grief and bereavement care, *Am J Nurs* 103:42, 2003.

Goldberg JF: Bipolar disorder with comorbid substance abuse: diagnosis, prognosis, and treatment, *J Psychiatr Pract* 7:109, 2001.

Jamison KR: Suicide and bipolar disorder, *J Clin Psychiatry* 61:47, 2000.

Jarrett RB et al: Preventing recurrent depression using cognitive therapy with and without a continuation phase: a randomized clinical trial, *Archives Gen Psychiatry* 58:381, 2001.

Kahn D et al: Medication treatment of bipolar disorder 2000: a summary of the expert consensus guidelines, *J Psychiatr Pract* 6:197, 2000.

Keller MB: Past, present and future directions for defining optimal treatment outcome in depression: remission and beyond, *JAMA* 289:3152, 2003.

Kessler RC et al: The epidemiology of major depressive disorder: results from the National Comorbidity Survey Replication, *JAMA* 289:3095, 2003.

Kirmayer LJ: Cultural variations in the clinical presentation of depression and anxiety: implications for diagnosis and treatment, *J Clin Psychiatry* 62:22, 2001.

Klein DN et al: Five-year course and outcome of dysthymic disorder: a prospective, naturalistic follow-up study, *Am J Psychiatry* 157:931, 2000.

Lewinsohn P et al: Reinforcement and depression. In Depue R, editor: *The psychobiology of the depressive disorders*, New York, 1979, Academic Press.

Mazure CM et al: Adverse life events and cognitive-personality characteristics in the prediction of major depression and antidepressant response, *Am J Psychiatry* 157:896, 2000.

Meredith LS et al: Are better ratings of the patient-provider relationship associated with higher quality care for depression? *Medical Care* 39:349, 2001.

Merikangas KR et al: Future of genetics of mood disorders research, *Biol Psychiatry* 52:457, 2002.

Miranda J et al: Ethnic minorities, *Ment Health Serv Res* 4:231, 2002a.

Miranda J et al: Gender issues and socially disadvantaged women, *Ment Health Serv Res* 4:249, 2002b.

Moorhead S, Johnson M, Maas M, editors: *Nursing outcomes classification (NOC)*, ed 3, St Louis, 2004, Mosby.

Nathan P, Gorman J: *A guide to treatments that work*, ed 2, New York, 2002, Oxford University Press.

Piper WE et al: Prevalence of loss and complicated grief among psychiatric outpatients, *Psychiatr Serv* 52:1069, 2001.

Raingruber B: Client and provider perspectives regarding the stigma of and nonstigmatizing interventions for depression, *Arch Psychiatr Nurs* 16:201, 2002.

Ranga K: Comorbidity of depression with other medical diseases in the elderly, *Biol Psychiatry* 52:559, 2002.

Rickelman, B: Demoralization as a precursor to serious depression, *J Am Psychiatr Nurs Assoc* 8:9, 2002.

Seligman M: *Helplessness: on depression, development, and death*, San Francisco, 1975, WH Freeman.

Sullivan PF, Neale MC, Kendler KS: Genetic epidemiology of major depression: review and meta-analysis, *Am J Psychiatry* 157:1552, 2000.

von Ammon Cavanaugh S et al: Medical illness, past depression, and present depression: a predictive triad for in-hospital mortality, *Am J Psychiatry* 158:43, 2001.

Wells K et al: Overcoming barriers to reducing the burden of affective disorders, *Biol Psychiatry* 52:655, 2002.

Zuroff DC et al: Relation of therapeutic alliance and perfectionism to outcome in brief outpatient treatment of depression, *J Consult Clin Psychol* 68:114, 2000.

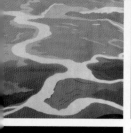

Out, out brief candle! Life's but a walking shadow, a poor player That struts and frets his hour upon the stage And then is heard no more. It is a tale Told by an idiot, full of sound and fury, Signifying nothing.

WILLIAM SHAKESPEARE, MACBETH, ACT V

20 | SELF-PROTECTIVE RESPONSES AND SUICIDAL BEHAVIOR

Gail W. Stuart

LEARNING OBJECTIVES

After studying this chapter, the student should be able to:

1. Describe the continuum of adaptive and maladaptive self-protective responses (I).
2. Identify behaviors associated with self-protective responses (II).
3. Analyze predisposing factors, precipitating stressors, and appraisal of stressors related to self-protective responses (II).
4. Describe coping resources and coping mechanisms related to self-protective responses (II).
5. Formulate nursing diagnoses related to self-protective responses (III).
6. Examine the relationship between nursing diagnoses and medical diagnoses related to self-protective responses (III).
7. Identify expected outcomes and short-term nursing goals related to self-protective responses (IV).
8. Develop a patient education plan to promote compliance with health-care treatment (V).
9. Analyze nursing interventions related to self-protective responses (VI).
10. Evaluate nursing care related to self-protective responses (VII).

TOPICAL OUTLINE

I. Continuum of Self-Protective Responses
   A. Epidemiology of Suicide
II. Assessment
   A. Behaviors
   B. Predisposing Factors
   C. Precipitating Stressors
   D. Appraisal of Stressors
   E. Coping Resources
   F. Coping Mechanisms
III. Diagnosis
   A. Nursing Diagnoses
   B. Medical Diagnoses
IV. Outcome Identification
V. Planning
VI. Implementation
   A. Protection and Safety
   B. Increasing Self-Esteem
   C. Regulating Emotions and Behaviors
   D. Mobilizing Social Support
   E. Patient Education
   F. Suicide Prevention
VII. Evaluation

evolve Visit Evolve for additional resources related to the content of this chapter.
http://evolve.elsevier.com/Stuart/principles/

Life is full of risk. People must choose the amount of danger to which they are willing to expose themselves. Sometimes these choices are conscious and rational. For instance, the elderly person who decides to stay in the house on an icy day has chosen not to risk falling and possibly fracturing a bone. Other risk-taking behavior is unconscious. Soldiers who volunteer for a suicide mission are probably unaware of their motivation. If asked, they would probably cite patriotism or concern for comrades. Most people go through life accepting some risks as part of their daily routine while carefully avoiding others.

Even though life is risky, most societies have a norm that defines the degree of danger to which people may expose themselves. This norm varies according to age, gender, socioeconomic status, and occupation. In general, the very young, the old, and women are seen as needing to be protected from harm. Some risk takers are admired, particularly athletes, military personnel, those with dangerous occupations, and those who place themselves in danger to help others. At the same time,

feelings of admiration may be accompanied by fear and perplexity about the danger-seeking behavior.

◼ CONTINUUM OF SELF-PROTECTIVE RESPONSES

Protection and survival are fundamental needs of all living things. A continuum of self-protecting responses would have **self-enhancement** and **growth-promoting risk taking** as the most adaptive responses, whereas indirect **self-destructive behavior, self-injury**, and **suicide** would be maladaptive responses. Self-destructive behavior may be direct or indirect.

Direct self-destructive behavior includes any form of suicidal activity, such as suicide ideation, threats, attempts, and completed suicide. The intent of this behavior is death, and the person is aware of the desired outcome.

Indirect self-destructive behavior is any activity detrimental to the person's physical well-being that potentially may result in death. However, the person may be unaware of this potential and deny it if confronted. Examples include eating disorders (see Chapter 25) and abuse of alcohol and other drugs (see Chapter 24). Other examples include cigarette smoking, reckless driving, gambling, criminal activity, sexual promiscuity, socially deviant behavior, stress-seeking behavior, participation in high-risk sports, and noncompliance with medical treatment.

Theories of self-destructive behavior overlap with those of self-concept and disturbances in mood. Careful study of Chapters 18 and 19 will help the reader understand the behaviors discussed in this chapter. To think about or attempt destruction of the self, the person must have low self-regard. Low self-esteem leads to depression, which is always present in self-destructive behavior. The range of self-protective responses is shown in Figure 20-1.

The levels of behavior in the continuum may overlap. For instance, the girl who learns and excels at gymnastics is building her self-esteem and projecting a positive self-concept. However, if she tries movements she is not prepared for and does not take safety measures, her behavior becomes self-injurious or indirectly self-destructive. Similarly, a diabetic man who has never complied completely with his prescribed diet and medication regimen may become discouraged and intentionally take an overdose of insulin. Thus the nurse must be alert to subtle shifts in the mood and behavior of patients when assessing maladaptive self-protective responses.

Where do you think patients' requests for assisted-suicide falls in the continuum of self-protective responses? ■

Epidemiology of Suicide

About 31,000 people complete the act of suicide each year, an average of one person every 18 minutes. Suicide is the eleventh leading cause of death in the United States. Suicides outnumber homicides in the United States; homicide is the fourteenth leading cause of death (American Association of Suicidology, 2002). The actual number of suicides may be two to three times higher because of the underreporting that occurs. In addition, many single-car accidents and homicides are, in fact, suicides.

Worldwide, at least 1000 suicides occur each day, and it is the leading cause of death, outnumbering homicide or war-related deaths. This loss of productive life in the United States each year amounts to 645,680 lost years. The United States now has one of the highest suicide rates for young men in the world, surpassing Japan and Sweden, countries long identified with high rates of suicide.

Suicide is the third leading killer of young people. The rate of suicide among youth has tripled in the past 30 years and has increased by 25% for the elderly. **The highest suicide rate for any group in this country is among people over age 65, especially white men over 85.** Although this group constitutes 12.6% of the total U.S. population, it accounts for about 18.1% of suicide deaths. White males over the age of 50 represent the greatest number of these deaths (Figure 20-2).

Teen suicide in the United States is nearly five times as common among boys as among girls. Suicide is also more common among whites than blacks at all ages. **The overwhelming majority of completed suicides are committed by males.** Well over half of these males shoot themselves, and the use of guns in suicide is increasing rapidly. **Women attempt suicide twice as often as men.** They use potentially less lethal means, such as medications and wrist slashing. However, one third of all women and over half of those 15 to 29 years of age who complete suicide use guns.

Reports of suicide among young children are rare, but suicidal behavior is not. As many as 12,000 children ages 5 to 14 may be hospitalized in this country every year for deliberate self-destructive acts.

What factors might contribute to the high rate of suicide among white elderly males? ■

ASSESSMENT

Behaviors

Noncompliance. It has been estimated that one half of patients do not comply with their health care treatment plan. This level of noncompliance is the same for those with both physical and psychiatric illnesses. Noncompliance accounts for 125,000 deaths annually and contributes to 10% to 25% of hospital and nursing home admissions.

People who do not comply with recommended health care activities are generally aware that they have chosen not to care for themselves. They usually have a reason for noncom-

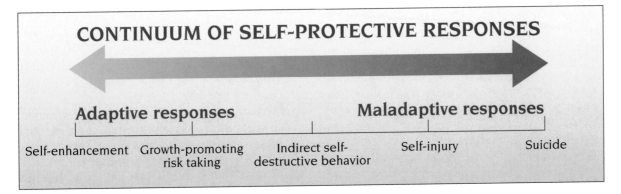

Figure 20-1   Continuum of self-protective responses.

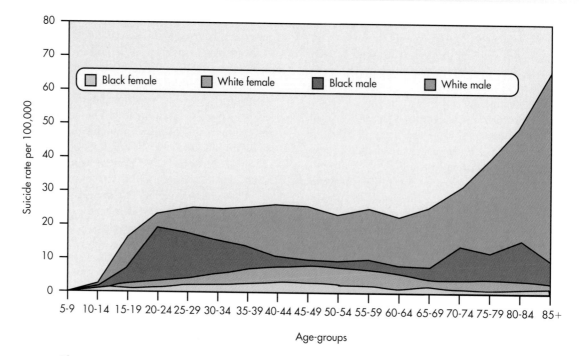

Figure 20-2   U.S. suicide rates by age, gender, and racial group, 2001. (From Centers for Disease Control and Prevention, National Center for Health Statistics, Washington, DC, 2003, National Institute of Mental Health.)

pliance, such as being asymptomatic, not being able to afford the treatment they need, not understanding the treatment, or not having time. Patients also may minimize the seriousness of their problems. Many chronic illnesses are characterized by long periods of stability, during which the person may not be aware of discomfort. This reinforces the noncompliant behavior.

The most prominent behavior associated with noncompliance is refusal to admit the seriousness of the health problem. This denial interferes with acceptance of treatment. Another aspect of noncompliance is that **guilt** about not following health care recommendations also may interfere with obtaining regular care. Noncompliant people are also struggling for **control.** Serious illness is often seen as an attack on the person and a betrayal by the body. Patients need to reassert their control and prove that they are still the master of their fate. Most chronically ill people need to test the limits of their control and the validity of the prescribed self-care regimen. The following clinical example illustrates the problem of noncompliance with a prescribed health care regimen.

CLINICAL EXAMPLE

Mrs. C was a 61-year-old, white married woman who had been in good health most of her life. She had three grown children who had left home and established their own families. She and her husband were both looking forward to his retirement in 6 months. They planned to buy a recreational vehicle and travel around the United States.

The nurse practitioner did a complete physical examination each time Mrs. C was seen. On her most recent visit, laboratory studies revealed an elevated blood glucose level. Her diagnosis was diabetes mellitus, adult onset. Mrs. C was told that her condition was not serious and could be controlled by diet. She was 20 pounds (9 kg) overweight and was advised that she needed to lose the excess weight. She was instructed about her diet, how to test her urine, and about possible complications of diabetes.

Mrs. C was frightened about her condition but did not mention this because no one else seemed very concerned. At first, she was conscientious about following her diet and testing her urine. She felt very well and was proud when she lost 5 pounds. As time went on, Mrs. C began to wonder whether she was really so sick. She had never felt ill. On her husband's birthday, she fixed a special dinner and baked a cake. She decided she deserved a reward for "being good" and did not follow her diet. She anxiously tested her urine at bedtime and it was negative. Then her son and his family visited for a week. She fixed all their favorite foods and ate with them. She still felt fine and decided she did not need to test her urine. When it was time for her next checkup, she postponed calling the nurse practitioner. She was very busy preparing for retirement travel.

Selected Nursing Diagnosis

- Noncompliance related to fear of the diagnosis of diabetes, as evidenced by lack of adherence to medical treatment plan ◼

Do you think that noncompliance can ever be an adaptive response? Why or why not? ◼

Self-Injury. Society accepts some forms of self-injury as normal. Examples of culturally sanctioned forms include body piercing, cosmetic eyebrow plucking, hair twisting, circumcision, nail biting, and tattoos. Various terms have been used to describe self-injurious behavior: self-abuse, self-directed aggression, deliberate self-harm, self-inflicted injury, and self-mutilation.

Self-injury can be defined as the act of deliberate harm to one's own body. The injury is done to oneself, without the aid of another person, and the injury is severe enough to cause tissue damage. Common forms of self-injurious behavior include cutting and burning the skin, banging the head and limbs, picking at wounds, and chewing fingers.

Many nurses mistake self-injury for potential suicide. In fact, these are two separate phenomena. Usually the lethality of self-injury is low, and patients who self-injure typically want relief from the tension they feel rather than to kill themselves (Gallop, 2002). Self-injury is also different from other self-destructive behaviors, such as bingeing, drug abuse, smoking, and high-risk activities. Self-injury is a contained event that occurs in a short time span and with an awareness of the consequences of the act.

Self-injurious behavior may be categorized by the type of patient and clinical context in which the behavior occurs:

- **People with mental retardation**. The mentally retarded may have outward-directed aggression along with self-injurious behavior.
- **Psychotic patients**. Self-injuring acts among psychotic patients tend to be sporadic and often occur in response to command hallucinations or delusions.
- **Prison populations**. Self-injury in prisons is difficult to assess because of poor documentation, drug use, and undiagnosed psychiatric disorders. Many self-injurious events among prisoners may be intentionally manipulative, designed to force transfer to a less restrictive facility.
- **Character disorders, particularly borderline personality disorder**. This group is often young and female with a poor tolerance of anxiety and anger; also included are patients with eating disorders.

Suicidal Behavior. Suicidal behavior is usually divided into the categories of suicide ideation, suicide threats, suicide attempts, and completed suicide. Suicide ideation is the thought of self-inflicted death, either self-reported or reported to others. Suicidal ideation may vary in seriousness. It can be *passive*, when there are only thoughts of suicide with no intent to act; or *active*, when there are plans or thoughts of causing one's own death. **All suicide behavior is serious, whatever the intent, and thus suicidal ideation deserves the nurse's highest priority care.**

A suicide threat is a warning, direct or indirect, verbal or nonverbal, that a person is planning to take one's own life. It may be veiled but usually occurs before overt suicidal activity takes place. The suicidal person may make a statement such as "Will you remember me when I'm gone?" or "Take care of my family for me." In the context of recent stressors and the person's life situation, statements such as these may be ominous.

Nonverbal communication often reveals the suicide threat. The person may give away prized possessions, make a will or funeral arrangements, or withdraw from friendships and social activities. Sometimes a person may make a direct verbal suicidal threat, but this occurs less often. The threat is an indication of the ambivalence that is usually present in suicidal behavior. It represents the hope that someone will recognize the danger and rescue the person from self-destructive impulses. It also may be an effort to discover whether anyone cares enough to prevent the person from harming himself or herself.

A suicide attempt is any self-directed actions taken by a person that will lead to death if not stopped. In the assessment of suicidal behavior, much emphasis is placed on the lethality of the method threatened or used. Although all suicide threats and attempts must be taken seriously, vigilant attention is indicated when the person is planning or tries a highly lethal method. Such methods include gunshot, hanging, or jumping. Less lethal means include carbon monoxide and drug overdose, which allow time for discovery once the suicidal action has begun.

Assessment of the suicidal person also includes whether the person has made a specific plan and whether the means to carry out the plan are available. The most suicidal person is one who plans a violent death (such as a gunshot to the head), has a specific plan (for example, as soon as his wife goes shopping), and has the means readily available (such as a loaded gun in a desk drawer). This person is exhibiting little ambivalence about a suicide plan. On the other hand, the person who contemplates taking a bottle of aspirin if the situation at work does not improve soon is communicating an element of hope. This person is really asking for help in coping with a poor work situation. The following clinical example illustrates the behavior of a suicidal person.

CLINICAL EXAMPLE

Mr. Y was a 52-year-old black man employed in the foundry of a large steel mill. He had worked for the company for 20 years. He lived in a rented room in a blue-collar neighborhood near the mill. Most of his neighbors were Appalachian white and southern black families who had moved to the community to work at the mill. The neighborhood had an undercurrent of racial tension, but Mr. Y was not involved in conflicts with his neighbors. He had separated from his wife before moving to the community and had no close friends or family. The separation resulted from his violent behavior related to drinking binges.

Mr. Y was seen by the occupational health nurse, Ms. G, when he came to the employee health clinic following a 6-week absence from work. He had been hospitalized for broken ribs and a concussion after he had been beaten and robbed by a gang of adolescents in an alley behind his home. Ms. G was familiar with this patient because he had participated in the company's employee assistance program for alcoholics. When she saw him in the clinic, she immediately noted that he appeared depressed. His face was expressionless, his posture was slumped, and he had lost weight. He appeared disheveled, which was a change from his usual neat appearance. His speech was slow and halting and so soft that he could barely be heard.

He told Ms. G that he had a request to make of her. He knew from past conversations that she was an animal lover. He wanted her to take his pet dog because he did not feel able to care for it adequately, and the neighbors who kept it while he was in the hospital had neglected it. Ms. G was very concerned about Mr. Y and asked him how he was spending his time. He said he kept the television on and he thought a lot. When asked, he said he felt "too shaky" to go outside unless he absolutely had to. He thought the boys who attacked him were still in the neighborhood.

Ms. G asked if he had thought about harming himself. Mr. Y looked startled, then admitted that he saw no other solution to his problem. "It makes sense. I don't have anybody. If you take Rover, I can go." With further questioning, he admitted that he had a loaded revolver at home and planned to use it after he left the clinic. Ms. G realized that Mr. Y needed help immediately and initiated plans for hospitalization.

Selected Nursing Diagnoses

- Risk for suicide related to impoverished social environment, as evidenced by intent to kill self with a gun
- Powerlessness related to recent neighborhood attack, as evidenced by expressed feelings of despair and hopelessness ■

Completed suicide, or simply suicide, is death from self-inflicted injury, poisoning, or suffocation where there is evidence that the decedent intended to kill himself or herself. Completed suicide may take place after warning signs have been missed or ignored. Some people do not give any easily recognizable warning signs.

Research done on completed suicide has of necessity been retrospective. However, it can be informative to interview survivors. This procedure is known as the psychological autopsy. It is a retrospective review of the person's behavior before the suicide. Table 20-1 compares the characteristics of suicide completers and suicide attempters based on this process.

Significant others of suicidal people, including survivors, have many feelings about this behavior. An element of hostility exists in suicidal behavior. Often the message to significant others, stated or implied, is "You should have cared more." At times, when the person survives the attempt, this message may be transmitted in a manipulative way.

An example is the adolescent girl who discovers that her boyfriend is dating someone else and takes an overdose of over-the-counter sleeping pills. If she sets the scene so that she will almost inevitably be discovered and makes sure that her boyfriend hears of her behavior, she is behaving in a hostile, manipulative way. A remorseful response by the boyfriend would be reinforcing and increase the likelihood that she will repeat the behavior.

It is important to treat all suicide attempts seriously and help the patient develop healthier communication patterns. People who do not really intend to die may do so if they are not discovered in time.

When suicide is successful, the survivors are left with many feelings that they cannot communicate to the involved object, the dead person (see A Family Speaks). This may lead to an unresolved grief reaction and depression (see Chapter 19). Some suicide prevention centers have become involved in postvention in which survivors are helped, either individually or in groups, to express their feelings and work through their grief.

In summary, the suicidal patient may have many different clinical behaviors. Mood disturbances are often present, as are somatic complaints. Feelings of hopelessness and helplessness are important in explaining suicidal ideation. Nurses should take a careful medical and psychiatric history, paying specific attention to the mental status examination described in Chapter 7 and the psychosocial history, and evaluate the patient for recent losses, life stresses, and substance use and abuse (see Critical Thinking about Contemporary Issues, on p. 370).

Contrary to common opinion, directly questioning the patient about suicidal thought and plans will not cause the patient to take suicidal action. Rather, most people want to be prevented from carrying out their self-destruction. Most patients are relieved to be asked about these feelings. One of the most important questions to ask of suicidal patients is whether they think they can control their behavior and refrain from acting on their impulses. If patients cannot do this, immediate psychiatric hospitalization is indicated.

Finally, the nurse should have some systematic way of evaluating a patient for the risk of suicide. The use of an assessment tool to explore self-protective responses, such as the one for inpatient settings presented in Figure 20-3, may be most helpful. Box 20-1 presents additional information for reference when using the suicide/self-harm assessment.

Table 20-1	Characteristics of Suicide Completers and Attempters	
SUICIDE COMPLETERS	SUICIDE ATTEMPTERS
Three times as likely to be men	Mainly women under age 40
Usually suffer from depression and/or alcohol or substance abuse	Less likely to have depression and other psychiatric conditions
	More likely to have personality disorders
Plan the suicide act	Act impulsively
Use highly lethal method	Use method with low lethality
Select setting unlikely to be interrupted	Act in the presence of or notify others

A FAMILY SPEAKS

My husband died last year. He didn't commit suicide, but he took his own life just as surely as if he had pulled the trigger of a gun. Only his weapon was a cigarette. You see, 2 years ago his doctor discovered a cancer lesion on his lung. At that time my husband was told he needed to lose weight, cut down on his drinking, and most of all, stop smoking. But my husband wasn't a very good patient.

Sometimes I blame myself for not doing more. I nagged for a while, but that only seemed to make our marriage worse. My husband said that what he did with his life was his own choice and that his father had smoked all of his life and had lived until he was 84. My husband died at age 62.

One good thing has come out of this tragedy, however. My son has stopped smoking and has vowed he will never touch another cigarette for as long as he lives. That small goodness gives me comfort and some sense of hope.

INPATIENT SUICIDE/SELF-HARM ASSESSMENT

Complete on admission, each shift, at discharge, and any time when suicidal or self-harm risk is suggested.

Directions:
1. Answer Question I.
2. Complete Section II by circling one of the three descriptors for each Key Factor that BEST describes the patient.
3. Complete Section III.
4. Add the points for each circled item in Sections I, II, and III to obtain the total score.

I.	Is the current admission precipitated by suicide attempt?	Yes 2	No 1

II. Key Factors	High Risk (1:1)	Moderate Risk (q15min observation)	No Precautions
Contract for safety	Unwilling to contract OR Unable to contract because of impaired reality testing (hallucinations, delusions, dementia, delirium, dissociation) 2	Contracts but is ambivalent or guarded 1	Reliably contracts for safety 0
Suicide plan	Has plan with actual or potential access to planned method 2	Has plan without access to planned method 1	No plan 0
Plan lethality	Highly lethal plan (gun, hanging, jumping, carbon monoxide) 2	Medium lethality of plan (sleeping pills, overdose of aspirin, barbiturates) 1	Low lethality of plan (superficial scratching, head banging, pillow over face, biting, holding breath) 0
Elopement risk	High elopement risk 2	Low elopement risk 1	No elopement risk 0
Suicidal ideation	Constant suicidal thoughts 2	Intermittent or fleeting suicidal thoughts 1	No current suicidal thoughts 0
Attempt history	Past attempts of high lethality 2	Past attempts of low lethality 1	No previous attempts 0
Symptoms (circle those that apply) hopelessness helplessness anhedonia guilt/shame anger/hostility impulsivity impaired problem solving	5-6 symptoms present 2	3-4 symptoms present 1	0-2 symptoms present 0
Current morbid thoughts (reunion fantasies, preoccupation with death, disturbing nightmares)	Constantly 2	Frequently 1	Rarely 0

III.	RN's Subjective Appraisal of Patient's Reliability:	Pt. replies not trustworthy; several nonverbal cues	4
		Pt. replies questionably trustworthy; at least one nonverbal cue	3
		Pt. replies trustworthy	0

IV. Scoring Key:	High Risk 10+ points	Moderate Risk 4–9 points	Low Risk 0–3 points

Total Score _____   Date/Time _____   RN Signature _____

Figure 20-3   Inpatient suicide/self-harm assessment.

Critical Thinking *About* Contemporary Issues

Are Health Care Professionals Missing Suicidal Behavior in Their Patients?

It has been reported that 8 of 10 patients who commit suicide talked about it with someone before completing the act. Often the person they talk with is a health care professional. The problem is that health care providers often miss the signs and symptoms of depression and the subtle indicators of self-destructive intentions.

There is evidence, for example, that 45% of people who complete suicide visit primary care providers within 1 month before their attempt, and 20% had contact with mental health services within 1 month before their suicide (Luoma, Martin, and Pearson, 2002). Among the elderly, more than 80% give clues of their intent. Of the elderly who commit suicide, 75% are known to have visited their personal physician in the month before they took their life (Blank et al, 2001).

Health care professionals report a surprisingly small amount of probing for depressive or suicidal symptoms, even when they are mentioned by the patient. It thus appears that much work needs to be done to alert health care providers to the severity and extent of this problem and to help them better evaluate patients for potential self-destructive responses.

Predisposing Factors

No one theory alone explains self-destructive responses or guides therapeutic intervention. Behavior theory suggests that self-injury is learned and reinforced in childhood or adolescence. Psychological theory focuses on problems in early stages of ego development, suggesting that early interpersonal trauma and unmanaged anxiety may provoke episodes of self-injury. Interpersonal theory proposes that self-injury may result from interactions that leave the child feeling guilty and worthless.

A history of abuse or incest also may precipitate self-destructiveness if negative perceptions have been internalized and acted on and secure attachments are lacking. Other predisposing factors related to self-destructive behavior include the inability to communicate needs and feelings verbally; feelings of guilt, depression, and depersonalization; and fluctuating emotions.

Five predisposing factors—psychiatric diagnosis, personality traits and disorders, psychosocial and environmental factors, genetic and familial variables, and biochemical factors—contribute to a biopsychosocial model for understanding self-destructive behavior over the life cycle.

BOX 20-1

Definitions and Examples of Terms Used in the Inpatient Suicide/Self-Harm Assessment

Section I: Is the Current Admission Precipitated by a Suicide Attempt?

Choose "YES" if:
- The patient states that suicide/self-harm was the intended outcome of his or her actions.
- The patient is unwilling/refuses to discuss the reason for admission.

Choose "NO" if:
- The patient states that suicide/self-harm was not the intended outcome of his or her actions.

Section II: Key Factors

Contract for safety
- Attempt to get patient to agree/promise to be safe.
- Use statements such as "I have to make sure you are going to be safe while you're here. Can you promise me that you won't try to hurt yourself?" and/or "If you start thinking about hurting yourself, will you tell us right away?"

High-Risk Behaviors:
- Unwilling to talk about being safe
- Refuses to agree/promise to be safe
- Demonstrates anger about failed suicide/self-harm attempt; statements such as "I wish I'd died"
- Unable to contract because of the thought processes not being consistent with reality (hallucinations, delusions, delirium and dementia)

Moderate-Risk Behaviors:
- Willing/able to talk about being safe but hesitant to agree; statements such as "I'll agree that right now I won't hurt myself, but I may change my mind"
- Willing/able to talk about being safe but agrees for only short periods of time

Low-Risk Behaviors:
- Able to verbally agree/promise to be safe
- Expresses regret about suicide/self-harm attempt

Suicide/self-harm plan
- Determine whether patient has a plan to attempt suicide/self-harm.
- Ask questions such as "Are you thinking about killing/hurting yourself now?" or "Are you feeling suicidal now?" and "Have you thought of how you would kill/hurt yourself?"

High-Risk Behaviors:
- Able to describe thoughts, plan, and method for suicide/self-harm that is accessible; statements such as "I'll get my father's gun from his closet and shoot myself in the head when nobody's home"

Moderate-Risk Behaviors:
- Thinking about or has a plan for suicide/self-harm, but has not identified a method, or the plan is not accessible; statements such as "I've thought about shooting myself but I don't have a gun," or "I've thought of taking a bunch of pills but I don't know which ones to take"

Low-Risk Behaviors:
- Has no plan for suicide/self harm

Plan lethality
- Determine how serious the injury would be if the patient's plan were carried out.
- Use patient statements to choose high, moderate, or low risk.

Elopement risk
- Determine whether patient is willing to accept hospital treatment. Use statements such as "Are you willing to stay here in the hospital for treatment?"

From Behavioral Health Services at Southwest Washington Medical Center, Vancouver, Washington, 2003. Used with permission.

Psychiatric Diagnosis. More than 90% of adults who end their lives by suicide have an associated psychiatric illness. There are four broad psychiatric disorders that put people at particular risk for suicide:

- Mood disorders
- Substance abuse
- Schizophrenia
- Anxiety disorders

Suicide is the most serious complication of mood disorders, with 15% of those with these illnesses ending their lives by suicide. Suicide is particularly common in depressed elderly men. Patients with bipolar disorder and psychotic depression are at greatest risk. Many who die from suicide have a prior history of attempts, have explicitly communicated their intent, and have been in psychiatric treatment during the months preceding their death (Sher et al, 2001).

Alcohol use is associated with 25% to 50% of suicides. Among patients who are alcohol dependent, suicide often occurs late in the disease and is often related to some interpersonal loss or the onset of medical complications (Goldberg, Singer, and Garno, 2001).

Schizophrenia, a disease that affects 1% of the population, is associated with a high incidence of suicide. Among these patients, 40% report suicidal thoughts, 20% to 40% make unsuccessful suicide attempts, and 10% to 15% end their lives by suicide. The risk is greatest for patients who are male, white, young, unmarried, unemployed, living alone, and depressed, with chronic recurring illness (American Psychiatric Association, 2003).

Anxiety disorders, particularly panic disorder and post-traumatic stress disorder, are associated with increased rates of suicidal ideation, suicide attempts, and completed suicide. Other groups that may be at high risk include those with eating disorders, attention deficit hyperactivity disorder, some personality disorders (borderline personality disorder and antisocial personality disorder), and conduct disorders in adolescents.

Personality Traits. The three aspects of personality that are most closely associated with increased risk of suicide are **hostility, impulsivity,** and **depression.** These traits are important because they cross diagnostic groups. The co-existence of antisocial and depressive symptoms appears to be a particularly

---

BOX **20-1**

Definitions and Examples of Terms Used in the Inpatient Suicide/Self-Harm Assessment—cont'd

High-Risk Behaviors:
- Expresses desire to leave the hospital.
- Attempting to leave.

Moderate-Risk Behaviors:
- Not sure about staying in the hospital.
- Agrees to stay for only a short or unrealistic period of time.

Low-Risk Behaviors:
- Agrees to stay in the hospital until discharged.

Suicidal ideation
- Determine how often the patient thinks about the act of suicide/self-harm.
- Use the same questions as described with suicide/self-harm plan and ask, "Have you thought about killing/hurting yourself?" "How often?" or "How often do you think about killing/hurting yourself?"

Attempt history
- Determine if the patient has attempted suicide/self-harm in the past and the seriousness of the attempt using the examples under plan lethality.
- Use questions such as, "Have you tried to hurt yourself before?" "How many times?" "How did you try to hurt yourself in the past?"

Symptoms
- Determine the symptoms that the patient displays from assessing answers to questions such as, "What thoughts/feelings do you have right now?" "What thoughts/feelings have you been having?"
- Hopelessness—Statements that reflect the patient's feeling that there is nothing to live for, that demonstrate belief that his or her life is over or will never get any better.

- Helplessness—Statements that reflect the patient's sense that nothing will help him, that there is nothing that will change his feelings/circumstances, or that he does not have the ability to change his feelings/circumstances.
- Anhedonia—The inability to derive pleasure from acts that are normally pleasurable, for example, "My favorite pastime used to be reading, but I don't seem to enjoy reading now." "Nothing is fun any more."
- Impulsivity—The inability to control urges to act without thinking through the consequences.
- Guilt, shame, anger, and rage—If the patient reports or displays these symptoms, they are to be noted in the patient's assessment record.

Current morbid thoughts
- Determine how often the patient thinks about death or being dead to be with a loved one who is dead. Use questions such as, "Do you think about being dead?" "Do you wish you could die to be with a loved one?" "Do you find yourself wishing you were dead?" "How often?"

Section III: RN's Subjective Appraisal of Patient's Reliability
- Choose the answer that best describes your clinical judgment of the patient.
- Nonverbal clues that **might** indicate lack of reliability include refusing to talk about or discuss his or her problems, avoiding eye contact, sarcasm, actions that are inconsistent with what is said.

lethal combination in both adults and young people. The association between hostility and suicide stems from the notion proposed by Freud that the suicidal person turns rage inward against the self. Other studies have found that suicidal people are more socially withdrawn, have lower self-esteem, are less trusting of others, expect bad things to happen to them, feel powerless over their lives, and have a rigid and inflexible way of thinking.

How might the personality traits of hostility, impulsivity, and depression contribute to the development of substance abuse? ■

Psychosocial Milieu. Predisposing factors for suicide include **loss, lack of social supports, negative life events,** and **chronic medical illnesses.** Recent bereavement, separation or divorce, early loss, and decreased social supports are all important factors related to potential suicide. Precipitants of suicidal behavior are often humiliating life events such as interpersonal problems, public embarrassment, loss of a job, or the threat of jail.

Evidence also shows that knowing someone who attempted or committed suicide or exposure to suicide through the media may make one more vulnerable to self-destructive behavior. This appears to be a particularly important factor in cluster suicides (Krysinska, 2003).

The strength of social supports is also important. Evidence has shown that the strength and quality of these supports are important to the etiology of psychiatric problems, compliance with treatment, and response to therapeutic interventions.

Finally, diseases with chronic and debilitating courses often precipitate self-destructive behavior. The prevalence of physical illness varies from 25% to 70% in those who commit

suicide and appears to be an important factor in 10% to 50% of completed suicides. The suicide rate in general hospital patients has been found to be almost three times higher than in the general population (Dhossche, Ulusarac, and Syed, 2001). Among the disorders most often associated with suicide are cancer, Huntington's chorea, epilepsy, musculoskeletal disorders, peptic ulcer disease, and HIV/AIDS.

Family History. A family history of suicide is a significant risk factor for self-destructive behavior. The offspring of mood-disordered suicide attempters are at a markedly greater risk for suicide attempts themselves. Explanations for this association include identification with and imitation of a family member who has committed suicide, family stress, and transmission of genetic factors (Brent et al, 2002; Brent et al, 2003; Runeson and Asberg, 2003). Families of suicide victims have a significantly higher rate of suicide than do families with members who are nonsuicidal but mentally ill. In addition, monozygotic twins have a higher concordance rate for suicide than dizygotic twins.

Biochemical Factors. Growing evidence of an association between suicide or suicidal tendencies and a low level of the brain neurotransmitter **serotonin (5-HT)** has been noted. Recent interest in the role of 5-HT levels as a factor in suicide activity stems from two main areas of study: an increase in the understanding of abnormal 5-HT transmission in the etiology of mental illness, particularly depression and schizophrenia, and a better appreciation that antidepressant drugs enhance the efficacy of serotonin.

This suggests that 5-HT must be in balance to facilitate adaptive emotional responses. This balance can be assessed by measuring the amounts of neurotransmitter produced, and the amount of its metabolites (the leftover products of neurotransmitter breakdown, or turnover). Thus the amount of the metabolite for serotonin, 5-hydroxyindoleacetic acid (5-HIAA), that can be measured in the blood and spinal fluid is an indication of the amount of 5-HT originally available in the brain.

The brain also attempts to regulate or balance neurotransmitter levels in another way. The number of postsynaptic 5-HT receptors in the brain is affected by the available levels of 5-HT. More of these receptors are present if there is too little 5-HT (up-regulation) and fewer are present if there is too much 5-HT (down-regulation) (Figure 20-4). Mood disorders are hypothesized to be the result of an imbalance or deficiency of neurotransmitters, particularly 5-HT. Antidepressant drugs generally increase the amount or efficiency of 5-HT, thus increasing the amount of metabolites and affecting the numbers of 5-HT receptors.

A deficiency in 5-HT and its metabolite, 5-HIAA, and an increase in one of the 5-HT postsynaptic receptors (5-HT_{2A}) are implicated in suicidal behavior. For example, depressed patients with low 5-HT levels have stronger suicidal tendencies than those with normal levels. Among people hospitalized for violent suicide attempts, those with low levels of 5-HIAA in their spinal fluid are 10 times more likely to kill themselves within a year. Similarly, schizophrenic patients

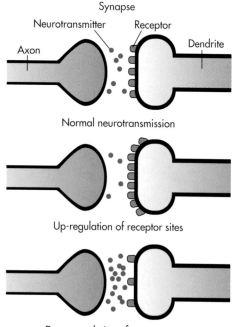

Synapse
Neurotransmitter   Receptor
Axon   Dendrite

Normal neurotransmission

Up-regulation of receptor sites

Down-regulation of receptor sites

Figure 20-4   Levels of postsynaptic serotonin (5-HT) receptors. More receptors are present when there is too little 5-HT (up-regulation) and fewer receptors when there is too much 5-HT (down-regulation).

who have attempted suicide have significantly lower 5-HIAA concentrations than those who have not.

In postmortem studies of the brains of suicide victims, researchers have discovered decreased 5-HT activity in the ventrolateral prefrontal cortex. Finally, a combination of impulsive aggressiveness and feelings of hopelessness, associated with 5-HT deficiency, is more common in men than in women. This may explain why men kill themselves much more often, even though women have a higher rate of depression.

Because of the increased rate of suicide globally and the high suicide risk in psychiatric patients, it would be beneficial to be able to identify high-risk people for suicide prevention and treatment. Thus a simple blood test that could provide a method for identifying those at greatest risk for suicide, in addition to demographic, psychosocial, personality, and behavioral indicators for suicide risk, would be a significant advantage for the mental health field.

Although currently no biological test shows a differentiation between people who commit suicide and those who do not, a great deal of interest has been shown in finding such a biological marker for suicide. Neuroimaging techniques, such as positron emission tomography (PET) scans, also offer an opportunity to visualize 5-HT function in vivo in more direct ways than has been previously available. This technology and emerging genetic research may provide the possibility of timely therapeutic intervention in patients at high risk for suicide.

Do you believe suicide is a fundamental human right and should be allowed by society? Why or why not? ■

Precipitating Stressors

Self-destructive behavior may result from any stress the person feels as overwhelming. Stressors are somewhat individualized, as is the person's ability to tolerate stress. All self-destructive behaviors may be seen as attempts to escape from uncomfortable or intolerable life situations. Anxiety is therefore central to self-destructive behavior.

The anxiety associated with a deliberate attempt at self-destruction is overwhelming. It is difficult to imagine if it has not been experienced. Most people cringe at merely contemplating their own deaths, much less actually initiating self-destruction. Self-death is experienced differently from the death of another because self-death literally cannot be experienced.

In contrast, people engaged in gradual self-destructive behavior tend to deny their eventual deaths, usually believing that they can assume control at any time. This fantasy of control, although it relieves anxiety, also helps to perpetuate the behavior. When the sense of self-worth is extremely low, self-destructive behavior reaches its peak. At this point, suicidal behavior is likely. Suicide implies a loss of the ability to value the self at all.

Appraisal of Stressors

The specific prediction of suicide is not possible. However, one may foresee the likelihood of a suicidal act based upon an assessment of a person's risk factors for suicide and his or her behavior. Therefore, it is essential for the nurse to assess each patient for the **suicidal risk factors** listed in Box 20-2. The best predictors is a previous suicide attempt. **Risk factors for suicide in special populations** are presented in Box 20-3.

BOX 20-2

Risk Factors in the Assessment of the Self-Destructive Patient

Assessing Circumstances of an Attempt
- Precipitating humiliating life event
- Preparatory actions: acquiring a method, putting affairs in order, suicide talk, giving away prized possessions, suicide note
- Use of violent method or more lethal drugs/poisons
- Understanding of lethality of chosen method
- Precautions taken against discovery

Presenting Symptoms
- Hopelessness
- Helplessness
- Self-reproach, feelings of failure and unworthiness
- Depressed mood
- Impaired problem solving
- Agitation and restlessness
- Persistent insomnia
- Weight loss
- Slowed speech, fatigue, social withdrawal
- Suicidal thoughts and plans

Previous suicide attempt

Psychiatric Illness
- Mood disorders
- Alcoholism or other substance abuse

- Borderline or antisocial personality disorder
- Schizophrenia
- Panic disorder
- Conduct disorders and depression in adolescents
- Early dementia and confusional states in the elderly
- Combinations of these illnesses

Psychosocial History
- Recently separated, divorced, or bereaved
- Lives alone
- Unemployed, recent job change or loss
- Multiple life stresses (relocation, early loss, breakup of important relationship, school problems, threat of disciplinary crisis)
- Chronic medical illness
- Excessive drinking or substance abuse

Personality Factors
- Impulsivity, aggressivity, hostility
- Cognitive rigidity and negativity
- Low self-esteem

Family History
- Family history of suicidal behavior
- Family history of mood disorder, alcoholism, or both

BOX 20-3

Risk Factors for Suicide in Special Populations

In Hospitalized Depressed Patients
- High levels of anxiety
- First week of admission
- First month after discharge

In Older Patients
- Death of a loved one

In Patients with Alcoholism
- Loss of a close relationship in the previous 6 weeks
- Concurrent use of other drugs
- Late in the course of illness

In Depressed Adolescents
- Comorbid substance abuse
- Prior suicide attempt
- Family history of major depression
- Previous antidepressant treatment
- History of legal problems
- Handgun available in the house

A PATIENT SPEAKS

The following are notes left by patients who committed suicide.
- *Please forgive me and please forget me. I'll always love you. All I have was yours. No one ever did more for me than you; oh please pray for me, please.*
- *To Whom It May Concern,*
  I, Mary Smith, being of sound mind, do this day make my last will as follows: I bequeath my rings, diamond and black opal to my daughter-in-law, Doris Jones, and any other of my personal belongings she might wish. What money I have in my savings account and my checking account goes to my dear father, as he won't have me to help him. To my husband, Ed Smith, I leave my furniture and car.
- *I hate you and all of your family and I hope you never have peace of mind. I hope I haunt this house as long as you live here and I wish you all the bad luck in the world.*
- *Dear Daddy:*
  Please don't grieve for me or feel that you did something wrong, you didn't. I'll leave this life loving you and remembering the world's greatest father. I'm sorry to cause you more heartache, but the reason I can't live anymore is because I'm afraid. Afraid of facing my life alone without love. No one ever knew how alone I am. No one ever stood by me when I needed help. No one brushed away the tears. I cried for "help" and no one heard. I love you Daddy, Jeannie.

Coping Resources

Patients with chronic, painful, or life-threatening illnesses may engage in self-destructive behavior. Often these people consciously choose to kill themselves. Quality of life becomes an issue that overrides quantity of life. An ethical dilemma

BOX 20-4

Protective Factors Against Suicide

- Effective and appropriate clinical care for mental, physical, and substance abuse disorders
- Easy access to a variety of clinical interventions and support for help-seeking
- Restricted access to highly lethal methods of suicide
- Family and community support
- Support from ongoing medical and mental health care relationships
- Learned skills in problem solving, conflict resolution, and nonviolent handling of disputes
- Cultural and religious beliefs that discourage suicide and support self-preservation instincts

From US Public Health Service: *The Surgeon General's call to action to prevent suicide*, Washington, DC, 1999, US Public Health Service.

may arise for nurses who become aware of the patient's choice to engage in this behavior, which is often called *rational suicide*. The question of how to resolve this conflict has no easy answer (Fontana, 2002; King and Jordan-Welch, 2003). Nurses must do so according to their own belief system.

Self-destructive behavior also is related to many social and cultural factors. The structure of society has a great influence on the individual. Society may either help or sustain individuals or lead them to self-destruction (see A Patient Speaks). Social isolation may lead to loneliness and increase the person's vulnerability to suicide (Sargent et al, 2002). People who are actively involved with others in their communities are more able to tolerate stress. Those who do not participate in social activities are more likely to turn to self-destructive behavior. Religious involvement is particularly supportive to many people during difficult times. **Factors that protect against suicide** are presented in Box 20-4.

Did you know that the U.S. suicide rate of over 31,000 people per year is higher than the homicide rate? That means once every 18 minutes an American commits suicide. Do you think this fact requires a reallocation of social resources? If so, in what way? ■

Coping Mechanisms

A patient may use a variety of coping mechanisms to deal with self-destructive feelings, including **denial, rationalization, regression,** and **magical thinking**. These coping mechanisms may stand between the person and self-destruction. They defend the person from strong emotional responses to life events that are a serious threat to the ego. If they are removed, underlying depression will become overt and may lead to suicidal behavior.

Suicidal behavior indicates the imminent failure of the coping mechanisms. A suicidal threat may be a last-ditch effort to get enough help to be able to cope. Completed suicide represents the total failure of adaptive coping mechanisms.

DIAGNOSIS

Nursing Diagnoses

When considering the nursing diagnosis of self-destructive behavior, the nurse must incorporate information about the seriousness and immediacy of the patient's harmful activity. The nurse must consider the information obtained in the assessment to identify accurately the patient's need for nursing intervention (Figure 20-5). Validation of the nursing diagnosis with the patient is essential. However, denial is a prominent defense associated with most self-destructive disorders. The patient may not be able to agree with a statement that confronts this behavior.

The primary concern is to communicate, through the diagnosis, the level of protection the patient needs. In the case of self-destructive behavior, caution is recommended in determining the level of risk. It is better to overestimate the patient's level of risk than to allow serious injury to occur.

Primary NANDA nursing diagnoses related to maladaptive self-protective responses are **risk for suicide**, **self-mutilation**, **noncompliance**, and **risk for self-directed violence**. Because of the nature of the disorders associated with self-destructive behavior, other nursing diagnoses are often applied in the care

of these patients. Nursing diagnoses related to the range of possible maladaptive responses are listed in the Medical and Nursing Diagnoses box (Box 20-5). Examples of expanded nursing diagnoses related to self-protective responses are presented in the Detailed Diagnoses table (Table 20-2).

Medical Diagnoses

Suicidal behavior is not identified as a separate diagnostic category in *DSM-IV-TR* (American Psychiatric Association, 2000). Several medical diagnostic classifications of the *DSM-IV-TR* include actual or potential self-destructive behavior among their defining criteria. The medical diagnoses in which this behavior is listed as possible include anxiety disorders, bipolar disorder, major depression, noncompliance with treatment, schizophrenia, and substance use disorders. Their essential features are described in the Detailed Diagnoses table (see Table 20-2).

OUTCOME IDENTIFICATION

The expected outcome when working with a patient with maladaptive self-protection responses is:

The patient will not physically harm himself or herself.

Careful setting of priorities is necessary with the self-destructive patient. Highest priority should be given to preser-

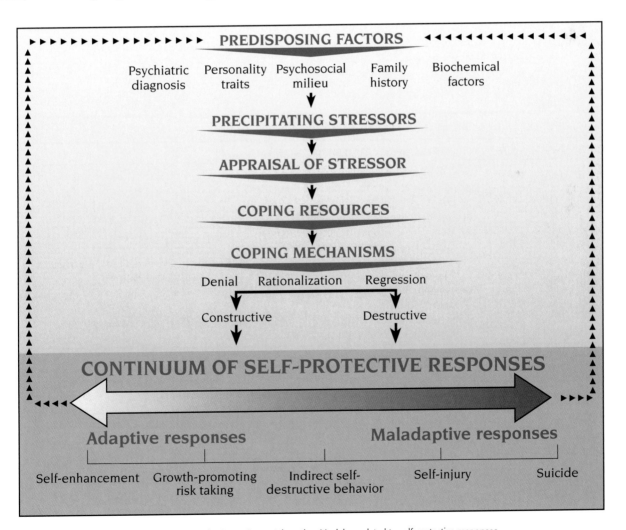

Figure 20-5   The Stuart Stress Adaptation Model as related to self-protective responses.

vation of life. The nurse must identify goals related to immediately life-threatening behavior. For example, the actively suicidal person must first be prevented from acting on impulses.

In dealing with self-destructive behavior, the nurse and the patient may appear to have incompatible goals. Suicidal patients may resist attempts to protect them and may actively try to evade their observers. However, most of these patients have some ambivalence. The nurse, in setting positive, life-preserving goals, is appealing to the healthy part of the person's self that wants to survive and be better able to cope with life. The very act of seeking help is an expression of this healthy aspect of the personality.

BOX 20-5 *Medical and Nursing Diagnoses Related to* **Self-Protective Responses**

RELATED MEDICAL DIAGNOSES (*DSM-IV-TR*)*	RELATED NURSING DIAGNOSES (NANDA)†
Anxiety disorders	Adjustment, Impaired
Bipolar disorder	Anxiety
Major depressive disorder	Coping, Ineffective
Noncompliance with treatment	Denial, Ineffective
Schizophrenia	Hopelessness
Substance use disorders	**Noncompliance‡**
	Powerlessness
	Self-esteem, Chronic low or Situational low
	Self-mutilation‡
	Spiritual distress
	Suicide, Risk for‡
	Violence, Risk for self-directed‡

*From American Psychiatric Association: *Diagnostic and statistical manual of mental disorders*, ed 4, text revision, Washington, DC, 2000, American Psychiatric Association.
†From North American Nursing Diagnosis Association: *NANDA nursing diagnoses: definitions and classification 2003-2004*, Philadelphia, 2003, The Association.
‡**Primary nursing diagnosis for self-destructive behavior.**

Table 20-2 *Detailed Diagnoses Related to* **Self-Protective Responses**

NANDA DIAGNOSIS STEM	EXAMPLES OF EXPANDED DIAGNOSIS
Risk for suicide	Risk for suicide related to loss of girlfriend, as evidenced by discussion of death and social withdrawal
Self-mutilation	Self-mutilation related to feelings of tension and worthlessness, as evidenced by cutting of arms and legs
	Self-mutilation related to command hallucinations, as evidenced by dissection of calf
Noncompliance	Noncompliance with taking antihypertensive medication related to asymptomatic behavior, as evidenced by unchanged elevation of blood pressure
	Noncompliance with 1800 calories/day diabetic diet related to denial of illness, as evidenced by gain of 10 pounds since last clinic visit
Risk for self-directed violence	Risk for self-directed violence related to loss of spouse, as evidenced by purchase of a gun and discussions of death
	Risk for self-directed violence related to phencyclidine (PCP) abuse, as evidenced by extreme psychotic disorganization and lack of body boundaries

DSM-IV-TR DIAGNOSIS	ESSENTIAL FEATURES*
Anxiety disorders	Presence of intense apprehension, fear, terror, worry, or increased arousal (see Chapter 16 for details)
Bipolar disorder	Presence of a manic episode and no past depressive episodes (see Chapter 18 for details)
Major depressive disorder	The presence of at least five symptoms nearly every day during the same 2-week period, with one being either depressed mood or loss of interest or pleasure (see Chapter 18 for details)
Noncompliance with treatment	Noncompliance with an important aspect of the treatment for a mental disorder or a general medical condition
Schizophrenia	Presence of two or more of the following symptoms for a 1-month period: delusions, hallucinations, disorganized speech, disorganized behavior, negative symptoms (see Chapter 21 for details)
Substance use disorders	Presence of substance dependence or substance abuse (see Chapter 24 for details)

*From American Psychiatric Association: *Diagnostic and statistical manual of mental disorders*, ed 4, text revision, Washington, DC, 2000, American Psychiatric Association.

The positive attitude of the nurse in setting constructive goals conveys a sense of hope to a patient who may be feeling hopeless. **Communicating hope** is often the most therapeutic element in any nursing intervention with a suicidal patient.

Outcome indicators related to "Suicide Self-Restraint" from the Nursing Outcome Classification (NOC) project are presented in Box 20-6 (Moorhead, Johnson, and Maas, 2004).

PLANNING

The nursing care plan for the person with self-destructive behavior must focus first on **protecting the patient from harm**. In addition, the plan must address the factors that contributed to the patient's dangerous behavior. Later, the nurse can attend to the development of insight into the suicidal behavior and substitution of healthy coping mechanisms.

Suicidal patients can be treated in a variety of settings. The decision about which setting is most appropriate for a given patient is based on the assessment of risk. The algorithm presented in Figure 20-6 begins with the issue of the nature of the suicidal ideation. People who seem very intent, have a specific plan for action, and cannot contract for safety should be admitted to an inpatient setting where they can be monitored closely.

Another important factor in determining the treatment setting is the patient's judgment. Anything that impairs a patient's judgment and rational decision-making capacity greatly increases the risk of a suicide attempt and is a good indication for inpatient treatment.

A final issue is the availability of a responsible family member or close friend willing to stay with the patient throughout the immediate crisis until the suicidal ideation abates. Sometimes this may require several family members taking shifts and watching the patient around the clock. In the final analysis, however, the safety of the patient is the top priority.

IMPLEMENTATION

Common elements exist in nursing intervention with all patients who exhibit self-destructive behavior. First, nurses must consider their own responses to people who are trying to harm themselves. It can be difficult for a person who is happy and involved in life to imagine the depth of despair that leads to suicidal impulses or the lack of caring for the self that results in physically, psychologically, and socially damaging behavior, even if not immediately lethal.

On the other hand, nurses who are depressed and dissatisfied with their own lives may be threatened by interacting with patients who are more upset because they may fear similar consequences for themselves. These nurses also may overidentify with the patient, which limits their ability to help. A therapeutic approach is empathic and nonjudgmen-

---

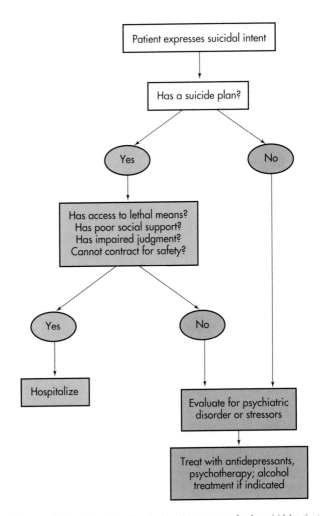

Figure 20-6   Clinical algorithm for planning treatment for the suicidal patient.

tal, with subjective responses limited by awareness of one's own attitudes.

All possible efforts must be made to protect patients and to motivate them to choose life. Nurses should align themselves with the patients' wish to live and then help them be responsible for their own behavior. However, nurses also must understand that some patients will choose death despite their best efforts to intervene. Nurses therefore must develop a realistic understanding of the patient's responsibility for his or her own life and accept the possibility of losing a suicidal patient even when the best nursing care is provided.

A friend tells you that suicidal patients are intent on dying and will ultimately succeed despite all intervention. How would you respond? ■

Protection and Safety

The highest priority nursing activity with self-destructive patients is to protect them from inflicting further harm on themselves and, if suicidal, from killing themselves. Lawsuits related to suicides began to increase in the 1980s and are now one of the most common reasons for litigation against nurses and hospitals.

Since implementation of the Sentinel Event Policy in 1995, suicide has become the number one type of sentinel event reviewed by the Joint Commission on Accreditation of Healthcare Organizations (JCAHO). Organizations that experienced inpatient suicides reviewed by JCAHO identified the following issues as root causes in order of frequency (Joint Commission Resources, 2001):

- Inadequate suicide assessment of the patient at intake, absent or incomplete reassessment, and lack of assessment at discharge
- Unsafe environment of care
- Insufficient orientation or training, incomplete competency review or credentialing, and inadequate staffing levels
- Incomplete communication among caregivers
- Inadequate care planning or care provision

All of these factors clearly speak to the need for psychiatric nurses to have a solid basis from which to approach risk reduction and suicide prevention (JCAHO, 2000).

The message of protection and safety is conveyed to patients verbally and nonverbally. Verbally, patients are informed of the nurse's intention not to allow harm to come to them. The nurse might say, "I understand that you are feeling impulses to harm yourself. I will be here with you to help you control those impulses. I will do whatever is necessary to protect you and keep you safe. I'd like to talk with you about how you are feeling whenever you are able to share that with me."

The nonverbal communication should reinforce and agree with the verbal. Obviously, dangerous objects such as belts, sharp implements, glass, and matches should be taken from the suicidal patient. It is impossible to make an environment perfectly safe. Even walls and floors can cause injury if patients throw themselves against them. However, the removal of dangerous objects gives a message of concern.

One-to-one observation of the suicidal patient also communicates caring. This observation should be carried out sensitively, with the nurse neither hovering over nor remaining aloof from the patient. The patient's nonverbal cues can guide the one-to-one interaction. It is important to remain alert until the mental health team and the patient agree that the self-destructive crisis is over.

Suicidal patients may appear to be feeling much better immediately before making an attempt. This is due to the feeling of relief experienced when the decision has been made and the plans finalized. Nurses have been fooled by this behavior pattern, subsequently relaxing their vigilance, only to have patients kill themselves when they are allowed to be alone for a moment.

An important aspect of protecting the patient involves coming to an agreement about the nature of the therapeutic relationship. Often this has involved the use of contracts in which the patient agrees not to inflict self-harm for a specified period of time. Typically, the patient further agrees to contact the clinician if he or she is tempted to act on self-destructive impulses and also agrees to give away any possibly lethal articles such as guns or pills.

Although no-suicide contracts have been used in clinical practice, there are no studies showing that they are effective. One of their major limitations is that they rely on subjective rather than objective evidence. In fact, studies of suicide attempters and inpatient suicides have shown that a significant number had a no-suicide contract in place at the time of their suicidal act (see Citing the Evidence). Thus, although no-suicide contracts may aid the therapeutic alliance, they are overvalued as a clinical or risk management technique and

---

CITING THE EVIDENCE ON
No-Suicide Contracts

BACKGROUND: Although negotiation of no-suicide contracts is common practice, research regarding the outcomes of contracting is inadequate. The purpose of this retrospective review of medical records was to examine how no-suicide contracting affected the likelihood of self-harm behavior in psychiatric inpatient settings.

RESULTS: Thirty one or 4.8% of 577 patients engaged in self-harm behavior during the 6-month period from which the data were collected. Approximately half of those patients expressed suicidal intent. Patients with no-suicide contracts and with higher levels of restriction had a significantly higher likelihood of self-harm behavior. Prevention of self-harm behaviors by the use of a no-suicide contract was not shown.

IMPLICATIONS: Negotiation of a no-suicide contract is likely a reflection of staff assessment that the patient was at high risk for suicide, but the contract did not prevent self-harm behavior. These findings confirm the need for thorough, ongoing assessment of suicidal risk, whether or not the patient has agreed to a no-suicide contract.

Drew BL: *Arch Psychiatr Nurs* 15:99, 2001.

should not take the place of a thorough suicide risk assessment (Farrow, 2002).

The nurse can take additional steps to ensure the safety of a suicidal patient. First, the patient should be supervised at all times. **The patient should never be left alone.**

Second, the nurse should **monitor any medications** the patient receives. For example, the tricyclic antidepressants are fatal in overdose. This suggests that the patient should have only a few days' supply if treated with them as an outpatient. In contrast, the newer selective serotonin reuptake inhibitor (SSRI) antidepressants are safer in the event of an overdose. The nurse also should understand that the benzodiazepines may disinhibit a patient, thereby supporting impulses and resulting in less control over self-destructive impulses (see Chapter 27).

Your depressed patient has been prescribed a tricyclic antidepressant because it is less expensive than the newer antidepressants. However, she lives in a rural area and cannot have the prescription filled every few days. You are worried about potential overdose. What alternatives can you identify? ∎

Increasing Self-Esteem

Self-destructive people have low self-esteem. The nurse may intervene by treating the patient as someone deserving attention and concern. Positive attributes of the patient should be recognized with genuine praise. An attempt to make up reasons to praise the patient is usually recognized as artificial and lowers the patient's self-esteem. The message is that the patient is so bad that one has to search for positive characteristics.

When getting to know the patient, the nurse should be alert to strengths that can be built on to provide the patient with positive experiences. It is also important to reinforce reasons for living and promote the patient's realistic expectations (Chesley and Loring-McNulty, 2003; Malone et al, 2000). Chapter 18 describes interventions the nurse can use to enhance a patient's self-esteem.

Regulating Emotions and Behaviors

Nursing care should be directed toward helping patients become aware of their feelings, label them, and express them appropriately. Anger is often a difficult feeling for these patients. The angry patient must be helped to deal constructively with anger through learning and using anger management skills. These are described in Chapter 30. Anxiety also can be overwhelming. Chapter 16 discusses anxiety-reducing interventions.

It may be helpful to assist patients with self-destructive responses to explore the predisposing and precipitating factors influencing their behavior. Once the acute crisis is over, the nurse can help the patient understand high-risk times and triggers, the feelings that are stimulated, dysfunctional thinking patterns, and resultant maladaptive coping responses. Plans can then be made to test out new coping mechanisms. For instance, during times of stress, the patient can do the following:

- Increase involvement with others
- Initiate a physical activity
- Engage in relaxation and tension-reducing activities
- Process feelings by talking with someone or writing in a journal

These and other examples of cognitive behavioral strategies are described in Chapter 31.

Mobilizing Social Support

Self-destructive behavior often reflects a lack of internal and external resources. Mobilization of social support systems is an important aspect of nursing intervention. Significant others have many feelings about the patient's self-destructive behavior. They need an opportunity to express their feelings and make realistic plans for the future. Family members must be made aware of control issues and helped to encourage self-control by the patient. Both the patient and the family may need help to see that caring can be expressed by fostering self-care, as well as by providing care.

Families of suicidal patients may be frightened of future suicidal activity. They need to be aware of behavioral clues that indicate suicidal thoughts and of community resources that can help with crises. Suicidal behavior often recurs. False reassurance should be avoided. A better approach is to foster improved communication and an ability to cope in the family. The nurse may help people sort out their feelings and may want to refer significant others for individual intervention or family therapy.

It has been estimated that each suicide intimately affects at least six other people. If a patient commits suicide, it is important to intervene with the survivors, who may themselves be at risk for suicidal behavior (Constantino et al, 2002; Mitchell et al, 2003). They need someone who can listen to them and let them know that their feelings are not abnormal. They need to be able to discuss their beliefs about why the death occurred and helped to find some meaning in the experience. Family members should be encouraged to support one another and seek help for their own feelings and responses. Survivors are often stigmatized and may need assistance in dealing with this.

Community resources are important for the long-term care of the self-destructive person. Self-help groups may provide the recovering patient with needed peer support. Family therapy may help in the reintegration of a family group that has been disrupted by the patient's recent experiences. Public health nurses, clergy, and other community-based helping people can provide the patient and family with day-to-day support. The nurse may be active in explaining resources to the patient and initiating referrals to other agencies.

Patient Education

Patient education is an important nursing intervention. Education must be timed carefully because patient readiness is essential if behavior change is to result. Patients who are noncompliant with prescribed health care regimens may not understand the nature of their problem. The nurse should assess the patient's knowledge and initiate appropriate teaching. A Patient Education Plan for a patient who is noncompliant with medical treatment is presented in Table 20-3.

| Table 20-3 | PATIENT EDUCATION PLAN | Compliance Counseling |

CONTENT	INSTRUCTIONAL ACTIVITIES	EVALUATION
Assess patient's knowledge of self-care activities.	Ask patient to describe usual diet, exercise, and medication patterns.	Patient describes unusual behavior.
	Validate whether described behaviors match self-care instruction received in the past.	Patient repeats directions.
Identify areas in which patient behavior differs from healthy self-care practices	Describe healthy self-care behavior to patient. Provide written patient education materials. Encourage patient to describe reasons for not performing recommended self-care.	Patient discusses compliance problems.
Discuss alternative approaches to self-care.	Help patient identify alternative self-care behaviors that would be more acceptable. Enable patient to talk about feelings related to illness and treatment regimen.	Patient decides on different approach and shares feelings related to illness.
Agree on a reward for compliant behavior.	Ask patient what reward he or she would choose for taking good care of himself or herself.	Patient identifies reward.
Reinforce.	Praise patient for making a commitment to a healthier lifestyle.	Patient recognizes renewed commitment to self-care.

Many patients are willing to participate in self-care if it makes sense to them. Teaching ways to monitor health status may be helpful. For example, if hypertensive patients learn to check their blood pressure, they can learn to associate their health care activities with their physiological response.

Patients following medication regimens, such as psychotropic medication for the previously suicidal patient, should know the prescribed dosage, frequency, and side effects. Information about how to handle any future crises should be provided to the patient. If the nurse has explained the possible reason for the patient's behavior, this may be reinforced at termination of the relationship to help the patient integrate the experience into his or her self-concept. Helping a patient work through self-destructive behavior can be an extremely rewarding aspect of psychiatric nursing.

Suicide Prevention

In 1999 the Surgeon General released a *Call to Action to Prevent Suicide*, (US Public Health Service) which introduced a blueprint for reducing suicide in the United States. Being both evidence-based and highly prioritized by leading experts, this report made 15 key recommendations. In 2002, the Institute of Medicine underscored suicide prevention as a significant health problem in its publication, *Reducing Suicide: A National Imperative*.

In addition, the National Strategy for Suicide Prevention (NSSP) (USDHHS) was developed in 2001 with the combined work of advocates, clinicians, researchers and survivors. It lays out a framework for action and guides development of an array of services and programs to be set in motion.

The NSSP strives to promote and provide direction toward efforts to modify the social infrastructure in ways that will affect the most basic attitudes about suicide and that will also change judicial, educational, social service, and health care systems. Its five basic steps are to:

1. Clearly define the problem.
2. Identify risk and protective factors.
3. Develop and test interventions.
4. Implement interventions.
5. Evaluate effectiveness.

As conceived, the NSSP requires a variety of organizations and individuals to become involved in suicide prevention and emphasizes coordination of resources and culturally appropriate services at all levels of government—Federal, State, tribal, and community—and with the private sector.

The NSSP represents the first attempt in the United States to prevent suicide through such a coordinated approach. The *New Freedom Commission on Mental Health* (2003) endorsed implementing the suicide prevention framework for action, goals, and objectives proposed by the NSSP as a promising blueprint for change. The aims and goals of the NSSP are listed in Box 20-7.

Nurses, in particular, need to be aware of several specific strategies that may help prevent suicide listed in Box 20-8. Educational measures and suicide programs in schools are other helpful interventions. These programs try to break down taboos about suicide and describe the symptoms of depression to students, teachers, and parents (Askland et al, 2003; Thompson et al, 2001). The development of prevention clinics in communities also may be helpful. Such clinics might offer expert clinical assessment and treatment combined with strong community links, increased social supports, family education, and hotlines staffed with mental health professionals.

Another effective suicide prevention strategy is telephone services that provide home assistance, need assessment, and

BOX **20-7**

Aims and Goals of the National Strategy for Suicide Prevention

Aims of the National Strategy for Suicide Prevention
Prevent premature deaths due to suicide across the life span
Reduce the rates of other suicidal behaviors.
Reduce the harmful after-effects associated with suicidal behaviors and the traumatic impact of suicide on family and friends.
Promote opportunities and settings to enhance resiliency, resourcefulness, respect, and interconnectedness for individuals, families, and communities.

Goals of the National Strategy for Suicide Prevention
Goal 1: Promote awareness that suicide is a public health problem that is preventable.
Goal 2: Develop broad-based support for suicide prevention.
Goal 3: Develop and implement strategies to reduce the stigma associated with being a consumer of mental health, substance abuse, and suicide prevention services.
Goal 4: Develop and implement suicide prevention programs.
Goal 5: Promote efforts to reduce access to lethal means and methods of self-harm.
Goal 6: Implement training for recognition of at-risk behavior and delivery of effective treatment.
Goal 7: Develop and promote effective clinical and professional practices.
Goal 8: Improve access to and community linkages with mental health and substance abuse services.
Goal 9: Improve reporting and portrayals of suicidal behavior, mental illness, and substance abuse in the entertainment and news media.
Goal 10: Promote and support research on suicide and suicide prevention.
Goal 11: Improve and expand surveillance systems.

From US Department of Health and Human Services: *National strategy for suicide prevention: goals and objectives for action,* Rockville, Md, 2001, USDHHS, Public Health Service.

BOX **20-8**

Suicide Prevention Strategies

Gun control and decreased availability of lethal weapons
Limitations on the sale and availability of alcohol and drugs
Increased public and professional awareness about depression and suicide
Less attention and reinforcement of suicidal behavior in the media
Establishment of community-based crisis intervention clinics
Campaigns to decrease the stigma associated with psychiatric care
Increased insurance benefits for psychiatric and substance abuse disorders

emotional support. In addition, education of the public and health care providers is needed to increase knowledge about the early warning signs of self-destructive behavior and implement effective treatment strategies (Grossman et al, 2003).

A Nursing Treatment Plan Summary for patients with maladaptive self-protective responses is presented in Table 20-4.

EVALUATION

Evaluation of the nursing care of the self-destructive patient requires careful daily monitoring of the patient's behavior. Patient involvement in evaluation of his or her progress can provide reinforcement and an incentive to work toward a goal. Modifications of the care plan are often necessary as patients reveal more of themselves and their needs to the nurse.

Unfortunately, self-destructive behavior tends to recur. Nurses sometimes become discouraged and angry with pa-

tients who return again and again with the same behavior. When this occurs, nurses may be caught in the trap of feeling responsible for patient behavior. Nurses who have given the best nursing care possible have done as much as they can for the patient. It is impossible to change the total life situation for the patient. The nurse can help only to identify alternative behaviors and provide encouragement for change. If the patient returns, the nursing process must begin again with an attitude of hope that this time the patient will learn and grow more and be better able to live a satisfying life.

A final issue related to suicidal behavior is the impact of a completed suicide on the clinical staff. Psychiatric nurses will inevitably experience a patient suicide sometime in their careers. When a patient commits suicide, staff response can split the interdisciplinary treatment team. Thus interventions must be aimed not only at helping the individual clinician heal but also at preserving the integrity of the treatment team (Joyce and Wallbridge, 2003; Valente, 2003; Valente and Saunders, 2002). The following activities can help this process (Bultema, 1994):

- Have an immediate review of the event by the treatment team to acknowledge feelings, and plan care for the other patients.
- If in an inpatient setting, hold a patient community meeting to help patients accept the reality of the loss.
- Call an additional meeting of the treatment team 2 to 3 days after the suicide to further process the suicide.
- Conduct an in-house memorial service to facilitate grieving.
- Participate in a continuous quality improvement critical incident review to help staff understand the suicide and objectively review the treatment.
- Identify opportunities for continuous process improvement.
- Acknowledge anniversary reactions.

If a variety of these activities are provided to promote healing of the treatment team, recovery can occur and growth can result.

Table 20-4	NURSING TREATMENT PLAN SUMMARY	Maladaptive Self-Protective Responses

Nursing Diagnosis: Risk for suicide
Expected Outcome: The patient will not physically harm himself or herself.

SHORT-TERM GOAL	INTERVENTION	RATIONALE
The patient will not engage in self-injury activities.	Observe closely. Complete a suicide risk assessment. Remove harmful objects. Provide a safe environment. Provide for basic physiological needs. Do not leave the patient alone. Monitor medications.	Highest priority is given to life-saving patient care activities. The patient's behavior must be supervised until self-control is adequate for safety.
The patient will identify positive aspects of oneself.	Identify patient's strengths. Encourage the patient to participate in activities that he or she likes and does well. Encourage good hygiene and grooming. Foster healthy interpersonal relationships.	Self-destructive behavior reflects underlying depression related to low self-esteem and anger directed inward.
The patient will implement two adaptive self-protective responses.	Facilitate the awareness, labeling, and expression of feelings. Help the patient recognize unhealthy coping mechanisms. Identify alternative means of coping. Reward healthy coping behaviors.	Maladaptive coping mechanisms must be replaced with healthy ones to manage stress and anxiety.
The patient will identify two social support resources that can be helpful.	Help significant others communicate constructively with the patient. Promote healthy family relationships. Identify relevant community resources. Initiate referrals to community resources.	Social isolation leads to low self-esteem and depression, perpetuating self-destructive behavior.
The patient will be able to describe the treatment plan and its rationale.	Involve patient and significant others in care planning. Explain characteristics of identified health care needs, nursing care needs, medical diagnosis, and recommended treatment and medications. Elicit responses to nursing care plans. Modify plan based on patient feedback.	Understanding of and participation in health care planning enhance compliance.

COMPETENT CARING   **A Clinical Exemplar of a Psychiatric Nurse**
PHILIP MACAIONE, BS, RN

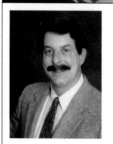

After 18 years of acute care nursing practice with a specialty in ICU, ER, and trauma nursing, I sought a new challenge and began psychiatric nursing practice. Having had the opportunity to associate professionally with hundreds of patients over the years who were experiencing critical and life-threatening situations, I felt well equipped to deal with psychiatric emergencies, until that seemingly routine day shift on an inpatient adult unit.

Ms. W had been committed to our unit as a dual-diagnosis patient. She was referred from our county emergency room. She had been found near-stuporous, wandering the city streets, and was thought to be homeless. She was addicted to heroin, cocaine, and alcohol. She also suffered from multiple personality disorder, anxiety disorder, major depression, and schizotypical disorder. She was 6'2" and weighed more than 300 pounds.

Her hospital course over the past few days was highlighted by her continued acting-out behaviors. These included disrupting the milieu; verbal, physical, and sexual threats to others; seeking the medication of other patients; noncompliance with her treatment plan; and defiance of unit rules and policies. Needless to say, she was a nursing challenge and required a firm, consistent approach by the staff and a constant vigil over her behavior.

One morning her behavior deteriorated to the point where staff intervened by placing her in scrubs and escorting her to the seclusion room to maintain her safety and that of the other patients. I explained to her that during this time-out I would help her begin processing her behavior and identify more effective coping strategies. I gave her a prn medication for her agitation and anxiety and suggested that she begin writing her thoughts

A Clinical Exemplar of a Psychiatric Nurse—cont'd
PHILIP MACAIONE, BS, RN

and feelings down in her journal. After about a half hour, she verbally contracted for safety, seemed aware of her actions, and was resting quietly on her mattress. She also said that she was "feeling much better now" and thanked me for my help. I decided to put her on 15-minute checks but leave her in open-door seclusion until we agreed that she was ready to return to the milieu. I remember thinking, "Wow, I did a good job with this patient, and she is really making progress."

After years of nursing practice, I notice that I have developed a sixth sense that tells me when something is just not right. On the surface Ms. W seemed to be in control, but my sixth sense drew me back to the seclusion room only minutes after I had left her. As I walked into the room I did a double take and thought to myself, "This can't be happening." Unfortunately, it was. Ms. W had managed, in the moments that had elapsed since I had left her side, to tear up her journal into small pieces, place the scraps between her legs, and ignite them with a cigarette lighter we later discovered she had hidden in her vagina.

She was madly waving the fire between her legs to produce more flames. Her scrub pants and mattress were now on fire. At this point I just reacted. I ran to her, pulled away the mattress, patted down the flames on her pants, and yelled for help. The smoke alarm had gone off, and within seconds other staff arrived. I instructed them to remove the patient to the corridor and give her first aid. This was no easy task given the patient's size and level of agitation. I then activated the fire procedure, grabbed the fire extinguisher, and returned to the seclusion room. By now the smoke was thick, but I pulled the pin of the fire extinguisher, aimed, and released the foam. Within seconds, the fire was extinguished. The fire department had now arrived and moved in to deal with the smoldering mattress. Ms. W suffered no injuries and was discharged to a boarding house about 1 week later.

I learned a great deal from this incident and think I am a better nurse because of it. The staff response and teamwork in reacting to this crisis were extraordinary. I also think that the many years of critical decision-making opportunities afforded me throughout my nursing practice made me well equipped to handle this seemingly routine shift on our unit. Most of all, I have a greater appreciation and respect for the sixth sense of nurses, which may be the mark of truly competent nursing care. ■

CHAPTER **FOCUS POINTS**

- The continuum of self-protective responses ranges from the most adaptive states of self-enhancement and growth-promoting risk taking to the maladaptive responses of indirect self-destructive behavior, self-injury, and suicide.

- Direct self-destructive behavior includes any form of suicidal activity, such as suicide ideation, threats, attempts, and completed suicide. Indirect self-destructive behavior is any activity detrimental to the person's physical well-being that potentially may result in death.

- Low self-esteem leads to depression, which is always present in self-destructive behavior.

- Suicide is the eleventh leading cause of death in the United States. The highest suicide rate for any group in this country is among people over age 65, especially white men over 85. The overwhelming majority of completed suicides are committed by males. Women attempt suicide twice as often as men.

- It has been estimated that one half of patients do not comply with their health care treatment plan. This level of noncompliance is the same for those with both physical and psychiatric illnesses.

- Self-injury can be defined as the act of deliberate harm to one's own body. Usually the lethality of self-injury is low, and patients who self-injure typically want relief from the tension they feel rather than to kill themselves.

- Suicide ideation is the thought of self-inflicted death, either self-reported or reported to others.

- A suicide threat is a warning, direct or indirect, verbal or nonverbal, that a person is planning to take one's own life.

- A suicide attempt is any self-directed actions taken by a person that will lead to death if not stopped. Although all suicide threats and attempts must be taken seriously, vigilant attention is indicated when the person is planning or tries a highly lethal method. Assessment of the suicidal person also includes whether the person has made a specific plan and whether the means to carry out the plan are available.

- Completed suicide, or simply suicide, is death from self-inflicted injury, poisoning, or suffocation where evidence indicates that the decedent intended to kill himself or herself. Contrary to common opinion, directly questioning the patient about suicidal thought and plans will not cause the patient to take suicidal action.

- There are four broad psychiatric disorders that put people at particular risk for suicide: mood disorders, substance abuse, schizophrenia, and anxiety disorders.

- The three aspects of personality that are most closely associated with increased risk of suicide are hostility, impulsivity, and depression.

- Predisposing factors for suicide include loss, lack of social supports, negative life events, and chronic medical illnesses. A family history of suicide is a significant risk factor for self-destructive behavior.

- A deficiency in serotonin (5-HT) and its metabolite, 5-HIAA, and an increase in one of the 5-HT postsynaptic receptors (5-HT$_{2A}$) are implicated in suicidal behavior.

- All self-destructive behaviors may be seen as attempts to escape from uncomfortable or intolerable life situations. People engaged in gradual self-destructive behavior tend to deny their eventual deaths, usually believing that they can assume control at any time.

- Patients with chronic, painful, or life-threatening illnesses may engage in self-destructive behavior. Self-destructive behavior is also related to many social and cultural factors.

- A patient may use a variety of coping mechanisms to deal with self-destructive feelings, including denial, rationalization, regression, and magical thinking. Suicidal behavior indicates the imminent failure of the coping mechanisms.

- When considering the nursing diagnosis of self-destructive behavior, the nurse must incorporate information about the seriousness and immediacy of the patient's harmful activity. It is better to overestimate the patient's level of risk than to allow serious injury to occur. Primary nursing diagnoses are risk for suicide, self-mutilation, noncompliance, and risk for self-directed violence.

- Suicide is not identified as a separate diagnostic category in the *DSM-IV-TR*. Medical diagnostic classifications of the *DSM-IV-TR* that include actual or potential self-destructive behavior are anxiety disorders, bipolar disorder, major depression, non-compliance with treatment, schizophrenia, and substance use disorders.

CHAPTER **FOCUS POINTS**—cont'd

- The expected outcome of nursing care is that the patient will not physically harm himself or herself.
- Communicating hope is often the most therapeutic element in any nursing intervention with a suicidal patient. The nursing care plan for the person with self-destructive behavior must focus first on protecting the patient from harm. Nurses also must consider their own responses to people who are trying to harm themselves.
- Nursing interventions include protecting the patient and providing for safety, increasing self-esteem, regulating emotions and behaviors, mobilizing social support, educating the patient, and suicide prevention.

- Although no-suicide contracts may aid the therapeutic alliance, they are overvalued as a clinical or risk management technique and cannot and should not take the place of a thorough suicide risk assessment. The patient should be supervised at all times and never left alone. The nurse also should monitor any medications the patient receives.
- Evaluating nursing care requires daily monitoring of the patient's behavior. The nurse must not become discouraged if self-destructive behavior recurs, but instead approach the patient with the hope that this time the patient will grow and be better able to live a satisfying life.

KEY TERMS

completed suicide, 368
denial, 366
direct self-destructive behavior, 364
indirect self-destructive behavior, 364

noncompliance, 365
postvention, 368
psychological autopsy, 368
self-injury, 367

suicide, 368
suicide attempt, 367
suicide ideation, 367
suicide threat, 367

CHAPTER REVIEW QUESTIONS

1. Indicate whether the following statements are true (T) or false (F).

_____ A. Suicide rates are highest for adolescent males.

_____ B. The most prominent behavior associated with non-compliance is refusal to admit the seriousness of the health problem.

_____ C. A suicide attempt is an attention-seeking behavior and should not be reinforced by focusing on it.

_____ D. Physical diseases with chronic and debilitating courses often precipitate self-destructive behavior.

_____ E. Currently no biological test is available that is an accurate predictor of suicide.

_____ F. The newer SSRI antidepressant medications have a higher rate of death by overdose than the older tricyclic antidepressants.

_____ G. Most people who commit suicide have sought medical help before their suicide attempt.

_____ H. Asking a person if he or she is planning to kill oneself will give the person the idea and lead to a suicide attempt.

2. Fill in the blanks.

A. The retrospective review of a person's behavior in the time preceding the suicide is called the _____.

B. The psychiatric disorders that put people at particular risk for suicide are _____,

_____, _____ and _____.

C. Mood disorders are hypothesized to be the result of an imbalance or deficiency of neurotransmitters, particularly

_____.

D. _____ is often the most therapeutic element in any nursing intervention with a suicidal patient.

E. The three personality traits most closely associated with increased risk of suicide are _____,

_____, and _____.

F. The _____ issued a *Call to Action to Prevent Suicide* in 1999.

3. Provide short answers for the following questions.

A. It has been observed that patients often act less depressed and seem to be in better spirits immediately before attempting suicide. Explain the reason for this behavior.

B. Identify the five factors to assess in the self-destructive patient.

C. Describe how you would determine the best treatment setting for a patient expressing suicidal thoughts.

D. Currently much discussion is ongoing concerning the wisdom and the ethics of assisted suicide. Discuss your position on this subject, first as a consumer of health care and then as a nurse.

Visit Evolve for additional resources related to the content of this chapter.

  http://evolve.elsevier.com/Stuart/principles/
- Topical Course Outline • Student Workbook Exercises • Critical Thinking Questions and Activities • Case Studies • Research Topics
- Monthly Content Updates • WebLinks

Student Study CD-ROM

Access the accompanying CD-ROM for animations, interactive exercises, review questions for the NCLEX examination, and an audio glossary.

REFERENCES

American Association of Suicidology: Suicide Sate Data, September 21, 2002.

American Psychiatric Association: *Diagnostic and statistical manual of mental disorders*, ed 4, text revision, Washington, DC, 2000, American Psychiatric Association.

American Psychiatric Association: Practice guideline for the assessment and treatment of patients with suicidal behaviors, *Am J Psychiatry* 160(suppl 11):1, 2003.

Askland K et al: A public health response to a cluster of suicidal behaviors: clinical psychiatry, prevention and community health, *J Psychiatr Pract* 9:219, 2003.

Blank K et al: Failure to adequately detect suicidal intent in elderly patients in the primary care setting, *Clin Geriatr* 9:26, 2001.

Brent DA et al: Familial pathways to early-onset suicide attempt: risk for suicidal behavior in offspring of mood-disordered suicide attempters, *Arch Gen Psychiatry* 59:801, 2002.

Brent DA et al: Peripubertal suicide attempts in offspring of suicide attempters with siblings concordant for suicidal behavior, *Am J Psychiatry* 160:1486, 2003.

Bultema J: The healing process for the multidisciplinary team: recovering post-inpatient suicide, *J Psychosoc Nurs Ment Health Nurs* 32:19, 1994.

Chesley K, Loring-McNulty N: Process of suicide: perspective of the suicide attempter, *J Am Psychiatr Nurs Assoc* 9:41, 2003.

Constantino R et al: Depression and behavioral manifestations of depression in female survivors of the suicide of their significant other and female survivors of abuse, *J Am Psychiatr Nurs Assoc* 8:27, 2002.

Dhossche DM, Ulusarac A, Syed W: A retrospective study of general hospital patients who commit suicide shortly after being discharged from the hospital, *Arch Intern Med* 161:991, 2001.

Farrow TL: Owning their expertise: why nurses use "no suicide contracts" rather than their own assessments, *Int J Ment Health Nurs* 11:214, 2002.

Fontana JS: Rational suicide in the terminally ill, *J Nurs Scholarsh* 34:147, 2002.

Gallop R: Failure of the capacity for self-soothing in women who have a history of abuse and self-harm, *J Am Psychiatr Nurs Assoc* 8:20, 2002.

Goldberg JF, Singer TM, Garno JL: Suicidality and substance abuse in affective disorders, *J Clin Psychiatry* 62(suppl 25):35, 2001.

Grossman J et al: Emergency nurses' responses to a survey about means restriction: an adolescent suicide prevention strategy, *J Am Psychiatr Nurs Assoc* 9:77, 2003.

Institute of Medicine: *Reducing suicide: a national imperative*, Washington DC, 2002, National Academies Press.

Joint Commission on Accreditation of Healthcare Organizations (JCAHO): *Preventing patient suicide*, Oakbrook Terrace, Ill, 2000, JCAHO.

Joint Commission Resources: *Front line of defense: the role of nurses in preventing sentimental events*, Oakbrook Terrace, Ill, 2001, JCAHO.

Joyce B, Wallbridge H: Effects of suicidal behavior on a psychiatric unit nursing team, *J Psychosoc Nurs Ment Health Serv* 41:14: 2003.

King P, Jordan-Welch M: Nurse-assisted suicide: not an answer in end-of-life care, *Issues Ment Health Nurs* 24:45, 2003.

Krysinska KE: Loss by suicide: a risk factor for suicidal behavior, *J Psychosoc Nurs Ment Health Serv* 41:34, 2003.

Luoma JB, Martin CE, Pearson JL: Contact with mental health and primary care providers before suicide: a review of the evidence, *Am J Psychiatry* 159:909, 2002.

Malone K et al: Protective factors against suicidal acts in major depression: reasons for living, *Am J Psychiatry* 157:1084, 2000.

Mitchell AM et al: The use of narrative data to inform the psychotherapeutic group process with suicide survivors, *Issues Ment Health Nurs* 24:91, 2003.

Moorhead S, Johnson M, Maas M, editors: *Nursing outcomes classification (NOC)*, ed 3, St Louis, 2004, Mosby.

New Freedom Commission on Mental Health, *Achieving the promise: transforming mental health care in America, final report*, DHHS Pub. No. SMA-03-3832, Rockville, Md, 2003, DHHS.

Runeson B, Asberg M: Family history of suicide among suicide victims, *Am J Psychiatry* 160:1525, 2003.

Sargent J et al: Sense of belonging as a buffer against depressive symptoms, *J Am Psych Nurs Assoc* 8:120, 2002.

Sher L et al: Risk of suicide in mood disorders, *Clin Neurosci Res* 1:337, 2001.

Thompson EA et al: Evaluation of indicated suicide risk prevention approaches for potential high school dropouts, *Am J Public Health* 91:742, 2001.

US Department of Health and Human Services (USDHHS): *National strategy for suicide prevention: goals and objectives for action*, Rockville, Md, 2001, USDHHS.

US Public Health Service: *Surgeon General's call to action to prevent suicide*, Washington, DC, 1999, US Public Health Service.

Valente SM: Aftermath of a patient's suicide: a case study, *Perspect Psychiatr Care* 39:17, 2003.

Valente SM, Saunders JM: Nurses' grief reactions to a patient suicide, *Perspect Psychiatr Care* 38:5, 2002.

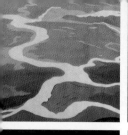

21 NEUROBIOLOGICAL RESPONSES AND SCHIZOPHRENIA AND PSYCHOTIC DISORDERS

Mary D. Moller

LEARNING OBJECTIVES

After studying this chapter, the student should be able to:

1. Describe the continuum of adaptive and maladaptive neurobiological responses (**I**).
2. Identify behaviors associated with maladaptive neurobiological responses (**II**).
3. Analyze predisposing factors, precipitating stressors, and appraisal of stressors related to maladaptive neurobiological responses (**II**).
4. Describe coping resources and coping mechanisms related to maladaptive neurobiological responses (**II**).
5. Formulate nursing diagnoses related to maladaptive neurobiological responses (**III**).
6. Examine the relationship between nursing diagnoses and medical diagnoses related to maladaptive neurobiological responses (**III**).
7. Identify expected outcomes and short-term nursing goals related to maladaptive neurobiological responses (**IV**).
8. Develop a family education plan to promote adaptive neurobiological responses (**V**).
9. Analyze nursing interventions related to maladaptive neurobiological responses (**VI**).
10. Evaluate nursing care related to maladaptive neurobiological responses (**VII**).

TOPICAL OUTLINE

I. Continuum of Neurobiological Responses
II. Assessment
   A. Behaviors
   B. Predisposing Factors
   C. Precipitating Stressors
   D. Appraisal of Stressors
   E. Coping Resources
   F. Coping Mechanisms
III. Diagnosis
   A. Nursing Diagnoses
   B. Medical Diagnoses
IV. Outcome Identification
V. Planning
VI. Implementation
   A. Interventions in the Crisis and Acute Phases
   B. Interventions in the Maintenance Phase
   C. Interventions in the Health Promotion Phase
VII. Evaluation

evolve Visit Evolve for additional resources related to the content of this chapter.
http://evolve.elsevier.com/Stuart/principles/

The word *psychosis* generally elicits the emotion of fear. Psychosis refers to the mental state of experiencing reality differently from others. During an episode of psychosis, the patient does not realize others are not experiencing the same things and wonders why others are not reacting in a similar manner. The overall goal of nursing care is to help the patient recognize the psychosis and develop strategies to manage the symptoms. The mutual confusion created by psychosis creates challenges when providing nursing care to patients with schizophrenia and other psychotic disorders. It is important to remember that these are complex neurobiological brain diseases affecting one's ability to perceive and process information and involving a number of syndromes.

The behaviors associated with these disruptions in brain function are difficult to understand, are usually severe, and can be long lasting. Patients who experience psychosis are often frightened by their experiences, have difficulty forming close relationships, are severely disabled, and tend to be alienated from society. Nurses should strive to connect with patients who are in a state of psychosis and help them toward rehabilitation and wellness. A Patient Speaks box describes one person's experience with psychosis.

Read the patient's description of psychosis a second time. Focus on identifying the feelings that might be associated with these experiences. ■

CONTINUUM OF NEUROBIOLOGICAL RESPONSES

The range of neurobiological responses includes a continuum from **adaptive responses, such as logical thought and accurate perceptions, to maladaptive responses, such as thought distortions and hallucinations.** The symptoms of **psychosis** are at the maladaptive end of this continuum (Figure 21-1). Schizophrenia is a serious and persistent neurobiological brain disease. It is a clinical syndrome of profoundly disrup-

A PATIENT SPEAKS

Psychosis is real. Its main feature is a loss of consciousness of the self in such a way that I can no longer discern my relationship to the reality that my body is in. This would not be destructive, except that I have done it inadvertently; I have done it without consciousness and have not provided for my body. My body, then, goes on without me. It wanders aimlessly and does not know to keep warm in the cold. It does not know how to avoid attack by violence. It does not know to protect itself from fire and deep water and the traffic that races down the highway.

My brain comes up with fantastical ideas about who I might be, since I am not there to tell it. Perhaps I am the Queen of Hearts, or a messenger from another planet, or even Jesus Christ himself. And why not? My brain distorts the reality of the senses: Is this burner hot or cold? Is this coat wet or dry? Is this chair a chair, or what exactly is this anyway, and for that matter, what in the world are you?

Maybe bugs are jumping out of my mind and onto that wall over there. Maybe there's a current coming up from the earth and into my feet and trying to pull me in. My brain can think of every kind of combination and definition, every kind of idea

that it can put together, for it has a nearly infinite number of choices. It has all it has ever experienced, all the sounds, all the sights, all the sensations, all the dreams, all the fantasies, all the nightmares.

My brain chooses its manifestation according to what emotions were available to it when I was in charge. Only I am not there to add my discernment, my wisdom, and my awareness according to what I have learned. My brain goes haywire then. It has no person to guide it, no captain, no helm, and no rudder. It has no fingers at the keyboard. It wanders through its inner space like the steel ball that is thrown into nothing and bounces at random from arbitrarily placed spots in the pinball machine.

What is this I, then, that is gone, and where did it go? It is consciousness. It is awareness. It is the presence of the I in me. It is ego. It is my separation. It is the part in me that tells me the difference between me and the world. It is the I-ness of me that holds me upright like a spine and says, "You will not fall into this tree, or this song, or this ocean of water or air, and it will not fall into you. The I that is gone is the intelligence that says I am me, and you are you."

From Corday R: *Psychosis, the inner experience*, Boulder, Colo, 1991, Common Loon Productions.

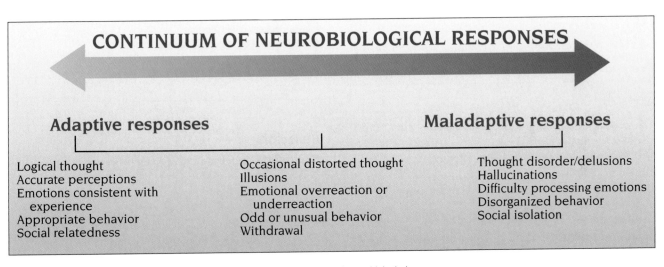

Figure 21-1   Continuum of neurobiological responses.

tive psychopathology that results in responses that severely impair the lives of individuals, their families, and communities. Box 21-1 presents information on the impact of schizophrenia on the individual and society.

ASSESSMENT

Schizophrenia is one of a group of related disorders that are heterogeneous in pathophysiology, predisposing factors, precipitating stressors, and related behaviors. Other psychotic disorders include schizophreniform disorder, schizoaffective disorder, delusional disorder, brief psychotic disorder, shared psychotic disorder (folie a deux), psychotic disorder due to a

general medical condition, and substance-induced psychotic disorder (American Psychiatric Association, 2000). In addition, psychosis is sometimes present in other disorders such as depression with psychotic features, manic episodes of bipolar disorder, substance abuse disorders, posttraumatic stress disorder, delirium, and organic mental disorders.

Although descriptions of the symptoms of what is called schizophrenia today are found throughout recorded history, the term *schizophrenia* was not introduced until 1911 by the Swiss psychiatrist Eugene Bleuler. He believed that the "schizophrenias" were multidimensional and organic in nature and that these illnesses were strongly influenced and

BOX **21-1**

Impact of Schizophrenia on the Individual and Society

- About one in every 100 people suffers from schizophrenia, or 2.5 million Americans, regardless of race, ethnic group, or gender.
- In three of every four cases it begins between the ages of 17 and 25 years.
- Of those with schizophrenia, 95% have it for their lifetime.
- The annual cost of family caregiving and crime- and welfare-related expenditures as a result of schizophrenia is $40 billion in the United States.
- More than 75% of taxpayer dollars spent on treatment of mental illness are used for people with schizophrenia.
- People with schizophrenia occupy 25% of all inpatient hospital beds.
- An estimated one third to one half of homeless people in the United States have schizophrenia.
- Schizophrenia is ranked fourth worldwide in terms of burden of illness. The top three are unipolar depression, alcohol use, and bipolar disorder.
- Schizophrenia is a chronic illness, five times more common than multiple sclerosis, six times more common than insulin-dependent diabetes, 60 times more common than muscular dystrophy, and 80 times more common than Huntington's disease.
- Of patients with schizophrenia, 25% do not respond adequately to traditional antipsychotic medication.
- Suicide is attempted by 20% to 50% of patients with schizophrenia; 9% to 13% succeed.
- Schizophrenia has been diagnosed in 16% of incarcerated persons.

BOX **21-2**

Positive and Negative Symptoms of Schizophrenia

Positive Symptoms
An exaggeration or distortion of normal function; usually responsive to traditional antipsychotic drugs
Psychotic disorders of thinking
Delusions (paranoid, somatic, grandiose, religious, nihilistic, or persecutory themes; thought broadcasting, insertion, or control)
Hallucinations (auditory, visual, tactile, gustatory, olfactory)
Disorganization of speech and behavior
Positive formal thought disorder (incoherence, word salad, derailment, illogicality, loose associations, tangentiality, circumstantiality, pressured speech, distractible speech, or poverty of speech)
Bizarre behavior (catatonia, movement disorders, deterioration of social behavior)

Negative Symptoms
A diminution or loss of normal function; usually unresponsive to traditional antipsychotics and more responsive to atypical antipsychotics
Problems of emotion
Affective flattening: Limited range and intensity of emotional expression
Anhedonia/asociality: Inability to experience pleasure or maintain social contacts
Impaired decision making
Alogia: Restricted thought and speech
Avolition/apathy: Lack of initiation of goal-directed behavior
Attentional impairment: Inability to mentally focus and sustain attention

could be shaped by psychological factors. The word schizophrenia is a combination of two Greek words, *schizein*, "to split," and *phren*, "mind." Bleuler's reference was not to a "split personality," which refers to separate identities, but to his belief that a split occurred between the cognitive and emotional aspects of the personality.

The symptoms of schizophrenia have been organized in various ways over time, depending on the evolving understanding of brain function in this disorder, as well as the increasing effectiveness of antipsychotic drugs. A common system for categorizing the symptoms of schizophrenia lists them as **positive symptoms (exaggerated behaviors)** and **negative symptoms (loss of behaviors)** (Box 21-2). Another useful categorization defines five core symptom clusters, presented in Figure 21-2. With minimum overlap, this model incorporates the positive and negative symptoms described above plus other aspects of schizophrenia, including cognitive symptoms, mood symptoms, and some of the social and occupational dysfunctions common in schizophrenia.

Assessment of this devastating and costly illness involves an understanding of the way in which the brain processes information from the senses and the resulting behavioral responses. These behaviors are organized into the following categories: cognition, perception, emotion, behavior and movement, and socialization.

Behaviors

Cognition. Cognition is the act or process of knowing. It involves awareness and judgment that enable the brain to process information in a way that ensures accuracy, storage, and retrieval. People with schizophrenia are often unable to produce complex logical thoughts and express coherent sentences because neurotransmission in the brain's information processing system is malfunctioning.

Information processing involves the organization of **sensory input** by **brain processes** into **behavioral responses** (Figure 21-3). Sensory input from both internal and external senses is screened according to the focus of the person's attention and ability to remember, learn, discriminate, interpret, and organize information. The result is evident in the person's thinking, perceiving, feeling, behavior, and relatedness to others.

Describe how your cognitive processing differs from that of a person of the opposite sex, an older generation, another race, and another socioeconomic class. What are the results of these differences? ■

The information processing of people with schizophrenia may be altered by brain deficits. However, interferences with cognitive function often keep people with schizophrenia

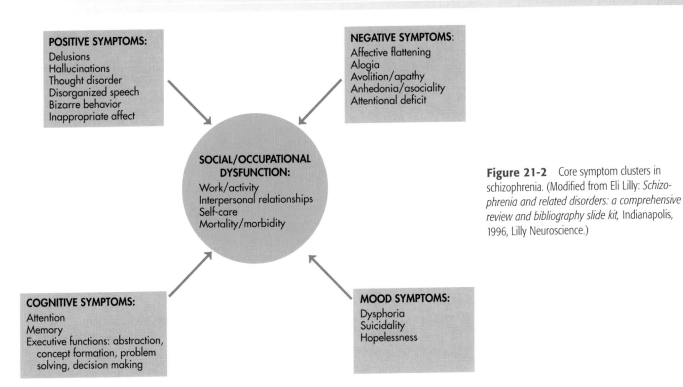

Figure 21-2   Core symptom clusters in schizophrenia. (Modified from Eli Lilly: *Schizophrenia and related disorders: a comprehensive review and bibliography slide kit,* Indianapolis, 1996, Lilly Neuroscience.)

from realizing that their ideas and behavior are different from others. This is particularly evident in their self-perception of worth and abilities and interpretation of hallucinations and delusions. People with schizophrenia tend to dramatically overestimate or underestimate their own capability. The abnormal brain dysfunction during an acute episode of schizophrenia makes it difficult for the patient to realize his or her need for help. This lack of insight is a neurological deficit involving the frontal and prefrontal lobes of the brain in which the patient does not recognize there is anything wrong or that there are deficits of any kind (Amador, 2000).

Symptoms related to problems in information processing associated with schizophrenia are often called **cognitive deficits.** They include problems in cognitive functioning in all aspects of memory, attention, form and organization of speech, decision making, and thought content (Box 21-3).

Memory is the retention or storage of knowledge about the world. Memory is a biological function carried out in several parts of the brain. Additional information about memory and its assessment can be found in Chapters 6, 7, and 23. Memory problems associated with schizophrenia can include **forgetfulness, disinterest, difficulty learning,** and **lack of**

BOX 21-3

Problems in Cognitive Functioning

Memory
Difficulty retrieving and using stored memory
Impaired short-term/long-term memory

Attention
Difficulty maintaining attention
Poor concentration
Distractibility
Inability to use selective attention

Form and Organization of Speech (Formal Thought Disorder)
Loose associations
Tangentiality
Incoherence/word salad/neologism
Illogicality
Circumstantiality
Pressured/distractible speech
Poverty of speech

Decision Making
Failure to abstract
Indecisiveness
Lack of insight (anosognosia)
Impaired concept formation
Impaired judgment
Illogical or concrete thinking
Lack of planning and problem-solving skills
Difficulty initiating tasks

Thought Content
Delusions
Paranoid
Grandiose
Religious
Somatic
Nihilistic
Thought broadcasting
Thought insertion
Thought control

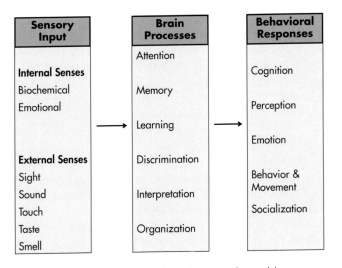

Figure 21-3   Brain information processing model.

compliance. It is important for the nurse to understand the frustration these symptoms cause patients. They commonly seek validation that they have done a task correctly, ask whether it is time to attend a group function or an appointment, and seek permission to make a telephone call just to verify whether they remember phone numbers. When people with schizophrenia repeatedly ask the same question, such as what time it is or how to get somewhere, it is important for the nurse to provide the requested information in a kind and matter-of-fact manner that does not cause embarrassment or decrease the person's self-worth.

Attention is the ability to focus on one activity in a sustained, concentrated manner. Disrupted attention is an impairment in the ability to pay attention, observe, focus, and concentrate on external reality. Disturbances in attention are common in schizophrenia and include **difficulty completing tasks, difficulty concentrating on work,** and **easy distractibility.** Distractibility refers to a patient's attention being drawn easily to irrelevant external stimuli such as noises, books out of order on a bookshelf, or people passing by. In addition, the patient who is experiencing auditory hallucinations often is distracted by them and thus has problems with attention.

These impairments are not constant and may fluctuate, depending on the brain activity required. This generates much frustration for the patient, who often complains about his inability to complete tasks because "my mind wanders." The nurse should be prepared to redirect the patient back to the task at hand. The nurse also will need to repeat directions often and in short, simple phrases.

The parents of a young man who has schizophrenia tell you that they are frustrated by their son's unwillingness to return to work. Based on your understanding of the cognitive disorders related to schizophrenia, how would you respond? ∎

Form and organization of speech are at the core of communication. Malfunctions in information processing produce disturbances in relaying thoughts that can result in incoherent communication. Problems with form and organization of speech (formal thought disorders) may include loose associations, word salad, **tangentiality, illogicality, circumstantiality, pressured speech, poverty of speech, distractible speech,** and **clanging.** These behaviors are described in Chapter 7. Box 21-4 presents nurse-patient dialogues that reflect problems in the form and organization of speech related to psychotic disorders.

Recognizing that speech is a reflection of cognitive processing helps the nurse appreciate the considerable difficulties a person with schizophrenia has in communicating clearly. The nurse will need to focus attention and use active listening to understand the patient. The nurse who is attempting to identify and clarify what a patient wants should not be afraid of offending the patient by clarifying his or her understanding. It is essential to remember that the patient is trying to answer, no matter how difficult or bizarre the answer is. The nurses' responsibility is to identify one or two key verbal or nonverbal responses and seek validation. This is usually achieved through simple trial and error.

Decision making means arriving at a solution or making a choice. Problems with decision making affect one's **insight, judgment, logic, decisiveness, planning, ability to carry out decisions,** and **abstract thought.** Lack of insight is probably one of the greatest problems in schizophrenia because patients generally do not believe that they are ill or different in any way. Unfortunately, many clinicians confuse lack of insight with denial and treat people who have schizophrenia as if their symptoms were willful and within conscious control. When decision making includes cognitive deficits, the patient makes decisions based on incorrect inferences, yet cannot understand that the judgment was faulty.

Some people with schizophrenia are simply unable to make a decision. For them, life is difficult at best. They wrestle with even simple decisions such as which coffee cup to use. Plans based on faulty decision making do not serve the intended purpose. This symptom creates much of the frustration related to schizophrenia. Following through on decisions is also a problem for people who have schizophrenia. Often this is mistaken for lack of motivation. Motivation involves having a desire, not having the ability to follow through. People with schizophrenia typically have difficulty initiating tasks of any kind because of problems related to decision making.

Concrete rather than abstract thinking is characteristic of schizophrenia, particularly during acute episodes. As a result, patients often have difficulty with multiple-step commands. In other words, if the nurse presents a patient with the daily schedule and, at the same time, gives directions about the time and place of group and occupational therapies, all of the information will not be processed because the brain perceives an overload. Thus the patient will probably miss one or more of the directions.

Another example of concrete thinking is difficulty with time management. People with schizophrenia describe this behavior as "trying to tell time with clocks that have no minute or second hands." This is why patients often are late or miss events and appointments altogether. This may create fear in patients who have to be alone for long periods of time or are required to be places at specific times. Some patients have developed clever ways to determine time, such as getting watches with built-in alarms and monitoring certain television programs.

Difficulty managing money is another result of concrete thinking. People with schizophrenia often lose their ability to understand the concept of dollars and cents and are exploited by other people as a result. A patient may agree to buy items without having enough money just because he sees *some* money in his wallet. He may not remember to pay for items he gets in a store or may leave a restaurant without paying for the meal. Unfortunately, many patients get into legal trouble because of this cognitive problem.

Literal interpretation of words and symbols is one of the most problematic behaviors related to concrete thinking. People with schizophrenia have difficulty abstracting the English language. Patients' descriptions of literal interpretation are presented in the following clinical examples.

"I was standing in the medication line and the nurse asked me to take my pills. So I took the medicine cup and held it

BOX 21-4

Form and Content of Speech Related to Psychotic Disorders

Loose Associations

Nurse: "Do you have enough money to buy that candy bar?"

Patient: "I have a real yen for chocolate. The Japanese have all the yen and have taken all our money and marked it. You know, you have to be careful of the Marxists because they are friends with the Swiss and they have all the cheese and all the watches and that means they have taken all the time. The worst thing about Swiss cheese is all the holes. People have to be careful about falling into holes."

Nurse: "It sounds like you are worried about your money."

Patient: "Yes, I have it all here in my wallet and you can't have it and the bank can't have it either."

Incoherence

Nurse: "What does your family like to do at Christmas?"

Patient: "I believe they took Christmas from the Russians to get all the cars into the ocean and make Jell-O. You could go and get the Christmas but you could not do it because the keylars have the fan."

Tangentiality

Nurse: "I'm interested in learning more about your landscape paintings."

Patient: "My interest in art goes back to my parents who lived on a farm in Indiana. They had lots of haystacks, kind of like they do in Ohio, but you know, the hay is different colors in different states so that gave me the ability to paint so many different colors of yellow. Some people do not really like bright yellow hay, but I do. If I make the hay really bright yellow, then I make the barns a dull red, because barns really should not be painted with bright red paint. Bright red should be saved for fire engines and fire hydrants and stop signs."

Illogical Speech

Nurse: "Do you think your medicine is helping you think more clearly?"

Patient: "I used to think my medicine helped me think. But I realized that it was me who took the medicine, so it wasn't the medicine that helped me think. Medicine cannot think, don't you realize that? Maybe you should take some medicine to help you think better. But if you do, I would have to give it to you because it is the fact I took it myself that my thinking is better, so, no, I do not think the medicine is helping me think better."

Distractible Speech

Nurse: "I would like to talk with you about your understanding of schizophrenia."

Patient: "I know it's got something to do with my brain. What perfume are you wearing? It must be from France. Is that where that picture was taken? Your hair is different than when that picture was taken. Was that about 4 years ago?"

Clang Associations

Patient: "I got a new shirt but the buttons became loose. Do you suppose Lucifer's buttons become lucent or are they lucid like Lucy's lucky ducky?"

"I want to sing ping pong that song wong kong long today hey way."

Poverty of Content of Speech

Nurse: "Do you want to go to the grocery store?"

Patient: "Yeah, uh huh, well what would I do with the, uh, the stuff that is over there on top of it? Do they, uh, have the, the, you know, the thing to do it with the wheels on the floor. I, uh, guess they should let me."

---

in my hand. The nurse asked me again to take my pills and I did not know what to do. She began to lose her patience as I stood there holding the medicine cup. She then told me to put the pills in my mouth and to swallow them with the water she handed me. I could follow each of the instructions and eventually 'took my pills.'"

An example of literal interpretation of symbols is described by this patient: "It took me at least 15 minutes to walk down the street because I stopped every time the light changed from green to red. I did not understand that the traffic signal was only for cars."

Sometimes this problem advances to the point where the patient interprets a metaphor literally, as seen in this example: "I remembered the expression 'step on a crack and break your mother's back.'" One day I was walking down the street and stepped on a crack in the sidewalk. That same day my mother had fallen off a step stool after getting a can of soup from the kitchen cupboard and fractured two vertebrae in her back. For 9 months I believed that I had caused this accident to happen. This is also called magical thinking.

Nursing implications regarding patient teaching for the person experiencing concrete thinking are profound. Consider this example: During the admission of a new patient, a nurse instructed the patient to collect a sterile urine specimen. The patient exhibited terror and strongly resisted. When the nurse gently asked him why he was so frightened, he replied, "I do not want to become sterile."

The role of the nurse is to help with decision making in a nonpunitive, supportive manner, recognizing that these symptoms represent neurological disabilities over which the patient has little control. The nurse functions in a rehabilitative role and needs to provide information as clearly and concretely as possible. The language used should involve simple words in short phrases that are easy to understand. The nurse also needs to seek validation regarding how instructions were heard to clarify confusion and misunderstanding.

It is important to involve the patient in planning nursing care. Describe how you would accomplish this if the patient has cognitive problems that interfere with decision-making ability. ∎

Thought content is the final domain for assessment of cognitive functioning and includes evaluation for the presence of delusions in persons with schizophrenia. A delusion is a personal belief based on an incorrect inference of external reality. One of the mind's primary functions is to produce thoughts. Thoughts provide a sense of identity. Thoughts are produced as a result of intricate processes that involve screening and filtering internal and external stimuli and the use of multiple feedback loops in the brain. Recognizing the complexity of this process helps the nurse appreciate the unyielding way in which a person defends personal beliefs.

Recalling the cognitive deficits already described helps the nurse understand why people with schizophrenia sometimes have beliefs different from those of other people. It is also important to realize that a delusion does not always last. It is common for a belief to be fixed for only a few weeks or few months, particularly in the less severe forms of schizophrenia. The inability of the brain to process data accurately can result in **paranoid, grandiose, religious, nihilistic,** and **somatic delusions**. The delusions can be complicated further by thought withdrawal, thought insertion, thought control, or thought broadcasting. Types of delusions are described in Chapter 7.

Delusions represent an elaborate interplay between brain physiology, current environmental stimuli, and the person's frame of reference regarding the world. Delusions have several characteristics that must be identified before effective interventions can be planned. Delusions can become intertwined with hallucinations. They may be a single thought or pervade the person's entire cognitive process. They can represent a complete thought or only a portion of an idea. Delusions may be systematized, which means they are restricted to a specific area of belief such as family or religion, or nonsystematized, meaning they extend into many areas of a person's life, so new people and new information are incorporated into the delusion. Many patients have reported the relief they experienced as their symptoms remitted and they realized the belief was really a delusion, just a symptom, not the actual truth.

Perception. Perception is identification and initial interpretation of a stimulus based on information received through sight, sound, taste, touch, and smell. Given the complex interplay of brain functions among brainstem, diencephalon, and cortex for each of the five senses, it is important to recognize that perceptual problems are often the first symptoms in many brain illnesses.

Hallucinations are false perceptual distortions that occur in maladaptive neurobiological responses. The patient actually experiences the sensory distortion as being real and responds accordingly. However, with a hallucination there is no identifiable external or internal stimulus. Although hallucinations are most commonly associated with schizophrenia, only about 70% of people with this illness experience them. They also can occur in those with a manic or depressive illness, delirium, organic mental disorders, and substance abuse disorders. It is essential to stress that hallucinations and delusions can occur in any illness that disrupts brain function.

In addition, the nurse should differentiate between auditory flashbacks that often occur in those with posttraumatic stress disorder, dissociative identity disorder, and borderline personality disorder, as well as in survivors of trauma and abuse, from the auditory hallucinations occurring in schizophrenia. Sensory **flashbacks** are hallmarks of the above disorders. Hallucinations can arise from any of the five senses as described in Table 21-1.

A young woman is hospitalized in a forensic psychiatric unit because she attempted to kill her preschool children. She says her dead mother's voice told her to do this because the devil would get them unless they were in heaven with her. Is this a delusion, a hallucination, or both? Would knowing the woman's sociocultural background influence your response? Why or why not? ■

Another category of perceptual behaviors involves **sensory integration** and includes **pain recognition, soft neurological signs, right/left recognition,** and **recognition and perception of faces.** Symptoms related to these perceptions are common in schizophrenia, yet often are assessed inaccurately within a behavioral instead of a perceptual context. Sensory integration disruptions often lead to deliberate acts of self-harm, as described in this clinical example.

Table 21-1	**Sensory Modalities Involved in Hallucinations**
SENSE	CHARACTERISTICS
Auditory	Hearing noises or sounds, most commonly in the form of voices. Sounds that range from a simple noise or voice, to a voice talking about the patient, to complete conversations between two or more people about the person who is hallucinating. Audible thoughts in which the patient hears voices that are speaking what the patient is thinking and commands that tell the patient to do something, sometimes harmful or dangerous.
Visual	Visual stimuli in the form of flashes of light, geometric figures, cartoon figures, or elaborate and complex scenes or visions. Visions can be pleasant or terrifying, as in seeing monsters.
Olfactory	Putrid, foul, and rancid smells such as blood, urine, or feces; occasionally the odors can be pleasant. Olfactory hallucinations are typically associated with stroke, tumor, seizures, and the dementias.
Gustatory	Putrid, foul, and rancid tastes such as blood, urine, or feces.
Tactile	Experiencing pain or discomfort with no apparent stimuli. Feeling electrical sensations coming from the ground, inanimate objects, or other people.
Cenesthetic	Feeling body functions such as blood pulsing through veins and arteries, food digesting, or urine forming.
Kinesthetic	Sensation of movement while standing motionless.

CLINICAL EXAMPLE

During an initial physical assessment a nurse noted many superficial scars on the left arm of a young woman who had just completed an 8-week education program on symptom management in schizophrenia. The nurse said, "Tell me about those scars," to which the patient replied: "Before I knew it was okay to talk about my symptoms I often lost sensation in my left arm and hand and thought my arm was poisoned or dead. I tried to determine if I was alive or not. I could see myself walking and see and feel my right arm, so I thought I was probably alive but I did not know for sure, so I used to take a knife and poke tiny holes in my skin. I could not feel the knife yet I saw blood. It was when I saw the blood that I knew I was still alive."

Selected Nursing Diagnoses

- Disturbed sensory perception, tactile, related to disrupted sensory integration, as evidenced by explanation of scars on right arm
- Risk for self-mutilation related to perceptual disturbance, as evidenced by scars from past episodes of cutting left arm ■

The concept of pain and pain recognition has been well studied. Knowing that the parietal lobe is the major site of pain recognition helps the nurse see this as a neurobiologically based symptom. Visceral pain recognition involves integration of stimuli from the spinal cord through the brainstem, diencephalon, and cortex using intricate feedback circuits. People with schizophrenia generally have poor visceral pain recognition and need to have an in-depth assessment of physical complaints, as described by the patient in the next clinical example.

CLINICAL EXAMPLE

"I told my case manager that I had a stomachache, some diarrhea, and vomiting and felt like I had the flu. I had a fever, so she took me to the doctor, who said I probably had the flu and should just go home and rest. After a few days I got real sick and had to be taken to the emergency room, where they discovered my appendix had ruptured, and I had to have a very long and complicated surgery." ■

It is not uncommon for people with schizophrenia to think they just have a bad cold and have it diagnosed as pneumonia. Unfortunately, the physical needs of psychiatric patients often can be neglected or disregarded by the individual, as well as by the health care system.

Sensory integration perceptions are included in standard neurological examinations under the category **soft signs**, meaning that they represent a neurological deficit in an undetermined location but are consistent with brain injury to the frontal or parietal lobes. These terms refer to the ability to identify objects by touch. Box 21-5 lists several neurological soft signs common in schizophrenia that should be assessed carefully during a baseline evaluation of each patient. Problems in these functions contribute to difficulty with fine motor actions of the hand, and the patient may appear clumsy. Problems with right/left discrimination also contribute to lack of coordination and ability to carry out directions involving concepts of right and left.

Misidentification and perception of faces can contribute to fear, aggressiveness, withdrawal from interactions, and hostility. This symptom also involves self-recognition and often is present when patients refuse to look in a mirror or avoid eye contact.

Environmental factors can stimulate hallucinations. In general, objects that are reflective, such as television screens, photo frames, and fluorescent lights can contribute to visual hallucinations. Auditory hallucinations can be caused by excessive noise and by sensory deprivation. The nurse should be acutely aware of environmental stimuli and the patient's response or lack of response. Patients may withdraw from sensory stimuli in an attempt to decrease sensory responses.

When perceptions are altered, concurrent symptoms in cognitive functions are common. Studies have shown that 90% of people who experience hallucinations also have delusions, whereas only 35% who experience delusions also have hallucinations. Approximately 20% of patients have mixed sensory hallucinations, usually auditory and visual.

Emotion. In psychiatry, emotions are described in terms of mood and affect. Mood is defined as an extensive and sustained feeling tone that can be experienced for a few hours or for years and can noticeably affect the persons' worldview (Chapter 19 includes a complete description of mood and mood disorders). Affect refers to behaviors such as hand and body movements, facial expression, and pitch of voice that can be observed when a person is expressing and experiencing feelings and emotions.

Terms related to affect include **broad, restricted, blunted, flat,** and **inappropriate.** What is considered normal varies greatly among cultures. Broad and restricted are usually considered within the range of normal, whereas blunted, flat, and inappropriate represent symptoms of an underlying problem.

BOX 21-5

Neurological Soft Signs: Prefrontal Cortical Dysfunction in Schizophrenia

- Astereognosis: Inability to recognize objects by the sense of touch (such as differentiating a nickel from a dime)
- Agraphesthesia: Inability to recognize numbers or letters traced on the skin
- Dysdiadochokinesia: Impairment of the ability to perform smooth, alternating movements (such as turning the hand face up and face down rapidly)
- Mild muscle twitches, choreiform and ticlike movements, grimacing
- Impaired fine motor skills and abnormal motor tone
- Increased rate of eye blinking
- Abnormal smooth pursuit eye movements (SPEM): Difficulty following movement of objects

Neurological hard signs: loss of function, weakness, diminished reflexes, paralysis caused by a CVA, tumor, traumatic injury, etc.

CVA, Cerebrovascular accident.

Disorders of affect refer to expression of emotion, not the experience of emotion. Patients describe affective symptoms in the following examples:

- "I remember trying to smile for 3 years, but my face did not work."
- "My face was as stiff as your fingers would be if you tied them to popsicle sticks for 3 months and then tried to use them to thread a needle."

Patients describe tremendous frustration with these affective symptoms because others assume that they do not experience any emotion. These descriptions demonstrate why patients are commonly misjudged as appearing bored, disinterested, and unmotivated.

Emotion refers to moods and affects that are connected to specific ideas. Emotions are generated from an interplay of neural activity between the hypothalamus, limbic structures (amygdala and hippocampus), and higher cortex centers such as the association cortices. The hypothalamus, in addition to its hormonal functions, is the emotional coordinating center.

Emotions can be hyperexpressed or hypoexpressed. People with schizophrenia commonly have symptoms of **hypoexpression**. Some patients perceive that they no longer have any feelings and that they have a decreased ability to feel intimacy and closeness. Problems of emotion usually seen in schizophrenia include the following:

- Alexithymia: Difficulty naming and describing emotions
- Anhedonia: Inability or decreased ability to experience pleasure, joy, intimacy, and closeness
- Apathy: Lack of feelings, emotions, interests, or concern

In addition to problems with emotions and affect, people with schizophrenia also can have mood disorders. A major depression may develop in up to 60% of people with schizophrenia. Nine percent to 13% of people with schizophrenia complete suicide (Pinikahana, Happell, and Keks, 2003). A diagnosis of schizoaffective disorder is given to the patient who meets the diagnostic criteria for schizophrenia as well as bipolar disorder or major depression.

Understanding the effect of brain malfunctions on the emotions and affect of the person with schizophrenia is important for promoting constructive communication and problem solving. One also should recognize that people with brain illnesses often have an uncanny ability to sense the emotions of others, yet they may have difficulty identifying their own emotions. This creates special problems in caring for the patient and requires the nurse to be aware of and in control of her own emotional reactions.

Caregivers often confuse feelings that are a direct result of brain malfunction and those that are an indirect product of social difficulties resulting from illness. Examples of feelings that are a direct result of brain malfunction include paranoid hostility and emotional flattening. An example of feelings that are an indirect product of social difficulties caused by illness is frustration over not being able to achieve one's potential. When patients and caregivers have difficulty identifying feelings and emotions, barriers to good communication usually result.

Behavior and Movement.   Definition of "normal" behavior and movement is based on culture, age appropriateness, and social acceptability. Maladaptive neurobiological responses cause behaviors and movements that are odd, unsightly, confusing, difficult to manage, dysfunctional, and puzzling to others. With exploration, many behaviors can be explained and movements can be understood. Some make sense in the context of information provided by the patient or of the patient's neurobiological illness.

Describe unusual behaviors or movements that you have observed in patients with maladaptive neurobiological responses. Were you able to discover the reason for the behaviors or movements? Can you think of possible explanations for wearing several layers of clothing in very hot weather? Refusing to bathe? Hugging oneself and rocking? ■

Maladaptive behaviors in schizophrenia include **deteriorated appearance, lack of persistence at work or school, avolition, repetitive or stereotyped behavior, aggression, agitation,** and **negativism.** Deterioration in appearance includes disheveled and dirty clothes, sloppy and unkempt appearance, poor or absent personal grooming, and lack of personal hygiene. This is often the first set of symptoms to occur and is a signal to the family that something is happening to their loved one.

Accompanying deterioration in appearance is lack of persistence at work or school. As problems in brain function begin to appear, the cognitive skills seem to "short circuit," and the person can no longer perform routine tasks. As deterioration continues, the person begins to experience avolition, which means lack of energy and drive. This is a result of the brain changes (which may be occurring rapidly) and frustration with the inability to accomplish tasks that required little effort in the past. Unfortunately, at this point most people with schizophrenia are mislabeled as lazy, disinterested, and unmotivated.

As deterioration continues, patients often engage in repetitive or stereotyped behaviors. These appear similar to obsessive-compulsive behavior but are related to a private meaning rather than to thoughts. Examples include having to eat foods in a certain way, wearing only certain clothes, walking four steps forward and one step back, or being able to drink only half a glass of water at a time.

Aggression, agitation, and the potential for violence unfortunately are often used to describe the person with schizophrenia. However, the person with schizophrenia generally is the victim rather than the aggressor (Brekke et al, 2001). People experiencing psychoses are sometimes violent, especially when their illness is out of control or they stop taking their medications (Torrey, 2001). Agitation is common for anyone who is living with a chronic illness for which there is no cure. It is important to identify and document situations that seem to be triggers for agitated behavior (see Chapter 30). People who have schizophrenia tend to become agitated when experiencing performance anxiety, particularly when they have difficulty carrying out tasks that previously were easy to do. Abnormal behaviors and movements in schizophrenia are summarized in Box 21-6.

Maladaptive movements associated with schizophrenia include **catatonia, abnormal eye movements, grimacing, apraxia/echopraxia, abnormal gait, mannerisms,** and **extrapyramidal side effects of psychotropic medications** (see Chapter 27). Catatonia is a stuporous state in which the patient may require complete physical nursing care, similar to that for a comatose patient, sometimes interspersed with unpredictable outbursts of aggressive behavior or strange posturing.

Abnormal eye movements include difficulty following a moving target, absence or avoidance of eye contact, decreased or rapid eye blinking, and frequent staring. These are common ocular motor symptoms found in 40% to 80% of people with schizophrenia.

Grimacing refers to abnormal facial movements that are beyond the patient's control and are not caused by psychotropic medications.

Apraxia is difficulty carrying out a purposeful, organized task that is somewhat complex, such as dressing. Echopraxia is defined as purposeless imitation of movements made by other people. This symptom may not always be purposeless but can illustrate a delusion, as described by the patient in the following clinical example.

🔔 CLINICAL EXAMPLE

"I thought the nurse was my mirror and I had to do what the mirror showed me, so I copied everything she did. As long as I could see her I could feel connected to myself and my surroundings, but she did not understand how important it was for me to be around her and watch what she did. Of course I could not explain what was happening to me at the time because I was psychotic, so she put me in seclusion and restraints."

Selected Nursing Diagnosis
• Disturbed thought processes related to maladaptive information processing, as evidenced by belief that the nurse was a mirror ∎

BOX 21-6

Abnormal Behaviors and Movements in Patients With Schizophrenia

Behaviors
Appearance
Aggression/agitation/violence
Repetitive or stereotyped behavior
Avolition
Lack of persistence at work or school

Movements
Catatonia, waxy flexibility, posturing
Extrapyramidal side effects of psychotropic medications
Abnormal eye movements
Grimacing
Apraxia/echopraxia
Abnormal gait
Mannerisms

Staggering, intentional stepping, and walking with the toes touching the ground first are abnormal gaits common in people with schizophrenia. Mannerisms involve gestures that seem contrived and are not appropriate to the situation, such as stopping in the middle of a sentence to whirl two fingers around.

Socialization. Socialization is the ability to form cooperative and interdependent relationships with others. This was placed last among the five major brain functions because problems with the others must be understood to appreciate the relational consequences of maladaptive neurobiological responses. Social problems are often the major source of concern to families and health care providers because these tangible effects of illness are often more prominent than the symptoms related to cognition and perception.

Social problems may result from the illness directly or indirectly. Direct effects occur when symptoms prevent the person from socializing within accepted sociocultural norms or when motivation deteriorates resulting in social withdrawal and isolation from life's activities. Behaviors directly causing these problems include **inability to communicate coherently, loss of drive and interest, deterioration of social skills, poor personal hygiene,** and **paranoia.**

Indirect effects on socialization are secondary consequences of the illness. An example is low self-esteem related to poor academic and social achievement. Significant social discomfort and further social isolation may result. Specific problems in the development of relationships include **social inappropriateness, disinterest in recreational activities, inappropriate sexual behavior,** and **stigma-related withdrawal by friends, families, and peers.**

Social inappropriateness relates directly to cognitive deficits and results in behaviors such as suddenly beginning loud, evangelistic prayer in public, toileting in public, standing in the middle of a street trying to direct traffic, dressing bizarrely, and engaging in intimate conversation with total strangers. Social inappropriateness often involves bizarre sexual behavior such as public masturbation, running nude in the street, or making inappropriate sexual advances. Sometimes bizarre sexual behavior is related to gender identity confusion. It is not uncommon, particularly with temporal lobe involvement, for people with schizophrenia to be unable to recognize their genitalia as their own. This often is the reason for sudden undressing and what appears to be public masturbation, when it actually may be a patient's futile attempt at reality testing.

Stigma also presents major obstacles to developing relationships and adversely affects quality of life. Stigma, which literally means mark of shame, is a major cause of the social isolation of people with schizophrenia. Stigma often spreads to the whole family, who may be having their own schizophrenia-related social problems stemming from embarrassment about having the illness in the family (see Chapters 11 and 15). They may avoid talking about it, or if they do want to talk, they may not know how to broach the subject. Stigma and rejection may discourage them from talking. Family members may feel like social outcasts for having this illness in the family. One family member explained, "For the rest of my life, I will be dealing not only with the heartbreak of my brother's illness but also with negative response, stigma, and ignorance in my hometown that will affect me deeply. I know, because the last 10 years of it already has been sheer hell."

Describe your own attitudes and behaviors and those of your peers toward people who have maladaptive neurobiological responses and their families. ■

Predisposing Factors

Biological. Behaviors related to maladaptive neurobiological responses have been described in writing and art since biblical times. Causes proposed for these strange behaviors ranged from demon possession, bad blood, and witchcraft to the full moon. Fortunately, modern science is now identifying many clues to the biological causes of these disorders (see Chapter 6).

Schizophrenia is a heterogeneous neurodevelopmental brain disorder. What accounts for the disruptions in brain function causing the many symptoms of schizophrenia is not known. Nonetheless, some interesting research results propose the hypothesize of an integrative model of schizophrenia as being a disorder of brain neural circuits.

Genetics. The aim of genetic research is to eventually map the genetic susceptibility for schizophrenia and then develop genetic interventions as treatment modalities. The specific genetic defects that cause schizophrenia have not yet been identified, but progress has been made toward identifying the mechanisms and potential gene locations. Two genetic hypotheses are as follows:

1. Trinucleotide repeat amplification-mutation in which a certain stretch of deoxyribonucleic acid (DNA) occurs more than once when genes are copied. This could explain some of the differential rates of occurrence of schizophrenia, even among monozygotic or identical twins. If one child in a family carrying a gene for schizophrenia happens to have more than one trinucleotide repeat than the others, that child could more easily be pushed over the threshold from health to mental illness.
2. Genome screens of entire families of individuals with schizophrenia support genetic linkage on chromosome 6, with additional genetic contributions associated with chromosomes 4, 8, 15, and 22 (Buchanan and Carpenter, 2000).

Although it is thought that schizophrenia is caused by the interaction of a variety of mechanisms that are biological, environmental, and experiential, family, twin, and adoption studies have long shown an increased risk for the disease in people with both a first-degree relative (parent, sibling, offspring) or a second-degree relative (grandparents, aunts and uncles, cousins, grandchildren) with schizophrenia (Table 21-2).

Children with a biological parent with schizophrenia who were adopted at birth by a family with no incidence of the disorder have the same risk as if they had been raised by their biological parents. Thus compelling evidence exists for both a genetic predisposition for the disorder and additional environmental or random factors, as evidenced by studies of identical twins, who share 100% of genes, but only a 50% risk for schizophrenia.

Neurobiology. Multiple studies show anatomical, functional, and neurochemical abnormalities in the living and postmortem brains of people with schizophrenia. Research suggests that the prefrontal cortex and the limbic cortex may never fully develop in the brains of persons with schizophrenia. The two most consistent neurobiological research findings in schizophrenia are imaging studies showing decreased brain volume and abnormal function, and neurochemical studies showing alterations of numerous neurotransmitter systems. The decreased brain volume reflects decreased white matter (neuronal axons). This has been recently attributed to faulty myelination occurring at about age 6 and again at about age 13 (Bartzokis, 2002). This also is thought to be determined by genetics.

Focus has been directed particularly on the frontal cortex, implicated in the negative symptoms of schizophrenia; the limbic system (in the temporal lobes), implicated in the positive symptoms of schizophrenia; and the neurotransmitter systems connecting these regions, particularly dopamine and serotonin, and more recently, glutamate. Therefore, psychotic behaviors may be related to **lesions in the frontal, temporal, and limbic regions of the brain,** and **dysregulation of neurotransmitter systems connecting these regions.**

Another theory describes a misconnection syndrome between the cortex and the cerebellum, mediated by the thalamus (this circuitry normally coordinates both motor and mental activity), as a theoretical framework for strategies to explore etiology, pathophysiology, intervention, and prevention of schizophrenia (Andreasen, 1999).

Imaging studies. Computed tomography (CT) and magnetic resonance imaging (MRI) studies of brain structure show decreased brain volume in people with schizophrenia. Findings include larger lateral and third ventricles; atrophy in the frontal lobe, cerebellum, and limbic structures (particularly the hippocampus and amygdala); and increased size of sulci (fissures) on the surface of the brain (Figure 21-4). These findings all suggest loss (atrophy) or underdevelopment of brain tissue. The trend is to associate enlarged ventricles with two indicators of poor prognosis: early age of onset and poor premorbid functioning (functioning before the first diagnosis).

Table 21-2	Genetic Risk for Schizophrenia	
PERSON AT RISK		**RISK (%)**
Monozygotic (fraternal) twin		50
Dizygotic (identical) twin		15
Sibling		10
One parent affected		15
Both parents affected		35
Second-degree relative affected		2-3
No affected relative		1

Positron emission tomography (PET) scans usually demonstrate decreased cerebral blood flow to the frontal lobes during specific cognitive tasks in people with schizophrenia. This frontal hypometabolism is thought to account for some problems with attention, planning, and decision making (Figure 21-5).

The thalamus (which lies in the center of the brain, near the temporal lobes and hippocampus, and regulates sensory input, serving as a filter or relay station between the cerebral cortex and the rest of the brain) also was found in several studies to be smaller than average and to have reduced activity in some schizophrenic patients. This may explain some of

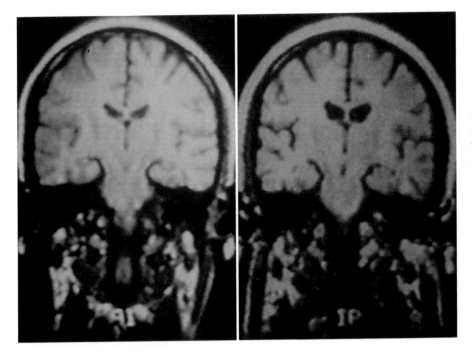

Figure 21-4   Magnetic resonance imaging (MRI) scans through the bodies of the lateral ventricles in a pair of monozygotic twins who are discordant for schizophrenia. Note the increase in the cerebrospinal fluid spaces in the twin with schizophrenia *(right)* as compared with the unaffected twin *(left)*. (From Roberts GS, Leigh PN, Weinberger DR: *Neuropsychiatric disorders*, London, 1993, Mosby-Wolfe.)

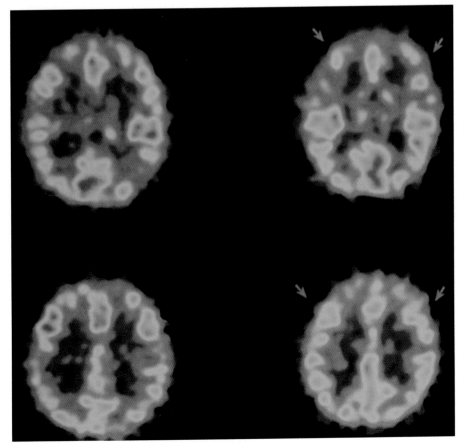

Figure 21-5   Blood flow demonstrated by a positron emission tomography (PET) scan during the performance of the Wisconsin Card Sort Task (a task that activates prefrontal cortex in normal subjects) in a twin with schizophrenia *(right column)* and an unaffected twin *(left column)*. The *arrows* indicate the relatively focused failure of activation in the affected twin compared with the unaffected twin. (From Roberts GS et al: *Neuropsychiatric disorders*, London, 1993, Mosby-Wolfe.)

the problems in sensory filtering and information processing in many people with schizophrenia.

The basal ganglia, part of the extrapyramidal system, are responsible for various aspects of movement, such as the inhibition of unwanted movement and the promotion of motor learning and planning, and also may play a role in cognitive function with their rich connectivity to the frontal lobes. The basal ganglia are overactive in people with schizophrenia, perhaps accounting for movement and speech abnormalities.

Neurotransmitter studies. During the past several decades, research in the area of neurotransmission has led to the **dysregulation hypothesis** of schizophrenia: a persistent impairment in one or more neurotransmitter or neuromodulator homeostatic regulatory mechanisms causing unstable or erratic neurotransmission. This theory proposes that the mesolimbic area has overactive dopamine pathways, whereas the dopamine pathways in the prefrontal mesocortical areas are hypoactive and that an imbalance exists between dopamine and serotonin neurotransmitter systems (and probably between others as well).

Dopamine has been implicated longer than any other chemical substance in neurotransmitter studies of schizophrenia. This is because it has long been known that mind-altering drugs such as amphetamines and cocaine increase brain levels of dopamine and produce psychosis, and because early on it was understood that the conventional antipsychotic drugs exerted their therapeutic effects by blocking dopamine receptors. Dopamine is important in responses to stress and has many connections to the limbic system. The prefrontal cortex has few dopamine receptors of its own, but it may regulate dopamine in other circuits in the brain. Also, dopamine is present in high levels in the brain during late adolescence, when schizophrenia usually first appears. Dopamine is found in three parts of the brain:

- **Substantia nigra** motor center, affecting movement and coordination
- **Midbrain**, involving emotion and memory
- **Hypothalamic-pituitary** connection, involving emotional responses and stress-coping patterns

Dopamine has four major pathways in the brain (Figure 21-6):

1. **Mesocortical**: Innervates the frontal lobes
   - *Function:* Insight, judgment, social consciousness, inhibition, and highest level of cognitive activities (reasoning, motivation, planning, decision making)
   - *Negative symptoms:* Affective flattening or blunting, poverty of speech or speech content, blocking, poor grooming, lack of motivation, anhedonia, social withdrawal, cognitive defects, and attention deficits
2. **Mesolimbic**: Innervates the limbic system
   - *Function:* Associated with memory, smell, automatic visceral effects, and emotional behavior
   - *Positive symptoms:* Hallucinations, delusions, disorganized speech, and bizarre behavior
3. **Tuberoinfundibular**: Originates in the hypothalamus and projects to the pituitary
   - *Function:* Endocrine function, hunger, thirst, metabolism, temperature control, digestion, sexual arousal,

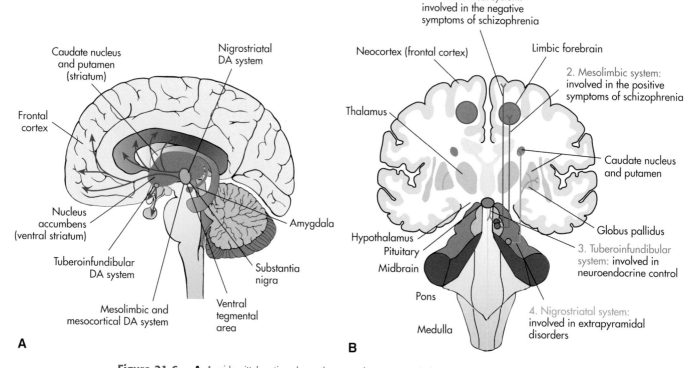

Figure 21-6 **A,** A midsagittal section shows the approximate anatomical routes of the four dopamine tracts. *DA,* Dopamine. **B,** A coronal section shows the sites of origin and the targets of all four tracts. (Modified from Kandel E, Schwartz J, Jessell T: *Principles of neural science,* ed 4, New York, 2000, Elsevier.)

and circadian rhythms (implicated in some of the endocrine abnormalities seen in schizophrenia and some of the side effects of antipsychotic drugs)

4. **Nigrostriatal**: Originates in the substantia nigra and terminates in the caudate nucleus–putamen complex (neostriatum)
   • *Function*: Innervates the motor and extrapyramidal systems (implicated in some of the movement side effects of antipsychotic drugs)

In addition to mediating many brain functions, **serotonin** also has been implicated in schizophrenia. It has a modulating effect on dopamine, and some atypical antipsychotic drugs (clozapine, risperidone, olanzapine, quetiapine, and ziprasidone) are combination serotonin/dopamine blocking agents, accounting for their improved efficacy over the typical antipsychotics used in the treatment of the negative symptoms of schizophrenia.

Aripiprazole, the first second-generation atypical drug is a dopamine/serotonin system stabilizer, and was introduced in the fall of 2002. It has both partial agonist and antagonist actions for dopamine and serotonin and the mesocortical as well as mesolimbic systems.

Glutamate is the major excitatory neurotransmitter in the brain. Research on the effect of PCP (phencyclidine), a drug that seems to mimic the symptoms of schizophrenia in normal volunteers, has led to a better understanding of how glutamate interacts with dopamine. The function of glutamates' major receptor complex, NMDA (N-methyl-D-aspartate), is interrupted by PCP.

This important brain communication system is abnormal in the prefrontal cortex and thalamus in postmortem studies of patients with schizophrenia. Experimental psychotropic agents that activate the NMDA receptor complex and its coagonist site for glycine are proposed as potential future treatments for schizophrenia.

Neurodevelopment. It is now clear that the multiple structural, functional, and chemical brain deviations seen in schizophrenia are usually present long before the symptoms appear, probably from the earliest years of life, and perhaps before birth. It is not clear yet whether these changes are caused by genetic programming defects or environmental injury, or both, creating a vulnerability that remains dormant until later developmental events occur.

Several brain structures are abnormal in patients with schizophrenia, as compared with control subjects, that interfere with working memory (prefrontal cortex and hippocampus), and these brains were found to have increased cortical folding (a sign of early developmental abnormality in the infant brain). Also, the volume of grey matter in the fusiform gyrus, a structure that participates in facial recognition and naming, a cognitive function commonly disturbed in psychosis, was 13% less in patients with schizophrenia as compared with control subjects (Lindsay, 2000).

Research has shown that some preschizophrenic children show subtle abnormalities involving attention, coordination, and emotional responses long before they exhibit overt symptoms of schizophrenia (Duzyurek and Wiener, 1999). In some

monozygotic twin pairs, the schizophrenic twin was noted to become permanently different from the unaffected identical twin by the age of 5 years, although symptoms of schizophrenia did not appear until young adulthood.

These early childhood differences included excessive shyness, hyperactivity, bed-wetting, aggressiveness, poor concentration and coordination, tantrums, hand-washing compulsions, reversion to baby talk, and delays in learning to walk and speak (Torrey, 2001). Identification of these prodromal symptoms in children at risk for adult schizophrenia can result in early intervention strategies, perhaps avoiding or delaying the onset of illness or minimizing its effects.

It has not been determined that the intrauterine environment or early infant events are linked to the development of schizophrenia (Cannon, Jones, and Murray, 2002). Some research has found a greater frequency of prenatal and perinatal complications among people with schizophrenia, including preeclampsia; trauma; oxygen deprivation at the time of delivery; extreme prematurity; and maternal problems such as poor nutrition, stress, use of tobacco, alcohol, street drugs, or caffeine, viral infection, hypertension, and use of teratogenic pharmacological agents.

This research suggests that some disruption in fetal neural development may change the way the brain matures throughout childhood and adolescence, affecting the myelination, migration, and interconnections of young neurons as they mature in utero and in the first few decades after birth and thus may contribute to brain abnormalities common in schizophrenia (Dalman et al, 1999).

Viral theories. Mixed evidence indicates that prenatal exposure to the influenza virus, particularly during the second trimester, may be one of the factors in the etiology of schizophrenia in some people but not in others. This theory is supported by research findings that more people with schizophrenia are born in the winter or early spring and in urban settings.

These findings suggest a potential season and place of birth impact on the risk for schizophrenia. Viral infections are more common in crowded places and in winter and early spring and may occur in utero or in early childhood in some vulnerable people (Battle et al, 1999).

Psychological. In the past, in the absence of identified biological causes for schizophrenia, psychological, sociological, and environmental influences became the focus of psychodynamic and other theories and beliefs about the illness. For most of the twentieth century schizophrenia was thought to be an illness caused partly by the family and partly by some individual character flaw. The mother was believed to be anxious, overprotective, or cold and unfeeling; the father was distant or overbearing. Marital conflict and families that stayed together for the sake of the children were blamed. Some theories described a "schizophrenogenic" mother and other theories described how communicating in double messages could "double bind" a person into developing schizophrenia.

Schizophrenia also was proposed by some to be a failure to accomplish an early stage of psychosocial development. For example, an infant's inability to form a trusting relationship could lead to a lifetime of intrapsychic conflict. Schizophrenia was seen as the most severe example of inability to cope with stress. Disturbances in identity, inability to attach to a love object, and inability to control basic drives also served as key theories.

It is important for psychiatric nurses and the health care community in general to realize that with the psychobiological discoveries of recent years, these psychodynamic theories have **no** scientific evidence to support them. In addition, they can have a very negative impact on patient and family alliances with mental health care professionals, perpetuate stigma associated with these illnesses, and contribute to a delay in obtaining appropriate treatment.

The "schizophrenogenic" mother was described as one who gave her child conflicting and confusing messages about their relationship, resulting in schizophrenia. How would this unsupported theory affect the mothers of people with schizophrenia, their relationships with their ill children, and their relationships with care providers? ■

Sociocultural and Environmental. Some theorists proposed that poverty, society, and cultural disharmony could cause schizophrenia or that people chose to become schizophrenic to cope with the insanity of the modern world. Others proposed that schizophrenia was caused by living in the city or living in isolation in the country. Although accumulated stress related to sociocultural and environmental factors is likely to be a contributing factor to the onset of schizophrenia and to relapses, neurobiological findings point to other causes for the etiology of psychotic disorders.

Precipitating Stressors

Biological. Interference in a brain feedback loop that regulates the amount of information that can be processed at a given time has been identified as one possible biological stressor. Normal information processing occurs in a predetermined series of neural activities. Visual and auditory stimuli are initially screened and filtered by the thalamus and sent for processing by the frontal lobe. If too much information is sent at once, or if the information is faulty, the frontal lobe sends an overload message to the basal ganglia.

The basal ganglia, in turn, send a message to the thalamus to slow down transmissions to the frontal lobe. The decreased function of the frontal lobe impairs the ability of this feedback loop to perform. Less ability to regulate the basal ganglia is available, and ultimately, the message to slow down transmissions to the frontal lobe never occurs. The result is **information-processing overload** and the neurobiological responses described in the beginning of this chapter.

Another possible biological stressor is the **abnormal gating mechanisms** that may occur in schizophrenia. Gating is an electrical process involving electrolytes. It refers to inhibitory and excitatory nerve action potentials and the feedback occurring within the nervous system related to completed nerve transmissions. Decreased gating is demonstrated by a person's inability to selectively attend to stimuli (Perry, Geyer, and Braff, 1999).

For example, at a baseball game the person with schizophrenia would be unable to differentiate the noise from the crowd, the music, the team, or the public address system. Normally, when people hear a loud noise they become startled; however, when the noise is repeated, the startle response is decreased. For example, if you hear a neighbor setting off firecrackers in celebration of the Fourth of July, you become startled. When you hear a second explosion soon after, you are generally less startled. The person with schizophrenia is just as startled the second time, and maybe even more so than the first. This inability to gate a noise stimulus causes people to become frightened in crowds or wherever they encounter increased noise.

Symptom triggers. Precursors and stimuli or combinations of them often precede a new episode of the illness. The word **trigger** is used to describe these stressors. Common triggers of neurobiological responses related to health, environment, attitudes, and behaviors are listed in Box 21-7. Patients

---

BOX 21-7

Neurobiological Response Symptom Triggers

Health
Poor nutrition
Lack of sleep
Out-of-balance circadian rhythms
Fatigue
Infection
Central nervous system drugs
Lack of exercise
Barriers to accessing health care

Environment
Hostile/critical environment
Housing difficulties (unsatisfactory housing)
Pressure to perform (loss of independent living)
Changes in life events, daily patterns of activity
Interpersonal difficulties, disruptions in interpersonal relationships
Social isolation
Lack of social support
Job pressures (poor occupational skills)
Stigmatization
Poverty
Lack of transportation (resources)
Inability to get/keep a job

Attitudes/Behaviors
"Poor me" (low self-concept)
"Hopeless" (lack of self-confidence)
"I'm a failure" (loss of motivation to use skills)
"Lack of control" (demoralization)
Feeling overpowered by symptoms
"No one likes me" (unable to meet spiritual needs)
Looks/acts different from others who are of the same age, culture
Poor social skills
Aggressive behavior
Violent behavior
Poor medication management
Poor symptom management

with schizophrenia can learn to recognize triggers that they are particularly reactive to, and they can be taught to avoid them, if possible, and to contact their mental health care provider for help if they cannot.

Appraisal of Stressors

Stress Diathesis Model. No scientific research has shown that stress causes schizophrenia, but it is increasingly clear that schizophrenia is a disorder that not only causes stress but also is made worse by stress (Corcoran et al, 2001). Studies of relapse and symptom exacerbation provide evidence that stress, one's appraisal of the stressor, and the problems associated with coping with the stress may predict the return of symptoms (Kennedy, Schepp, and O'Connor, 2000). The **stress diathesis model** described in a classic work by Liberman

and colleagues (1994) states that schizophrenic symptoms develop based on the relationship between the amount of stress that a person experiences and an internal stress tolerance threshold. This is an important model because it integrates biological, psychological, and sociocultural factors. In this way, it is similar to the Stuart Stress Adaptation Model, which is used as the organizing conceptual framework of this text (Figure 21-7). Wuerker (2000) provides an adaptation of a model that helps explain the integration of stress in this neurobiological brain disease (Figure 21-8).

Coping Resources

Coping skills tend to be learned from parents. Children and young adults with schizophrenia need to be actively taught these skills because they have difficulty internalizing them

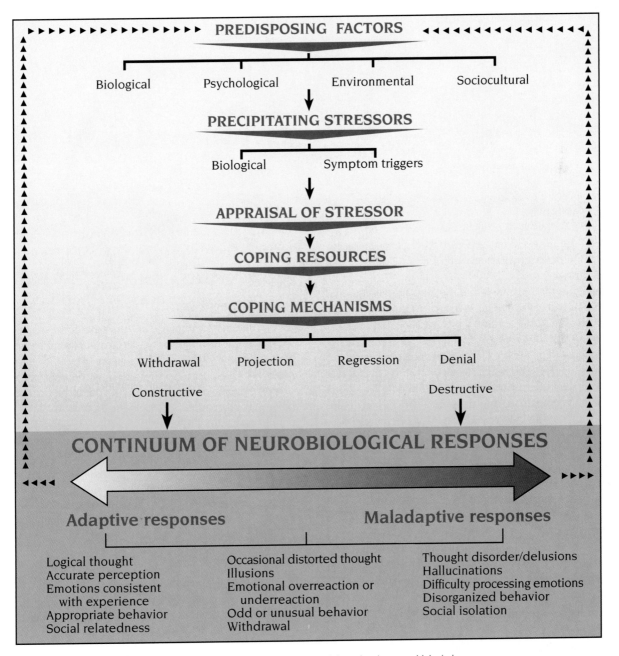

Figure 21-7   The Stuart Stress Adaptation Model as related to neurobiological responses.

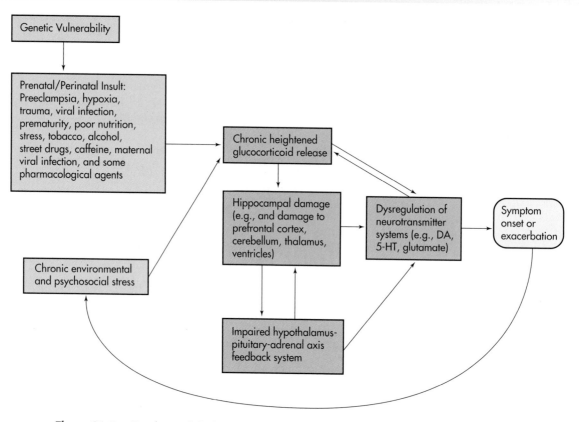

Figure 21-8   Neural stress diathesis model of schizophrenia. (Modified from Wuerker KA: *Issues Ment Health Nurs* 21:127, 2000.)

from observation. Family resources such as parental understanding of the illness, finances, availability of time and energy, and ability to provide ongoing support influence the course of illness.

It is important to remember that the mix of disabilities and resources of a particular patient is related to the type and location of the brain dysfunction. Thus it is essential to assess mental status carefully to identify the person's strengths. For instance, some people with maladaptive neurobiological responses are highly intelligent but unable to express themselves well. Others may be artistically talented but not skilled at verbal communication. Exploring these areas of strength helps the nurse in planning individualized nursing interventions.

Coping Mechanisms

Patients attempt to protect themselves from the frightening experiences caused by their illnesses. **Regression** is related to information-processing problems and expenditure of large amounts of energy in efforts to manage anxiety, leaving little for activities of daily living. **Projection** is an effort to explain confusing perceptions by assigning responsibility to someone or something. **Withdrawal** is related to problems establishing trust and preoccupation with internal experiences. Families often express **denial** when they first learn of their relative's diagnosis. This is the same as the denial that occurs whenever one receives information that causes fear and anxiety. It al-

lows the person time to gather internal and external resources and then adapt to the stressor gradually.

DIAGNOSIS

Nursing Diagnoses

In formulating the nursing diagnosis the nurse should review the complete nursing assessment as illustrated in the Stuart Stress Adaptation Model (see Figure 21-7). Nursing diagnoses take into account the functional level, stressors, and support systems of the patient and should be prioritized according to the patient's stage of illness (crisis, acute, maintenance, or health promotion). Nursing diagnoses associated with maladaptive neurobiological responses are presented in the Medical and Nursing Diagnoses box (Box 21-8). Primary NANDA nursing diagnoses include **impaired verbal communication, disturbed sensory perception, impaired social interaction,** and **disturbed thought processes.** Examples of expanded nursing diagnoses are presented in the Detailed Diagnoses table (Table 21-3).

Medical Diagnoses

The medical diagnoses associated with maladaptive neurobiological responses include **the schizophrenias, schizophreniform disorder, schizoaffective disorder, delusional disorder, brief psychotic disorder,** and **shared psychotic disorder.**

▪▪ **BOX 21-8** *Medical and Nursing Diagnoses Related to* **Maladaptive Neurobiological Responses**

RELATED MEDICAL DIAGNOSES (*DSM-IV-TR*)*	RELATED NURSING DIAGNOSES (NANDA)†

Schizophrenia
  Paranoid type
  Disorganized type
  Catatonic type
  Undifferentiated type
  Residual type
Schizophreniform disorder
Schizoaffective disorder
Delusional disorder
Brief psychotic disorder
Shared psychotic disorder
	Anxiety
	Body image, Disturbed
	Communication, Impaired verbal‡
	Confusion, Acute
	Coping, Compromised family
	Coping, Ineffective
	Decisional conflict
	Hopelessness
	Memory, Impaired
	Noncompliance
	Personal identity, Disturbed
	Role performance, Ineffective
	Self-care deficit (bathing/hygiene, dressing/grooming)
	Sensory perception, Disturbed‡
	Social interaction, Impaired‡
	Social isolation
	Suicide, Risk for
	Therapeutic regimen management, Ineffective
	Thought processes, Disturbed‡

*From American Psychiatric Association: *Diagnostic and statistical manual of mental disorders*, ed 4, text revision, Washington, DC, 2000, American Psychiatric Association.
†From North American Nursing Diagnosis Association: *NANDA nursing diagnoses: definitions and classification 2003-2004*, Philadelphia, 2003, The Association.
‡**Primary nursing diagnosis for maladaptive neurobiological responses.**

These diagnoses and related essential features are presented in the Detailed Diagnoses table (see Table 21-3).

◣ OUTCOME IDENTIFICATION

The expected outcome for nursing care of the patient with maladaptive neurobiological responses is:

The patient will live, learn, and work at a maximum possible level of success, as defined by the individual.

Prevention of relapse and early intervention are key components of a successful outcome. Relapse is the return of symptoms severe enough to interfere with activities of daily living. It can be prevented only by thorough, ongoing symptom monitoring (Herz, 1999). Planning therapeutic interventions depends on goals related to diagnosis and level of wellness.

Short-term goals identify the steps that will lead the patient to successfully accomplish the expected outcome. Examples include the following:

- The patient will initiate conversation with at least one person daily.
- The patient will participate in a medication education group weekly.
- The patient will identify medications and describe the prescribed dose, expected effects, possible side effects, and actions to take if questions arise.
- The patient will engage in a wellness lifestyle.
- The patient will describe preferred living situation following hospital discharge.

- The patient will practice community living skills such as food preparation, housekeeping, care of clothing, money management, and use of public transportation.

◣ PLANNING

When a person is in the crisis or acute stage of illness, care is often given in a hospital. The overall goal is to help the patient reach stability while establishing a foundation for rehabilitation and recovery. Because of the complex psychosocial needs of patients with maladaptive neurobiological responses, planning for discharge begins with admission. All patient resources must be studied. The family resources are particularly important because families are the providers of care for at least 65% of patients with schizophrenia (Berglund, Vahlne, and Edman, 2003).

Federal law requires that patients and, with patients' permission, family members be present at treatment planning meetings. This facilitates a smooth transition from the hospital to home. Recognizing the burden of caring for loved ones with schizophrenia, families must decide what resources they are able to use to assist the patient (Lukens et al, 1999). These resources may include time, energy, knowledge, and money. The discharge plan must be based on the reality of available resources.

Care of the patient in the maintenance phase occurs at home or in another community setting. The focus of this phase is to assist with rehabilitation and recovery. **Hope is an essential element in this process because regaining hope can be a turning point in a person's recovery** (Kirkpatrick et al, 2001).

Table 21-3	*Detailed Diagnoses Related to* **Maladaptive Neurobiological Responses**

NANDA DIAGNOSIS STEM	**EXAMPLES OF EXPANDED DIAGNOSIS**
Impaired verbal communication	Impaired verbal communication related to formal thought disorder, as evidenced by loose associations
Disturbed sensory perception	Disturbed sensory perception related to physiological brain dysfunction, as evidenced by verbal reports of "hearing voices that say bad things about me"
Impaired social interaction	Impaired social interaction related to inadequate social skills, as evidenced by inappropriate sexual advances toward members of both sexes
Disturbed thought processes	Disturbed thought processes related to physiological brain dysfunction, as evidenced by stated belief that staff members are really actors who were hired by parents to watch him

***DSM-IV-TR* DIAGNOSIS**	**ESSENTIAL FEATURES***
Schizophrenia	At least two of the following, each present for a significant portion of time during a 1-month period: Delusions Hallucinations Disorganized speech Grossly disorganized or catatonic behavior Negative symptoms For a significant portion of the time since the onset of the disturbance, one or more major areas of functioning such as work, interpersonal relations, or self-care is markedly below the level achieved before the onset. Continuous signs of the disturbance persist for at least 6 months.
Paranoid type	Preoccupation with one or more delusions or frequent auditory hallucinations.
Disorganized type	All of the following are prominent: disorganized speech, disorganized behavior, flat or inappropriate affect; does not meet the criteria for catatonic type.
Catatonic type	At least two of the following dominate the clinical picture: motor immobility as evidenced by catalepsy or stupor; excessive motor activity; extreme negativism or mutism; peculiarities of voluntary movement, as evidenced by posturing, stereotyped movements, prominent mannerisms, or prominent grimacing; echolalia or echopraxia.
Undifferentiated type	Symptoms meeting the first general criteria for schizophrenia are present, but criteria for other types are not met.
Residual type	Criteria for schizophrenia are not met, nor are those for any other subtype. There is continuing evidence of the disturbance, indicated by negative symptoms or attenuated presence of two or more symptoms included in the general criteria.
Schizophreniform disorder	Meets criteria for schizophrenia and an episode lasts at least 1 month but less than 6 months. Specify with or without good prognostic features based on at least two of the following: onset of prominent psychotic symptoms within 4 weeks of first noticeable change in behavior or functioning, confusion or perplexity at the height of the psychosis, good premorbid social and occupational functioning, and absence of blunted or flat affect.
Schizoaffective disorder	An uninterrupted period of illness including a major depressive episode or manic episode concurrent with symptoms of schizophrenia. During the same period of illness, there have been delusions or hallucinations for at least 2 weeks in the absence of prominent mood symptoms. Symptoms of a mood episode are present during a substantial part of the illness.
Delusional disorder	Nonbizarre delusions (situations that could occur, such as being followed, poisoned, or having a disease) lasting at least a month. Has never met criteria for schizophrenia. Apart from the impact of the delusion, functioning and behavior are not markedly affected.
Brief psychotic disorder	Presence of at least one of the following: delusions, hallucinations, disorganized speech, or grossly disorganized or catatonic behavior. (Behaviors are not culturally sanctioned.) Duration between 1 day and 1 month, with eventual return to premorbid functioning. The presence (brief reactive) or absence of marked stressors should be noted, as should onset within 4 weeks postpartum.
Shared psychotic disorder (folie a deux)	A delusion develops in a patient in the context of a close relationship with someone who already has a delusion. The delusions of the people involved are similar in content.

*From American Psychiatric Association: *Diagnostic and statistical manual of mental disorders*, ed 4, text revision, Washington, DC, 2000, American Psychiatric Association.

CITING THE EVIDENCE ON

Patterns of Usual Care

BACKGROUND: This survey of 719 persons with schizophrenia examined the current patterns of usual care they received as compared with the Schizophrenia Patient Outcomes Research Team (PORT) Treatment Recommendations.

RESULTS: The rates at which patients' treatment conformed to the recommendations were modest at best, generally below 50%. Specifically:

Only 29% of patients received the appropriate dose of antipsychotic medication over the long-term.

Fewer than half of people who also suffered symptoms of depression received antidepressant medication.

Only half of those suffering serious side effects of medication received appropriate and effective treatment to counteract those problems.

African Americans were almost twice as likely to be overmedicated with antipsychotic medications and suffer higher rates of side effects.

Fewer than 1 in 10 families received even minimal education and support.

Fewer than 1 in 4 patients who could have benefited from employment received any such support.

As few as 2% of patients received assertive community treatment (ACT), which is highly effective in preventing relapse (see Chapter 35).

IMPLICATIONS: The findings indicate that current usual treatment practices related to schizophrenia fall substantially short of what is recommended based on the best evidence on treatment efficacy. This disparity points to the need for greater efforts to ensure that treatment research results are translated into practice in order to improve the quality of care provided to patients.

Lehman A et al: *Schizophr Bull* 24:11, 1998.

The process of rehabilitation begins with learning to identify symptom triggers and early symptoms. Successful rehabilitation also involves the identification of symptom management techniques that reduce the potential for relapse and maintain stability. Additional information about the rehabilitation of people with maladaptive neurobiological responses is included in Chapter 15.

It is important for nurses to be aware that although effective treatments for schizophrenia are available, many people experiencing this serious brain disease are not receiving them (Sernyak et al, 2003) (see Citing the Evidence). Thus the nurse has a significant responsibility to patients, families, and communities to educate, advocate, and promote effective treatment strategies for neurobiological illnesses.

When stability has been attained, the health promotion phase begins. The goal is to collaboratively develop and implement symptom management techniques that prevent relapse and promote recovery. When patients and families recognize that relapse prevention is possible, they become empowered and can enjoy a quality of life that places the patient rather than the illness in control.

IMPLEMENTATION

Intervention modalities encompass the full range of psychosocial and psychobiological treatments and must include the patient, family, and caretaker if possible (American Psychiatric Association, 2004; Pharoah et al, 2002; Lehman and Steinwachs, 1998). The modality chosen should be based on predisposing factors, precipitating stressors, coping resources, coping mechanisms, and the patient's responses.

The core problems related to cognition, perception, emotion, behavior and movement, and socialization create significant difficulties for people with schizophrenia. These problems affect the implementation of the nursing treatment plan. Table 21-4 outlines areas of difficulty and related nursing in-

Table 21-4	Behavioral Strategies for People With Psychosis
CORE PROBLEMS	**NURSING INTERVENTIONS**
Anxiety	Teach patient the symptoms related to anxiety.
	Help patient identify what triggers anxiety.
	Help patient use symptom management techniques to cope with anxiety.
	Assess whether anxiety is a relapse trigger and, if so, make a plan to reduce anxiety while still in the moderate stage.
Depression	Teach patient the symptoms related to depression.
	Help patient use symptom management techniques to cope with depression.
	Assess whether depression is a relapse trigger and, if so, make a plan to reduce depression while still in a mild stage because there is a high correlation between depression and being able to perform activities of daily living.
Inability to learn from experience	Review both positive and negative experiences.
	Identify what was successful in helping the patient achieve the desired goal and what was not successful.
Problems with cause-and-effect reasoning	Analyze each experience to see what went well and what did not.
	Help reasoning patient sequence events leading to the outcome in each experience.
	Rehearsal may be helpful in enacting an event before it occurs.

Continued

Table 21-4	Behavioral Strategies for People With Psychosis—cont'd
CORE PROBLEMS	**NURSING INTERVENTIONS**
Difficulty assessing passage of time	Teach patient how to use clocks to tell time.
	Teach patient to use environmental cues such as the sun going down or a certain radio program to orient oneself to time of day.
	Help patient create and maintain a calendar of scheduled activities.
Concrete thinking	Realize that the patient sees every problem as having one solution.
	Teach patient to look at other possible solutions to problems.
	Realize that the patient often thinks there is only one way to do a task.
	Create alternative ways to approach situations.
Difficulty telling background from foreground information	Teach patient to distinguish between important and unimportant information.
	Teach patient to focus on only the important information.
	Help patient learn to avoid or minimize confusion caused by excess stimulation from noise and large crowds.
Slowed information processing	Give patients time to process and respond to information.
	Minimize anxiety because this increases information processing difficulties.
	Demonstrate genuine interest in trying to understand what the patient is saying.
	Be clear and simple when communicating with patient.
Difficulty screening information to share	Teach patient to identify people who are safe to talk to about one's illness.
	Teach patient to go to these people when the symptoms are creating problems.
	Let patient know that you understand the illness and are a safe person to talk with.
Communication difficulties	Use active listening to understand the patient.
	Clarify what the patient is trying to tell you.
	Listen for the theme.
	Seek validation from patient on what is communicated.
	Help patient with vocabulary as needed.
	Use the literal meaning of words.
	Have patient repeat back what was heard.
	Help patient understand the words and phrases used.
Problems expressing needs	Help patient identify and prioritize needs.
	Help patient express needs in ways that others will understand.
	Role play conversations and practice negotiating with others.
Low self-concept	Help patient identify and maximize his or her strengths and positive characteristics.
	Use role play to handle common situations patients face.
	Give positive feedback when patient handles a situation well.
	Analyze a problem to determine how it could have been better handled.
Forced isolation due to stigma	Maximize patient's understanding of his or her illness.
	Teach patient to minimize stigmatizing behaviors when possible.
	Identify comments that are difficult to handle.
	Teach ways to handle stigma and rude comments.
	Develop concrete humorous comebacks.
	Role play various situations with the nurse being the patient.
Difficulty with perception and interpretation of sensory stimuli	Review problematic situations with the patient.
	List and assess the thought processes in interpreting events.
	Help patient reality test and reframe problematic interpretations.
	Reinforce positive and productive processes.
Poor attention span and difficulty completing tasks	Help patient break tasks into small sequential steps.
	Help the patient keep focused on a single task, a step at a time.
	Do not emphasize completing the task.
	Give directions to patient one step at a time.
Inappropriate social behaviors	Identify the patient's thought processes that lead to the behavior.
	Ask patient about the behavior.
	Help correct inaccurate perceptions.
	Help patient identify undesirable outcomes of the behavior.
	Teach appropriate social skills.
Difficulty with decision making	Help patient determine desired outcomes.
	Help patient prioritize goals and categorize them into short and long term.
	Help patient establish a time line for attainment of each goal.
	Help establish small, concrete steps to achieve desired goals.
	Ensure that these small steps are achievable by the patient and are culturally and value congruent.

terventions in working with a patient who is psychotic. These issues must be addressed in order to maximize the patient's recovery and enhance compliance with the treatment plan. **Empirically validated treatments** related to schizophrenia are summarized in Box 21-9 (Nathan and Gorman, 2002).

Interventions in the Crisis and Acute Phases

Unstable neurobiological responses require constant observation and monitoring of health, behavior, and attitudes. Research has shown that aggressive early intervention improves both prognosis and quality of life (Stephenson, 2000). Nursing interventions in this phase should focus on restoring adaptive neurobiological responses while providing for the safety and well-being of the patient.

Patient Safety. Patient safety is the most important issue during the crisis and acute phases, particularly in light of the fact that 9% to 13% of patients with schizophrenia commit suicide, and 20% to 40% attempt suicide. Environmental safety factors should be attended to, including the availability of sharp and dangerous objects, as well as the placement of furniture, art objects, and pictures (see Chapter 20).

It is important to maintain constant vigilance with the patient and carefully explain all actions involving the patient. Patients may accidentally harm themselves because of impaired judgment or as a response to their hallucinations or delusions. For example, a patient with a badly abscessed tooth refused to go to the dentist. He was afraid the dentist would plant a radio in his tooth that would broadcast his thoughts to those who were trying to harm him. The concern of the health care providers was that the infection was interfering with the patient's health and making the psychosis worse. Unfortunately, patients often have difficulty distinguishing between people who are trying to help them and those who they believe seek to harm them.

Staff can create safety issues for patients when they fail to respond to patient needs in a caring and appropriate manner. Patients should not feel threatened, belittled, anxious, ignored, rejected, boxed in, or controlled by staff. Helping the patient reduce anxiety and feel safe and accepted decreases the incidence of harmful behaviors toward self and others.

Managing Delusions. Patients cope with delusions in several ways. Some adapt by learning to live with them. Others deny the presence of these troublesome symptoms. Still others seek to understand the symptom and become empowered to manage delusions when they occur. The art of communicating with people who have delusions requires the development of trust. Patients with cognitive disorders have difficulty processing language; therefore, the beginning of trust is more readily accomplished through nonverbal communication.

Patients with delusions perceive the environment as much more stimulating than others do. It is essential for the nurse to approach the patient with calmness, empathy, and gentle eye contact. Patients report they can literally "feel the vibrations" of others and can "sense if the nurse is with me or against me." Once trust is established, the use of clear, direct, and simple statements becomes significant in communicating with people who have delusions.

> *Describe nonverbal nursing approaches that would foster the development of trust between a nurse and a delusional patient.* ■

Patients with schizophrenia are keenly sensitive to rejection. When they sense anxiety and avoidance in the nurse, they often feel annoyed, inadequate, and hopeless. Sensing rejection by health care professionals also can lead to anger on the part of the patient.

If patients perceive that the nurse is going along with the delusion, they become confused, particularly if they sense that the nurse is trying to get their cooperation. The nurse should not attempt a logical explanation of the delusion because it will not be possible to identify one. Only the patient understands the logic behind the delusion and is not able to express it until after the delusion has reached conscious awareness (Myin-Germies, Nicolson, and Delespaul, 2001). On gaining insight into the illness and symptoms, the patient can differentiate experiences with delusions from those that are reality based. In the meantime, the nurse should not underestimate the power of a delusion and the patient's inability to differentiate the delusion from reality.

It is normal for the nurse to feel confused by a delusion. The nurse must carefully assess the content of the delusion without appearing to probe. It is also important to assess the context and

---

BOX **21-9**	SUMMARIZING THE EVIDENCE ON **Neurobiological Responses**
Disorder	Schizophrenia
Treatment	◆ Behavioral therapy and social-learning-token-economy programs help structure, support, and reinforce prosocial behavior in persons with schizophrenia. ◆ Structured, educational family interventions help patients with schizophrenia maintain gains achieved with medication and case management. ◆ Social skills training has enabled persons with schizophrenia to acquire instrumental and affiliative skills to improve functioning in their communities. ◆ Pharmacological treatment has had a profoundly positive impact on the course of schizophrenia. The introduction of atypical antipsychotics is promising because of their reduced side effects and enhanced efficacy in some patients.

From Nathan P, Gorman J: *A guide to treatments that work,* ed 2, New York, 2002, Oxford University Press.

environmental triggers for the delusional experience. The nurse must avoid becoming incorporated into the delusion. However, this is difficult if the nurse has achieved a trusting relationship with the patient, because people who are significant to the patient in reality also may become part of the delusional world.

Box 21-10 identifies strategies helpful in working with the patient who is delusional. Box 21-11 identifies barriers to intervening. The intervention plan should be followed consistently by the entire treatment team. If the nurse resorts to "trying anything" to gain compliance, care will be inconsistent and will create an even more chaotic environment for the patient, who already has great difficulty identifying reality.

Managing Hallucinations. Approximately 70% of hallucinations are auditory, 20% are visual, and the remaining 10% are gustatory, tactile, olfactory, kinesthetic, or cenesthetic. Therapeutic nursing interventions for hallucinations involve understanding the characteristics of the hallucination and identifying the related anxiety level (Trygstad, et al, 2002). Table 21-5 describes intensity levels, characteristics, and observable behaviors commonly associated with hallucinations.

The goal of intervention with patients who are hallucinating is to help them increase awareness of these symptoms so that they can distinguish between the world of psychosis and the world of reality experienced by others without schizophrenia. The first step toward achieving this goal is facilitative communication. Unfortunately, patients experiencing these symptoms are often avoided, laughed at, belittled, or ignored when these symptoms emerge.

Learning about a person's hallucinations helps avoid the roadblocks to communication these symptoms can create when unrecognized. Left unattended, hallucinations will continue and may escalate. Nurses may become so involved in planning what to say that they forget about the impor-

---

BOX 21-10

Strategies for Working With Patients With Delusions

Place the Delusion in a Time Frame and Identify Triggers
Identify all of the components of the delusion by placing it in time and sequence.
Identify triggers that may be related to stress or anxiety.
If delusions are linked to anxiety, teach anxiety management skills.
Develop a symptom management program.

Assess the Intensity, Frequency, and Duration of the Delusion
Fleeting delusions can be worked out in a short time frame.
Fixed delusions, endured over time, may have to be temporarily avoided to prevent them from becoming stumbling blocks in the relationship.
Listen quietly until there is no need to discuss the delusion.

Identify Emotional Components of the Delusion
Respond to the underlying feelings rather than the illogical nature of the delusions.
Encourage discussion of fears, anxiety, and anger without assuming that the delusion is right or wrong.

Observe for Evidence of Concrete Thinking
Determine whether the patient takes you literally.
Determine whether you and the patient are using language in the same way.

Observe Speech for Symptoms of a Thought Disorder
Determine whether the patient exhibits a thought disorder (is talking in circles, going off on tangents, easily changing subjects, and unable to respond to your attempts to redirect).
It may not be the appropriate time to point out discrepancy between fact and delusion.

Observe for the Ability to Accurately Use Cause-and-Effect Reasoning
Determine whether the patient can make logical predictions based on past experiences.
Determine whether the patient can conceptualize time.
Determine whether the patient can access and use meaningfully his or her recent and long-term memory.

Distinguish Between the Description of the Experience and the Facts of the Situation
Identify false beliefs about real situations.
Promote the patient's ability to reality test.
Determine whether the patient is hallucinating, because this will strengthen the delusion.

Carefully Question the Facts as They are Presented and Their Meaning
Sometimes talking with the patient about the delusion will help him or her see that it is not true.
If you take this step before the previous steps are completed, it may reinforce the delusion.

Discuss Consequences of the Delusion When the Person Is Ready
When the intensity of the delusion lessens, discuss the delusion when the patient is ready.
Discuss the consequences of the delusion.
Allow the patient to take responsibility for his or her behavior, daily activities, and decision making.
Encourage the patient's personal responsibility for and participation in wellness and recovery.

Promote Distraction as a Way to Stop Focusing on the Delusion
Promote activities that require attention to physical skills and will help the patient use time constructively.
Recognize and reinforce healthy and positive aspects of the personality.

tance of listening. Listening and observing are the keys to successful intervention with the person who is hallucinating.

Hallucinations are very real to the person having them, just as dreams during sleep are very real. The hallucinating person may have no way to determine whether these perceptions are real. It usually does not even occur to the person to verify the experience. An analogy might be hearing an ordinary weather report on the radio and not thinking to question whether the voice is from a real person.

Inability to perceive reality accurately makes life difficult. Therefore, hallucinations can be considered problems needing a solution. This is best accomplished when the person can talk freely about the hallucinations. Nurses also need to be able to talk about hallucinations because they are useful indicators of the current level of symptoms in ongoing monitoring of a psychotic illness. To facilitate monitoring, the patient needs to be comfortable telling the nurse about symptoms.

BOX 21-11

Barriers to Successful Intervention for Delusions

Becoming Anxious and Avoiding the Person
Anxiety leads to annoyance, anger, a sense of hopelessness and failure, feelings of inadequacy, and potentially laughing at or discounting the patient.

Reinforcing the Delusion
Do not go along with the delusion, especially to get the cooperation of the patient.

Attempting to Prove the Person Is Wrong
Do not attempt a logical explanation.

Setting Unrealistic Goals
Do not underestimate the power of a delusion and the patient's need for it.

Becoming Incorporated into the Delusional System
This will cause great confusion for the patient and make it impossible to establish boundaries of the therapeutic relationship.

Failing to Clarify Confusion Surrounding the Delusion
If the complexity and many intricacies of the delusion are not clearly understood, the delusion will become more elaborate.

Being Inconsistent in Intervention
The intervention plan must be firmly adhered to; if you resort to "trying anything," approaches will become inconsistent and the patient will be less able to identify reality.

Seeing the Delusion First and the Person Second
Avoid making references such as "the person who thinks he's being poisoned."

Table 21-5   Levels of Intensity of Hallucinations

LEVEL	CHARACTERISTICS	OBSERVABLE PATIENT BEHAVIORS
Stage I: Comforting **Moderate level of anxiety** Hallucination is generally pleasant.	The hallucinator experiences intense emotions such as anxiety, loneliness, guilt, and fear and tries to focus on comforting thoughts to relieve anxiety. The person recognizes that thoughts and sensory experiences are within conscious control if the anxiety is managed. **Nonpsychotic**	Grinning or laughter that seems inappropriate. Moving lips without making any sounds. Rapid eye movements. Slowed verbal responses as if preoccupied. Silent and preoccupied.
Stage II: Condemning **Severe level of anxiety** Hallucination generally becomes repulsive.	Sensory experience is repulsive and frightening. The hallucinator begins to feel a loss of control and may attempt to distance self from the perceived source. Person may feel embarrassed by the sensory experience and withdraw from others. It is still possible to redirect the patient to reality. **Mild psychotic**	Increased autonomic nervous system signs of anxiety such as increased heart rate, respiration, and blood pressure. Attention span begins to narrow. Preoccupied with sensory experience and may lose ability to differentiate hallucination from reality.
Stage III: Controlling **Severe level of anxiety** Sensory experiences become omnipotent.	Hallucinator gives up trying to combat the experience and gives in to it. Content of hallucination may become appealing. Person may experience loneliness if sensory experience ends. **Psychotic**	Directions given by the hallucination will be followed rather than objected to. Difficulty relating to others. Attention span of only a few seconds or minutes. Physical symptoms of severe anxiety such as perspiring, tremors, inability to follow directions.
Stage IV: Conquering **Panic level of anxiety** Generally becomes elaborate and interwoven with delusions.	Sensory experiences may become threatening if person does not follow commands. Hallucinations may last for hours or days if there is no therapeutic intervention. **Severe psychotic**	Terror-stricken behaviors such as panic. Strong potential for suicide or homicide. Physical activity that reflects content of hallucination such as violence, agitation, withdrawal, or catatonia. Unable to respond to complex directions. Unable to respond to more than one person.

Patients often learn not to discuss their unusual experiences with anyone because they have received negative responses from people who think their ideas are strange. The experience of hallucinations can be especially troublesome for the patient who does not have anyone to talk to about them. Being able to talk about one's hallucinations is a greatly reassuring and self-validating experience. This discussion can take place only in an atmosphere of genuine interest and concern.

For those who have never experienced a hallucination, it can be difficult to understand that the person has no control over it. People with true psychosis have no direct voluntary control over the brain malfunction that causes hallucinations. This means that they cannot just will them away. Ignoring hallucinations may increase the confusion of the already chaotic brain filled with delusional ideas and disjointed thoughts.

If the person is left alone to sort out reality without the input of trusted health care providers, the symptoms may overwhelm available coping resources. Interactive discussion of hallucinations is a vital element in the development of reality-testing skills. Communicating right at the time of the hallucination is particularly helpful. Honesty, genuineness, and openness are the foundation for effective communication during hallucinations.

Modulation of sensory stimulation to an optimal level is another useful technique for helping the patient minimize the perceptual confusion. Some patients do well with minimal environmental stimulation, whereas others find that noise and distraction help drown out the hallucinations. It is essential to find out how the patient has previously managed hallucinations.

Command hallucinations are hallucinations that tell the patient to take some specific action, such as to kill oneself or harm another. As such, they are potentially dangerous. They may lead a person to perform harmful acts such as cutting off a body part or striking out at someone at the instruction of voices. Fear caused by these often frightening hallucinations also can lead to dangerous behaviors such as jumping out of a window. Because of the potential seriousness of this symptom, intervention is crucial.

Intervening during the acute phase of hallucinations requires patience and the ability to spend time with the patient. Box 21-12 outlines strategies useful in working with patients who experience hallucinations. Adhering to the following four basic principles is helpful during this phase: maintain eye contact, speak simply in a slightly louder voice than usual, call the patient by name, and use touch. The patient needs sensory validation to override the abnormal sensory processes that are occurring in the brain.

Traditional interventions have often focused on isolating the patient. However, isolating a person during this time of intense sensory confusion often reinforces the psychosis and thus is not a recommended intervention. As with delusions, consistency is the essential ingredient to a successful intervention plan.

Psychopharmacology. Psychopharmacology as a treatment for maladaptive neurobiological responses is described in Chapter 27. Drugs that are more site and symptom specific and provide a better response with fewer side effects will ultimately improve patient adherence and patient outcome.

Typical antipsychotics have provided some measure of symptom relief for the majority of patients for the past 50 years, but these drugs have problematic side effects and are not effective for all symptoms of schizophrenia. Clozapine was the first of the newer **atypical antipsychotic** drugs. Because of the potential for it to cause agranulocytosis, its use is usually limited to the treatment of those patients who are treatment resistant to several trials of antipsychotic drugs. It is estimated that clozapine is effective for approximately 30% of the 20% not responding to the traditional antipsychotics.

Other atypical antipsychotic medications, such as risperidone, olanzapine, quetiapine, ziprasidone, and aripiprazole, do not have the potentially life-threatening side effects associated with clozapine and are more efficacious and have fewer side effects than the typical antipsychotics. Thus they are considered by most experts to be cost-effective, first-line treatments for schizophrenia (Citrome and Volavka, 2002).

Table 21-6 summarizes the medications most often prescribed for maladaptive neurobiological responses.

Cognitive-Behavioral Therapy. Cognitive-behavioral therapy (CBT), originally developed and evaluated with affective disorders, has been used successfully to treat persistent hallucinations and delusions as an adjunct to medication (Seckinger and Amador, 2001). This treatment also has been shown to be effective in patients with schizophrenia who were resistant to medication.

CBT is a method of changing patients' thought processes, behavior, and emotion. Implementing CBT using a psychoeducational approach in addition to routine care can reduce the common positive psychotic symptoms of hallucinations and delusions in patients with chronic schizophrenia.

Interventions in the Maintenance Phase

Nursing interventions that focus on teaching self-management of symptoms and identifying symptoms indicative of relapse are most useful in the maintenance phase. Patient teaching should involve caregivers whenever possible (see A Family Speaks) (Jungbauer et al, 2003). A Family Education Plan

Table 21-6	Antipsychotic Drugs
Generic Name (Trade Name)	**Usual Adult Daily Dosage Range (mg/day)**
Atypical Drugs	
Clozapine (Clozaril)	100-900
Risperidone (Risperdal)	2-8
Olanzapine (Zyprexa)	5-20
Quetiapine (Seroquel)	150-750
Ziprasidone (Geodon)	40-160
Aripiprazole (Abilify)	10-15
Typical Drugs	
Thiothixene (Navane)	5-30
Haloperidol (Haldol)	2-20
Loxapine (Loxitane)	20-100
Molindone (Moban)	50-225
Pimozide (Orap)	2-6

BOX **21-12**

Strategies for Working With Patients Who Have Hallucinations

Establish a Trusting, Interpersonal Relationship
If the nurse is anxious or frightened, the patient will be anxious or frightened.
Be patient, show acceptance, and use active listening skills.

Assess for Symptoms of Hallucinations Including Duration, Intensity, and Frequency
Observe for behavioral clues that indicate the presence of hallucinations.
Observe for clues that identify the level of intensity and duration of the hallucination.
Help the patient record the number of hallucinations that are experienced each day.

Focus on the Symptom and Ask the Patient to Describe What Is Happening
Empower the patient by helping him or her understand the symptoms experienced or demonstrated.
Help the patient gain control of the hallucinations, seek helpful distractions, and minimize intensity.

Identify Whether Drugs or Alcohol Have Been Used
Determine whether the person is using alcohol or drugs (over-the-counter, prescription, or street drugs).
Determine whether these may be responsible for or exacerbate the hallucinations.

If Asked, Point Out Simply That You Are Not Experiencing the Same Stimuli
Respond by letting the patient know what is actually happening in the environment.
Do not argue with the patient about differences in perceptions.
When an hallucination occurs, do not leave the person alone.

Suggest and Reinforce the Use of Interpersonal Relationships as a Symptom Management Technique
Encourage the patient to talk to someone trusted who will give supportive and corrective feedback.
Help the patient in mobilizing social supports.

Help the Patient Describe and Compare Current and Past Hallucinations
Determine whether the patient's hallucinations have a pattern.
Encourage the patient to remember when hallucinations first began.
Pay attention to the content of the hallucination; it may provide clues for predicting behavior.
Be especially alert for command hallucinations that may compel the patient to act in a certain way.
Encourage the patient to describe past and present thoughts, feelings, and actions as they relate to hallucinations.

Help the Patient Identify Needs That May Be Reflected in the Content of the Hallucination
Identify needs that may trigger hallucinations.
Focus on the patient's unmet needs and discuss the relationship between them and the presence of hallucinations.

Determine the Impact of the Patient's Symptoms on Activities of Daily Living
Provide feedback regarding the patient's general coping responses and activities of daily living.
Help the patient recognize symptoms, symptom triggers, and symptom management strategies.

A FAMILY SPEAKS

When our daughter, Sue, was in college, she began to change quite suddenly. She had been almost a perfect child. She got good grades all the way through high school, and we never worried that she would get into trouble. In fact, we used to feel sorry for our friends who suspected that their children were experimenting with drugs and sex, hanging out with wild friends, and failing at school.

What a shock it was when we visited Sue and she had completely changed. Her room was a mess. She was wearing sloppy clothes and obviously needed a bath. When we asked what was wrong, she denied there was a problem and then became angry and refused to say anything more to us at all. When we got home, we called a counselor at the college, who told us that Sue was about to flunk out. She had not been attending classes, and other students had been reporting that she was "living in her own world."

We returned to the college to take our daughter home. We immediately took her to a psychiatrist who said that she was schizophrenic and referred her to a hospital. We were frightened, confused, and depressed. We had little understanding of schizophrenia, except that it is a terrible disease that people never recover from and they usually end up being in a hospital forever. We also felt guilty that we had perhaps failed Sue in some way. What a relief it was to talk with her primary nurse. She immediately scheduled us for a family education group that met at the hospital. Every time that she was working when we visited, she made sure to spend time with us so we could ask questions, and we had a million of them. Most important, she told us about the Alliance for the Mentally Ill. It was so reassuring to meet and talk with other family members who knew what we were going through. We know now that our daughter may never achieve the potential that we thought she once had, but she can lead a productive life. We continue to learn with her about how that will happen for her.

for understanding the world of psychosis is presented in Table 21-7.

Behavioral interventions that teach patients skills for coping with psychotic symptoms include cognitive reframing regarding the cause of symptoms, gaining control over symptoms, and behavioral coping strategies. Patients and families also should be taught the following classic stages of relapse (Docherty et al, 1978).

Stages of Relapse. The first two of these five stages of relapse do not involve symptoms that indicate psychosis. This is relevant because during these two stages is the crucial time to intervene. In the first two stages, the patient is able to seek and use feedback constructively.

Stage one is **overextension**. In this stage the patient complains of feeling overwhelmed. Symptoms of anxiety are intensified and great energy is used to overcome them. Patients describe feeling overloaded, being unable to concentrate on or complete tasks, and tend to forget words in the middle of sentences. Other symptoms of overextension include increasing mental efforts to perform usual activities, decreasing performance efficiency, and easy distractibility.

Stage two is **restricted consciousness**. The previous symptoms of anxiety are joined by symptoms of depression. The depression is more intense than usual daily mood variations. There are added dimensions of appearing bored, apathetic, obsessional, and phobic. Somatization may occur. The patient seems to withdraw from everyday events and limits ex-

Table 21-7	**FAMILY EDUCATION PLAN**	Understanding Psychosis
CONTENT	**INSTRUCTIONAL ACTIVITIES**	**EVALUATION**
Describe psychosis.	Introduce participants and leaders. State purpose of group. Define terminology associated with psychosis.	The participant will describe the characteristics of psychosis.
Identify the causes of psychotic disorders.	Present theories of psychotic disorders. Use audiovisual aids to explain brain anatomy, brain biochemistry, and major neurotransmitters.	The participant will discuss the relationship between brain anatomy, brain biochemistry, and major neurotransmitters and the development of psychosis.
Define schizophrenia according to symptoms and diagnostic criteria.	Lead a discussion of the diagnostic criteria for schizophrenia. Show a film on schizophrenia.	The participant will describe the symptoms and diagnostic criteria for schizophrenia.
Describe the relationship between anxiety and psychotic disorders.	Present types and stages of anxiety. Discuss steps in reducing and resolving anxiety.	The participant will identify and describe the stages of anxiety and ways to reduce or resolve it.
Analyze the impact of living with hallucinations.	Describe the characteristics of hallucinations. Demonstrate ways to communicate with someone who is hallucinating.	The participant will demonstrate effective ways to communicate with a person who has hallucinations.
Analyze the impact of living with delusions.	Describe types of delusions. Demonstrate ways to communicate with someone who has delusions. Discuss interventions for delusions.	The participant will demonstrate effective ways to communicate with a person who has delusions.
Discuss the use of psychotropic medications.	Provide and explain handouts describing the characteristics of psychotropic medications that are prescribed for schizophrenia.	The participant will identify and describe the characteristics of medications prescribed for self/family member.
Describe the characteristics of relapse and the role of compliance with the therapeutic regimen.	Help the participants describe their own experiences with relapse. Discuss symptom management techniques and the importance of complying with the therapeutic regimen.	The participant will describe behaviors that indicate an impending relapse and discuss the importance of symptom management and compliance with the therapeutic regimen.
Analyze behaviors that promote wellness.	Discuss the components of wellness. Relate wellness to the elements of symptom management.	The participant will analyze the effect of maintaining wellness on the occurrence of symptoms.
Discuss ways to cope adaptively with psychosis.	Lead a group discussion focused on coping behaviors and the daily problems in living with psychosis. Propose ways to create a low-stress environment.	The participant will describe ways to modify lifestyle to crease a low-stress environment.

ternal stimulation as a way to protect against the upcoming loss of control.

The first appearance of psychotic features occurs in stage three, **disinhibition**. Symptoms may resemble those of hypomania and usually include the emergence of hallucinations and delusions that the patient is no longer able to control. Previously successful defense mechanisms tend to break down.

In stage four, **psychotic disorganization**, clearly psychotic symptoms occur. Hallucinations and delusions intensify and the patient ultimately loses control. This stage is characterized by three distinct phases:

1. The patient no longer recognizes familiar environments or people and may accuse family members of being impostors. Extreme agitation is possible. This phase is called **destructuring of the external world**.
2. The patient loses personal identity and may refer to oneself in the third person. This is called **destructuring of the self**.
3. Total fragmentation is the total loss of the ability to differentiate reality from psychosis and may be called **loudly psychotic**. The patient experiences complete loss of control. Hospitalization is usually required at this point, and family members may have to enlist law enforcement officers to take the patient to the hospital. When this happens, it is extremely devastating and embarrassing to both the patient and the family.

Stage five, **psychotic resolution**, usually occurs in the hospital. The patient is generally medicated and still experiencing psychosis, but the symptoms are "quiet." The person may appear to follow instructions in a robotic manner and often looks dazed. Unfortunately, many patients are discharged while in this stage because they are compliant or they no longer have insurance benefits.

Identify how you would approach a patient and family regarding the need for a change in the treatment plan at each stage of the relapse process. Why is it important to identify relapse as soon as possible? ■

An example of how well patients can recognize their symptoms compared with staff and families is described in the following clinical example.

◣ CLINICAL EXAMPLE

During a class on relapse and symptom management, a patient was asked what symptoms caused his return to the hospital. The patient responded, "It was my red dots." When asked to explain, he said, "I see red dots all the time, but when they change in a way that I can no longer tell the difference between my red dots, brake lights of the car in front of me, or stop lights, I know it's time to go back to the hospital for a medication check." A staff member said, "So that's why you are always staring at the exit sign, because it's red?" The patient nodded, and the staff member continued with, "So why didn't you tell us?" The patient simply said, "You didn't ask."

This example clearly demonstrates the need to not only teach patients about symptoms indicative of relapse but also to ask what they already know about their own symptoms. ■

Managing Relapse. The key to managing relapse is awareness of the onset of behaviors indicating relapse. About 70% of patients and 90% of families are able to notice symptoms of illness recurrence, and almost all patients know when symptoms are intensifying.

A prodromal phase occurs before relapse. A prodromal phase is the time between the onset of symptoms and the need for treatment. With the majority of patients and families indicating a prodromal period lasting longer than 1 week, it is essential that nurses collaborate with the patient, family, and residential staff regarding the onset of relapse (Lamberti, 2001). Box 21-13 presents a guide for patients on how to best handle a potential relapse.

Identifying and managing symptoms help decrease the number and severity of relapses. Teaching this to patients and families is a cost-effective intervention that can give them control over their lives and decrease the number or length of hospitalizations. A growing number of studies have demonstrated a significant reduction in relapse rates as a result of psychoeducational interventions (Lukens et al, 1999).

Tools such as the Moller-Murphy Symptom Management Assessment Tool (MM-SMAT) (Murphy and Moller, 1993) can help the patient self-report symptoms, difficulties in activities of daily living, problems with medications, and ways of managing symptoms. Once patients can validate their experiences, they are empowered to manage symptoms rather than have the symptoms rule their lives.

In what ways is self-assessment of symptoms an empowering experience for patients? How might it positively affect the nurse-patient relationship? ■

BOX **21-13**

A Patient Guide for Handling Potential Relapse

- Go to a safe environment with someone who can help you if help is needed. This person should be able to monitor behavior that indicates the relapse is getting worse.
- Reduce the stress and demands on yourself. This includes reducing stimuli. Some people find a quiet room where they can be alone, perhaps with soft music. Relaxation techniques or distraction techniques may work for you. A quiet place where you can talk with one person you trust is often helpful.
- Take medications if this is part of your program. Work with your prescriber to determine whether medications may be useful in reducing relapse. Medications are most helpful when used with a safe, quiet environment and stress reduction.
- Talk to a trusted person about what the voices are saying to you or about the thoughts you are having. This person needs to know ahead of time that you will call him or her if you need help.
- Avoid negative people who say such things as, "You are thinking crazy" or "Stop that negative talk."

When assessing symptom stability of any chronic illness, it is important to evaluate whether daily symptoms are better, about the same, or worse than usual. Some patients with schizophrenia have psychotic symptoms daily yet are able to maintain adaptive responses and carry out activities of daily living. Relapse for these patients is usually indicated by an increase in symptom intensity.

The nurse conducting discharge teaching or working in an outpatient or residential setting must stress the lengthy recuperation process, with special emphasis on the sedative qualities of the medication used to prevent relapse. When families and residential supervisors who do not understand the length of time needed for recuperation complain that the patient just wants to sit around, smoke, and watch television, the nurse is encouraged to provide information. This clinical example illustrates this behavior.

CLINICAL EXAMPLE

A 26-year-old man with a medical diagnosis of schizophrenia, who had experienced a lengthy relapse, was discharged from the acute care setting and admitted to a residential group home affiliated with a local mental health center. He was later asked to leave both community-based treatment programs because he was not able to actively engage in the required therapies. He was discharged to the care of his parents, who were to motivate him to take his medications and engage him in some type of therapy, eventually leading to a job. The parents were active in the National Alliance for the Mentally Ill (NAMI). After months of frustration the parents attended a program on relapse and learned about the lengthy rehabilitation period required. They were encouraged to make sure their son ate well and kept up daily hygienic practices, to stop trying to force him to go out, and to support his basic needs based on the wellness model. After 6 months, one day he said that he wanted to play a sport at which he had previously excelled. He was encouraged to practice and then entered competition. After that positive experience he was able to reenter life within the limits of his neurobiological responses.

Selected Nursing Diagnoses
- Impaired social interaction related to low energy during recovery, as evidenced by resistance to involvement in activities
- Caregiver role strain related to parents' unrealistic expectations for rapid recovery, as evidenced by positive response to education about relapse and recovery ∎

Anxiety and depression are often overlooked as major contributors to poor health-related practices of people with schizophrenia. Common observable behaviors related to anxiety include pacing, restlessness, irritability, quickness to anger, or withdrawal. The high incidence of suicide in people with schizophrenia mandates the importance of assessing lethality, potential dangerousness toward self, and risk of discontinuing treatment against medical advice. Because of impaired information processing, patients also should be assessed for potential dangerousness to others.

Finally, a variety of symptom management techniques have been found useful by patients. Box 21-14 categorizes these techniques. Patients who have found other symptom management techniques should be encouraged to use them as long as the technique is not harmful to self or others. The fol-

---

BOX 21-14

Symptom Management Strategies

Category I: Distraction
Watch TV
Concentrate on my hobby
Read
Take a walk/go swimming/go for a ride
Go to the forest, mountains, beach, or park
Use humor
Dance
Go to a party or concert
Sing/play a musical instrument
Work
Write
Listen to music

Category II: Fighting Back
Talk to myself (self-talk)
Don't pay attention to the thoughts
Yell back at the voices
Try to think positively
Avoid situations that cause the symptoms to get worse
Rehearsal (problem solve an upsetting incident)

Category III: Isolation
Stay home
Go to bed
Try to live with my symptoms

Category IV: Attempts to Feel Better
Pray
Eat
Take prescription medication
Use relaxation/meditate
Take a shower/bath
Take herbs
Hug pillow/stuffed animal

Category V: Help-Seeking
Talk to my family members/friend(s)
Go to a hospital/emergency room
Go to a mental health center/clinic
Talk to the doctor/nurse
Talk to my case manager/therapist

lowing six steps can serve as a guide to the teaching of effective symptom management techniques:

1. Identify problem symptoms.
2. Identify current symptom management techniques.
3. Identify specific support systems.
4. Discuss additional symptom management techniques.
5. Eliminate nonproductive symptom management.
6. Develop new symptom management plan.

Relapse and Medications. The most common causes of relapse relate in some way to medications. Patients will most likely stop taking their medications some time in the first year after diagnosis. They will stop taking them because the medication worked and symptoms are gone or because they didn't work and symptoms didn't go away. Patients frequently stop taking medication because of problematic side effects, or because they feel the medication increases stigma.

Unfortunately, one of the first things nurses often do in assessing relapse is to blame the patient for not taking medications without determining the reason the patient stopped. Patients may think nothing is really wrong and may take the medications just to follow orders. The nurse should realize that relapse is likely to occur whether the patient is taking medications or not, particularly if the patient has poor health practices. However, a distinct difference in the onset, quality, and length of relapse will be present based on adherence to the treatment regimen.

Caffeine and nicotine can affect the action of psychotropic medications (see Critical Thinking About Contemporary Issues). Predicting the success of any medication is impossible if the patient consumes alcohol or other drugs. Research on a variety of ethnic groups also has determined that enzyme variations among population groups cause medications to act and metabolize differently in people of different ethnic or racial backgrounds.

Studies consistently show that without medication, people with schizophrenia relapse at a rate of 60% to 70% within the first few years of diagnosis. For those who are faithful to the medication regimen, the relapse rate is approximately 40%, but drops to 15.7% with a combination of medications, group education, and support (Olfson et al, 2000). This statistic has tremendous implications for the role of patient education.

Patients who adhere to their medication regimen, yet still experience relapse, tend to have a rapid onset of mood-related symptoms and recover quickly with minimal or no change in their antipsychotic medications. These patients usually volunteer for treatment and are generally able to trace the onset of their relapse to an identifiable stressor.

Noncompliant patients tend to have a gradual onset of relapse with prominent psychotic features and generally enter treatment through an involuntary hospital commitment. They usually require a longer hospitalization and a change in medication. Typically they cannot trace the onset of the relapse to any specific trigger.

Even with support, education, and adherence to the treatment regimen, relapse still occurs. This emphasizes the need for ongoing symptom monitoring and identification of factors leading to nonadherence (Jarboe, 2002; Zygmunt et al, 2002). Cooperative medication management can be fostered if the patient is included as an equal partner in treatment. This only occurs when the patient is taught about the effects and side effects of the medication and when staff and family are sensitive to feedback from the patient concerning how the medication makes him or her feel.

Even with education, medication noncompliance still occurs. In a classic study of 253 psychiatric inpatients inter-

---

Critical Thinking *About* Contemporary Issues

Should Inpatient and Residential Mental Health Care Facilities Be Caffeine and Nicotine Free?

Many patients are faithful to their treatment regimens, but because of a daily intake of over 250 mg of caffeine, experience a decrease in effectiveness of most antipsychotic and antianxiety drugs, as well as lithium. In addition, a nicotine intake of more than 10 to 20 cigarettes daily dramatically decreases the effectiveness of antipsychotic drugs (Lyon, 1999).

Because of the effects of nicotine and caffeine on maladaptive neurobiological responses and the effectiveness of medications, many inpatient psychiatric units have eliminated use of these substances. Smoking also has been banned because of the direct and indirect impact on health (El-Guebaly et al, 2002; Forchuk et al, 2002).

This is a major change in psychiatric settings. Previously, coffee and cigarettes were an important part of the inpatient culture. Cigarettes, in particular, were used as rewards in token economy behavioral management plans. Patients often measured the course of the day from one cigarette break to the next. Nicotine may be particularly reinforcing in schizophrenia because it stimulates the subcortical reward system and the prefrontal cortex, which both appear to have decreased functioning in schizophrenia (Spring, Pingitore, and McChargue, 2003).

Given this history of reinforcement of these habits, some believe that it is cruel to deprive chronically hospitalized people of one of their few pleasures. Others believe that these restrictions are not in keeping with the philosophy of individual choice and the value that adults should make their own health-related decisions.

Limits on smoking and caffeine are based on the obligation of a health care program to promote healthful behavior. Careful attention should be paid to patient education and programs that help with withdrawal. An issue that needs more attention is the impact on a newly admitted person of sudden withdrawal from these highly addictive substances. Nurses need to assess preadmission use of caffeine and nicotine carefully. The impact of withdrawal must be considered when evaluating response to medications. In addition, the nurse should be aware of the possibility of withdrawal symptoms, help the patient understand them, and design alternatives to sudden withdrawal from these substances if the patient is addicted to them.

viewed on the day of discharge from a short hospital stay, more than half did not know the name and dosage of the psychiatric medications prescribed for them or why they were supposed to take them; 38% of the patients knew the names of all their psychiatric medications, but only 53% of this group knew when to take them (Clary, Dever, and Schweizer, 1992). These results are surprising because all of the patients had attended both group and individual medication instruction classes during the hospitalization. Considering the cognitive symptoms of an acute episode of schizophrenia, the results are less surprising and implications for ongoing postdischarge medication instruction become clear.

Interventions in the Health Promotion Phase

Teaching in the health promotion phase focuses on prevention of relapse and symptom management through engaging the patient in a healthy lifestyle. Patient teaching methods that involve simple, clear, and concrete instructions including repetition and return demonstrations are the most helpful. One of the keys to preventing relapse includes identifying symptom triggers and strategies for managing them. Box 21-15 summarizes nursing interventions intended to prevent relapse.

Relatives often do not know how to react to more autonomous functioning and need as much teaching and support as the patient. Psychotherapy also may be helpful in the rehabilitative phase of recovery as patients deal with the neurobiological deficits that often become apparent to them only then. The focus of the psychotherapy is usually supportive and nonconfrontational.

Many families make comments such as, "When we learned our son's diagnosis was schizophrenia, it was like he had died." Thus it is understandable that schizophrenia remains a closely held secret in many households. These attitudes often prevent families from effectively coping with schizophrenia.

The situation may be complicated by incorrect advice from health professionals who tell or imply to families that they caused or perpetuated the illness. Parental guilt stemming from self-blame further blocks communication within the family. Parents often do not know how to talk with their ill child and perhaps even fear him or her. Clearly this situation does not help parents face the many problems they encounter in their additional roles of case manager, residential supervisor, and legal guardian.

Parents also must act as negotiators between the assigned case manager, guardian, and an adult child. No one knows a person better than the family, but it can be emotionally painful and draining to be a loving, nurturing, advocating parent in one situation, a treatment-enforcing case manager in another, and residential supervisor to an outside case manager in yet another. Simultaneous patient/family teaching about symptom management and medication compliance is useful at this stage. Patient and family education also may dispel myths and provide suggestions for improving communication with the treatment team.

Research shows that structured rehabilitation programs provide significant improvement in function and coping skills (see Chapter 15). Four programs with structured curricula and participant manuals have been developed that have as their main goal either to rehabilitate the patient or to help the family cope more effectively with chronic mental illness.

The **Three Rs Psychiatric Rehabilitation Program** is for patients with chronic mental illness and their families (Moller and Murphy, 1997; 2002). The three Rs are **relapse, recovery**, and **rehabilitation**. The aim of the program is to teach patients to use a wellness model to manage their illness and integrate back into the community. Developed by advanced practice psychiatric rehabilitation nurses, this program has shown a significant decrease in hospitalization of its participants.

Liberman's **Skill Training Program** has as its aim the rehabilitation of patients by teaching life skills (Liberman, 1994). The patient is taken through a structured set of modules that teach coping strategies in order to effect life changes.

McFarlane's **Family Education Program** is aimed at teaching families about schizophrenia and helping them cope with the illness (McFarlane, 1992). This is the only program that is exclusively for families and uses professionals specifically trained to conduct the program.

Family to Family is a self-help program developed by the National Alliance for the Mentally Ill (NAMI) for families of people with chronic mental illness. It is a scripted program that uses family members trained to facilitate the program. It is further described in Chapter 11.

A Nursing Treatment Plan Summary for the patient with maladaptive neurobiological responses is presented in Table 21-8.

EVALUATION

Evaluation of the nursing care provided to patients who have maladaptive neurobiological responses includes input from the patient and family. Because these are serious, long-term illnesses, care is often episodic. Relapse should not be interpreted as a failure of the nursing intervention but should be considered in the context of the patient's life situation.

To evaluate the nursing intervention, the following questions may be asked:

- Is the patient able to describe the behaviors that characterize the onset of a relapse?
- Is the patient able to identify and describe the medications prescribed, reason for taking them, frequency of taking them, and possible side effects?

BOX **21-15**

Nursing Interventions To Prevent Relapse

- Identify symptoms that signal relapse.
- Identify symptom triggers.
- Select symptom management techniques.
- Identify coping strategies for symptom triggers.
- Identify support system for future relapse.
- Document action plan in writing and file with key support people.
- Facilitate integration into family and community.

- Does the patient participate in relationships with other people at a comfortable level?
- Is the patient's family aware of the characteristics of the illness and able to participate in a supportive relationship with the patient?

- Are the patient and family informed about available community resources such as rehabilitation programs, mental health care providers, educational programs, and support groups, and do they use them?

Table 21-8	NURSING TREATMENT PLAN SUMMARY	Maladaptive Neurobiological Responses

Nursing Diagnosis: Disturbed thought processes
Expected Outcome: The patient will live, learn, and work at a maximum possible level of success, as defined by the individual.

SHORT-TERM GOAL	INTERVENTION	RATIONALE
The patient will participate in brief, regularly scheduled meetings with the nurse.	Initiate a nurse-patient relationship contract mutually agreed on by nurse and patient. Schedule brief (5- to 10-minute), frequent contacts with the patient. Consistently approach the patient at the scheduled time. Extend length of sessions gradually based on patient's agreement.	The establishment of a trusting relationship is fundamental to developing open communication. A patient with disturbed thought processes cannot tolerate extended, intrusive interactions and functions best in a structured environment.
The patient will describe delusions and other disturbed thought processes.	Demonstrate attitude of caring and concern. Validate the meaning of communications with the patient. Help the patient identify the difference between reality and internal thought processes.	Patients are very sensitive to others' responses to their symptoms. A respectful, interested approach will enable the patient to discuss unusual and frightening thoughts. Identification of reality by a trusted person is helpful.
The patient will identify and describe the effect of brain disease on thought processes.	Provide information about causes of psychoses. Discuss the relationship between the patient's behaviors and brain function. Involve significant others in educational sessions.	Understanding of the physiological basis for disturbed thought processes helps the patient recognize symptoms and feel in control of the illness. Significant others can provide support and experience less stigma if they are informed about the illness.
The patient will identify signs of impending relapse and describe actions to take to prevent relapse.	Help patient and significant others identify behaviors related to disturbed thought processes that indicate threatened relapse. Identify community resources and mutually plan actions directed toward prevention of relapse.	Relapse can be predicted if the patient and family are alert to warning signs. Early intervention allows the patient to control the course of the illness. Family members can help the patient identify symptoms and provide support for seeking assistance.
The patient will describe symptom management techniques that are helpful in living with disturbed thought processes.	Describe symptom management techniques that other patients have used. Ask the patient to describe techniques used to manage symptoms. Encourage the patient to take control of the illness by using symptom management techniques. Discuss the advantages of engaging in a wellness lifestyle.	Many patients with psychoses continue to have delusions after the acute phase of the illness has passed. Patients can function better if they learn ways to manage the symptom. Symptom self management promotes personal empowerment. Elimination of substances that interfere with healthy CNS function improves cognition and perception.
The patient will engage in a trusting relationship with the nurse.	Initiate a nurse-patient relationship contract mutually agreed on by nurse and patient. Establish mutual goals related to social interaction. Establish trust by consistently meeting the elements of the plan and engaging in open and honest communication.	Patients who have maladaptive neurobiological responses often have difficulty trusting others. Difficulty with information processing causes problems with interpreting the communication of others.

CNS, Central nervous system.

Continued

Table 21-8	NURSING TREATMENT PLAN SUMMARY	Maladaptive Neurobiological Responses—cont'd

Nursing Diagnosis: Disturbed thought processes
Expected Outcome: The patient will live, learn, and work at a maximum possible level of success, as defined by the individual.

SHORT-TERM GOAL	INTERVENTION	RATIONALE
The patient will discuss personal goals related to social interaction.	Encourage the patient to describe current relationship patterns. Discuss past relationship experiences. Identify problems associated with social interaction. Explore goals.	The patient may be unaware of the characteristics of mutually satisfying interpersonal relationships. Honest feedback from the nurse can help the patient identify the reasons for past problems. Knowledge of the patient's relationship goals leads to the development of realistic behavioral change.
The patient will identify behaviors that interfere with social relationships.	Share observations about the patient's behavior in social situations.	Identification of problematic behavior helps the patient and nurse target changes.
The patient will practice alternative social behaviors with the nurse.	Discuss possible behavioral changes that will facilitate the establishment of social relationships. Role play alternative behaviors. Provide feedback.	Practice will help the patient gain comfort with new behaviors. Feedback provides reinforcement for successful behavioral change.
The patient will select one person and practice social interaction skills.	Discuss experience of practicing new behavior with another person. Discuss ways of maintaining a relationship.	The patient will need ongoing feedback and support related to maintaining behavioral change.

COMPETENT CARING

A Clinical Exemplar of a Psychiatric Nurse
MICHAEL BRODY, RN, PMHNP

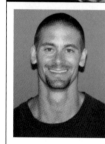

As an undergraduate student at the University of California at Berkeley, I became enamored with a bumper sticker mounted on the door of a popular philosophy professor: 'Reality is a Crutch.' The phrase always made me think. Like a Zen *koan*, it bends the mind in on itself, calling into question that which we often take for granted. Those of us working in the field of psychiatry rely on our ability to draw a line between sanity and psychosis, in order to make sound diagnostic decisions and to plan, initiate, and evaluate effective interventions. In my first year as a psychiatric mental health nurse practitioner in a college health center, I worked with a student who forced me to abandon the comfort of this distinction and to reconsider the nature of reality and psychosis.

AB had recently arrived in this country from his childhood home in Europe. He was an exceptionally talented 18-year old freshman scholar, a gifted singer, scientist, and linguist who excelled in just about every academic subject. The family nurse practitioner who worked in our health center referred AB to me early in the fall semester when AB became tearful during a routine health assessment.

On our first meeting, AB entered my office somewhat sheepishly, meeting my eyes only momentarily, then shifting his attention to his surroundings, seeming to pay careful attention to every detail in the room. When I asked him to please sit wherever he felt comfortable, he hesitated for some time. He eventually settled cross-legged on the floor in front of the couch on which most students usually sat, adding to my impression that AB was, in many ways, different. AB was guarded and seemed apprehensive about our meeting, saying that he didn't know why he had been sent to talk to a therapist. He stated in flawless English that he had little faith in the practice of psychotherapy, would refuse under any circumstances to take psychotropic medication, and was adamant that I could be of no use to him.

As we talked about his views on psychotherapy, he intimated that he had some personal experience with psychiatrists in Europe, but refused to elaborate. He began to draw a timeline on graph paper in order to clarify for me the chronology of his history. As he gradually became more comfortable in that first session, his emotions began to seep through the barrier of his intellect. Somewhat abruptly, AB began to cry. He told me that he felt totally alone, and while he felt sure that this feeling was exacerbated by culture shock and myriad changes that had taken place in his life recently, he pointed at the timeline he had drawn and said that he had felt isolated and confused for years.

We began by discussing AB's immediate social and academic concerns. My initial diagnostic impressions led me to believe that AB was suffering from an adjustment disorder with depressive features. As I got to know him better, he began to discuss his childhood and his relationship with his parents, as well his exceptionally close connection to a group of friends he had left behind in Europe. While he often complained that a language barrier prevented him from connecting with his peers here in the United States and made it difficult for him to participate effectively in his seminar classes, he expertly wielded a vast English vocabulary and spoke very articulately during our sessions. He often diverged somewhat from our conversations to pursue one or another related philosophical tangent, some of which were difficult for me to follow. This tendency was particularly noticeable when I tried to discuss AB's feelings, and it was not uncommon in my experience for intellectually gifted students to retreat into abstractions at the first sign of a discussion about their emotions.

AB seemed to be thinking as clearly as any displaced, depressed 18-year-old. He denied any auditory or visual hallucinations and demonstrated no clear evidence of disordered thought. However, he did describe several occasions in his past when he had experienced a kind of vague dissociation, including one episode when he found himself on the floor of his bedroom grasping a piece of paper upon which he read line after line of jumbled text that he knew he must have written, but could not recognize as his own. He denied any symptoms that would indicate a manic or hypomanic episode, or any kind of brief psychosis. He did not use any drugs or alcohol and had never had a seizure or head injury.

I had been working with AB for about a month, consulting closely with my clinical supervisor. I was surprised, however, when she asked me about the potential psychotic nature of AB's condition. Psychotic? AB was emotionally labile and eccentric to be sure, but psychotic? As a relatively inexperienced clinician, and one who had spent very little time working with the severely and persistently mentally ill, I had an image in my mind of how a psychotic patient would look and act, and AB did not fit the picture. I felt compelled to defend my patient against this "accusation" of insanity. AB denied any psychotic symptoms and my supervisor encouraged me to keep working with him, but to keep my mind open to the full spectrum of diagnostic possibilities. Over time, despite the fact that he continued to attend classes and participate actively in therapy, I began to see the extent to which AB's thinking was impaired.

As he gradually developed an ability to describe his thought processes, it became clear that AB was not thinking like the rest of us. He tended to analyze in a very systematic way each moment of his day, just as the moment passed, in order to understand and assign meaning to the moment and decide how to respond. This process was exceedingly labor intensive, leaving AB mentally and emotionally exhausted, and robbing him of any authentic, spontaneous emotional experience or interpersonal connection. Mired in this lonely and often confusing internal reality, AB was painfully isolated from his external environment.

It was my impression that in addition to regular therapy, he would benefit from low-dose atypical antipsychotics. However, AB maintained his initial stance—he would have nothing to do with medication. He continued to feel lonely on campus, but eventually came to see me as someone who understood him. This 'feeling understood' was a spontaneous emotional experience for AB, and he delighted in the brief and fleeting moments when he felt connected.

Unfortunately, despite his considerable intellectual powers, his inability to organize his thoughts in the moment eventually made it impossible for him to function in the academically demanding environment of his college classes. In addition, the social isolation outside my office became unbearable. Eventually, AB chose to return to Europe in hopes of finding an environment in which he could function more effectively.

In retrospect, AB clearly met criteria for a psychosis. However, the fact that his thought disorder existed in the context of an otherwise finely tuned intellectual machine, along with my inexperience and misconceptions regarding the sometimes subtle nature of psychosis, temporarily blinded me to the extent of his disability. If there is any truth to the philosopher's bumper sticker, if reality is indeed a crutch, AB taught me that life can be very difficult and very lonely for even the brightest and most privileged of those who have no crutch at all. ■

CHAPTER **FOCUS POINTS**

- The range of neurobiological responses includes a continuum from adaptive responses such as logical thought and accurate perceptions to maladaptive responses, such as thought distortions, hallucinations, and psychosis.
- A common system for categorizing the symptoms of schizophrenia lists them as "positive symptoms" (exaggerated behaviors) and "negative symptoms" (loss of behaviors).
- Symptoms related to problems in information processing associated with schizophrenia include problems in cognitive functioning in all aspects of memory, attention, form and organization of speech, decision making, and thought content.
- Memory problems associated with schizophrenia can include forgetfulness, disinterest, difficulty learning, and lack of compliance.
- Disturbances in attention are common in schizophrenia and include difficulty completing tasks, difficulty concentrating on work, and easy distractibility.
- Problems with form and organization of speech (formal thought disorders) may include loose associations, word salad, tangentiality, illogicality, circumstantiality, pressured speech, poverty of speech, distractible speech, and clanging.
- Problems with decision making include insight, judgment, logic, decisiveness, planning, ability to carry out decisions, and abstract thought.
- The inability of the brain to process data accurately can result in paranoid, grandiose, religious, nihilistic, and somatic delusions.
- Hallucinations are false perceptual distortions that can arise from any of the five senses.

- Problems with sensory integration include pain recognition, soft neurological signs, right/left recognition, and recognition and perception of faces.
- Terms related to affect include broad, restricted, blunted, flat, and inappropriate.
- Problems of emotion usually seen in schizophrenia include alexithymia, apathy, and anhedonia.
- Maladaptive behaviors in schizophrenia include deteriorated appearance, lack of persistence at work or school, avolition, repetitive or stereotyped behavior, aggression and agitation, and negativism.
- Maladaptive movements associated with schizophrenia include catatonia, abnormal eye movements, grimacing, apraxia/echopraxia, abnormal gait, mannerisms, and extrapyramidal side effects of psychotropic medications.
- Symptoms may prevent the person from socializing within accepted sociocultural norms resulting in social withdrawal and isolation from life's activities. Specific problems in the development of relationships include social inappropriateness, disinterest in recreational activities, inappropriate sexual behavior, and stigma-related withdrawal by friends, families, and peers.
- Evidence shows that maladaptive neurobiological responses are complex illnesses that include genetics, dysregulated neurochemistry, and abnormal structure and function of the brain.
- Precipitating stressors include biological characteristics, environmental stress, and symptom triggers.
- Coping resources are individualized and depend on the nature and extent of the neurobiological disruption. Family resources are very important.

CHAPTER FOCUS POINTS—cont'd

- Coping mechanisms may include regression, projection, withdrawal, and denial and represent the person's attempt to control the illness.
- Primary NANDA nursing diagnoses are impaired verbal communication, disturbed sensory perception, impaired social interaction, and disturbed thought processes.
- Primary *DSM-IV-TR* diagnoses are the schizophrenias, schizophreniform disorder, schizoaffective disorder, delusional disorder, brief psychotic disorder, and shared psychotic disorder.
- The expected outcome of nursing care is that the patient will live, learn, and work at a maximum possible level of success as defined by the individual.

- The nursing care plan must be based on an understanding of the patient's disabilities, strengths, and preferences. Patient and family education about symptom management and relapse prevention is a critical element of the plan.
- Primary nursing interventions for patients with maladaptive neurobiological responses include intervention in delusions, intervention with hallucinations, medication management, and patient and family education about symptom management and relapse.
- Evaluation is based on the patient's satisfaction with the level of functioning and on the ability to communicate improvement or impending relapse.

KEY TERMS

affect, 393
alexithymia, 394
anhedonia, 394
apathy, 394
apraxia, 395
attention, 390
avolition, 394
catatonia, 395
cognition, 388
command hallucinations, 410
computed tomography (CT), 396

delusion, 392
echopraxia, 395
hallucinations, 392
insight, 389
loose associations, 390
magical thinking, 391
magnetic resonance imaging (MRI), 396
memory, 389
mood, 393
neurotransmitter, 396

noncompliance, 415
perception, 392
positron emission tomography (PET), 397
prodromal phase, 413
psychosis, 386
recovery, 403
rehabilitation, 403
relapse, 403
stigma, 395
word salad, 390

CHAPTER REVIEW QUESTIONS

1. Match each term in Column A with the correct definition in Column B.

Column A

_____ Attention
_____ Perception
_____ Hallucinations
_____ Mood
_____ Cognition
_____ Anhedonia
_____ Affect
_____ Decision making
_____ Memory
_____ Soft signs

Column B

A. The act or process of knowing
B. The retention and storage of knowledge learned
C. The ability to focus on one activity in a sustained, concentrated manner
D. Identification and initial interpretation of a stimulus based on information from the senses
E. Perceptual distortions
F. Neurological deficits consistent with frontal or parietal lobe damage
G. An extensive and sustained feeling tone affecting the person's worldview
H. Inability to experience pleasure, joy, intimacy, and closeness
I. Behaviors and expressions that show during experiences of feelings
J. Insight, judgment, logic, decisiveness, planning, and abstract thought

2. Fill in the blanks.

A. The five areas affected by maladaptive neurobiological responses related to disruptions in brain functioning are

_____, _____,

_____, _____,

and _____.

B. Difficulty carrying out a purposeful, organized, complex task is called _____.

C. One of the current dominant biological theories of schizophrenia that proposes abnormal neurotransmission is the

_____.

D. _____ are precursors and stimuli that often precede a new episode of schizophrenia and can serve as warnings to the patient and mental health care provider.

E. The five stages of relapse in schizophrenia are

_____, _____,

_____, _____,

and _____.

3. Indicate whether the following statements are true (T) or false (F).

_____ A. Studies show multiple abnormalities in the brains and behaviors of many people with schizophrenia before they become symptomatic.

_____ B. The majority of hallucinations experienced by people with schizophrenia are visual.

_____ C. Atypical antipsychotic drugs should be used only when the patient does not respond to typical (conventional) treatments.

_____ D. Teaching during the health promotion phase focuses on relapse prevention and symptom management.

_____ E. The self-help program developed by the National Alliance for the Mentally Ill is called the Three Rs.

4. Provide short answers for the following questions.

A. Review the positive and negative symptoms of schizophrenia. How would their presence or absence affect the treatment plan you design for your patient?

B. One of your patients with schizophrenia and her husband tell you they would like to have children. They ask you to explain the risk factors for having children with the disorder. How would you respond?

C. Spend some time in a crowded place and make a detailed list of the things you notice about people that make them stand out or blend into the crowd. How can you use this knowledge to help your socially isolated patients?

 Visit Evolve for additional resources related to the content of this chapter.
http://evolve.elsevier.com/Stuart/principles/
• Topical Course Outline • Student Workbook Exercises • Critical Thinking Questions and Activities • Case Studies • Research Topics
• Monthly Content Updates • WebLinks

 ### Student Study CD-ROM

Access the accompanying CD-ROM for animations, interactive exercises, review questions for the NCLEX examination, and an audio glossary.

REFERENCES

Amador X: *I'm not sick, I don't need help!* Peconinc, New York, 2000, VidaPress.

American Psychiatric Association: *Diagnostic and statistical manual of mental disorders,* ed 4, text revision, Washington, DC, 2000, American Psychiatric Association.

American Psychiatric Association: Practice guideline for the treatment of patients with schizophrenia, *Am J Psychiatry* 161 (suppl):1, 2004.

Andreasen N: A unitary model of schizophrenia: Bleuler's "fragmented phrene" as schizencephaly, *Arch Gen Psychiatry* 56:781, 1999.

Battle Y et al: Seasonality and infectious disease in schizophrenia: the birth hypothesis revisited, *J Psychiatr Res* 33:501, 1999.

Bartzokis G: Schizophrenia: breakdown in the well-regulated lifelong process of brain development and maturation, *Neuropsychopharmacology* 27:672, 2002.

Berglund N, Vahlne JO, Edman A: Family intervention in schizophrenia: impact on family burden and attitude, *Soc Psychiatry Psychiatr Epidemiol* 38:116, 2003.

Brekke JS et al: Risks for individuals with schizophrenia who are living in the community, *Psychiatr Serv* 52:1358, 2001.

Buchanan R, Carpenter W: Schizophrenia: introduction and overview. In Saddock B, Saddock V, editors: *Comprehensive textbook of psychiatry,* Philadelphia, 2000, Williams & Wilkins.

Cannon M, Jones PB, Murray RM: Obstetric complications and schizophrenia: historical and meta-analytic review, *Am J Psychiatry* 159:1080, 2002.

Citrome L, Volavka J: Atypical antipsychotics: revolutionary or incremental advance? *Expert Rev Neurotherapeutics* 2:69, 2002.

Clary C, Dever A, Schweizer E: Psychiatric inpatients' knowledge of medication at hospital discharge, *Hosp Comm Psychiatry* 43:140, 1992.

Corcoran C et al: The neurobiology of the stress cascade and its potential relevance for schizophrenia, *J Psychiatr Pract* 7:3, 2001.

Dalman C et al: Obstetric complications and the risk of schizophrenia: a longitudinal study of a national birth cohort, *Arch Gen Psychiatry* 56:234, 1999.

Docherty JP et al: Stages of onset of schizophrenic psychosis, *Am J Psychiatry* 135:420, 1978.

Duzyurek S, Wiener JM: Early recognition in schizophrenia: the prodromal stages, *J Pract Psychiatr Behav Health* 5:187, 1999.

El-Guebaly N et al: Smoking cessation approaches for persons with mental illness or addictive disorders, *Psychiatr Serv* 53:1166, 2002.

Forchuk C et al: Schizophrenia and the motivation for smoking, *Perspect Psychiatr Care* 38:41-49, 2002.

Herz MI: Early intervention in different phases of schizophrenia, *J Pract Psychiatry Behav Health* 5:197, 1999.

Jarboe K: Treatment nonadherence: causes and potential solutions, *J Am Psychiatr Nurs Assoc* 8:S18, 2002.

Jungbauer J et al: Subjective burden over 12 months in parents of patients with schizophrenia, *Arch Psychiatr Nurs* 17:126, 2003.

Kennedy MG, Schepp KG, O'Connor FW: Symptom self-management and relapse in schizophrenia, *Arch Psychiatr Nurs* 15:266, 2000.

Kirkpatrick H et al: How people with schizophrenia build their hope, *J Psychosoc Nurs Ment Health Serv* 39:46, 2001.

Lamberti JS: Seven keys to relapse prevention in schizophrenia, *J Psychiatr Pract* 7:253, 2001.

Lehman AF, Steinwachs DM: Translating research into practice: the Schizophrenia Patient Outcomes Research Team (PORT) treatment recommendations, *Schizophr Bull* 24:1, 1998.

Liberman R et al: Biobehavioral treatment and rehabilitation of schizophrenia, *J Behav Ther* 25:89, 1994.

Lindsay H: Neurodevelopment of schizophrenia revealed, *Clin Psychiatr News* 3:34, 2000.

Lukens E et al: Family psychoeducation in schizophrenia: emerging themes and challenges, *J Pract Psychiatr Behav Health* 5:314, 1999.

Lyon ER: A review of the effects of nicotine on schizophrenia and antipsychotic medications, *Psychiatr Serv* 50:1346, 1999.

McFarlane W: From research to clinical practice: dissemination of New York State's family psychoeducation project, *Hosp Community Psychiatry* 44:265, 1992.

Moller MD, Murphy M: *Recovering from psychosis: a wellness approach,* Nine Mile Falls, Wash, 2000, Psychiatric Resource Network.

Moller MD, Murphy M: The three R's rehabilitation program: a prevention approach for the management of relapse symptoms associated with psychiatric diagnoses, *J Psychiatr Rehab* 20:42, 1997.

Murphy MF, Moller MD: Relapse management in neurobiological disorders: the Moller-Murphy Symptom Management Assessment Tool, *Arch Psychiatr Nurs* 7:226, 1993.

Myin-Germeys I, Nicolson NA, and Delespaul PA: The context of delusional experiences in the daily life of patients with schizophrenia, *Psychol Med* 31:489-498, 2001.

Nathan PE, Gorman JM, editors: *A guide to treatments that work,* ed 2, New York, 2002, Oxford University Press.

Olfson M et al: Predicting medication noncompliance after hospital discharge among patients with schizophrenia, *Psychiatr Serv* 51:216, 2000.

Perry W, Geyer MA, Braff DL: Sensorimotor gating and thought disturbance measured in close temporal proximity in schizophrenic patients, *Arch Gen Psychiatry* 56:277, 1999.

Pharoah F et al: Family intervention for schizophrenia, *Cochrane Library* 3, 2002.

Pinikahana J, Happell B, Keks NA: Suicide and schizophrenia: a review of literature for the decade (1990-1999) and implications for mental health nursing, *Issues Ment Health Nurs* 24:27, 2003.

Seckinger RA, Amador XF: Cognitive behavioral therapy in schizophrenia, *J Psychiatr Pract* 7:173, 2001.

Sernyak MJ et al: Prescribers' nonadherence to treatment guidelines for schizophrenia when prescribing neuroleptics, *Psychiatr Serv* 54:246, 2003.

Spring B, Pingitore R, McChargue DE: Reward value of cigarette smoking for comparably heavy smoking schizophrenic, depressed, and nonpatient smokers, *Am J Psychiatry* 160:316, 2003.

Stephenson J: Delay in treating schizophrenia may narrow therapeutic window of opportunity, *JAMA* 283:2091, 2000.

Torrey EF: *Surviving schizophrenia: a manual for families, consumers, and providers,* ed 4, New York, 2001, Harper Collins.

Trygstad L et al: Behavioral management of persistent auditory hallucinations in schizophrenia: outcomes from a 10-week course, *J Am Psychiatr Nurs Assoc* 8:84, 2002.

Wuerker AK: The family and schizophrenia, *Issues Ment Health Nurs* 21:127, 2000.

Zygmunt A et al: Interventions to improve medication adherence in schizophrenia, *Am J Psychiatry* 159:1653, 2002.

> The emptiness caused by dissatisfaction with mere achievement and the helplessness that results when the
> channels of relation break down have brought forth a loneliness of soul such as never existed before.
>
> KARL JASPERS, *EXISTENZPHILOSOPHIE*

SOCIAL RESPONSES AND PERSONALITY DISORDERS

22

Gail W. Stuart ▪ *Carol K. Perlin*

LEARNING OBJECTIVES

After studying this chapter, the student should be able to:

1. Describe the continuum of adaptive and maladaptive social responses (**I**).
2. Identify behaviors associated with social responses (**II**).
3. Analyze predisposing factors, precipitating stressors, and appraisal of stressors related to social responses (**II**).
4. Describe coping resources and coping mechanisms related to social responses (**II**).
5. Formulate nursing diagnoses related to social responses (**III**).
6. Examine the relationship between nursing diagnoses and medical diagnoses related to social responses (**III**).
7. Identify expected outcomes and short-term nursing goals related to social responses (**IV**).
8. Develop a patient education plan to promote adaptive social responses (**V**).
9. Analyze nursing interventions related to social responses (**VI**).
10. Evaluate nursing care related to social responses (**VII**).

evolve Visit Evolve for additional resources related to the content of this chapter.
http://evolve.elsevier.com/Stuart/principles/

To find satisfaction in life, people must be able to establish positive and healthy interpersonal relationships. Such people experience closeness with others while keeping their own separate identities. This closeness is called **intimacy** and is characterized by sensitivity to the other person's needs. Other classic characteristics of healthy relatedness include open communication of feelings, acceptance of the other person as valued and separate, and empathic understanding (Rogers, 1961).

To become intimately involved with another person, an individual must be willing to risk revealing private thoughts and feelings. This can be frightening, especially if one has had past difficulty sharing feelings with other people. Fear of exposing private feelings makes some people reluctant to become involved in intimate relationships. People who have extreme difficulty in relating intimately to others may have behaviors that are characteristic of a personality disorder.

■ CONTINUUM OF SOCIAL RESPONSES

Every person has the potential to be involved in many levels of relationships, from intimacy to casual contact. Intimate and interdependent relationships provide security and instill the self-confidence necessary to cope with the demands of daily life. A lack of intimacy with family members and friends leaves only superficial encounters, thereby excluding many of life's most meaningful experiences.

Relatedness can be analyzed based on the levels of one's involvement, comfort and well-being. Doing so suggests four

423

dimensions (Figure 22-1). The state of **connectedness** indicates that the person is actively involved in satisfying relationships. **Disconnectedness** relates to a lack of involvement that is not satisfactory to the person. **Parallelism** is a lack of involvement that is comfortable and acceptable to the individual. **Enmeshment** occurs when the person is involved in relationships but is unable to maintain one's own unique sense of self and ego boundaries. Connectedness involves high levels of belonging, mututality, reciprocity, and interdependence.

Adaptive and Maladaptive Responses

Within a relationship the participants usually develop a continuum of dependent and independent behavior. Ideally, these behaviors are balanced, which is described as interdependence. The interdependent person can decide when to rely on others and when it is appropriate to be independent. An interdependent person can let another be dependent or independent without needing to control that person's behavior.

All people are responsible for controlling their own behavior while receiving support and help from significant others as needed. Adaptive social responses therefore include the ability to tolerate **solitude** and the expression of **autonomy, mutuality,** and **interdependence.**

Interpersonal relationship behaviors may be represented on a continuum that ranges from healthy interdependent in-

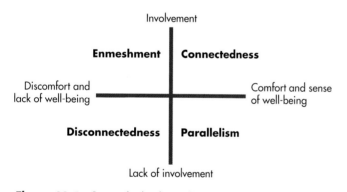

Figure 22-1 States of relatedness. (From Hagerty BMK et al: *Image* 25:291, 1993.)

teractions to those involving no real contact with other people (Figure 22-2). At the midpoint of the continuum, a person experiences **loneliness, withdrawal,** and **dependence.** The maladaptive end of the continuum reflects the dominance of **manipulation, impulsiveness,** and **narcissism.** People with these responses often have a history of problematic relationships in the family, on the job, and in the social arena.

Based on your experiences, compare the relationships you have had with family, with friends, and with patients in a nurse-patient relationship. How are they alike and different? ▪

Development Through the Life Cycle

Researchers agree that personality is shaped by biology and social learning, and that whether it develops a healthy or pathological form depends on the nature, timing, and interaction of these influences. As more is learned about child development and the structure and function of the brain, it is clear that the seed of personality is "temperament"—hereditary biological dispositions, evident almost from birth, that affect mood and activity level, attention span, and responsiveness to stimulation (Grinspoon, 2000). It is also true that establishing a strong affective bond with an important other and repairing this bond's inevitable ruptures are crucial to personality maturation across the lifespan (Lewis, 2000).

Infancy. From birth until 3 months of age the infant does not perceive physical separation between self and mother. Although physical differentiation occurs at about 3 months, psychological differentiation does not begin until 18 months. **The period between 3 and 18 months is the symbiotic stage of development.** The infant is completely dependent on others. Trust develops as needs are met consistently and predictably. The infant experiences the environment as unconditionally loving, nurturing, and accepting. Feelings of positive self-worth result from the infant's complete dependence on an environment that is good and loving. This creates a capacity for empathic understanding in future relationships.

Preschool Years. The period between 18 months and 3 years of age is the separation-individuation stage of devel-

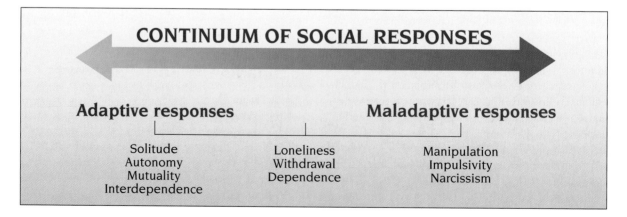

Figure 22-2 Continuum of social responses.

opment. **Separation** includes all the experiences, events, and developmental achievements that promote self-differentiation and a sense of being separate and unique. **Individuation** is the evolution of the child's internal psychological structure and growing sense of separateness, wholeness, and capability. In this developmental stage the toddler ventures away from the mother to explore the environment and a sense of object constancy develops. This means that the child knows that a valued person or object continues to exist when it cannot be directly perceived. Games such as peek-a-boo teach object constancy.

At the beginning of the separation-individuation process, the child seeks the parents' reassurance, support, and encouragement. If the response to autonomous behavior is positive and reinforcing, there is a foundation for building a solid sense of self and future relationships characterized by interdependence, commitment, and a capacity for interpersonal growth.

Childhood.
The internal development of morality and empathic feelings occurs between the ages of 6 and 10 years. During this period a supportive environment that encourages the budding sense of self fosters development of a positive, adaptive self-concept. Conflict occurs as adults set limits on behavior, often frustrating the child's efforts toward independence. However, loving, consistent limit setting communicates caring and helps the child develop interdependence.

The older child adopts the parents' guidelines for behavior and a value system begins to emerge. In school the child begins to learn cooperation, competition, and compromise. Peer relationships and approval of adults from outside the family, such as teachers, community leaders, and friends' parents become important.

Preadolescence.
By preadolescence the person becomes involved in an intimate relationship with a friend of the same sex, a best friend. This relationship involves sharing. It offers another chance to clarify values and recognize differences in people. This is usually a very dependent relationship, and it is often accompanied by active efforts to exclude others.

Adolescence.
As adolescence develops, the dependence on a close friend of the same sex usually yields to a dependent heterosexual relationship. While young people are involved in these dependent relationships with peers, they are asserting independence from their parents. Friends support each other in this struggle, which often includes rebellious behavior. Parents can help the adolescent grow by providing consistent limits and a caring tolerance of rebellious outbursts. Another step toward mature interdependence is taken as the person learns to balance parental demands and peer group pressures.

Young Adulthood.
Adolescence ends when the person is self-sufficient and maintains interdependent relationships with parents and peers. Decision making is independent, taking the advice and opinions of others into account. The person may marry and begin a new family. Occupational plans are made and a career begun. The mature person demonstrates self-awareness by balancing dependent and independent behavior. Others are allowed to be dependent or independent as appropriate. Being sensitive to and accepting the feelings and needs of oneself and others is critical to this level of mature functioning. Interpersonal relationships are characterized by mutuality.

Middle Adulthood.
Parenting and adult friendships test the person's ability to foster independence in others. Children gradually separate from parents, and friends may move away or drift apart. The mature person must be self-reliant and find new supports. Pleasure can be found in the development of an interdependent relationship with children as they grow. Decreased dependent demands by children create freedom that can be used for new activities.

Late Adulthood.
Change continues during late adulthood. Losses occur, such as the physical changes of aging, the death of parents, loss of occupation through retirement, and later the deaths of friends and one's spouse. The need for relatedness still must be satisfied. The mature person grieves over these losses and recognizes that the support of others can help resolve the grief.

However, new possibilities arise, even with a loss. Old friends and relatives cannot be replaced, but new relationships can be developed. Grandchildren may become important to the grandparent, who may delight in spending time with them. The aging person also may find a sense of relatedness to the culture as a whole. Life has deeper meaning in relation to one's perception of personal accomplishments and contributions to the welfare of society.

The mature older person can accept whatever increase in dependence is necessary but also strives to retain as much independence as possible. Even loss of physical health does not necessarily force the person to give up all independence. The ability to maintain mature relatedness throughout life enhances one's self-esteem (Masterson, 1985).

ASSESSMENT

Behaviors

"Personality" is a set of deeply ingrained, enduring patterns of thinking, feeling, and behaving. A personality disorder is a set of patterns or traits that hinder a person's ability to maintain meaningful relationships, feel fulfilled, and enjoy life. It is an enduring pattern of inner experience and behavior that deviates markedly from the expectations of the individual's culture, is pervasive and inflexible, has onset in adolescence or early adulthood, is stable over time, and leads to distress or impairment (Shea et al, 2002).

Personality disorders are attitudes toward self, others, and the world expressed in everything a person thinks, feels, and does. They often decrease in severity of expression as a person ages, mainly due to corrective life experiences

(Agronin and Maletta, 2000). Personality disorders are **continuous** rather than episodic, and they are **pervasive** across a wide range of circumstances in the individual's life, although the appearance and severity of a particular symptom can vary at times.

The concept of personality "disorder" implies that one knows what a normal personality is even though it is very difficult to define. It is doubtful that research and therapeutic efforts to date have significantly increased clinical insights into personality or succeeded in modifying it (Blashfield and Intoccia, 2000). It is clear, however, that although a healthy individual is able to adjust and adapt to the demands or expectations of different people and different situations, individuals with personality disorders have a persistent impairment in their interpersonal relationships and other aspects of functioning.

It can be difficult to separate the differences between "personality" and mood, anxiety, responses to stress, demands of social roles, or situational reactions. Although the border between normal and abnormal personality can be elusive, the distinction involves significant maladaptation.

A limitation of the current medical diagnostic system is that the criteria for the different personality disorders overlap. Two thirds of patients with one personality disorder meet criteria for another personality disorder (Grinspoon, 2000). This can confuse efforts to determine etiologies, make a diagnosis, select specific treatments, and measure outcomes. Regardless, because patients with these problems are among the most challenging in the health care system, nurses should develop the skills needed to identify the different personality disorders in their patients, which will enable them to intervene appropriately (see Citing the Evidence).

The three features of personality disorders are as follows (Millon and Davis, 1995):

1. The individual has acquired few strategies for relating and his or her approach to relationships and to the environment is inflexible and maladaptive.
2. The individual's needs, perceptions, and behavior have a tendency to foster vicious cycles that continue unhelpful patterns and provoke negative reactions from others.
3. The individual's adaptation skills are characterized by tenuous stability, fragility, and lack of resilience when faced with stressful situations.

Prevalence estimates of personality disorders in the general population range from 10% to 18%, and at least some of these disorders are associated with a high mortality rate due to suicide. Suicide victims with personality disorders almost always also have a depressive illness, substance abuse disorder, or both.

The fixed, enduring quality of specific personality disorder symptoms is an essential element of the diagnosis. Even with treatment, it is not possible to completely change someone's personality. However, it is possible to help people with personality disorders improve the quality of their life. Research shows that specific treatment modalities may lead to significant improvement in the symptoms, distress, and general functioning of patients with personality disorders (Bateman and Fonagy, 2000; Perry, Banon, and Ianni, 1999; Zanarini et al, 2003).

The behaviors observed in people with personality disorders are characterized by chronic, maladaptive social responses. The *DSM-IV-TR* (American Psychiatric Association, 2000) has grouped the personality disorders into three clusters based on descriptive similarities:

1. **Cluster A includes personality disorders of an odd or eccentric nature** (paranoid, schizoid, and schizotypal personality disorders).
2. **Cluster B disorders are of an erratic, dramatic, or emotional nature** (antisocial, borderline, histrionic, and narcissistic personality disorders).
3. **Cluster C includes disorders of an anxious or fearful nature** (avoidant, dependent, and obsessive-compulsive personality disorders).

Two additional personality disorder diagnoses are under consideration for inclusion in the *DSM-IV-TR* (passive-

▌CITING THE EVIDENCE ON
Mental Health Treatment Utilization

BACKGROUND: This study compared utilization of mental health treatment by patients with personality disorders with use of treatment by patients with major depressive disorder who did not have personality disorder.

RESULTS: Patients with personality disorders had more extensive histories of psychiatric outpatient, inpatient, and psychopharmacological treatment than patients with major depressive disorder. Compared with the depression group, patients with borderline personality disorder were significantly more likely to have received every type of psychosocial treatment except that related to self-help groups, and patients with obsessive-compulsive personality disorder reported greater utilization of individual psychotherapy. Patients with borderline personality disorder also were more likely to have used antianxiety, antidepressant, and mood stabilizer medication, and those with borderline or schizotypal personality disorder had a greater likelihood of having received antipsychotic medications. Patients with borderline personality disorder had received greater amounts of treatment, with the exception of family/couples therapy and self-help, than the depressed patients and patients with other personality disorders.

IMPLICATIONS: These results underscore the importance of considering personality disorders in diagnosis and treatment of psychiatric patients. Borderline and schizotypal personality disorders are associated with extensive use of mental health resources, and other less severe personality disorders may not be addressed sufficiently in treatment planning. More work is needed to determine whether patients with personality disorders are receiving adequate and appropriate mental health care.

Bender D et al: *Am J Psychiatry* 158:295, 2001.

aggressive and depressive). A specific classification of interpersonal and behavioral characteristics associated with each of the personality disorders is presented in Table 22-1. The patient usually reports or exhibits more than one of these traits in the course of the nursing assessment.

People with cluster B personality disorders have unique character features that can make the provision of nursing care complicated and difficult. Studies have found that patients with borderline personality disorder and antisocial personality characteristics are more likely to have attempted suicide (Hawton et al, 2003). Furthermore, a diagnosis of borderline personality disorder and the total number of cluster B personality traits in depressed inpatients has been found to correlate with the number and lethality of previous suicide attempts.

For these reasons, the nursing assessment and implementation of care for people with antisocial, borderline, and narcissistic personality disorders are emphasized in this chapter. Common maladaptive responses of people with cluster B personality disorders include manipulation and narcissism and the impulsivity that often overlaps both.

Manipulation. People who use manipulative behaviors present a particularly difficult nursing problem. Manipulation is a behavior in which people treat others as objects, and form relationships that center around control issues. Their behavior is easily misunderstood, as illustrated in the following clinical example.

CLINICAL EXAMPLE

Mr. Y was a 20-year-old single man who was committed to an inpatient psychiatric unit by a judge for a psychiatric evaluation. He had been charged with the sale of illicit drugs, statutory rape of his 15-year-old pregnant girlfriend, and contributing to the delinquency of a minor. He had been arrested on the grounds of a junior high school, where he was selling PCP and barbiturates to a group of young teenagers.

In jail Mr. Y had been observed to be "crazy" by the guards. He paced his cell, chanted, and threw his food on the floor. Because of this behavior, the judge agreed to order a psychiatric evaluation. On arrival at the psychiatric unit Mr. Y continued to behave in the same manner. However, his behavior did not seem typical of psychosis. There was no evidence of hallucinations or disorders of thought or affect. When unaware that he was being observed,

Table 22-1 Classification and Features of DSM-IV-TR Personality Disorders

DISORDERS	FEATURES/BEHAVIORS
Cluster A: Odd, Eccentric, General Tendency Toward Social and Emotional Withdrawal	
Paranoid	Distrust: persistent suspiciousness, secretive, withholding, hypervigilant, jealous, envious; suspects without sufficient basis that others are exploiting, harming, or deceiving them.
Schizoid	Social detachment: self-absorbed; restricted emotionality; cold and indifferent; neither desires nor enjoys close relationships; anhedonic, indifferent to others; less disturbed than schizotypal.
Schizotypal	Interpersonal deficits; cognitive distortions; eccentricities; paranoid; difficulty feeling understood and accepted; odd beliefs, magical thinking, unusual perceptual experiences; social isolation.
Cluster B: Overemotional, Dramatic, Erratic, Impulsive	
Antisocial	Disregard for rights of others; lies; manipulates; exploitative; seductive; repeatedly performs acts that are grounds for arrest.
Borderline	Instability; impulsivity; hypersensitivity; self-destructive behavior; profound mood shifts; unstable and intense interpersonal relationships.
Histrionic	Excessive emotionality; attention seeking; superficial and stormy relationships; lively; uncomfortable when not the center of attention.
Narcissistic	Arrogance; need for admiration; lack of empathy; seductive; socially exploitative; manipulative; grandiose sense of self-importance.
Cluster C: Anxious, Fearful	
Avoidant	Social inhibition; withdraw from social and occupational situations that involve significant interpersonal contact; longs for relationships; inadequacy; hypersensitivity to negative criticism, rejection, or shame.
Dependent	Submissive behavior; low self-esteem; dependency in relationships; extreme self-consciousness; urgently and indiscriminately seeks another relationship when close relationship ends; inadequate; helpless.
Obsessive-compulsive	Unable to express affection; overly cold and rigid; crippling preoccupation with trivial detail, orderliness, perfectionism, and control (i.e., attends to rules, lists, organization, schedules, to the extent that the major point of the activity is lost); superior attitude.
Suggested Personality Diagnoses in DSM-IV-TR Needing Further Study	
Passive-aggressive	**Negativistic Attitudes:** Sullen and argumentative, resents others, resists fulfilling obligations, complains of being unappreciated
Depressive	**Depressive Cognitions:** Gloomy, brooding, pessimistic, guilt-prone, highly critical of self and others, cheerless

From American Psychiatric Association: *Diagnostic and statistical manual of mental disorders*, ed 4, text revision, Washington, DC, 2000, American Psychiatric Association; Kay J, Tasman A: *Psychiatry: behavioral science and clinical essentials*, Philadelphia, 2000, WB Saunders.

Mr. Y seemed relaxed and was noted at one time to be talking with another patient.

By the day after admission he seemed to be free of his symptoms. At this point the staff began to describe him as a "nice guy." He complimented female staff members and behaved toward them in a pleasantly seductive manner. He was respectful to the physicians and agreed to abide by all the rules. He was helpful with other patients. In group meetings he admitted that he had behaved badly in the past and described how he had been led astray by his friends. He said he became involved in drugs because he wanted to be "one of the gang" and he needed money so he "had to" start selling drugs. By the end of his first week in the hospital he had received the sympathy of all the other patients and the staff.

Nine days after admission, after visiting hours, it was noted that Mr. Y and two other patients looked lethargic. Their speech was slurred and their gaits ataxic. The nursing staff immediately collected urine and blood specimens for toxicological analysis. The unit was searched for hidden drugs, but none were found. The results of the toxicology screening tests were positive for barbiturates.

Suspicion was immediately focused on Mr. Y because the other patients involved were young adolescents with no history of drug abuse. When confronted, Mr. Y seemed amazed that he could be suspected and pointed out his past behavior as a model patient. He admitted that he had behaved strangely and wondered whether someone had "slipped" him some drugs. He was convincing but was warned that if he was involved in any way with drugs, he would be sent directly back to jail.

Mr. Y convinced his family of his good intentions, and they agreed to allow him to move into their house. On the basis of these indications of positive behavioral change, Mr. Y received a recommendation for probation, which was carried out by the judge.

Three months after discharge from the hospital, Mr. Y and a friend were arrested for operating a PCP manufacturing laboratory in a friend's garage.

Selected Nursing Diagnoses
* Impaired social interaction related to need for control, as evidenced by illegal behavior and treating people like objects
* Defensive coping related to inability to identify relationship problems, as evidenced by manipulation of others ∎

These patients usually have little motivation to change because manipulative behavior often has rewards for them, facilitating the accomplishment of a desired goal. The manipulator is goal-oriented or **self-oriented, not other-oriented.** However, the person is skilled at giving the impression of involvement with others. In this clinical example, Mr. Y was able to gain the confidence of the staff in order to have support in court. This is typical of a person with an antisocial personality disorder.

Antisocial personality disorder is a complex disorder that is particularly difficult to diagnose and treat (Reid, 2001). To meet *DSM-IV-TR* criteria, an individual must be at least 18 years old but must demonstrate a pattern of breaking rules since the age of 15 (American Psychiatric Association, 2000). The diagnosis is applied when an individual consistently ignores social rules; is manipulative, exploitative or dishonest; lacks remorse for actions; and is frequently involved in criminal activity. Although this diagnosis occurs in only 3% of men and 1% of women, these individuals are responsible for a large proportion of crime, violence, and social distress.

The manipulative person is unaware of a lack of relatedness and assumes that all interpersonal relationships are formed to **take advantage of others.** This person cannot imagine an intimate, sharing relationship. The manipulator believes in maintaining control at all times to avoid being controlled. Patients with borderline personality disorder are often manipulative. This results in their inability to participate in mature interpersonal relationships, as illustrated in the next clinical example.

CLINICAL EXAMPLE

Ms. S is a 23-year-old woman who was admitted to a general hospital psychiatric unit. She had lacerated her wrists superficially three times during the week before admission. Each time she cut herself, she had telephoned her therapist, a psychiatric advanced practice nurse. Because her therapist was about to leave for vacation and she was concerned about the safety of Ms. S, the nurse decided to hospitalize her.

On admission Ms. S appeared mildly depressed. She gave the impression of a guilty child who had been punished. She denied any current self-destructive thoughts. During the physical assessment, the nurse noted that there were many scars on the patient's body. When asked about these, she claimed she was abused as a child. Her therapist's records described the scars as the result of much self-mutilation since the age of 16 years. This had been her main reason for seeking therapy. There was also a history of sexual promiscuity.

Ms. S described herself as a failure, stating that she had "the best parents in the world, but they did not get the daughter they deserve." She said she was a drifter who had never been able to settle on a career, a lifestyle, or any consistent friends. She didn't know who or what she was. When asked how she felt, she responded, "Most of the time, I don't feel anything, just empty." She had no signs of psychosis.

Ms. S was placed on constant observation to prevent further cutting. All sharp objects were removed from the room. At first she was very cooperative and superficially friendly to other patients. Because of her smooth adjustment, constant observation was discontinued after 3 days. She was also given a schedule of activities and informed that she was responsible for following it. The next day, an X-Acto knife was missing from the activities therapy room. Ms. S was found in the bathroom, bleeding from several small cuts on her ankles. This sequence was repeated several times. Each time the constant observation was discontinued, she found a sharp object and cut herself.

Ms. S was also very labile emotionally. She had unpredictable outbursts of anger, similar to temper tantrums. However, these outbursts passed as quickly as they came, never lasting more than a few minutes. She also began to categorize the staff as "good guys and bad guys." When she was with staff members she liked, she was pleasant, complimenting them on their kind and understanding attitudes toward her. With staff she disliked, she was sullen and uncooperative, comparing them unfavorably to the others. Eventually the staff began to bicker about her care, some believing she was spoiled and others that she was neglected.

Ms. S remained in the hospital during her therapist's absence. When the therapist returned, Ms. S refused to see her. The frequency of angry outbursts increased dramatically. However, following frequent visits from her therapist, Ms. S began to request discharge. Behavioral criteria for discharge were set, including no self-mutilation and no temper tantrums. She met the criteria and was discharged back to outpatient treatment.

Selected Nursing Diagnoses
- Risk for self-mutilation related to anxiety about her therapist's vacation, as evidenced by lacerating her wrists
- Chronic low self-esteem related to unclear goals and expectations, as evidenced by describing herself as a failure
- Impaired social interaction related to inability to tolerate close relationships, as evidenced by splitting staff into "good guys" and "bad guys" ∎

The diagnosis of borderline personality disorder occurs in 2% to 3% of the general population and is the most prevalent personality disorder in clinical settings. The diagnosis is made three times more often in women than in men. Theories that may explain this include the following:

- Women may be more biologically vulnerable than men.
- Sociocultural expectations of perceived roles and attitudes may contribute to this problem in women.
- Similar symptoms may generate a diagnosis of narcissistic personality disorder in men.

Research shows that women with borderline personality disorder feel that the label is difficult to live with, that their self-destructive behavior is seen as manipulative, and that they have limited access to care.

Developmental theory (Masterson, 1985) proposes that the borderline person fails to achieve object constancy during the separation-individuation stage of psychosocial development. Because of this, the person relates to another as a series of disconnected parts rather than as a whole. The borderline person cannot recall the image of someone who is absent. He or she is not able to mourn the loss of another person. When someone fails to meet the borderline person's needs, the relationship is likely to end.

People who fail to complete separation from the mother (or primary caretaker) and develop autonomy in childhood often repeat this developmental crisis at adolescence. Behaviors characteristic of this phase include the following:

- Clinging
- Depression accompanied by rage and defended by acting out or neurotic behavior
- Detachment and withdrawal

Many of these behaviors can be seen in the preceding clinical example. Borderline personality disorder, in particular, has one of the highest suicide rates (3% to 10%) of all the personality disorders (Paris, 2002). **Impulsive aggression is the hallmark of borderline personality disorder, and it plays a pivotal role in the borderline person's self-mutilation, unstable relationships, violence, and completed suicides** (Stanley et al, 2001).

Because of their inability to become involved in reciprocal interpersonal relationships and the related manipulativeness, these patients are frustrating for nursing staff to interact with and treat. It must be remembered that their behavior is not consciously planned, but is a defense against a fear of loneliness.

Narcissism. The term narcissism comes from the Greek myth of Narcissus, who fell in love with his own reflection in the waters of a spring and died. The flower that bears his name sprang up at the site of his death. Many successful people are narcissistic. Acting, modeling, professional sports, and politics are usually attractive occupations to people with this personality trait. In these contexts, self-centeredness is usually expected.

However, problems occur when the person does not gain the status he or she thinks is deserved or loses status or tries to have interpersonal relationships. The frustration caused by lack or loss of recognition may be expressed as anger, depression, substance abuse, or other maladaptive behaviors.

People with narcissistic personality disorders have **fragile self-esteem**, driving them to search constantly for praise, appreciation, and admiration. The clinical example that follows demonstrates narcissistic entitlement, which describes an egocentric attitude, envy, and rage when others are seen as critical or not supportive.

◢ CLINICAL EXAMPLE

Mr. T, the psychiatric nurse, was called to the emergency room to see a new patient, Mr. F, who was accompanied by his wife. The nurse knew from the intake form that Mr. F was a 44-year-old man with no psychiatric history. His chief complaint was that he had gone into a "blind rage" when he had an argument with his wife earlier in the evening and he had punched her in the arm. He was frightened by his loss of control and said that he felt like a failure. Both Mr. and Mrs. F denied any history of violence, although Mr. F said that his first marriage ended "because of my anger."

Mr. F appeared quite anxious; he was tapping his foot and wringing his hands, and he avoided eye contact with Mr. T. After a short time, however, he became more verbal, and he willingly explained what had led to the "blow up." He had been self-employed for the past 10 years and had been "highly successful," expanding his company nationally. He told Mr. T that his father was a "multimillionaire" and that he had been on his way to exceeding his father's wealth. It seemed important to impress Mr. T by dropping the names of well-known people, whom he described as his friends.

Mrs. F angrily interrupted him, saying "that's important to you—who you know and how it looks." Mrs. F then explained that business began slipping 2 years ago. Despite several profitable years, he had never invested or saved money. When sales fell, instead of cutting expenses and downsizing the company, he continued to live lavishly, making extravagant purchases. It was this situation that led to their argument. When Mrs. F accused her husband of taking them to the brink of financial collapse, he went into a rage and punched her.

Mrs. F began sobbing, and Mr. F seemed not to notice. He said he felt like his life was falling apart and that he must be the failure his father always said he was. He angrily referred to his "rich brother," who, in his father's eyes, was the perfect son. He became tearful, and Mrs. F then turned to her husband, attempting to provide support and reassurance.

Selected Nursing Diagnoses
- Impaired social interaction related to the need for approval by others, as evidenced by attempts to impress others and inability to respond to wife's distress
- Risk for other-directed violence related to impulsivity, as evidenced by acts engaged in during "blind rage"

- Interrupted family processes related to inconsistency between goals of husband and wife, as evidenced by wife's reaction to patient's description of his problem
- Defensive coping related to fear of failure, as evidenced by bragging and name-dropping
- Chronic low self-esteem related to perceived lack of caring and approval from father, as evidenced by stated need to exceed his father's success and description of himself as "a failure" in his father's eyes ■

Mr. F's impulsiveness was demonstrated by his extravagance, inability to establish and follow a life plan, failure to learn by experience, poor judgment, and unreliability.

The behaviors related to maladaptive social responses are summarized in Table 22-2. Patients often exhibit combinations of these behaviors. The nurse should be able to identify the complex behaviors associated with high levels of stress and anxiety. In some cases, a usual mode of behavior, such as manipulation, may be exaggerated or combined with a change in behavior. For instance, manipulative people may withdraw when confronted about their manipulations and may be rejected by those they have been trying to manipulate. In other instances, the behavior resulting from stress may be different from the person's usual style of relatedness. A person who is usually agreeable may become critical and defensive when under great stress. It is thus helpful to include a description of the patient's usual relationships in the nursing assessment. This provides a baseline of behavior for that person against which the nurse measures the patient's progress.

Predisposing Factors

Current research supports the multifactorial origins of personality disorders, including a variety of predisposing neurobiological, early developmental, and sociocultural factors (Pally, 2002). The nurse should explore all relevant areas during the nursing assessment.

Biological Factors. Many researchers believe that for severe mental illness, such as borderline personality disorder or antisocial personality disorder, to develop, an inherited biological vulnerability or a genetic susceptibility must be part of the "equation," which then sets the stage for environmental influences. Studies suggest a genetic link for antisocial personality disorder and a biological hypothesis that impulsive and violent behavior may be caused by brain dysfunction, a low threshold of excitability of the limbic system, low levels of serotonin, or toxic chemical substances.

Other studies have found that people with antisocial personality disorder have reduced prefrontal gray matter volume and lower than average activity in the frontal lobes of their brain (Raine et al, 2000; Miller, 2001). This results in low arousal, poor fear conditioning, lack of conscience, and decision-making deficits.

Personality disorders also have been linked to alcohol and drug abuse. Findings reveal that first-degree relatives of people with personality disorders have a higher than normal rate of being substance abusers, thus they are considered to have a probable genetic link. Borderline personality disorder and antisocial personality disorder in particular are associated with a wide variety of substance use disorders, and the combination results in severe global impairment (Miller, 2000).

Researchers are looking for the biological basis of very early infant and childhood characteristics. For instance, about 20% of children are inhibited from an early age and can be upset easily by the age of $4\frac{1}{2}$ months. Evidence shows that these children have an accelerated heart rate, even in the womb, and that their amygdalas (the brain region that governs learned fear and emotion) may be more excitable than average.

In contrast, antisocial personality appears to be correlated with abnormal brain processing of emotionally charged words, an unusually low heart rate, and slow responses to experimental rewards and punishments from an early age (Grinspoon, 2000). Further research is needed to clarify the role of inheritance and brain structure and function in the development of personality disorders.

Developmental Factors. Early studies of the childhood experiences of patients with personality disorders focused on the etiological role of early separations and disturbed parental involvement. More current research has focused specifically on the developmental consequences of early traumatic experiences, losses suffered by the attachment figure and childhood abuse, in the etiology of cluster B personality disorders, particularly borderline personality disorder (Liotti and Pasquini, 2000).

Research has shown that patients with borderline personality disorder compared with patients with other personality disorders were significantly more likely to report having been emotionally and physically abused by a caretaker and sexually abused by a noncaretaker. However, the results suggest that sexual abuse by itself is neither necessary nor sufficient for the etiology of borderline personality disorder, therefore other predisposing factors also must be involved.

About 25% of patients with borderline personality disorder are also given a diagnosis of posttraumatic stress disorder,

Table 22-2	Behaviors Related to Maladaptive Social Responses
BEHAVIOR	**CHARACTERISTICS**
Manipulation	Others are treated as objects
	Relationships center around control issues
	Person is self-oriented or goal-oriented, not other-oriented
Narcissism	Fragile self-esteem
	Constant seeking of praise and admiration
	Egocentric attitude
	Envy
	Rage when others are not supportive
Impulsivity	Inability to plan
	Inability to learn from experience
	Poor judgment
	Unreliability

a condition that results from an overwhelming psychological assault (Brown and Dodson, 1999). Similarly, childhood histories of people with antisocial personality disorder often reveal abuse, neglect, and the absence of an early emotional attachment. Based on these findings, it has been theorized that lack of parental caring is internalized, and the individual becomes incapable of bonding with others. People with antisocial personality disorder thus do not develop a sense of trust or a capacity for guilt or remorse (Kaylor, 1999).

In a longitudinal study of childhood behaviors that preceded a diagnosis of personality disorders in adolescence, four childhood conditions were found: conduct problems, depressive symptoms, anxiety or fear, and immaturity. Thus antecedents of adolescent personality disorder may be able to be identified in childhood through an accurate assessment of emotional and behavioral problems. It also has been reported that cluster A and cluster B personality disorders and paranoid, narcissistic, and passive-aggressive personality disorder symptoms during adolescence may increase risk for violent behavior that persists into early adulthood (Johnson et al, 2000).

Theories of family impact on personality are controversial. Some research supports the fact that, apart from genetic similarity, children raised in the same family do not resemble one another more closely than strangers. Thus influences outside the family (i.e., peer groups) are greater than parental influences during childrearing. Other theorists support the notion that many people with maladaptive social responses are enmeshed in a family system that blocks further development and makes change difficult and hazardous.

Families of borderline and narcissistic people often operate with the unspoken ground rule that independence and separation from the family imply rejection of family values. The parents often re-enact their own developmental conflicts through their children, and role reversals (for example, parent as child) are common. Features of these families include various degrees of restrictiveness from the extra-familial world, absence of clear-cut lines of authority, confusion of parental executive and nurturing roles, blurred generational boundaries, generations of family patterns in which people are labeled as good and bad, and the generational transmission of irrational forms of thinking and relating (see Chapter 33).

The nurse should therefore assess the nature of family interactions and gather information related to early child behaviors, child abuse, and alcohol abuse as part of a comprehensive data collection.

Sociocultural Factors. Sociocultural factors also can influence the person's ability to establish and maintain relatedness. Many forces in American culture make people feel isolated and lonely. Friendships are often short term because of the mobility involved in many occupations. Family relationships are more distant as adult children move away and see their parents only occasionally. Friends are often closer than siblings.

Involuntary social isolation also affects the disabled and chronically ill of any age. People with chronic or terminal illnesses or disfiguring disorders are often stigmatized and avoided by others. This is also true for people with long-term psychiatric problems. Although an effort has been made to decrease chronic institutionalization, many people continue to resist integrating disabled people into 'their' community. This involuntary isolation may result in a variety of maladaptive social responses as the person tries to cope with loneliness.

Immigration continues to be an active cultural force in the United States and many other parts of the world. As people move into entirely different cultures, they may feel alienated and frightened about customs they do not understand. Sometimes immigrants form separate communities to preserve their traditions. These close-knit communities help meet relationship needs but create barriers to broader community participation and integration. Unfortunately, they also focus attention on the group, often attracting discriminatory behavior by others.

Closeness is the ideal in American culture. At the same time, people are given the message that they need to be careful in deciding whom to trust. This can cause confusion and a feeling of insecurity. Rising crime rates cause fear and reluctance to risk closeness or contact with strangers. Some urban residents, particularly the elderly, often become lonely prisoners in their own homes.

Identify a novel, a popular song, or a work of art that would have meaning for a person who is trying to cope with an interpersonal loss. How do such things help you? ■

Precipitating Stressors

Maladaptive social responses are the result of experiences that negatively influence the person's emotional growth. In most instances a series of life events predisposes a person to have relationship problems. Many people cope with their interpersonal problems and say they are reasonably satisfied with their relationships. However, additional stress can cause a somewhat satisfying interpersonal life to become disrupted. Response to stressors is highly individual, and the nurse should remember that the person experiences an increase in anxiety as a result of the stressor, and this is often at the root of behavioral disruption. Precipitating stressors may be sociocultural or psychological in nature.

Sociocultural Stressors. One sociocultural stressor may be instability in the family. Divorces are common. Mobility has broken up the extended family, depriving people of all ages of an important support system. Less contact occurs between the generations. Tradition, which provides a powerful link with the past and a sense of identity, is less observable when the family is fragmented. Interest in ethnicity and "roots" may reflect the efforts of isolated people to associate themselves with a specific identity. The many stresses on the family have made it more difficult for family members to accomplish the developmental tasks related to intimacy.

Nurses who work in general hospitals often encounter patients with maladaptive social responses. Even a reasonably well-adjusted person may have difficulty maintaining a satisfying level of intimacy while hospitalized. The patient's feeling of isolation is enhanced by the impersonal hospital environment. Sometimes patients need to be isolated because of infection or, in the psychiatric setting, to control behavior. They are then susceptible to the effects of sensory deprivation. Creative nursing care is needed to minimize this problem.

For instance, a patient who is in isolation for infection control could be given a schedule of times when staff will be present. This should include time to talk. Family members should be encouraged to visit, telephone, and share current activities. On the other hand, sensory overload may be a problem for patients in critical care units. This also can lead to loneliness and separation from others.

Psychological Stressors. Many psychological theories have been proposed to explain problems in establishing and maintaining satisfying relationships. It is known that high anxiety levels result in impaired ability to relate to others. A combination of prolonged or intense anxiety with limited coping ability is believed to cause severe relationship problems.

It has been suggested that the person with borderline personality disorder is likely to experience an incapacitating level of anxiety in response to life events that represent increased autonomy and separation (such as high school or college graduation, going away to camp, marriage, birth of a child, employment, job promotion). The person who has narcissistic personality disorder tends to experience high anxiety, causing relationship difficulties, when the significant other no longer adequately nourishes the person's fragile self-esteem. These relationships often move through predictable stages:

1. Idealization and overvaluation
2. Disappointment when unrealistic needs for maintaining self-esteem are not met
3. Rationalization and devaluation
4. Rejection of the other person based on "narcissistic injury"

Typically, these people go through life repeating this pattern on the job, in marriages, and in friendships.

Appraisal of Stressors

The mature person who can participate in healthy relationships is still vulnerable to the effects of psychological stress. A person's appraisal of the stressor is critically important in this regard. A series of losses or a single significant loss may lead to problems in establishing future intimate relationships. The pain of a loss can be so great that the person avoids future involvements rather than risk more pain. This response is more likely if the person had difficulty with developmental tasks pertinent to relatedness.

Losses of significant others may cause difficulty with future relationships, but other types of losses may do the same. For example, the loss of a job decreases a person's self-esteem. This can also result in future withdrawal and emo-

tional problems unless the person has a well-established support system.

Coping Resources

When a person is having problems with relationships, it is important for the nurse to assess the person's coping resources. For many people, when one relationship is troublesome or lost, others are available to offer support and reassurance. Those who have broad networks of family and friends have many resources to draw upon. Sometimes they need encouragement to reach out for help.

Some people do not have readily available human supports but have other ways of managing interpersonal problems. Pets can be an important way of expressing relatedness. Isolated elderly people often focus their need to give and receive affection on a dog or cat. Sometimes a person who is troubled about a relationship will use creative ways to express feelings. Use of expressive media such as art, music, or writing allows the person to explore and resolve an upsetting experience. Others are helped by reading, exercise, looking at art, dancing, or listening to music.

Coping Mechanisms

Coping mechanisms associated with maladaptive social responses are attempts to cope with anxiety related to threatened or actual loneliness (Booth, 2000; Sargent et al, 2002). However, they are not healthy and sometimes have the unintended effect of driving people away. Thus the person is always caught in the approach-avoidance conflict of the need-fear dilemma, searching for some degree of human contact on one hand and pushing people away on the other.

Manipulative people view other people as objects. Their defenses protect them from potential psychological pain related to the loss of a significant other. People with antisocial personality disorder often use the defenses of projection and splitting.

Projection places responsibility for antisocial behavior outside oneself. For instance, a patient may rationalize using drugs by saying, "Everybody I know uses cocaine. Why shouldn't I?"

Splitting is characteristic of people with borderline and narcissistic personality disorders as well. It is the inability to integrate the good and bad aspects of oneself and objects. An object is anything outside of the self, animate or inanimate, to which the person has an attachment. An object could be a parent, a friend, or a teddy bear. The process of splitting by a borderline patient in an inpatient setting results in different staff members seeing the borderline patient in very different ways.

Projective identification is a complex defense mechanism. When the borderline patient projects parts of himself or herself onto others, these people are often not consciously aware of this. However, they may begin to behave like the projected parts. For example, a patient projects onto a nurse cruel, punishing parts of himself. The projection reverberates with something in the nurse that had been submerged, and the nurse will tend to react to the patient in a cruel, punishing manner. Likewise, staff who have received idealized projected parts of the patient will tend to respond in an overly involved, protective, indulgent manner. An example of projective identification is demonstrated by Ms. T in the following clinical example.

CLINICAL EXAMPLE

A nurse, Ms. M, was describing her relationship with a borderline patient, Ms. T, who had been on the unit for approximately 2 weeks. She explained that Ms. T had become negativistic and increasingly demanding to the point that her demands had no bounds. For the past week Ms. T had been calling Ms. M "Nurse Ratchet." If that was not difficult enough, Ms. T was also telling new patients on the unit about what a tyrant Ms. M was. Further inquiry made it clear that soon after Ms. T had cast Ms. M as "Nurse Ratchet," she started to react to the patient far more rigidly than was typical for her. Indeed, most of her interactions with Ms. T were now focused on policy adherence and strict limit setting. Without knowing it, Ms. M was on her way to repeating a script straight out of the movie *One Flew Over the Cuckoo's Nest.*

Selected Nursing Diagnosis
• Chronic low self-esteem related to use of the defense mechanism of splitting, as evidenced by need to belittle the nurse ■

Finally, the defense mechanisms of splitting and projective identification help explain why different staff members often see the same patient in very different ways, as illustrated in Figure 22-3.

Compare the processes of empathic understanding and projective identification. Give some examples of each from your experience. ■

DIAGNOSIS

Nursing Diagnoses
When diagnosing maladaptive social responses, the nurse should consider the extent and nature of maladaptive behaviors, coping mechanisms, and the predisposing factors and precipitating stressors leading to the behaviors. The nurse may formulate a nursing diagnosis by using the Stuart Stress Adaptation Model (Figure 22-4) as a guide. Nursing diagnoses associated with maladaptive social responses and related medical diagnoses are presented in the Medical and Nursing Diagnoses box (Box 22-1). Primary NANDA diagnoses include **defensive coping, chronic low self-esteem, risk for self-mutilation, impaired social interaction,** and **risk for violence (self-directed or other-directed).** Examples of expanded nursing diagnoses are presented in the Detailed Diagnoses table (Table 22-3).

Medical Diagnoses
Personality is composed of temperament, which is inherited, and character, which is learned. In general, distinguishing elements of personality disorders include that they tend to be:
• Chronic and long-standing.
• Not based on a sound personality structure.
• Difficult to change.

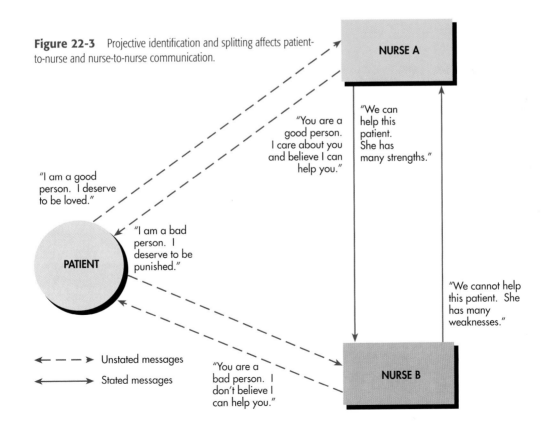

Figure 22-3 Projective identification and splitting affects patient-to-nurse and nurse-to-nurse communication.

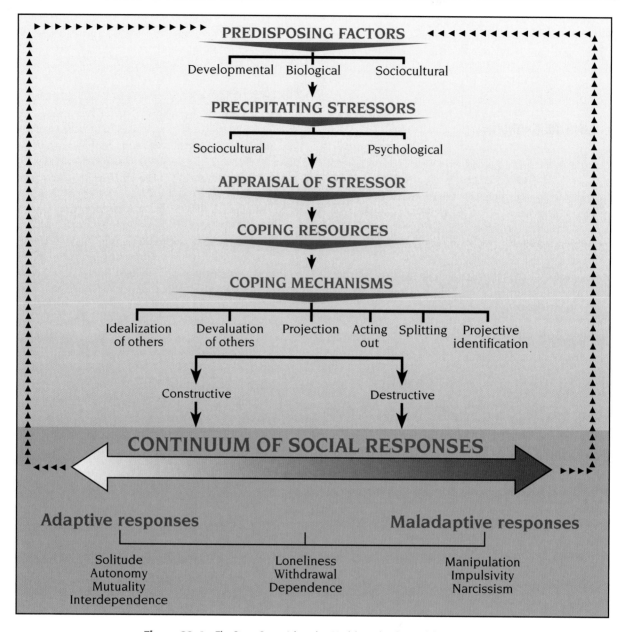

Figure 22-4   The Stuart Stress Adaptation Model as related to social responses.

Medical diagnoses related to maladaptive social responses include **paranoid, schizoid, schizotypal, histrionic, antisocial, narcissistic, borderline, obsessive-compulsive, dependent,** and **avoidant personality disorders**. They are described in the Detailed Diagnoses table (see Table 22-3).

Describe one of your own personality traits that is due to temperament and one that is due to character. How have each affected your life? ■

■ OUTCOME IDENTIFICATION

The expected outcome for nursing care of the patient with maladaptive social responses is:

The patient will obtain maximum interpersonal satisfaction by establishing and maintaining self-enhancing relationships with others.

Short-term goals are more specific to the patient's problems. They may progress from simpler to more complex changes in behavior. It can be difficult to set mutual nursing care goals with a patient who has problems with relatedness. This is partly because mutuality must be based on a strong nurse-patient relationship. It is difficult to develop a strong relationship with a patient who fears intimacy.

In addition, setting a goal implies a commitment to change. Many patients who have maladaptive social responses are reluctant to commit themselves to change. Because most of these behavioral problems also serve as coping mechanisms, resistance to change can be quite pronounced. For these reasons, even though it is desirable to have the patient's full participation, it may be necessary for the nurse to set more immediate initial goals that will eventually lead to

■ **BOX 22-1** *Medical and Nursing Diagnoses Related to* **Maladaptive Social Responses**

RELATED MEDICAL DIAGNOSES (*DSM-IV-TR*)*

Paranoid personality disorder
Schizoid personality disorder
Schizotypal personality disorder
Antisocial personality disorder
Borderline personality disorder
Histrionic personality disorder
Narcissistic personality disorder
Avoidant personality disorder
Dependent personality disorder
Obsessive-compulsive personality disorder

RELATED NURSING DIAGNOSES (NANDA)†

Anxiety
Coping, Defensive‡
Family processes, Interrupted
Role performance, Ineffective
Self-esteem, Chronic low‡
Self-mutilation, Risk for‡
Social interaction, Impaired‡
Social isolation
Violence, Risk for self-directed or other-directed‡

*From American Psychiatric Association: *Diagnostic and statistical manual of mental disorders*, ed 4, text revision, Washington, DC, 2000, American Psychiatric Association.
†From North American Nursing Diagnosis Association: *NANDA nursing diagnoses: definitions and classification 2003-2004*, Philadelphia, 2003, The Association.
‡**Primary nursing diagnosis for maladaptive social responses.**

Table 22-3 *Detailed Diagnoses Related to* **Maladaptive Social Responses**

NANDA DIAGNOSIS STEM	EXAMPLES OF EXPANDED DIAGNOSIS
Defensive coping	Defensive coping related to early traumatic losses, as evidenced by grandiosity and superior attitudes toward others
Chronic low self-esteem	Chronic low self-esteem related to physical abuse during childhood, as evidenced by verbalized unhappiness with personal accomplishments
Risk for self-mutilation	Risk for self-mutilation related to fear of rejection, as evidenced by cutting self after visits from parents
Impaired social interaction	Impaired social interaction related to rejection of sociocultural values, as evidenced by stated belief that rules do not pertain to self
Risk for self-directed violence	Risk for self-directed violence related to need to punish self, as evidenced by repeated burning of hands and feet when criticized
Risk for other-directed violence	Risk for other-directed violence related to use of projection, as evidenced by blaming, argumentativeness, and recent purchase of a handgun

DSM-IV-TR DIAGNOSIS	ESSENTIAL FEATURES*
Paranoid personality disorder	A pervasive distrust and suspiciousness of others such that their motives are interpreted as malevolent, beginning in early adulthood and present in a variety of contexts
Schizoid personality disorder	A pervasive pattern of detachment from social relationships and a restricted range of expression of emotions in interpersonal settings, beginning in early adulthood and present in a variety of contexts
Schizotypal personality disorder	A pervasive pattern of social and interpersonal deficits marked by acute discomfort with disorder and reduced capacity for close relationships and by cognitive and perceptual distortions and eccentricities of behavior, beginning in early adulthood and present in a variety of contexts
Antisocial personality disorder	A pervasive pattern of disregard for and violation of the rights of others occurring since age 15 years
Borderline personality disorder	A pervasive pattern of instability of interpersonal relationships, self-image, and affects, and marked impulsivity beginning by early adulthood and present in a variety of contexts
Histrionic personality disorder	A pervasive pattern of excessive emotionality and attention-seeking, beginning by early adulthood and present in a variety of contexts
Narcissistic personality disorder	A pervasive pattern of grandiosity (in fantasy or behavior), need for admiration, and lack of empathy beginning by early adulthood and present in a variety of contexts
Avoidant personality disorder	A pervasive pattern of social inhibition, feelings of inadequacy, and hypersensitivity to negative evaluation, beginning by early adulthood and present in a variety of contexts
Dependent personality disorder	A pervasive and excessive need to be taken care of that leads to submissive and clinging behavior and fears of separation, beginning by early adulthood and present in a variety of contexts
Obsessive-compulsive personality disorder	A pervasive pattern of preoccupation with orderliness, perfectionism, and mental and interpersonal control, at the expense of flexibility, openness, and efficiency, beginning by early adulthood and present in a variety of contexts

*From American Psychiatric Association: *Diagnostic and statistical manual of mental disorders*, ed 4, text revision, Washington, DC, 2000, American Psychiatric Association.

mutual care goals. To overcome a problem with relatedness, the person must be involved with others. At first, the other person may be the nurse, but eventually others will take the nurse's place.

Short-term goals for these patients may focus on reducing acting-out behaviors and modifying specific communication patterns. Examples include the following:

- The patient will use verbal communication as an alternative to acting out.
- The patient will verbally identify angry feelings when they occur during a one-to-one interaction.

These goals should be developed with the patient's active participation.

Learning to relate more directly and openly causes anxiety. Therefore, the patient's ability to tolerate anxiety must be considered when setting goals. Increasing the anxiety level before the patient has increased coping ability and environmental supports may reinforce use of maladaptive coping behaviors (Klonsky, Oltmanns, and Turkheimer, 2003).

PLANNING

The nursing treatment plan provides a guide for intervention and promotes consistency among the treatment staff who provide care to the patient. This is particularly important when working with patients with maladaptive social responses. Planning also includes attending to the patient's educational needs. A Patient Education Plan for modifying impulsive behavior is presented in Table 22-4. It is an important and challenging part of the nurse's responsibility to

help patients and their families understand the nature and treatment of any of the disorders that cause maladaptive social responses.

IMPLEMENTATION

Patients with personality disorders come to treatment for help with depression, anxiety, alcoholism, or difficulties in work or personal relationships, not to have their personalities changed. In fact, they often regard any attempt to change their personality as unnecessary and intrusive. The focus of therapy therefore is to help patients change the thinking and the behavior that result from personality traits or limit the consequences and also to treat their symptoms of depression or other disorders.

Empirically validated treatments for some of the medical diagnoses related to personality disorders are summarized in Box 22-2 (Nathan and Gorman, 2002). The various therapies include corrective learning experiences in which the patient's relationship with the therapist serves as a model.

Protection From Self-Harm

The deliberate self-destructive or self-mutilating behavior of the borderline patient is very difficult to treat (see Chapter 20). Often the nursing staff must **observe the patient constantly** to prevent serious physical harm. At the same time, these patients have intense dependency needs related to an unresolved separation-individuation developmental phase. This makes it extremely difficult to wean them from constant

Table 22-4 PATIENT EDUCATION PLAN	Modifying Impulsive Behavior	
CONTENT	**INSTRUCTIONAL ACTIVITIES**	**EVALUATION**
Describe characteristics and consequences of impulsive behavior.	Select a situation in which impulsive behavior occurred. Ask the patient to describe what happened. Provide the patient with paper and a pen. Instruct the patient to keep a diary of impulsive actions, including a description of events before and after the incident.	The patient will identify and describe an impulsive incident. The patient will maintain a diary of impulsive behaviors. The patient will explore the causes and consequences of impulsive behavior.
Describe behaviors characteristic of interpersonal anxiety and relate anxiety to impulsive behavior.	Discuss the diary with the patient Help the patient to identify interpersonal anxiety related to impulsive behavior.	The patient will connect feelings of interpersonal anxiety with impulsive behavior.
Explain stress-reduction techniques.	Describe the stress response (see Chapter 16). Demonstrate relaxation exercises (see Chapter 31). Help the patient to return the demonstration.	The patient will perform relaxation exercises when signs of anxiety appear.
Identify alternative responses to anxiety-producing situations.	Using situations from the diary and knowledge of relaxation exercises, help the patient to list possible alternative responses	The patient will identify at least two alternative responses to each anxiety-producing situation. Practice using alternative responses to anxiety-producing situations.
Role-play each of the identified alternative behaviors.	Discuss the feelings associated with impulsive behavior and the alternatives.	The patient will describe the relationship between behavior and feelings. The patient will select and perform anxiety-reducing behaviors.

staff attention, and contact must be decreased very gradually. Observation may need to be increased again if the patient seems out of control.

Patient involvement in planning for decreased observation may be helpful. The patient must be reassured that less contact does not equal no contact. Consistent, scheduled time with a staff member is recommended. Primary nursing is particularly effective with a patient who needs to work through these separation issues (see Critical Thinking About Contemporary Issues).

Establishing a Therapeutic Relationship

No matter what type of maladaptive social response the patient is experiencing, nursing care is based on accessibility. The nurse must be **physically present** with the patient on a regular basis to foster an opportunity for interaction. **Psychological accessibility** must be a component of this regular interaction. This means that the nurse shows genuine interest in the patient. The nurse tries to understand the patient by clarifying meanings and validating perceptions. The nurse is also empathic.

BOX 22-2 | **SUMMARIZING THE EVIDENCE ON Personality Disorders**

Disorder	Avoidant personality disorder
Treatment	◆ Group administered behavioral interventions are effective in improving social skills. ◆ Antidepressants may be helpful as well.
Disorder	Borderline personality disorder
Treatment	◆ Dialectical behavioral therapy (DBT) produces lower attrition, fewer and less severe episodes of parasuicidal behavior, and fewer days of hospitalization. ◆ Partial hospitalization involving group and individual psychotherapy for 18 months decreases the number of suicidal attempts, acts of self-harm, psychiatric symptoms, and inpatient days and increases the quality of social and interpersonal functioning. ◆ Noradrenergic agents tend to improve mood but not irritability or dyscontrol. ◆ Serotonergic agents may act to decrease impulsivity.
Disorder	Mixed personality disorder (excluding cluster A disorders)
Treatment	◆ An average of 40 weeks of brief dynamic therapy yields substantial symptomatic improvement at both the end of treatment and after 1.5 years. ◆ Medications may be useful for several of these disorders, although many methodological problems remain to be worked out.
Disorder	Schizotypal personality disorder (and other cluster A disorders)
Treatment	◆ Antipsychotic medications may be useful in reducing some of the symptoms of these disorders.

From Nathan P, Gorman J: *A guide to treatments that work*, ed 2, New York, 2002, Oxford University Press.

Critical Thinking *About* Contemporary Issues

Should Constant Close Observation Be the Primary Nursing Approach for Borderline Patients With Impulsive Self-Harming Behavior?

Patients with borderline personality disorder are most often hospitalized because of impulsive attempts at self-mutilation or suicide. The nursing intervention of constant close observation is usually initiated to protect the patient from impulsive behavior. This intervention activates the patient's conflicts about close relationships. Splitting may become evident as the patient establishes preferences for the staff assigned to observation. The patient is challenged to outwit the staff and find opportunities to act out. When efforts are made to decrease the level of observation, the patient's attachment conflicts become evident. Behavior intended to maintain the undivided attention of staff by renewed self-harming behavior is often exhibited.

Much attention in the media recently has been directed toward an exploration of the use of restrictive environments, such as restraint and seclusion, in psychiatric settings. The focus has been on alternative interventions that are less restrictive or intrusive, staff training regarding the use of these interventions, and careful documentation. It is important to assist the patient in understanding the purpose of these interventions, enlisting the patient's help whenever possible, and encouraging the patient to participate in the steps necessary to change to a less restrictive modality as soon as he or she is ready. The nurse should encourage the patient's help in defining and describing the harmful behavior.

Identification of cues and triggers allows the patient to request assistance, thereby becoming an active participant in the therapeutic process. Nurses are less judgmental about the patient if they understand the source of the behaviors and if they are in touch with the patient's feelings. The challenges to nurses are to maintain the patient's safety, facilitate the patient's participation in care, select the least restrictive intervention, facilitate behavioral change, and help the patient assume responsibility for his behaviors.

In working with patients with personality disorders, the nurse must closely focus on monitoring appropriate levels of concern and monitoring the boundaries of the relationship (Nehls, 2000). If the nurse-patient relationship is a healthy one, the patient can learn how to find satisfaction in other human relationships (see A Patient Speaks).

Family Involvement

Because intimate relationships are always affected by maladaptive social responses, significant others must be involved in the plan of care (see A Family Speaks). This is especially important for manipulative patients, who often shift attention away from themselves by creating conflict between the family and the staff. For instance, the patient may complain to family members about poor nursing care. At the same time, the patient may tell the staff about mistreatment by the family. Staff and family are then in conflict. Attention is distracted from the patient, who then can avoid the discomfort of self-examination. When the staff finally realizes what is happening, the result is usually anger directed toward the patient. Nurses should be aware of this tendency and avoid a punitive response. When manipulative patients are hospitalized, this behavior is apt to occur many times. The patient returns home, still relating to others as objects. Family involvement is also important in promoting and maintaining positive change for the patient and family.

How would you help family members participate in the treatment of a person with a personality disorder? ■

Milieu Therapy

Because it is difficult and takes a long time to change maladaptive social responses, most patients are treated in the community rather than in an inpatient setting. However, sometimes hospitalization is needed. For instance, the person with a borderline personality disorder may be self-destructive, or the antisocial person may require a structured environ-

ment with limit setting. Day treatment or partial hospitalization programs can be advantageous in treating patients with borderline personality disorder; they offer them an acceptable level of intensiveness and containment, resulting in less regressive dependency and acting-out behavior (Smith, Ruiz-Sancho, and Gunderson, 2001).

The milieu, as found in hospitals, residential treatment, or outpatient programs, can effectively provide patients with an opportunity to gain insight into their behavior. Aside from staff limit setting, patients with maladaptive social responses learn from other patients about how much acting out will be tolerated. The patient responds well to a therapeutic milieu in which mature, responsible behavior is expected.

Milieu work with these patients is most effective if it focuses on realistic expectations and the processes of decision making and interactional behaviors in the here and now. Nursing functions when working with patients with personality disorders in milieu therapy are intended to:

- **Provide a structured environment.**
- **Serve as an emotional sounding board.**
- **Clarify and diagnose conflicts and consequences of actions.**
- **Facilitate adaptive change in behavior.**

Consistent clinical supervision is also very important because **transference** (intense emotional attachment or rejec-

---

A PATIENT SPEAKS

When I was hospitalized, the nurses were my link to the outside world. They were with me more than anyone else. They were also my link to the treatment that was prescribed by my psychiatrist. The doctor left prn orders because he thought I was a mature woman who could decide when I needed medication. I often felt a loss of dignity when the nurse questioned my need for the prn medication. Because the medicine decreased my anxiety, I think I was the best judge of when I needed it. Because the doctor made me responsible for requesting the medication, it was not the nurse's job to question my need for it unless I asked for more than was prescribed. Even if someone is in the hospital, she needs to be treated with dignity and respect. She is sick, not a child and not stupid. Nothing hurts more than being treated like a second-class citizen by people who are in a more powerful position. It is much easier to work with a nurse who is kind and supportive.

A FAMILY SPEAKS

It seems like my brother was always a problem. When we were growing up, he got us both into trouble all the time. Finally I learned to ignore his schemes and stay away from him. As he got older, the situation got worse. Our parents kicked him out of the house, but he would come back and promise to change, and they would let him back in. Then it would start all over again. He began to get into trouble with the law. First there was vandalism for spray-painting graffiti on a building; then he was with a gang of kids who stole a car. He said he was just along for the ride, but I didn't really believe him.

The rest of the family was pretty embarrassed about his behavior. I thought about telling people I was adopted so they wouldn't think I was like him. I didn't do that because I knew it would hurt my parents and they had enough trouble already. I'll never forget the night when the phone rang at 4:00 AM, and it was my brother saying he was in jail. He had been caught with drugs in a stolen car and also had resisted arrest. My parents refused to bail him out and he didn't have any money. The next day he called again to say that he was at the local psychiatric hospital. He had threatened to kill himself in jail, so they sent him to the hospital to see whether he was really mentally ill. My parents were really upset about this development. I think it was actually a good thing because the doctors and nurses at the hospital explained to us that he has a personality disorder. It did help to know that there might be a reason for his behavior, although he hasn't really changed much. I think my parents are beginning to accept this, but I know it's really hard for them.

tion derived from feelings about earlier personal relationships) and **countertransference** (the therapist's strong reaction to the patient, such as feelings of excessive sympathy, impatience, anger, or contempt; fantasies of rescue; moralistic distain; impulses to accept compliments from or identify with or hurt the patient) are often an issue when caring for these patients (see Chapter 2).

Positive countertransference by some staff members, and negative by others, leads to splitting and staff conflict. Whenever these behavioral patterns emerge while a manipulative patient is on the psychiatric unit, the staff must examine their level of involvement with the patient.

The principles of milieu treatment for patients with cluster B personality disorders include the following:

- Establish control with no option to escape involvement.
- Provide an experienced, consistent staff.
- Implement a clear structure with rules that are fair, firm, and consistently enforced.
- Provide support while the patient learns to experience painful feelings and try out new behavioral responses.

Limit Setting and Structure

The way the nurse approaches limit setting can make the difference between a productive hospital experience and one that is nonproductive or counterproductive. Angry, punitive limit setting confirms the patient's expectations. Suppressive and rigid limits create obstacles to self-exploration and therapeutic change. This approach also confirms the patient's belief of having little or no control over life situations. It is essential that the nurse not view limits as a way of controlling the patient. Rather, **limit setting must occur in the context of the patient and nurse working together toward the process of change.**

For example, a patient with antisocial personality structure engages in physically aggressive acting-out behavior. One way of dealing with this might be to emphasize the need for medications and to tighten up restrictions. The treatment team also might issue an ultimatum, such as "One more similar episode, and we're going to have to transfer you to another hospital."

A more positive way of approaching the situation could be worded as follows: "You seem to want to put the treatment team in the position of having to reassess continuation of your stay in this hospital. Has there been some change about wanting to help yourself?" The difference in the latter approach is emphasis on the idea that the patient has responsibility for life situations and that the control and the decisions belong to the patient (Suchman 2001). It also communicates an attitude of respect, which could boost the patient's self-esteem. The more the nurse is able to align with the nonregressed aspects of the patient's ego, the better are the chances for improved functioning.

Manipulative patients also should be held responsible for their behavior. They are skilled at placing responsibility on others. Staff members should communicate with each other so that consistent messages are given. These patients recognize any inconsistency and use it to focus attention on others. They usually resist rules. Staff and family members should collaborate in enforcing clear limits. Manipulative patients

sometimes lie. It is important to confront the patient who consciously lies.

Availability of staff attention combined with structured discipline is a definite need (Kerr, 2002). There must be an expectation that the patient will meet standards of healthy behavior. Failure to meet the standard is identified, and acting out is confronted. Loss of control may be dealt with by room restriction, with the patient instructed to think about the episode so that it may be discussed in therapy. The length of the restriction should be based on the seriousness of the behavior.

These approaches may lead to depression. The depressed feelings should be dealt with in formal psychotherapy sessions; but the staff also can act as role models for appropriate behavior. A school program, occupational therapy, and the milieu may be used to teach age-appropriate social skills and achievement skills. Reality orientation also may be necessary.

> *You believe that a manipulative adolescent patient is exploiting another patient by "borrowing" money, clothing, and snacks. When confronted, the first patient claims that the items were gifts, "because we're friends." Do you think that limit setting is needed? If so, how would you set appropriate limits?* ∎

Focusing on Strengths

Patients with maladaptive social responses often are effective leaders within the patient group. A useful nursing approach is to encourage them to **identify and use their strengths**. They may be given responsibilities within the patient care unit and can be helpful to other patients. They are often intelligent and can participate actively in planning their own care. However, they are extremely resistant to recognizing or dealing with feelings and need consistent encouragement to verbalize these emotions.

Nurses become frustrated with these patients because they seem to be so aware of what is happening and so in control of most situations, yet so unaware of others' needs. Nurses should remember that these patients have little tolerance for intimacy. Their maneuvering of others is a way to keep them at a safe distance. These patients are often charming, and it is easy to become involved with them. However, as soon as other people make demands or show signs of emotional closeness, the patients dilute the relationship by withdrawing, frustrating others, or distracting attention from themselves.

Journal writing is a nursing intervention that can be helpful to patients who have difficulty with close relationships. Keeping a diary of their thoughts and feelings helps them identify the various aspects of their interpersonal experiences and review them over time. It gives them an opportunity to see continuity of people and relationships. Interpersonal strengths can be identified and reinforced. The nurse also can note behavioral strengths that the patient has not yet identified and help the patient in recognizing these as well.

Behavioral Strategies

Various behavioral strategies can help decrease antisocial behavior (Stanley, Bundy, and Beberman, 2001). These can include **social skills training** and **anger management** among

Table 22-5	NURSING TREATMENT PLAN SUMMARY	Maladaptive Social Responses

Nursing Diagnosis: Impaired social interaction
Expected Outcome: The patient will obtain maximum interpersonal satisfaction by establishing and maintaining self-enhancing relationships with others.

SHORT-TERM GOAL	INTERVENTION	RATIONALE
The patient will participate in a therapeutic nurse-patient relationship.	Initiate a nurse-patient relationship contract mutually agreed on by patient and nurse. Develop mutual behavioral goals. Maintain consistent behavior by all nursing staff. Communicate honest responses to the patient's behavior. Provide honest, immediate feedback about behavioral change. Maintain confidentiality. Demonstrate accessibility.	An atmosphere of trust facilitates open expression of thoughts and feelings. A trusting relationship enables the patient to risk sharing feelings. Honest responses reinforce openness. Staff consistency creates a predictable environment that creates trust.
The patient will describe interpersonal strengths and weaknesses.	Provide opportunities to demonstrate strengths, such as helping other patients, assuming leadership roles. Help to analyze experiences that are perceived as failures. Communicate acceptance of the patient as a person while not accepting maladaptive social behavior.	Patients with maladaptive social responses are unable to identify accurately their interpersonal strengths and weaknesses, leading to fear of closeness and fear of failure. It is important to help the patient separate behavioral incidents from total self-worth and recognize that one can be liked even if imperfect.
The patient will establish or reestablish one interpersonal relationship that is mutually satisfying and adaptive.	Provide consistent feedback about adaptive and maladaptive social behavior. Encourage patient to describe successful and unsuccessful relationship experiences orally or in a written journal. Help patient in initiating or resuming a relationship with one other person. Review aspects of this relationship with the patient. Reinforce the patient's adaptive social responses. Evaluate with the patient alternatives to maladaptive social responses.	Describing and evaluating one's behavior requires taking responsibility for the behavior and its consequences. Patients need to go beyond understanding or insight to engaging in actual behavioral change. It is important for the nurse to help the patient evaluate whether one's responses are adaptive or maladaptive. Alternatives can then be identified to further the patient's goal achievement.

others (see Chapters 30 and 31). The patient is usually impatient with delays in gratification. Material rather than emotional rewards are preferred. Thus reinforcers used in a behavior modification program should be concrete and readily available.

Ignoring undesirable behavior is the least reinforcing but is not always possible. If behavior is disruptive and there must be a response, it should be matter-of-fact and one not desired by the patient. For instance, removal from contact with others for a specific period of time may discourage undesirable behavior, whereas a lecture that attracts attention may be a reinforcer.

A specific form of cognitive-behavioral therapy called **dialectical behavior therapy (DBT)** is an empirically validated treatment approach for patients with borderline personality disorder (Linehan, 1993; Alper and Peterson, 2001; APA, 2001). DBT uses behavioral and cognitive techniques that include psychological education, problem solving, training in social skills, exercises in monitoring moods, modeling by the therapist, homework assignments, and meditation. It is based on the assumption that temperament and an unresponsive

environment have made them unable to trust their own emotional responses or soothe themselves.

Dialectical behavior therapy has shown a high rate of effectiveness in decreasing hospital stays, suicide attempt frequency, visits to emergency rooms, and therapy attrition among patients with borderline personality disorder.

Medications

Medications have a limited role in the treatment of personality disorders (see Box 22-2). They are used primarily to relieve symptoms (anxiety, mood swings, impulsive aggression, psychotic delusion, hallucinations), thus facilitating other treatments (APA, 2001). The patient must be stable enough to take the medications as prescribed. Personal attention and reassurance by the nurse and the rest of the health care team are important.

A Nursing Treatment Plan Summary for the patient with impaired social interaction is presented in Table 22-5. A Nursing Treatment Plan Summary for the patient at risk for self-mutilation is presented in Table 22-6.

| Table 22-6 | NURSING TREATMENT PLAN SUMMARY | Maladaptive Social Responses |

Nursing Diagnosis: Risk for self-mutilation
Expected Outcome: The patient will select constructive rather than self-destructive ways of coping with interpersonal anxiety.

SHORT-TERM GOAL	INTERVENTION	RATIONALE
The patient will not engage in self-mutilation.	Develop a contract with the patient to notify staff when anxiety is increasing. Provide close 1:1 observation of the patient when necessary to maintain safety. Remove all potentially dangerous objects from the patient and the environment. Provide prescribed medications.	When the patient is unable to cope with anxiety, safety is the nurse's highest priority. A contract helps the patient assume responsibility and explore healthier coping responses.
The patient will describe self-mutilating episodes.	Help the patient review these events. Identify cues and triggers that precede self-mutilating behavior. Help the patient explore feelings related to these episodes.	Self-mutilation is often a way of relieving extreme anxiety. Structured interpersonal support can help the patient review these events.
The patient will describe alternatives to self-mutilation.	Suggest alternative behaviors such as seeking interpersonal support or engaging in an adaptive anxiety-reducing activity.	The nurse can help the patient review the full range of adaptive responses. Supportive but critical evaluation is necessary for behavioral change.
The patient will implement one new adaptive response when experiencing high interpersonal anxiety.	Help the patient select new adaptive responses. Reinforce the patient's adaptive behavior. Identify positive consequences of the adaptive responses. Discuss ways these may be generalized to other situations.	The nurses should take an active role in setting limits, examining patient behaviors, and reinforcing adaptive actions. These new learned responses also can be reviewed for their applicability to other life events.

EVALUATION

Evaluating the success of nursing interventions is difficult when the focus is on the quality of the therapeutic relationship. Because the relationship is central to effective nursing care, it is threatening for many nurses to examine their ability to relate to others. This type of evaluation must take place on two levels.

One level of evaluation focuses on the nurse and the nurse's participation in the relationship. Self-examination may be useful in accomplishing this, especially if the nurse reviews an interaction immediately. Blind spots about one's own feelings that may be present while involved with the patient may become clearer in retrospect.

However, self-evaluation is colored by self-perceptions. Supervision by an experienced nurse therapist can thus be very helpful in identifying aspects of the nurse-patient relationship that may be less obvious to the nurse. Constructive supervision can help nurses identify the dynamics of the relationship. It also can help them deal with patients' resistance to change. No matter how experienced, nurses' perceptions of their participation in a relationship are affected by their self-concept. The need for supervision continues throughout their career.

The second level of evaluation focuses on the patient's behavior and the behavioral changes that the nurse works to facilitate. The patient is the primary source of input about these changes. Perceived changes in behavior should be validated with the patient to see whether the patient is also aware of change. Sharing feelings and intimate thoughts denotes increased trust and a willingness to risk self-revelation.

Nonverbally the patient also reveals responses to the therapeutic relationship. Accessibility to the nurse for scheduled meetings indicates trust and involvement in the relationship. Eye contact usually occurs more often when one person is comfortable with another. Initiation of activities with others indicates more openness to relatedness. Increased decision making and assumption of leadership roles imply improved self-esteem and increasing self-confidence. Such behaviors can be observed, documented, and validated with other staff members. Therefore, these are useful evaluation criteria.

Significant others also may contribute to the evaluation. They can provide valuable information about the patient's baseline behaviors. It also helps them understand new, more adaptive behaviors learned by the patient, and it gives them an idea of reasonable expectations.

Several questions may help the nurse evaluate the outcomes of interventions with the patient who has maladaptive social responses:

- Has the patient become less impulsive, manipulative, or narcissistic?
- Does the patient express satisfaction with the quality of his or her relationships?
- Can the patient participate in close relationships?
- Does the patient express recognition of positive behavioral change?

COMPETENT CARING

A Clinical Exemplar of a Psychiatric Nurse
REATHA L. RYAN, PMHNP, RN, CS, CHT

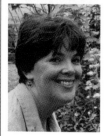

A patient with the diagnosis of borderline personality disorder is often branded and labeled with the letter "B" by the treatment staff. This diagnosis may be inappropriately assigned to an inpatient because staff are irritated and judgmental of the patient's behavior. Some psychiatric nurses apply this "diagnosis" without ever consulting the *DSM-IV-TR* to see if the criteria are actually met. Perhaps the frustrated nurse is stuck in his or her own projections and countertransference. The nurse also may be reacting to defensive, immature, or regressive behavior displayed by the patient. This less than adequate functioning by the patient is often part of the very reason for the patient's admission for care.

I saw the many dimensions of this problem in my first job as a nurse on the adult unit of a private psychiatric hospital. I was practicing active listening, validation, reflection, and many other of my newly learned communication skills when the head nurse got a call from admissions, advising her that "Jane Don't" would be brought to the ward in 30 minutes. As word spread among the staff nurses, there were many groans, heads shaking, and negative comments such as "She's a sickie." "Look out, she's a manipulator." "She's stuck in the revolving door and she'll never get better anyway." My stomach turned and twisted inside as I heard such negative comments and expectations for this yet-to-be admitted patient. Did she stand a chance of getting better if the staff expected her to fail? I made a mental note to myself to bring this up in a staff meeting. I wanted to talk about the power of our words, thoughts, and expectations. I wanted to talk about how I felt when I heard that kind of talk.

I closed my ears to the negative comments, as I heard myself volunteering to admit this patient. As I went through the process of admission with "Jane Don't," I was warm and empathetic, listening and professional. When she barked at me, "I don't want anyone touching me," I was surprised. Yet soon I was able to shift to a neutral space internally, with the help of a deep breath and the determination to ground my energy squarely over my feet. "I will not take this personally," I said to myself. I calmly continued, letting Jane know that I would not touch her without her permission. I let her know that I respected her but that there were times when certain tasks required touching. I explained that checking her blood pressure and pulse would require some touching. I let her choose when that would happen. "Would you like to have your blood pressure checked now, or after lunch, in about an hour?" Jane responded, "You may as well go ahead." By giving her two acceptable choices, she could make a decision and feel empowered, and I could still get done what I needed to do. I explained each thing I was going to do, before I touched her. She cooperated. This cooperation increased as she learned to trust me. Though she would still have her outbursts, by maintaining my professionalism and shifting to neutral, I was able to accept her and work with her as she was, without being emotionally reactive to her. I kept my expectations for her positive, and pointed out places of improvement, no matter how small.

What I learned from this patient was that the social and interactive functioning of the hospitalized patient may not meet the norm. The patient is ill and behavioral functioning is often compromised. The nurse does well to maintain professionalism in working with this type of patient. He or she can choose to "shift into neutral" in regard to one's own judgments, reactions, and personal projections. Only by consciously making this shift can the nurse truly function professionally. Instead of joining in with the negative comments of other staff, the professional nurse can be therapeutic, functioning with respect, clarity, and positive regard for all patients, including those with borderline traits or a borderline personality disorder. ■

CHAPTER FOCUS POINTS

- In a healthy relationship, people experience intimacy with each other while maintaining their own separate identities. Adaptive social responses include the capacity for solitude, autonomy, mutuality, and interdependence. Maladaptive responses include manipulation, impulsivity, and narcissism.
- Personality is shaped by biology and social learning including hereditary biological dispositions and the influence of affective bonds with important others.
- A personality disorder is a set of patterns or traits that hinder a person's ability to maintain meaningful relationships, feel fulfilled, and enjoy life. The fixed, enduring quality of specific personality disorder symptoms is an essential element of the diagnosis.
- Three features of personality disorders are (1) the individual has acquired few strategies for relating and their approach to relationships and to the environment is inflexible and maladaptive; (2) there is a tendency for the individual's needs, perceptions, and behavior to foster vicious cycles that continue unhelpful patterns and provoke negative reactions from others; and (3) the individual's adaptation is characterized by tenuous stability, fragility, and lack of resilience when faced with stressful situations.
- Cluster A includes personality disorders of an odd or eccentric nature (paranoid, schizoid, and schizotypal personality disorders). Cluster B disorders are of an erratic, dramatic, or emotional nature (antisocial,

borderline, histrionic, and narcissistic personality disorders). Cluster C includes disorders of an anxious or fearful nature (avoidant, dependent, and obsessive-compulsive personality disorders).
- The diagnosis of antisocial personality disorder is applied when an individual consistently ignores social rules; is manipulative, exploitative, or dishonest; lacks remorse for actions; and is frequently involved in criminal activity.
- Impulsive aggression is the hallmark of borderline personality disorder, and it plays a pivotal role in the borderline person's self-mutilation, unstable relationships, violence, and completed suicides.
- People with narcissistic personality disorders have fragile self-esteem, driving them to search constantly for praise, appreciation, and admiration.
- It is helpful to include a description of the patient's usual relationships in the nursing assessment.
- Current research supports the multifactorial origins of personality disorders, including a variety of predisposing neurobiological, early developmental, and sociocultural factors.
- Precipitating stressors that affect social responses include sociocultural values and norms and psychological pressures.
- A wide array of relationships and interests provide coping resources.
- Coping mechanisms associated with maladaptive social responses are attempts to cope with anxiety related to threatened or actual

CHAPTER FOCUS POINTS—cont'd

- loneliness and may include idealization of others, devaluation of others, projection, acting out, splitting, and projective identification.
- Primary NANDA nursing diagnoses are defensive coping, chronic low self-esteem, risk for self-mutilation, impaired social interaction, and risk for violence (self-directed or directed at others).
- Primary *DSM-IV-TR* diagnoses are paranoid, schizoid, schizotypal, histrionic, antisocial, narcissistic, borderline, obsessive-compulsive, dependent, and avoidant personality disorders.
- The expected outcome of nursing care is that the patient will obtain maximum satisfaction by establishing and maintaining self-enhancing relationships with others.

- The plan of nursing care must be realistic, considering the patient's ability to tolerate anxiety, and promote consistency of interventions.
- Primary nursing interventions for patients with maladaptive social responses include protection from self-harm, establishing a therapeutic relationship, family involvement, milieu therapy, limit setting and structure, focusing on strengths, and behavioral interventions.
- One level of evaluation focuses on the nurse and the nurse's participation in the relationship. Another level is based on the patient's recognition of improvement in the quality and quantity of interpersonal relationships.

KEY TERMS

antisocial personality disorder, 428
borderline personality disorder, 429
manipulation, 427

narcissism, 429
narcissistic personality disorder, 429
personality disorder, 425

CHAPTER REVIEW QUESTIONS

1. For each personality disorder listed in Column A, select the cluster from Column B to which it belongs.

Column A

_____ Antisocial personality disorder
_____ Avoidant personality disorder
_____ Borderline personality disorder
_____ Dependent personality disorder
_____ Histrionic personality disorder
_____ Narcissistic personality disorder
_____ Obsessive-compulsive personality disorder
_____ Paranoid personality disorder
_____ Schizoid personality disorder
_____ Schizotypal personality disorder

Column B

A. Cluster A
B. Cluster B
C. Cluster C

2. Fill in the blanks.

A. Personality disorders are usually recognizable by

_____ and continue throughout

much of _____.

B. Patients with _____ are high users of psychiatric treatment and are particularly at risk for suicidal behavior, depression, and substance use disorders.

C. Low levels of the neurotransmitter _____ have been reported in people prone to aggressive and impulsive behaviors.

D. The inability to integrate the good and bad aspects of oneself

and of objects is called _____.

E. _____ occurs when one projects part of oneself onto different people.

F. Clinical supervision is important for the psychiatric nurse working with patients with personality disorders because

_____ is often an issue when working with these patients.

3. Provide short answers for the following questions.

A. Identify the three distinguishing characteristics of personality disorders.

B. Describe the two levels of evaluation necessary when working with patients with personality disorders.

C. In the United States, the diagnosis of borderline personality is most often given to females; males most often are given the diagnosis of antisocial personality disorder. Discuss the impact of American culture on this issue. Explore how these diagnoses are made in other cultures.

D. Analyze yourself and members of your family in respect to their states of relatedness: connectedness, disconnectedness, parallelism, and enmeshment.

E. Analyze yourself and members of your family in respect to their states of relatedness and their developmental life stage.

Visit Evolve for additional resources related to the content of this chapter.

http://evolve.elsevier.com/Stuart/principles/
• Topical Course Outline • Student Workbook Exercises • Critical Thinking Questions and Activities • Case Studies • Research Topics
• Monthly Content Updates • WebLinks

Student Study CD-ROM

Access the accompanying CD-ROM for animations, interactive exercises, review questions for the NCLEX examination, and an audio glossary.

REFERENCES

Agronin ME, Maletta G: Personality disorders in late life: understanding and overcoming the gap in research, *Am J Geriatr Psychiatry* 8:4, 2000.

Alper G, Peterson SJ: Dialectical behavior therapy for patients with borderline personality disorder, *J Psychosoc Nurs Ment Health Serv* 39:38, 2001.

American Psychiatric Association: *Diagnostic and statistical manual of mental disorders*, ed 4, text revision, Washington, DC, 2000, American Psychiatric Association.

American Psychiatric Association: Practice guideline for the treatment of patients with borderline personality disorder, *Am J Psychiatry* 158:4, 2001.

Bateman AW, Fonagy P: Effectiveness of psychotherapeutic treatment of personality disorder, *Br J Psychiatry* 177:138, 2000.

Blashfield RK, Intoccia V: Growth of the literature on the topic of personality disorders, *Am J Psychiatry* 157:472, 2000.

Booth R: Loneliness as a component of psychiatric disorders, *Medscape Ment Health* 5:1, 2000.

Brown A, Dodson K: Borderline personality disorder, *NARSAD Research Newsletter* 153:3, 1999.

Grinspoon L: Personality disorders, *Harvard Mental Health Letter* 16:1, 2000.

Hawton K et al: Comorbidity of axis I and axis II disorders in patients who attempted suicide, *Am J Psychiatry* 160:1494, 2003.

Johnson JG et al: Adolescent personality disorders associated with violence and criminal behavior during adolescence and early adulthood, *Am J Psychiatry* 157:1406, 2000.

Kaylor L: Antisocial personality disorder: diagnostic, ethical, and treatment issus, *Issues Ment Health Nurs* 20:247, 1999.

Kerr N: Clinical management of "entitled" clients, *J Psychsoc Nurs Ment Health Serv* 40:40, 2002.

Klonsky ED, Oltmanns TF, Turkheimer E: Deliberate self-harm in a nonclinical population: prevalence and psychological correlates, *Am J Psychiatry* 160:1501, 2003.

Lewis JM: Repairing the bond in important relationships: a dynamic for personality maturation, *Am J Psychiatry* 157:1375, 2000.

Linehan M: *Skills training manual for treating borderline personality disorder*, New York, 1993, The Guilford Press.

Liotti G, Pasquini L: Predictive factors for borderline personality disorder: patients' early traumatic experiences and losses suffered by the attachment figure, *Acta Psychiatr Scand* 102:282, 2000.

Masterson J: *Treatment of the borderline adolescent: a developmental approach*, New York, 1985, Brunner/Hazel.

Miller M: Antisocial personality—part I, *The Harvard Mental Health Letter* 17:1, 2000.

Miller M: Antisocial personality—part II, *The Harvard Mental Health Letter* 17:1, 2001.

Millon T, Davis R: *The development of personality disorders*, New York, 1995, Wiley.

Nathan PE, Gorman JM, editors: *A guide to treatments that work*, ed 2, New York, 2002, Oxford University Press.

Nehls N: Being a case manager for persons with borderline personality disorder: perspectives of community mental health center clinicians, *Arch Psychiatr Nurs* 14:12, 2000.

Pally R: The neurobiology of borderline personality disorder: the synergy of "nature and nurture," *J Psychiatr Pract* 8:133, 2002.

Paris J: Chronic suicidality among patients with borderline personality disorder, *Psychiatr Serv* 53:738, 2002.

Perry JC, Banon E, Ianni F: Effectiveness of psychotherapy for personality disorders, *Am J Psychiatry* 156:1312, 1999.

Raine A et al: Reduced prefrontal gray matter volume and reduced autonomic activity in antisocial personality disorder, *Arch Gen Psychiatry* 57:119, 2000.

Reid WH: Antisocial personality, psychopathy, and forensic psychiatry, *J Psychiatr Pract* 7:55, 2001.

Rogers C: *On becoming a person*, Boston, 1961, Houghton Mifflin.

Sargent J et al: Sense of belonging as a buffer against depressive symptoms, *J Am Psychiatr Nurs Assoc* 8:120, 2002.

Shea MT et al: Short-term diagnostic stability of schizotypal, borderline, avoidant, and obsessive-compulsive personality disorders, *Am J Psychiatry* 159:2036, 2002.

Smith GW, Ruiz-Sancho A, Gunderson JG: An intensive outpatient program for patients with borderline personality disorder, *Psychiatr Serv* 52:532, 2001.

Stanley B et al: Are suicide attempters who self-mutilate a unique population? *Am J Psychiatry* 158:427, 2001.

Stanley B, Bundy E, Beberman R: Skills training as an adjunctive treatment for personality disorders, *J Psychiatr Pract* 7:324, 2001.

Suchman A: Control and relation: two foundational values and their consequences, *Issues Interdisc Care* 3:145, 2001.

Zanarini MC et al: The longitudinal course of borderline psychopathology: 6-year prospective follow-up of the phenomenology of borderline personality disorder, *Am J Psychiatry* 160:274, 2003.

Cogito, ergo sum. I think, therefore I am.

DESCARTES

COGNITIVE RESPONSES AND ORGANIC MENTAL DISORDERS

23

Michele T. Laraia

LEARNING OBJECTIVES

After studying this chapter, the student should be able to:

1. Describe the continuum of adaptive and maladaptive cognitive responses (**I**).
2. Identify behaviors associated with cognitive responses (**II**).
3. Analyze predisposing factors, precipitating stressors, and the appraisal of stressors related to cognitive responses (**II**).
4. Describe coping resources and coping mechanisms related to cognitive responses (**II**).
5. Formulate nursing diagnoses related to cognitive responses (**III**).
6. Examine the relationship between nursing diagnoses and medical diagnoses related to cognitive responses (**III**).
7. Identify expected outcomes and short-term nursing goals related to cognitive responses (**IV**).
8. Develop a family education plan to help caregivers cope with maladaptive cognitive responses (**V**).
9. Analyze nursing interventions related to cognitive responses (**VI**).
10. Evaluate nursing care related to cognitive responses (**VII**).

TOPICAL OUTLINE

I. Continuum of Cognitive Responses
II. Assessment
   A. Behaviors
   B. Predisposing Factors
   C. Precipitating Stressors
   D. Appraisal of Stressors
   E. Coping Resources
   F. Coping Mechanisms
III. Diagnosis
   A. Nursing Diagnoses
   B. Medical Diagnoses
IV. Outcome Identification
V. Planning
VI. Implementation
   A. Intervening in Delirium
   B. Intervening in Dementia
VII. Evaluation

evolve Visit Evolve for additional resources related to the content of this chapter.
http://evolve.elsevier.com/Stuart/principles/

The ability to think and reason and to behave accordingly is a distinguishing feature of human beings. This ability created civilization and allowed the progression from the Stone Age to the Space Age and beyond. Information is growing at such a rapid rate that there is an overwhelming demand for each person to assimilate new information daily. Society has moved from the time when power meant physical strength, to the use of money to acquire power, to an era in which power lies in having the latest information.

Intellectual functioning is highly valued in Western society. Most people fear the possibility of losing their cognitive abilities of reasoning, memory, judgment, orientation, perception, and attention. These functions allow a person to make sense of experience and interact productively with the environment. Maladaptive cognitive responses leave the affected person in a state of confusion—unable to understand and learn from experience and unable to relate current to past events or to interact reasonably with the people in his or her life. Maladaptive cognitive responses change the way in which individuals think of themselves and the world in which they find themselves, as well as how the world thinks of and relates to them in return.

■ CONTINUUM OF COGNITIVE RESPONSES

Learning may be defined as any relatively permanent change in behavior that results from experience. Learning involves biological changes in the brain that are affected by external environments (the experience of the world in which humans are raised) and internal environments (genetic characteristics, developmental events, neurotransmission). All organisms can modify their behavior by instinctive, reflexive, and maturational responses to the environment, but human behavior is particularly affected by the ability to learn from experience, to remember what is learned, and to modify behavior in response.

Memory is defined as the storage and retrieval of past experience and, like learning, is a neurochemical process mediated by the brain. Memory is a key cognitive ability; to exercise judgment, make decisions, or even be oriented to time and place, a person must remember past experiences. Therefore memory loss is a particularly frightening symptom.

There are several types of memory, each with specific biological correlates and clinical implications; these different types of memory work together in most learning situations. Figure 23-1 depicts different types of learning and memory and their behavioral and biological correlates.

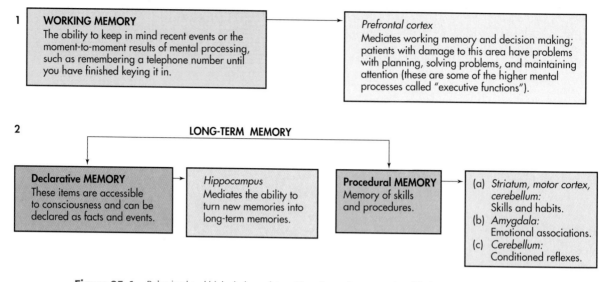

1

WORKING MEMORY
The ability to keep in mind recent events or the moment-to-moment results of mental processing, such as remembering a telephone number until you have finished keying it in.

Prefrontal cortex
Mediates working memory and decision making; patients with damage to this area have problems with planning, solving problems, and maintaining attention (these are some of the higher mental processes called "executive functions").

2   **LONG-TERM MEMORY**

Declarative MEMORY
These items are accessible to consciousness and can be declared as facts and events.

Hippocampus
Mediates the ability to turn new memories into long-term memories.

Procedural MEMORY
Memory of skills and procedures.

(a) *Striatum, motor cortex, cerebellum:*
Skills and habits.
(b) *Amygdala:*
Emotional associations.
(c) *Cerebellum:*
Conditioned reflexes.

Figure 23-1   Behavioral and biological correlates of learning and memory. (Modified from Nolte J: *The human brain: an introduction to its functional anatomy,* ed 4, St Louis, 2000, Mosby.)

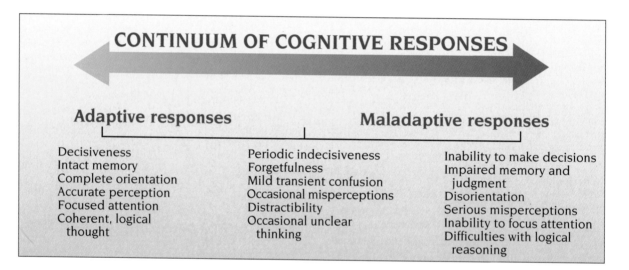

CONTINUUM OF COGNITIVE RESPONSES

Adaptive responses   **Maladaptive responses**

Decisiveness	Periodic indecisiveness	Inability to make decisions
Intact memory	Forgetfulness	Impaired memory and
Complete orientation	Mild transient confusion	judgment
Accurate perception	Occasional misperceptions	Disorientation
Focused attention	Distractibility	Serious misperceptions
Coherent, logical	Occasional unclear	Inability to focus attention
thought	thinking	Difficulties with logical
		reasoning

Figure 23-2   Continuum of cognitive responses.

In some people with brain dysfunction, cognitive responses either do not develop fully or deteriorate once they have developed. In general, maladaptive cognitive responses that occur during childhood are called *developmental disabilities* or *mental retardation.* The reader is referred to a textbook of pediatric nursing for a discussion of these disorders.

This chapter considers maladaptive cognitive responses in the adult. Although maladaptive cognitive responses may occur at any age, they are most common in the elderly. It is recommended that this chapter be read in conjunction with Chapter 38, because the content of these two chapters is complementary.

Maladaptive cognitive responses include **an inability to make decisions, impaired memory and judgment, disorientation, misperceptions, decreased attention span,** and **difficulties with logical reasoning.** They may occur episodically or be present continuously. Depending on the stressor, the condition may be reversible or characterized by a progressive

deterioration in functioning. Figure 23-2 illustrates the continuum of cognitive responses.

The knowledge of how to get to school or work is a mixture of learned habits, attention, procedures, and remembered facts. Explain this using the biological and behavioral model of learning and memory to the caregiver of a patient with Alzheimer's disease. ■

ASSESSMENT

Behaviors

Maladaptive cognitive responses are most apparent in people who have a psychiatric diagnosis of delirium, dementia, and amnestic and other cognitive disorders as described in the *DSM-IV-TR* (American Psychiatric Association, 2000). Such responses are classified as cognitive because they feature as a cardinal symptom an impairment in important functions such as memory, language, or attention.

Discussions in this chapter focus primarily on delirium and dementia because these are the psychiatric diagnostic categories related to cognitive impairment that nurses encounter most often. Assessment relies heavily on both biological findings (see Chapter 6) and on the results of the mental status examination (see Chapter 7).

Cognitive activity is dependent on **intelligence, education, life experience,** and **culture.** These variables among patients can affect test scores, but not all rating scales of cognitive function or raters take them into account. The nurse should consider that some measures may have these shortcomings when assessing patients with varied abilities and from varied sociocultural backgrounds.

Associated With Delirium. Delirium is the behavioral response to widespread disturbances in cerebral metabolism, effecting 2 million patients a year in the United States. **It represents a sudden decline from a previous level of functioning and is usually considered a medical emergency that can lead to death or permanent cognitive decline in some cases if not treated.**

Delirium should be considered any time there is an acute change in mental status. It is a syndrome with many possible causes and is thought to be the result of the interaction of a vulnerable patient and several risk factors. Although delirium can occur at any age, advanced age is probably the greatest risk factor. It often occurs in hospitalized patients, but also can occur after hospitalization and in many cases may result from medications or medical procedures.

Delirium results in disturbances in the following areas:

- **Consciousness**—Reduced clarity or awareness of the environment
- **Attention**—Impaired ability to direct and maintain mental focus, resulting in problems with processing stimuli into information
- **Cognition**—Recent memory impairment, disorientation to time and person, or language disturbance
- **Perception**—Misinterpretations, illusion, or hallucinations
- **Motor ability**—Poor balance, ambulation, or coordination

Thus the patient experiences a diminished awareness of the environment that involves sensory misperceptions and disordered thought (disturbed attention, memory, thinking, and orientation) and also experiences disturbances of psychomotor activity and the sleep-wake cycle. These disturbances develop rapidly (over hours to days) and tend to fluctuate over the course of the day, with occasional periods of mental clarity. The disturbances usually worsen at night. The clinical example that follows illustrates the behavior typical of a patient who is delirious.

CLINICAL EXAMPLE

Ms. S was brought to the emergency department of a general hospital by her parents. This 22-year-old single woman was described as having been in good health until 2 days before admission, when she complained of malaise

and a sore throat and stayed home from work. She worked as a typist in a small office and had a stable employment record. According to her parents, she had an active social life, and there were no significant conflicts at home.

On admission, Ms. S was extremely restless and had a frightened facial expression. Her speech was garbled and incoherent. When approached by an unfamiliar person, she would become agitated, try to climb out of bed, and strike out aimlessly. Occasionally she would slip into a restless sleep. Her temperature on admission was 104° F (40° C) rectally, her pulse was 108 beats per minute, and her respirations were 28 per minute. Her skin was hot, dry, and flushed. According to her mother, Ms. S had only a few sips of water in the last 24 hours and had not urinated at all, but she had experienced several episodes of profuse diaphoresis.

Ms. S's ability to cooperate with a mental status examination was limited. She would respond to her own name by turning her head. When her mother asked her where she was, she said "home," but she could not say where her home was. She would give only the month when asked for the date and said it was January (the actual date was February 19). She also refused to give the day of the week. A neurological examination was negative for signs of increased intracranial pressure or for localized signs of central nervous system (CNS) disease.

The tentative medical diagnosis was delirium secondary to fever of unknown origin. Symptomatic treatment of the fever, including intravenous fluids, an aspirin suppository, and a cool water mattress, was begun immediately while further diagnostic studies were performed. Nurses caring for Ms. S noticed that she continued to be restless and disoriented and that her speech was still incoherent. They also noticed that she was picking at the bed clothing. Suddenly she became extremely agitated and tried to get out of bed while crying out, "Bugs, get away, get bugs away!" She was brushing and slapping at herself and the bed. As her mother and the nurse talked with her and held her, she gradually became calmer but periodically continued to slap at "the bugs" and needed reassurance and reorientation.

Additional laboratory results became available later in the day. A lumbar puncture was normal, as was magnetic resonance imaging (MRI) of the head. Results of a toxicological screening of the blood were also negative. However, the electroencephalogram revealed diffuse slowing. In addition, the elevated white blood count and electrolyte imbalance were consistent with severe dehydration. Cultures of Ms. S's throat and blood were both positive for beta-hemolytic streptococci, and intravenous antibiotic therapy was begun at once while other supportive measures were continued.

Ms. S's mental state improved as the infection gradually came under control and the fever decreased. Her cognitive functioning was completely normal when she was discharged from the hospital a week later, with the exception of amnesia for the time during which she was delirious.

Selected Nursing Diagnoses

- Hyperthermia related to infection, as evidenced by elevated temperature; hot, dry, flushed skin; and diaphoresis
- Deficient fluid volume related to decreased fluid intake, as evidenced by anuria for 24 hours and hot, dry, flushed skin
- Risk for injury related to fear and disorientation, as evidenced by agitated behavior
- Impaired verbal communication related to altered brain chemistry, as evidenced by garbled and incoherent speech
- Disturbed sensory perception (visual) related to altered brain chemistry, as evidenced by the hallucination of bugs
- Disturbed thought process related to altered brain chemistry, as evidenced by disorientation ■

BOX 23-1

Reversible Causes of Dementia

- Subdural hematoma
- Tumor (especially meningioma)
- Cerebral vasculitis
- Hydrocephalus

Table 23-1   Types and Occurrence Rates of Dementia

Type of Dementia	Rate (%)
Vascular dementias Multi-infarct dementia	5%
Vascular dementias with Alzheimer's disease	10%
Alzheimer's disease	**65%**
Alzheimer's disease plus dementia with Lewy bodies	5%
Dementia with Lewy bodies Parkinsonian dementia	7%
AIDS dementia complex Frontal lobe dementia Creutzfeldt-Jakob disease Corticobasal degeneration Supranuclear palsy	8%

Data from Zurad E: New treatments of Alzheimer's disease: a review, *Behavioral Health Trends*, 2002.

Ms. S demonstrates many behaviors often seen in patients with delirium. These behaviors have a sudden onset and are related to alterations in neurochemical and electrical responses in the brain as a result of the stressor that causes the maladaptive response. Disorientation is generally present and sometimes is present in all three spheres of time, place, and person. Thought processes are usually disorganized. Judgment is poor, and little decision-making ability exists.

Stimuli may be misinterpreted, resulting in illusions or distortions of reality. An example of such an illusion is the perception that a polka-dot drape is actually covered with cockroaches. Delirious patients may **hallucinate.** These hallucinations are usually visual and often take the form of animals, reptiles, or insects. They are real to the person experiencing them and are very frightening. Assaultive or destructive behavior may be the patient's attempt to strike back at a hallucinated image.

At times, patients with delirium also exhibit a labile affect, changing abruptly from laughter to tearfulness and vice versa for no apparent reason. A loss of usual social behavior also may be noted, resulting in acts such as undressing, playing with food, and grabbing at others. Delirious patients tend to act on impulse.

Other behaviors may be specifically related to the cause of the behavioral syndrome. For example, Ms. S's brain syndrome and the fever and dehydration she experienced were a result of her systemic streptococcal infection. It is very important that observations of behavior be described carefully, because this helps identify the stressor. Treatment is usually conservative until a specific stressor has been isolated. Although most patients recover, it is possible for the person to develop long-term disabilities or to die as a result of the severity of the stressor.

Delirium is commonly found in hospitalized patients, particularly in intensive care units, geriatric psychiatry units, emergency departments, alcohol treatment units, and oncology units. In addition, a diagnosis of delirium can be missed because the symptoms are assumed to be caused by depression. If adequate intervention does not take place, delirium may become chronic and irreversible.

Associated With Dementia. Dementia is a maladaptive cognitive response that features a loss of intellectual abilities and interferes with the patient's usual social or occupational activities. The loss of intellectual ability includes an impairment of memory, judgment, and abstract thought. The patient with dementia does not have the clouding of awareness or the rapid onset that is seen with delirium.

The onset of dementia is usually gradual. It may result in progressive deterioration, or the condition may become stable. Personality changes often occur and may appear either as an alteration or as an accentuation of the person's usual character traits. In some cases the process of dementia can be reversed, and the person's intellectual functioning improves if the underlying stressors are identified and treated. Reversible sources of dementia are listed in Box 23-1.

However, in many cases dementia involves a continual and irreversible decline in mental function and behavior. **Senility** or **senile** are nonspecific terms with negative connotations, and therefore the use of these terms to describe persons with diminished cognitive responses is discouraged.

Dementia may occur at any age but most often affects the elderly. This condition results from structural and neurochemical changes in the brain as a result of trauma, infection, cerebrovascular disruptions, substance use, or an unknown cause. **Alzheimer's disease** (AD) is the most common type of dementia and accounts for approximately 65% of cases of dementia. There are several other types of dementia, and these are listed in Table 23-1.

It is estimated that 4.8 million people in the United States have AD at an annual cost of $80 billion. The prevalence of AD doubles every 5 years in those between 65 and 85 years of age and is present in every race and ethnic group. The onset of symptoms occurs after 40 years of age in 96% of cases and between 45 and 65 years of age in 80% of cases.

Early-onset AD is associated with a more rapid course and genetic predisposition as compared with late-onset AD. AD is the fourth leading cause of death after 75 years of age. Figure 23-3 graphically presents the estimated numbers of new AD cases that will occur in the United States. The following clinical example demonstrates the behaviors associated with dementia.

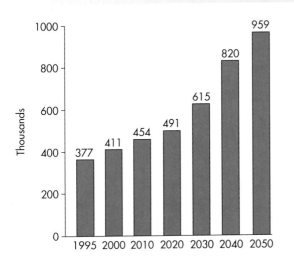

Figure 23-3   Estimated number of new Alzheimer's disease cases (in thousands). (From National Institute of Aging: Alzheimer's disease: unraveling the mystery, NIH pub number: 02-3782, 2002, US Department of Health and Human Services, National Institutes of Health.)

CLINICAL EXAMPLE

Mr. B is a 73-year-old widower who has resided in a retirement home for 3 years. He chose to move to the retirement home after his wife's death even though his son encouraged him to live with him and his family. Mr. B stated that he did not want to burden his family and would be happier with others of his same age. He did well for the first 18 months. He was an active participant in social groups both in the home and in his church, which he continued to attend regularly. He also visited his son once a week and enjoyed seeing his grandchildren and puttering around his son's house.

Approximately 18 months ago Mr. B began to seem forgetful. He would ask the same question several times and on occasion prepared for church on a Friday or Saturday. He also became irritable and accused his son of not caring about him and of abandoning him in "that place." Mr. B spent many hours taking papers from his desk and studying them. When asked what he was doing, he would say, "Attending to my business." He began to withdraw from activities and make flimsy excuses to avoid playing his favorite card game, gin rummy. When persuaded to play, he usually quit in frustration because he could not remember which cards had been played. Mr. B was quite anxious at times. He seemed well oriented periodically and expressed great concern about the changes he was experiencing, wondering if he was "going crazy."

Because of the concern of the retirement home staff, Mr. B was scheduled for a complete physical examination by his family physician and for a psychiatric evaluation by the geriatric psychiatric nurse consultant who came to the retirement home each week. The physical examination revealed Mr. B to be in generally good health for a man his age. He had a mild hearing loss and slight prostatic hypertrophy. Hypertension had been diagnosed 10 years before this examination but was well controlled by diuretics. A neurological examination revealed normal reflexes, normal muscle strength, a slight intention tremor, normal responses to sensation, normal cranial nerves, and no disturbance of gait. An electroencephalogram was normal, as were the results of laboratory studies of blood and urine. Computed tomography studies of the brain revealed some atrophy of the cerebral cortex.

The mental status examination confirmed the deficits in cognitive functioning observed by the nursing home staff and Mr. B's son. He was oriented to person and place but stated the date as April 6, 1958 (the real date was January 21, 2004). He also thought the day of the week was Friday, and it was actually Wednesday. He correctly identified the season of the year as winter. Mr. B was able to state correctly his birth date, the date of his son's birth, and the year he began to work at his first job. He spoke at length and with great detail about his exploits as a young man. His vocabulary was excellent, as was his fund of general information. However, he could not repeat the names of three objects after 5 minutes and could not remember what he had eaten for lunch or the last name of the man who shared his room. He became distressed while trying to answer these questions. He was unable to remember the names of the two most recent presidents but could recite the names of the eight presidents preceding them.

Mr. B's judgment was somewhat impaired. When asked what he would do if he found a stamped, addressed, sealed envelope, he said he would "read it, then mail it." His ability for abstract thinking was slightly concretized, as was demonstrated by his difficulty in interpreting proverbs. His attention span and ability to concentrate were normal. His eye-hand coordination was disrupted, as demonstrated by his difficulty in copying simple figures. A hand tremor was evident both when he was drawing and when he was signing his name.

Mr. B's affect was appropriate to the content of the discussion both in quality and in quantity. He appeared depressed when talking about his memory loss but cheerful and proud when describing his grandchildren. No abrupt mood swings were noted. His flow of speech was of a normal rate and volume. The content of his speech was logical and coherent but became somewhat disjointed when he tried to remember and describe recent events.

As a result of the data gathered in the physical and mental status examinations, Mr. B was diagnosed as having dementia not otherwise specified. Over the next several months his condition continued to deteriorate gradually. He became increasingly forgetful and began to confabulate and fabricate stories. He was less conforming to social norms and needed to be reminded about hygiene and appropriate dress. He also became seductive with female residents and staff, making suggestive remarks and occasionally fondling someone. Visits to his son's home became impossible as his behavior deteriorated. His memory of the identity of family members was sometimes confused. He would misidentify his daughter-in-law as his wife and his grandson as his son. His conversation increasingly consisted of rambling reminiscences about his life in his youth. His son and health care providers began to discuss plans to move him to the Assisted Living Program associated with his retirement home. Because he was surrounded by caring people, Mr. B continued to live with dignity and respect despite his progressively limited ability to communicate and to take care of himself.

Selected Nursing Diagnoses

- Impaired verbal communication related to cognitive impairment, as evidenced by recent memory loss and confabulation
- Impaired social interaction related to altered thought processes, as evidenced by a loss of conformity to social norms
- Self-care deficit (bathing/hygiene) related to cognitive impairment, as evidenced by a failure to perform personal hygiene activities without reminders
- Self-care deficit (dressing/grooming) related to cognitive impairment, as evidenced by a need for assistance in selecting appropriate clothing
- Disturbed thought processes related to cognitive impairment, as evidenced by disorientation and memory loss ∎

Table 23-2	Association of Areas of Brain Pathology to Behavioral Changes in Dementia	
ANATOMICAL STRUCTURE	FUNCTION	DYSFUNCTION
Occipital lobe	Visual processing	Blindness, loss of depth perception, color agnosia (lack of recognition), persistent after-images
Frontal lobe	Organization of words into fluent speech	Difficulty using "little words" (e.g., in , on, he, she, or); changes in personality, judgment, and behavior
Parietal lobe	Association area for integrating sensory input	Alexia (inability to read), agraphia (inability to write), neglect syndrome, inability to perceive pain, agnosia, apraxia, aphasia, visual-spatial disturbances, loss of executive functions, psychosis
Temporal lobe	Recognition and comprehension of sensory input, hearing, memory consolidation, association of memory, thought, perception, and emotion	Agnosia, apraxia, aphasia, visual-spatial disturbances, loss of executive functions, disorientation in space and time, psychosis, memory loss, misinterpretation of emotional events, misinterpretation of relationships
Limbic system	Emotions, storage of short-term memory, mood	Memory dysfunction, no affective dimension to memory, apathy, unstable affect, personality changes, poor learning ability, memory loss

Modified from Garand L et al: *Issues Ment Health Nurs* 21:91, 2000.

BOX 23-2

The Three Stages of Alzheimer's Disease

Stage I: Mild
- Impaired memory
- Insidious loses in activities of daily living (ADL)
- Subtle personality changes
- Socially normal

Stage II: Moderate
- Obvious memory impairment
- Overt ADL impairment
- Prominent behavioral difficulties
- Variable social skills
- Supervision needed

Stage III: Severe
- Fragmented memory
- No recognition of familiar people
- Assistance needed with basic ADL
- Fewer troublesome behaviors (usually)
- Reduced mobility

The behaviors associated with dementia reflect the brain tissue alterations that are taking place (Table 23-2). **Behavioral change occurs slowly in the early and late stages of AD and rapidly in the middle stage.** The three stages of AD are listed in Box 23-2.

Cognitive changes are related to the actions of stressors that interfere with the functioning of the cerebral cortex and the hippocampus. Other areas of the brain also are affected, which is one reason for performing a complete medical and neurological examination. Another reason is that although the condition may be irreversible, progression may be stopped or slowed by identifying the stressor and treating the underlying dysfunction. For example, the treatment of hypertension may prevent a further occurrence of one large or many small brain hemorrhages, which are possible causes of vascular dementia.

Depression in the elderly is often misinterpreted as dementia and therefore is not treated appropriately. **Pseudodementia** is a cognitive impairment secondary to a functional psychiatric disorder such as depression, characterized by lapses in memory and judgment, poor concentration, and seemingly diminished intellectual capacity. This condition is reversible with appropriate treatment of the depression.

On the other hand, **depression associated with AD** may be among the most common mood disorders of older adults (Zubenko et al, 2003). Aggression in patients with dementia is strongly linked to the presence of depressive symptoms; appropriate treatment of the depression may be a means of preventing and managing the physically aggressive behavior. AD behaviors related to delirium, dementia, and depression are compared in Table 23-3.

Race, culture, and ethnicity also may be important factors when calculating the impact of AD. In one study of race and AD, black men were found to have more anxiety and depression and less formal education than white men, but were no different in terms of actual memory performance. However, significant differences *were* found in the subjective aspects of memory evaluation, which affected the ability of black men in this study to know whether they were maintaining memory function or declining with age (McDougall and Holston, 2003). This information may have important implications for the manner in which patients and families are evaluated and understood.

Elderly adults with depression are often misdiagnosed as having dementia; the diagnosis of delirium is often missed too. What nursing observations help determine whether a patient's mental disorder is primarily affective or cognitive, and how would this affect treatment?

Table 23-3	Comparison of Delirium, Depression, and Dementia		
	DELIRIUM	DEPRESSION	DEMENTIA
Onset	Rapid (hours to days)	Rapid (weeks to months)	Gradual (years)
Course	Wide fluctuations; may continue for weeks if cause is not found	May be self-limited or may become chronic without treatment	Chronic; slow but continuous decline
Level of consciousness	Fluctuates from hyperalert to difficult to arouse	Normal	Normal
Orientation	Patient is disoriented, confused	Patient may seem disoriented	Patient is disoriented, confused
Affect	Fluctuating	Sad, depressed, worried, guilty	Labile; apathetic in later stages
Attention	Always impaired	Difficulty concentrating; patient may check and recheck all actions	May be intact; patient may focus on one thing for long periods
Sleep	Always disturbed	Disturbed; excess sleeping or insomnia, especially early-morning waking	Usually normal
Behavior	Agitated, restless	Patient may be fatigued, apathetic; may occasionally be agitated	Patient may be agitated or apathetic; may wander
Speech	Sparse or rapid; patient may be incoherent	Flat, sparse, may have outbursts; understandable	Sparse or rapid; repetitive; patient may be incoherent
Memory	Impaired, especially for recent events	Varies day to day; slow recall; often short-term deficit	Impaired, especially for recent events
Cognition	Disordered reasoning	May seem impaired	Disordered reasoning and calculation
Thought content	Incoherent, confused, delusional, stereotyped	Negative, hypochondriac, thoughts of death, paranoid	Disorganized, rich in content, delusional, paranoid
Perception	Misinterpretations, illusions, hallucinations	Distorted; patient may have auditory hallucinations; negative interpretation of people and events	No change
Judgment	Poor	Poor	Poor; socially inappropriate behavior
Insight	May be present in lucid moments	May be impaired	Absent
Performance on mental status examinations	Poor but variable; improves during lucid moments and with recovery	Memory impaired; calculation, drawing, and following directions usually not impaired; frequent "I don't know" answers	Consistently poor; progressively worsens; patient attempts to answer all questions

Modified from Holt J: *Am J Nurs* 93:32, 1993; Henry M: *Am J Nurs* 102:49, 2002.

A common behavior related to dementia is **disorientation**. Time orientation is usually affected first, then place and, finally, person. This behavior can be distressing to the patient, who may be aware of this difficulty and embarrassed or frightened by it. This is particularly true if the person's mental acuity is fluctuating. In these instances the person is aware, during periods of lucidity, of the confusion and disorientation experienced at other times.

Memory loss is another prominent characteristic of dementia. There are five abstract concepts of memory:

1. Sensory memory (visual or auditory)
2. Primary memory (immediate or short-term)
3. Secondary memory (storage of information that one intends to retain)
4. Tertiary memory (long-term)
5. Working memory (operates with primary memory and includes the simultaneous storage and processing of information over a short time).

These abstract concepts of memory do not correlate with brain structures but can be predictably demonstrated with functional testing and are evaluated during a mental status examination.

In the last clinical example, Mr. B had trouble remembering the three objects he heard named 5 minutes before and what he had eaten for lunch, but he gave accurate dates for significant events earlier in his life. Most aging people dwell on the past, but people with recent memory loss have difficulty shifting to the present and at advanced stages may seem to live in the past. This is exemplified by Mr. B's misidentification of his grandson and his daughter-in-law.

Another behavior related to memory loss is confabulation. Confabulation is a confused person's tendency to make up a response to a question when he or she cannot remember the answer. For instance, when Mr. B was asked whether he knew one of the female residents of the home, he replied, "Of course I know her. I used to play gin with her husband." Actually, the woman's husband had been dead for many years, and Mr. B had never met him.

Confabulation should not be viewed as lying or as an attempt to deceive but rather as a way of trying to save face in an embarrassing situation. Mr. B is aware that he should know the answer to the question and gives an answer that seems reasonable, not entirely disbelieving it himself. It is not unlike the situation in which a person meets an acquaintance and cannot recall the other's name or where they met. The person acts as if these facts are remembered, hoping that the other will offer clues about his or her identity. Denial of memory loss also may be related to the effect of dementia on the cognitive abilities needed for awareness of the problem.

As AD progresses, patients often develop aphasia, apraxia, agnosia, and amnesia:

- Aphasia is difficulty finding the right word.
- Apraxia is an inability to perform familiar skilled activities.
- Agnosia is a difficulty in recognizing well-known objects, including people.
- Amnesia is significant memory impairment in the absence of clouded consciousness or other cognitive symptoms.

These behaviors are related to the effect of the illness on the temporal-parietal-occipital association cortex.

Vocabulary and general information may be less affected by dementia until its late stages and depends on when the information was learned. Facts learned early in life may be recalled well, whereas those learned recently may be quickly forgotten, as demonstrated by Mr. B's performance in listing the last 10 presidents.

Patients with dementia may have labile affective behavior, particularly if the limbic system has been affected by the disease process. Some deterioration in social skills may be present as well. Impulsive sexual advances may occur, which reflects decreased inhibition and impaired judgment, as well as deterioration in the limbic system. Often this behavior is an attempt to establish interpersonal contact and is a way of asking for caring from others. It is also a way of reinforcing an important part of the person's identity—a part that becomes less secure as mental functioning declines.

Alterations in sexual functioning associated with AD causes great concern for patients and their partners. Loss of erection ability is a common problem among men with AD, and it is uncertain whether this is physiological or psycho-logical in origin. However, often both the patient and the sexual partner can benefit from continued sexual intimacy.

Restlessness and agitation are other behaviors that occur with dementia. Extreme agitation may occur at night; this is sometimes called the sundowning syndrome. Sundowning syndrome probably results from tiredness at the end of the day combined with fewer orienting stimuli, such as planned activities, meals, and contact with people.

Based on your understanding of sundowning syndrome, describe nursing interventions that would decrease the severity of this problem in patients with dementia at home, in the hospital, or in the nursing home. ∎

Disorientation can result in fear and agitation when individuals have cognitive impairment. Behavior that becomes extremely agitated is called a **catastrophic reaction** and is a medical emergency. The following are precipitating factors related to catastrophic reactions:

- A change in cognitive status that results in difficulty organizing and interpreting information; sensory or cognitive overload or misinterpretation of sensory stimuli may be contributing factors
- Side effects of medications
- Psychosocial factors that result in increased demands to remember, such as fatigue, changes in routines or caregivers, and disorienting stimuli
- Environmental factors, including environmental changes, noise, and decreased light

The term **confusion** is often used when referring to a person with cognitive impairment. Although widely accepted as nursing and medical jargon, this term has not been specifically defined. It is better to use specific terms when describing a patient's behavior. Five types of disturbing behaviors characteristic of dementia are summarized in Table 23-4.

Some people with maladaptive cognitive responses function at a level that is lower than would be expected on the basis of objective measurements of their impairment. This

Table 23-4	Disturbing Behaviors Characteristic of Dementia	
BEHAVIOR	**DESCRIPTION**	**EXAMPLES**
Aggressive psychomotor behavior	An increase in gross motor movement that has the effect of harming or repelling another	Hitting, kicking, pushing, scratching, assaultiveness
Nonagressive psychomotor behavior	An increase in gross motor movement that does not have an apparent negative effect on others but draws attention because of its repetitive nature	Restlessness, pacing, wandering
Verbally aggressive behavior	Vocalizations that have the effect of repelling others	Demanding, disruptive, manipulative behaviors; screaming; complaining; negativism
Passive behavior	A diminution of behavior, that is, a decrease in gross motor movement accompanied by apathy and a lack of interaction with the environment	Decreased activity, loss of interest, apathy, withdrawal
Functionally impaired behavior	Loss of ability to perform self-care, the expression of which may be aversive and burdensome	Vegetative behaviors, incontinence, poor personal hygiene

Modified from Kolanowski AM: *Arch Psychiatr Nurs* 9:188, 1995; Geldmacher D: *Contemporary diagnosis and management of Alzheimer's dementia*, Newton, Pa, 2003, Handbooks in Health Care Company.

type of functional deficit is classically called **excess disability**. This problem adds to the frustration of the patient and to the burden placed on caregivers. Caregivers may contribute to the development of excess disability by performing activities for the patient rather than coaching and assisting when needed. Functional abilities are lost more rapidly as the patient becomes more passive in his or her self-care routines.

Patients with a cognitive impairment are often referred to a clinical psychologist for psychological testing. This referral should be made for a specific purpose because the testing is time consuming, expensive, and tiring for the patient. Reasons for psychological testing include measuring the extent of the disability, identifying the stressors causing the disruption, understanding the dynamics of the problem, developing guidelines for therapeutic intervention, and obtaining a prognosis for recovery.

Predisposing Factors

Maladaptive cognitive responses are usually caused by a biological disruption in the functioning of the central nervous system (CNS). The CNS requires a continuous supply of nutrients, including oxygen, in order to function. Any interference with the provision of supplies to the brain or with the removal of waste products will cause functional disruptions in cognition.

Aging. In the United States, the number of people over 65 years of age is projected to reach almost 80 million by 2045; in 1990 there were just over 30 million in this age-group. Although aging itself predisposes the person to maladaptive cognitive responses, it is now accepted that a loss of mental abilities is not automatically associated with aging. Although a cumulative degeneration of brain tissue *is* associated with aging, it is not extensive enough to be particularly noticeable in most people.

As people age normally, their cognitive functions slow down but remain intact. If other stressors are added, the person may experience difficulty. Exposure to a toxic chemical or heavy metal, disease, or injury may result in maladaptive cognitive responses, which disrupts normal cognitive responses at any age. However, advanced age is one of the risk factors for dementia associated with AD.

Neurobiological. AD is the most prevalent cause of maladaptive cognitive responses. Intensive research has focused on identifying its causes, characteristics, and treatment. Investigators have found that characteristic alterations occur in brain tissue:

- **Neuritic plaques,** which consist of beta-amyloid (a starchlike protein) and remains of dying nerve cells. Plaques also contain altered glial cells.
- **Neurofibrillary tangles,** which are twisted clumps of protein fibers. Tangles contain a substance called *tau protein,* which seems to interfere with internal transport in neurons.

It is not known how excessive amyloid and tau protein deposits lead to the plaques and tangles that cause extensive structural and biochemical changes in axons, dendrites, and neuronal cell bodies. These changes reduce synaptic function by as much as 40% in affected regions and reduce protein synthesis and cellular processes. However, there is no doubt that this buildup of amyloid protein, combined with the formation of neurofibrillary tangles and other structural changes in neurons, contributes to a progressive breakdown of neuronal circuits necessary for communication in the brain.

It is as if the limbic system, particularly the hippocampus, amygdala, and the association cortices (which are affected early in the AD process and are necessary to the organization of mental processes), becomes isolated and out of touch with other brain regions, hence the gradual impairment of memory, judgment, abstraction, and language. Eventually, motor and sensory regions also are affected, and the patient with AD becomes totally disabled.

These phenomena are found in the cortex (cognition, judgment), the amygdala (emotion), and the hippocampus (consolidation of short-term memory). This is consistent with the emotional changes and short-term memory loss characteristic of AD. In addition, atrophy of the associational areas of the cortex is noted.

Alterations also have been noted in the neurotransmitter systems, in particular, a significant deficiency of the neurotransmitter **acetylcholine.** The cholinergic system originates in the basal forebrain, which is positioned at the interface between the limbic system and the cerebral cortex, where it plays a role in emotion and memory. Acetylcholine (ACh) is produced in a region of the basal forebrain that is selectively devastated by AD. It is thought that too little ACh may allow a buildup of amyloid protein, implicated in the pathophysiology of AD.

Although correlations can be drawn between neurotransmitter deficits and the pathology and clinical symptoms of AD, they seem to reflect damage specific to affected regions and specific structures rather than entire neurotransmitter systems throughout the brain. Table 23-5 lists the relationships between neurotransmitters and behavior in dementia.

Up to one third of people who are infected with HIV develop an organic brain syndrome, AIDS dementia complex, usually in the late stages of the disease, which affects several brain structures (Table 23-6). Symptoms include very slowed thinking and severe forgetfulness, difficulty performing multistage complex tasks (such as dressing and other activities of daily living [ADL]), muscle control problems, and eventually, social withdrawal, apathy, and depression.

Vascular dementia was previously called *multi-infarct dementia* because of the underlying cause—disruptions in the cerebral blood supply. Causes include hemorrhage, hypoperfusion (cardiac arrest, hypotension), ischemic stroke, postsurgical complications, vasculitis from autoimmune (lupus) and infectious (neurosyphilis, Lyme) diseases. Patients with hypertensive vascular disease may experience this type of dementia as a result of the sudden closure of the lumen of arterioles related to pressure changes. Atherosclerosis may lead to the formation of thrombi or emboli. In either case, the outcome is infarction of the brain tissue in the area supplied by

Table 23-5	Relationships Between Neurotransmitters and Behavior in Dementia		
NEUROTRANSMITTER SYSTEM/ NEUROTRANSMITTER	ANATOMICAL ORIGIN	FUNCTION	DYSFUNCTION AND BEHAVIOR
Cholinergic system/ acetylcholine (Ach)	Synthesized by an enzyme, choline acetyltransferase, in the nucleus basalis of Meynert in the basal forebrain	Promotes hippocampal and cerebral cortex function; necessary for selective attention, learning, memory, and the sleep-wake cycle	Diminished levels of Ach lead to amnesia, agitation, and psychotic symptoms Possible direct relationship to severity of disease Imbalance in the DA system
Noradrenergic system/ norepinephrine (NE)	The locus ceruleus in the rostral pons of the brainstem	Modulates mood and stress response; produces psychotic symptoms	Increased NE: hypervigilance, decreased appetite, insomnia, anxiety, agitation, psychosis Decreased NE: depressed mood Imbalance in the 5-HT system
Serotonergic system/ serotonin (5-HT)	The raphe nuclei in the brainstem	Regulates body temperature, cardiovascular system, respiratory system, sleep/alertness, mood, aggression, sensory perception, sexual behavior, and feeding behavior	Decreased 5-HT: anxiety, agitation, psychomotor activity, insomnia, psychosis, depressed mood, possibly suicidal behavior Imbalance in the NE system
Dopaminergic system/ dopamine (DA)	The substantia nigra in the brainstem, with projections directly communicating with the frontal lobe, limbic system, and motor areas	Regulates emotional responses (limbic system), executive functions (frontal lobes), and complex movements (motor striatum)	Decreased DA: difficulty initiating movement, rigidity, postural abnormalities, parkinsonian tremor (akinesia or bradykinesia), blunted affect, apathy Imbalance in the Ach system

Modified from Garand L et al: *Issues Ment Health Nurs* 21:91, 2000; Cummings J et al: *Am Fam Phys* 65:2263, 2002.

Table 23-6	HIV Symptoms Related to Brain Structures and Functions
BRAIN STRUCTURE	CLINICAL SYMPTOMS
Frontal lobes	Apathy, trouble concentrating and planning, loss of organizational skills, depression
Basal ganglia	Impaired movement, tremor
Limbic system	Emotional lability, memory loss, language impairment
Brainstem	Disturbances of gait, vision, and eye movement
Demyelination	Impaired fine motor skills, delayed information processing, impaired response time, incontinence

the affected blood vessels. The resulting cognitive problems are related to the area of the brain involved.

Dementia with Lewy bodies (DLB) represents the second most common form of degenerative dementia. Lewy bodies are neurofilament material found in the brainstem, thalamus, and basal ganglia of patients with dementia associated with atypical Parkinson's disease and in the cerebral cortex of patients with dementia with Lewy bodies. In AD, 50% to 75% of patients also have Lewy bodies present in their brains.

Frontotemporal dementia (FTD), previously called *Pick's disease*, is the accumulation of cytoplasmic collections in the brain, leading to a progressive loss of judgment, disinhibition, social misconduct, apathy, and loss of expressive language and comprehension. It is the third most common cause of cortical dementia affecting the frontal and/or temporal lobes of the brain (Yeaworth and Burke, 2000).

Creutzfeldt-Jakob disease (CJD) and other prion dementias are relatively rare in humans; however, they can be transmitted via infections (organ transplants or growth hormone injections from contaminated sources), food (kuru, transmitted during cannibalism when contaminated human brains are consumed), or inherited (DNA mutation). The normal cell protein, prion, is transformed in these disorders into an abnormal isoform of prion, causing varying clinical symptoms and a spongy appearance of the brain at post mortem. Symptoms usually include rapidly progressing motor and behavioral disturbances, dementia, and abnormal electroencephalogram (EEG) activity.

Brain imaging. Positron emission tomography (PET) scans and performance tests indicate that the brains of healthy people in their 80s are almost as active and function nearly as well, although slower, on tests of memory, perception, and language as people in early adulthood. Patients with early onset AD may show **cortical atrophy, ventricular enlargement,** and **loss of temporal lobe volume** (particularly the hippocampus) with computed tomography (CT) or magnetic resonance imaging (MRI), as well as a marked loss in brain weight. Patients with late-onset AD who develop the disease after the age of 75 usually show only age-related changes.

PET scans in patients with either kind of AD show a typical pattern of frontal, association, and temporal **hypometabolism.** However, these changes must be correlated with the clinical picture in order to reach a tentative diagnosis in living persons (Figure 23-4).

Sultzer and colleagues (2003) studied the relationship between delusional thoughts and regional cortical metabolism

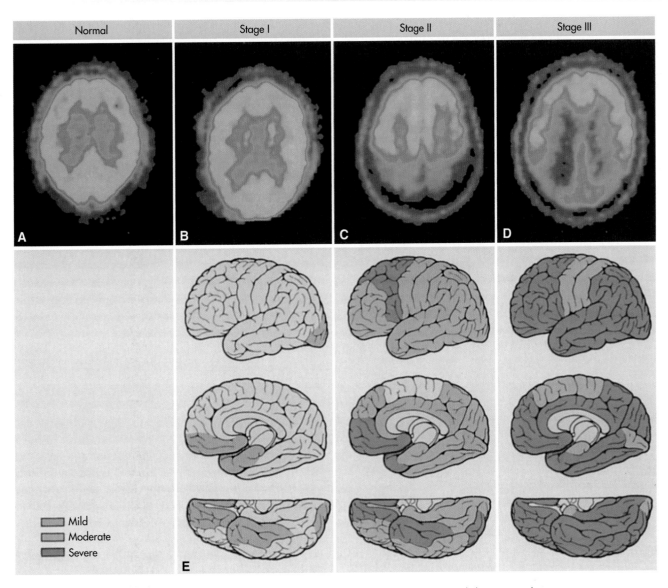

| Normal | Stage I | Stage II | Stage III |

□ Mild
□ Moderate
■ Severe

Figure 23-4   Pathological spread of Alzheimer's disease as shown by positron emission tomography scans. **A,** Normal brain. **B,** Brain in stage I Alzheimer's disease. **C,** Brain in stage II Alzheimer's disease. **D,** Brain in stage III Alzheimer's disease. **E,** Diagrams show the spread of the pathology in Alzheimer's disease. (From Roberts GS et al: *Neuropsychiatric disorders*, London, 1993, Mosby-Wolfe.)

using PET imaging technology in patients with AD. They found that delusional thoughts in these patients were highly correlated with hypometabolism in specific regions of the right prefrontal cortex. This study illustrates the continuing effort to determine the relationship between specific brain regions and human behavior.

Genetic. Genetic predisposition also may be a cause of maladaptive cognitive responses. Progress has been made in identifying the genetic markers that indicate a potential for developing AD. The risk for development of AD is greater for relatives of people with the illness than it is for those with no family history of AD (Wolozin, 2003). **The risk is greatest for relatives of people who developed AD before age 55 (early-onset AD).** An individual with one parent with early-onset AD has a 50% chance of developing it before the age of 55 as well.

Those offspring who do not inherit early-onset AD do not pass it on to their own children and presumably have the same risk of developing AD much later in life, as does the general population. Early-onset AD also occurs more often in people with Down syndrome (who have three rather than two copies of chromosome 21), another genetic brain disorder that affects normal growth and development and cognitive abilities.

Chromosomes 1 and 14 are involved in activities that prevent amyloid precursor protein (beta-APP) from elongating and accumulating in the brain. Chromosome 21 is the gene that forms the protein beta-APP, the substance from which the protein beta amyloid is formed. Although the function of beta amyloid is not fully understood, its production is accelerated in AD; excessive deposits form the senile plaques cluster outside each affected neuron, and the amyloid is deposited in the walls of cerebral blood vessels. It is also probably related to the production of the neurofibrillary tangles seen within the neurons of patients with AD.

In early-onset Alzheimer's disease, which accounts for only 10% of the incidence of AD, the genes are located on the following chromosomes (NSW, 2003):

- Chromosome 14: The presenilin-1 gene, a mutation that is thought to be implicated in over 50% of these relatively rare familial cases.
- Chromosome 1: The presenilin-2 gene, a mutation implicated in a group of families from an ethnic group known as the Volga Germans, who now live mostly in the United States and Canada.
- Chromosome 21: The amyloid precursor protein (APP) gene, known to be implicated in about 20 families in the world.
- Chromosome 17: The *tau* gene, a mutation reported to result in dementia affecting the brain at the front of the skull.

In cases where a strong family history of early-onset AD is noted and a mutation on one of these genes is identified as causing AD in the family, genetic testing may be available. Such testing is called *pre-symptomatic testing* because the test is usually done before the onset of any symptoms of the condition. Counseling that examines the implications of the testing is essential (see Citing the Evidence).

Alzheimer's disease that occurs in later life is associated with several genes:

- The first gene to be identified that is associated with AD in later life is called *apoe*, located on chromosome 19. Everyone has two copies, one from each parent. The apoe gene tells the cell to produce apolipoprotein e, which guides cholesterol through the blood stream. It is thought that the e4 form of the apoe gene increases the risk for AD (perhaps making people somehow more susceptible to some other influence, which then causes the disease). The e2 form appears to be somewhat protective against developing AD; e4 is the chief known genetic risk factor for later-life AD.
- The *K variant* gene is located on chromosome 3, and its interaction with e4 is thought to increase the risk of developing late onset AD.
- About 10 % to 15% of cases of late onset AD are thought to be related to mutations in a gene called *a2m* (alpha-2–macroglobulin), located on chromosome 12. This mutation is thought to break down beta amyloid protein. Although the function of this protein is not fully understood, its production is accelerated in AD.

The search for other genes is continuing, as is the search for risk factors and factors that may protect a person from developing AD. Studies of identical twins (monozygotic twins) have found that often when one twin develops AD, the other twin remains unaffected, implying that non-genetic factors for AD also must be involved. Although more information is discovered almost daily, until more is known about the role of apoe and the interactions of brain proteins in AD, genetic testing for this gene is not indicated.

Underlying Psychiatric and Medical Disorders. A degree of cognitive impairment may be found along with other maladaptive psychiatric responses. For instance, people with delusions may seem disoriented because they misidentify their location. People who have affective disorders may have short attention spans. Depression also may result in memory disorders, although it is often difficult to determine whether the problem is related to memory loss or to a lack of motivation.

Patients with mental disorders resulting from a general medical condition also can exhibit symptoms of cognitive impairment. Such medical conditions include thyroid disease, adrenal dysfunction, hypoglycemia, brain lesions, and degenerative disorders. The predisposing factors related to maladaptive cognitive responses as a result of psychiatric and medical disorders are related to the underlying primary problem.

Precipitating Stressors

Associated With Delirium. Any major dysregulation in the balance of body functions can disrupt cognitive functioning. The most commonly recognized risk factor for the evolution of delirium is **drug and/or substance use.** Medications associated with delirium can be found in Box 23-3.

Delirium related to alcohol or sedative hypnotic withdrawal is most commonly recognized by an agitated hyperactive/hyperalert motoric state. The use of polypharmacy and the frequent addition of over-the-counter drugs to prescribed drug regimens, particularly in the elderly, has received much attention recently, as has the mixing of drugs with alcohol in various populations.

CITING THE EVIDENCE ON
Genetic Testing

BACKGROUND: This was a general population survey of 314 people that asked about their attitudes toward genetic testing for Alzheimer's disease.

RESULTS: Of respondents who participated in the survey, 79% stated they would take a hypothetical test to predict whether they would eventually develop Alzheimer's disease. The proportion fell to 45% for a "partially predictive" test that had a 1 in 10 chance of being correct. Inclination to obtain testing was similar across age-groups. Respondents were willing to pay $324 for the completely predictive test. Respondents stated that if they tested positive, 84% would sign advance directives, 74% would get their finances in order, and 69% would purchase long-term care insurance. Only a third of the respondents expressed concern about confidentiality.

IMPLICATIONS: These results suggest that people value genetic testing for personal and financial reasons, but they also underscore the need to counsel potential recipients carefully about the accuracy and implications of test information.

Neumann P et al: *Health Affairs* 20:252, 2001.

The underlying medical conditions most commonly associated with delirium can be categorized into five major groups: **CNS disorders, metabolic disorders, cardiopulmonary disorders, systemic illnesses,** and **sensory deprivation or stimulation** (Table 23-7). The psychiatric nurse should be alert for possible causes of delirium when evaluating each patient with maladaptive cognitive responses and when assessing a change of cognitive status from a previous level of functioning for each patient.

Central nervous system disorder. Any major assault on the brain is likely to disrupt cognitive functioning. Severe head trauma and other brain diseases and infections such as meningitis and encephalitis cause changes in the normal function of the brain. When these disorders occur in areas of the brain responsible for cognitive function, the patient exhibits symptoms that are indicative of maladaptive cognitive responses.

Metabolic disorder. Metabolic disorders often affect mental functioning, especially when they are severe or of long duration. **Endocrine malfunctioning,** whether it involves underproduction or overproduction of hormones, can adversely affect cognition. For example, thyroid hormone greatly influences mental alertness. People with hypothyroidism are sluggish and dysfunctional in their thinking. Those with severe hypothyroidism (myxedema) may develop psychotic behavior characterized by delusional thinking. Other endocrine disorders that may cause cognitive disruptions include hypoglycemia, hypopituitarism, and adrenal disease.

Hypoxia can result in cognitive dysfunction because the brain is not getting its normal oxygen supplies. Hypoxia resulting from anemia may be insidious in onset. Possible stressors include aspirin ingestion that results in occult bleeding; other occult blood loss; or deficiencies of iron, folic acid, or vitamin B_{12}. Other causes of hypoxia can include dehydration, hyperthermia, hypothermia, or increased intracranial pressure resulting from a tumor, subdural hematoma, or normal pressure hydrocephalus.

Nutrition in general can affect cognitive functioning. Malnutrition increases a person's risk of organic brain disease and is often a problem in the elderly, who may lack the physical or financial resources needed for an adequate diet. Young people with anorexia nervosa or bulimia nervosa are also at risk for cognitive impairment. Vitamin B–complex deficiency, particularly thiamine, is believed to cause the Wernicke-Korsakoff syndrome found in some chronic alcoholics. A prominent feature of this syndrome is a severe deficit in cognitive functioning.

Based on a review of neurophysiology, compare the effects of hypoxia, hypothyroidism, and hypoglycemia on cerebral functioning. ■

Cardiopulmonary disorder. Heart disease that compromises the flow of blood to the brain or to the lungs to ex-

---

BOX 23-3

Medications Associated With Delirium

Narcotics
- Meperidine

Sedative Hypnotics
- Benzodiazepines
- Barbiturates

Cardiac Medications
- Antiarrythmics
- Antihypertensives

Anticholinergics
- Antihistamines
- Antiparkinsonian agents
- Antispasmodics
- Tricyclic antidepressants

Miscellaneous
- Anticonvulsants
- Steroids
- Nonsteroidal antiinflammatories
- Caffeine
- Cold and sinus preparations

Modified from Henry M: *Am J Nurs* 102:49, 2002; Clary G et al: *J Psychiatric Pract* 7:310, 2001.

Table 23-7	Underlying Conditions Commonly Associated With Delirium	
TYPE	**DISORDER**
Central nervous system disorders	Head trauma, seizures, postictal state, vascular disease (e.g., hypertensive encephalopathy), degenerative disease, tumor, brain abscess, meningitis, encephalitis
Metabolic disorders	Renal failure, hepatic failure, anemia, hypoxia, hypoglycemia, vitamin deficiency (thiamine, folate, B_{12}, nicotinic acid), endocrinopathy, fluid or electrolyte imbalance, acid-base imbalance, low albumin, malnutrition
Cardiopulmonary disorders	Myocardial infarction, congestive heart failure, cardiac arrhythmia, shock, respiratory failure, severe hypertension
Systemic illnesses	Substance intoxication or withdrawal (e.g., alcohol, antidepressants, antipsychotics, anesthetics, benzodiazepines, opiates, anticholinergics, nonsteroidal anti-inflammatory drugs [NSAIDs], corticosteroids), toxins (insecticides, carbon monoxide, fuel, paint), infections (urinary tract, pneumonia, HIV, septicemia), neoplasm (primary and metastatic tumors), severe trauma (burns, surgery, and fractures, especially hip), sensory deprivation, temperature dysregulation, postoperative state
Sensory deprivation or stimulation	Sensory deprivation (underload), sensory stimulation (overload)

Modified from American Psychiatric Association: *Am J Psychiatry* 156(5 suppl):1, 1999.

change carbon dioxide for oxygen is likely to cause maladaptive cognitive responses. Respiratory illnesses, such as chronic obstructive lung disease, acute respiratory infection, and cardiac conditions, such as congestive heart failure, atherosclerosis, hypotension, and hypertension, are common problems and may be underlying causes of changes in cognitive function.

Systemic illness. Substances such as **alcohol** and **drugs**, even many drugs commonly used in the treatment of psychiatric disorders, can cause changes in sensorium during ingestion. Some substances may cause these changes during withdrawal. Prescription and over-the-counter drugs can be potential toxic stressors.

A thorough assessment of drug use is critical with all patients. It is especially critical with elderly patients because of their increased sensitivity to drugs associated with normal aging and because confusion can lead to difficulty in following the directions for taking drugs. Interactions between drugs or between drugs and other substances, particularly alcohol, also may lead to disruptions in cognitive functioning.

Toxic and **infectious agents** also may result in the behavior typical of maladaptive cognitive responses. Toxins may originate within the patient or in the external environment. An example of an internally generated toxin is the elevated blood level of urea found in a patient with renal failure. Environmental toxins include various poisonous substances, such as toxic wastes and animal venoms. Infections in any body system also may impair the CNS if body temperature is extremely elevated.

Sensory deprivation or stimulation. Sensory deprivation or sensory overload can result in cognitive dysfunction. People who are placed in environments with minimal stimuli seem to develop internally produced stimuli in the form of hallucinations. In contrast, the constant light and activity in intensive care units (ICUs) can lead to confusion, delusions, and hallucinations; this is sometimes called *ICU psychosis*.

It is difficult to determine the extent to which the cognitive impairment results from the sensory experience as opposed to other concurrent stressors, such as the introduction of multiple drugs into the system, the result of massive assaults on physical integrity, immobilization from the use of physical restraints, and changes in the normal sleep cycle imposed upon ICU patients.

Sensory overload or sensory deprivation may lead to maladaptive cognitive responses. In what way is this information significant in planning the nursing care of a patient who is confined to a seclusion room on a psychiatric unit? ∎

Associated With Dementia. The underlying conditions most commonly associated with dementia are the subject of much research and conjecture. In addition to age, family history of AD, and Down syndrome, the most common underlying conditions associated with dementia across the life span are listed in Box 23-4.

Factors that may precede AD are depression, mild cognitive impairment, hippocampal atrophy, and delayed paragraph recall on neurocognitive testing. Box 23-5 lists the risk factors and proposed protective factors for AD.

BOX 23-4

Underlying Conditions Commonly Associated With Dementia Across the Life Span

Elderly
Degenerative brain disorders
Alzheimer's disease
Frontotemporal dementia
Dementia with Lewy bodies
Parkinson's disease
Huntington's disease
Pick's disease
Late-onset extrapyramidal symptoms
Cerebrovascular dementia
Multi-infarct dementia
Binswanger's disease
Cerebral hemorrhage
Toxic-metabolic disturbances
Iatrogenic drug-induced dementia
Alcoholism
Poisons
Inhalants
Heavy metals
Cardiopulmonary disease
B_{12} deficiency
Hypothyroidism
Central nervous system infections
Chronic meningitis
Neurosyphilis
Creutzfeldt-Jakob disease

AIDS
Kuru
Subacute sclerosing panencephalitis
Miscellaneous
Traumatic brain injury
Brain tumors
Hydrocephalus
Depression
Thyroid disease

Adolescents
Huntington's disease (juvenile type)
Wilson's disease (hepatolenticular degeneration)
Subacute sclerosing panencephalitis
AIDS
Substance abuse (especially inhalants)
Head trauma

Children
Head trauma (including child abuse)
Subacute sclerosing panencephalitis
AIDS

Modified from Kay J, Tasman A: Dementia, delirium, and cognitive disorders. In Kay J, Lieberman JA, Tasman A: *Psychiatry: behavioral science and clinical essentials*, Philadelphia, 2000, WB Saunders.

Appraisal of Stressors

Unfortunately, the specific stressor related to cognitive impairment often cannot be identified. Understanding the biochemical process of the brain and the response of the brain and nervous tissue to stressors is the subject of intense research. As knowledge advances, specific biological components may be identified as part of the etiology of all psychiatric disorders.

For example, severe deficiency in the neurotransmitter acetylcholine has been observed in patients with AD. It is not known whether this is a cause or an effect of the illness, but psychopharmacological treatment approaches include drugs such as the cholinesterase inhibitors, designed to preserve this neurotransmitter in the brain.

In general, when assessing maladaptive cognitive responses, physiological causes are ruled out first, and then psychosocial stressors are considered. Even when physiological

BOX 23-5

Risk Factors and Proposed Protective Factors for Alzheimer's Disease

Risk Factors

Definitive
- Age
- Family history
- Gene apoe e4 genotype
- Down syndrome
- Specific mutations on chromosomes 1, 14, and 21

Possible
- Female gender
- Low level of education
- Head injury with loss of consciousness
- Vascular brain lesions
- Aluminum
- Insulin-dependent diabetes mellitus

- Solvent exposure
- Electromagnetic exposure
- Elevated thyrotropin
- Hypertension
- Myocardial infarction

Proposed Protective Factors
- Estrogen
- Gene apoe e2 and e3 genotypes
- Higher education
- Anti-inflammatory medications
- Vitamin E
- Lifestyle issues: social, physical, and intellectual activity

Modified from American Psychiatric Association: *Am J Psychiatry* 156(5 suppl):1, 1999; Geldmacher D: *Contemporary diagnosis and management of Alzheimer's dementia*, Newton, Pa, 2003, Handbooks in Health Care Company.

factors are present, psychosocial stress may further compromise the person's thought process; therefore appraisal of this stressor is critically important. Each patient should receive a complete assessment so that nursing care can be planned in a competent and thorough manner.

Coping Resources

Individual and interpersonal resources are important to the person who is attempting to cope with maladaptive cognitive responses. A person who has a varied repertoire of skills may be able to substitute for functional losses. For instance, it has been noted that people with AD who have attained higher levels of education and who have remained active and involved in their lives deteriorate less rapidly than those who have less education and have remained sedentary and socially isolated.

Interpersonal resources are extremely important to the person with a cognitive impairment. Family members and friends often have a calming influence on the agitated person. They can provide the nurse with information about the person's usual lifestyle and ensure that the environment contains familiar objects. Caregivers also need coping resources, which often can be found by attending self-help groups such as the Alzheimer's Disease and Related Disorders Association. The importance of family involvement is illustrated in A Family Speaks.

Coping Mechanisms

How a person copes with maladaptive cognitive responses is greatly influenced by past experience. A person who has developed many effective coping mechanisms is better able to handle the onset of a cognitive problem than one who has not.

A FAMILY SPEAKS

My mother, Margaret, is 78 years old and has been in a nursing home for the past 3 years. She is diagnosed with dementia. There are days when she does not recognize me and there are some days when she does, but even then her mood may not be very pleasant. Many days she just sits in her chair and responds to nothing. Often she cannot feed herself or express her needs. I visit her nearly every day.

The nurses in the home are my only link to my mother. The doctor visits weekly but rarely communicates with me unless there is an emergency. The nurses give me information about my mother's condition and listen to me when I have concerns about her. In the beginning the nurses were indifferent to me, and I worried that they were the same with my mother. I brought pictures of the family to the nursing home and shared them with the nurses. These pictures allowed the nurses to see a person instead of a patient. They began to see that her past life had been very different, and this helped them treat her with more respect and dignity. Now I really depend on the nurses to let me know how my mother is doing from day to day.

Associated With Delirium. Because the basic behavioral disruption in those with delirium is altered awareness (which reflects the severe biological disturbance in the brain), psychological coping mechanisms are not generally used. Therefore the nurse must protect the patient from harm and provide a substitute for the patient's previous coping mechanisms by constantly reorienting him or her and reinforcing reality during the treatment process.

Associated With Dementia. The patient's response to the onset of dementia often mirrors his or her basic personality. For instance, a person who usually reacted to stress with anger toward other people and the environment before developing dementia will probably react similarly when limitations in intellectual abilities occur. A person who is more apt to direct anger inward and become depressed will be more likely to respond with depressive behaviors. A person who has relied on a mechanism such as intellectualization will be even more threatened by the loss of intellectual ability than a person who has used a mechanism such as reaction formation.

One characteristic of early dementia is the mechanism of denial. Those with dementia attempt to pursue their usual daily routine and make light of memory lapses. They may be able to use some environmental resources to help them cope. For instance, a businessman who is experiencing difficulty with recent memory might ask his secretary to remind him of all his appointments and to provide him with the names of the people with whom he is meeting and the meeting's purpose. As the impairment progresses, the person may become very resistant to any limitations on independence. For example, the family of a woman with AD might become very concerned about her ability to continue to drive a car safely. She probably would be very reluctant to give up her driver's license and would deny having any problem.

Regression is often used to cope with advanced dementia and may be caused in part by a deterioration in mental function. It probably also results from the behavioral manifestations of dementia, which cause the patient to become more dependent on others for the fulfillment of basic needs such as nutrition and hygiene. Encouraging patients to perform self-care also supports their use of healthier coping mechanisms.

As cognitive ability decreases, efforts to cope become more obvious. For instance, a family member may complain that a relative has "always been irritable but is now belligerent when he doesn't get his way." In other cases the person's behavior may be perceived as a personality change.

Behaviors that are likely attempts to cope with a loss of cognitive ability include suspiciousness, hostility, joking, de-pression, seductiveness, and withdrawal. Because it is threatening to admit that a close relative has dementia, family members may focus on the coping mechanism instead of on the real problem, thus participating in the denial of the underlying cognitive impairment.

DIAGNOSIS

Nursing Diagnoses

The nursing diagnosis of the patient with cognitive impairment should consider both the possible underlying stressors and the patient behaviors. Figure 23-5 summarizes the Stuart Stress Adaptation Model as related to maladaptive cognitive responses.

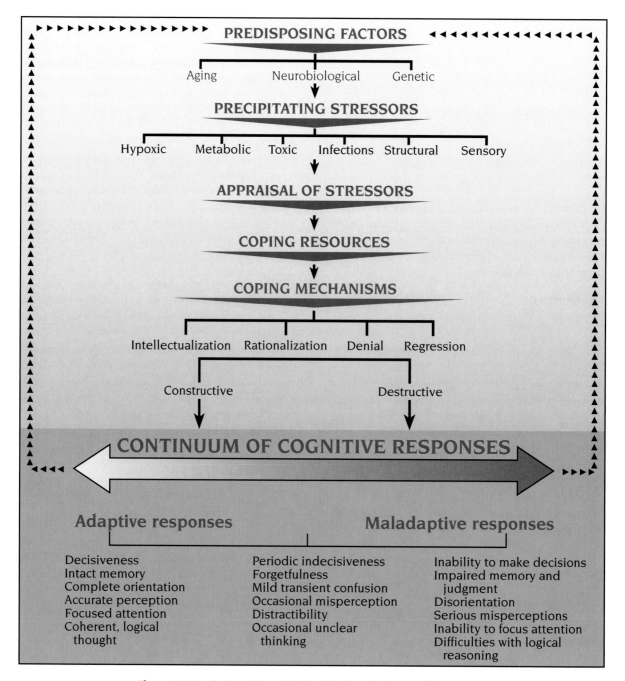

Figure 23-5 The Stuart Stress Adaptation Model as related to cognitive responses.

Most cognitive impairment disorders are physiological in origin. Therefore the nurse should consider both the patient's physical needs and the psychosocial behavioral problems. For example, a delirious patient may be reacting to an infection, a drug overdose, or a drug reaction. The identified problem and all its effects should be reflected in an expanded nursing diagnosis.

Many people with dementia are also elderly. They experience many effects of the aging process in addition to impaired cognitive functioning. A thorough nursing diagnosis reflects all of these influences on the patient's behavior.

In addition, the nature of a cognitive impairment may inhibit the patient's ability to participate in the care-planning process. The nurse should rely on observational skills and on the input of significant others to arrive at an accurate, relevant diagnosis. If the nursing diagnosis cannot be validated with the patient, a family member familiar with his or her behavioral patterns should be involved.

The primary NANDA nursing diagnoses related to maladaptive cognitive response are **acute or chronic confusion** and **disturbed thought processes**. The range of common NANDA nursing diagnoses and the *DSM-IV-TR* psychiatric diagnoses are included in the Medical and Nursing Diagnoses box (Box 23-6). The primary NANDA diagnoses and examples of expanded nursing diagnoses are presented in the Detailed Diagnoses table (Table 23-8).

Medical Diagnoses

Medical diagnoses related to maladaptive cognitive responses are most apparent in people who have a psychiatric diagnosis of **delirium, dementia,** and **amnestic disorders**. Their essential features are described in the Detailed Diagnoses table (see Table 23-8).

OUTCOME IDENTIFICATION

The expected outcome related to the patient who has maladaptive cognitive responses is:

The patient will achieve optimum cognitive functioning.

Goals may be directed toward an improved ability to process information (if this is realistic) or toward optimum use of the abilities the patient retains (if the impairment is irreversible). For example, a goal for a patient who is disoriented because of drug withdrawal might be to verbalize the complete date within 3 days.

In contrast, a goal for a patient who is disoriented because of chronic alcoholism and who is not in withdrawal might be to find his or her own bed every night without assistance after 1 month.

The second patient may never be able to remember the exact date, but he or she may not need that information if he or she will be functioning in a protected setting. However, the first patient will need that information. In addition, the nurse can use the assessment of the patient's orientation to time to assess the current status of mental functioning.

Goals should be realistic to avoid discouragement. If the second patient is required to learn the date, frequent confrontation with deteriorated cognitive skills might result and lead to frustration, higher anxiety, and possibly less effective coping.

If an identified stressor is causing the patient's behavioral disruption, goals that focus on that stressor also should be developed. For instance, if a person is delirious because of a

---

BOX 23-6 *Medical and Nursing Diagnoses Related to* **Maladaptive Cognitive Responses**

RELATED MEDICAL DIAGNOSES (*DSM-IV-TR*)*	RELATED NURSING DIAGNOSES (NANDA)†
Delirium due to a general medical condition	Anxiety
Substance-induced delirium	Caregiver role strain
Delirium due to multiple etiologies	Communication, Impaired verbal
Dementia of the Alzheimer's type	**Confusion, Acute or chronic‡**
Vascular dementia	Health maintenance, Ineffective
Dementia due to other general medical conditions	Home maintenance, Impaired
Substance-induced persisting dementia	Injury, Risk for
Dementia due to multiple etiologies	Noncompliance
Amnestic disorder due to a general medical condition	Role performance, Ineffective
Substance-induced persisting amnestic disorder	Self-care deficit (specify: bathing/hygiene, dressing/grooming, feeding, toileting)
	Sensory perception, Disturbed (specify: visual, auditory, kinesthetic, gustatory, tactile, olfactory)
	Sleep pattern, Disturbed
	Social interaction, Impaired
	Thought processes, Disturbed‡
	Trauma, Risk for

*From American Psychiatric Association: *Diagnostic and statistical manual of mental disorders*, ed 4, text revision, Washington, DC, 2000, American Psychiatric Association.
†From North American Nursing Diagnosis Association: *NANDA nursing diagnoses: definitions and classification 2003-2004*, Philadelphia, 2003, The Association.
‡**Primary nursing diagnosis for maladaptive cognitive responses.**

Table 23-8	*Detailed Diagnoses Related to* **Maladaptive Cognitive Responses**

NANDA DIAGNOSIS STEM	EXAMPLES OF EXPANDED DIAGNOSIS
Acute confusion	Acute confusion related to severe dehydration, as evidenced by hypervigilance, distractibility, visual hallucinations, and disorientation to time, place, and person
Disturbed thought processes	Disturbed thought processes related to barbiturate ingestion, as evidenced by altered sleep patterns, delusions, disorientation to time and place, and decreased ability to grasp ideas
	Disturbed thought processes related to brain disorder, as evidenced by inaccurate interpretation of environment, deficit in recent memory, impaired ability to reason, and confabulation

DSM-IV-TR DIAGNOSIS	ESSENTIAL FEATURES*
Delirium (general criteria) (to be applied to all other categories of delirium)	Disturbed consciousness accompanied by a cognitive change that cannot be accounted for by dementia
	Impaired ability to focus, sustain, or shift attention
	Cognitive changes that include impaired recent memory, disorientation to time or place, language disturbance, or perceptual disturbance
	Develops over a short time; tends to fluctuate during the course of a day
Delirium due to a general medical condition	Evidence that the cognitive disturbance is the direct result of a general medical condition
Substance-induced delirium	Evidence of substance intoxication or withdrawal, medication side effects, or toxin exposure judged to be related to the delirium
Delirium due to multiple etiologies	Evidence of multiple causes for the delirium
Dementia (general criteria) (to be applied to all other categories of dementia)	Development of multiple cognitive deficits, including memory impairment and at least one of the following: aphasia, apraxia, agnosia, or disturbed executive functioning (ability to think abstractly and plan, initiate, sequence, monitor, and stop complex behavior)
	Must cause severe impairment in social or occupational functioning
Dementia of the Alzheimer's type	Gradual onset with continuing cognitive decline; all other causes of dementia must be ruled out
Vascular dementia	Focal neurological signs and symptoms or laboratory evidence of cerebrovascular disease that are judged to be related to the dementia
Dementia due to other general medical conditions	Evidence that the general medical condition (such as HIV, traumatic brain injury, Parkinson's disease, Huntington's disease, Pick's disease, Creutzfeldt-Jakob disease, normal-pressure hydrocephalus, hypothyroidism, brain tumor, vitamin B_{12} deficiency) is etiologically related to the dementia
Substance-induced persisting dementia	Deficits do not occur exclusively during delirium and persist beyond the usual duration of substance intoxication or withdrawal
	Evidence that the deficits are related to persisting effects of substance use (e.g., drug of abuse, medication)
Dementia due to multiple etiologies	Evidence that the dementia has more than one etiology
Amnestic disorder (general criteria)	Development of memory disorder, as evidenced by impaired ability to learn new information or to recall previously learned information
	Disturbance causes significant impairment in social or occupational functioning and represents a significant decline from a previous level of functioning
	Does not occur exclusively during the course of delirium or dementia
Amnestic disorder due to a general medical condition	Evidence that the disturbance is directly related to a general medical condition (including physical trauma)
Substance-induced persisting amnestic disorder	Evidence that the memory disturbance is etiologically related to the persisting effects of substance use (e.g., drug of abuse, medication)

*From American Psychiatric Association: *Diagnostic and statistical manual of mental disorders*, ed 4, text revision, Washington, DC, 2000, American Psychiatric Association.

fever, a goal might state that the patient's temperature will be maintained below 100° F (37.8° C).

When the cause of the elevated temperature is identified, appropriate goals are written to address that problem. For example, dehydration may be a stressor that contributes to an elevated temperature. A related nursing goal would be that the patient's fluid intake is at least 3000 ml in each 24-hour period. As the various elements of the patient's behavior are explored and documented, nursing goals must be updated and modified, new goals must be added, and accomplished goals must be deleted.

PLANNING

The nursing care plan for a patient with maladaptive cognitive responses must address all of his or her **biopsychosocial** needs. In most cases, the patient either has or is at risk for physiological problems in addition to the psychosocial disruption. **Life-threatening problems always receive the high-**

Table 23-9	FAMILY EDUCATION PLAN	Helping a Family With a Cognitively Impaired Member
CONTENT	**INSTRUCTIONAL ACTIVITIES**	**EVALUATION**
Explain possible causes of maladaptive cognitive responses.	Describe predisposing factors and precipitating stressors that may lead to impaired cognition. Provide printed reference materials.	The family identifies possible causes of the patient's disorder.
Define and describe orientation to time, place, and person.	Define the three spheres of orientation. Role play interpersonal responses to disorientation.	The family identifies disorientation and provides reorientation.
Relate level of cognitive functioning to ability to communicate.	Describe the impact of maladaptive cognitive responses on communication. Demonstrate effective communication techniques. Videotape and discuss return demonstration.	The family adjusts communication approaches to the patient's ability to interact.
Describe effect of maladaptive cognitive responses on self-care behaviors.	Describe the usual progression of the gain or loss of self-care ability related to the nature of the disorder. Encourage the family to help in providing care to patient. Provide written instructional materials.	The family helps with activities of daily living as required by the patient's level of biopsychosocial functioning.
Refer to community resources.	Provide a list of community resources. Arrange to meet with staff members of selected community programs. Visit meetings of selected programs and self-help groups.	The family describes various programs that provide services relevant to the patient's and family's needs and contacts appropriate programs or self-help groups when needed.

est priority for nursing intervention. Protection of safety is almost always a concern with these patients.

Mental health education related to patients with impaired cognition is often directed toward the family, who are often the caregivers for these patients. The nurse can help caregivers cope with this difficult and demanding responsibility by providing them with information about problematic behaviors and problem solving. A Family Education Plan for the families of cognitively impaired people is presented in Table 23-9.

Another strategy to facilitate family involvement in caring for individuals with dementia is to develop a formal protocol. This approach details a negotiated partnership with staff caregivers and family and includes education about caregiving, negotiation of a partnership agreement, and evaluation and renegotiation of the partnership as needed (Kelley et al, 2000).

◀ IMPLEMENTATION

Practice guidelines have been developed to treat delirium and dementia (American Psychiatric Association, 1999; Doody et al, 2001; Knopman et al, 2001; Peterson et al, 2001). These are excellent references for comprehensive clinical care.

Intervening in Delirium

Physiological Needs. Highest priority is given to nursing interventions that will maintain life. If the patient is too disoriented or agitated to attend to his or her basic physiological needs, nursing care should be planned to meet those needs. **Nutrition** and **fluid balance** may be maintained by intravenous therapy. If the patient is very agitated or restless,

restraint may be necessary to keep the intravenous line open. However, restraints can increase agitation and anxiety and thus should be used only when absolutely necessary. A disoriented patient should never be restrained and left alone.

Sleep deprivation may be another problem. Intervention is important because a lack of sleep can add to an already existing cognitive dysfunction. Because sedative medications may complicate attempts to identify the original stressor, the physician or advanced practice nurse prescriber may be reluctant to prescribe a sedative.

Nursing measures such as a back rub, a glass of warm milk, and gentle but persistent orientation so that patients are continually reminded of their surroundings are low-tech interventions that decrease the incidence of delirium in elderly patients (Inouye, 1999; Geldmacher, 2003).

The presence of a family member is also reassuring to the patient. Disoriented patients need to be in a lighted room. Shadows may be misinterpreted and add to the patient's fear. Environmental objects also help the patient orient to place and person.

Do you think it is safer and more effective to use physical (mechanical) restraints than to use chemical restraints (medication) with an agitated, delirious patient? ■

Hallucinations. Disoriented patients may need to be protected from hurting themselves or others, particularly when they are having hallucinations. Visual hallucinations of delirium are often very frightening. Patients may try to run away or even jump out of a window. Patients' rooms must be safe, with security screens and a minimum of extra furniture or other objects that might cause harm. These patients often require one-on-one nursing observation and repetitive verbal reorientation.

It is tempting to help a frightened patient eliminate the hallucinated object. For instance, the patient might request help in brushing the bugs off the sheets. Agreeing to do this is not usually therapeutic. By participating in this activity, the nurse is nonverbally communicating to the patient that the hallucinated objects are real. This can make the patient even more frightened.

In reality the hallucinations will continue until the underlying stressor is eliminated. A more appropriate response is to orient the patient continually to the reality of being sick and hospitalized. In addition, the patient can be assured that the nursing and medical staff are there to help and to keep the patient safe. Family members also should be helped to respond in a supportive way. Nursing interventions for hallucinations are further discussed in Chapter 21.

Communication. Patients with maladaptive cognitive responses need clear messages and instructions. Choices should be kept to a minimum. Independent decision making can be introduced into the plan of nursing care as the patient improves. Decisions related to orientation may be especially difficult for the patient. Responding appropriately to the question "What time would you like to take your bath?" requires knowledge of the present time and some idea of the usual routine.

Simple, direct statements are reassuring and are most likely to result in an appropriate response. Orienting phrases such as "here at the hospital" or "now that it's June" can be woven into a conversation. Patients who have difficulty dressing or feeding themselves need matter-of-fact, specific directions.

Confused patients need to be fed or dressed in a manner that allows them to maintain their dignity. Families often can help with this. Helping the patient can lessen the family's anxiety, and the patient may be reassured by the family's physical closeness and concern.

Patient Education. While recovering, patients may be concerned about what has happened to them. The health care team needs to discuss this issue and arrive at a conclusion about the disruption in functioning that occurred. This should then be explained to patients and their families.

The nurse should assess the patient's understanding of the nature of the problem, the stressors that were involved, any ongoing therapy that is required, and preventive measures that will decrease the probability of a recurrence.

Teaching may need to be repeated several times before the patient can cope with personal feelings and understand the information. Written materials can be helpful to patients who are having residual problems processing information. The teaching should include at least one responsible family member so that the information will be reinforced when the patient goes home.

A community health nursing referral may be helpful if the patient is discharged from the hospital with a residual deficit in cognitive functioning. The community health nurse can then continue to implement the nursing care plan and validate the patient's compliance with the treatment plan.

Intervening in Dementia

Nursing care of the patient with dementia is similar in some respects to that of the patient with delirium. In dementia, the stressors involved usually do not present an immediate threat to life; thus highest priority is given to nursing care that will help the patient maintain an optimum level of functioning. This will differ for each patient.

An attitude of hopelessness often evolves in those who work with chronically ill people. This can lead to stereotyping and a decreased ability to see and appreciate the uniqueness of each person. It is challenging to search for this uniqueness and rewarding to find it. Individualized nursing care is probably most important for those who will be institutionalized for a long time.

Nursing approaches should address the patient's need for social interaction. Interventions that may be helpful include

Table 23-10 Cholinesterase Inhibitor Therapy for Alzheimer's Disease			
CHARACTERISTIC	DONEPEZIL (ARICEPT)	GALANTAMINE (REMINYL)	RIVASTIGMINE (EXELON)
Dosage	5-10 mg/day	16-32 mg/day	6-12 mg/day
Mechanism of action	Selective AChE inhibition	AChE inhibition + nicotinic modulatory receptor effect	Butyryl ChE + AChE inhibition
Plasma $\frac{1}{2}$ life	5-7 hr	5-7 hr	0.6-2.0 hr
Elimination pathway	Hepatic	Renal + hepatic	Renal
Metabolism	CYP 2D6 CYP 3A4	CYP 2D6 CYP 3A4	ChE mediated hydrolysis
Protein binding	96%	18%	40%
Doses per day	1	2	2
Net proportion of subjects improved relative to placebo in clinical trials at 6 months	23%-24%	20%-25%	10%-29%

Data from Geldmacher D: *Contemporary diagnosis and management of Alzheimer's dementia*, Newton, Pa, 2003, Handbooks in Health Care Co.
AChE, Acetylcholinesterase; *ChE*, cholinesterase.

discussion groups with structured agendas, exercise groups to promote physical activity, reality orientation groups, sensory stimulation, and parties that are appropriate to the time of year or that recognize important events such as birthdays.

Arranging for visits from community volunteer groups provides stimulation as well as an opportunity to socialize. Referral to other members of the treatment team, especially the occupational, recreational, art, music, and dance therapists, may be indicated.

Pharmacological Approaches. The goal of AD research is to identify agents that prevent the occurrence, defer the onset, slow the progression, or improve the symptoms of disease. Pharmacological approaches to the treatment of dementia are related to theories about the cause of the disorder. Cholinesterase inhibitors improve cognitive symptoms or temporarily reduce the rate of cognitive decline (Cummings, 2000).

The acetylcholinesterase inhibitor class of drugs have shown proven efficacy in the treatment of some of the symptoms of AD. The three approved agents most often used are listed in Table 23-10. This class of drugs maximizes the function of cholinergic neurons by inhibiting the enzyme acetylcholinesterase (AChE); such inhibition prevents the metabolism of acetylcholine, the neurotransmitter that is associated with memory and learning and is found to be lower than normal in those with AD. Thus these drugs allow a greater concentration of acetylcholine in the brain, thereby improving cholinergic function.

Tacrine (Cognex), a fourth agent, was the first cholinesterase inhibitor to receive approval as a specific treatment for the cognitive symptoms of AD. It is used only occasionally now because of liver toxicity problems. Because AChE is the primary gastrointestinal motility-enhancing transmitter, nausea, anorexia, and diarrhea are common and are the primary limiting factors in practice when using these drugs.

Medications in general must be used with care when treating persons with dementia. Elderly people are very sensitive to medications and combinations of medications. Drugs with anticholinergic effects and benzodiazepines (which interfere with learning) should be avoided. Table 23-11 lists the categories of pharmacological treatment options for symptoms of AD.

Schultz and colleagues (2003) studied daily functioning in nursing home settings and found that, after cognitive effects were accounted for, behavioral dysregulation was a major cause of functional impairment. The use of the antipsychotic drugs (Table 23-12), particularly the atypicals, has been shown to decrease the agitation in patients with dementia, and several of them have received approval from the Food and Drug Administration for this purpose (Masand, 2000; Brodaty et al, 2003).

Much current research is focused on identifying pharmacological agents that can protect neurons from the progressive death caused by AD. Brain functions involving glutamate, calcium, and free radicals are being targeted in this research. Other brain research related to cognitive disorders involves investigating the role of phospholipid metabolism and the usefulness of anti-inflammatory drugs, nerve growth factor, and estrogen (Geldmacher, 2003).

Orientation. **Disorientation** is a common problem of people with cognitive impairment. Nursing interventions should help the patient function in the environment. In an institution it is helpful to mark patient rooms with large, clearly printed signs indicating the occupant's name. This also reminds forgetful people of others' names. Everyone needs a personal space. A favorite rocking chair, a handmade afghan, or a family picture gives the patient a sense of identity and helps to identify a personal area of the institution. Personal possessions also can be orienting devices.

A light in the room at night helps the patient remain oriented and decreases nighttime agitation. Clocks with large

Table 23-11	Pharmacological Treatment Options in Alzheimer's Disease
CATEGORY	TARGET SYMPTOMS
Cholinesterase inhibitors	Apathy, psychosis (delusions, hallucinations), agitation, anxiety, nighttime behavior; positive effects have been shown on cognition, activities of daily living, and global functioning
Antipsychotics	Psychosis (delusions, hallucinations), hostility, aggression, agitation, violent behavior
Antidepressants	Depressive symptoms, anxiety disorders
β-Blockers	Agitation
Benzodiazepines	Anxiety, agitation
Estrogen	Agitation
Anticonvulsants	Agitation, aggression, mood swings
Serotonergic agents	Psychosis, agitation

Modified from *J Clin Psychiatry* 61:307, 2000.

Table 23-12	Antipsychotic Agents Used in Elderly Patients With Behavioral Disturbances and Dementia		
AGENT	INITIAL DOSE (DAILY DOSE, IN MG)	AVERAGE TARGET DOSE (MG)	HIGHEST RECOMMENDED DOSE (MG)
Risperidone *	0.25-0.5	0.5-1.5	2-6
Olanzapine *	2.25-5.0	5.0-7.5	12.5-15
Quetiapine,* †	12.5-25	50-100	150-300
Haloperidol‡	0.5-1.0	1.5-2.0	2-7

Data from Geldmacher D: *Contemporary diagnosis and management of Alzheimer's dementia*, Newton, Pa, 2003, Handbooks in Health Care Company.
*Atypical antipsychotic agents. †Quetiapine usually requires at least twice daily dosing. ‡Typical antipsychotic agent.

faces help with orientation to time. A digital clock is not recommended because the confused person may not identify it as a clock. Calendars with large writing and a separate page for each day also help with time orientation. Newspapers provide other orienting stimuli and help to stimulate interest in current events. An institutional newspaper provides a creative outlet that focuses on patient strengths and helps patients maintain an awareness of their environment.

In general, reality orientation is helpful to patients with cognitive impairments. Systematic reality orientation includes attention to the dimensions of time, place, and person. This approach often takes place in a group and is most effective if the group meets daily, if possible, and at a consistent time. A pattern of group activity should be established.

For instance, the group might begin with each person introducing himself or herself, after which everyone is informed of the date and time. A review of the schedule for the day is often helpful. A brief time is allowed for questions. In general, this type of group meeting should last only 15 to 20 minutes. If the members become fatigued, their cognitive ability will deteriorate.

Communication. Recent memory loss is another common problem. Patients may be frustrated when constantly confronted with evidence of failing memory. Conversational focus can be directed toward topics that the patient initiates. Most patients feel more comfortable talking about remote memories and may derive pleasure from discussing past experiences. Misperceptions of the present can be dealt with gently and diplomatically.

For example, if an elderly woman who has been widowed for 10 years says that she expects her husband to come home soon, the nurse might reply, "You must have loved your husband very much. Sometimes it seems to you that he's still here." Explicitly or implicitly agreeing that her husband will "come home" fosters false hope, perhaps leading to a disappointment and distrust. Abrupt confrontation with the reality of her husband's death is cruel and will increase her anxiety. Considerations about reality orientation are discussed in Critical Thinking About Contemporary Issues.

The nurse should introduce herself at each interaction with the patient. The nurse's attitude should reflect unconditional positive regard. Empathy, warmth, and caring are important, and verbal communication should be clear, concise, and unhurried. A pleasant, calm, supportive tone of voice should be used, with the voice modulated in relationship to the patient's ability to hear. Shouting may be interpreted as anger by a person who hears well.

The use of pronouns should be avoided. Questions that require "yes" and "no" answers are best. Behavior should be requested one step at a time; if repetition is required, it should be stated in exactly the same way as the first time.

Nonverbal communication skills are also important, and verbal and nonverbal communication must be congruent. Nonverbal techniques, especially touch, are sometimes reassuring to the patient.

The nurse should try to understand who the patient was in the past. This can be accomplished by encouraging reminiscence and talking with family members. Pictures or music may help the patient remember past experiences. The patient's daily schedule should be predictable and unhurried. Distraction or diversion, along with decreased stimulation, should be used if a patient appears to become agitated. An appropriate use of humor and flexibility by the nurse helps the patient function in the environment.

Reinforcement of Coping Mechanisms. Previously helpful coping mechanisms are often used by patients with maladaptive cognitive responses. Sometimes these attempts to cope may be hard to understand unless placed in the appropriate context. An older man who pats and pinches nurses and makes lewd remarks may have had past success dealing with his anxiety by behaving seductively. An elderly woman who hoards food in her room may equate food with security. An aging person who has been suspicious of others in the past may become more suspicious over time.

These behaviors have a protective nature and therefore should not be actively confronted. The nurse should instead try to discover the source of the patient's anxiety and attempt to alleviate it, thus allowing the person to behave less defensively.

Wandering. Wandering is a behavior that causes great concern to caregivers. In fact, it often leads to institutionalization or to the use of restraints. Nurses should observe patients care-

---

> ### Critical Thinking *About* Contemporary Issues
>
> **Is Reality Orientation Always the Best Nursing Intervention for Patients Who Are Experiencing Progressive Memory Loss?**
>
> Reality orientation is often recommended as a nursing intervention for patients who are disoriented. The rationale is that patients are reassured by being in touch with where they are in time and place. For the same reason, clocks and calendars are placed where patients can see them.
>
> Reality orientation is appropriate for patients who can process the information given to them. However, in the case of progressive memory loss related to dementia, the question arises regarding whether repeated efforts at reality orientation serve patients' needs.
>
> For example, consider a situation in which a patient was distressed at attempts by the nursing staff to convince him that he was in a hospital. When a nurse participated in his life situation as he was experiencing it and responded as if she were in his workplace with him, he was much happier. The nurse's rationale for this intervention was that she was helping him to reminisce, which is an important developmental task for the elderly.
>
> Nurses must maintain a delicate balance between providing the patient with needed information about the environment and denying the patient's inability to process that information in a meaningful way. This means that nurses must question the automatic use of reality orientation as the best intervention for every disoriented patient.

fully in order to understand such behavior, identify the situations that contribute to it, and plan appropriate interventions.

In some cases medications may cause agitation and restlessness. Some patients are extremely sensitive to stress and tension in the environment, and their wandering may be an attempt to get away. Similarly, if patients are aware that an activity they dislike is about to occur (e.g., bathing or medication administration), they may try to avoid it. If wandering meets a patient's need for attention, efforts to control the behavior may actually reinforce it.

The nurse should decrease stress in the patient's environment, especially at night, when many people have decreased stress tolerance. Eliminating distracting background noise or shadows may help. Safe areas should be provided where patients can move about freely. If possible, this should include an outside area with adequate staff supervision to ensure safety.

Environmental design can be used to camouflage doorways or to incorporate distractions. Any method of increasing orientation also can decrease the need to wander. However, it is important to base nursing interventions on observations and an analysis of the motivation for the patient's behavior.

Decreasing Agitation. Patients may become agitated when pushed to do something unfamiliar or unclear. Expectations should be explained simply and completely. If the patient can make choices, the appropriate choices should be offered. An individual daily schedule of activities can help the person prepare for and plan his or her day. If a patient refuses to participate in an activity, continued insistence usually leads to increased agitation and sometimes to a loss of behavioral control, resulting in a catastrophic response.

The best approach may be to wait a few minutes and then return to see if the patient will agree to the request. Meanwhile the approach to the patient can be examined to see if the nurse might have contributed to the problem. Perhaps the patient thought the nurse was too controlling and a power struggle developed, or perhaps the nurse initiated the request abruptly and did not allow the patient a time for transition.

Family and Community Interventions. Many people with dementia live in the community with their families. It is important to support the caregivers, because the patient usually derives great benefit from being with them. When hospitalization occurs, careful discharge planning is needed to help the family prepare to receive the patient back home. Box 23-7 provides practical recommendations that may be helpful to caregivers.

Families of patients with AD may need support in identifying and coping with feelings such as denial, anger, and guilt—feelings much like those experienced by individuals who are grieving over a dying loved one. **Loneliness** and **depression** were found to be significantly higher in the caregiving wives of husbands with AD than in caregiving husbands of wives with AD and in the general spousal population (Beeson, 2003).

BOX **23-7**

Practical Recommendations for Caregivers of Agitated and Aggressive Patients With Dementia

Decrease Escalation
Decrease environmental stimuli and modify the environment.
Approach in a calm manner.
Use distraction: food, drink, music.
Maintain eye contact and a comfortable posture with arms/hands relaxed.
Use more than one sensory modality to send a calm message.
Match verbal and nonverbal signals.
Identify the affect observed in the patient; verbalize this for him or her.
Do not add more demands at this time.
Slow down pace and simplify your actions.
Maintain physical comfort.
Identify what is fueling the fire (e.g., triggers and reactions).
Maintain safety.

Communicate Effectively
Capture the patient's attention; stay in view.
Use simple, direct statements.
Limit choices.
Use gestures to assist with verbal directions.
Use one-step commands.
Speak clearly and slowly; allow time for response.

Use lower tone if voice needs to be raised because of hearing deficit.
Communicate your desire to help.

Review the Basics
Behavior is symptomatic of the illness; separate the behavior from the person.
A damaged mind gets stuck in one activity and has trouble shifting gears; what worked an hour ago may not work now.
The caregiver is the only security in a shrinking world.
Persons with dementia lose the ability to plan.
Know the person and structure his or her environment accordingly.
Having a daily pattern of repetitive behaviors at predictable times and by familiar persons helps those with memory impairment to help themselves.
A loving voice, attentiveness, touch, and consistency are enormously important.
Remember, a caregiver is not always an angel; there are times when frustration and anger are expressed; no one is perfect.
The caregiver's needs also must be recognized and respected.
Maintain the patient's religious/spiritual identity.
Humor can help.

From Tariot P: *J Clin Psychiatry* 60(suppl 8):11, 1999.

It is important for nurses to be aware of the mental health needs of family members, particularly of the caregiver, who often is female, the wife, daughter, or daughter-in-law of the afflicted person. Families may need assistance in providing 24-hour care for the patient. Home care agencies may provide nursing and homemaking services to enable patients to remain in their own homes.

If family members are not available during the day, adult day-care centers are available in some communities. These programs provide help with activities of daily living, recreation, health supervision, rehabilitation, exercise, and nutrition. Families also receive support and assistance, particularly during the first few weeks of attendance, when the patient may be resistant because he or she is having difficulty adapting to a new experience.

The National Chronic Care Consortium and the Alzheimer's Association (Borgenicht K, et al, 2001) have developed a model for helping families with Alzheimer's disease (Table 23-13). This model identified critical issues and helpful nursing interventions to implement with families at each phase of the illness.

A Nursing Treatment Plan Summary for patients who have maladaptive cognitive responses is presented in Table 23-14.

EVALUATION

Expectations of the patient who has cognitive difficulty must be realistic but not pessimistic. One evaluation criterion is the appropriateness of the nursing goal to the patient. The nurse should assess whether the expectation is too high or too low. Levels of expectation can be increased until the patient is clearly unable to function and then lowered to the realistic level.

The evaluation of the nursing care of the patient who has maladaptive cognitive responses is based on achievement of the identified nursing care goals. If these goals are not achieved, the nurse should ask the following questions:

- Was the assessment complete enough to correctly identify the problem?
- Were the goals individualized for the patient?
- Was enough time allowed for goal achievement?
- Did I have the skills needed to carry out the identified interventions?
- Were there environmental factors that affected goal achievement?
- Did additional stressors affect the patient's ability to cope?
- Was the goal achievable for this patient?
- What alternative approaches could be tried?

Table 23-13	Six-Phase Model for Helping Families With Alzheimer's Disease	
PHASE	DESCRIPTION	NURSING INTERVENTIONS
1: Prediagnostic	There is a growing awareness in the family that something is wrong.	Provide information and educational materials to help families understand their situation.
2: Diagnostic	Families must deal with the fear, emotions, and lost dreams related to the diagnosis.	Provide a one-session family consultation meeting to help family process the information and facilitate communication.
3: Role change	The person with dementia needs increasing care, the family must learn his/her abilities and adapt situations to maximize participation, family tasks must be reassigned, the entire family deals with issues of loss.	Provide family educational programs, support groups, counseling; also, services to the person with dementia in order to maintain a sense of self and morale.
4: Chronic caregiving	With increasing needs of the person with dementia, the family must stave off the exhaustion, burnout, and depression associated with caregiving. Respite must be provided, appropriate community services must be accessed. Normal family life is crowded out by the disease.	Provide psycho-educational programs to minimize caregiver stress; connect family with services such as day care and caregiver skills training programs to provide concrete guidance in caring for the person with dementia, the caregiver, and the family.
5: Transition to alternative care	The person with dementia often must eventually be placed in a nursing home or other care facility. The family needs help to identify this time and find a placement. This marks the end of personal caregiving and a shift into collaborative caregiving with appropriate role expectations.	Provide services that address the demoralization families experience with placement; facilitate the development of collaborative care relations between family and facility staff.
6: End of life	Ethical dilemmas faced in making end of life decisions must be resolved. The family must be helped to develop an image of a "good death", including rituals and legacies, to bring closure and meaning at the point of death.	Provide a bridge to the primary medical provider to educate the family on treatment options and offer support as the family anticipates death and faces repeated discussions involving decision making.

Modified from Educational Support Advisory Group: Tools for the assessment and treatment of dementia in managed care settings, 2001, a publication of the Chronic Care Networks for Alzheimer's Disease Initiative.

Colleagues are helpful in evaluating the nursing care plan. They may suggest alternative interventions or provide feedback about transference and countertransference issues. For instance, nurses who work with aging patients with dementia may respond to concerns about their own aging or that of their parents and have difficulty seeing patients as unique persons. Hallucinating patients often arouse anxiety in nurses, who may then respond with their own defense mechanisms. Regular supervision can help nurses develop enhanced self-awareness and determine when a particularly anxiety-provoking situation has bothered them and why.

The population of individuals suffering from alterations of cognitive responses is growing. By approaching care for these patients in a multidimensional manner, nurses convey competence, respect, and understanding, and build an interactional relationship with patients and their families. This includes the understanding of links between cognitive, behavioral, and functional abilities of the patient, the effects of their decline over time, and the understanding of the emotional, psychological, physical, and social needs of patients and families (Hendry and Douglas, 2003). Multidimensional, comprehensive, competent, and empathetic care focuses on the person caught in fading cognitive function, potentially lost in the growing needs caused by potentially devastating illness.

Table 23-14	NURSING TREATMENT PLAN SUMMARY	Maladaptive Cognitive Responses

Nursing Diagnosis: Disturbed thought processes
Expected Outcome: The patient will achieve optimum cognitive functioning.

SHORT-TERM GOAL	INTERVENTION	RATIONALE
The patient will meet basic biological needs.	Maintain adequate nutrition, monitor fluid intake and output, and monitor vital signs. Provide opportunities for rest and stimulation. Help with ambulation if necessary. Help with hygiene activities as needed.	Basic biological integrity is necessary for survival. Interventions related to survival are given high priority for nursing intervention.
The patient will be safe from injury.	Assess sensory and perceptual functioning. Provide access to items such as eyeglasses, hearing aids, canes, and walkers. Observe and remove safety hazards (e.g., obstacles, slippery floors, open flames, and inadequate lighting). Supervise medications if necessary. Protect from injury during periods of agitation with one-to-one nursing care; use restraints only if absolutely necessary.	Maladaptive cognitive responses usually involve sensory and perceptual disorders that can endanger the patient's safety.
The patient will experience an optimum level of self-esteem.	Provide reality orientation. Establish a trusting relationship. Encourage independence. Identify interests and skills; provide opportunities to use them. Give honest praise for accomplishments. Use therapeutic communication techniques to help patient communicate thoughts and feelings.	Cognitive impairment is a threat to self-esteem. A positive nurse-patient relationship can help the patient express fears and feel secure in the environment. The recognition of accomplishments also raises self-esteem.
The patient will maintain positive interpersonal relationships.	Initiate contact with significant others. Encourage patient to interact with others; involve in group activities. Teach family and patient about the nature of the problem and the recommended health care plan. Allow significant others to help with patient care if they wish. Meet with significant others regularly and provide them with an opportunity to talk. Involve patient and family in discharge planning.	Caring relationships with others promote a positive self-concept. Communication from significant others often can be understood more easily than communication from strangers. Family and friends can provide help in knowing the patient's habits and preferences. Involvement of significant others in caregiving often helps them cope with the stress of the patient's health problems.

COMPETENT CARING

A Clinical Exemplar of a Psychiatric Nurse
ALISON MEEKS, RN, MS

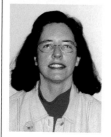

I worked on a unit that was set up to care for patients with behavioral problems that develop as a result of their dementia. I vividly remember one call we received about a patient who was described as violent, explosive, confused, and in need of total care in regard to activities of daily living. When the patient arrived on the unit, I discovered that Ms. S weighed 90 pounds, had long beautiful hair arranged up in a bun-style hairdo, and was ambulatory. She thought she was going to a hotel, so we took her bags and served her lunch while we interviewed her husband, who was her primary caregiver.

His was a very sad story. Tearfully he reported that his wife no longer loved him, that she was very malicious, and that she became physically violent at least once a day. He wanted to go on vacation while she was in the hospital, which some of the staff felt was probably the reason for this admission. However, he had been caring for his wife for 5 years with little or no help from the community or family members, and it was clear that he needed a break. It would be hard on him, however, because this would be the first time they had been apart from each other in their 58 years of marriage.

Ms. S had a Mini-Mental State Examination score of 12 and had great difficulty visually interpreting her environment. For example, she thought a comb was a knife and the garbage can, her purse. She was also very sensitive to her environment. If the unit was loud and a lot of people were walking around, she became more active and often had the potential for getting hurt or hurting someone else. During periods of activity on the unit, such as a shift change, we escorted Ms. S to her room, where she would fold clothes or go through one of four pocketbooks we put together for her. We needed four pocketbooks because she would misplace one and we would not be able to find it. This symptom presented great problems at home for the caregiver because anything left out would be moved and often never found. Our solution was to set up several baskets of safe items for Ms. S to rummage through.

Ms. S became physically violent three times during her 8-day hospitalization. Each incident occurred when staff members entered her room and she accused them of breaking into her home. We started to knock on her door before entering and would have something for her such as a pocketbook, a book, or her stockings in our hands. That seemed to solve that problem. Another intervention that worked for Ms. S was music. She always liked ballet and now thought she was a retired dancer. We never challenged this and listened to her wonderful stories about dance and other dancers.

Ms. S did not recognize her husband when he came back from vacation. He was hurt and said we had done nothing to help her. We worked extensively with her husband by having him come and observe our interventions with Ms. S. Our goal was to help him realize the level of her impairment. He soon realized that her actions were not malicious. We diagnosed a urinary tract infection during her admission, which we treated, and we prescribed 0.5 mg of haloperidol each morning, which helped to decrease her explosive episodes. We also enlisted the help of family members, friends, and a home health provider to care for Ms. S. I made one home visit after discharge and gave suggestions on how to make the home safe for Ms. S.

Four weeks after discharge Mr. S mailed the nurses a letter thanking us for giving him his life back. He explained that he felt he should have been better able to care for his wife on his own before her hospitalization and that he had even contemplated suicide because of the overwhelming burden of caring for his wife. It seemed to us that in this case, we touched the lives of two rather than one. ∎

CHAPTER FOCUS POINTS

- The continuum of cognitive responses is related to behavioral and biological models of learning and memory. Cognitive activity depends on intelligence, education, life experience, and culture.
- Behaviors related to cognitive responses vary depending on whether the maladaptive response is acute and likely to resolve (as in delirium) or progressive and chronic (as in dementia).
- Maladaptive cognitive responses include an inability to make decisions, impaired memory and judgment, disorientation, misperceptions, decreased attention span, and difficulties with logical reasoning.
- Delirium is the behavioral response to widespread disturbances in cerebral metabolism, represents a sudden decline from a previous level of functioning, and is usually considered a medical emergency.
- Dementia is a maladaptive cognitive response that features a loss of intellectual abilities and interferes with the patient's usual social or occupational activities. Alzheimer's disease (AD) is the most common type of dementia and accounts for approximately 65% of the cases of dementia.
- Pseudodementia is a cognitive impairment secondary to a functional psychiatric disorder. Depression associated with AD may be among the most common mood disorders of older adults.
- Predisposing factors related to impaired cognition are aging, neurobiological functioning, changes in brain structures, genetic factors, and underlying psychiatric and medical conditions.

- Precipitating stressors related to delirium are categorized as CNS disorders, metabolic disorders, cardiopulmonary disorders, systemic illness, and sensory deprivation or stimulation.
- Precipitating stressors related to dementia are categorized as degenerative brain disorders, cerebrovascular causes, toxic-metabolic disturbances, CNS infections, and miscellaneous causes.
- Coping resources are largely based on individual and interpersonal supports.
- Coping mechanisms include intellectualization, rationalization, denial, and regression.
- The primary NANDA nursing diagnoses are acute or chronic confusion and disturbed thought processes.
- The primary *DSM-IV-TR* diagnoses are categorized as delirium, dementia, and amnestic disorders.
- The expected outcome of nursing care is that the patient will achieve the optimum level of cognitive functioning.
- Interventions related to delirium include caring for physiological needs, responding to hallucinations, therapeutic communication, and patient education.
- Interventions related to dementia include pharmacological approaches, orientation, therapeutic communication, reinforcement of coping mechanisms, responding to wandering, decreasing agitation, and family and community approaches.
- Evaluation of nursing care is based on goal accomplishment and involves feedback from the patient, significant others, peers, and supervisors.

KEY TERMS

agnosia, 452
AIDS dementia complex, 453
amnesia, 452
aphasia, 452
apraxia, 452
confabulation, 451
countertransference, 469

delirium, 447
dementia, 448
denial, 459
empathy, 466
hallucinations, 463
hypoxia, 457
learning, 445

memory, 445
polypharmacy, 456
pseudodementia, 450
reality orientation, 466
regression, 460
sundowning syndrome, 452
transference, 469

CHAPTER REVIEW QUESTIONS

1. Match each term in Column A with the correct definition in Column B.

Column A

_____ Delirium
_____ Denial
_____ Dementia
_____ Agnosia
_____ Pseudodementia
_____ Sundowning syndrome
_____ Amygdala
_____ Aphasia
_____ Apraxia
_____ Excess disability

Column B

A. Responsible for emotion and emotional memory
B. Difficulty recognizing well-known objects
C. Disturbed consciousness and cognitions developing over a short time
D. May ignore memory loss, interfering with treatment planning
E. Depressed, missed in the elderly, not treated appropriately
F. Gradual onset with continuing cognitive decline
G. Difficulty finding the right word
H. Extreme agitation, occurring at night
I. Cognitive responses functioning at a lower level than one would expect
J. Inability to perform familiar skilled activities

2. Fill in the blanks.

A. The brain lesions that are characteristic of Alzheimer's disease are _____ and _____.
B. Cholinesterase inhibitors are pharmacological interventions for _____.
C. The term _____ refers to extreme agitation related to dementia.
D. _____ is usually sudden and a medical emergency.

3. Provide short answers for the following questions.

A. Describe the behavioral and biological differences between working memory and long-term memory.
B. List three coping strategies that you would suggest to the caregiver of a person who has a moderate level of cognitive impairment resulting from dementia.
C. Describe a discharge plan for a person who has been hospitalized for the treatment of delirium related to combining prescription medicine and alcohol.

Visit Evolve for additional resources related to the content of this chapter.
http://evolve.elsevier.com/Stuart/principles/
• Topical Course Outline • Student Workbook Exercises • Critical Thinking Questions and Activities • Case Studies • Research Topics
• Monthly Content Updates • WebLinks

Student Study CD-ROM

Access the accompanying CD-ROM for animations, interactive exercises, review questions for the NCLEX examination, and an audio glossary.

REFERENCES

American Psychiatric Association: *Diagnostic and statistical manual of mental disorders*, ed 4, text revision, Washington, DC, 2000, American Psychiatric Association.

American Psychiatric Association: Practice guideline for the treatment of patients with delirium, *Am J Psychiatry* 156:1, 1999.

Beeson RA: Loneliness and depression in the spousal caregivers of those with Alzheimer's disease versus non-caregiving spouses, *Arch Psychiatr Nurs* 17:135, 2003.

Borgenicht K et al: *Tools for the assessment and treatment of dementia in managed care settings*, 2001, a publication of the Chronic Care Networks for Alzheimer's Disease Initiative.

Brodaty H et al: A randomized placebo-controlled trial of risperidone for the treatment of aggression, agitation, and psychosis of dementia, *J Clin Psychiatry* 64:134, 2003.

Cummings JL: Cholinesterase inhibitors: a new class of psychotropic compounds, *Am J Psychiatry* 157:4, 2000.

Doody RS et al: Practice parameter: management of dementia (an evidence-based review). Report of the Quality Standards Subcommittee of the American Academy of Neurology, *Neurology* 56:1154, 2001.

Geldmacher DS: *Contemporary diagnosis and management of Alzheimer's dementia*, Newtown, Pa, 2003, Handbooks in Health Care Company.

Hendry K and Douglas D: Promoting quality of life for clients diagnosed with dementia, *J Am Psychiatr Nurs Assoc* 9:96, 2003.

Inouye SK: A multicomponent intervention to prevent delirium in hospitalized older patients, *N Engl J Med* 340:669, 1999.

Kelley L et al: Family involvement in care for individuals with dementia protocol, *J Gerontol Nurs* 2:13, 2000.

Knopman DS et al: Practice parameter: diagnosis of dementia (an evidence-based review). Report of the Quality Standards Subcommittee of the American Academy of Neurology, *Neurology* 56:1143, 2001.

Masand P: Atypical antipsychotics for elderly patients with neurodegenerative disorders and medical conditions, *Psychiatr Ann* 30:202, 2000.

McDougall GJ Jr, Holston EC: Black and white men at risk for memory impairment, *Nurs Res* 52:42, 2003.

NSW: Genetics Fact Sheet: Alzheimer's Disease, NSW Genetic Education Program, 281:33, 2003, http://www.genetics.com.au.

Peterson RC et al: Practice parameter: early detection of dementia (an evidence-based review). Report of the Quality Standards Subcommittee of the American Academy of Neurology, *Neurology* 56:1133, 2001.

Schultz SK et al; The influence of cognitive impairment and behavioral dysregulation on daily functioning in the nursing home setting, *Am J Psychiatry* 160:582, 2003.

Sultzer DL et al: Delusional thoughts and regional frontal/temporal cortex metabolism in Alzheimer's disease, *Am J Psychiatry* 160:341, 2003.

Wolozin B: Cyp46 (24S-cholesterol hydroxylase): a genetic risk factor for Alzheimer's disease, *Arch Neurol* 60:16, 2003.

Yeaworth R, Burke W: Frontotemporal dementia: a different kind of dementia, *Arch Psychiatr Nurs* 14: 249, 2000.

Zubenko GS et al: A collaborative study of the emergence and clinical features of the major depressive syndrome of Alzheimer's disease, *Am J Psychiatry* 160:857, 2003.

Sleepmonger, deathmonger, with capsules in my palms each night, eight at a time from sweet pharmaceutical bottles I make arrangements for a pint-sized journey. I'm the queen of this condition. I'm an expert on making the trip and now they say I'm an addict. Now they ask why. Why!

ANNE SEXTON, THE ADDICT

CHEMICALLY MEDIATED RESPONSES AND SUBSTANCE-RELATED DISORDERS

24

Michele T. Laraia ■ Linda V. Jefferson

LEARNING OBJECTIVES

After studying this chapter, the student should be able to:

1. Describe the continuum of adaptive and maladaptive chemically mediated responses (**I**).
2. Identify behaviors associated with chemically mediated responses (**II**).
3. Analyze predisposing factors, precipitating stressors, and appraisal of stressors related to chemically mediated responses (**II**).
4. Describe coping resources and coping mechanisms related to chemically mediated responses (**II**).
5. Formulate nursing diagnoses related to chemically mediated responses (**III**).
6. Examine the relationship between nursing diagnoses and medical diagnoses related to chemically mediated responses (**III**).
7. Identify expected outcomes and short-term nursing goals related to chemically mediated responses (**IV**).
8. Develop a patient education plan to promote patients' adaptive chemically mediated responses (**V**).
9. Analyze nursing interventions related to chemically mediated responses (**VI**).
10. Evaluate nursing care related to chemically mediated responses (**VII**).

 Visit Evolve for additional resources related to the content of this chapter.
http://evolve.elsevier.com/Stuart/principles/

Psychoactive substances have been used by people in almost all cultures since prehistoric times. Psychoactive substances affect the brain. They alter the mind, the way reality is perceived, and the way people feel. These substances have been seen by many as enhancers of individual and social functioning. People continue to use them for relief of negative emotional states, such as depression, fear, and anxiety; relief from fatigue or boredom; and as a break from daily routines by way of producing altered states of consciousness. Alcohol and drugs also continue to be used in various religious ceremonies.

Ethical and legal considerations aside, moderate use for any of these purposes would probably not result in major social or individual harm. However, all cultures also have recognized the negative effects of alcohol and drug use. Excessive use of these substances has contributed to profound individual and social problems.

Any drug that affects the pleasure centers of the brain and thus can produce pleasurable changes in mental or emotional states has potential for abuse. Drugs that cause the most marked and immediate desirable effects have the greatest abuse potential. Alcohol and cocaine are very popular because they produce effects on the brain within minutes. Drugs of potential abuse include legal drugs, such as alcohol and prescription drugs; illegal drugs, such as heroin, cocaine, and marijuana; and household products, such as inhalants.

CONTINUUM OF CHEMICALLY MEDIATED RESPONSES

Definition of Terms

A person may achieve a state of relaxation, euphoria, stimulation, or altered awareness in several ways. The range of these chemically mediated coping responses is illustrated in Figure 24-1. Although there is a continuum from **occasional drug use** to **frequent drug use** to **abuse** and **dependence**, not everyone who uses drugs becomes an abuser, nor does every abuser become dependent. The definitions of the terms *use, abuse,* and *dependence* have changed through the years and vary greatly in the addiction literature. The nurse should realize that what one person or health care professional means by addiction is not necessarily meant by another. Reading and discussion should start with agreement about the meanings of terms.

Substance abuse, as described in the *Diagnostic and Statistical Manual of Mental Disorders*, fourth edition, text revision (*DSM-IV-TR*) (American Psychiatric Association, 2000) refers to continued use despite related problems. The term substance dependence, related to either drugs or alcohol, indicates a severe condition, usually considered a disease. There may be physical problems as well as serious disruptions in the person's work, family, and social life.

The psychosocial behaviors related to substance dependence are often called addiction. For most purposes, the terms dependence and addiction are used interchangeably. Dual diagnosis is the co-existence of substance abuse and psychiatric disorders within the same person.

Withdrawal symptoms and tolerance are signs that the person has physical dependence on the drug. Withdrawal symptoms result from a biological need that develops when the body becomes adapted to having the drug in the system. Characteristic symptoms occur when the level of the substance in the system decreases. Tolerance means that with continued use, more of the substance is needed to produce the same effect.

Physical dependence can occur independently from the symptoms of substance dependence. For example, a patient who receives narcotics for chronic pain may develop both tolerance and withdrawal, yet not have any of the other problems related to substance dependence, such as preoccupation with getting the drug, loss of control, or use despite problems. This person would be described as physically dependent on the narcotic but would not be called a drug addict.

Many people progress from use to abuse at some time in their lives. However, only about 1 in 10 people progress from use to abuse to dependence. Once use has begun, the risk of becoming dependent is influenced by many biological, psychological, and sociocultural factors.

Attitudes Toward Substance Abuse

Substance abuse is viewed differently depending on the substance used, the person using it, and the setting in which it is used. Nurses should be aware of these social and cultural attitudes and recognize their impact on individual users and people close to them. For instance, a businessman who starts arguments after a few drinks with his associates would not usually be considered an alcohol abuser. If the same person was caught nipping from a bottle in his desk, he would probably be considered to have a drinking problem.

Tobacco abuse is still accepted in the United States despite convincing evidence of medical problems related to smoking, the effects of secondary smoke inhalation, and the release of a number of practice guidelines for the treatment of patients with nicotine dependence. On the other hand, a person who smokes opium would be considered deviant, even if the behavior took place in private.

Can you describe other examples of sociocultural mixed messages regarding the use of tobacco, caffeine, alcohol, and marijuana? How would you, as a health professional, go about changing these attitudes? ■

Changing laws related to consumption, sale, and serving of alcohol and drugs may reflect changing attitudes toward their use. **Driving while intoxicated (DWI)** laws are becom-

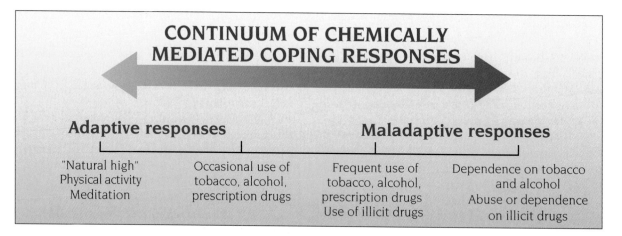

CONTINUUM OF CHEMICALLY MEDIATED COPING RESPONSES

Adaptive responses		Maladaptive responses	
"Natural high" Physical activity Meditation	Occasional use of tobacco, alcohol, prescription drugs	Frequent use of tobacco, alcohol, prescription drugs Use of illicit drugs	Dependence on tobacco and alcohol Abuse or dependence on illicit drugs

Figure 24-1 Continuum of chemically mediated coping responses.

ing tougher. When groups of friends go out, it is common for one person to be chosen as the designated driver who will not drink. Places where alcoholic beverages are served can be held liable if a customer overindulges and then causes an accident. Mandatory sentencing for certain drug offenses is intended to show an unaccepting attitude toward drug abuse.

Many nurses have negative attitudes toward alcoholics and other drug abusers. Some have had negative experiences with family members or friends who have had substance-related problems. This may influence the nurse's ability to assess and care for these patients. Nurses often see substance abusers at their worst, during a medical or psychiatric crisis. They see these patients returning repeatedly for alcohol- or drug-related health problems. Nurses rarely have contact with alcoholics and drug addicts who have recovered from their addiction because once they have recovered, they are ill less often. When they do seek health care, these patients may try to hide their substance abuse history.

Substance abuse is a chronic, relapsing, disabling health condition with both genetic and societal implications. Substance abusers may be in treatment multiple times before they are successful at prolonged recovery. The best way for nurses to change their negative attitudes is to attend open meetings of self-help groups, where they will meet recovering alcoholics and addicts who have overcome tremendous odds to remain sober and lead healthy, productive lives.

Prevalence

The United States has one of the **highest levels of substance abuse in the world.** Substance abuse is involved in many medical illnesses, hospitalizations, emergency room visits, and deaths. Substance abuse is a **chronic, relapsing health problem.** Substance abusers may be in treatment many times, or make repeated attempts to quit, before they are successful.

Adolescence is the most common period for the first experience with drugs. Although teenagers who use psychoactive substances tend to progress from nicotine to alcohol to marijuana and then to drugs that are perceived to be more dangerous, drug use patterns seem to be most related to availability.

According to the National Institute on Drug Abuse, about 81% of people in the United States age 12 and older have used alcohol sometime in their lives (Johnson et al, 2003). Among 8th graders, 50% have had at least one drink of alcohol, 20% of them report having been drunk, 17% describe their alcohol use as "heavy," 41% have smoked cigarettes, and 20% have used marijuana. Among 12th graders, 50% had consumed alcohol in the past 30 days, 30% reported drinking on four or more occasions during the past month, and about 6% reported heavy alcohol consumption, called "binge drinking" (at least five or more drinks on one occasion within the past 2 weeks).

Apart from being illegal, underage drinking poses a high risk for injury and social consequences, such as increased motor vehicle accidents, suicide, sexual assault, and high risk sexual behavior. Underage alcohol use is also more likely to kill young people than is all the illegal drugs combined (Al-

cohol Alert, 2003). Information about substance abuse by adolescents is provided in Chapter 37.

In 2001 an estimated 15.9 million or 7.1% of Americans age 12 years or older used an illicit drug, compared to 6.3% in 2000. The largest increase in regular drug use was for "club drugs"—MDMA or ecstasy—whose regular use among high school seniors has more than doubled in recent years. Heroin overdoses in teenagers also have increased in the past decade. When examined by age-groups, in 2001 10.8 % of youths ages 12 to 17 were current drug users, compared with 9.7 % in 2000. Among adults ages 18 to 25 years, current drug use increased between the years 2000 and 2001 from 15.9% to 18.8%. No significant changes in the rates of drug use among adults age 26 or older were noted (SAMHSA, 2003).

Overall, use of alcohol and illicit drugs appears to increase into a person's mid-20s, level off, and then decrease with age (Figure 24-2). **If use begins before age 15, the individual is 4 times more likely to have abuse problems as an adult** compared with individuals who begin using alcohol after age 21 (DeWit et al, 2000).

It has been reported that both the lifetime prevalence and the intensity of alcohol use is greater among males, who are

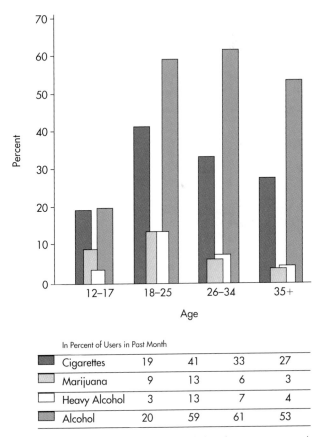

In Percent of Users in Past Month	12–17	18–25	26–34	35+
Cigarettes	19	41	33	27
Marijuana	9	13	6	3
Heavy Alcohol	3	13	7	4
Alcohol	20	59	61	53

Note: Heavy alcohol use is having five or more drinks on the same occasion on each of five or more days in the past 30 days.

Figure 24-2   Use of substances by age group. (Data from US Substance Abuse and Mental Health Services Administration, Office of Applied Studies. *Summary of findings from the 1998 National Household Survey on Drug Abuse,* Rockville, Md, 1999, USDHHS.)

4 times more likely to be heavy drinkers than females. In addition, whites and Hispanics reported higher levels of alcohol use than blacks, yet deaths from alcohol use are highest for black males. Those with more education were more likely to use alcohol, but heavy use was more common among the less educated and unemployed (Horgan, 2001).

At least half of adults arrested for **major crimes,** including homicide, theft, and assault, test positive for drugs at the time of their arrest. Among those convicted of violent crimes, approximately half of state prison inmates and 40% of federal prisoners had been drinking or taking drugs at the time of their offense.

One of the most troubling effects of alcohol is its effect on marriage, which is reflected in the relationship between heavy drinking and marital violence. Illicit drugs and alcohol play a role in **domestic violence,** affecting both married and unmarried couples. More than three-quarters of female victims of nonfatal domestic violence report that their assailant had been drinking or using drugs (Horgan, 2001).

Most people with alcohol use disorders do not seek treatment (Weisner and Matzger, 2002). It is estimated that from 75% to 93% of adults in the United States who need alcohol treatment do not actually receive it. The most frequently cited reasons for not seeking alcohol treatment are shown in Figure 24-3.

Multiple Substance Use. Simultaneous or sequential use of more than one substance is very common. People do this to enhance, lessen, or otherwise change the nature of their intoxication or to relieve withdrawal symptoms. Use of alcohol with cocaine or use of alcohol with heroin, also known as **speedballing,** is especially common. Heroin users often combine alcohol, marijuana, and benzodiazepines with heroin.

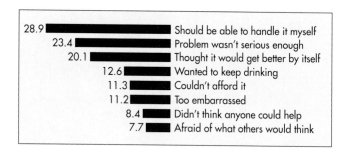

28.9	Should be able to handle it myself
23.4	Problem wasn't serious enough
20.1	Thought it would get better by itself
12.6	Wanted to keep drinking
11.3	Couldn't afford it
11.2	Too embarrassed
8.4	Didn't think anyone could help
7.7	Afraid of what others would think

Figure 24-3 Reasons why people (%) do not seek alcohol treatment. (From Grant B: NLAES identifies treatment beliefs as barriers to access, 1999.)

Multiple drug use is particularly dangerous if synergistic drugs, such as barbiturates and alcohol, are used. It also complicates substance abuse assessment and intervention because the patient may be demonstrating effects of or withdrawal from several drugs at the same time.

Dual Diagnosis. In the addicted population, prevalence of psychiatric illness is no greater than in the general population. However, up to 51% of individuals with a serious mental illness are also dependent on or addicted to alcohol or illicit drugs (Table 24-1). Thus they are referred to as having a **dual diagnosis**.

For example, people with schizophrenia are more than 4 times as likely to have a substance use disorder during their lifetimes, and those with bipolar disorder are more than 5 times as likely to have such a diagnosis than are people in the general population. Nearly 60% of male and 70% of female alcohol abusers are thought to have at least one other psychiatric disorder. This poses unique challenges for clinicians, because these patients can be more difficult to diagnose and are often treatment-resistant with high relapse rates.

Despite their prevalence, substance-related disorders are frequently underdetected and underdiagnosed in primary care settings, as well as in acute-care psychiatric and medical settings, particularly in hospital emergency services (Reynaud et al, 2001). Failure to detect substance abuse disorders results in misdiagnosis of the psychiatric disorder, suboptimal pharmacological treatment, neglect of appropriate interventions for substance abuse, and inappropriate treatment planning and referral.

This underdetection can be caused by a combination of factors including (1) clinicians' lack of awareness of the symptoms or the high rates of substance disorders in psychiatric populations; (2) the difficulty in differentiating substance disorders from psychiatric disorders; (3) patients' denial, minimization, and failure to acknowledge their substance-related problems; and (4) patients' cognitive, psychotic, and other impairments related to their psychiatric illness. Studies have shown that dual disorders are especially common among the homeless (50% of the homeless mentally ill have a substance abuse problem), prisoners (56% of prisoners have a substance abuse problem and/or another psychiatric illness), and patients in psychiatric facilities (34%) (Harvard Mental Health Letter, 2003).

Substance-Related Disorders in Nurses. Disciplinary records from state boards of nursing provide information

Table 24-1	Lifetime Prevalence of Substance Abuse and Psychiatric Disorders			
PSYCHIATRIC DISORDER	**ALCOHOL ABUSE**	**ALCOHOL DEPENDENCE**	**DRUG ABUSE**	**DRUG DEPENDENCE**
Schizophrenia	10%	24%	15%	13%
Antisocial personality	22%	52%	11%	31%
Panic disorder	7%	22%	3%	11%
Major depression	5%	12%	7%	11%

From EPA Study Data: *Harvard Mental Health Letter* 20:1, 2003.

about impaired nurses. According to the National Council of State Boards of Nursing, 53% of all disciplinary actions taken against registered nurses in 1995 were drug related (down from 94.4% in 1987 and 68% in 1991). These figures could reflect a decrease in the problem, a decrease in reporting of the problem, earlier and more effective treatment, or an increase in the reporting of non–substance-related competency problems.

Unfortunately, it is still a common practice to deal with a nurse who has a drug problem by ignoring the problem, firing the nurse, or asking for the nurse's resignation rather than reporting it to the state licensing board and facilitating treatment for the nurse. Therefore, these data may only reflect a small segment of the problem. Alternative approaches facilitate impaired nurses receiving treatment that is more effective and humane (see Citing the Evidence).

Alcohol is the drug of choice for nurses, as it is in the general population. Also, as in the general population, the nurse's choice of substance is influenced by availability and exposure. Of all health care professionals, physicians and nurses use parenteral narcotics the most in their practices. Therefore, they are more likely to choose these drugs for their own use.

Among narcotics, the drug of choice for nurses is meperidine (Demerol). Anesthesiologists and nurse anesthetists who abuse substances tend to favor fentanyl, a potent, short-acting narcotic. In general, health care professionals tend to abuse prescription drugs rather than "street" drugs, whether they acquire them by prescription or diversion.

CITING THE EVIDENCE ON
State Policies and Impaired Nurses

BACKGROUND: This longitudinal comparative 6-month study evaluated the outcomes for two groups of RNs and LPNs with substance use problems. A group of 100 had disciplinary actions taken against their licenses by four U.S. regulatory boards using a traditional, disciplinary approach. The alternative approach consisted of a group of 119 from three U.S. states in which the regulatory boards supported nurses and diverted them to programs of treatment, and subsequent to program completion, determined their suitability to return to practice.

RESULTS: The alternative group had more nurses with active licenses, fewer with criminal convictions, and more nurses employed in nursing than the traditional group at the end of 6 months. No difference in relapse rate was found.

IMPLICATIONS: Alternative policies were as effective as disciplinary policies and were a more humane and rehabilitative approach. Regulatory state boards of nursing should be consistent with approaches that rehabilitate nurses and return them to the work force as well as being consistent with the principles of Healthy People 2010 in eliminating financial barriers limiting access to treatment.

Haack M, Yocom C: *J Nurs Scholarsh* 34:89, 2002.

ASSESSMENT

Although accurate assessment of a patient's patterns of drug and alcohol use is important, it is sometimes very difficult to accomplish. Alcohol and drug addicts may use many defense mechanisms when discussing their chemical use. They tend to deny how much they use and its relationship to problems in their lives. They often rationalize their substance use. Patients should not be criticized for these unconscious mechanisms. They are often not aware of the extent or effects of their use.

It is also true that some patients purposely distort the truth about drug use to avoid feared consequences. The nurse should be aware of these behaviors and take them into account. On the other hand, the nurse should be aware that only about 1 in 10 people who drink develop substance dependence at some point in their lives. Thus one should not jump to the conclusion that a person is in denial if he or she relates no alcohol-related problems.

Screening for Substance Abuse

One must first be asking the right questions. People who drink, take drugs, or do both tend to be around others who drink and use drugs as they do. They do not have a good idea of what "normal" use patterns are. However, even people who deny drug and drinking problems are apt to answer certain questions truthfully. These questions are included in screening tools, which are the first level of assessment for alcohol and drug dependence.

Simple screening tools are available that are useful in identifying people who may have problems with substance use. Because screening tools are only suggestive, findings from them should be followed by a full diagnostic assessment.

CAGE. The simplest tool that can be used in any health setting to screen for alcoholism is the CAGE questionnaire. CAGE is an acronym for the four questions it contains (Box 24-1). Answering "yes" to two or more questions indicates probable alcohol abuse. Further assessment would be needed to make a diagnosis. The CAGE questionnaire is recommended as an initial screening tool for alcohol abuse because its questions and scoring can be remembered easily and included in any interview.

Given that CAGE is such a simple screening tool, why do you think it is not used more often in routine nursing assessments?

BOX 24-1

The CAGE Questionnaire

- Have you ever felt you ought to **C**ut down on your drinking?
- Have people **A**nnoyed you by criticizing your drinking?
- Have you ever felt bad or **G**uilty about your drinking?
- Have you ever had a drink first thing in the morning to steady your nerves or get rid of a hangover (**E**ye-opener)?

Scoring: Two "yes" answers indicates probable alcohol abuse and warrants further assessment.

From Schiffer R et al: *Neuropsychiatry*, ed 2, Philadelphia, 2003, Lippincott, Williams, and Wilkins.

B-DAST. The Brief Drug Abuse Screening Test (B-DAST) is the quickest drug abuse screening tool (Box 24-2). Each item has a one-point value. Scores of 6 or more suggest significant drug-abuse problems. Patients who score above established cutoff scores are considered to be addicted.

Breathalyzer. The simplest biological measure to obtain is blood alcohol content (BAC) by use of a Breathalyzer. Alcohol in any amount has an effect on the central nervous system (CNS). The behaviors that can be expected from a nontolerant person at different concentrations of alcohol in the blood are shown in Table 24-2.

Table 24-2	Comparison of Blood Alcohol Concentrations With Behavioral Manifestations of Intoxication	
BLOOD ALCOHOL LEVEL	**BEHAVIORS**
0.05 to 0.15 g/dl	Euphoria, labile mood, cognitive disturbances (decreased concentration, impaired judgment, loss of sexual inhibitions)
0.15 to 0.25 g/dl	Slurred speech, staggering gait, diplopia, drowsiness, labile mood with outbursts
0.3 g/dl	Stupor, aggressive behavior, incoherent speech, labored breathing, vomiting
0.4 g/dl	Coma
0.5 g/dl	Severe respiratory depression, death

A person who has developed tolerance to alcohol would not demonstrate these behaviors and could have a high BAC without showing any signs of impairment. A level greater than 0.10% without associated behavioral symptoms indicates the presence of tolerance. **The higher the level without symptoms, the more severe the tolerance. High tolerance** is usually a sign of **physical dependence.**

Blood and Urine Screening. Blood and urine are the body fluids most often tested for drug content, although saliva, hair, breath, and sweat analysis methods have been developed. Identification and measurement of drug levels in the blood are useful for treating drug overdoses or complications in emergency room and other medical settings. Otherwise, urine drug screening is the method of choice because it is noninvasive.

Urine drug screening is sometimes used to test prospective employees and athletes for evidence of drug use. Drug treatment personnel also use it to determine whether patients have used drugs while in treatment. Urine drug screening is often used in court to validate a person's drug use related to criminal activity.

The person being tested may try to alter the sample to hide drug use. The most common ways to do this are diluting the specimen with water from the toilet or substituting a "clean" specimen donated by a friend for the "dirty" specimen. To help prevent these practices, the specimen is often collected on random days under direct observation of a same-

BOX 24-2

Brief Drug Abuse Screening Test (B-DAST)

Instructions: The following questions concern information about your involvement and abuse of drugs. Drug abuse refers to (1) the use of prescribed or over-the-counter drugs in excess of the directions and (2) any nonmedical use of drugs. Carefully read each statement and decide whether your answer is yes or no. Then circle the appropriate response.

YES NO   1. Have you used drugs other than those required for medical reasons?
YES NO   2. Have you abused prescription drugs?
YES NO   3. Do you abuse more than one drug at a time?
YES NO   4. Can you get through the week without using drugs (other than those required for medical reasons)?
YES NO   5. Are you always able to stop using drugs when you want to?
YES NO   6. Have you had "blackouts" or "flashbacks" as a result of drug use?
YES NO   7. Do you ever feel bad about your drug abuse?
YES NO   8. Does your spouse (or parents) ever complain about your involvement with drugs?
YES NO   9. Has drug abuse ever created problems between you and your spouse?
YES NO 10. Have you ever lost friends because of your use of drugs?
YES NO 11. Have you ever neglected your family or missed work because of your use of drugs?
YES NO 12. Have you ever been in trouble at work because of drug abuse?
YES NO 13. Have you ever lost a job because of drug abuse?
YES NO 14. Have you gotten into fights when under the influence of drugs?
YES NO 15. Have you engaged in illegal activities in order to obtain drugs?
YES NO 16. Have you ever been arrested for possession of illegal drugs?
YES NO 17. Have you ever experienced withdrawal symptoms as a result of heavy drug intake?
YES NO 18. Have you had medical problems as a result of your drug use (e.g., memory loss, hepatitis, convulsions, bleeding)?
YES NO 19. Have you ever gone to anyone for help for a drug problem?
YES NO 20. Have you ever been involved in a treatment program specifically related to drug use?

Items 4 and 5 are scored in the "no," or false, direction; each item is 1 point; 6 or more points suggest significant problems.

From Skinner HA: *Addict Behav* 7:363, 1982.

sex staff member. Another way is to have the person leave jackets, sweaters, purses, and so forth outside the stall, place drops of dye in the toilet water to alter its color, and test the specimen for temperature. Fresh, undiluted urine should feel warm through the cup and should be approximately 37° C.

The length of time that drugs can be found in blood and urine varies according to dosage and the metabolic properties of the drug. All traces of the drug may disappear within 24 hours or may still be detectable several weeks later.

Random urine testing for drugs is required for members of some occupations, including some nurses. This practice has been challenged as an invasion of privacy and an intrusion on professional integrity. What is your opinion about random urine testing for nurses? ■

Behaviors of Abuse and Dependence

Using alcohol and drugs can have many consequences. Some of these consequences are very serious and have led to great social concern. Lifestyles associated with substance abuse carry risks. Accidents are frequent, and violence is common. Self-neglect is the norm, contributing to physical and mental illnesses. Substances of abuse and associated lifestyle also can lead to complications during pregnancy and the risk of fetal abnormalities and fetal substance dependence.

Intravenous drug users and their sexual partners are at high risk for infection with blood-borne pathogens, particularly hepatitis B (HBV) and the human immunodeficiency virus (HIV), which causes the acquired immunodeficiency syndrome (AIDS). More recently, hepatitis C (HCV) has become recognized in the drug abuse population and has become one of the leading causes of chronic hepatitis in the United States (Box 24-3) (CDC, 2003; Scheel, 2003). It is common for addicts to share needles when they are using drugs in a group. Because the needles are not cleaned, blood is transferred from one person to the others. This is an ideal situation for the transmission of HIV or hepatitis.

BOX 24-3

The Hepatitis C Virus (HCV)

- HCV is one of the most significant causes of chronic liver disease in the United States.
- HCV accounts for 20% of acute viral hepatitis, 60% to 70% of chronic hepatitis, 30% of cirrhosis, end stage liver disease.
- Four million Americans, or 1.8% of the U.S. population, have the antibody to HCV, indicating ongoing or previous infection with the virus.
- HCV can remain dormant for many years; when activated, initial symptoms include nausea, poor appetite, weight loss, fatigue, tenderness in the right upper quadrant, and muscle and joint pains.
- Hepatitis C causes an estimated 10,000 deaths annually in the United States.

Modified from Centers for Disease Control and Prevention website, 2003: http://www.cdc.gov/ncidod/diseases/hepititis/resource/index.htm and Scheel K: *Counselor* 4:22, 2003.

CNS Depressants. The term *CNS depressant* is used for any drug that depresses excitable tissues at all levels of the brain. These drugs are also called *sedative-hypnotics.* Their primary effects are to reduce anxiety (the calming, antianxiety, or sedative effect), induce sleep (the hypnotic effect), or both. Included in this class are alcohol, barbiturates, and benzodiazepines. The signs and symptoms of the use of, overdose by, and withdrawal from CNS depressants are listed in Table 24-3.

It should be noted that **cross-tolerance** develops among most drugs in this category. This means that as tolerance develops to one drug, it develops to other drugs in this category as well. For example, a chronic alcoholic will need very high doses of benzodiazepines to control signs of withdrawal.

Alcohol. Although alcohol is a sedative, it creates an initial feeling of euphoria. This is probably related to decreased inhibitions. Symptoms of sedation of different CNS structures increase as the amount of alcohol ingested increases.

Approximately 15% of drinkers progress to alcoholism. A person's drinking may begin like everyone else's, or a person may be able to drink more alcohol than others before feeling intoxicated. In either case, the person likes the feeling of intoxication and continues to drink whenever possible. Gradually, drinking occurs more often and in larger quantities. As this happens, drinking begins to cause problems in the person's life, which he or she may quickly explain away. The problems increase, the drinking increases, **physical and psychological dependence** develops, and then the person begins to drink to avoid withdrawal symptoms. Or, the person drinks in binges.

Not everyone progresses in the same way or displays all of these characteristics, and the time period over which the progression occurs varies widely. The following clinical example illustrates many of the behaviors described. Mr. H has the medical diagnoses of alcohol dependence and alcohol withdrawal delirium.

⑤ CLINICAL EXAMPLE

Mr. H was admitted to the detoxification center of a large metropolitan hospital in acute alcohol withdrawal. He was delirious and having visual hallucinations of bugs in his bed. He was extremely frightened, thrashing around in bed, and mumbling incoherently. Because he had a long and well-documented history of alcohol abuse, family members were contacted and confirmed that he had recently stopped drinking after a 2-week binge.

The patient had been a successful lawyer with a large practice. He specialized in corporate law and conducted much business over lunch or dinner. He also kept a well-stocked bar in his office to offer clients a drink. Without his really being aware of it, Mr. H's drinking had gradually increased. After a few years he was drinking almost nonstop from lunchtime to bedtime. He then began to have a Bloody Mary with breakfast "just to get myself going."

His wife reported that he had become irritable, particularly if she questioned his drinking. On two occasions he had hit her during their arguments. She was seriously considering divorce. He also had become alienated from his children, who appeared frightened of him. Infrequently he would feel guilty about his neglect of his family and plan a special outing. Most of the time, though, he was too drunk to carry out his plans. The family also had become less involved in activities with friends. Mrs. H and the children felt

| Table 24-3 | Characteristics of Substances of Abuse |

SUBSTANCE	ROUTE (MOST COMMON FIRST)	COMMON STREET NAMES	DEPENDENCE: PHYSICAL/ PSYCHOLOGICAL	USE SIGNS AND SYMPTOMS OF CLASS
Depressants				
Alcohol	Ingestion	Booze, brew, juice, spirits	Yes/Yes	Depression of major brain functions such as mood, cognition, attention, concentration, insight, judgment, memory, affect, and emotional rapport in interpersonal relationships
Barbiturates	Ingestion, injection	Barbs, beans, black beauties, blue angels, candy, downers, goof balls, G.B., nebbies, reds, sleepers, yellow jackets, yellows	Yes/Yes	Extent of depression is dose dependent and ranges from lethargy through anesthesia and death
Benzodiazepines	Ingestion, injection	Downers	Yes/Yes	Psychomotor impairment, increased reaction time, interruption of hand-eye coordination, motor ataxia, nystagmus
				Decreased REM sleep leading to more dreams and sometimes nightmares
Stimulants				
Amphetamines	Ingestion, injection	A, AMT, bam, bennies, crystal, diet pills, dolls, eye-openers, lid poppers, pep pills, purple hearts, speed, uppers, wake-ups	Yes/Yes	Sudden rush of euphoria, abrupt awakening, increased energy, talkativeness, elation
				Agitation, hyperactivity, irritability, grandiosity, pressured speech
				Diaphoresis, anorexia, weight loss, insomnia
Cocaine	Inhalation, smoking, injection, topical	Bernice, bernies, big C, blow, C, charlie, coke, dust, girl, heaven, jay, lady, nose candy, nose powder, snow, sugar, white lady. Crack = conan, freebase, rock, toke, white cloud, white tornado	Yes/Yes	Increased temperature, blood pressure, and pulse
				Tachycardia, ectopic heartbeats, chest pain
				Urinary retention, constipation, dry mouth
				High dose: Slurred, rapid, incoherent speech
				Stereotypic movements, ataxic gait, teeth grinding, illogical thought processes, headache, nausea, vomiting
				Toxic psychosis: Paranoid delusions in clear sensorium; auditory, visual, or tactile hallucinations; very labile mood
				Unprovoked violence
Opiates				
Heroin	Injection, ingestion, inhalation	H, horse, harry, boy, scag, shit, smack, stuff, white junk, white stuff	Yes/Yes	Euphoria, relaxation, relief from pain, "nodding out" (apathy, detachment from reality, impaired judgment, and drowsiness); constricted pupils, nausea, constipation, slurred speech, respiratory depression
Morphine	Injection		Yes/Yes	
Meperidine	Injection, ingestion		Yes/Yes	
Codeine	Ingestion, injection		Yes/Yes	
Opium	Smoking, ingestion		Yes/Yes	
Methadone	Ingestion		Yes/Yes	
Marijuana				
	Smoking, ingestion	Acapulco gold, aunt mary, broccoli, dope, grass, grunt, hay, hemp, herb, J, joint, joy stick, killer weed, maryjane, pot, ragweed, reefer, smoke, weed	No/Yes	Altered state of awareness, relaxation, mild euphoria, reduced inhibition, red eyes, dry mouth, increased appetite, increased pulse, decreased reflexes, panic reaction

OVERDOSE SIGNS AND SYMPTOMS OF CLASS	WITHDRAWAL SIGNS AND SYMPTOMS OF CLASS	SPECIAL CONSIDERATIONS/ CONSEQUENCES OF USE OF CLASS
Unconsciousness, coma, respiratory depression, death	*General depressant withdrawal syndrome*: Tremors, agitation, anxiety, diaphoresis, increased pulse and blood pressure, sleep disturbance, hallucinosis, seizures, delusions, delirium tremens (DTs) *High-dose sedative-hypnotic withdrawal*: For short-acting sedative hypnotics (including alcohol), symptoms begin between several hours to 1 day after the last dose and peak after 24-36 hours. For long-acting sedative hypnotics, symptoms peak after 5-8 days. *Low-dose sedative-hypnotic withdrawal*: Usually transient "symptom rebound" effects (anxiety, insomnia) for 1-2 weeks; may have more severe symptoms: perceptual hyperacusis, psychosis, cerebellar dysfunction, seizures *Postacute (protracted) withdrawal*: Irritability, anxiety, insomnia, mood instability may occur for months.	Chronic alcohol use leads to serious disruptions in most organ systems: malnutrition and dehydration; vitamin deficiency leading to Wernicke's encephalopathy and alcoholic amnestic syndrome; impaired liver function, including hepatitis and cirrhosis; esophagitis, gastritis, pancreatitis; osteoporosis; anemia; peripheral neuropathy; impaired pulmonary function; cardiomyopathy; myopathy; disrupted immune system; and brain damage High susceptibility to other dependencies Dependence on barbiturates and benzodiazepines may develop insidiously; users may underreport the actual amount taken because of guilt about multiple prescriptions and abuse
Seizures; cardiac arrhythmias, coronary artery spasms, myocardial infarctions, marked increase in blood pressure and temperature that can lead to cardiovascular shock and death	*Acute withdrawal (after periods of frequent high-dose use)*: Intense and unpleasant feelings of depression and fatigue and sometimes suicidal ideation *Otherwise*: Milder symptoms of depression, anxiety, anhedonia, sleep disturbance, increased appetite, and psychomotor retardation, which decrease steadily over several weeks Sometimes a user stops stimulants purposely to decrease tolerance, decreasing the amount needed to get high	Certain amphetamines prescribed for ADHD in children because of a paradoxical depressant action Sometimes these medications are stolen and abused; may be used alternately with depressants Cocaine use may lead to multiple physical problems: destruction of the nasal septum related to snorting, coronary artery vasoconstriction, seizures, cerebrovascular accidents; transient ischemic episodes, sudden death related to respiratory arrest, and myocardial infarction Intravenous use of stimulants may lead to the serious physical consequences described under "Opiates"
Unconsciousness, coma, respiratory depression, circulatory depression, respiratory arrest, cardiac arrest, death; anoxia can lead to brain abscess	*Initially*: Drug craving lacrimation, rhinorrhea, yawning, diaphoresis *In 12-72 hr*: Sleep disturbance, mydriasis, anorexia, piloerection, irritability, tremor, weakness, nausea, vomiting, diarrhea, chills, fever, muscle spasms, flushing, spontaneous ejaculation, abdominal pain, hypertension, increased rate and depth of respirations *Protracted withdrawal*: Hypersensitivity to sensory stimuli, paresthesias, perceptual distortions, muscle pains, twitching tremors, headache, and sleep disturbances; tension, irritability, lack of energy, impaired concentration, derealization, and depersonalization May last for several months	Intravenous use leads to risk for infection with blood-borne pathogens, such as HIV or hepatitis B; other infections (skin abscesses, phlebitis, cellulitis, and septic emboli causing pneumonia, pulmonary abscess, or subacute bacterial endocarditis) may occur as a result of lack of asepsis or contaminated substances Chronic use leads to lack of concern about physical well-being, resulting in malnutrition and dehydration; criminal behavior may occur as a means of acquiring money for drugs
Toxic psychosis	No acute symptoms, but irritability and difficulty sleeping may last for a couple days	Pulmonary problems; interference with reproductive hormones; may cause fetal abnormalities

Continued

| Table 24-3 | Characteristics of Substances of Abuse—cont'd |

SUBSTANCE	ROUTE (MOST COMMON FIRST)	COMMON STREET NAMES	DEPENDENCE: PHYSICAL/ PSYCHOLOGICAL	USE SIGNS AND SYMPTOMS OF CLASS
Hallucinogens				
LSD	Ingestion, smoking	Acid, big D, blotter, blue heaven, cap, D, deeda, flash, L, mellow yellows, microdots, paper acid, sugar, ticket, yello	No/No	Distorted perceptions and hallucinations in the presence of a clear sensorium
DMT			No/No	
Mescaline			No/No	Distortions of time and space, illusions, depersonalization, mystical experiences, heightened sense of awareness
MDMA		Ecstasy	No/No	Extreme mood lability
				Tremor, dizziness, piloerection, paresthesias, synesthesia, nausea, and vomiting
				Increased temperature, pulse, blood pressure, and salivation
				Panic reaction, "bad trip"
Phencyclidine (PCP)				
	Smoking, ingestion	Angel dust, DOA, dust, elephant, hog, peace pill, supergrass, tic tac	No/No	Intensely psychotic experience characterized by bizarre perceptions, confusion, disorientation, euphoria, hallucinations, paranoia, grandiosity, agitation
				Anesthesia
				Apparent enhancement of strength and endurance
				Rage reactions
				May be agitated and hyperactive with tendency toward violence or catatonic and withdrawn or vacillate between the two conditions
				Red, dry skin; dilated pupils, nystagmus, ataxia, hypertension, rigidity, and seizures
Inhalants				
Gasoline, glue, aerosol sprays, paint thinner	Inhalation	Spray, rush, bolt, huffing, bagging, sniffing	Yes/Yes	*Psychological:* Belligerence, assaultiveness, apathy, impaired judgment
				Physical: Dizziness, nystagmus, incoordination, slurred speech, unsteady gait, depressed reflexes, tremor, blurred vision, euphoria, anorexia
Nicotine				
	Smoking, chewing, buccal	Cigarettes, cigars, bidis, kreteks, pipe tobacco, snuff, chewing tobacco	Yes/Yes	Feelings of pleasure, increased alertness, enhanced mental performance, increased heart rate, increased blood pressure, restricts blood flow to heart muscle

ADHD, Attention deficit/hyperactivity disorder; DMT, N,N-dimethyl-tryptamine; LSD, lysergic acid diethylamide; MDMA, methylenedioxymethamphetamine.

embarrassed about his behavior and did not invite anyone to their home. On two occasions, Mr. H had tried to stop drinking. The first time he went to a private hospital, where he was detoxified. He abstained from drinking for about 1 month after discharge.

He then lost an important case and decided to have "just one drink" to carry him through the crisis. Soon his drinking was again out of control. His second hospitalization was at a general hospital with an active alcoholism rehabilitation program. He was introduced to Alcoholics Anonymous (AA) and started taking disulfiram (Antabuse). This program worked until he decided that he could manage without medication. A couple of weeks later his co-workers persuaded him to "help celebrate" at an office party. This was the start of a binge that ended when he had an automobile accident on the way home from a bar. A passenger in the other car was killed, and Mr. H was charged with vehicular homicide and driving under the influence of alcohol.

Overdose Signs and Symptoms of Class	Withdrawal Signs and Symptoms of Class	Special Considerations/ Consequences of Use of Class
Rare with LSD: convulsions, hyperthermia, death	None	Flashbacks may last for several months; permanent psychosis may occur
Seizures, coma, death	None	If flashbacks occur, they are mild and usually not disturbing
Lethargy, stupor/coma, respiratory arrest, cardiac arrhythmia	Symptoms similar to alcohol withdrawal	Death from inhalants can occur in different ways: • Sudden death is caused by cardiac arrhythmia—sometimes this happens the first time the child uses inhalants • Suicide may be a result of impaired judgment Injury: Under the influence of inhalants, youth feel invulnerable Burns and frostbite also can be caused by these chemicals Permanent cognitive impairment may require an individual to reside in a structured setting
N/A	Anger, anxiety, depressed mood, difficulty concentrating—all of which subside within 3-4 weeks; increased appetite and craving for nicotine, which may persist for months	Smoking by pregnant women contributes to low birth weight, increased incidence of stillborn and premature babies

He stopped drinking abruptly, which resulted in his current hospital admission 3 days later.

Selected Nursing Diagnoses
• Disturbed sensory perception (visual) related to neurobiological changes induced by acute alcohol withdrawal, as evidenced by hallucinations of bugs in the bed

• Ineffective coping related to repeated drinking, as evidenced by work and family problems and denial of drinking problems
• Risk for injury related to drinking and driving, as evidenced by recent automobile accident
• Risk for other-directed violence related to lack of control of behavior when drunk, as evidenced by past pattern of violent behavior ■

Barbiturates. Barbiturates include barbital, amobarbital (Amytal), phenobarbital, pentobarbital (Nembutal), secobarbital (Seconal), and butabarbital. These drugs were once widely prescribed for their sedative and hypnotic effects. However, many problems were associated with their use, and they have been the major cause of **overdose death** from accidental poisonings and suicide.

They produce excessive drowsiness, even at therapeutic doses. Also, **tolerance** to them develops rapidly. Like alcohol, barbiturates are depressants that cause an initial response of euphoria. Thus they are popular street drugs.

Barbiturate use leads to both **physical and psychological dependence**. The combination of **alcohol and barbiturates produces a synergistic effect**, meaning that either drug potentiates the effects of the other. For this reason, combinations of these drugs are particularly dangerous and can lead to accidental overdose and death, and their use as sedative hypnotics has decreased.

Despite these drawbacks, barbiturates are very useful for the treatment of epilepsy and general depressant withdrawal syndromes.

Benzodiazepines. In the 1960s benzodiazepines replaced barbiturates as the preferred treatment for anxiety and related disorders. They are as effective as barbiturates but are safer to use. Benzodiazepines cause decreased anxiety and drowsiness (although less than barbiturates). They also can be addictive, causing both **physical and psychological dependence.** In addition, they lead to the same withdrawal symptoms as alcohol.

Because benzodiazepines are longer acting, the symptoms are less intense and continue over a longer period. They are less harmful in cases of overdose. Despite these drawbacks, they are commonly prescribed in the United States, generally with few resulting problems if used as directed. The clinical uses of benzodiazepines are described in Chapter 27.

Stimulants. Stimulants are drugs known to stimulate the CNS at many levels. The most common of these are the amphetamines and cocaine. People use these drugs for the feelings of euphoria, relief from fatigue, added energy, and alertness that they provide. The signs and symptoms of use, overdose, and withdrawal are basically the same for all drugs in this class (see Table 24-3).

Amphetamines. The amphetamine drugs include amphetamine, methamphetamine, dextroamphetamine, and benzphetamine. Amphetamines are thought to act by crowding norepinephrine and dopamine out of storage vesicles and into the synapse. The increase of these catecholamines at the receptors causes increased stimulation.

Clear patterns of **tolerance** and **withdrawal** have been described. Tolerance develops to the euphoria and the pleasant effects of these drugs but not to the wakefulness effects. Prolonged or excessive use of amphetamines can lead to **psychosis**, which is almost identical to paranoid schizophrenia.

In the 1950s and 1960s, amphetamines were widely prescribed for weight loss and relief of fatigue and depression. Their effectiveness for both conditions was only temporary

and often led to dependency. In 1970 the Food and Drug Administration (FDA) restricted the legal use of amphetamines to three types of conditions: narcolepsy, attention deficit hyperactivity disorder (ADHD) in children and adults, and short-term weight reduction programs.

Today it is clear that the abuse potential of amphetamines outweighs the benefit of their medical use for almost any reason. Safer treatments for these conditions are generally preferred, although amphetamines are still used in the treatment of ADHD.

Cocaine. Cocaine may be a drug of recent popularity, but it has been around for thousands of years. Cocaine is inhaled as a powder, injected intravenously, or smoked.

The form of cocaine that is smoked is produced by a process called **freebasing**. The "crack" form of freebase cocaine is produced by "cooking" street-grade cocaine in a baking soda solution. Its name is derived from the cracking sound it makes when it is smoked.

The euphoria caused by cocaine is short acting, starting with a 10- to 20-second rush and followed by 15 to 20 minutes of less intense euphoria. A person who is high on cocaine feels euphoric, energetic, self-confident, and sociable.

Cocaine produces **physical dependence**, and a pattern of **withdrawal** symptoms very similar to that seen in amphetamine users has been observed, beginning with intense craving and drug-seeking behavior. The **relapse rate** for patients who try to discontinue cocaine use is very high. Cocaine use has been known to result in **sudden death**.

Biochemically, cocaine blocks the reuptake of norepinephrine and dopamine. Because more neurotransmitter is present at the synapse, the receptors are continuously activated. It is believed that this causes the euphoria. At the same time, presynaptic supplies of dopamine and norepinephrine are depleted. This causes the "crash" that happens when the effect of the drug wears off.

Cocaine use has been glamorized by the publicity given to it by movie stars, sports figures, and other well-known people. This makes it particularly inviting to adolescents who regard famous people as role models.

Addiction to barbiturates ("downers") and stimulants ("uppers"), particularly the amphetamines, often occurs simultaneously. Sometimes a patient who has been using downers develops a need for uppers to provide enough energy to function. The next clinical example illustrates this pattern. Ms. W's pattern is not uncommon. Aside from street use, many people slip into drug abuse without being aware of the consequences of their behavior.

CLINICAL EXAMPLE

Ms. W was a 34-year-old woman who was moderately overweight. She had tried various diets on her own with little success. A friend told her about a "diet doctor" who had a reputation for helping his patients lose weight with minimum deprivation. Ms. W decided to see the physician and was accepted for treatment. She was given a diuretic and appetite suppression medication. The latter contained amphetamines. She began to lose weight as soon as she started the prescribed regimen and was delighted. She also liked the additional burst of energy she felt every time she took her medication. She completed projects that she had been planning to work on for months. However, her family began to complain because she was irritable and very restless. In addition, she developed insomnia and roamed about the house at night.

On the urging of her husband, she went to her family physician. She felt guilty about seeing another physician for her weight problem, so did not tell her regular physician about this. With the history of insomnia, irritability, and recent weight loss, her physician thought she might be depressed. He ordered an antidepressant medication and a barbiturate sedative. Ms. W soon found that she was able to sleep well with her sedative. However, she felt slightly hung over in the morning and still wanting to lose more weight, she continued with her diet pills as well. For a while she was able to function well. Gradually, however, she found that she needed two sedatives, and then she also began to use extra stimulants. Her husband questioned her drug use. Ms. W had read about drug abuse and with her husband's help identified that she had a problem. She decided to see her family physician again and this time told him the whole story. He then advised a brief hospitalization so that she could be withdrawn from both drugs under medical supervision. Ms. W was very embarrassed by her addiction. While in the hospital, she needed a great deal of nursing support to integrate this experience.

Selected Nursing Diagnoses
- Ineffective coping related to dependence on stimulants and depressants, as evidenced by inability to function without the drugs and the development of tolerance
- Ineffective role performance related to drug dependence, as evidenced by family concern over her behavior
- Imbalanced nutrition: more than body requirements related to repeated dieting failures, as evidenced by seeking out a doctor who would help her lose weight with minimal deprivation ■

Opiates. The opiates include opium, heroin, meperidine, morphine, codeine, and methadone. Meperidine, morphine, and codeine are commonly used analgesics. Methadone is used to treat addiction to other opiates. It can be used either to aid withdrawal or to provide maintenance at a stable dose. It is useful because it does not interfere with the ability to function productively, as other narcotics do. Patients taking a maintenance dose of methadone may work and live normally, although they are still addicted to narcotics.

Opiate use is less widespread than depressant or stimulant use but is still a serious social problem. Although some people use opiates for years with few problems, people with opiate addiction often deteriorate mentally and physically until they are unable to function productively. One characteristic of narcotic addiction is the development of **tolerance,** which also increases the expense of the habit. Physiological effects of narcotics are included in Table 24-3. Illegal behavior, such as stealing or prostitution to acquire money for drugs, may result from addiction. Obtaining and using drugs becomes an all-consuming passion.

The most important psychological response to opiate use is euphoria, or feeling high. This powerful, pleasurable response causes the person to use the drug repeatedly, leading to addiction. Other psychological effects of narcotics include apathy, detachment from reality, and impaired judgment. The phrase "nodding out" describes this group of behaviors combined with drowsiness. The next clinical example demonstrates the behaviors associated with opiate abuse.

CLINICAL EXAMPLE

Mr. C was a 35-year-old man who had been jailed for auto theft. He was believed to be a member of a large ring of automobile thieves in a major metropolitan area. His arrest record included several episodes of armed robbery and breaking and entering. A few hours after he had been jailed, Mr. C complained of abdominal cramps and appeared very anxious. His nose and eyes were running, there were beads of perspiration on his brow, and he was rocking back and forth on his bunk. The guard called Ms. V, the correctional health nurse.

Ms. V observed Mr. C and performed a brief physical assessment. She noted that his pupils were dilated, his blood pressure was elevated, and he had gooseflesh. In addition, there were multiple needle tracks on his arms. She asked him directly about drug use, and he admitted that he had been addicted to heroin. He stated that his addiction began in 1967 while he was stationed with the army in Vietnam. When he returned to the United States, he remained in the army for 18 months and was able to stop using drugs altogether. He planned to get a job and attend school after leaving the service. He related that he was disturbed by the attitude of people toward Vietnam veterans. While he was still in the service, he was able to use peer support to cope with his feelings. However, after his discharge, he was reluctant to talk about his military experience. Others seemed disinterested, embarrassed, or hostile when he talked about it.

Mr. C had difficulty finding a civilian job. He was an artillery specialist in the army and found that it was difficult to apply this experience to civilian life. He began to have nightmares and flashbacks of his combat experiences. Because of the anxiety associated with this, he returned to drugs. Without a job, he used illegal means to finance his habit and therefore was repeatedly sent to jail.

Ms. V discussed Mr. C's problem with the physician in the prison health department. They decided to assess Mr. C's eligibility for a methadone drug treatment program and to request consultation from a counselor at the local veterans counseling center.

Selected Nursing Diagnoses
- Ineffective coping related to inability to obey the law, as evidenced by repeated arrests
- Ineffective role performance related to difficulty adjusting to civilian life, as evidenced by inability to find a job or seek out peer support
- Social isolation related to unresolved stressful military experiences, as evidenced by reliance on drugs rather than people
- Risk for other-directed violence related to compelling need for drugs, as evidenced by history of armed robbery ■

Withdrawal from narcotics is extremely uncomfortable but is not usually life threatening. Overdosage of narcotics, on the other hand, is very dangerous. It can rapidly lead to **coma, respiratory depression,** and **death.** Accidental overdoses among narcotic addicts sometimes occur, particularly because the user is uncertain of the drug's strength. Drugs are usually cut with inert (and sometimes toxic) substances before they are sold, resulting in the availability of varied strengths on the streets.

Natural opiates. In 1975 natural substances that acted very much like morphine were isolated in the brain. It was later learned that these biochemicals, known as **endorphins** and **enkephalins**, were neurotransmitters that bond with opiate receptors in the brain and pituitary gland. Release of these "natural opiates" results in a feeling of euphoria.

This understanding has led to a theory of **drug cravings**: When large amounts of artificial opiates are taken over a long period, the brain responds by cutting off production of endorphins in an attempt to restore homeostasis. As the artificial opiates leave the system, there are no natural opiates to take their place. This deprivation is experienced as craving. Details of these mechanisms continue to be studied.

Marijuana. Marijuana is sometimes classified as a hallucinogenic drug, but it rarely causes hallucinations. It causes sedation, but is not primarily a CNS depressant. The active ingredient in marijuana is tetrahydrocannabinol (THC).

The marijuana cigarette can be smoked as it is or through a water-pipe, or "bong," to cool the hot vapors. Marijuana generally produces an altered state of awareness accompanied by a feeling of relaxation and mild euphoria. Effects depend on the potency of the drug, as well as the setting and the experience of the user. Strength can vary widely from 1% to 30%.

Prolonged use may lead to apathy, lack of energy, loss of desire to work or be productive, diminished concentration, poor personal hygiene, and preoccupation with marijuana. This cluster of symptoms is known as the amotivational syndrome. Although study findings are controversial, there seems to be general support for the existence of such a syndrome.

Use of very large doses can lead to a *toxic psychosis* that clears as the substance is eliminated from the body. Marijuana also may precipitate psychosis when used by people with schizophrenia, whose symptoms are otherwise controlled with antipsychotic drugs. It does not appear to lead to psychosis in people without schizophrenia.

The main physiological effects of marijuana are mild (see Table 24-3). **Tolerance** develops in heavy users, but no withdrawal pattern is noted. Marijuana has been reported to have medicinal benefits in alleviating glaucoma and the nausea and vomiting associated with chemotherapy used in cancer treatment.

Supporters of legalization of marijuana use say that the penalties for using it are too severe and that marijuana is no more harmful than legal substances such as alcohol and nicotine. What is your position on the legalization of marijuana? ◼

Hallucinogens. Drugs that create experiences very similar to those typical of a psychotic state have been called hallucinogens, although they generally produce **perceptual distortions**, not true hallucinations. They also have been called psychedelic or mind-revealing drugs. Lysergic acid diethylamide (LSD), peyote, mescaline, and psilocybin are commonly used hallucinogens.

LSD is generally swallowed. It is colorless and tasteless and is often added to a drink or food, such as a sugar cube. It may be given to a person without that person knowing. Pleasurable effects of hallucinogen use include intensification of sensory experiences. Colors are described as more brilliant, and sounds, smells, and tastes are heightened. Sometimes users of these drugs report synesthesia, or a crossover of sensory experiences during which music may be seen or colors may be heard. Space and time are distorted.

The hallucinogens do not appear to cause physical dependence, but **tolerance** develops if they are used regularly. Hallucinogens also can lead to self-destructive behavior because they cause impaired judgment. Vulnerable people who take these drugs may experience "bad trips," sometimes resulting in psychotic episodes. They may experience paranoid, grandiose, or somatic delusions, usually accompanied by vivid hallucinations. The hallucinatory experience may be pleasant or frightening.

Patients who are psychotic are not in contact with reality and often misinterpret environmental events. They may be unable to attend to any of their biological needs and may inadvertently hurt themselves or others in response to hallucinations or while trying to escape from the frightening experience.

Because no physical dependence develops, withdrawal symptoms do not occur. Usually psychotic behavior decreases gradually, although the patient may have **flashbacks** for several months. These brief recurrences of the hallucinogenic experience can be frightening. Patients may express the fear that they are crazy and will never be free of the after effects of the drug.

A college classmate who is not a nursing major tells you that she overheard her 12-year-old brother talking with a friend about "doing microdots." You suspect that he was talking about LSD. What would you advise her to do? ◼

Phencyclidine. As a street drug, phencyclidine (PCP) may be ingested, but it is often smoked in a mixture with another substance, such as marijuana. Severity of symptoms are dose dependent. At low doses (less than 5 mg) the user experiences a euphoric, floating feeling, along with heightened emotionality and incoordination. Distorted perceptions such as objects floating or growing in size, inability to judge distance, or feelings of being outside one's body are common. At higher doses, PCP use may precipitate an intensely **psychotic experience** characterized by extreme agitation. **Patients may become violent** toward themselves or others.

Because the drug is an anesthetic, PCP-intoxicated people **feel little or no pain** and may pound their heads into a wall or strike out violently, causing serious injury to themselves or others. Physical manifestations of PCP intoxication are noted in Table 24-3. PCP may cause or exacerbate a previously controlled psychosis. The unpredictability of the reaction to PCP makes it an extremely dangerous drug.

Inhalants. Approximately 1400 products are known that can be inhaled. The most common inhalants include butane (lighter fluid), gas, air fresheners, rubber cement, correction fluid, and nitrous oxide (whippets). It is estimated that approximately 21% of 8th graders in the United States have used inhalants at least once in their lives. Children and adolescents choose inhalants as a means of obtaining a euphoric effect because of the quality of the high, the rapid onset of the effect, the low cost, and the ease of availability.

The nurse should be alert to the physical indicators of inhalant abuse when completing an assessment. These signs include residue from paint, glue, or substances noted on the clothes, hands, or face, especially around the nose. Youth also may have symptoms of a cold, such as a runny nose, or pimples or sores around the mouth. These are caused by the abrasive effect of the chemicals on the skin. Finally, it is essential that nurses take a leadership role in educating children and adults about the nature of inhalant abuse.

You are working as a nurse in a local high school in which a 15-year-old student recently died while inhaling butane. The principal approaches you requesting that students not be told that inhalants were involved in the death because it might "give other students ideas." How would you respond? ■

Nicotine. Nicotine is the active substance found in cigarettes, cigars, pipe tobacco, snuff, bidis (small brown cigarettes with up to 7 times the nicotine of regular cigarettes), and kreteks (clove cigarettes that anesthetize the throat thus promoting deeper inhalation). It is both a stimulant and a depressant.

Because smoke is a lung irritant, a person must learn how to inhale and must adjust to the body's natural rejection of this substance. Once inhaled, the nicotine in tobacco is readily absorbed into the blood stream and has an almost immediate effect on the reward systems in the brain.

Nicotine mimics the neurotransmitter, acetylcholine, binding to and activating a subset of receptors called the *nicotinic acetylcholine receptors*. Nicotine affects the brain in much the same way as cocaine, opiates, and amphetamines. Nicotine not only stimulates the release of dopamine; it also prolongs the actions of dopamine by decreasing the metabolizing enzyme, monoamine oxidase, and increases the expression of nitric oxide, which inhibits dopamine reuptake, so even more dopamine is available in the synapse.

Because the brain adjusts to the presence of nicotine, the individual who consumes this substance experiences **withdrawal** if the substance is discontinued (Morgan, 2003). Smoking is associated with increased morbidity and mortality and thus poses a serious public health problem (Box 24-4).

Caffeine. Caffeine is the active ingredient in coffee, tea, chocolate, and many carbonated beverages. Major effects of use are increased alertness and increased blood pressure. Overuse can cause jitteriness. Although caffeine increases alertness, it does not affect the dopaminergic brain structures related to reward, motivation, and addiction, as do the drugs of abuse and nicotine. Therefore, it is not addictive.

However, heavy use of caffeine can lead to **withdrawal** symptoms, a sign of physical dependence. These symptoms

---

BOX 24-4

Effects of Smoking in the United States

- There are 48 million smokers in the United States.
- Between 1990 and 1994, cigarette smoking accounted for 2.2 million deaths—an average of 430,700 deaths a year, or 20% of all U.S. deaths.
- Each year, more than 5 million years of life would have been saved if every person who died that year of cigarette smoking had lived to his or her average life expectancy.
- Ninety percent of lung cancer deaths result from smoking, accounting for 28% of all deaths attributable to smoking.
- Smoking contributes to deaths from coronary heart disease, chronic bronchitis and emphysema, stroke, and other cancers (pancreas, trachea, bronchus, and larynx).
- Smoking promotes tumor growth, ages the skin, stalls wound healing, and may alter the chemical structure of proteins.
- Secondary smoke results in 3000 lung cancer deaths among nonsmokers.
- Smoking is the single most preventable cause of poor pregnancy outcome. Six thousand deaths among children, primarily from low birth weight, respiratory infections, and sudden infant death syndrome are attributed to parental smoking each year.
- Although the prevalence of smoking in the United States has decreased in most population groups (adults, people with a college education, and those without a high school education) from 1990 to 2000, it has increased among high school seniors.

Modified from Fogarty M: *The Scientist* 17:6, 2003; Morgan K: *Sci News* 163:184, 2003.

---

include headache, sleepiness, fatigue, problems in attention and concentration, and decreased vigor. They are generally transient and mild, with relatively little interference in a person's daily life. However, the presence of these withdrawal symptoms may be the main factor for the continued use of the substance.

Co-Dependence. When the term *co-dependency* was first coined in 1979, it referred to people who had become dysfunctional as a result of living in a committed relationship with an alcoholic. It was said that the alcoholic was addicted to the bottle, and the co-dependent was addicted to the alcoholic. The major focus was initially on the spouse of the alcoholic.

Al-Anon was created in the 1930s specifically to help family members of alcoholics cope with their own problems that stem from living with an alcoholic. However, the co-dependency movement stresses the lasting effects of growing up in an alcoholic home. Adult children of alcoholics (ACOA) are believed to share certain characteristics as adults because they all struggled to survive the chaos of growing up with an alcoholic parent. The major aspects of the condition are as follows:

- Overinvolvement with a dysfunctional person
- Obsessive attempts to control the dysfunctional person's behavior

- A strong need for approval from others
- Constantly making personal sacrifices to help the dysfunctional person become "cured" of the problem behavior
- Enabling behavior, which inadvertently reinforces the drinking of the alcoholic person

As the movement has grown, however, the definition has broadened to include almost anyone who has had anything to do with a dysfunctional person, either while growing up or as an adult. Anyone who can identify with the laundry list of symptoms associated with co-dependency (most notably low self-esteem, need to please others, and over-responsibility for others) can identify with the term. Many researchers note that the construct of co-dependency is still poorly researched, and the nurse should be cautious before referring to a patient as "co-dependent" (Stafford, 2001).

The positive aspect of this movement is that it may allow many people who are unhappy with themselves to reframe their life situation and improve their functioning in very significant ways, with or without formal counseling. In fact, many people who otherwise would never have recognized their own dysfunction identify with the characteristics of co-dependency and are motivated to seek specific counseling and self-help groups.

ACOA and co-dependency self-help groups, based on the 12-step recovery program of Alcoholics Anonymous (AA), have sprung up all over the country. Dozens of self-help books have been published by people who self-identify with the concept and who offer recommendations about how to recover from it. Clinicians also have developed specific recovery programs for co-dependents. The negative side of the movement is that some people use the label to blame problems on current or past relationships without taking responsibility for their own part in the process.

Despite the popularity of this movement, no evidence has been found to support the existence of a clinical syndrome distinct for ACOA. A number of studies have shown that adults raised in alcoholic homes share many characteristics with adults raised in nonalcoholic but otherwise seriously dysfunctional homes. Furthermore, symptoms of adults raised in dysfunctional alcoholic or nonalcoholic homes vary from none to very severe. Thus the environment, family system, and individual all must be assessed when working with ACOA.

Whether a clearly identifiable and unique syndrome exists or not, it is easy to understand how children who grow up in alcoholic homes can develop low self-esteem. As an adult this is often expressed in a preoccupation with the lives, feelings, and problems of others. Although co-dependents want their loved ones to stop drinking or using drugs, their behavior may have the opposite effect and enable the person to continue drug or alcohol use.

The nurse may observe some of these behaviors in family members of substance-dependent patients, in the patients themselves, or in nurses and other professionals. Simple questions asked of family members about efforts they have made to try to control the addict's use may uncover the pattern. Questions asked of patients about their relationships with others may indicate that growing up in an alcoholic home may have contributed to their own substance abuse problem.

Listening to colleagues talk about their family and friends may reveal similar patterns in their relationships. Nurses tend to find great satisfaction in caring for others. When this behavior is the person's only source of self-esteem, it is done at the expense of personal health and welfare. It takes on a compulsive quality that is evidence of co-dependence.

Dual Diagnosis

A patient may have a substance use disorder, a psychiatric disorder, or both concurrently. The co-occurrence of psychiatric and substance use disorders, or **dual diagnosis**, is very common. The reasons for this are varied and are listed in Box 24-5. One disorder can precede and cause the other, such as when the alcoholic becomes severely depressed or when the depressed person uses alcohol to treat the depression.

It is often very difficult to distinguish between the two disorders, especially early in the assessment process. To complicate matters further, substance abuse may cause psychiatric symptoms such as hallucinations or paranoia, even though the person has no separate psychiatric diagnosis.

Data analyzed from the Healthcare for Communities Survey found that even though effective treatments were available, patients with a dual diagnosis were not receiving appropriate mental health and comprehensive substance abuse treatments (Watkins et al, 2001). Because substance use problems are so common among psychiatric patients, mental health clinicians should routinely assess all patients for these problems and use evidence-based treatments for the patient with dual diagnosis.

Detection of substance abuse in patients with psychiatric illness is most effective when multiple types of assessment are used. A combination of interview, screening tools, information from collateral sources, and laboratory tests including urine drug screens should be used. Diagnostic assessment is done according to *DSM-IV-TR* criteria.

BOX 24-5

Relationships Between Substance Use and Psychiatric Disorders

- Substances may be used to "self-medicate" the symptoms of the psychiatric disorder (alcohol may alleviate the distress associated with social anxiety or panic disorder).
- Substance use may be causing the psychiatric disorder (alcohol-induced depressive disorders, cocaine-induced psychotic disorders, stimulant-induced anxiety disorders).
- Substances may be used to counter the side effects of prescribed medications (stimulants or cocaine may counter the lethargy and sedation or the extrapyramidal side effects caused by some antipsychotic drugs).
- The individual may have a genetic predisposition to both a substance use disorder and a psychiatric disorder.
- There may be no relationship between the substance use and the psychiatric disorders.

The nurse should be aware that psychiatric patients may be especially vulnerable to small amounts of substances. For example, even small amounts of cocaine may precipitate a psychotic episode in a patient with schizophrenia. Specialized assessment can follow the more general diagnostic assessment to obtain more detailed information necessary for treatment planning. The special problems posed by patients who are dually diagnosed can be seen in the following clinical example.

CLINICAL EXAMPLE

Robbie is a 25-year-old, single, white male who began using alcohol and drugs at age 16, around the time he dropped out of school. He continued to live with his mother and spent most of his time in his room, although there were long periods of time when she did not know where he was. His mother reported that he increasingly isolated himself and acted so strangely that others did not feel comfortable around him.

Over the next couple of years, Robbie's behavior became increasingly bizarre until one day his mother observed him pacing, talking to himself, saying strange and threatening things aloud, and pounding his fists together. She obtained an emergency petition, and the police took him to the emergency room for an evaluation. He was diagnosed with schizophrenia, stabilized with medication, and returned to his mother's home with an appointment for outpatient follow-up. However, he did not return to the clinic, stopped taking his medication, and was rehospitalized 1 month later. This time, he was prescribed fluphenazine (Prolixin) and promised to return to the clinic as scheduled in 2 weeks. He seemed to do well for a few days until he resumed drinking and smoking marijuana. He disappeared for several weeks, then was found by his mother wandering the city streets, dirty, unkempt, reeking of alcohol, and talking to himself again. During the subsequent rehospitalization, he admitted also using cocaine and heroin occasionally. He was referred to AA and assigned to a social worker, who helped him obtain social services.

Soon he was getting a disability check every month, which exacerbated his problems. Every month he cashed his check as soon as he got it and went on a binge of drug and alcohol use until his money was gone, usually in about 1 week. Unable to afford such heavy use for the remainder of the month, Robbie approached people on the streets and demanded money. Eventually, he was picked up by the police for aggressive panhandling. By the time he was 24, Robbie was well-known by the police and emergency rooms in town. He'd been hospitalized at least a dozen times and arrested for numerous petty crimes. His mother, doctor, and social worker were totally exasperated by his failure to comply. When the new Dual Diagnosis Clinic opened in the Mental Health Center, Robbie was one of the first referrals. ■

Predisposing Factors

Several models or etiological factors have been proposed for substance abuse. Belief in a particular model influences the assessment and intervention. Awareness of the differences between these models helps the nurse understand why patients, as well as other professionals, hold many different views about substance abuse treatment. Much research has been conducted concerning the factors that predispose a person to becoming chemically dependent. These factors may be biological, psychological, or sociocultural.

Biological. A key biological factor is the tendency of substance abuse to run in families. More than half of current drinkers have a family history of alcoholism. Most genetic research has focused on alcoholism, but the body of knowledge on the genetics of other drugs of abuse is growing as well. Much evidence from adoption, twin, and animal studies indicates that heredity is significant in the development of alcoholism (Kendler et al, 2000b).

Some research has identified subtypes of alcoholism that differ in heritability. One type of alcoholism is associated with an early onset, inability to abstain, and an antisocial personality. This type appears to be limited to males and is primarily genetic in origin. Another type tends to be associated with onset after age 25, inability to stop drinking once started, and a passive-dependent personality. This type seems to be influenced much more by the environment. However, controversy in the field has caused some to question whether such subtypes actually exist and if so, what the precise nature of their characteristics is.

Fifty years after the discovery of DNA, and 3 years after the sequence of DNA was published as a result of the Human Genome Study, **genomics** (the study of genes and their functions) has begun to transform medicine. Mental illnesses seem to occur as an interplay of genes and environmental factors. Genes for mental illness and substance abuse (and many common illnesses like heart disease and diabetes and prostate cancer) will likely confer risk (susceptibility, or vulnerability) rather than be "causative" (the genes for Huntington's disease and cystic fibrosis are causative—all those who inherit the gene will eventually develop the disease) (Patoine, 2003). Thus it will continue to be important to understand the role of the environment and our response to it to better understand how one becomes "high risk" for mental illness or substance use disorders.

The discovery in 1990 that the A1 allele of the DRD2 gene appeared to be associated with alcoholism, and other substance abuse disorders gave rise to much subsequent genetic research. It is theorized that genetic abnormalities may block feelings of well-being. This results in a tendency toward anxiety, anger, low self-esteem, and other negative feelings, as well as a craving for a substance that will take the bad feelings away. People with such a disorder need alcohol or some other psychoactive drug just to feel "normal." These genetic findings are still preliminary and are only one of many predisposing factors in the etiology of substance abuse. It is important to understand that a larger role appears to be played by environmental factors and still unidentified genes.

If genetic factors are clearly identified as major influences on the development of alcoholism in some people, what ethical issues are likely to be debated? ■

Biological differences in the response to alcohol ingestion also may influence susceptibility. For example, many Asian people experience a physiological response to alcohol including flushing, tachycardia, and an intense feeling of discomfort. This appears to be related to the tendency for Asians to have a genetically inactive form of the enzyme aldehyde dehydrogenase. This leads to a buildup of the toxic substance acetaldehyde, an alcohol metabolite, which causes the symptoms. This response may help explain why Asian Americans have the lowest level of alcohol consumption and alcohol-related problems of any of the major racial and ethnic groups in the United States.

Psychological. Many psychological theories have attempted to explain the factors that predispose people to developing substance abuse. Psychoanalytic theories see alcoholics as being fixated at the oral stage of development, thus seeking need satisfaction through oral behaviors such as drinking. Behavior or learning theories view addictive behaviors as overlearned, maladaptive habits that can be examined and changed in the same way as other habits. Cognitive theories suggest that addiction is based on a distorted way of thinking about substance use. Family system theory emphasizes the pattern of relationships between family members through the generations as an explanation for substance abuse.

Clinicians have observed a link between substance abuse and several psychological traits such as depression, anxiety, antisocial personality, and dependent personality. Little evidence has been found to indicate that these psychological problems existed before or caused substance abuse. It is just as likely that they resulted from drug and alcohol use and dependence.

Many studies have tried to find common personality traits among people addicted to alcohol or drugs. No addictive personality has been identified to date. Studies show a wide variety of personality types among alcoholics. Observed personality patterns result from the effects of the alcohol or drug on previously normal psychological functions, combined with ineffective responses to these effects.

Another theory of substance abuse focuses on the human tendency to seek pleasure and avoid pain or stress. Drugs create pleasure and reduce physical or psychological pain. Because pain returns when the effect of the drug wears off, the person is powerfully attracted to repeated drug use. It has been suggested that some people are more sensitive to the euphoric effects of drugs and are more likely to repeat their use. This repeated drug use leads to more problems and initiates the downhill spiral of substance use.

Some substance abusers have psychological problems related to adverse childhood experiences and parental alcohol abuse (Anda et al, 2002). Many have histories of childhood physical or sexual abuse (Kendler et al, 2000a). Most have low self-esteem and difficulty expressing emotions. These problems may have influenced the initial use of drugs and the progression toward dependence.

Sociocultural. Several sociocultural factors influence a person's choice of whether to use drugs, which drugs to use, and how much to use. Attitudes, values, norms, and sanctions differ according to nationality, religion, gender, family background, and social environment. Assessment of these factors is necessary to understand the whole person. Combinations of factors may make a person more susceptible to drug abuse and interfere with recovery.

Nationality and ethnicity influence alcohol use patterns. For example, it has been found that northern Europeans have higher alcoholism rates than southern Europeans. Values may influence the way in which addiction is viewed. Some believe that addiction results from moral weakness or lack of willpower. Unfortunately, a moralistic approach may cause the person to feel guilty, often resulting in drinking to alleviate the guilt.

Formal religious belief also can affect drinking behavior. Members of religions that discourage the use of alcohol have much lower rates of alcohol use and alcoholism than members of those that accept or encourage its use. Of the major religious groups in the United States, Roman Catholics have the highest rate of alcoholism and Jews the lowest. During assessment, however, the nurse should not assume certain use or nonuse patterns related to ethnic or religious factors.

Gender differences also have been noted in the prevalence of substance abuse. Research is needed to determine the influence of biological as opposed to sociocultural reasons for this. However, powerful gender-related cultural factors do help shape substance-using behaviors. Alcoholism in females is much less accepted by society, which is one reason this abuse problem is often hidden, even though it has been increasing in the past decade. Women tend to deny having a drinking problem even longer than men do. In the United States more women than men abuse prescription drugs, such as benzodiazepines. This is more socially acceptable and sometimes even encouraged. In contrast, use of antianxiety drugs is viewed as weak and unmasculine behavior in men, whereas the ability to drink large amounts of alcohol is considered manly.

Finally, sociocultural factors influence drug use, abuse, and treatment. Multiple social crises can contribute to the risk for drug abuse in poor neighborhoods. Affordable and decent housing and shelter are difficult to find. Job opportunities are limited, and many jobs are low paying. Social programs often inadvertently foster development of single-parent families. The dropout rate in inner-city schools is high, and advanced education is difficult to obtain.

Living in neighborhoods dominated by these problems, along with poor health care access, crime, and violence, creates vulnerability to the escape some people find in drugs and alcohol. However, it is important to recognize that the majority of people living in these circumstances are not addicted to drugs, which further supports the belief that many factors influence the development of drug use patterns, not just the social environment.

What sociocultural factors have you observed that encourage the use of drugs and alcohol? ▪

Precipitating Stressors

Withdrawal. If a person becomes physically dependent on a substance, substance abuse may continue simply to avoid withdrawal symptoms. The person may no longer get much effect from the substance other than its ability to prevent withdrawal. Symptoms of withdrawal from specific drugs of abuse are listed in Table 24-3.

Debate is ongoing as to whether drug cravings also should be considered part of the withdrawal syndrome. However they are categorized, it is clear that the emergence of withdrawal symptoms and cravings together serve as powerful precipitating stressors for continued drug use.

General depressant drug withdrawal. Withdrawal from all depressant drugs (including alcohol) is similar and sometimes is referred to as the **general depressant withdrawal syndrome**. The main difference in the **time course of symptoms** depends on the **half-life** of the particular drug. The main difference in the **severity of symptoms** depends on the **drug dose and length of use**.

For example, substances with short half-lives, such as alcohol and the short-acting benzodiazepines and barbiturates, lead to earlier appearance of withdrawal symptoms and a shorter withdrawal syndrome. The shorter-acting drugs are considered to be more addictive because the effect is felt quicker. However, these drugs also leave the system more quickly, increasing the chance of withdrawal.

Prescribed depressants/sedative-hypnotics withdrawal. The use of depressants at higher-than-therapeutic doses for more than 1 month can produce physical dependence and can result in "high dose withdrawal syndrome." Symptoms may peak within 24 hours for the short-acting drugs but take as long as 8 days for long-acting ones.

Patients who have taken regular, therapeutic doses of sedative-hypnotics for at least 4 months (or less with higher doses) may experience a "low-dose withdrawal syndrome" when the dosage is decreased or discontinued. These effects

may be due to an intensified return of the symptoms for which the drug was prescribed in the first place, a phenomenon called **symptom rebound**. Although many patients have no symptoms or only mild symptoms after cessation of therapeutic doses, a few may experience a more severe syndrome.

Alcohol withdrawal. When a large amount of alcohol is ingested, unpleasant symptoms usually occur. If overindulgence is short-lived, symptoms are caused by the direct effect of alcohol on body cells. This results in headache and stomach and intestinal distress—the typical hangover.

However, if heavy drinking occurs over a long time, a decrease in blood alcohol level may cause symptoms of withdrawal. Alcohol sedates the CNS. When alcohol is withdrawn, the symptoms resemble a rebound reaction in the CNS. Figure 24-4 presents information on the alcohol withdrawal syndrome (Mayo-Smith et al, 1997).

Neurobiology. Most abused drugs interact with specific nerve cell receptors, either imitating or blocking the actions of normally working neurotransmitters in the brain. Heroin and other opiates, for example, activate opioid receptors that normally respond to the brain's natural opioid-like neurotransmitters (such as endorphin, enkephalin, and dynorphin).

Alcohol both activates some receptors (for the neurotransmitter gamma-aminobutyric acid [GABA]) and blocks others (for the neurotransmitter glutamate). In contrast, cocaine and other stimulants block the reuptake of various neurotransmitters, including dopamine, serotonin, and norepinephrine, with the effect of prolonging the action of these brain chemicals on target cells.

Other aspects of neurobiology account for the reinforcing and addicting aspects of drugs of abuse. The mesolimbic dopamine system is a pathway in the brain that originates

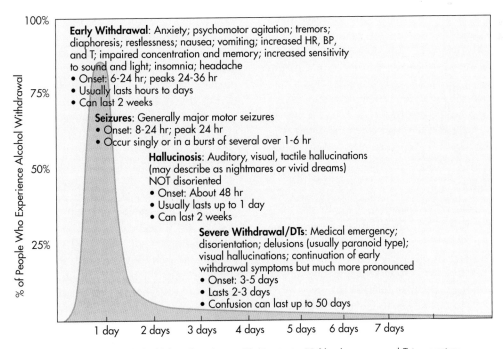

Figure 24-4   Alcohol withdrawal syndrome. *HR,* Heart rate; *BP,* blood pressure; and *T,* temperature.

from dopamine-producing cells in the brainstem and targets higher regions of the brain (see Chapter 6). This brain pathway regulates natural drives such as the desire for food, drink, and sex. Taking drugs of abuse repeatedly produces long-lasting changes in these areas of the brain, leading to the negative feelings during withdrawal and strong drug cravings. They also produce cognitive changes, making the risk of relapse over many years and even a lifetime quite high.

Most drugs also inhibit the cyclic adenosine monophosphate (cAMP) pathway, which is an intracellular messenger system. cAMP is one of the chemicals within target cells that can either be activated or inhibited when a neurotransmitter locks onto a receptor. Most drugs of abuse inhibit the cAMP response, and this is thought to contribute to the reinforcing actions of the drugs.

As the person continues to use drugs, the brain cells try to compensate for the lack of cAMP by making more cAMP and other molecules involved with its action. This is what leads to drug tolerance. Because of changes in gene expression, the brain cells continue to overproduce cAMP, which leads to withdrawal symptoms, such as dysphoria and lack of motivation. These unpleasant feelings are countered by taking more drug, thus leading to drug dependence.

With chronic drug exposure, certain other nerve cells become more excitable, making the drug user more sensitive to the drugs or to conditioned cues associated with drug exposure, or even to stress. This sensitization is thought to be a powerful factor in drug relapse and thus a powerful precipitating stressor for the continued use of drugs.

Appraisal of Stressors

The reasons a person initiates use of substances vary widely. Curiosity, desire to be grown up, desire to rebel against authority, peer pressure, desire to ease the pains of living, desire to feel good—all of these are stressors and may apply. If use of the substance brings about the desired effects, then use is likely to continue.

As the amount and frequency of substance use increase, so do the perceived stressors, which lead to more use. If substance use becomes associated with relief from emotional and social pain in the person's mind, then these stressors will lead to more substance use. Perceiving the substance as the answer to these problems, the person fails to develop healthier coping mechanisms. Gradually it takes more and more of the substance to get the same effect.

Coping Resources

Comprehensive assessment of a patient with a substance abuse problem must include assessment of the personal, social, and material assets available to the person. Assessment of motivation and social supports is particularly important.

- What is the patient's **motivation to change** the substance use pattern? It could be that the patient is sick and tired of being sick and tired, or may have been ordered to complete a treatment program after receiving a DWI charge.

- What **social supports** does the patient have? Family, friends, and co-workers may be available for support, or the patient may be homeless and have no family or friends.
- What is the status of the patient's **health?** The health status may be perfect, or the patient may have hepatitis, AIDS, or other complications of abuse.
- What **social skills** does the patient have? Some patients are very adept in social interactions, and some are withdrawn, quiet, and isolated.

Patients may not have developed problem-solving skills in other areas of their lives. They may not have other social, material, and economic assets to support recovery (Kelly, Blacksin, and Mason, 2001). They may not have intellectual skills and personality traits that contribute to positive change.

Coping Mechanisms

Although the patient may have used substances in response to certain stressors, the substance use may have escalated to the point at which it has become an additional stressor. Patients who use problem-focused coping mechanisms will take responsibility for the substance-use problem and either find ways to change or seek help in doing so (Committee on Addictions, 2002). These are constructive coping mechanisms.

Patients also may use destructive coping mechanisms, such as when they change the meaning of the substance-abuse problem so that it becomes a nonproblem, saying that there is no problem ("It's just the thing to do") or devaluing a desired object ("I didn't want that job anyway").

Patients also may try to decrease emotional stress by **minimization** of the extent of use ("I only had a couple of beers") or the consequences of use ("We don't fight about it too much"), **denial** ("I don't have a problem. I can quit anytime I want"), **projection** ("Tom's the one who can't deal with his family or hold his liquor"), and **rationalization** ("If you had the problems I have, you'd drink, too").

It is impossible in the initial assessment to sort out the facts from the distortions caused by these coping mechanisms. This is one reason why assessment is an ongoing process. Information from collateral sources and continued observation of behavior over time are essential.

DIAGNOSIS

Nursing Diagnoses

After completion of the nursing assessment, the nurse synthesizes the data regarding the patient's drinking or drug use behavior. Using the Stuart Stress Adaptation Model (Figure 24-5) and the NANDA classification system, appropriate nursing diagnoses are identified.

Addiction problems are very complex. They affect nearly every aspect of the patient's functioning. The nurse should be sure that the nursing diagnoses selected reflect the whole person. Nursing diagnoses related to chemically mediated responses and medical diagnoses for substance-related disorders are listed in the Medical and Nursing Diagnoses box (Box 24-6).

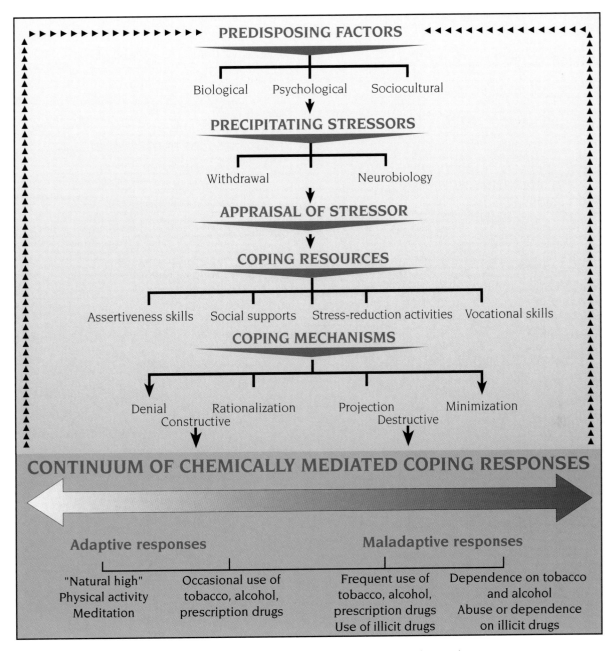

Figure 24-5   The Stuart Stress Adaptation Model as related to substance abuse.

The primary NANDA diagnoses include **disturbed sensory perception, acute confusion, ineffective coping,** and **dysfunctional family processes: alcoholism**. Examples of expanded nursing diagnoses are presented in the Detailed Diagnoses table (Table 24-4).

Medical Diagnoses

Disorders that are related to substance abuse are included in *DSM-IV-TR* in two ways. First, diagnoses that are primarily related to alcohol or drug use are categorized as substance-related disorders. The essential features of these are presented in the Detailed Diagnoses table (see Table 24-4). A patient with a substance-related disorder who is also diagnosed with another Axis I psychiatric disorder is considered to be **dually diagnosed**.

Second, if substance-induced intoxication or withdrawal is associated with another type of mental disorder, the diagnosis is located in the substance-induced category. For example, if a person is depressed related to alcohol withdrawal, the medical diagnosis would be substance-induced (withdrawal) mood disorder. The categories that include substance-induced diagnoses are delirium, dementia, amnestic, psychotic, mood, anxiety, sex, and sleep.

How would you respond to a patient who prefers street drugs over prescribed medication because of the side effects of the medication? ■

■ BOX 24-6 *Medical and Nursing Diagnoses Related to* **Chemically Mediated Responses**

RELATED MEDICAL DIAGNOSES (*DSM-IV-TR*)*	RELATED NURSING DIAGNOSES (NANDA)†

RELATED MEDICAL DIAGNOSES (*DSM-IV-TR*)*

Alcohol abuse
Alcohol dependence
Alcohol intoxication
Alcohol withdrawal
Amphetamine (or related substance) abuse
Amphetamine (or related substance) dependence
Amphetamine (or related substance) intoxication
Amphetamine (or related substance) withdrawal
Caffeine intoxication
Cannabis abuse
Cannabis dependence
Cannabis intoxication
Cocaine abuse
Cocaine dependence
Cocaine intoxication
Cocaine withdrawal
Hallucinogen abuse
Hallucinogen dependence
Hallucinogen intoxication
Hallucinogen persisting perception disorder (flashbacks)
Inhalant abuse
Inhalant dependence
Inhalant intoxication
Nicotine dependence
Nicotine withdrawal
Opioid abuse
Opioid dependence
Opioid intoxication
Opioid withdrawal
Phencyclidine (or related substance) abuse
Phencyclidine (or related substance) dependence
Phencyclidine (or related substance) intoxication
Sedative, hypnotic, or anxiolytic abuse
Sedative, hypnotic, or anxiolytic dependence
Sedative, hypnotic, or anxiolytic intoxication
Sedative, hypnotic, or anxiolytic withdrawal
Polysubstance dependence

RELATED NURSING DIAGNOSES (NANDA)†

Anxiety
Communication, Impaired verbal
Confusion, Acute‡
Coping, Ineffective‡
Family processes, Dysfunctional: alcoholism‡
Hopelessness
Injury, Risk for
Noncompliance
Nutrition, Imbalanced
Parenting, Impaired
Powerlessness
Self-care deficit
Self-esteem, Chronic or Situational low
Sensory perception, Disturbed‡
Sexual dysfunction
Sleep pattern, Disturbed
Spiritual distress
Therapeutic regimen management, Ineffective: individuals or families
Thought processes, Disturbed
Violence, Risk for

*From American Psychiatric Association: *Diagnostic and statistical manual of mental disorders*, ed 4, text revision, Washington, DC, 2000, American Psychiatric Association.
†From North American Nursing Diagnosis Association: *NANDA nursing diagnoses: definitions and classification 2003-2004*, Philadelphia, 2003, The Association.
‡**Primary nursing diagnosis for chemically mediated responses.**

▨ OUTCOME IDENTIFICATION

The expected outcome for patients in **withdrawal** from drugs or alcohol is:

The patient will overcome withdrawal safely and with minimum discomfort.

Short-term goals related to this phase of recovery may include the following:

- The patient will withdraw from dependence on the abused substance.
- The patient will be oriented to time, place, person, and situation.
- The patient will report symptoms of withdrawal.

- The patient will correctly interpret environmental stimuli.
- The patient will recognize and talk about hallucinations or delusions.

The expected outcome for patients **dependent** on drugs or alcohol is:

The patient will abstain from all mood-altering chemicals.

Studies have shown that most people who are dependent on a drug or alcohol cannot safely return to any level of use of any addictive drug. If they do, eventually the vast majority return to their old addictive patterns. However, patients of-

Table 24-4	*Detailed Diagnoses Related to* **Chemically Mediated Responses**

NANDA DIAGNOSIS STEM	EXAMPLES OF EXPANDED DIAGNOSIS
Disturbed sensory perception	Disturbed sensory perception related to hallucination, as evidenced by visual hallucination of snakes in the bed
Acute confusion	Acute confusion related to alcohol withdrawal, as evidenced by disorientation to time, person, and place
Ineffective coping	Ineffective coping related to cocaine abuse of 6 months' duration, as evidenced by loss of job and lack of personal goals
Dysfunctional family processes: alcoholism	Dysfunctional family processes related to alcoholism, as evidenced by marital conflict and avoidance of the family and home by the children

DSM-IV-TR DIAGNOSIS	ESSENTIAL FEATURES*
Substance dependence	Maladaptive pattern of substance use characterized by any three of the following within 12 months: tolerance; withdrawal; using more of the substance or using for longer than planned; persistent desire or unsuccessful efforts to cut down or control use; much time spent in efforts to obtain, use, or recover from use; interference with social, occupational, or recreational activities; continued use despite knowledge of use-related recurrent physical or psychological problems
Substance abuse	Maladaptive pattern of substance use characterized by one or more of the following within 12 months: recurrent use resulting in failure to meet role obligations, recurrent use in physically hazardous situations, recurrent use-related legal problems, continued use despite persistent or recurrent use-related social or interpersonal problems; has never met the criteria for dependence for this class of substance

From American Psychiatric Association: *Diagnostic and statistical manual of mental disorders*, ed 4, text revision, Washington, DC, 2000, American Psychiatric Association.
*The essential features of intoxication and withdrawal vary according to the substance and are listed in Table 24-3.

ten become very anxious at the thought of never again using the substance to which they are addicted. Therefore it may be helpful to focus on short-term goals. Short-term goals related to abstinence may include the following:

- The patient will agree to remain drug and alcohol free for 1 week, with the agreement to be renewed weekly.
- The patient will make a daily commitment to abstain.
- The patient will attend at least two support group meetings weekly.
- The patient will contact a supportive person if he or she experiences an urge to use an addictive substance.

Development of some kind of support system is an essential expected outcome for drug-dependent patients. Once abstinence and support system goals are established, attention can turn to learning about dependence and recovery and developing alternative coping skills.

Goals related to the person's job, relationships, or education should be deferred until later, unless any are a roadblock to recovery. For instance, a person is usually encouraged to focus on self and not on a relationship. However, if the person's spouse is an alcoholic and violence in the home is common, then the priority shifts to finding a safe place to live.

Goals should be worded so that it is clear that the patient is responsible for behavior. Addicted patients often want others to do the work for them. Nurses sometimes comply because they want to be helpful. However, such behavior does not help in the long run. Writing the goals and a specific plan of action into a contract and providing the patient with a copy of the contract will reinforce the patient's responsibility. The contract should be signed by both the nurse and the patient.

PLANNING

Long-range goals of treatment for patients with substance use disorders include the following:

1. Abstinence or reduction in the use and effects of substances
2. Reduction in the frequency and severity of relapse
3. Improvement in psychological and social functioning

Priority must be given to the most immediate needs. For patients who are experiencing drug withdrawal, **the highest priority is given to patient safety,** which involves the stabilization of the patient's physiological status until the crisis of withdrawal has subsided. Once safety needs are met, **abstinence** and **support system** issues must be addressed.

Plans related to these needs must be made in collaboration with the patient with consideration of the overall assessment and the patient's current life situation and desires. Family members and supportive friends should be included in the planning process. This will help them understand the problems that the patient may encounter as recovery continues.

The nurse should be aware that it is rare for an addicted person to suddenly stop substance use forever. Most addicts try at least once and usually several times to use the substance in a controlled way. It is important for addicts to know that they should return to treatment after these relapses. They can learn from what they did and try to prevent further relapses. These issues should be addressed openly in the planning process.

IMPLEMENTATION

The nurse encounters patients with substance abuse problems in all health care settings. The types of interventions recommended depend largely on the setting in which the nurse works. When encountering these patients outside addiction treatment programs, the nurse may be able to refer the person to treatment.

If a patient has a history of seizures or serious withdrawal symptoms or is at risk for developing symptoms because of a heavy, chronic use pattern, the first referral should be to a detoxification program. Otherwise, referral should be to the program that appears to match the patient's level of severity. Studies to determine which kinds of treatment programs are best for which kinds of patients have found similar efficacy rates for various alcohol treatment strategies (Project MATCH Research Group, 1997; Rychtarik et al, 2000).

Substance abusers often come into contact with the health care system because of a physiological crisis. It may be related to overdose, withdrawal, allergy, or toxicity. Physical deterioration caused by the damaging effects of drugs may be noted, including conditions such as malnutrition; dehydration; and various infections, including HIV.

When an acute physical condition is present, it takes priority over the other health needs of the patient. It is particularly important to attend to the condition that the patient has identified as the problem. The nurse is then seen as potentially helpful and will have more credibility when other aspects of the addiction are addressed.

Empirically validated treatments related to substance-related disorders are summarized in Box 24-7 (Nathan and Gorman, 2002).

Intervening in Withdrawal

Interventions depend on the current and potential withdrawal symptoms that the patient may experience. **Substances with potentially life-threatening courses of withdrawal include alcohol, benzodiazepines, and barbiturates.** Withdrawal from the general depressants and opiates is generally treated by substitution with a longer-acting drug in the same class, which is then gradually tapered. Withdrawal from opiates and stimulants can be extremely uncomfortable but is generally not dangerous, although a patient may become suicidal during the acute phase of cocaine withdrawal. Symptom-specific medications may be used to treat symptoms of stimulant withdrawal. Phenobarbital may be prescribed for inhalant withdrawal symptoms. No acute withdrawal pattern associated with marijuana, hallucinogens, or PCP has been identified.

Withdrawal symptoms may occur despite efforts to prevent them. Substance abusers do not always give accurate drug use histories, although it is extremely important to obtain as specific an assessment as possible. If the amount of substance used has been understated or if multiple abuse is undetected, withdrawal symptoms may occur unexpectedly.

The possibility of **seizures** should always be anticipated. Emergency equipment should be at hand. Drug abuse should always be considered possible when unexpected seizures occur. If drug abuse is suspected, the physician should be informed so that blood and urine specimens can be collected for laboratory analysis and an appropriate treatment plan initiated.

The process of helping an addict safely through withdrawal is called detoxification. Actually, the liver detoxifies the substance. Medications and nursing actions only help to relieve the symptoms.

Detoxification is best accomplished in a setting in which there can be close monitoring of the patient. This can be an inpatient medical or psychiatric unit or a crisis stabilization unit. Outpatient detoxification also may be possible.

It is best to maintain a quiet, calm environment for patients experiencing the general depressant withdrawal syndrome. This helps the patient relax and decreases nervous system irritability. Reassurance in a calm, quiet tone of voice is also helpful.

To help maintain the patient's orientation, the nurse should place a clock within sight and give frequent, low-key

---

BOX **24-7**	SUMMARIZING THE EVIDENCE ON **Chemically Mediated Responses**
Disorder	Alcohol use disorder
Treatment	◆ Cognitive behavioral treatments help patients shape and adapt to their life circumstances. ◆ 12-step treatment may be as effective as cognitive behavioral treatments. ◆ Therapist characteristics may have a stronger impact on outcome than type of treatment. ◆ Lower intensity treatment for a longer duration may be an effective treatment strategy. ◆ There appears to be little difference in outcome between inpatient and outpatient treatment. ◆ Naltrexone is effective in preventing full-blown relapses in alcoholics who have had a "slip" after achieving abstinence.
Disorder	Substance use disorders
Treatment	◆ The nicotine patch and nicotine gum significantly increase nicotine abstinence. ◆ Maintenance treatment using methadone for heroine dependence is effective. ◆ LAAM, a longer-acting opioid, is also effective.

From Nathan P, Gorman J: *A guide to treatments that work,* ed 2, New York, 2002, Oxford University Press.
LAAM, L-alpha acetyl methadol.

reminders about who he or she is, where the patient is, the nurse's name, and the day of the week. If possible, another patient who is further along in detoxification may be assigned as a buddy so that the patient is not left alone. A family member may help also.

The patient in withdrawal should be treated symptomatically. Fluids should be encouraged only if the person is dehydrated. Eating should be encouraged, and vitamins are usually ordered. Acetaminophen (Tylenol) or attapulgite (Kaopectate), if ordered, may be given for discomfort or diarrhea. A small amount of milk may be offered frequently to help manage epigastric distress. Seizure precautions should be taken. A cool washcloth can be offered for use on the forehead if the patient is feeling warm or diaphoretic. Position changes, assistance with ambulation, and changing damp clothing are also indicated.

Evidence suggests that offering this type of intense, supportive care can reduce withdrawal symptoms rapidly and often dramatically without medications. If the patient is receiving large doses of benzodiazepines, the nurse should monitor for signs of toxicity, such as ataxia (difficulty walking) and nystagmus (involuntary rhythmic movement of the eyeball). The patient always should be treated with respect and dignity.

Management of Alcohol Withdrawal.
The principles of **alcohol detoxification**, according to evidence-based practice guidelines, are as follows (Mayo-Smith et al, 1997):

- The long-acting **benzodiazepines** are the drugs of choice in treating alcohol withdrawal because they effectively reduce signs and symptoms of withdrawal, prevent seizures, and have a better margin of safety than many other drugs. The dosing regimens recommended in the practice guidelines are listed in Box 24-8.
- A symptom-triggered dosing regimen is preferred over fixed-schedule dosing because it is effective, requires significantly less medication, and appears to prevent seizures as well as fixed schemes.
- The use of a clinically valid and reliable withdrawal assessment tool such as the Clinical Institute Withdrawal Assessment–Alcohol, Revised (CIWA–AR) is recommended as the basis for medication determinations. This reduces overmedication resulting from patient over-reporting of symptoms or fixed regimens and undermedication resulting from staff reluctance to treat.
- A fixed schedule, with prn dosing, may be indicated if used on a unit where the staff have no training in the use of a withdrawal assessment tool.
- Although neither magnesium nor thiamine reduces seizures, administration of thiamine is recommended to prevent Wernicke's disease and Wernicke-Korsakoff syndrome (see Chapter 6).

Symptoms of alcohol withdrawal do not always progress from mild to severe in a predictable manner. A grand mal seizure may be the first sign of acute withdrawal. How-

---

BOX 24-8

Management of Alcohol Withdrawal

Monitor patient q4-8h with the CIWA–AR until score has been less than 8 to 10 for 24 hr. Use additional assessments as needed.

Symptom-Triggered Regimen
Administer one of the following every hour when CIWA-AR scores are >8-10:
  Chlordiazepoxide, 50-100 mg
  Diazepam, 10-20 mg
  Lorazepam, 2-4 mg
Repeat CIWA-AR 1 hr after every dose to assess need for further medication.

Fixed-Schedule Regimen
Chlordiazepoxide, 50 mg q6h for 4 doses, then 25 mg q6h for 8 doses
Diazepam, 10 mg q6h for 4 doses, then 5 mg q6h for 8 doses
Lorazepam, 2 mg q6h for 4 doses, then 1 mg q6h for 8 doses
Provide additional medication as needed when symptoms not controlled (i.e., CIWA-AR >8-10) with above measures.
Other benzodiazepines may be used at equivalent doses.

---

ever, initial assessment and ongoing monitoring with the CIWA–AR may be effective in preventing the onset of more severe symptoms. A score of 9 or less on the CIWA–AR indicates mild withdrawal, 10 to 18 indicates moderate withdrawal, and a score greater than 18, severe withdrawal.

The CIWA–AR should be used with caution in patients with co-occurring medical or psychiatric illnesses and in those with concurrent withdrawal from other drugs because it rates signs and symptoms that may be caused by the other conditions and not by the alcohol withdrawal.

The CIWA–AR should be repeated every 1 to 2 hours. Increasing scores signify the need for additional medication according to a predetermined scale, whereas decreasing scores indicate a therapeutic response to the treatment regimen. Scores less than 10 do not generally require use of medication.

Some evidence indicates that symptom-triggered medication shortens the length of treatment and requires significantly less medication. There is also evidence that the use of the CIWA–AR as a basis for medication need results in significantly less medication being given with no reduction in efficacy.

Management of Benzodiazepines, Barbiturates, and Other Sedative-Hypnotics Withdrawal.
These drugs are generally prescribed for therapeutic purposes, sometimes for long periods of time. When this occurs, development of physical dependence on the drug is sometimes unavoidable. As long as the drug is taken as prescribed, such a physical de-

pendence is not considered substance abuse and the term **detoxification** should be replaced by the term **therapeutic discontinuation**.

Heroin and stimulant users sometimes use these drugs as part of their drug abuse pattern. When individuals use the drug other than prescribed, obtain the drug by illegitimate means, or when the drug use interferes with their lives, then such use can lead to dependence, which requires detoxification. Whether used therapeutically or abused, abrupt cessation from these drugs can lead to severe withdrawal and even death. Therefore, careful medical management is required.

High-dose withdrawal may be treated by a gradual reduction of the drug being used, or **phenobarbital** may be substituted during the detoxification process. The dosing regimen starts with the patient's average daily dose (as self-reported) of all sedative-hypnotic drugs, including alcohol. This dose is then converted to phenobarbital equivalents, and the daily amount is divided into three doses.

Before each dose, the nurse checks for signs of phenobarbital toxicity (sustained nystagmus, slurred speech, or ataxia). Because nystagmus is the most reliable sign, if present, the dose is withheld. If all three signs are present, the next two doses of phenobarbital are withheld, and the daily dosage of phenobarbital for the following day is reduced by half.

If the patient is in acute withdrawal and is at risk for withdrawal seizures, the first dose of phenobarbital is administered intramuscularly (IM). If nystagmus and other signs of intoxication develop 1 to 2 hours after IM dosing, then the patient is in no immediate danger from barbiturate withdrawal. In this case, patients continue to receive the initial dosing schedule for 2 days. Then, if the patient displays neither signs of withdrawal nor toxicity nor has an unsteady gait, doses are decreased by 30 mg/day.

If toxicity develops, the daily dose is decreased by 50% and the 30 mg/day withdrawal is continued from the reduced dose. If the patient has objective signs of withdrawal, the daily dose is increased by 50%, and the patient is restabilized before continuing withdrawal.

Low-dose withdrawal depends on the patient's symptoms. Seizures are uncommon unless the patient has an underlying seizure disorder, in which case anticonvulsants should be administered and other medications that lower the seizure threshold should be avoided. If symptoms are severe, 200 mg of phenobarbital is given per day initially, then slowly tapered over several months.

Management of Opiate Withdrawal. All opiates produce similar withdrawal signs and symptoms, but the time of onset and the duration vary. Treatment is aimed at alleviating the acute symptoms. This may be done by substitution of the long-acting opiate methadone or by management of the withdrawal symptoms with medications such as clonidine.

- **Methadone** substitution involves initial administration of methadone—an opiate agonist—to stabilize symptoms of heroin withdrawal, usually 10 to 40 mg in the first 24 hours. Once the patient is stabilized, the dose can be slowly tapered to 0. Tapering by 5 mg/day is common, but slower tapering may be more comfortable for the patient. The detoxification of patients from longer-acting opioids, such as methadone, requires an even longer period of time.

- **Clonidine** is available in oral, sublingual, or transdermal patch preparations. The protocol for clonidine administration usually involves 0.1 to 0.3 mg in three divided doses on the first day (perhaps higher doses for inpatients who can be closely monitored). The dose is then adjusted until withdrawal symptoms are reduced. The blood pressure should initially be checked every 45 minutes, because some patients are extremely sensitive to clonidine and experience profound hypotension, even at low doses. If the blood pressure drops below 90/60 mm Hg, the next dose should be withheld and subsequent doses adjusted according to patient response. Although clonidine effectively relieves several symptoms of opiate withdrawal, it is not helpful for muscle aches, insomnia, or drug craving, which then require additional medication.

Just as the CIWA–AR is useful in rating alcohol withdrawal, the Clinical Institute Narcotic Assessment (CINA) rating scale may be helpful in the assessment and monitoring of opiate withdrawal.

Management of Nicotine Withdrawal. Nicotine gum and the **nicotine patch** both provide mechanisms for nicotine to be delivered into the body without the carcinogens and carbon monoxide present in cigarettes. Nicotine in these forms serves to replace the nicotine in cigarettes, thus relieving withdrawal symptoms and allowing for tapering of the dose to 0 over time.

The optimum length of treatment before tapering is 4 to 6 weeks. Dosing is most effective at 2 to 4 mg/hour for the gum, which comes in 2- and 4-mg sticks. Patches are available in a 21- to 22-mg/24-hour patch and a 15-mg/16-hour patch (for use while awake). Other available, but less popular, forms of nicotine are nasal sprays and inhalers.

Bupropion is the first FDA approved non-nicotine replacement therapy for treating nicotine dependence. Dosage should include 150 mg every morning for 3 days, then 150 mg twice daily. Treatment should begin 1 to 2 weeks before the initial quit date and should last for 8 to 12 weeks with 6 months maintenance. Clonidine and nortriptyline are second-line medications (Cataldo, 2001).

Management of Caffeine Withdrawal. Although not classified as a drug of abuse, caffeine has a well-defined physical withdrawal syndrome. Symptoms are relieved with caffeine. There is no published regimen of caffeine administration for the purpose of relieving withdrawal. The recommendation is to gradually decrease caffeine intake over as much time as it takes to avoid most withdrawal symptoms.

Intervening in Toxic Psychosis. Users of LSD, PCP, and stimulants often come to the emergency room in acute toxic psychosis. Their behavior may be quite similar to that of the patient with schizophrenia. However, there may be no history of abnormal behavior.

Careful assessment of an acute psychotic reaction, particularly in an adolescent or young adult, should include exploration of drug use. It may be necessary to interview friends of the patient to obtain this information. An attempt should be made to identify the specific drug used, although LSD and PCP may be taken without the knowledge of the person involved.

The nursing approach to users of PCP and amphetamine has one important difference as opposed to those who have an adverse reaction to LSD. Unless the psychiatric symptomatology is severe, LSD users experiencing a "bad trip" often respond to reassurance and may be "talked down." Patients should be oriented frequently and discouraged from closing their eyes because this may make the symptoms worse.

However, victims of PCP-induced psychosis do not respond well to attempts at interaction. Agitated PCP and amphetamine users are more likely to strike out in response to their misperceptions and panic. They are potentially more harmful to themselves and others. This aggression may be totally unprovoked.

In addition, because PCP is also an anesthetic, these patients feel little or no pain. For this reason, they seem to have enormous strength. They do not feel pain when they exceed the limits of their muscular capability and may continue pushing, pulling, or hitting until they seriously injure themselves or others.

Other elements of treatment are basically the same for acutely agitated LSD and PCP users. Both require **a safe environment that has minimum stimulation.** Staff should not perform any procedures without a thorough explanation, should not touch the patient without permission, and should avoid rapid movements in the patient's presence. Adequate staff should be present to control impulsive behavior.

Vital signs should be monitored, and other physiological needs should be met. Although restraints may exacerbate muscle damage and agitation, they may be necessary, especially if a seclusion room is not available. **Benzodiazepines** are the treatment of choice, followed by high-potency **antipsychotic medications** if benzodiazepines are ineffective. Gastric lavage may be necessary for persistent symptoms or if an overdose has been taken, although this is not recommended for PCP users because it increases agitation.

Intervening To Maintain Abstinence

The immediate short-term goal of pharmacological treatment of substance abuse is the safety of the patient, because many intoxication and withdrawal syndromes are potentially life threatening. Once the individual is through the initial withdrawal phase, interventions to maintain abstinence can begin. **The first months after cessation of substance use represent the highest risk for relapse** and offer the greatest opportunity for pharmacological interventions that can help patients decrease cravings and maintain abstinence. However, the drugs currently available are limited in number, and patients often stop taking them. Thus the effects are often

temporary unless the drugs are used as part of a broader program of psychosocial treatment.

The goals for the pharmacological maintenance of abstinence in substance abuse treatment are as follows (Welsh and Liberto, 2001):

- **The individual:** Either total abstinence or a reduction in drug consumption that will allow the person to function better in all facets of life, including educational, occupational, and family domains.
- **The dually diagnosed person:** Reduce symptoms that are exacerbated by substance abuse as well as enhance compliance with medications needed for the management of the psychiatric condition.
- **Society:** Reduction of crime, violence, family discord, the spread of HIV and other infectious diseases associated with IV drug use and other risky behaviors and other health complications associated with substance abuse.

A number of strategies are used in the pharmacological treatment of substance abuse (Box 24-9). Each substance of abuse requires a different pharmacological approach in the maintenance phase of relapse prevention.

Alcohol

Naltrexone. Naltrexone (ReVia) was approved by the FDA in 1994 for the treatment of alcohol dependence. Nal-

---

BOX 24-9

Strategies in the Pharmacological Treatment of Substance Abuse

- Use of a drug with pharmacological properties similar to the substance of concern (benzodiazepines in the management of alcohol/sedative/hypnotic withdrawal; methadone in the long-term treatment of opioid dependence)—referred to as agonist or substitution therapy
- Use of receptor antagonists to block or lessen the effects of the drug of concern (naltrexone in the acute and chronic treatment of opioid overdose and dependence)
- Use of a drug that produces a conditioned aversive reaction to the substance of concern in order to reduce the positive reinforcement properties of the substance, decreasing use (disulfiram in the treatment of alcohol dependence)
- Use of a drug to reduce the reinforcing properties of the drug of concern by altering neuronal mechanisms associated with the pleasure pathway to produce a reduced subjective craving for the substance (naltrexone in the treatment of alcohol dependence)
- Use of a substance to increase the metabolism or clearance of the drug of concern from the body (butylcholinesterase to accelerate the metabolism of cocaine)
- Although still in development, the use of blood-borne peripheral blockers or "vaccines" to bind drugs of concern before they reach the brain, preventing them from activating the receptors that are usually responsible for their actions

trexone, an opiate antagonist, has demonstrated effectiveness in helping the alcoholic patient maintain abstinence. It diminishes craving during the early stages of abstinence and works best when accompanied by psychosocial interventions.

It is believed to act in the following way: Alcohol intake increases the number of endorphins (naturally occurring opioids) in the brain. Naltrexone, in doses of approximately 50 mg/day, appears to block the effects of these endorphins, thus reducing the reinforcing effects of alcohol (Welsh and Liberto, 2001). Limitations of this medication include discontinuation from side effects (primarily nausea) and dose-dependent hepatotoxic effects, which are particularly concerning considering the damaging effects of alcohol on the liver.

Antabuse. A long-term biological approach to substance abuse is the prescription of disulfiram (Antabuse) for alcoholics. This drug interrupts the metabolism of alcohol, causing a buildup of a toxic substance in the body if the person uses alcohol in any form. The physiological response may include a severe headache, nausea and vomiting, flushing, hypotension, tachycardia, dyspnea, diaphoresis, chest pain, palpitations, dizziness, and confusion. Rarely, it can lead to respiratory and cardiac collapse, unconsciousness, convulsions, and death.

Antabuse should never be given without the patient's stated willingness to comply. It is also important that the patient agree to take Antabuse only after careful instruction about the potential consequences of drinking while taking the drug. This instruction should include a written list of alcohol-containing preparations to be avoided, including cough medicines, rubbing compounds, vinegar, aftershave lotions, and some mouthwashes.

Drinking must be avoided for 14 days after Antabuse has been discontinued. This medication cannot prevent someone who is determined to drink from drinking. This person can simply wait until the Antabuse has been excreted. However, it does help prevent impulsive drinking because the person has to wait for the Antabuse to clear the body to be able to drink safely. This treatment should be used in conjunction with other supportive therapies, not by itself.

Describe the information that should be provided to a patient who is to be treated with Antabuse. What issues related to informed consent should be considered in the use of this drug? ■

Nalmefene. Nalmefene (Revex) is a newer opioid antagonist that is structurally similar to naltrexone but with a number of pharmacological advances for the treatment of alcohol dependence. These include no dose-dependent association with toxic effects to the liver, greater oral bioavailability, longer duration of antagonist action, and more complete binding with opioid receptor subtypes that are thought to reinforce drinking. It has been found to be effective in preventing relapse to heavy drinking and has few side effects.

Acamprosate. Acamprosate (Campral), (calcium acetylhomotaurine) is a synthetic compound, similar in chemical structure to GABA. It is used extensively in Europe, exerts agonist activity at the GABA receptors and antagonist (in-

hibitory) activity at the N-methyl-D-aspartate (NMDA) glutamate receptors. It has demonstrated increased abstinence through decreased alcohol craving.

It has been shown to positively affect length of total abstinence, time to relapse, number of total nondrinking days, and retention in treatment. It is associated with few side effects (diarrhea and headache), and organ toxicity does not appear to be a problem. It is renally excreted so must be used with caution in patients with renal insufficiency. Dosage ranges from 1300 mg to 4000 mg/day.

Citalopram. Citalopram (Celexa) is a selective serotonin reuptake inhibitor (SSRI) that augments central serotonergic function approved for the treatment of depression. It has been shown to decrease desire and the sense of "liking" alcohol.

Ondansetron. Ondansetron (Zofran) is a serotonin (5-HT3) receptor antagonist that has been shown to reduce alcohol consumption and craving in patients with early-onset alcohol dependence.

Opiates. Long-term opiate addicts who meet federal criteria for opiate dependence may be eligible for maintenance with methadone or L-alpha acetyl methadol (LAAM). Patients in maintenance programs take stable doses of one of these substitute drugs for years—possibly even for the rest of their lives. They must report to the clinic daily (for methadone) or every other day (for LAAM) to have their medication dispensed to them. Because these medications are Schedule II drugs, they can be distributed only in special clinics that are heavily government regulated, and often these clinics are excluded by local zoning laws. The result is a national shortage of these treatment facilities.

These medications are also controversial because they are narcotics. However, addiction to them does not cause impaired functioning; thus the person can be productive while being addicted. Those in favor of methadone or LAMM maintenance point out the benefits of avoiding the debilitating effects of heroin addiction and the lifestyle associated with obtaining illegal drugs on the streets (Clarke, 2003).

LAAM. LAAM is a long-acting opiate agonist. Because LAAM has not been approved for take-home dosing, if LAAM patients cannot get through the weekend free of withdrawal symptoms, they may be given a Sunday take-home dose of methadone (Welsh and Liberto, 2001).

Methadone. Methadone hydrochloride is a mμ-opioid receptor agonist used since 1960 for the treatment of opioid dependence. At adequate doses it can relieve symptoms of opioid withdrawal and craving for opioids and can block the effect of illicitly used opioids. It is well absorbed orally and has a long half-life and duration of action, thus once daily dosing is usually sufficient.

For maintenance treatment of opioid dependence, the patient is started on 20 to 30 mg/day, increasing the dose by 5 mg every 1 to 2 days until symptoms of opioid withdrawal are relieved and the patient reports an absence of craving. Evidence shows that many patients will need up to 80 or more mg per day for effective treatment. Side effects include constipation, drowsiness, diaphoresis, and decreased libido.

Methadone is primarily metabolized by the liver (cytochrome P450 3A4); medications that induce liver enzymes may lower methadone blood levels (rifampin, phenytoin, phenobarbital, and carbamazepine). Medications that inhibit this liver enzyme system may raise blood levels of methadone (erythromycin, fluoxetine, fluvoxamine, indinavir, ketoconazole, nefazodone, paroxetine, and sertraline, among others).

> *Methadone maintenance is essentially substituting a legal narcotic for an illegal one. Do you believe that this is a responsible practice? State the reasons for your position.* ■

Buprenorphine. Buprenorphine (Temgesic) is a partial rather than full agonist at opioid nerve receptors. That means that it mimics the effects of opioids in some situations but blocks or reverses those effects in other situations by displacing opioids when they are present in excessive amounts.

Buprenorphine has several advantages over methadone and LAAM. It generally produces a less serious withdrawal reaction. Because it is less likely to cause respiratory arrest, the risk of an accidental or intentional overdose is lower. Another advantage is that it needs to be taken only three times a week instead of daily, like methadone. Most important, buprenorphine can be administered in other settings besides formal narcotics treatment programs, thus allowing more addicts to receive treatment (O'Connor, 2000).

Cocaine

Vaccine in development. An exciting breakthrough in the field is the development of a cocaine vaccine that is designed to be part of a comprehensive approach to treating cocaine addiction. A therapeutic vaccine that induces anticocaine antibodies and prevents the drug from crossing the blood-brain barrier is being used in experimental animal trials with some success. It may prove to be a powerful tool for inhibiting the reinforcing activity of the drug.

Nicotine

Nicotine replacement. The various nicotine replacement therapies (transdermal patch, gum, nasal spray, and inhaler) all appear to be effective in reducing withdrawal from nicotine and subsequent use. Despite this, the 1-year relapse rates are very high.

Bupropion. Bupropion sustained release (Zyban) is a novel antidepressant (called Wellbutrin when used for this indication) with effects on norepinephrine, serotonin, and dopamine reuptake. Evidence for why it affects smoking cessation is not clear, but it does not appear that it is simply treating an underlying depression. It is well tolerated and has few side effects (dry mouth, insomnia, and headache). It also may reduce the weight gain that is associated with smoking cessation. It can lower the seizure threshold and is contraindicated in patients with a seizure disorder or an eating disorder and should be used cautiously with patients at increased risk for head trauma and seizures (alcoholics). As with nicotine replacement therapy, relapse in patients is common.

Effects of Use During Pregnancy. Because most of the drugs that are abused cross the placental barrier, women should be counseled about the possible effects of substance use during pregnancy. Congenital abnormalities have occurred in infants of mothers who have taken drugs. A fetal alcohol syndrome has been identified, which involves a pattern of physical growth and mental deficiencies.

In addition, during pregnancy use of drugs that cause physical dependence can result in the birth of an addicted baby who must be withdrawn from the drug. The safest pregnancy is one in which the mother is **totally drug and alcohol free** with one exception: For pregnant women addicted to heroin, methadone maintenance is safer for the fetus than acute opiate detoxification.

> *Some policymakers have proposed that pregnant women who abuse substances should be jailed, placed under house arrest, or committed to a mental hospital until the baby is born. Do you agree with this? Support your position. Do you have the same opinion related to all abused substances, including alcohol and nicotine?* ■

Finally, medications alone have less effectiveness in the treatment of drug and alcohol dependence. Most patients have optimum benefit with a comprehensive treatment program that includes the addition of psychological, social, and spiritual treatments.

Psychological Interventions

Before initiating nursing intervention with a substance-abusing patient, the nurse must develop self-awareness of feelings and attitudes about the problem (see A Patient Speaks). It is recommended that a value clarification approach be used, as described in Chapter 2.

Most people have had personal contact with substance abuse by family, friends, or colleagues. This may create negative feelings and attitudes. It is important that the nurse be able to differentiate feelings associated with past situations from those aroused by contacts with patients and their families. A supervisor, teacher, or senior clinical nurse can be of

---

A PATIENT SPEAKS

I have abused drugs and alcohol for many years. One thing that has been important is for nurses to spend time with me so I can learn to trust them. It helps when they make sure I schedule treatment appointments and keep them. Substance abuse education is very important, and it has to be repeated over and over.

I've been through detoxification many times. Some of the nurses in those programs have coddled me. This makes it easy for me to dance around issues of sobriety. I've had the best success with the nurse who will hang in there with me and not let me make excuses, get in my face, and cut me no slack. The nurses who have high expectations leave me enough room to help myself, but not enough to be dishonest. There needs to be a balance of empathy and toughness. It's not easy, but that's the role for the nurse to establish.

assistance when a nurse is having difficulty sorting out these feelings.

Traditional addiction treatment is based on the concepts of addiction as a disease, total abstinence from all substances, immersion in 12-step recovery programs, direct confrontation of denial and other defense mechanisms (generally in group sessions), and a lifelong recovery process. Groups are usually led by recovering alcoholic/addict counselors. Ambivalence, resistance, and denial are viewed as characteristics of the disease of addiction. Confrontation is viewed as being necessary to break through these defenses.

Through the years, a practice of using very harsh and confrontational counseling techniques has evolved. Although some people respond well to these approaches, others do not. Despite their popularity, clinical outcome studies do not support such confrontational strategies, and some of the traditional programs consequently have adopted gentler approaches.

In the past, traditional addiction treatment was offered in specialized programs, whereas psychiatric patients with substance abuse problems were treated in psychiatric and mental health programs. Many psychiatric professionals viewed alcoholism and other drug addictions as being secondary to psychiatric disorders. They believed that the substance abuse would cease when the person's primary psychiatric disorder was resolved. Psychiatric patients often were given tranquilizers to treat what was believed to be their underlying pathology.

However, instead of abstaining from their substance of choice, many of these patients became addicted to the tranquilizers as well. Psychiatric treatment models operated from a different philosophical base, which was effective in dealing with psychiatric problems but less effective in dealing with addiction. Differences in treatment philosophies and backgrounds of providers contributed to a developing rift between psychiatric clinicians and addiction counselors. Dually diagnosed patients often were caught in the middle.

However, over the years, approaches have been developed for the treatment of addictions that incorporate knowledge of both addictions and mental health strategies. Addiction counselors now include motivational interviewing, family counseling, and cognitive behavioral techniques in their treatment strategies (Barrowclough et al, 2001). So too, psychiatric clinicians better understand addiction as a separate disorder. Dual diagnosis programs have been developed, and mental health approaches have been adapted for the primary treatment of addiction.

Although these newer approaches vary, they generally involve creation of an alliance between the therapist and the patient, inclusion of the patient in the setting of treatment goals (even if the patient's goal is not total abstinence), avoidance of confrontation, brevity of treatment, and use of professional therapists. More than just a series of techniques, they offer a new type of relationship between clinician and patient. Even more important, they have demonstrated efficacy in the treatment of patients with substance abuse disorders. Some of these newer approaches are described here.

Motivational Approaches. Motivational counseling is a relatively new approach to helping patients with substance abuse problems (Carey et al, 2002). It is based on the concept that motivation for change is not static but dynamic and that the clinician can influence change by developing a therapeutic relationship that respects and builds on the patient's autonomy and by making the patient a partner in the change process (SAMHSA, 2003; Joe et al, 2001). Although many different techniques can be used, the most important element of treatment is the attitude of the clinician. Five basic principles are used with this approach:

- **Express empathy through reflective listening**. This communicates respect for and acceptance of patients and their feelings. It also establishes a safe and open environment that helps in examining issues and exploring personal reasons for change.
- **Develop discrepancy between patients' goals or values and their current behavior**. Focus patients' attention on how current behavior differs from behavior described as ideal or desired.
- **Avoid argument and direct confrontation**. Trying to convince a patient that a problem exists or that change is needed could precipitate even more resistance. Arguments can rapidly degenerate into a power struggle and do not enhance motivation for beneficial change.
- **Roll with resistance**. Resistance is a signal that the patient views the situation differently. There are four types of resistance: arguing, interrupting, denying, or ignoring. The clinician's job is to ask questions in a way that helps the patient understand and work through resistance.
- **Support self-efficacy**. This requires the clinician to recognize the patient's strengths and bring these to the forefront whenever possible. It involves supporting hope, optimism, and the feasibility of accomplishing change.

Critical components of effective motivational interventions include the FRAMES approach and decisional balance exercises. FRAMES is an acronym for the basic elements of motivational counseling as described below:

- **F**eedback regarding personal risk or impairment is given to the patient after assessment of substance use patterns and related problems.
- **R**esponsibility for change is placed explicitly on the patient, with respect for the patient's right to make his or her own choices.
- **A**dvice about changing substance use behavior is given to the patient clearly and nonjudgmentally by the clinician.
- **M**enus of self-directed change options and treatment alternatives are offered.
- **E**mpathic counseling—showing warmth, respect, and understanding—is emphasized.
- **S**elf-efficacy—or optimistic empowerment—is engendered in the patient to encourage change.

Decisional balance exercises are specific ways that the clinician can assist the patient to explore the **pros and cons of old and new behaviors** for the purpose of tipping the scales toward a decision for positive change. The items are identified by the patient with gentle assistance from the clinician and then written in blocks, as in Figure 24-6. The four blocks add a new twist to the traditional two-column "pros and cons" list.

One advantage of the four-block grid is recognition that there are positive elements about the old behavior that must be acknowledged. For example, if drinking helps the patient relax, part of recovery may include finding other ways to relax without alcohol. Even more important than the number of items in each block is the weight of each item. For example, the negative impact on the family may more than outweigh the social pleasures of drinking.

The clinician then summarizes the list of concerns and presents them to the patient in a way that expresses empathy, develops discrepancy, and weights the balance toward change. The objective is to meet the patients where they are, concerning mental attitude, and walk with them through the process.

All of these motivational approaches are designed to help improve patient participation in the treatment process. They are based on the **stages of change** model, which identifies five stages of change (Figure 24-7): **precontemplation, contemplation, preparation, action,** and **maintenance** (Prochaska and DiCelemente, 1986).

DECISIONAL BALANCE GRID	
Old Behavior	**New Behavior**
<u>Pros/Benefits</u> Like the taste of alcohol Helps me to relax Source of fun and socialization Makes me forget my problems	<u>Pros/Benefits</u> Better relationship with spouse No more DWIs Save money Feel better about myself More time for other activities and people in my life

<u>Cons/Costs</u>
Costs a lot of money
Led to DWI—costly, embarrassing, and
  inconvenient
Spouse gets upset
Poor role model for children
Feel bad about myself
If I lose my driver's license, I could lose
  my job
	<u>Cons/Costs</u>
	Will miss my drinking friends
	Don't know how to have fun without it
	It will be harder to face my problems
	I'll feel left out, "different"
	I'll be more up-tight, less relaxed

Figure 24-6   Decisional balance grid.

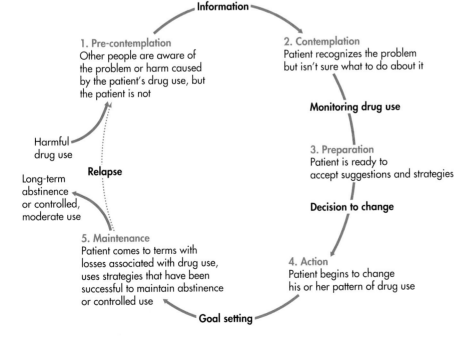

Figure 24-7   A model of change in substance use disorders. (Modified from Prochaska J, DiClemente C: Towards a comprehensive model of change. In Miller W, Heather N, editors: *Treating addictive behaviors: process of change,* New York, 1986, Plenum.)

Goals and approaches differ for each stage. For instance, if a patient is in the precontemplation stage of change, the decisional-balance would be an appropriate tool to use to help patients recognize they have a problem. Presenting these patients a menu of treatment options, however, would not be helpful because they are not ready to accept help for a problem they do not yet acknowledge having. However, options would be appropriate during the preparation stage.

Cognitive-Behavioral Strategies.

Cognitive-behavioral approaches are aimed at improving self-control, self-efficacy, and social skills in order to reduce drinking.

- **Self-control strategies** include goal-setting, self-monitoring, functional analysis of drinking antecedents, and learning alternative coping skills.
- **Social-skills training** focuses on learning skills for forming and maintaining interpersonal relationships, assertiveness, and drink refusal.
- **Contingency management** is another behavioral approach in which rewards (often in the form of vouchers that can be exchanged for desired items) are given for adaptive behavior (such as compliance with treatment or clean urine).
- **Behavioral contracting** involves creating a written agreement with the patient that specifies targeted patient behavior and consequences.

In general, cognitive-behavioral strategies can be adapted well to the briefer interventions that have been necessitated by managed care programs (Washington, 2001). They appear to be as effective as longer-term therapies. Cognitive-behavioral treatment strategies are discussed in more detail in Chapter 31.

Discuss the significance of the substance abuser's level of self-esteem to the recovery process. Describe nursing interventions designed to enhance self-esteem. ■

Working With Co-Dependency.

Whether or not co-dependency exists as an independent phenomenon is not important in treatment planning. However, it is important not to discount the patient's identification with the co-dependency movement or the syndrome. Having a label for problems makes them more legitimate and easier to accept for some people.

The co-dependency label has popular appeal. It is nonstigmatizing because the cause does not lie within the self, but with another person. The nurse should accept the patient's view of the problem as a legitimate starting point for a therapeutic alliance. Then the patient can be helped to understand how behavior that once allowed survival in a dysfunctional family no longer serves this purpose. The nurse can help the patient move gradually away from anger and fear and toward responsibility for self-fulfillment.

Interventions center around the patient's primary identified problems and may include assertiveness training, challenging cognitive distortions, teaching self-affirmations, and relaxation training. Because physical and sexual abuse are common in alcoholic families, specific assessment and intervention strategies must be implemented to identify and help patients with these types of problems. Referral to specialized programs may be useful. Additional information about appropriate interventions for survivors of abuse and violence is in Chapter 39.

ACOA self-help groups may be useful. The nurse should suggest that the patient try several self-help groups before deciding to be actively involved in any one group. The nurse also should monitor how the patient responds to participation in these groups. Some groups are more positive and forward-focused than others.

Alcoholism is known to run in families. People who grew up in an alcoholic home often develop alcohol problems themselves or may marry alcoholics. It is clear that both biological and environmental factors contribute to generational transmission of this disorder. Thus it is common for a patient to be alcoholic and have an alcoholic parent. Intervention is most effective if it addresses intergenerational patterns.

Intervening in Relapse.

Behavior change is always difficult, but change related to addiction is even more difficult because of the chemical imbalance in the brain induced by the substance. It is rare, therefore, for a person to make a sudden and drastic behavioral change and maintain it with no return to the old behaviors.

Because there are very few medications to counteract the effects on the brain, the patient must be assisted to make behavioral and lifestyle changes in spite of extremely powerful chemical forces in the brain luring him or her to return to the substance that would temporarily restore the chemical brain balance.

Relapse prevention strategies have been widely used in substance abuse recovery programs and have been shown to be effective in assisting patients to stay clean and sober (Irvin et al, 1999). However, most people who try to stop using an addictive substance are not successful on the first attempt. The nurse who is a smoker can generally identify with this phenomenon. The nurse who has never used an addictive substance but may have tried dieting can understand through this experience the difficulty of making behavioral changes that have strong physiological forces pulling in the opposite direction. Such personal identifications can help the nurse empathize with the patient and reduce negative judgments, which are essential to being a credible counselor.

In a sense, it would be better to abandon the notion of relapse altogether because it represents dichotomous thinking that does not fit well with the complexities of human behavior (such as a person is either abstinent or relapsed, sober or drinking). **Behavior change is actually a process that occurs over time.** Nurses can help those who are trying to change by helping them learn from whatever works and does not work in their behavior change efforts. This seems to have a more positive focus than a focus on failures or "relapses."

In these strategies, relapse, or the return of symptoms, is seen as a process, not an event. **Rather than being viewed as an indicator of treatment failure, it is dealt with as an**

error from which to learn—a temporary setback on the road to recovery. Recovery is not an all-or-nothing proposition. Rather "success" is measured by improvements—such as increasing lengths of time being clean between relapses and shorter time periods of relapse.

It is important for the nurse to accept the patient without judging and to assist the patient in learning from the relapse. The nurse should help the patient identify external and internal triggers that may precipitate cravings and thus lead to drug use.

External triggers include the people, places, and things that have been associated with previous drug use. The nurse helps the patient figure out ways to avoid these triggers. Situations that include one or all of these triggers are called *high-risk situations.* Because these cannot always be avoided, the nurse should assist the patient in managing them successfully. For example, if alcohol will be served at a family wedding and it is important to the patient to attend, the nurse can encourage the patient to attend the wedding with a relative who will support his or her decision to remain abstinent. Major lifestyle changes—such as making new friends, moving to a different neighborhood—may have to happen to avoid these triggers.

Internal triggers are the thoughts and feelings contributing to past drug use, such as loneliness, boredom, or anger. The nurse can help the patient identify internal triggers and develop healthy coping skills to deal with these negative emotional states without using substances.

The nurse generally will need to help patients restructure their time. So much time may have been spent in obtaining and using drugs that patients may have no idea what to do with their newly found free time. Lastly, the nurse should teach patients how to identify and deal with cravings. At the time they occur, it sometimes seems that the only way to satisfy cravings is to use the substance of choice. However, the nurse can reassure patients that the cravings will pass if they get involved in some other nondrug-related activity.

Patients also should be taught that there are many decision points on the road to relapse—one being before using, others being after the first use, and so on. This can help patients avoid the abstinence violation effect, in which patients feel so guilty about violating a period of abstinence that they figure they may as well keep using and "start again tomorrow. . . Monday. . . next week. . . after this run." The goal is for the patient to want to avoid the use altogether, but if it happens, to minimize the amount of substance abuse and the length of time involved.

Social Interventions

Family Counseling. Reliable support from caring people is crucial to the recovery of substance abusers. However, the family is often frustrated with the patient's behavior and finds it difficult to be supportive. The family seldom understands the nature of addiction and generally does all the wrong things in its attempt to help the substance abuser.

The family often tries to protect the patient from consequences. Many times, family members cover up by making excuses to employers and other family members for the person's erratic behavior. They also tend to blame themselves for the behavior and go to great lengths to avoid confrontation with the user.

All of these behaviors are called **enabling** behaviors, and family members who have these behaviors are called enablers. By shielding the person from the consequences of drug use, the family enables the person's continued use of the drug.

Addiction is a family problem (see A Family Speaks). Everyone in the family suffers, not just the alcoholic or drug addict. Some problems that families experience include guilt, shame, resentment, insecurity, delinquency, financial troubles, isolation, fear, and violence.

Families think their problems would be solved if their loved one simply stopped using drugs or alcohol. However, they can get help even if the user refuses to do so. They also should realize that without help, many of the negative pat-

---

A FAMILY SPEAKS

When I met Jim in 1983, I knew he dabbled in drugs, but I still married him. I had no idea how his growing drug abuse problem would affect my life over the next decade. In 1986 Jim entered treatment for his heroin addiction for the first time. I was impressed with the nurses in that program. They were compassionate, understanding, and knowledgeable about addiction. They taught Jim the first steps in the recovery process and supported him through the difficult changes that he had to make to maintain a drug-free lifestyle.

One nurse was particularly helpful to me as a family member of a newly recovering addict. She stood out because she consistently showed genuine concern for Jim and me. She always asked about Jim by name. She talked like he was an individual, not just one of the patients in the program. This allowed me to open up to her. I was finally able to ask if some of the things he was going through were normal, and I was very relieved to find out that they were! In contrast, another nurse on the staff talked down to all the patients. Neither the patients nor the family members felt they could talk to her.

Despite all the help he received, Jim relapsed after a few months of being clean. I was disappointed, but I had learned about relapse and I refused to give up on him. After 5 more years, Jim entered a methadone maintenance program. By then our marriage was falling apart. A nurse in the program had special training in working with families. We saw her together. With her help, Jim was able to recognize that he, not I, was responsible for his addiction. He became more responsible for himself. I learned about how I had enabled his addiction and how I would have to change for our drug-free marriage to succeed. It seemed like each of us could hear what the nurse said better than we could hear each other. Now, 4 years later, Jim is still taking methadone, and we are still together. I want nurses to know that little kindnesses as well as bigger interventions can make a positive difference in the lives of drug addicts and their families.

terns of behavior developed over years of dysfunctional family life will continue after sobriety.

The nurse should encourage family members to seek counseling from a professional experienced in addiction treatment. Referral to **Al-Anon**, a support group for friends and family of alcoholics, or **NarAnon,** for friends and family of narcotic addicts, is also helpful. These groups are based on the same 12 steps as AA and Narcotics Anonymous (NA) except that they are powerless over their alcoholic/addict family member instead of the substance itself.

These families must learn to pay attention to their own needs. They should stop covering up for the addict. They need to be direct in their communication. They also need to know that they are not alone. These issues are evident in the following clinical example.

CLINICAL EXAMPLE

Mr. B was a 45-year-old man who was admitted to the medical unit of a general hospital with a diagnosis of gastritis. He complained of abdominal pain, nausea, and vomiting. He had a slightly elevated temperature of 37.5° C (100° F). When the admitting nurse who was completing the nursing assessment asked Mr. B about alcohol use, he said he had "a couple of beers" after work every day. He also reported that his wife had left him the day before admission. He said he was not sure why she left, but he was sure she would be back. Mrs. B did come to the hospital to visit her husband. His primary nurse met with them together and asked Mrs. B why she left. She said she was tired of putting Mr. B to bed every night after he passed out from drinking and did not want to continue to call his employer saying he was sick when he was really hung over. She had threatened to leave before, but Mr. B had always begged her to stay and she had relented. She had married him because she felt sorry for him. He had been living alone and was not taking good care of himself. She revealed that her first husband was also an alcoholic and her father had been one as well. She would agree to try again to make the marriage a success if he would agree to stop drinking and seek counseling. Mr. B said to the nurse, "I'll be good and do what she says. You tell her I'll be good."

Selected Nursing Diagnoses
- Ineffective coping related to reluctance to be responsible for his behavior, as evidenced by denial of why his wife left
- Dysfunctional family processes related to alcoholism, as evidenced by cycles of drinking, threats to leave, and promises to change ■

Mr. B used alcohol to avoid responsibility for his actions and his life. He used his wife in a similar way. When Mrs. B confronted him with her expectations, he responded in a childlike way and tried to place the nurse in the parental role.

Mrs. B appears to be drawn to dependent men. She is probably a very maternal person who likes to take care of others. This increases the possibility that she will assume the role of enabler. The enabler perpetuates the substance abuse problem by not confronting the substance abuser and by helping to cover up the problem. When Mrs. B called Mr. B's employer to say he was sick, she was being an enabler. When significant others play an enabling role, family counseling or family support groups help the family accept and support the changing behavior of the patient.

Group Therapy. Group psychotherapy is the usual method of treatment in traditional substance abuse treatment programs. Chapter 32 provides detailed information about therapeutic groups.

History sharing and feedback are important elements in traditional program groups. Patients share their substance abuse histories and talk about their daily efforts to stop drinking or taking drugs. The therapist and group members listen closely and give feedback to patients about their recovery efforts. Feedback is the honest reaction of group members to what the speaker says. It is based on the content of what the person says and on previous experiences with the speaker.

Although feedback from one person, especially the therapist, may be discounted, it is difficult for the addict to ignore feedback from several group members, especially if they have experienced the same type of behavior at some point. The style of giving feedback varies from person to person. It may be gentle and facilitative or direct and confrontational. The best feedback is that which is focused and shows respect for the person.

In traditional programs, another major group focus is participation in 12-step self-help programs. Patients may be required to attend a certain number of AA or NA meetings each week in order to remain in the group. Patients share their reactions to the meetings that they have attended and are encouraged to obtain a sponsor, do service work (such as set up the chairs or make coffee for meetings), and actively work the steps of the program.

Successes and difficulties with maintaining abstinence during the past week are shared and discussed. Less traditional groups may encourage trials or active involvement with 12-step programs but not require it. Expectations for work done outside of the group are more individualized. In all groups, homework may be assigned that emphasizes an important recovery topic.

A group member says he has read that studies have found that some alcoholics can learn to drink in a controlled way. How would you respond? ■

Self-help groups. The most common type of self-help group for substance abusers is the 12-step group. **Alcoholics Anonymous (AA)** is the model for 12-step support groups. It is composed entirely of alcoholics who have a desire to stop drinking. They believe that mutual support can give the alcoholic strength to abstain.

AA aims for total abstinence. The member must admit to alcoholism openly and publicly by introducing himself or herself at meetings, saying, "My name is (John) and I am an alcoholic." At speaker meetings, one or more members share their life histories with the group. This shows that members are more alike than different, removing a common resistance to involvement.

AA members commit themselves to helping each other. Some AA members serve as sponsors, a role that involves availability and accessibility to another member whenever a member feels the need to drink. The sponsor also teaches the person how to work the 12 steps of the program. This reciprocal relationship gives the new member caring support and the sponsor improved self-esteem.

AA also involves a strong spiritual orientation that is experienced as supportive by some alcoholics. The 12 steps of AA are listed in Box 24-10. It is easy to see the therapeutic benefit of these steps (Morgenstern et al, 2002). For example, admitting the problem, making amends for past behavior, and reaching out to others who need help are sound therapeutic processes.

Some aspects of 12-step programs do not appeal to everyone. One of these is the powerlessness that must be acknowledged. Many people believe that the power to change lies within oneself. Some people are upset by the need to turn over one's will to a higher power. Members are told that this higher power can be the AA group, the sponsor, or anything else they want. Although the higher power does not have to be God in the religious sense, the meetings generally have a religious overtone and usually end with the Lord's Prayer. Some members have formed AA groups especially for agnostics.

Other self-help groups have emerged. One of these is Women for Sobriety (WFS) (Kirkpatrick, 1999). This program shows women how to change their way of life through a change of thinking. The program serves women's needs by teaching them to overcome depression, guilt, and low self-esteem. WFS helps women overcome their drinking problems with the support of other group members who have the same problems and needs. The difference from AA is evident in the first statement of the WFS acceptance program: "I have a drinking problem that once had me." All of the 13 statements of WFS are worded positively.

Another very popular self-help program is the Rational Recovery (RR) movement, which is based on Albert Ellis' Rational Emotive Therapy (see Chapter 3). This program asserts that alcohol dependence is not biologically determined nor beyond our control. Rather, it is seen as a way of thinking. Irrational thoughts keep the alcoholic drinking. Rational thoughts can get and keep the alcoholic sober.

RR philosophy is one of personal power; no reference is made to a higher power. RR groups have professional advisors who provide occasional rational input and observe members for problems that indicate a need for a higher level of care. Group meetings operate by discussion, also known as *cross-talking*. This is in contrast to AA, which strongly discourages interrupting or responding to others. Group members read rational literature, learn to think rationally, and become rational counselors to themselves and others.

It should be noted that total abstinence is the goal of each of these programs. Patients who choose to try controlled drinking will get no support for this goal from these programs. Controlled drinking for a person who has experienced the loss of control characteristic of addiction has mixed support in the research literature (see Critical Thinking About Contemporary Issues).

Community Treatment Programs. A variety of community programs are available for drug abusers. Medical detoxification is most often done in hospitals, either on medical,

---

BOX **24-10**

The Twelve Steps of Alcoholics Anonymous

1. We admitted we were powerless over alcohol—that our lives had become unmanageable.
2. Came to believe that a Power greater than ourselves could restore us to sanity.
3. Made a decision to turn our will and our lives over to the care of God as we understood Him.
4. Made a searching and fearless moral inventory of ourselves.
5. Admitted to God, to ourselves, and to another human being the exact nature of our wrongs.
6. Were entirely ready to have God remove all these defects of character.
7. Humbly asked Him to remove our shortcomings.
8. Made a list of all persons we had harmed, and became willing to make amends to them all.
9. Made direct amends to such people wherever possible, except when to do so would injure them or others.
10. Continued to take personal inventory, and when we were wrong, promptly admitted it.
11. Sought through prayer and meditation to improve our conscious contact with God, as we understood Him, praying only for knowledge of His will for us and the power to carry that out.
12. Having had a spiritual awakening as the result of these Steps, we tried to carry this message to alcoholics and to practice these principles in all our affairs.

The Twelve Steps are reprinted with permission of Alcoholics Anonymous World Services, Inc. Permission to reprint this material does not mean that AA has reviewed or approved of the contents of this publication. AA is a program of recovery from alcoholism only; use of the 12 Steps in connection with programs and activities that are patterned after AA, but address other problems, does not imply otherwise.

 Critical Thinking *About* Contemporary Issues

Is Abstinence Necessary?

For several decades, experts have been debating about whether alcoholics can return to moderate drinking after detoxification. According to AA and many mental health professionals, abstinence is necessary because alcoholics will inevitably lose control once they start to drink. Advocates of controlled drinking believe that most alcoholics are not powerless over the drug and that they can change their drinking behavior without giving up alcohol entirely.

One way to approach the issue is to distinguish between degrees of severity. Perhaps dependent alcoholics need to quit cold, but those with milder cases of abuse can possibly handle controlled drinking. Aiming for abstinence also can be a way to achieve moderation, just as a lower speed limit causes people to drive more slowly even if they still break the law.

psychiatric, or special substance abuse units. Criteria for admission to these programs may be strict because of managed care restrictions. Length of stay is generally very short—just long enough to stabilize the person medically. Attempts to secure the patient's agreement to participate in aftercare programs is a major part of the intervention.

Detoxification also can be done safely on an outpatient basis. For patients not requiring intense medical monitoring, but still in need of strict environmental controls, there are residential, free-standing rehabilitation programs that provide services for weeks to months. Some patients receive court orders to enter into these treatment programs after drug-related arrests, with the costs being covered by the state.

The next level of care after inpatient and residential care is day or evening partial hospitalization. In these programs, the patient spends most of the day in treatment and returns home at night, or spends the day at work and several evenings a week in treatment.

Methadone maintenance programs offer methadone maintenance or withdrawal for opiate addicts. Patients must attend daily to obtain their methadone. Methadone programs must have special licensure to operate and follow federal guidelines. For the very stable patient on methadone mainte-

nance, a policy change to monthly visits to the provider have been suggested and may be approved in the future.

Regular outpatient programs that are attended once or twice per week are even less intensive. Most programs provide a mix of group, individual, and family therapy; vocational counseling; drug and health education; and involvement with 12-step self-help programs; 12-step programs such as AA may be an adjunct to or substitute for professionally run programs.

Employee Assistance Programs. Another potential resource for the substance-abusing patient is employee assistance programs (EAPs) that may be part of an employee health service (see Chapter 9). Many businesses have found that it is profitable for them to help substance-abusing employees. These programs generally offer counseling and health education. Employees with a substance abuse problem are usually required to participate in the program to retain their jobs. Nurses are often key staff members in employee assistance programs.

A Nursing Treatment Plan Summary for ineffective coping related to substance-abusing behaviors is presented in Table 24-5. A Nursing Treatment Plan Summary for a patient with disturbed sensory perception is presented in Table 24-6.

Table 24-5	NURSING TREATMENT PLAN SUMMARY	Chemically Mediated Responses

Nursing Diagnosis: Ineffective coping
Expected Outcome: The patient will abstain from using all mood-altering chemicals.

SHORT-TERM GOAL	INTERVENTION	RATIONALE
The patient will substitute healthy coping responses for substance-abusing behavior.	Help the patient identify the substance-abusing behavior and its consequences. Help the patient identify the substance abuse problem. Involve the patient in describing situations that lead to substance-abusing behavior. Consistently offer support and the expectation that the patient has the strength to overcome the problem.	Motivation for change is related to recognition of a problem that is upsetting to the patient. Identification of predisposing factors and precipitating stressors must precede planning for more adaptive behavioral responses.
The patient will assume responsibility for behavior.	Encourage the patient to participate in a treatment program. Develop with the patient a written contract for behavioral change that is signed by the patient and nurse. Help the patient identify and adopt healthier coping responses.	Denial and rationalization are dysfunctional coping mechanisms that can interfere with recovery. Personal commitment will enhance the likelihood of successful abstinence.
The patient will identify and use social support systems.	Identify and assess social support systems that are available to the patient. Provide support to significant others. Educate the patient and significant others about the substance abuse problem and available resources. Refer the patient to appropriate resources and provide support until the patient is involved in the program.	Substance abusers are often dependent and socially isolated people who use drugs to gain confidence in social situations. Substance-abusing behavior alienates significant others, thus increasing the person's isolation. It is difficult to manipulate people who have participated in the same behaviors. Social support systems must be readily available over time and acceptable to the patient.

Table 24-6	NURSING TREATMENT PLAN SUMMARY	Chemically Mediated Responses

Nursing Diagnosis: Disturbed sensory perception
Expected Outcome: The patient will overcome addiction safely and with a minimum of discomfort.

SHORT-TERM GOAL	INTERVENTION	RATIONALE
The patient will withdraw from dependence on the abused substance.	Supportive physical care: vital signs, nutrition, hydration, seizure precautions. Administer medication according to detoxification schedule.	Detoxification of the physically dependent person can be dangerous and is always uncomfortable for the patient. The patient's physical safety must receive high priority for nursing intervention.
The patient will be oriented to time, place, person, and situation.	Assess orientation frequently, orient the patient if needed, and place a clock and calendar where they can be seen by the patient.	Cognitive function is usually affected by addiction; disorientation is frightening.
The patient will report symptoms of withdrawal.	Observe carefully for withdrawal symptoms and report suspected withdrawal immediately.	Withdrawal symptoms provide powerful motivation for continued substance abuse; judgment may be impaired by substance use.
The patient will correctly interpret environmental stimuli.	Explain all nursing interventions, assign consistent staff, keep soft light on in room, avoid loud noises, and encourage trusted family and friends to stay with the patient.	Sensory and perceptual alterations related to use of drugs or alcohol are frightening; consistency reduces the need to interpret stimuli.
The patient will recognize and talk about hallucinations or delusions.	Observe for response to internal stimuli, encourage patient to describe hallucinations or delusions, and explain the relationship of these experiences to withdrawal from addictive substances.	Helping the patient identify delusional or hallucinatory experiences and relating them to withdrawal is reassuring.

Working With Dually Diagnosed Patients

The dually diagnosed patient needs treatment for both disorders. The problem is that the substance abuse and mental health fields have developed approaches that appear to conflict with each other. For instance, many substance abuse counselors rely on direct confrontation of behavior. Such an approach could be detrimental to a person with severe mental illness. Substance abuse counselors also tend to have a limited understanding of the medications used for psychiatric disorders. In fact, the chronically mentally ill are often excluded from substance abuse programs.

Mental health clinicians, on the other hand, often do not understand substance abuse and may overlook symptoms of continued use. They tend to think that the substance abuse will stop when the person's psychiatric illness is under control. Patients can suffer from these differences in providers, either by missing out on some important treatments or by getting caught in the middle of two different approaches with two different clinicians (called *parallel treatment*). To avoid this, treatment is sometimes offered in sequence (first psychiatric treatment, then substance abuse treatment or vice versa).

The best possible treatment is an integrated one, with both services offered by program staff qualified in both areas and excellent coordination of other community services (Drake, et al, 2001; Jerrell et al, 2000; Herman et al, 2000). The chronically mentally ill can benefit more from these programs, which generally are less confrontational and more supportive than traditional substance abuse programs.

They have professional staff to prescribe and follow medication effectiveness. They often practice assertive case management, in which case workers seek out patients when they fail to show up for treatment and help patients meet multiple psychosocial needs, including basic living arrangements.

Such specialized treatment programs offer special treatment groups for the mentally ill, chemically addicted (MICA) patient (also called *mentally ill, substance abusing,* or *MISA*) and refer patients to community self-help groups developed for such people, called *double trouble groups*. Nurses who understand both conditions are in an ideal position to work with dually diagnosed patients.

Appropriate treatment is linked to correct assessment of co-existing conditions. If the causative disorder can be isolated, it should be the focus of initial treatment unless the secondary disorder has become life-threatening, as when the alcoholic develops a suicidal depression. However, it should not be assumed that resolution of primary psychiatric problems will automatically resolve associated substance abuse problems.

If substances are used chronically, substance abuse can develop into a primary disorder, taking on a life of its own. In these cases, the initial emphasis of treatment must be on the most serious problem at the time. Although the relative importance of symptoms may vary with time and influence the focus of treatment, both disorders must be treated.

Comprehensive treatment for co-occurring disorders usually requires a combination of pharmacological treatment,

psychosocial treatment, and supportive services (Akerele and Levin, 2002). Successful psychosocial programs for patients with psychiatric and substance abuse disorders provide behavioral skill-building interventions as the primary ingredient of active treatment, which has been shown to be more effective than case management or 12-step intervention (Jordan, et al, 2002). In addition, the following five therapeutic tasks or steps that can serve as guidelines for structuring treatment of dual-diagnosis patients have been identified (Carey, 1996):

1. Establish a therapeutic alliance with the patient.
2. Help the patient evaluate the costs and benefits of continued substance use.
3. Individualize goals for change with the patient that include harm reduction as an alternative to total abstinence.
4. Help the patient build an environment and lifestyle supportive of abstinence.
5. Acknowledge that recovery is a long process, and help the patient cope with crises by anticipating triggers of relapse and coping with setbacks as they occur.

Because both mental illness and substance abuse are chronic, relapsing conditions, the course of treatment can be expected to take considerable time. Stages of treatment have been identified and are used as the basis for treatment planning in many dual-diagnosis treatment programs today. Interventions appropriate to each stage have been identified and are listed along with goals in Table 24-7 (Drake et al, 1996). Counselors and interdisciplinary teams are also useful, as can be seen in the following clinical example.

CLINICAL EXAMPLE

Bobby was a 17-year-old who was admitted to the hospital in an acutely psychotic state with a history of recent use of PCP. The emergency room nurse noted scarring of the veins in Bobby's arm and surmised that he also used heroin. Blood and urine testing confirmed this suspicion. Bobby recovered from his psychotic episode in 24 hours but was extremely uncomfortable because of opiate withdrawal. The decision was made to use titrated doses of methadone to help with the withdrawal. Mr. L, a young nurse, established a close relationship with Bobby during this time. Bobby requested the nurse's help in planning for his future, but doubted that he had the strength to stay away from drugs. He was advised to take a day at a time. Mr. L took Bobby on a visit to a drug treatment program, and he agreed to try membership in one of the groups at this center. Bobby did well in the group and was very helpful to new members, describing his experiences and encouraging them to "take 1 day at a time." Bobby expressed an interest in finishing school and said he would like to become a drug counselor. The staff of the drug treatment program agreed that Bobby seemed to have an aptitude for that role and encouraged him to pursue his goal.

Selected Nursing Diagnoses
- Disturbed thought processes related to PCP use, as evidenced by uncontrolled behavior in the emergency room
- Situational low self-esteem related to pessimism about ability to stop using drugs, as evidenced by expressed self-doubt ∎

Mr. L used his relationship with Bobby to communicate his belief that he could successfully give up drugs. This message has a core of positive regard for Bobby's potential strength. The staff of the drug treatment program added to this seed of self-esteem by encouraging Bobby to help others in the program and then to aim higher at becoming a counselor himself. This taught Bobby that there were rewards in life other than those attached to drug use. Gradually, he learned to value the interpersonal rewards more than the drug rewards while making positive use of his past difficulties.

Intervening With Impaired Colleagues

It is usually difficult for nurses to respond to a colleague who is showing signs of a substance abuse problem. This is true of supervisors as well as peers. For the safety of the nurse, as well as the nurse's patients, it is necessary to identify such a problem and take action. In addition, many states have laws that require health care professionals to report colleagues who show signs of working while impaired. In these states, reporting is both an ethical and a legal obligation.

Usually it is not easy to be sure that a nurse's practice is impaired by drug or alcohol use. However, particular patterns of behavior and signs are characteristic of this problem (Box 24-11). The concerned colleague should **report incidents of this nature to the supervisor.** It is also important that these incidents be **documented in writing,** with the time, date, place, description of the incident, and the names of others who were present. This documentation will make it easier to intervene.

If the pattern of behavior indicates that impairment exists, an intervention should be planned. An advisor should be selected who has expertise in the area of impaired nursing practice. This advisor could be someone from the state nurse rehabilitation committee, if there is one.

A team of people who have meaningful relationships with the nurse should be asked to prepare written statements demonstrating their observations of probable impaired practice. The team should consist of co-workers, the supervisor or other nurse administrator, and perhaps a family member. The team rehearses the statements in a meeting without the suspected nurse being present so that any details can be worked out and a nonmoralistic tone can be ensured. They also anticipate various reactions the nurse may have and decide how to respond to these. Treatment options are discussed and plans are made to escort the nurse directly from the meeting to a treatment facility.

After this preparation, a meeting is called in which the team members read their statements to the nurse, who is informed of the disciplinary action recommended by the team, which usually requires that the nurse enter treatment or resign from nursing and potentially lose the license to practice. The nurse is escorted to either an inpatient treatment program or an outpatient appointment. Because the suicide risk for nurses who have just gone through an intervention is great, the nurse should not be left alone after the intervention.

Table 24-7	Treatment Stages, Goals, and Interventions for Dually Diagnosed Patients	
STAGE OF TREATMENT	SUGGESTED GOALS	INTERVENTIONS
Engagement	Development of working relationship between patient and nurse	Intervene in crises, help with practical living problems, establish rapport with family members, demonstrate caring and support, listen actively
Persuasion	Patient acceptance of having a substance abuse problem and the need for active change strategies	Help analyze pros and cons of substance use, educate patient and family, arrange peer group discussions, expose patient to double trouble self-help groups, adjust medication, persuade patient to comply with medication regimen (motivational interviewing skills are particularly helpful during this stage)
Active treatment	Abstinence from substance use and compliance with medication	Help change thinking patterns, friends, habits, behaviors, and living situations as necessary to support goals; teach social skills; encourage patient to develop positive social supports through double trouble self-help groups; enlist family support of changes; monitor urine and breath for substances; offer medications
Relapse prevention	Absence or minimization of return to substance abuse	Reinforce abstinence, compliance, and behavioral changes; identify risk factors and help patient practice preventive strategies; encourage continued involvement in double trouble groups; continue laboratory monitoring

BOX 24-11

Signs of Impaired Nursing Practice

Job Performance Changes

Controlled drug handling/records (potential drug diversion)
- Drug counts incorrect
- Excessive errors
- Excessive wastage, often not countersigned
- Medicine signed out to patient who has not been in pain
- Two strengths of drug signed out to same patient, same time
- Packaging appears to be tampered with
- Patient complaints of ineffective pain control
- Volunteers to give controlled drugs
- Comes in early or stays late
- Disappears into the bathroom after handling controlled drugs
- Unexplained absences from the unit

General performance
- Medication errors
- Poor judgment
- Euphoric recall for involvement in unpleasant situations, or confrontations on the job
- Illogical or sloppy charting
- Absenteeism, especially in conjunction with days off
- Requesting leave time just before the assigned shift
- Tardiness with elaborate excuses
- Job shrinkage (does the minimum work required to get by)
- Missed deadlines

Behavior/Personality Changes
- Sudden changes in mood
- Periods of irritability
- Forgetfulness
- Wears long sleeves, even in hot weather
- Socially isolates from co-workers
- Inappropriate behavior
- Has chronic pain condition
- History of pain treatment with controlled substances

Signs of Use
- Alcohol on the breath
- Constant use of perfumes, mouthwash, and breath mints
- Flushed face, reddened eyes, unsteady gait, slurred speech
- Hyperactivity, accelerated speech
- Increasing family problems that interfere with work

Signs of Withdrawal
- Tremors, restlessness, diaphoresis, pupil changes
- Watery eyes, runny nose, stomach aches, joint pains, gooseflesh

During treatment the supervisor should maintain contact with the treatment program to see how the nurse is progressing. It is strongly advised that a return-to-work contract be written that clearly describes the nurse's responsibilities upon return. If the state has a nurse rehabilitation or peer assistance program, it can assume some responsibility for monitoring the nurse's progress and in developing treatment and return-to-work contracts. This type of intervention makes it possible for the chemically dependent nurse to get the treatment needed, yet remain employed, a situation in which everyone benefits.

An enabler is a person who supports someone in maintaining an addiction. Describe behaviors that would enable a colleague to continue drug or alcohol use that impairs performance of nursing roles. What alternative behaviors would be more helpful? ■

Preventive Interventions

The best approach to prevention is to begin early to reduce emerging behavioral and emotional problems in youth. Longer lasting results can be obtained from changing school, community, and family environments that promote and maintain drug problems in youth. Communities need nurses and other health care providers who are knowledgeable about substance abuse prevention and who can advocate for the implementation of prevention programs with proven effectiveness (Kumpfer, 2002).

Many communities across the country have taken positive steps to combat the problem of substance abuse. Examples include alcohol and drug-free school parties, smoke-free buildings, and drug courts. Reducing access and demand are important public health strategies. Raising the minimum drinking age to 21 was found to decrease alcohol use by 25% in those 18 to 20 years old, along with a reduction in related accidents and problems. In contrast, laws prohibiting cigarette sales to minors have not resulted in decreased use. Youth simply get older friends to make purchases for them.

Media campaigns provide needed information and can slowly affect community norms. Efforts spearheaded by citizen groups, such as Mothers Against Drunk Driving (MADD), can have a positive impact as well, whereas warning labels on alcohol or tobacco appear to have little impact on behavior change.

Primary Prevention. Primary prevention programs aimed at preventing drug use among children are in place in many elementary schools in this country. School nurses can be involved in education efforts in the schools. Family strengthening strategies are key to preventing problems, as are social competency programs. Nurses also can support legislation designed to reduce the incidence of use and abuse, and serve as public speakers in the community on drug abuse issues.

The millions of Americans enrolled in managed care organizations could significantly benefit from effective preventive behavioral health services. In a comprehensive review of the evidence-based literature, Dorfman and Smith (2002) found the following types of preventive interventions to be effective for smoking, alcohol, and substance use problems:

1. Targeted cessation education and counseling for smokers, especially pregnant smokers. Although success was modest, significant outcomes were achieved. Successful techniques included:
   a. 15-minute counseling session with a nurse or health educator supplemented by written materials and two follow-up phone calls.
   b. 15-minute counseling and skill development session, supplemented by patient reinforcement, social support, newsletter, and mention in prenatal class.
   c. 4 minutes of clinician advice to quit smoking, supplemented by a self-help book and a 1-year follow-up visit.
2. Self-care education for adults addressing substance use and mental health. Significant improvements were

noted in health-risk behaviors, including smoking, alcohol use, and reported stress. Successful techniques included:
   a. Group education workshops led by a nurse practitioner, supplemented by a self-care guide and videotapes, a nurse-run telephone information service and individual health evaluation and planning conference.
   b. Computer-based serial, personal health-risk reports augmented by individualized recommendation letters and written materials.
   c. Access to a self-care center.
   d. One-on-one education centers with a clinician.
   e. Slide-tape shows.
3. Brief counseling and advice to reduce alcohol use. Physicians, nurses, psychologists, and other health care providers in the United States and in Europe provided 5 to 15 minutes of advice or counseling on reducing alcohol consumption. Supplemental workbooks or informational or self-help materials were sometimes used. Reinforcement strategies included follow-up visits or telephone calls. Results showed significant reductions in alcohol consumption.

Secondary Prevention. Secondary prevention efforts are aimed at people with mild to moderate drinking problems. For every person with a severe drinking problem, there are several more people with mild to moderate drinking problems. Several brief therapies have evolved to address their special needs. These range from simple advice to stop drinking to more elaborate programs involving early identification, presentation of assessment findings, education (see Patient Education Plan, Table 24-8), advice regarding the need to reduce drinking with an emphasis on personal responsibility, self-help manuals, and periodic follow-up. People with mild to moderate drinking problems are increasingly being referred to treatment programs through the courts after DWI charges.

Tertiary Prevention. Tertiary prevention involves decreasing the complications of addiction. Medical and psychiatric treatment settings still serve a major role here, as do more current case management, community outreach, and dual-diagnosis programs.

Policy approaches often include legislation to reduce the negative consequences of using drugs, rather than the use itself. This approach is called **harm reduction.** It includes efforts to reduce the effects of drunkenness on oneself and others such as that occurring through car accidents, drowning, and family disputes. It also can include providing public education to increase the number of designated drivers, offering rides to incapacitated friends, using seat belts and arranging sleep-overs after parties involving alcohol.

Under development are cars whose ignition locks if the driver cannot pass a quick sobriety test. In Europe and Australia, harms associated with drug use have been reduced by developing needle exchanges, offering drug-testing stations, and offering water at raves.

Table 24-8 PATIENT EDUCATION PLAN	Promoting Adaptive Chemically Mediated Responses	
CONTENT	INSTRUCTIONAL ACTIVITIES	EVALUATION
Elicit perceptions of substance use.	Lead group discussion regarding knowledge about chemical use and experience with it; correct misperceptions.	The patient will describe accurate information about substance use.
Demonstrate negative effects of substance abuse.	Show films of physical and psychological effects of substance abuse; provide written materials.	The patient will identify and describe physical and psychological effects of substance abuse.
Interaction with peer who has abused chemicals.	Small group discussion with peer group member who has abused substances and quit because of negative experiences.	The patient will compare advantages and disadvantages of using mind-altering substance.
Obtain agreement to abstain from use of mind-altering substances.	Discuss future plans for refusing abused chemicals if offered.	The patient will verbally agree to abstain from using mind-altering substances.

EVALUATION

The evaluation of substance abuse treatment is based on accomplishment of the expected outcomes and short-term goals. The nurse and patient together should evaluate progress toward these goals on a regular basis. If progress is not being made, together they should reevaluate both the goal and the progress to see where the problem lies and what needs to be done about it.

Relapse does not mean failure. Progress toward a lifelong goal of abstinence from substances of abuse can be measured in many ways. For example, a significant increase in the periods of time that a chronic alcoholic patient stays sober between binges or relapses can be viewed as improvement. A decrease in the amount of time that the alcoholic patient remains in relapse before returning to sobriety can likewise indicate improvement.

The patient who returns to treatment after relapse should be commended for previous successes and for the decision to keep trying. Then the nurse and patient together can analyze what worked and what did not work in the patient's attempts to maintain sobriety. This information should be used to modify the patient's relapse prevention plan.

It is also recommended that several measures of success toward abstinence goals be used, not just patient self-report. Objective measures such as breath analysis and urinalysis should be used as well as information from collateral sources such as spouses and employers (with a signed release of information). Success toward goals in other areas of living such as obtaining or keeping a job, improvements in health, and improvements in family relationships are interrelated with abstinence goals and important in the total recovery process.

COMPETENT CARING

A Clinical Exemplar of a Psychiatric Nurse
S.W. JERNIGAN, BS, RN, C

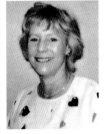

One Sunday morning I was doing a dressing change on a patient in for her third admission. This patient's right knee had been injured during a "bust" for possession of narcotics. Though the dressing change was a simple one, she seemed talkative and jumped at the chance to complete the procedure in the treatment room. She talked at length about her Baltimore neighborhood where she had lived all her life, her deep roots in the community, and her mother's recent death.

At the time I had perhaps the easiest job in the world—saying "mmm hum," and "uh-huh," to an interesting person who wanted to talk. But it wasn't long before she got to the subject of her repeated failures to stay off drugs. Then she began to speak more slowly and with intense feeling, obviously looking for answers—of which I had few. The old standards, she'd already heard, "Keep try-

ing," "Don't give up," "Go to NA," and her facial expressions confirmed this. A silence ensued. Quietly she said, "This is going to kill me. What can I do?" Another silence. Finally I said to her, "I have heard from some who said the only way they could 'stay clean' was to move; to get totally away from the old neighborhood, leave all the old friends, and start a new life. It is a radical, shocking change, but for some people it is the only way." Her shoulders straightened. She nodded.

She was discharged several days later, and hasn't "reappeared"—maybe because she moved to another state.... maybe because of being "clean"—or so we heard. In retrospect, I think this patient didn't just have something to say—there was something she wanted to hear, and on some level she knew what she needed to hear. Patients in difficulty often have a sort of homing instinct about what they need in order to be well—it might be attention; it might be solitude; it might be, as in this case, permission to take the next step. ■

CHAPTER FOCUS POINTS

- Adaptive chemically mediated responses include "natural highs," which may be related to physical activity or meditation. Maladaptive responses include dependence on tobacco and alcohol and abuse of or dependence on illicit drugs.
- Substance abuse refers to continued use despite related problems.
- Substance dependence, related to either drugs or alcohol, indicates a severe condition, usually considered a disease.
- The psychosocial behaviors related to substance dependence are often called *addiction*.
- Dual diagnosis is the co-existence of substance abuse and psychiatric disorders within the same person.
- Withdrawal symptoms and tolerance are signs that the person has physical dependence on the drug. Withdrawal symptoms result from a biological need that develops when the body becomes adapted to having the drug in the system.
- Tolerance means that with continued use, more of the substance is needed to produce the same effect.
- The United States has one of the highest levels of substance abuse in the world. Most people with substance use disorders do not seek treatment.
- Despite their prevalence, substance-related disorders are frequently underdetected and underdiagnosed in acute-care psychiatric and medical settings.
- Screening for substance abuse can involve the use of the CAGE or B-DAST questionnaires, a breath analysis, or blood and urine testing.
- Patient behaviors related to chemically mediated responses are related to dependence, intoxication, or overdose and vary according to the abused substances. Abused substances may include CNS depressants (alcohol, barbiturates, benzodiazepines), marijuana, stimulants, opiates, hallucinogens, PCP, inhalants, and nicotine.
- Consequences of abuse and dependence include accidents, violence, self-neglect, fetal abnormalities, fetal substance dependence, and infection with blood-borne pathogens.
- Predisposing factors that lead to maladaptive chemically mediated responses include biological, psychological, and sociocultural perspectives.

- The emergence of withdrawal symptoms and drug cravings are powerful precipitating stressors for continued drug use. Most abused drugs interact with specific nerve cell receptors, either imitating or blocking the actions of normally working neurotransmitters in the brain.
- Coping resources include motivation, social supports, health, social skills, problem-solving skills, material and economic assets, and intellectual and personality traits.
- Maladaptive coping mechanisms include denial, rationalization, projection, and minimization.
- Primary NANDA nursing diagnoses related to maladaptive chemically mediated responses are disturbed sensory perception, acute confusion, ineffective coping, and dysfunctional family processes: alcoholism.
- Primary *DSM-IV-TR* diagnoses are dependence, abuse, intoxication, or withdrawal related to a particular substance.
- The expected outcome for patients in withdrawal from drugs or alcohol is that the patient will overcome withdrawal safely and with minimum discomfort.
- The expected outcome for patients dependent on drugs or alcohol is that the patient will abstain from all mood-altering chemicals.
- Planning is based on first providing for safe withdrawal, followed by developing ways to maintain abstinence. Support systems, including family, friends, and self-help groups, should be involved whenever possible.
- Substances with potentially life-threatening courses of withdrawal include alcohol, benzodiazepines, and barbiturates.
- Long-range goals of treatment for patients with substance use disorders include (1) the abstinence or reduction in the use and effects of substances; (2) reduction in the frequency and severity of relapse; and (3) improvement in psychological and social functioning.
- Interventions include biological, psychological, and social interventions; working with dually diagnosed patients; intervening with impaired colleagues; and preventive interventions.
- Evaluation criteria for nursing care related to chemically mediated responses include goal achievement, increases in amount of sober time, negative breath and urinalysis tests, and improved psychosocial dimensions.

KEY TERMS

addiction, 474
amotivational syndrome, 486
ataxia, 497
detoxification, 496
dual diagnosis, 474

employee assistance programs (EAPs), 508
enablers, 505
hallucinogens, 486
methadone maintenance, 508
nystagmus, 497

physical dependence, 474
relapse, 504
substance abuse, 474
substance dependence, 474
tolerance, 474
withdrawal symptoms, 474

CHAPTER REVIEW QUESTIONS

1. Indicate whether the following statements are true (T) or false (F).

_____ A. Race is an important determinant of substance dependence.

_____ B. Substance abuse invariably leads to substance dependence.

_____ C. Opioids are known to have an acute withdrawal syndrome.

_____ D. Patients with psychiatric disorders have more substance abuse problems than the general population.

_____ E. Mental illness is a primary cause of substance dependence.

_____ F. More genetic research has been focused on alcoholism than on other substances of abuse.

_____ G. The longer the half-life of the abused drug, the more intense the withdrawal symptoms will be.

_____ H. Newer psychological treatment approaches to substance use disorders emphasize a therapeutic alliance with the patient, avoidance of confrontation, and brevity of treatment.

_____ I. Most patients succeed in abstaining from drugs in their first attempt.

_____ J. Alcoholics Anonymous (AA) uses the 12-step model for recovery from alcoholism.

2. Fill in the blanks.

A. The main principle in the treatment of detoxification is

_____.

B. Co-existence of psychiatric disorder and substance-related disorder within the same person is called _____.

C. Among adolescents, nicotine, alcohol, and marijuana often act as _____ drugs to substances that are perceived to be more dangerous.

D. The simplest screening tool consisting of only four questions related to alcohol abuse is the _____.

E. The simplest biological measure to obtain a blood alcohol content is by use of a _____.

F. The term _____ was first used to describe people who had become dysfunctional as a result of living in a committed relationship with an alcoholic.

G. The brain's natural opiates are the neurotransmitters called

_____.

H. Medically, withdrawal from the _____ drugs is the most dangerous.

I. The process of helping an addict safely through withdrawal is called _____.

J. _____ was the first drug to be approved more than 40 years ago for treatment of alcohol dependence, and it has been followed by the more recent approval of _____.

3. Provide short answers for the following questions.

A. Methadone treatment is available across the country and allows a person to maintain drug abstinence. Why do you think more people do not take advantage of it? Relate your answer to the overall dynamics of addiction and abstinence.

B. Some people believe that treatment programs should only employ as counselors people who have recovered from substance abuse. How would you respond to this?

C. You suspect that one of your friends has a problem with alcohol. How would you go about helping her?

D. Carefully read the 12 steps of Alcoholics Anonymous. Evaluate their content as a treatment approach. How would you respond to a patient who did not believe in a higher power?

E. Design a comprehensive treatment plan for a patient who is dually diagnosed with both bipolar disorder and alcoholism.

Visit Evolve for additional resources related to the content of this chapter.
http://evolve.elsevier.com/Stuart/principles/
• Topical Course Outline • Student Workbook Exercises • Critical Thinking Questions and Activities • Case Studies • Research Topics
• Monthly Content Updates • WebLinks

Student Study CD-ROM

Access the accompanying CD-ROM for animations, interactive exercises, review questions for the NCLEX examination, and an audio glossary.

REFERENCES

Alcohol Alert: Underage drinking: a major public health challenge, NI-AAA, no 59, April, 2003, DHHS, PHS, NIH.

Akerele EO, Levin FR: Substance abuse among patients with schizophrenia, *J Psychiatr Pract* 8:70, 2002.

American Psychiatric Association: *Diagnostic and statistical manual of mental disorders*, ed 4, text revision, Washington, DC, 2000, American Psychiatric Association.

Anda RF et al: Adverse childhood experiences, alcoholic parents, and later risk of alcoholism and depression, *Psychiatr Serv* 53:1001, 2002.

Barrowclough C et al: Randomized controlled trial of motivational interviewing, cognitive behavior therapy and family intervention for patients with comorbid schizophrenia and substance use disorders, *Am J Psychiatry* 158:1706, 2001.

Carey KB: Treatment of co-occurring substance abuse and major mental illness, *New Dir Ment Health Serv* 70:19, 1996.

Carey KB et al: The feasibility of enhancing psychiatric outpatients' readiness to change their substance abuse, *Psychiatr Serv* 53:602, 2002.

Cataldo JK: The role of advanced practice psychiatric nurses in treating tobacco use and dependence, *Arch Psychiatr Nurs* 15:107, 2001.

Centers for Disease Control and Prevention (CDC) website, 2003: http://www.cdc.gov/ncidod/diseases/hepititis/resource/index.htm

Clarke J: The most misunderstood medical treatment, *Counselor* 4:68, 2003.

Committee on Addictions of the Group for the Advancement of Psychiatry: Responsibility and choice in addiction, *Psychiatr Serv* 53:707, 2002.

DeWit DJ et al: Age at first alcohol use: a risk factor for the development of alcohol disorders, *Am J Psychiatry* 157:745, 2000.

Dorfman SL, Smith SA: Preventive mental health and substance abuse programs and services in managed care, *J Behav Health Serv Res* 29:233, 2002.

Drake RE, et al: The course, treatment, and outcome of substance disorder in persons with severe mental illness, *Am J Orthopsy* 66:42-51, 1996.

Drake RE et al: Implementing dual diagnosis services for clients with severe mental illness, *Psychiatr Serv* 52:469, 2001.

Harvard Mental Health Letter: Duel diagnosis, *Harvard Health Publications* 20:1, 2003.

Herman SE et al: Longitudinal effects of integrated treatment on alcohol use for persons with serious mental illness and substance use disorders, *J Behav Health Serv Res* 27:286, 2000.

Horgan C: Substance abuse: the nations number one health problem, *Schneider Institute for Health Policy*, Princeton, NJ, 2001, Brandeis University, the Robert Wood Johnson Foundation.

Irvin JE et al: Efficacy of relapse prevention: a meta-analytic review, *J Consult Clin Psychol* 67:563, 1999.

Jerrell JM, Wilson JL, Hiller DC: Issues and outcomes in integrated treatment programs for dual disorders, *J Behav Health Serv Res* 27:303, 2000.

Joe GW et al: Relationships between counseling rapport and drug abuse treatment outcomes, *Psychiatr Serv* 52:1223, 2001.

Johnson LD et al: *Monitoring the future: national results on adolescent drug use*, NIH pub no 03-5374, Bethesda, Md, 2003, NIDA.

Jordan LC et al: Involvement in 12-step programs among persons with dual diagnoses, *Psychiatr Serv* 53:894, 2002.

Kelly PJ, Blacksin B, Mason E: Factors affecting substance abuse treatment completion for women, *Issues Men Health Nurs* 22:287, 2001.

Kendler KS et al: Childhood sexual abuse and adult psychiatric and substance use disorders in women: an epidemiological and co-twin control analysis, *Arch Gen Psychiatry* 57:953, 2000a.

Kendler KS et al: Illicit psychoactive substance use, heavy use, abuse, and dependence in a US population-based sample of male twins, *Arch Gen Psychiatry* 57:261, 2000b.

Kirkpatrick J: *Turnabout: new help for the woman alcoholic*, New York, 1999, Barricade Books.

Kumpfer K: Prevention of alcohol and drug abuse: what works? *Substance Abuse* 23:25, 2002.

Mayo-Smith MF et al: Pharmacological management of alcohol withdrawal: a meta-analysis and evidence-based practice guideline, *JAMA* 278:144, 1997.

Morgan K: More than a kick, *Sci News* 163:184, 2003.

Morgenstern J et al: Examining mechanisms of action in 12-step treatment: the role of 12-step cognitions, *J Stud Alcohol* 63:665, 2002.

Nathan P, Gorman J: *A guide to treatments that work*, ed 2, New York, 2002, Oxford University Press.

O'Connor PG: Treating opioid dependence—new data and new opportunities, *N Engl J Med* 343:1332, 2000.

Patoine B: Mental illness and addiction genes, The Dana Foundation Neuroscience Newsletter, *Brain Work* 13:1, 2003.

Prochaska J, DiClemente C: Towards a comprehensive model of change. In Miller W, Heather N, editors: *Treating addictive behaviors: process of change*, New York, 1986, Plenum.

Project MATCH Research Group: Matching alcoholism treatments to client heterogeneity: project MATCH post-treatment drinking outcomes, *J Stud Alcohol* 58:7, 1997.

Reynaud M et al: Patients admitted to emergency services for drunkenness: moderate alcohol users or harmful drinkers? *Am J Psychiatry* 158:96, 2001.

Rychtarik RG et al: Treatment settings for persons with alcoholism: evidence for matching clients to inpatient versus outpatient care, *J Consult Clin Psychol* 68:277, 2000.

SAMHSA website 2003: www.samhsa.gov/oas/nhsda/2k1nhsda/vol1/highlights.htm.

Scheel K: Hepatitis C: What every counselor should know, *Counselor* 4:22, 2003.

Stafford LL: Is codependency a meaningful construct? *Issues Ment Health Nurs* 22:273, 2001.

Substance Abuse and Mental Health Services Administration: Enhancing motivation for change in substance abuse treatment, *Treatment Improvement Protocol Series*, no 35, Rockville, Md, 1999, USDHHS

Washington OG: Using brief therapeutic interventions to create change in self-efficacy and personal control of chemically dependent women, *Arch Psychiatr Nurs* 15:32, 2001.

Watkins KE et al: A national survey of care for persons with co-occurring mental and substance use disorders, *Psychiatr Serv* 52:1062, 2001.

Welsh C, Liberto J: The use of medication for relapse prevention in substance dependence disorders, *J Psychiatr Pract* 1:15, 2001.

Weisner C, Matzger H: A prospective study of the factors influencing entry to alcohol and drug treatment, *J Behav Health Serv Res* 29:126, 2002.

EATING REGULATION RESPONSES AND EATING DISORDERS

25

Carolyn E. Cochrane

LEARNING OBJECTIVES

After studying this chapter, the student should be able to:

1. Describe the continuum of adaptive and maladaptive eating regulation responses (I).
2. Identify behaviors associated with eating regulation responses (II).
3. Analyze predisposing factors, precipitating stressors, and the appraisal of stressors related to eating regulation responses (II).
4. Describe coping resources and coping mechanisms related to eating regulation responses (II).
5. Formulate nursing diagnoses related to eating regulation responses (III).
6. Examine the relationship between nursing diagnoses and medical diagnoses related to eating regulation responses (III).
7. Identify expected outcomes and short-term nursing goals related to eating regulation responses (IV).
8. Develop a family education plan to promote adaptive eating regulation responses (V).
9. Analyze nursing interventions related to eating regulation responses (VI).
10. Evaluate nursing care related to eating regulation responses (VII).

TOPICAL OUTLINE

I. Continuum of Eating Regulation Responses
  A. Prevalence of Eating Disorders
II. Assessment
  A. Behaviors
  B. Predisposing Factors
  C. Precipitating Stressors
  D. Appraisal of Stressors
  E. Coping Resources
  F. Coping Mechanisms
III. Diagnosis
  A. Nursing Diagnoses
  B. Medical Diagnoses
IV. Outcome Identification
V. Planning
  A. Choice of Treatment Setting
  B. Nurse-Patient Contract
VI. Implementation
  A. Nutritional Stabilization
  B. Exercise
  C. Cognitive Behavioral Interventions
  D. Body Image Interventions
  E. Family Involvement
  F. Group Therapies
  G. Medications
VII. Evaluation

 Visit Evolve for additional resources related to the content of this chapter.
http://evolve.elsevier.com/Stuart/principles/

Food is essential to life because it supplies needed nutrients and sources of energy. As such, eating is a crucial self-regulatory activity. However, it also can assume importance and meaning beyond that of nutrition and become associated with biopsychosocial processes that promote or inhibit adaptive functioning.

CONTINUUM OF EATING REGULATION RESPONSES

As a pattern of self-regulation, properly controlled eating contributes to psychological, biological, and sociocultural health and well-being. Adaptive eating responses are characterized by **balanced eating patterns, appropriate caloric intake,** and **body weight that is appropriate for height**. Although eating is a common occurrence, society appears to have difficulty under-standing the idea of unregulated eating. Everyone has at times overeaten, skipped one or more meals, or seen adolescent boys consume large amounts of food at a single meal. Many women have premenstrual cravings for salty, sweet, or other types of foods. These eating behaviors are not viewed as problematic.

However, food also can be used to satisfy unmet emotional needs, to moderate stress, and to provide rewards or punishments. People can have unrealistic images of their ideal body size and desired body weight. Research has shown that most people think they should weigh less than they do, and this can result in behaviors that range from fasting fads to severe dieting. The inability to regulate eating habits and the frequent tendency to overuse or underuse food interferes with biological, psychological, and sociocultural integrity.

Illnesses associated with maladaptive eating regulation responses include **anorexia nervosa, bulimia nervosa, binge eat-**

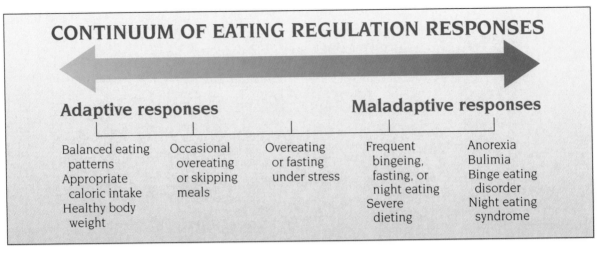

Figure 25-1   Continuum of eating regulation responses.

CITING THE EVIDENCE ON

Ethnicity and Eating Disorders

BACKGROUND: This community-based study describes the relationship between race and clinical functioning in black and white women with and without binge eating disorder.

RESULTS: As compared with women without the disorder, women who had binge eating disorder were more likely to be obese, with obesity being more common among black women. However, black women with the disorder had significantly lower scores on surveys of eating concerns, shape concerns, and weight concerns. Black and white women with binge eating disorder did not differ in the age that they first met criteria for having an eating disorder. However, white women were more than 8 times more likely than black women to also meet criteria for bulimia nervosa. Both black and white women with the disorder were likely to have been treated for a weight problem, but black women were less likely to have been treated for an eating problem. Although women with binge eating disorder also reported higher levels of psychiatric distress, more white women than black women met criteria for multiple Axis I disorders of the *DSM-IV-TR.*

IMPLICATIONS: For both black and white women, binge eating disorder was associated with significant impairment in clinical functioning. Findings suggest that screening for binge eating disorder in obese patients may be indicated and that the likelihood of receiving mental health care is low for racial minority groups.

Pike K et al: *Am J Psychiatry* 158:1455, 2001.

ing disorder, and **night eating syndrome** (Figure 25-1). Eating disorders are more commonly seen among females, with a male-to-female ratio ranging from 1:6 to 1:10. The gender differences in the prevalence of eating disorders may result from biological, sociocultural, and psychodynamic factors, as well as the fact that men may be more reluctant to seek treatment.

Racial differences related to eating disorders do exist (see Citing the Evidence). In the United States, eating disorders appear to be about as common in young Hispanic women as in whites, more common among Native Americans, and less common among blacks and Asians. Black women are more likely to develop bulimia nervosa than anorexia nervosa and are more likely to purge with laxatives than by vomiting (American Psychiatric Association, 2000a; Striegel-Moore et al, 2003).

These disorders can cause biological changes that include altered metabolic rates, profound malnutrition, and possibly death. Obsessions about eating can cause psychological problems that include depression, isolation, and emotional lability. Sociocultural ideals concerning body size can lead to an eating disorder by influencing a person to perceive his or her body size as being larger or smaller than it actually is. This distorted body image may lead to an attempt to attain an unrealistic body size.

Before working with patients with maladaptive eating regulation responses, nurses must closely examine their own feelings and prejudices about weight and body size. It may be helpful for nurses to think about the following questions:

- What do I believe is the ideal body size and shape?
- How do I feel about people who are overweight?
- Can a person ever really be too thin?
- Do I worry about my weight a lot?
- Do I have biases about eating and weight that will interfere with my ability to take care of patients with eating disorders?

A nurse who suspects that he or she has an eating disorder may not be able to provide care for patients who cannot regulate their eating responses. The nurse should seek out professional help for himself or herself before attempting to care for others.

Identify three sociocultural factors that influence the type and amount of food you eat and your perception of the ideal body size. ■

Prevalence of Eating Disorders

Anorexia Nervosa. Anorexia nervosa occurs in approximately 0.5% to 1% of the female population. Its onset usually occurs between 13 and 20 years of age, but the illness can occur in any age-group, including the elderly and prepubertal children. Anorexia nervosa is also seen in males, who are thought to make up only 5% to 10% of the anorectic population. The mortality from anorexia nervosa is estimated to be approximately 5% of those with the disorder.

Anorexia nervosa is a chronic illness for many. A review of studies that followed up patients who had been hospitalized with anorexia found that after 4 years the outcome of treatment was good for 44%, moderate for 28%, and poor for 24%. Two thirds were still preoccupied with food and weight; 40% still had symptoms of bulimia; and 5% had died (Vitiello and Lederhendler, 2000).

Vomiting, bulimia, purging, and obsessive-compulsive personality symptoms are associated with the least favorable prognosis (Steinhausen 2002). An additional predictor of mortality is severity of alcohol use disorder during the course of care (Keel et al, 2003).

Bulimia Nervosa. Bulimia nervosa is more common than anorexia, with an estimated occurrence of 1% to 4% of the population and 4% to 15% of female high school and college students (Pritts and Susman, 2003). The age of onset is typically 15 to 18 years of age. The female-to-male ratio for bulimia nervosa is about 11:1, but males with eating disorders have clinical features that are indistinguishable from females with eating disorders (Woodside et al., 2001).

For patients with bulimia nervosa, a 5-year prospective follow-up study revealed that 35% of patients treated for their eating disorder continue to meet full criteria for the disorder, with relapse occurring in one-third of patients. Remission was attained by approximately one-third of the patients for each year of the follow-up (Fairburn et al, 2000).

Another study found that 72% of patients with bulimia recover and that a good outcome was associated with a shorter duration between onset of symptoms and the first treatment intervention (Reas et al, 2000). This finding suggests that early identification of bulimia nervosa may be important in preventing a chronic eating disorder.

Bulimia and anorexia both may be present in the same patient. As many as 50% of individuals with anorexia develop bulimic symptoms, and some people with bulimia develop anorexia. Bulimia usually occurs in people of normal weight, but it also may occur in obese people and thin people.

Binge Eating Disorder. Individuals with binge eating disorder consume large amounts of calories but do not attempt to prevent weight gain. This disorder has a prevalence of approximately 2% to 4% of the population. It has been estimated that 19% to 40% of obese people who seek treatment for weight control have binge eating disorder. This suggests that assessing for eating disorders should be an important part of weight management programs (Grilo, 1998).

Night Eating Syndrome. Night eating syndrome is a severe eating problem that is under consideration for inclusion in the *DSM-IV-TR* as a separate eating disorder. Individuals with night eating syndrome have symptoms of morning anorexia and difficulty staying asleep and experience depression mostly in the evening. Night eaters average two awakenings per night and these awakenings are associated with food intake. The prevalence of night eating syndrome has been estimated to be 1.5% in the general population, 8.3% in the obese population, and 27% among severely obese populations seeking surgical treatment (Strunkard and Allison, 2003).

The overlapping relationships among the various maladaptive eating responses are seen in Figure 25-2.

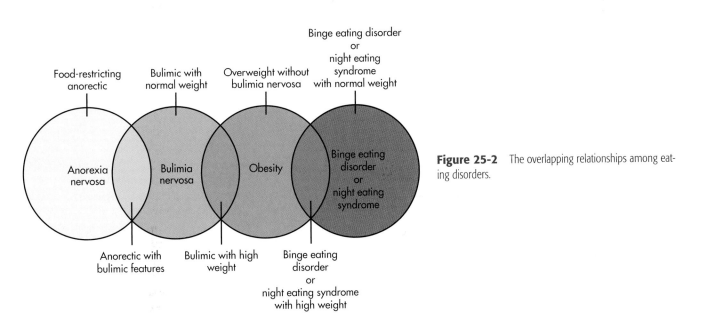

Figure 25-2   The overlapping relationships among eating disorders.

ASSESSMENT

Patients with maladaptive eating regulation responses need to receive a comprehensive nursing assessment that includes complete biological, psychological, and sociocultural evaluations. A **full physical examination** should be performed, with particular attention given to vital signs, weight for height and age, skin, the cardiovascular system, and evidence of laxatives, diet pills, or diuretic abuse and/or vomiting. A **dental examination** may be indicated, and it is useful to assess growth, sexual development, and general indicators of physical development. A **psychiatric history** including dieting history, substance use history, family assessment, and medication history also are needed.

Specific attention should focus on the assessment of eating regulation responses. Several questionnaires and rating scales have been developed to screen for the presence of eating disorders. However, asking only the following two questions may be as effective as using more extensive questionnaires in identifying women with eating disorders:

- Are you satisfied with your eating patterns?
- Do you ever eat in secret?

These two questions can be easily incorporated into the nursing assessment of all patients. If a patient is being evaluated for an eating disorder, additional information should be obtained, including the following:

- Actual and desired weight and weight history
- Onset and pattern of menstruation
- Food avoidances, restrictions, dieting, and fasting patterns
- Frequency, extent, and timing of binge eating and/or purging
- Unusual beliefs about nutrition
- Use of laxatives, diuretics, diet pills, and other methods of purging
- Chewing and spitting food
- Weight and shape preoccupations
- Body image disturbances
- Food preferences and peculiarities
- Compulsive exercise patterns

It is also helpful to ask the patient how the illness developed and what impact it has had on school, work, and social relationships so that a holistic view of the patient's world can be obtained.

Behaviors

Binge Eating. Binge eating involves the rapid consumption of large quantities of food in a discrete period of time, although there is no agreement on exactly how many calories constitutes a binge. Patients with anorexia who binge may describe a binge of several hundred calories. Patients with bulimia who are not also anorectic may ingest several thousand calories at a sitting. An emphasis on the patient's perception of loss of control and perceived excessive caloric intake is more important to the nursing assessment than the total number of calories consumed during a binge. Therefore it is important that the nurse carefully assess exactly what each patient means by a binge.

People usually binge secretively, whether during the day or in the middle of the night. Considerable shame is often associated with their bingeing behavior. A person with bulimia typically is of average weight or is slightly overweight and has a history of unsuccessful dieting. The severity of the bingeing can vary greatly, ranging from several times a week, to more than 10 times a day, to only occasional binges related to stressful situations.

Fasting or Restricting. People with anorexia often do not consume more than 500 to 700 calories daily and may ingest as few as 200 calories daily, yet they see their intake as adequate for their energy needs. They may follow an unbalanced vegetarian diet, eliminating all meat, poultry, fish, and dairy products without substituting nonanimal sources of protein and other important nutrients. They may be obsessive-compulsive about their eating habits and food choices, such as eating the same foods repeatedly, eating foods in a predetermined order, or eating at the same time every day. They may have bizarre food preferences, avoid foods that are considered fattening, and fast for days at a time.

Despite these restrictions, many people with anorexia are preoccupied or obsessed with food and may do much of the family cooking or be employed in a food-related occupation. The following clinical example describes the fasting behavior seen in people with anorexia.

CLINICAL EXAMPLE

Barbara is a 15-year-old white female who has been restricting her food intake for 6 months because she feels too fat. Her weight at the beginning of her food restriction was 128 pounds. This weight was appropriate for her age, her height (5 feet, 5 inches), and her small body frame. Her current weight is 102 pounds, which is approximately 80% of what she should weigh. The patient denies having any eating problems and believes that her family is overreacting to her weight loss. She is willing to come for treatment only because her family wants her to do so.

Barbara was age 13 at menarche and had regular periods until they stopped 2 months ago. She says she never tried or planned to lose weight but admits to becoming a vegetarian 6 months ago. Despite her low weight, Barbara thinks she needs to lose another 10 pounds because she thinks her thighs are too large. She is an avid ballet dancer and practices dancing 2 to 3 hours a day. Her family describes her as the perfect daughter.

Selected Nursing Diagnoses
- Imbalanced nutrition: less than body requirements related to restricted food intake, as evidenced by weight loss
- Disturbed body image related to eating disorder, as evidenced by continued desire to lose weight
- Ineffective denial related to eating problems, as evidenced by a lack of acceptance of realistic weight parameters ■

Purging. A variety of purging behaviors may be used by people with maladaptive eating regulation responses to prevent weight gain. These behaviors include excessive exercise, forced vomiting, and over-the-counter or prescription diuretics, diet pills, laxatives, and steroids. Laxatives are commonly abused by people with eating disorders, yet they are one of the most inefficient ways to lose calories.

Laxative abuse often begins gradually but can increase to 60 doses per week in some people. Less well-known substances used to counteract weight gain include insulin, cocaine, heroin, thyroid replacements, nicotine, hallucinogens, analgesics, benzodiazepines, antidepressants, ipecac, and sorbitol. Many patients engage in more than one purging behavior.

For these patients, exercising often becomes a grueling, time-consuming affair. Running or participating in high-impact aerobics for 2 to 3 hours each day is typical of the compulsive exerciser. Many patients with an eating disorder exercise so much that they sustain major skeletal injuries, but this still does not deter them from continuing this maladaptive behavior. Such behavior is seen in the following clinical example.

CLINICAL EXAMPLE

Bill is a 30-year-old single man with a 7-year history of anorexia nervosa and bulimia nervosa. Bill exercises compulsively at least 3 hours daily; from age 23 until age 29 he exercised 6 to 7 hours daily. Examples of current and previous exercise rituals include running 25 miles followed by a 2- to 3-mile swim and bicycling 25 miles before allowing himself to eat a meal. His athletic abilities have been rewarded with numerous trophies. He is receiving fewer trophies lately because of damage to his knees from overuse.

In addition to exercising compulsively, Bill also vomits after bingeing and has periods of fasting that last 2 to 3 days. When he does eat a regular meal, he eats only certain foods and eats them in a certain order. Bill also writes obsessively and is methodical about the order of his personal hygiene. He is depressed about the fact that his life revolves around his eating, hygiene, and exercise rituals, and he is eager to receive treatment.

Selected Nursing Diagnoses

* Imbalanced nutrition: less than body requirements related to anxiety about body size, as evidenced by bingeing and fasting
* Disturbed body image related to fears of gaining weight, as evidenced by excessive exercise and food restrictions
* Risk for injury related to excessive exercise, as evidenced by knee injuries ▪

Bingeing, fasting, and purging are sometimes described as addictive behaviors. Compare these behaviors to smoking, gambling, and substance abuse. ▪

Medical Complications. Every person with a maladaptive eating regulation response usually has some type of associated physical problem. The various complications associated with eating disorders are listed in Box 25-1.

BOX **25-1**

Medical Complications of Eating Disorders

Central Nervous System
* Cortical atrophy
* Decreased rapid eye movement and shortwave sleep
* Fatigue
* Seizures
* Thermoregulatory abnormalities
* Weakness

Renal
* Hematuria
* Proteinuria
* Renal calculi

Hematological
* Anemia
* Leukopenia
* Thrombocytopenia

Gastrointestinal
* Dental caries and erosion
* Diarrhea (laxative abuse)
* Esophagitis, esophageal tears
* Gastric dilation
* Hypercholesterolemia
* Pancreatitis
* Parotid swelling

Metabolic
* Acidosis
* Dehydration
* Hypocalcemia
* Hypochloremic alkalosis
* Hypokalemia
* Hypomagnesemia
* Hypophosphatemia
* Osteoporosis

Endocrine
* Amenorrhea
* Decreased luteinizing hormone and follicle-stimulating hormone
* Decreased triiodothyronine, increased reverse triiodothyronine, rT3, abnormal thyroxin and thyroid-stimulating hormone
* Irregular menses
* Regression of secondary sex characteristics

Cardiovascular
* Bradycardia
* Dysrhythmia, sudden death
* Postural hypotension
* Ventricular enlargement

An assessment of the patient's physical status can reveal the seriousness of the eating problem. For example, patients 20% below or 40% above their ideal body weight demonstrate more physical abnormalities than those who are closer to their ideal weight. Patients who are 30% below or 100% above their ideal body weight will have clinical and laboratory findings that are often life threatening. People who vomit and use laxatives or diuretics, regardless of their weight, usually have significant and sometimes life-threatening clinical findings and laboratory abnormalities.

In anorexia nervosa, metabolic and endocrine abnormalities result from the reaction of the body to the malnutrition associated with **starvation**. All body systems are affected. Most commonly seen are amenorrhea, osteoporosis, and hypometabolic symptoms such as cold intolerance and bradycardia. Starvation may cause hypotension, constipation, and acid-base and fluid-electrolyte disturbances, including pedal edema.

In bulimia nervosa, **potassium depletion** and **hypokalemia** often are seen as a result of vomiting and laxative or diuretic abuse. Symptoms of potassium depletion include muscle weakness, cardiac arrhythmias, conduction abnormalities, hypotension, and other problems associated with electrolyte imbalance. Gastric, esophageal, and bowel abnormalities are common complaints in patients with bulimia. Those who vomit are subject to erosion of the dental enamel and enlargement of the parotid glands.

Serious health problems caused by excess weight or prior health problems exacerbated by increased weight are common for individuals with binge eating disorder and concurrent morbid obesity. Many have hypertension, cardiac problems, sleep apnea, difficulties with mobility, and diabetes mellitus. Some of the medical consequences of eating disorders are seen in the following clinical example.

⚕ CLINICAL EXAMPLE

Audrey is a 25-year-old black woman with a 4-year history of restrictive intake and a 3-year history of binge eating and laxative abuse. Audrey has been concerned about her weight since high school, when she was a star basketball player, a competitive swimmer, and a participant in track, volleyball, and tennis. She bypassed her senior year in high school. She began to diet at age 20, and her severe restriction of food at age 21 led to a 20-pound weight loss and amenorrhea. At age 22 she began to binge and use laxatives. Since that time she has binged two to three times each week and uses an average of 30 to 60 laxatives each week.

Audrey is constantly preoccupied with food and her weight and has periods of mood lability, sadness, lack of energy, social isolation, anxiety, irritability, and difficulty concentrating. Audrey also reports chronic constipation; bloating; edema of the hands, feet, legs, and face; and lightheadedness. She recently consulted a gastroenterologist for her severe constipation and was advised that her large intestine is grossly oversized. Audrey became very frightened by the report and immediately called a local eating disorder program for help.

Selected Nursing Diagnoses
- Imbalanced nutrition: less than body requirements related to fear of gaining weight, as evidenced by bingeing
- Disturbed body image related to anxiety about body size, as evidenced by excessive use of laxatives

- Constipation related to maladaptive eating patterns, as evidenced by pain, bloating, and enlarged intestine ■

Psychiatric Complications. Many patients seeking treatment for eating disorders show evidence of other psychiatric disorders as well, most particularly **depression, anxiety disorders,** and **substance abuse** (American Psychiatric Association, 2000a). Comorbid major depression or dysthymia has been reported in 50% to 75% of people with anorexia and bulimia, and obsessive-compulsive disorder may be found in as many as 25% of patients with anorexia nervosa.

Among patients with bulimia are found increased rates of anxiety disorders, posttraumatic stress disorder, substance abuse, and mood disorders. People with antisocial personality disorders are 6 to 7 times more likely to have bulimia than the general population.

Binge eating disorder has been found to be associated with higher rates of major depression, panic disorder, bulimia nervosa, borderline personality disorder, and avoidant personality disorder. Night eating syndrome is associated with increased rates of mood disorders characterized by a circadian pattern.

Predisposing Factors

Researchers have identified biological, psychological, and sociocultural factors that may predispose a person to the development of an eating disorder (Klump et al, 2002). These factors are involved in the regulation and control of food intake and reflect a combination of genetic, neurochemical, developmental, personality, social, cultural, and familial factors (Figure 25-3).

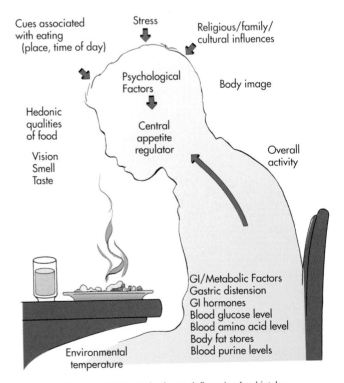

Figure 25-3 Major factors influencing food intake.

Biological. Both anorexia nervosa and bulimia nervosa are familial (Strober et al, 2000). The risk for eating disorders is higher in first-degree female relatives of people with eating disorders than in the general population. The concordance rates for eating disorders are 52% in monozygotic twins and 11% in dizygotic twins. The risk for other eating disorders, depression, and substance abuse also are higher in first-degree relatives of people with eating disorders (Wade et al, 2000). Current genetic studies are exploring the chromosomal location of the genes responsible for contributing to the development of eating disorders (Bulik et al., 2003a). In time, these findings may lead to better prevention programs for eating disorders.

Biological models of the etiology of eating disorders focus on the appetite regulation center in the **hypothalamus**, which controls specific neurochemical mechanisms for feeding and satiety. It has been hypothesized that the neurotransmitters, neuromodulators, and hormones that control feeding and satiety are dysregulated in patients with eating disorders.

Studies in animals and humans indicate that reduced **serotonin** is associated with reduced satiety, increased food intake, and dysphoric mood. When dietary tryptophan (the amino acid necessary for the brain to manufacture serotonin) is reduced, women with bulimia show a marked increase in eating behavior and mood changes such as irritability, lability, and fatigue; this suggests a disturbance of serotonin activity.

SPECT studies in humans have continued to support the animal model of serotonin dysregulation in eating disorders (Frank et al., 2002; Audenaert et al., 2003). It also has been reported that 3-methoxy-4-hydroxyphenylglycol (MHPG), the major metabolite of norepinephrine, is reduced in eating disorders, which suggests a role for this neurotransmitter as well.

A role for brain **dopamine** in eating disorder patients has been found in obese individuals with binge eating disorder. It is hypothesized that decreases in dopamine receptors in this subset of eating disorder patients perpetuate pathological eating as a way to compensate for the decreased activation of reward circuits that are modulated by dopamine (Wang et al., 2001). Leptin, a protein that inhibits food intake, and gherlin, also may have a role in the neurobiology of eating disorders (Jimerson D, 2002; Tanaka et al., 2002).

All of these models are still in the development stage. Ongoing research promises to shed more light on the biological factors that may predispose a person to maladaptive eating regulation responses.

Analyze the hypothesized role of serotonin in the development of both eating disorders and depressive disorders, as well as the implications this has for the use of selective serotonin reuptake inhibitors as a medication strategy for treating both disorders. ■

Psychological. Most patients with eating disorders exhibit psychological symptoms such as rigidity, ritualism, and meticulousness, often deriving from childhood (Anderluh et al, 2003; Bulik et al, 2003b). Women who have recovered continue to show an obsessive need for perfectionism, exactness, and symmetry, as well as greater risk avoidance, restraint, and impulse control.

Early separation and individuation conflicts, a pervasive sense of ineffectiveness and helplessness, difficulty interpreting feelings and tolerating intense emotional states, and a fear of biological or psychological maturity may predispose a person to an eating disorder. Women who binge also report great fluctuations of self-esteem, negative affect, shame, and guilt (Greeno, Wing, and Shiffman, 2000; Stein and Corte, 2003).

Environmental. A variety of environmental factors may predispose a person to developing an eating disorder. Early histories of patients with eating disorders are often complicated by medical and surgical illnesses, separations, and family deaths. Women with bulimia also describe growing up in a detached family environment and experiencing more behavioral disturbances such as drug abuse, suicide attempts, truancy, and other emotional problems. Sexual abuse has been reported in 20% to 50% of patients with bulimia and anorexia—a rate higher than in the general population (Wonderlich et al, 2001).

Parents who overemphasize athletics, reward slimness, or express disapproval of overweight people are placing their children at risk for developing eating disorders (Brink, Ferguson, and Sharma, 1999). Parents who continually skip meals, eat when distressed, and otherwise model poor nutritional habits are not teaching children about the appropriate value of food as nourishment. An important preventive nursing intervention involves educating the parents of young children regarding healthy eating behaviors (White, 2000) (see the Family Education Plan, Table 25-1).

Sociocultural. In the past 50 years the incidence of diagnosed eating disorders, subclinical eating problems, and body image disturbances has steadily increased. Eating disorders are thought to be rare in cultures where plumpness is accepted or valued. Shifting cultural norms for young women have forced them to face multiple, ambiguous, and often contradictory role expectations.

Thinness is highly valued, culturally rewarded, and associated with achievement. The contemporary American ideal woman is lean, strong, graceful, and feminine. One advantage to this profile is its emphasis on fitness and health. A disadvantage is the demand this norm places on women to focus on and control their bodies, often as a means for achieving desired goals. This leads to intense social pressure on women for self-discipline, rigorous exercise, dieting, and often obsessive concern about weight and body image (McKnight Investigators, 2003). The result is that at least 50% of American women are on a diet at any given time, with Americans spending more than $5 billion on dieting products.

Children, adolescents, and young adults living in communities or going to schools where emphasis is placed on weight and size are often prone to developing eating disorders. Activities or occupations that emphasize beauty or fitness also promote a preoccupation with weight and eating behaviors. Ballet dancers, models, actors, athletes, fashion retailers, cooks, and flight attendants have demands placed on them concerning body weight and size. Although these occupations and activities in themselves do not cause eating disorders, they do attract people who may measure their self-esteem, self-worth, and at-

Table 25-1	FAMILY EDUCATION PLAN	Preventing Childhood Eating Problems
CONTENT	**INSTRUCTIONAL ACTIVITIES**	**EVALUATION**
Describe self-demand feeding and its importance in healthy eating behaviors.	Explore parents' current feeding practices and understanding of healthy eating. Provide information to enhance knowledge of healthy eating behaviors.	Parents will identify healthy eating behaviors and self-demand feeding and begin to explore how their relationship with food influences their children's eating.
Describe the physiological and psychological signs of hunger and satiety, as well as the meaning and difference of both types of signs.	Explore parents' own signs of hunger and satiety, and have parents describe children's signs.	Parents will keep a hunger diary to record physical and psychological signs of hunger and satiety for themselves and their children.
Describe the danger of psychological hunger.	Explain the use of a hunger diary, which is a daily journal regarding signs of hunger.	Parents will be able to distinguish between psychological and physical hunger.
Explore myths about feeding, such as "cleaning the plate" and "eating because other children are starving."	Describe the importance of allowing children to determine their feeding needs and the relationship of healthy eating to the children's ability to differentiate between physical and psychological signs of hunger and satiety. Give a homework assignment for each parent to interview three other adults about their current eating practices and memories of eating.	Parents will complete homework assignment, discuss interview experiences, and describe how perpetuating myths about feeding can harm their children.
Implement self-demand feeding at particular developmental stages of children.	Review the eating stages children experience and the potential problems they may have at each stage.	Parents will discuss the developmental stages of their children and plan to implement self-demand feeding.
Discuss parental experiences related to implementing self-demand feeding.	Review parents' expectations and experiences with implementing self-demand feeding.	Parents will relate any problem with implementing self-demand feeding. Nurse will evaluate family for further education and plan for follow-up if necessary.

BOX **25-2**

Psychosocial Predisposing Factors for the Development of Eating Disorders

Personal Factors
- Weight
- Puberty/maturation
- Restrained eating/dieting
- Body image dissatisfaction
- Problems regulating affect
- Depression
- Perfectionism
- Low self-esteem
- Stress
- Low resiliency/confidence
- Poor coping skills
- Alcohol and substance use
- Sexual/physical abuse
- Early dating

Family Factors
- Parental attitudes
- Family functioning

Peers
- Attitudes about weight
- Behaviors
- Teasing

Culture
- Media influences

Activities
- Gymnastics
- Professional dance
- Modeling

tractiveness by their body parameters rather than by their accomplishments and personal satisfaction. Psychosocial predisposing factors for the development of eating disorders are summarized in Box 25-2.

Watch television for an evening and count the number of men and women who are overweight. Explain any sociocultural bias you observe. ■

Precipitating Stressors

Having one or more predisposing factors puts a person at risk for an eating disorder. People who are predisposed are especially vulnerable to environmental pressures and stress. Lacking an integrated self-concept and realistic body image, they rely on external feedback such as the reactions of others to their appearance and actions.

They are unable to perceive or interpret stimuli from within the body, have difficulty describing their feelings and self-concepts, and lack an internal center of initiative and regulation. Thus they must rely on external cues to regulate themselves. Food becomes one of these cues and is used as an external replacement for a deficient internal regulator and an inadequate integration of the body and mind.

Appraisal of Stressors

The person with an eating disorder is very susceptible to the impact of life stressors, such as the loss of a significant other, interpersonal rejection, and failure. Some researchers have suggested that people predisposed to eating disorders exercise not as a way to lose weight but as an attempt to experience the reality of their bodies.

Controlling their eating or vomiting is another attempt to avoid the anguish of emptiness, boredom, or tension. Although binge eating may momentarily release this tension, it sets in motion a cycle of bingeing and purging that, once begun, is very difficult to stop. The importance of a person's appraisal of stressors related to eating disorders is seen in the following clinical example.

■ ⑤ CLINICAL EXAMPLE

Lydia is a 15-year-old female with a 6-year history of bingeing, a 9-month history of purging, and a 2-year history of restricting food intake. She is the only child of parents who separated when she was 3 and divorced when she was 6. Her father has a history of frequent mood swings and has been diagnosed with and treated for bipolar disorder. He has always been overly concerned not only about his bodily appearance but also about the appearance of his family. When Lydia was 9, her father moved to a city 500 miles away, and 2 years later he remarried. Lydia's mother remarried several months later, but her marriage lasted less than a year. Her new husband had concealed an alcohol problem, and Lydia and her mother were verbally abused by this man on many occasions.

After her second divorce, Lydia's mother socialized very little and became overprotective of Lydia. She has often criticized Lydia's father for his extramarital behavior during their marriage. She supported him through college and dental school and was angry about her lowered standard of living since their divorce.

Lydia's parents continue to have a stormy relationship, and she feels caught between them at times. She avoids conflict by siding with her custodial parent (her mother) and by avoiding any discussion about her mother with her father. Lydia tries to be the perfect daughter and strives to avoid displeasing either parent. She has become very overprotective of her mother and secretly despises her father. She feels that a number of people have hurt her mother and that she and her mother must protect each other. She is afraid to grow up because her mother will be left alone. She states, "I'm the center of my mom's universe. If she's alone, her world will crumble.... I'm happiest when I'm worrying about my mom." Lydia does not think she has any eating problems and is very resistant to treatment. Her parents feel otherwise.

Selected Nursing Diagnoses
- Imbalanced nutrition: less than body requirements related to unrealistic self-image, as evidenced by bingeing, purging, and restricting food
- Ineffective denial related to family conflict, as evidenced by overprotection of mother and ambivalence toward father ■

Coping Resources

One of the most important parts of the assessment of patients with maladaptive eating regulation responses is their **motivation to change their behavior** (Geller, 2002). This may be determined by asking patients to rate their desire for treatment on a scale of 1 to 10, with 10 representing high motivation and 1 representing low motivation for change. Patients also may be asked to identify the advantages and disadvantages of giving up the behavior. This information can be used to evaluate a patient's insight, to identify coping resources, and to stimulate therapeutic issues for future discussion.

Four specific areas have been found to be crucial in engaging patients who are reluctant to treat their eating disorder. These are (Vitousek, Watson, and Wilson, 1998):
1. The provision of psychoeducational material.
2. An examination of the advantages and disadvantages of symptoms.
3. The use of focused strategies.
4. An exploration of personal values.

The nurse might ask patients how their bingeing, fasting, and purging serve as a form of coping. Asking patients what precedes these episodes and how they feel afterward are important elements of the nurse's assessment. The patient also should be asked how stress and tension have been handled adaptively in the past and what supports in the environment are available to help in the treatment process. Such supports may include family members, friends, work, and leisure activities.

Coping Mechanisms

People with anorexia nervosa are happiest when fasting, losing weight, or achieving their weight goals. Their use of **denial** is severely maladaptive, and they are unlikely to seek help on their own. Concerned family members, primary practitioners, nurses, or school counselors are usually the ones who identify a problem and attempt to obtain help.

People with anorexia are usually angry or impatient with the concern shown by others. Interestingly, as the family becomes more distraught about the loss of weight or signs of malnutrition, the insistence of normalcy by the person with anorexia increases.

For people with anorexia, the issue is not really about weight—it is about **controlling life and fears.** Those who fear maturity, independence, failure, sexuality, or parental demands believe they have found a solution to the problem by controlling their food intake and their bodies. As family concerns increase, people with anorexia are then able to gain control over the focus of significant others as well. For them, anorexia seems to be the perfect solution for gaining control.

The defense mechanisms used by people with bulimia include **avoidance, denial, isolation of affect,** and **intellectualization.** Regardless of their weight, people with bulimia are usually very upset about their bingeing and purging behavior. They realize that their behavior is a sign that they are not in control or coping adaptively, but they do not know why. They are more likely to acknowledge that they have a problem than are patients with anorexia. However, they may regard the symptoms as preferable to the prospect of weight gain, and it may be years before they accept treatment.

People with binge eating disorder share the bulimic patient's distress about bingeing, but it is unclear how motivated they are to seek treatment. Obese binge eaters are more likely to seek assistance on their own or be willing to be referred by their primary practitioner. Night eating syndrome patients are also very distressed, especially if obese. They will readily seek treatment.

DIAGNOSIS

Nursing Diagnoses

In formulating the nursing diagnosis, the nurse should review all aspects of the assessment phase as identified in the Stuart Stress Adaptation Model (Figure 25-4). Nursing diagnoses related to eating disorders encompass biological, psychologi-

cal, and sociocultural concerns. Because of the complexity of these disorders, many NANDA nursing diagnoses may be appropriate.

The primary NANDA diagnoses for working with patients with maladaptive eating regulation responses include **anxiety, disturbed body image, imbalanced nutrition, powerlessness, chronic or situational low self-esteem** and **risk for self-mutilation**. The Medical and Nursing Diagnoses box (Box 25-3) presents nursing diagnoses and medical diagnoses associated with the range of possible maladaptive eating regulation responses. Primary NANDA nursing diagnoses and examples of complete nursing diagnoses are presented in the Detailed Diagnoses table (Table 25-2).

Patients with moderate to extreme nutritional deficiencies exhibit symptoms of malnutrition that may be mistakenly related to other causes. Irritability, apathy, depression, obsessiveness, difficulty with concentration, anxiety, decreased in-

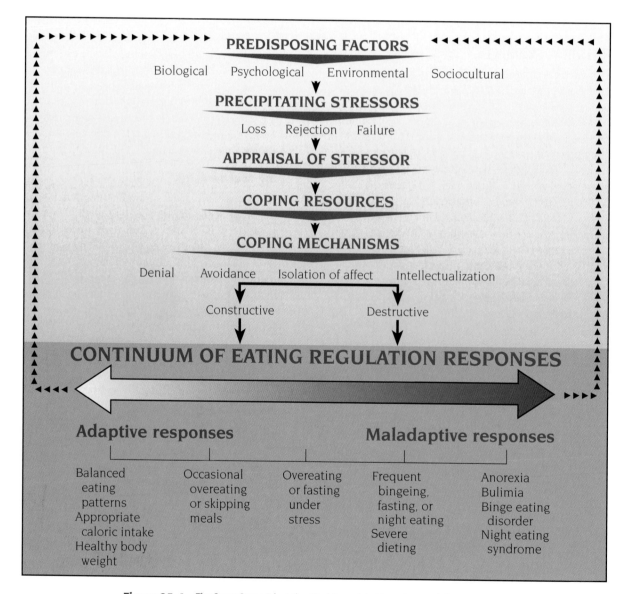

Figure 25-4   The Stuart Stress Adaptation Model as related to eating regulation responses.

■ **BOX 25-3** *Medical and Nursing Diagnoses Related to* **Eating Regulation Responses**

RELATED MEDICAL DIAGNOSES (*DSM-IV-TR*)*	RELATED NURSING DIAGNOSES (NANDA)†
Anorexia nervosa Binge eating disorder Bulimia nervosa	**Anxiety**‡ **Body image, Disturbed**‡ Coping, Ineffective Denial, Ineffective Family processes, Interrupted Fatigue Fluid volume, Deficient Hopelessness Injury, Risk for **Nutrition, Imbalanced: less than body requirements or more than body requirements**‡ **Powerlessness**‡ Role performance, Ineffective **Self-esteem, Chronic or Situational low**‡ **Self-mutilation, Risk for**‡ Sexual dysfunction

*From American Psychiatric Association: *Diagnostic and statistical manual of mental disorders*, ed 4, text revision, Washington, DC, 2000, American Psychiatric Association.
†From North American Nursing Diagnosis Association: *NANDA nursing diagnoses: definitions and classification 2003-2004*, Philadelphia, 2003, The Association.
‡**Primary nursing diagnosis for eating problems.**

Table 25-2 *Detailed Diagnoses Related to* **Eating Regulation Responses**

NANDA DIAGNOSIS STEM	EXAMPLES OF EXPANDED DIAGNOSIS
Anxiety	Anxiety related to fear of weight gain, as evidenced by rituals associated with food preparation and eating
Disturbed body image	Disturbed body image related to fear of weight gain, as evidenced by verbalization of being "fat" while actually being 30% below ideal body weight
Imbalanced nutrition: more than body requirements	Imbalanced nutrition: more than body requirements related to excessive intake of calories, as evidenced by being 40% above ideal body weight, sleep apnea, and difficulty with mobility
Powerlessness	Powerlessness related to perceived lack of control over eating behaviors, as evidenced by inability to stop binge eating and the avoidance of food-related settings
Chronic low self-esteem	Chronic low self-esteem related to feelings of low self-worth, as evidenced by verbalization of sole standard of success being related to physical attractiveness
Risk for self-mutilation	Risk for self-mutilation related to feelings of inadequacy, as evidenced by injuries caused by excessive exercise and self-induced vomiting

DSM-IV-TR DIAGNOSIS	ESSENTIAL FEATURES*
Anorexia nervosa	An intense fear of gaining weight, even when underweight. There is a disturbance in the way the body is experienced and a refusal to maintain body weight above a minimal normal weight for age and height; this leads to a body weight 15% below expected. In females menstrual cycles are also absent for at least three consecutive cycles. Two subtypes of anorexia nervosa are (1) restricting type, and (2) binge-eating/purging type.
Bulimia nervosa	Recurrent episodes of binge eating with a feeling of lack of control over the eating behavior and a persistent overconcern with body shape and weight. The person also regularly engages in self-induced vomiting; the misuse of laxatives, diuretics, enemas, or other medications; fasting; or excessive exercise.
Binge eating disorder	Recurrent episodes of bingeing that are a cause of distress, with a feeling of lack of control over the eating behavior but with no behaviors used to prevent weight gain.

*From American Psychiatric Association: *Diagnostic and statistical manual of mental disorders*, ed 4, text revision. Washington, DC, 2000, American Psychiatric Association.

terest in sex, and negativism are psychological symptoms that usually reverse with adequate nutrition.

The nurse may see a very different outward presentation in a patient who is no longer malnourished. Family members may offer important insights into the patient's premorbid functioning and be able to give a clearer picture of the patient's personality before the eating disorder developed.

Medical Diagnoses

The medical diagnoses associated with maladaptive eating regulation responses include **anorexia nervosa, bulimia nervosa,** and **binge eating disorder** (American Psychiatric Association, 2000b). Night eating syndrome is not yet a validated medical diagnosis but it is under consideration for identification as a separate eating disorder. These medical diagnoses and their essential features are described in the Detailed Diagnoses table (see Table 25-2). The key features distinguishing anorexia nervosa from bulimia nervosa are listed in Box 25-4.

OUTCOME IDENTIFICATION

The expected outcome for the patient with maladaptive eating regulation responses is:

> *The patient will restore healthy eating patterns and normalize physiological parameters related to body weight and nutrition.*

For patients with anorexia nervosa or bulimia nervosa, this means eating 100% of all meals without bingeing, purging, or engaging in other compensatory behavior. Obese patients with binge eating disorder or night eating syndrome should be encouraged to leave something (no more than 5% and no less than 2%) on their plate at the end of the meal.

Short-term goals may further specify the steps the patient needs to take to demonstrate adaptive eating regulation responses. These steps might include the following:

- The patient will identify cognitive distortions about food, weight, and body shape.
- The patient will develop a week's worth of menus for nutritionally balanced meals.
- The patient will accurately describe body dimensions.
- The patient will exercise in moderate amounts only when nutritionally and medically stable.
- The patient will demonstrate positive family interactions and successful movement toward the achievement of separation and individuation issues.
- The patient will be able to describe the complications and medical sequelae of his or her eating disorder behavior.

PLANNING

Choice of Treatment Setting

Nursing care varies to some degree based on the treatment setting of the patient with maladaptive eating regulation responses. A number of factors affect the choice of treatment setting, including the patient's physical and psychological condition, financial resources, availability of treatment specialists, and patient preference. Clinical criteria for inpatient treatment of eating disorders are listed in Box 25-5.

Outpatient treatment is often the best choice because it allows the patient the greatest opportunity for self-control

---

BOX 25-4

Key Features of Anorexia Nervosa and Bulimia Nervosa

Anorexia Nervosa (Without Bingeing or Purging)	Bulimia Nervosa
Rare vomiting or diuretic/laxative abuse	Frequent vomiting or diuretic/laxative abuse
More severe weight loss	Less weight loss
Slightly younger	Slightly older
More introverted	More extroverted
Hunger denied	Hunger experienced
Eating behavior may be considered normal and a source of esteem	Eating behavior considered foreign and source of distress
Sexually inactive	More sexually active
Obsessional and perfectionist features predominate	Avoidant, dependent, or borderline features as well as obsessional features
Death from starvation (or suicide, in chronically ill)	Death from hypokalemia or suicide
Amenorrhea	Menses irregular or absent
Fewer behavioral problems (these increase with level of severity)	Drug and alcohol abuse, self-mutilation, and other behavioral problems

---

BOX 25-5

Clinical Criteria for Hospitalization of Patients With an Eating Disorder

Medical
- Need for extensive diagnostic evaluation
- Weight loss greater than 25% of body weight over 3 months
- Heart rate less than 40 beats/min or greater than 110 beats/min
- Temperature less than 97.0° F
- Systolic blood pressure 70 mm Hg or marked orthostatic hypotension 20 mm Hg/minute standing
- Serum potassium less than 2.5 mEq/L despite oral potassium replacement
- Severe dehydration or vomiting of blood
- Concurrent somatic illnesses (e.g., infection)

Psychiatric
- Risk of suicide or self-mutilation
- Severe depression
- Substance abuse
- Psychosis
- Family crisis
- Failure to comply with treatment contract or poor motivation
- Inadequate response to outpatient treatment

and autonomy. It requires a high level of patient motivation, the active support and involvement of family members, and ongoing physiological monitoring. Contingencies for outpatient treatment should be mutually agreed on expectations of behavioral change, including weight gain and decreased bingeing or purging, as well as the acceptance of inpatient or more intense day treatment programs if the patient is not making progress.

Outpatient settings, including day treatment, intensive outpatient, and partial hospitalization programs, as well as weekly outpatient office care, are the current standard treatment settings. Unfortunately, the setting for treatment and the number of treatment episodes is often restricted by resources, particularly health insurance (Striegel-Moore et al, 2000). Reimbursement for inpatient programs except under dangerous or severe conditions, such as suicidal intent, is often difficult to obtain.

An advantage to inpatient treatment, however, is the availability of 24-hour nursing care to ensure patient safety, to support needed behavioral change, and to monitor physiological responses. Patients with eating disorders can present a unique challenge to staff, and care requires a high level of interdisciplinary collaboration, coordination, and consistency.

Empirically validated treatments for bulimia nervosa are summarized in Box 25-6 (Nathan and Gorman, 2002).

Nurse-Patient Contract

Nurse-patient contracts can be formulated for patients with eating disorders who are seen in either inpatient or outpatient settings. The terms of the contract may vary, but the goal is the same—to engage the patient in a therapeutic alliance and to obtain commitment to the treatment process.

Before a patient is admitted to an eating disorder treatment program, the patient's cooperation should be obtained with a nurse-patient contract. By signing such a contract, patients will show they understand what treatment they will be receiving and will be able to make informed decisions about their commitment to the treatment process and their ability to honor the contract.

How would you respond to a patient who wants to receive treatment for an eating disorder but does not want to sign the nurse-patient contract because it is "too restrictive"? ∎

IMPLEMENTATION

Nutritional Stabilization

Stabilizing the patient's nutritional status is a high priority for nursing intervention. Healthy target weights and expected rates of controlled weight gain or loss should be set. In life-threatening circumstances, patients who are malnourished may need refeeding interventions (see Critical Thinking About Contemporary Issues), but these cases are exceptional.

Specific nursing interventions to promote weight stabilization and restore healthy eating patterns can be facilitated by program protocols that identify treatment goals, program components, and patient and staff responsibilities. These protocols may include some of the following:

- The time, frequency, and procedure for weighing the patient and whether the patient may view the weight reading
- The time when meals will be served and the number of meals that are to be eaten each day

Critical Thinking *About* Contemporary Issues

Should Tube Feeding Be a Part of an Eating Disorders Treatment Program?

The positive and negative consequences of nasogastric tube feeding or even total parenteral nutrition for patients with an eating disorder have been debated among clinicians and researchers. Current guidelines recommend that refeeding interventions be used only rarely and in life-threatening situations (American Psychiatric Association, 2000a). Specifically, there is recognition of the danger of rapid refeeding, which includes severe fluid retention and cardiac failure, and of forced nasogastric or parenteral feeding. Therefore these procedures should not be used routinely. However, some severely malnourished patients with anorexia may accept nasogastric feeding more willingly than eating, especially in the early stages of renourishment.

If forced feeding is being considered, careful thought should be given to the patient's clinical condition, the patient's and family's opinion of this intervention, and the legal and ethical dimensions of the patient's treatment. Each of these areas merits a full discussion by the interdisciplinary health care team, and treatment decisions should include specific timelines, outcomes, and alternatives.

BOX 25-6	SUMMARIZING THE EVIDENCE ON Eating Disorders
Disorder	Bulimia nervosa (BN)
Treatment	◆ Several different classes of antidepressant drugs produced significant, short-term reductions in binge eating and purging. ◆ Manual-based cognitive-behavioral therapy (CBT) was most effective in eliminating the core features of BN; roughly half the patients receiving CBT reduced binge eating and purging; long-term maintenance of improvement was good.

From Nathan P, Gorman J: *A guide to treatments that work,* ed 2, New York, 2002, Oxford University Press.

- How the staff is to interact with the patient during mealtimes to maximize the therapeutic value of their presence
- The amount of time the patient will be allotted to eat each meal, and the consequences if the meal is not completed in that time
- Whether diet foods, condiments, or food substitutions are to be allowed
- The amount of water the patient may drink each day
- The frequency of obtaining the patient's vital signs, intake and output, and required laboratory work
- Conditions regarding bathroom privileges
- Indications for close observation by staff

Once patients are able to master eating their meals, they can move toward having more independence over scheduling their meals and food selection. Selecting their own menus with assistance is next. The patient can then progress to shopping for and cooking food with supervision. By the time of discharge, the patient should have gained a high level of comfort with food and its preparation.

For outpatients with anorexia nervosa, stabilizing nutrition and promoting weight gain usually require a motivated patient and cooperative family. Obtaining the patient's agreement to stop trying to lose weight is the first obstacle the nurse must overcome; patients are often very resistant to such an idea.

Getting a patient with anorexia to gain weight is an even more difficult task. Nurse-patient contracts can be effective tools in working with these patients because their need for control of food is so great. For example, the nurse and patient may set a realistic goal of gaining 1 pound per week. If the patient fails to gain 4 pounds in a month, the contract would stipulate that the patient would agree to enter a hospital, day treatment program, or some other more intensive type of care.

Counseling about healthy eating patterns and behaviors is an essential aspect of nursing care for all patients, regardless of whether they need to gain, lose, or maintain weight. The nurse should also clarify with patients the effect of poor nutrition on the body. Collaboration with a dietitian may be helpful in teaching patients about proper eating habits and in planning menus with patients.

Nurses should teach, clarify, and reinforce knowledge about proper nutrition and the importance of planning healthy meals. Patients should be encouraged to make their own shopping lists; the nurse may even accompany the patient to the grocery store. Nutritional assessment, education, and ongoing support are essential nursing care activities.

The patient who is struggling with major issues regarding food will not be ready for intensive psychological interventions. As the patient feels less need to be in control of food and eating, issues underlying the eating disorder may start to surface. This can be a difficult time for the patient, who may actually begin to feel worse than at the time treatment began.

Patients in a hospital or a partial hospitalization program always have someone available to talk with, but this is not always true for the outpatient. Thus the outpatient may need more frequent sessions with the nurse or more phone con-

tacts between sessions. When sufficient progress has been made toward nutritional rehabilitation, the patient will be better prepared both cognitively and emotionally to begin the next phase of treatment.

Exercise

As the patient's eating increases, the need to increase exercise or engage in a new purging or compensatory behavior also may increase. Patients on an inpatient or partial hospitalization unit can be closely monitored to prevent such compensatory activity. It is often appropriate to have the patient begin a gradual exercise program as he or she stabilizes and responds to treatment.

For patients who previously exercised compulsively, this time of restricted exercise can be the most difficult period of treatment. The nurse should initially allow patients limited amounts of exercise, with gradual increases over time. The focus of the exercise program should be on physical fitness rather than on working off calories. Consultation with a recreational therapist or exercise physiologist may be helpful to maximize the therapeutic value of the exercise regimen.

Cognitive Behavioral Interventions

Cognitive-behavioral therapy has been found to be the single most effective treatment for patients with eating disorders (Fairburn, Shafran, and Cooper, 1999; Whittal et al, 1999). It is important for the nurse to work with patients in regard to their **cognitive distortions** or their faulty thinking about body shape, weight, and food. Box 25-7 presents a list of cognitive distortions common among patients with eating disorders, as well as an example of each. Cognitive distortions and cognitive behavioral therapy is discussed in detail in Chapter 31.

Helping the patient become aware of his or her cognitive distortions is the first step in changing them. The patient should be asked to monitor and record eating, bingeing, and purging behavior and his or her thoughts and feelings regarding weight, shape, and food. The goal of these exercises is for the patient to better understand the following aspects of his or her behavior:

- Cues that trigger problematic eating responses
- Thoughts, feelings, and assumptions associated with the specific cues
- Connection between these thoughts, feelings, and assumptions and eating regulation responses
- Consequences resulting from the eating responses

Cues. Cues that trigger maladaptive eating behavior can be social, situational, physiological, and psychological. Examples of social cues are loneliness, interpersonal conflict, social awkwardness, and holiday celebrations. Examples of situational cues include diet advertisements and walking by a store that sells snack food that can easily accommodate bingeing behavior. Hunger and fatigue are the two most common physiological cues. Memory and mental images are two examples of psychological cues.

Specific cues such as these can trigger cognitive distortions and lead to maladaptive eating regulation responses.

For example, when stepping on the scale, a patient may see that she has gained a pound. She then may use dichotomous thinking: "Since I've gained 1 pound, I will probably gain 20 pounds in the next week. I'd better take a package of laxatives so that I can lose the pound by tomorrow."

- Stepping on the scale is the cue.
- Believing she will gain 20 pounds is the related irrational thought.
- Taking the laxatives is the maladaptive eating regulation response connected to the cognitive distortion.
- Beginning another purge cycle is the consequence resulting from the maladaptive response.

Cues can be used as a strategy for change. Rearranging cues, avoiding a cue, and changing the response to a cue are ways of altering maladaptive responses. After continued learning about eating, bingeing, and purging behavior, as well as thoughts and feelings about food, shape, and weight, it is hoped that the patient will begin to see the connections between thoughts and behaviors and recognize the consequences of the harmful activity.

Thoughts, Feelings, and Assumptions. The nurse helps patients challenge their faulty thoughts, feelings, and assumptions by questioning the evidence supporting or challenging a particular belief. In the previous example, the nurse might ask the patient what specifically happened in the past when she gained a pound. Did she gain 19 more pounds in the same week? If so, how often has it happened in the past? If not, why does the patient believe it will happen this time?

It is also important for the nurse to ask the patient about the implications of this type of thinking. Do other people have the same problem if they gain a pound? If so, how do they deal with it? The nurse can help the patient consider alternative explanations for his or her thoughts, thereby gradually modifying the irrational assumptions that underlie these beliefs. These and other cognitive behavioral techniques may be successfully used in patients with maladaptive eating regulation responses (see A Patient Speaks).

Eating Regulation Responses. The patient with an eating disorder needs help in **solving problems** and in **making decisions**. Rather than resorting to maladaptive responses, the patient must be helped to distinguish between adaptive and maladaptive coping responses and to find alternative solutions.

One way of doing this is to encourage the patient to make a list of high-risk situations that cue maladaptive eating and purging behaviors. The high-risk situation may be a certain day of the week, time of the day, season of the year, person, group, event, or emotional response, such as anger or frustration. The nurse can then help the patient identify specific, alternative, and more adaptive ways of handling these high-risk situations.

Decision-making strategies also may need to be reviewed and modified. Many patients with eating disorders know what they need to do in a given situation but may feel inadequate or shy about carrying out a certain plan of action. These people may benefit from assertiveness training and role modeling sessions with the nurse.

BOX 25-7

Cognitive Distortions Related to Maladaptive Eating Regulation Responses

Magnification: Overestimating the significance of undesirable events. Stimuli are embellished with meaning not supported by objective analysis. "I've gained 2 pounds, so I can't wear shorts any more."

Superstitious thinking: Believing in the cause-effect relationship of noncontingent events. "If I eat a sweet, it will instantly be turned into stomach fat."

Dichotomous or all-or-none thinking: Thinking in extreme or absolute terms, such as that events can only be black or white, right or wrong, good or bad. "If I gain 1 pound, I'll go on to gain 100 pounds."

Overgeneralization: Extracting a rule on the basis of one event and applying it to other dissimilar situations. "I used to be of normal weight and I wasn't happy. So I know gaining weight isn't going to make me feel better."

Selective abstraction: Basing a conclusion on isolated details while ignoring contradictory and more important evidence. "The only way I can be in control is through eating."

Personalization and self-reference: Egocentric interpretations of impersonal events or overinterpretation of events related to the self. "Two people laughed and whispered something to each other when I walked by. They were probably saying that I looked unattractive. I have gained 3 pounds."

From Garner D et al: *Handbook of treatment for eating disorders,* New York, 1997, Guilford.

A PATIENT SPEAKS

Learning to separate my feelings from my eating has been the hardest part but has been the greatest benefit of treatment for my eating disorder. From early childhood, food had been my main outlet for almost every emotion. When I was sad, I comforted myself by eating. When I was happy, I celebrated by eating. Feelings of loneliness could be diminished by gathering up all my "food friends" and eating. Feeling angry at anyone other than myself was unacceptable, so I would eat and then had a "good reason" to be angry and focus it all on myself.

Discovering that everything in life is not black or white, good or bad, perfect or imperfect, or hungry or full has enabled me to be kinder to myself and more accepting of my imperfections and humanity. I now realize that shades of gray do exist when making a decision, performing a task, feeling an emotion, and even experiencing hunger. Another benefit of this insight is a decrease in my level of anxiety and in my feelings of worthlessness.

Each day is no longer a battle to control all aspects of my life, especially my food consumption. The struggle with food and my weight still remains, but now it doesn't completely overshadow everything else that happens in my life. Food is no longer the only friend and enemy life offers. I learned all of this from a nurse who took the time to get to know me and in turn helped me to get to know myself.

Consequences. It is particularly important for the nurse and patient to explore the positive and negative consequences that result from cognitive distortions and maladaptive responses. These consequences can be biological, psychological, and sociocultural, with positive and negative consequences resulting from each behavior. Some of these consequences are presented in Table 25-3. A maladaptive behavior such as bingeing is maintained because the positive consequences are more immediate or are more valued than the negative consequences.

Strategies for change that focus on consequences involve the use of rewards that increase the likelihood of behavior change. In the example in which laxatives were taken in response to a 1-pound weight gain, rewards would be given if the person was able to resist taking the laxative. The reward should be received immediately following the desired behavior change. It should be something pleasurable and can be either a material item or a psychological reinforcer, but it should not involve food.

Should overweight nurses be assigned to care for patients with eating disorders? Why or why not? ▪

Body Image Interventions

Body image distortions are one of the most difficult-to-treat aspects of the eating disorder. This is partly because researchers disagree on what exactly constitutes a body image distortion. The only agreement is that body image distortion in the eating disorders involves perceptual, attitudinal, and behavioral features (Cash and Pruzinsky, 2002) (Figure 25-5).

A distinction between body image distortion and body dissatisfaction must be made. **Body image distortion** is a discrepancy between the patient's actual size and his or her perceived body size. **Body dissatisfaction** is the degree of unhappiness that a person feels in relation to his or her body size.

All people may express dissatisfaction with their bodies at some point in their lives, but such dissatisfaction is constant in persons with anorexia or bulimia. People with eating disorders place so much value on their appearance that it begins to define their self-worth to an exclusive degree.

Behavioral features of body image disturbance are manifested in a lifestyle that revolves around a self-concern about the body. Examples of such behaviors include constantly measuring body weight, wearing baggy clothes, and avoiding social situations in which appearance might be scrutinized. Overestimation of body size or of a body part is a common perceptual distortion in anorexia and bulimia.

When intervening in body image problems, the nurse should first determine whether the patient has problems with perception, attitude, or behavior and then devise a treatment program targeting the specific problem area. Cognitive behavioral interventions are effective, as are dance and move-

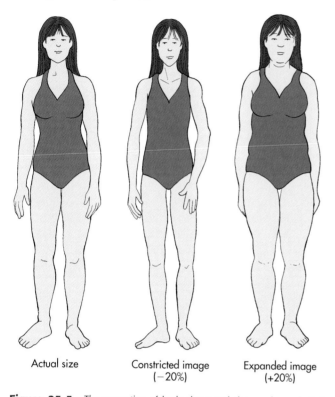

Actual size   Constricted image   Expanded image
                        (−20%)   (+20%)

Figure 25-5   The perception of body shape and size can be evaluated through the use of special computer drawing programs that allow a subject to distort the width of an actual picture of a person's body by as much as 20%, larger or smaller. Both anorectic and normal subjects adjusted the figures of other people's bodies to normal dimension. However, anorectic subjects consistently adjusted their own body picture to a size 20% larger than its true form, which suggests they have a major problem with the perception of self-image.

Table 25-3	Consequences of Maladaptive Eating Regulation Responses	
	POSITIVE CONSEQUENCES	NEGATIVE CONSEQUENCES
Biological	Reduced fear of fatness	Weakness, fatigue, dizziness
	Reduced perception of hunger	Poor concentration
	Avoidance of biological maturity	Electrolyte disturbance
		Dental problems
Psychological	Relief from tension, anger, and stress	Depression, guilt, shame
	Relief from boredom	Tendency to overreact emotionally
	Emotional anesthesia	Increase in negative self-reference or guilt-related behavior
	Feelings of nurturance or pleasure	
	Thoughts about avoiding weight gain	
Sociocultural	Avoidance of interpersonal conflict	Social withdrawal
	Social reinforcement for not gaining weight	Lying and lack of trust in relationships
	Distraction from unpleasant tasks	Occupational problems
	Avoidance of responsibility and independence	Financial problems
		Legal problems

ment therapies, which create pleasant body experiences and can enhance the integration of mind and body, clarify body boundaries, and modulate negative feelings about the body (Cash and Pruzinsky, 2002). Other therapeutic approaches include the use of imagery and relaxation, working with mirrors, and depicting the self through art.

Family Involvement

Families should be engaged from the beginning of treatment and included in family meetings and treatment planning sessions. The nurse should gather information about the family system and explore how the maladaptive eating response might serve a specific function within the family. Questions the nurse might ask include the following:

- What part does the eating disorder serve in stabilizing the family system?

A FAMILY SPEAKS

We have a 19-year-old daughter who has had an eating disorder for 8 years. These past 8 years have been most painful for our family—we went from doctor to doctor, counselor to counselor, and therapist to therapist, all with little or no results. What clinicians don't realize is how hard the day-to-day struggle is for families who want so much for their child to be healthy and happy but who feel so helpless in knowing how to make this happen.

Then we were referred to a nurse who specialized in eating disorders, and slowly our lives began to change. Clearly, this nurse knew about our daughter's illness, and together we went about treating it. We went through individual and family therapy, all in an attempt to help our daughter recover. At times it was painful and even frustrating. In the family sessions the nurse helped family members be aware of the part they had to play in our daughter's struggle and helped us realize that it would take a family team effort to help her get well. The most important part is that all of the hard work of our daughter, each family member, and our nurse has been worth it. Our daughter now knows how to control her eating disorder. She has had very few problems in the last 6 months, and our family has become even closer as we look back on the past with relief and into the future with hope.

- How has the family attempted to deal with the eating disorder?
- What is the central theme surrounding the eating behavior?
- What would be the consequences of change for each family member?
- What is the underlying therapeutic issue from a family perspective?

Many young patients need intensive family therapy after successfully completing the refeeding stage. The initial issue of such therapy is centered on the separation and individuation of the patient within the context of the family. This process requires much openness on the part of the family, and not every family may be able to complete the process. However, the nurse should work with identified family strengths and help involved family members work toward change (see A Family Speaks). Family therapy is described in more detail in Chapter 33.

Group Therapies

Many models of group therapy are used for patients with eating disorders, including cognitive-behavioral, psychoeducational, psychodynamic, and interpersonal models. Reality testing, support, and communicating with peers are essential therapeutic factors provided by group intervention. In addition, outpatient support groups may be helpful if they reinforce social alliances and encourage members to identify and express feelings. Therapeutic groups are described in detail in Chapter 32.

Medications

Patients with anorexia often resist medication, and no drugs have been found to be completely effective for this disorder. Medications should not be used as the sole or primary treatment for anorexia. The role of antidepressants is usually best assessed following weight gain, when the psychological effects of malnutrition are resolving (American Psychiatric Association, 2000a).

An antidepressant medication may be helpful with comorbid depression, mood swings or irritability, and obsessions about food and fat. Clinical trials of the atypical antipsychotic olanzapine to promote weight gain in anorexia nervosa are underway (Table 25-4).

Table 25-4	Strength of Evidence of Randomized Pharmacological Trials in Eating Disorders		
	ANTIPSYCHOTICS	ANTIDEPRESSANTS (ACUTE TREATMENT) (SSRIs)	ANTIDEPRESSANTS (RELAPSE PREVENTION) (SSRIs)
Anorexia nervosa	Not recommended	Not recommended	Modest
Bulimia nervosa	Not recommended	Considerable	Modest
Binge eating disorder (BED)*	Modest	Modest	None
Atypical eating disorder (e.g., night eating syndrome)	None	None	None

Modified from Fairburn, CG, Harrison, PH: *Lancet* 361: 407:2003.
None, no control trials done; *Modest,* slight beneficial effect based on more than four studies of less than superior quality; *Considerable,* some beneficial effect based on between 2 to 10 trials of superior quality.
*Limited (slightly modest) evidence (more than three controlled studies) for the use of mood stabilizer topiramate (Topamax) to control bingeing in BED.

Table 25-5	NURSING TREATMENT PLAN SUMMARY	Eating Regulation Reponses

Nursing Diagnosis: Imbalanced nutrition: more than body requirements
Expected Outcome: The patient will restore healthy patterns and normalize physiological parameters related to body weight and nutrition.

SHORT-TERM GOAL	INTERVENTION	RATIONALE
The patient will engage in treatment and acknowledge having an eating disorder.	Help the patient identify maladaptive eating responses. Discuss the positive and negative consequences of maladaptive eating responses. Contract with the patient to engage in treatment.	The first step of treatment is for the patient to acknowledge the illness and see the need for help.
The patient will be able to describe a balanced diet based on the five food groups.	Complete a nutritional assessment, including eating-related behaviors and preferences. Teach, clarify, and reinforce the patient's knowledge of proper nutrition.	Knowledge of healthy nutrition is essential to establishing and maintaining adaptive eating responses.
The patient's nutritional status will be stabilized by a specified date.	Monitor physiological status for signs of compromised nutrition. Administer medications and somatic treatments for the management of symptoms. Monitor and evaluate the patient's response to somatic treatments. Implement nursing activities as specified in the program contract and protocol.	Weight stabilization must be a central and early goal for the nutritionally compromised patient. Medications may assist the appetite regulation center and neurochemical response to feeding and satiety.
The patient will participate in a balanced exercise program on a daily basis.	Review established exercise routines. Modify exercise patterns, focusing on physical fitness rather than on weight reduction. Reinforce new exercise and fitness behaviors.	The focus of a balanced exercise program should be on physical fitness rather than on caloric reduction to lose weight.

Table 25-6	NURSING TREATMENT PLAN SUMMARY	Eating Regulation Reponses

Nursing Diagnosis: Disturbed body image
Expected Outcome: The patient will express clear and accurate descriptions of body size, body boundaries, and ideal weight.

SHORT-TERM GOAL	INTERVENTION	RATIONALE
The patient will correct body image distortions.	Modify body image misperceptions through cognitive and behavioral strategies. Use dance and movement therapies to enhance the integration of mind and body. Use imagery and relaxation interventions to decrease anxiety related to body perceptions.	Body image distortions involve perceptions, attitudes, and behaviors that place so much emphasis on appearance that they define self-worth.
The patient will modify cognitive distortions about body weight, shape, and eating responses.	Help the patient identify cues that trigger problematic eating responses and body image concerns; the thoughts, feelings, and assumptions associated with each cue; the connections between these thoughts, feelings, assumptions, and eating regulation responses; and the consequences of the eating responses.	Cognitive distortions result in lowered self-esteem. Behavioral change results from an increased awareness of feelings and faulty cognitions.
The patient will identify social support systems that will reinforce accurate body perceptions and adaptive eating responses.	Include family members in the evaluation and treatment planning process. Assess the family as a system and the impact of the eating disorder on family functioning. Initiate group therapy to mobilize social support and reinforce adaptive responses.	Patients with eating disorders benefit from the involvement of family members and supportive group work.

In the treatment of bulimia, studies have shown that antidepressant medications have a therapeutic effect on many patients (Nakash-Eisenvits et al, 2002). Medication-induced benefits include decreases in the frequency of binge eating and weight regulatory behaviors such as vomiting. The mood stabilizer topiramate also may have some positive effects (McElroy et al., 2003). Chapter 27 discusses these medications in detail. They are most effective when used with other psychotherapeutic interventions.

A Nursing Treatment Plan Summary for a patient with imbalanced nutrition is presented in Table 25-5. A Nursing Treatment Plan Summary for a patient with disturbed body image is presented in Table 25-6.

EVALUATION

Patients with maladaptive eating regulation responses present special challenges to psychiatric nursing care. The evaluation of their care should begin with a focus on the therapeutic nurse-patient relationship. Nurses should determine whether they have provided effective role modeling, emotional support, biological monitoring, and reinforcement of the patient's attempts to explore and experiment with new cognitive and behavior patterns. Evaluation activities can then address three specific aspects of care:

1. Have normal eating patterns been restored?
2. Have the biological and psychological sequelae of malnutrition been corrected?
3. Have the associated sociocultural and behavioral problems been resolved so that relapse does not occur?

In answering these questions, the nurse should review each aspect of the nursing process and modify care as needed to achieve the identified outcomes.

COMPETENT CARING

A Clinical Exemplar of a Psychiatric Nurse
LEIGH ALEXANDER, RN, MSN, ARNP

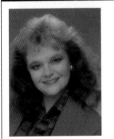

I entered the community meeting to find only one seat open—beside a newly admitted patient. Little did I realize how this opportunity would impact my understanding of how a person with anorexia survives each day.

The patient, L, was pale and thin and had open sores on her extremities from self-harm actions. She had short brown hair that had lost its luster and was broken off at the ends. Long lashes fringed her blue eyes, which darted about the room. Her appearance was like a frail rag doll with very little muscle tone. I could see the protruding veins in her hands and noted the slow pulse beating in her temple. She was 30 years old and currently unemployed. Her diminished physical status no longer allowed her to work as a day care attendant in a senior citizen center. In addition, the complexity of her illness had caused her to drop the college courses she was taking towards earning a degree in health education. The meeting began and so did our therapeutic relationship.

Each day, L would struggle with consuming adequate calories to meet her physiological demands. Her obsession to overexercise and restrict her intake was the major treatment battle. With intense inpatient supervision, L was able to progress to a day treatment program. She returned to part-time employment working with the elderly and also began to enter local and regional sporting events. Her name began to appear in the newspaper—she took first, second, or third place in many of the competitive sporting events she enjoyed.

Our treatment goals focused on caloric levels, exercise, self-esteem, body image, and relationships. L had been overweight at one time in her life and was terrified that she would be fat once again. Using cognitive behavioral therapy, we focused on eliminating self-harm behaviors. I often wondered how this unique person, who was so bright, giving, and creative, could survive with minimal nutritional intake and the relentless compulsions to be thin and to hurt herself. Her cracked, dry lips were often my first indicator that she was restricting her intake too much—sometimes to the degree that periodic hospitalizations were necessary to provide safety, stabilization, and further education.

I am pleased to say that L has survived this harrowing experience with anorexia. She is now in her mid 30s. Periodically, she writes me of her progress. She continues weekly individual therapy and has entered a university to further her education. Her appearance has changed. Her features are tanned and trim. Her slight build now has well defined muscles. She styles her hair, and the self-harm episodes have decreased in frequency. Her eyes now shine with the increased knowledge of her self-worth and positive body image. Her love of sports is rarely impeded by her eating disorder, although occasional lapses of appropriate caloric intake do still occur. But, over time, L has learned to individualized her dietary regimen to accommodate her physiological and psychological demands.

I knew she was following the path to recovery when the letters she sent me no longer closed with "Love, L." She now closes her letters without the word "love" and confidently uses her entire name. ■

CHAPTER **FOCUS POINTS**

- Adaptive eating regulation responses include balanced eating patterns, appropriate caloric intake, and body weight that is appropriate for height.
- Maladaptive responses include anorexia nervosa, bulimia nervosa, binge eating disorder, and night eating syndrome.

- Eating disorders are more commonly seen among females, with a male-to-female ratio ranging from 1:6 to 1:10. They occur in 1% to 4% of adolescent and young adult women.
- These disorders can cause biological changes that include altered metabolic rates, profound malnutrition, and possibly death. Obses-

Continued

CHAPTER FOCUS POINTS—cont'd

- sions about eating can cause psychological problems that include depression, isolation, and emotional lability. Sociocultural norms may result in a distorted body image.
- Assessment of patients should include a full physical examination, dental examination, and psychiatric history.
- Patient behaviors related to eating regulation responses include binge eating, fasting or restricting, and purging. Medical complications can include starvation, potassium depletion, and hypokalemia. Psychiatric complications include comorbid depression, anxiety disorders, and substance abuse.
- Both anorexia nervosa and bulimia nervosa are familial. Models of biological predisposing factors are focused on the hypothalamus and serotonin and dopamine levels.
- Psychological, environmental, and sociocultural factors also can predispose an individual to the development of an eating disorder.
- Precipitating stressors that affect eating responses include peer pressure, interpersonal rejection, and daily solitude.
- The patient's level of motivation to change his or her behavior is an important coping resource to assess.

- A variety of maladaptive coping mechanisms may be used, including denial, avoidance, intellectualization, and isolation of affect.
- Primary NANDA nursing diagnoses are anxiety, disturbed body image, imbalanced nutrition, powerlessness, chronic or situational low self-esteem and risk for self-mutilation.
- Primary *DSM-IV-TR* diagnoses are anorexia nervosa, bulimia nervosa, and binge eating disorder. Night eating syndrome is under consideration for inclusion in the *DSM-IV-TR* as a separate disorder.
- The expected outcome of nursing care is that the patient will restore healthy eating patterns and normalize physiological parameters related to body weight and nutrition.
- Planning activities involve decisions related to choice of treatment setting and the formulation of a nursing care plan contract.
- Interventions include nutrition stabilization, exercise, cognitive behavioral interventions, body image interventions, family involvement, group therapies, and medications.
- The nurse and patient together should evaluate whether normal eating patterns have been restored and whether associated biopsychosocial problems have been resolved.

KEY TERMS

anorexia nervosa, 519
binge eating, 520

bulimia nervosa, 519
purging, 520

CHAPTER REVIEW QUESTIONS

1. Match each term in Column A with the correct definition in Column B.

Column A

_____ Maladaptive eating regulation responses

_____ SSRIs

_____ Adaptive eating regulation responses

_____ Predisposing factors

_____ Serotonin

Column B

A. Balanced eating patterns, caloric intake, and weight

B. Neurotransmitter implicated in eating disorders

C. Anorexia, bulimia, binge eating disorder, night eating syndrome

D. Treatments for eating disorders

E. Biological, psychological, environmental, sociocultural

2. Fill in the blanks.

A. The majority of eating disorders occur in _____, and they may range from _____% to _____% of adolescents and young adults.

B. _____ is the rapid consumption of large quantities food in a discrete period of time.

C. Maladaptive coping mechanisms that may affect motivation for change in eating patterns and therefore must be assessed by the nurse include _____, _____, _____, and _____.

D. A patient states, "If I eat one piece of cake at my brother's wedding, I'll never be able to stop." This is an example of

_____.

E. The most effective treatment for eating disorders is

_____.

3. Provide short answers for the following questions.

A. What are the differences between individuals with anorexia nervosa and bulimia in the areas of weight loss, hunger, and personality features?

B. What is the expected outcome of nursing care for the patient with an eating disorder?

C. Keep a food diary for 1 week and list your thoughts about each meal. Ask a friend/classmate to evaluate it.

D. Design an eating disorder treatment contract that would help improve your eating patterns and one that you think would be helpful for one of your friends or colleagues. What are the essential differences between the two?

E. How would you explain the differences in cultural support and stigma for the person with obesity and for the person with anorexia nervosa?

Visit Evolve for additional resources related to the content of this chapter.
http://evolve.elsevier.com/Stuart/principles/
• Topical Course Outline • Student Workbook Exercises • Critical Thinking Questions and Activities • Case Studies • Research Topics
• Monthly Content Updates • WebLinks

Student Study CD-ROM

Access the accompanying CD-ROM for animations, interactive exercises, review questions for the NCLEX examination, and an audio glossary.

REFERENCES

American Psychiatric Association: Practice guidelines for the treatment of patients with eating disorders (revision), *Am J Psychiatry* 157:1, 2000a.

American Psychiatric Association: *Diagnostic and statistical manual of mental disorders*, ed 4, text revision, Washington, DC, 2000b, American Psychiatric Association.

Anderluh MB et al: Childhood obsessive-compulsive personality traits in adult women with eating disorders: defining a broader eating disorder phenotype, *Am J Psychiatry* 160:242, 2003.

Audenaert K et al: Decreased 5-HT2a receptor binding in patients with anorexia nervosa, *J Nucl Med* 44:163, 2003.

Brink PT, Ferguson K, Sharma A: Childhood memories about food: the Successful Dieters Project, *J Child Adolesc Psychiatr Nurs* 12:17, 1999.

Bulik CM et al: Significant linkage on chromosome 10p in families with bulimia nervosa, *Am J Hum Genet* 72:200, 2003a.

Bulik CM et al: The relation between eating disorders and components of perfectionism, *Am J Psychiatry* 160:366, 2003b.

Cash TF, Pruzinsky T, editors: *Body image: a handbook of theory, practice and research*, Carlsbed, 2002, Gurze Books.

Fairburn CG, Shafran R, Cooper Z: A cognitive behavioural theory of anorexia nervosa, *Behav Res Ther* 37:1, 1999.

Fairburn C et al: The natural course of bulimia nervosa and binge eating disorder in young women, *Arch Gen Psychiatry* 57:559, 2000.

Frank GK et al: Reduced 5-HT2A receptor binding after recovery from anorexia nervosa, *Biol Psychiatry* 52:896, 2002.

Geller J: Estimating readiness for change in anorexia nervosa: comparing clients, clinicians, and research assessors, *Int J Eat Disord* 31:251, 2002.

Grilo C: The assessment and treatment of binge eating disorder, *J Pract Psychiatr Behav Health* 4:191, 1998.

Greeno CG, Wing RR, Shiffman S: Binge antecedents in obese women with and without binge eating disorder, *J Consult Clin Psychol* 68:95, 2000.

Jimerson DC: Leptin and the neurobiology of eating disorders, *J Lab Clin Med* 139:70, 2002.

Keel PK et al: Long-term outcome of bulimia nervosa, *Arch Gen Psychiatry* 56:63, 1999.

Keel PK et al: Predictors of mortality in eating disorders, *Arch Gen Psychiatry* 60:179, 2003.

Klump KL et al: Does environment matter? A review of nonshared environment and eating disorders, *Int J Eat Disord* 31:118, 2002.

McElroy SL et al: Topiramate in the treatment of binge eating disorder associated with obesity: a randomized, placebo-controlled trial, *Am J Psychiatry* 160:255, 2003.

McKnight Investigators: Risk factors for the onset of eating disorders in adolescent girls: results of the McKnight longitudinal risk factor study, *Am J Psychiatry* 160:248, 2003.

Nakash-Eisenvits O et al: A multidimensional meta-analysis of pharmacotherapy for bulimia nervosa: summarizing the range of outcomes in clinical trials, *Harv Rev Psychiatry* 10:193, 2002.

Nathan PE, Gorman JM: *A guide to treatments that work*, ed 2, New York, 2002, Oxford University Press.

Pritts SD, Susman J: Diagnosis of eating disorders in primary care, *Am Fam Physician* 67:297, 2003.

Reas DL et al: Duration of illness predicts outcome for bulimia nervosa: a long-term follow-up study, *Int J Eat Disord* 27:428, 2000.

Stein KF, Corte C: Reconceptualizing causative factors and intervention strategies in the eating disorders: a shift from body image to self-concept impairments, *Arch Psychiatr Nurs* 17:57, 2003.

Steinhausen HC: The outcome of anorexia nervosa in the 20th century, *Am J Psychiatry* 159:1284, 2002.

Striegel-Moore RH et al: One-year use and cost of inpatient and outpatient services among female and male patients with an eating disorder: evidence from a national database of health insurance claims, *Int J Eat Disord* 27:381, 2000.

Striegel-Moore RH et al: Eating disorders in white and black women, *Am J Psychiatry* 160:1326, 2003.

Strober M et al: Controlled family study of anorexia nervosa and bulimia nervosa: evidence of shared liability and transmission of partial syndromes, *Am J Psychiatry* 157:393, 2000.

Strunkard A, Allison K: Two forms of disordered eating in obesity, binge eating and night eating, *Int J Obes Related Metab Disord* 27:1, 2003.

Tanaka M et al: Increased fasting plasma gherlin: Levels in patients with bulimia nervosa, *Eur J Endocrinol* 146:R1, 2002.

Vitiello B, Lederhendler I: Research on eating disorders: current status and future prospects, *Biol Psychiatry* 47:777, 2000.

Vitousek K, Watson S, Wilson GT: Enhancing motivation for change in treatment-resistant eating disorders, *Clin Psychol Rev* 18:391, 1998.

Wade TD et al: Anorexia nervosa and major depression: shared genetic and environmental risk factors, *Am J Psychiatry* 157:469, 2000.

Wang G et al: Brain dopamine and obesity, *Lancet* 357:354, 2001.

White JH: The prevention of eating disorders: a review of the research on risk factors with implications for practice, *J Child Adolesc Psychiatr Nurs* 13:76, 2000.

Whittal M et al: Review: medication and cognitive behaviour therapy control symptoms of bulimia nervosa, *Behav Ther* 30:117, 1999.

Wonderlich SA et al: Eating disturbance and sexual trauma in childhood and adulthood, *Int J Eat Disord* 30:401, 2001.

Woodside DB et al: Comparisons of men with full or partial eating disorders, men without eating disorders, and women with eating disorders in the community, *Am J Psychiatry* 158:570, 2001.

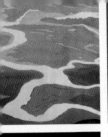

I locked myself away from you Too long, Tossing aside my feelings For you. Looking for a way out, an excuse Not to touch you; Because I want to, Inciting a riot within me. To reach out for you Is difficult, But less difficult Than turning away.

LESLIE BERTEL

26 SEXUAL RESPONSES AND SEXUAL DISORDERS

Susan G. Poorman

LEARNING OBJECTIVES

After studying this chapter, the student should be able to:
1. Describe the continuum of adaptive and maladaptive sexual responses (I).
2. Identify behaviors associated with sexual responses (II).
3. Analyze predisposing factors, precipitating stressors, and appraisal of stressors related to sexual responses (II).
4. Describe coping resources and coping mechanisms related to sexual responses (II).
5. Formulate nursing diagnoses related to sexual responses (III).
6. Examine the relationship between nursing diagnoses and medical diagnoses related to sexual responses (III).
7. Identify expected outcomes and short-term nursing goals related to sexual responses (IV).
8. Develop a patient education plan to promote adaptive sexual responses (V).
9. Analyze nursing interventions related to sexual responses (VI).
10. Evaluate nursing care related to sexual responses (VII).

evolve Visit Evolve for additional resources related to the content of this chapter.
http://evolve.elsevier.com/Stuart/principles/

Sexuality broadly refers to all aspects of being sexual and is one dimension of the personality. It includes more than the act of intercourse and is an integral part of life. It is evident in the person's appearance and in beliefs, behaviors, and relationships with others. Four aspects of sexuality are as follows:

- **Genetic identity,** which is a person's chromosomal gender
- **Gender identity,** which is a person's perception of his or her own maleness or femaleness
- **Gender role,** which is the cultural role attributes of one's gender, such as expectations regarding behavior, cognitions, occupations, values, and emotional responses
- **Sexual orientation,** which is the gender to which one is romantically attracted

Accepting a broad concept of sexuality allows nurses to explore ways in which people are sexual beings and understand more fully their feelings, beliefs, and actions. Nurses are often called on to intervene in the sexual concerns of pa-

tients when providing holistic patient care. Therefore it is important to develop skills and competence in addressing sexual issues by increasing awareness through education.

As nurses become educated in the basic principles of sexuality, they will better understand sexual needs and problems. If nurses are comfortable with sexual issues, they will convey this to the patient, who will feel more comfortable in discussing these issues. Patients are often experiencing pain and change as a result of threats to health or even as a part of normal growth and development. Thus it is important that the nurse-patient relationship allow for honest discussions about sexuality.

In answering the question, **What do nurses need to know about sexuality?,** several factors emerge (Lamp et al, 2000). First, nurses need to know themselves and be aware of their feelings and values regarding sexuality. If nurses are not aware of their feelings, they cannot help patients meet their needs. Second, nurses need to understand that other people's feelings and values about sexuality may be different from their own. Third, all nurses can become educated about sexual health and use sound counseling methods with patients. Specifically, nurses can:

- Develop confidence in their ability to discuss sexual issues with patients.
- Learn interviewing skills for sexual assessment and history taking.
- Counsel or refer patients for counseling.

Education can be gained through nursing courses and continuing education programs. Some nurses pursue additional education and may become sex educators in schools, outpatient clinics, and planned parenthood agencies. Nurses prepared at the graduate level may become sex therapists through postgraduate work in human sexuality and extensive clinical supervision.

■ CONTINUUM OF SEXUAL RESPONSES

Adaptive and Maladaptive Sexual Responses

Experts in sexuality do not agree on what is normal sexual behavior. For years many people believed that only sexual relations between married heterosexual partners for procreation were normal. Today people view sexual behavior with a wider range of attitudes. Sexuality, on a continuum, ranges from adaptive to maladaptive (Figure 26-1). The most adaptive responses meet the following criteria: **between two consenting adults, mutually satisfying to both, not psychologically or physically harmful to either, lacking in force or coercion, and conducted in private.**

Sometimes, however, sexual behavior can meet the criteria for adaptive responses and yet be altered by what society deems acceptable and unacceptable. Unfortunately, society often decides this based on fear, prejudice, and lack of information rather than on data and facts (see Critical Thinking About Contemporary Issues). For example, the homosexual person may have the potential for healthy responses but be impaired by anxiety concerning societal disapproval.

Maladaptive sexual responses include **behaviors that do not meet one or more of the criteria for adaptive responses.** The degree to which these behaviors are maladaptive varies. Some sexual behaviors may not meet any of the criteria mentioned. For example, incest may include force and be psychologically harmful. However, other sexual responses may meet four of the five criteria for adaptive responses but still be maladaptive.

Caution must be used when attempting to label sexual behaviors as adaptive or maladaptive. There will always be disagreements and exceptions to the rule. The continuum shown in Figure 26-1 is free of moral judgment and was developed to help the nurse in developing self-awareness and in understanding the range of sexual responses.

How do you define "normal" sexuality? Compare your views with those of a friend, a family member, and a health care provider. ■

Critical Thinking *About* Contemporary Issues

Does Sex Education in Schools Promote Teenage Promiscuity?

Some people believe that teenagers are sexually active because they are taught sex education in their schools. The issue of sex education for youth in this country has raised a storm of questions and controversy. Unfortunately, much of the controversy is based on values, beliefs, and personal opinion instead of facts. People who oppose sex education fight against comprehensive sex education programs in public schools. They believe some topics should be excluded. In contrast, many parents believe that their children are indeed receiving comprehensive sex education in school when often they are not being given all the facts.

Research provides some answers to this controversial question. Studies have demonstrated that comprehensive sex education programs can delay the initiation of first intercourse, reduce unprotected intercourse, and decrease unwanted teen pregnancy. Based on these findings, along with the rising incidence of teen pregnancy and sexually transmitted diseases, the more important question this country faces is whether we can afford *not* to provide comprehensive sex education in our schools.

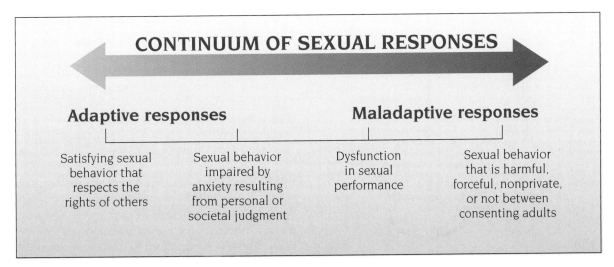

Figure 26-1   Continuum of sexual responses.

Self-Awareness of the Nurse

The nurse's level of self-awareness is a critical component of discussions with patients regarding sexual issues. The first step in developing self-awareness involves clarification of values regarding human sexuality. Figure 26-2 illustrates four phases of the nurse's growth: cognitive dissonance, anxiety, anger, and action (Foley and Davies, 1983).

Cognitive Dissonance. The first phase of growth in developing sexual self-awareness is cognitive dissonance, which arises when two opposing beliefs exist at the same time. For example, nurses grow up learning what society, family, and friends believe about sexual issues. If a nurse is raised in an environment that teaches "it is impolite to talk about sex; it's too personal a subject," the nurse will carry that belief into nurs-

ing practice. When a patient wants to discuss a sexual concern, the nurse may feel two opposing reactions simultaneously: "I should not ask questions about a subject as personal as sex" and "As a professional, I should be able to discuss any problem, including sexual problems, with my patient."

These opposing thoughts, based on differing role expectations, make the nurse uncomfortable. However, the discomfort can be positive because it forces the nurse to examine feelings about the issue. The nurse resolves the cognitive dissonance in one of two ways: by continuing to believe that sexual concerns are too personal to discuss with patients or by examining the fact that sexuality is an integral part of being human.

Both of these beliefs have consequences that involve how the nurse relates to patients who voice sexual concerns. If the nurse continues to believe that sex is too personal to discuss with the patient, the nurse may become uncomfortable and choose not to follow up on sexual issues. This discomfort may be projected onto the patient, with the nurse stating, "The patient seemed too upset to talk about that right now." In this case, the nurse should explore personal values and beliefs about sexuality and ask, "Do I believe these ideas about discussing sexual concerns because I have researched the facts and have accurate, current information?" Only when the nurse has examined the available information and made an informed choice on values will clarification of those values occur. If the nurse examines personal and professional values and believes that sexuality is an integral part of being human, a second phase of growth occurs.

Anxiety. Most people think that anxiety is a negative emotion. However, a mild level of anxiety can be positive because it can promote an awareness of danger, give extra energy, or stimulate professional growth by creating enough discomfort to initiate some type of action. In this second phase, the nurse realizes that uncertainty, insecurity, questions, and problems regarding sexuality are normal. The nurse begins to understand that everyone is capable of a variety of sexual feelings and behaviors and that anyone can have a sexual dysfunction or question sexual identity.

The nurse experiencing anxiety may exhibit behaviors that hinder the discussion of sexual issues, such as talking too much (not allowing patients to express their feelings), failing to listen (not picking up on patients' cues and messages), and diagnosing and analyzing (becoming preoccupied with facts rather than feelings). As the anxiety level rises, the nurse becomes more uncomfortable and tries to reduce that feeling. Learning about sexuality and facing conflicting values bring the nurse to the third phase of growth.

Anger. Anger generally arises after anxiety, fear, and shock subside. It is generally self-directed or directed toward the patient or society. The nurse begins to recognize that issues associated with sex or sexuality are emotional and sometimes highly volatile. Rape, abortion, birth control, equal rights, child abuse, pornography, and religious issues all are related to sexuality and give rise to controversy and debate. This re-

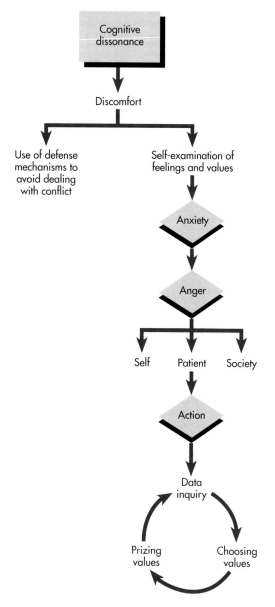

Figure 26-2   Phases of the nurse's growth in developing awareness of human sexuality.

alization often breeds anger and contempt in the nurse. For example, the nurse may become angry at a colleague or a friend who makes judgmental remarks about pro-life or pro-choice activists.

During this phase of anger the nurse tends to choose words and actions that may be as judgmental as the attitudes the nurse is fighting against. The nurse may lecture other nurses about the need for sex education or critically judge a teenager who does not fear the consequences of having unprotected sex with someone known to be human immunodeficiency virus (HIV) positive. The nurse also may be angry with society for perpetuating ignorance about sexuality. Toward the end of this phase, the nurse begins to understand that blaming self or society for lack of proper awareness does not help patients with sexual concerns. This realization helps defuse the anger, and the nurse is then ready for the final phase.

Action. The final step in the growth experience is the action phase. Several behaviors emerge during this final phase of the growth experience: **data inquiry, choosing values,** and **prizing values.** Data inquiry occurs when the nurse seeks out additional information about sexual issues. Once the information is obtained, the nurse may discuss and debate the issues. These are healthy ways of exploring and deciding what to believe, and the nurse will eventually make some choices about a value position.

The final behavior is prizing the value position, which is an awareness and cherishing of feelings and values and being willing to share them publicly. Although prizing values is the final step in a positive growth experience, it does not mean that what is valued will not change. Values are never static; they evolve and shift as a person changes, grows, and acquires new experiences. Thus a person who once opposed abortion may later become understanding and empathetic toward women who have abortions.

The following clinical example shows the growth health professionals experience while increasing their awareness about sexuality. Chapter 2 has additional content on developing self-awareness and the nurse's therapeutic use of self.

CLINICAL EXAMPLE

Carol was a new staff nurse at a rehabilitation hospital. At the monthly staff meeting the nursing supervisor asked whether there were any concerns the staff would like to discuss. Carol offered, "I wonder if any of you could help me with a suggestion. Over the past several weeks I've seen a number of patients masturbating. One patient was in the lounge and another was in his room when I came in to give him his meds. I was so embarrassed I didn't know what to do. I just ignored it both times, but part of me wanted to say 'stop that you dirty old man—that's not appropriate for a hospital!' I guess I could use some help with this one." Another staff nurse followed up and said, "That's what I feel like saying when I see that kind of behavior." Several other staff in the room began to snicker. The nursing supervisor interrupted and asked, "Can anyone give Carol some suggestions on how to handle this situation therapeutically?" After several moments of silence, other staff members admitted that they too were uncomfortable dealing with patients who were masturbating.

With the help of the supervisor, the staff began to brainstorm about how to handle this situation. Staff agreed that dealing with patients who are masturbating is a difficult issue for many nurses, and that the problem is most often the nurses' rather than the patients' because masturbation is a normal form of sexual expression. They decided that when they observe a patient masturbating in a public area, an appropriate nursing response would be to have the patient return to his or her room for privacy. If a nurse walks in on a patient masturbating in his or her room, the nurse should ensure the patient's privacy by excusing himself or herself and telling the patient he or she will return at a later time. ■

In which phase of growth are you in relation to the development of awareness of human sexuality? ■

ASSESSMENT

Any basic health history must include questions about sexual history. A nurse who is comfortable discussing sexuality conveys the message that it is normal to talk about sexual health in a health assessment interview. If nurses can be composed and professional, they can ask questions about patients' sexual health naturally. The patient can then discuss sexual matters openly and without embarrassment.

Effective interviewing skills are an essential part of a sexual assessment. At times, nurses may be uncomfortable when addressing sexual issues. However, the principles of effective interviewing are the same even when addressing sexual issues. **Open-ended questions** are one of the most effective ways of promoting a discussion on sexual issues, although some nurses report that direct questions also can be helpful in opening up the subject. Regardless, it is important to remember that questions must be asked at the patient's level of understanding, with sensitivity to the patient's cultural background, because each person is unique.

The time and number of questions needed to discuss a problem vary depending on the patient. Often just a few questions during an interview will obtain the relevant information. Examples of questions nurses may ask related to a patient's sexual health include the following:

- Tell me what you understand about (menstruation, intercourse, sexual changes with aging, menopause).
- Since you've been diagnosed, what questions have you had regarding your sexuality?
- Are there any changes you've noticed in your sexual patterns since becoming ill?
- Have you noticed any differences or problems in your sexual responses since taking this medication?
- Often people have questions about (masturbation, sexual frequency, safe sex, alternate positions).
- Sometimes it is uncomfortable to talk about sexual issues with your partner. How is this for you and your partner?

Behaviors

There are many modes of sexual expression. In a classic work, Kinsey (1953) suggested that most people are not exclusively heterosexual or homosexual. His studies indicated that a substantial percentage of men and women had experienced both heterosexual and homosexual activity.

Heterosexuality. Heterosexuality can be defined as sexual attraction to members of the opposite sex. It is the predominant sexual orientation among people in American society. The coupling of a man and a woman in a sexual partnership has both legal and religious sanctions. As such, it influences the culture, values, and norms of contemporary American life.

Homosexuality. Homosexuality can be defined as sexual attraction to members of the same sex. The term **gay** is used to refer to both male and female homosexuals; however, some use the term to refer only to male homosexuals and use the term **lesbian** to refer to female homosexuals. A person's attraction to people of the same sex, opposite sex, or both sexes is called sexual orientation or *sexual preference*. Some prefer the term *sexual orientation* over *sexual preference* because preference implies that homosexuals choose to be homosexual. Although sexual behaviors do involve choice, research has indicated that sexual orientation is affected by genetics and biochemical events (Altemeyer, 2001).

It is difficult to estimate the actual incidence of homosexuality in this country. The estimates have ranged from 3% to 10% of the population (King, 1999). However, many people have had a sexual experience with a member of the same sex at one time in their lives, and this is typically not identified when surveys are taken. One of the reasons that it is difficult to obtain an accurate incidence of homosexuality is that considerable social stigma is still attached to labeling oneself as homosexual, so it is possible that many individuals do not report their true sexual identity.

Throughout history many theories have been postulated concerning the origin of homosexuality. Although there is no conclusive evidence to support any one specific cause, most researchers agree that both biological and social factors influence the development of sexual orientation. Some sexuality experts question our need to find a cause for homosexuality rather than simply accepting the fact that it exists. If current estimates of homosexuality are accurate, nurses come into contact with homosexuals daily but often know little about homosexuality and often assume that all patients are heterosexual.

How are health care providers' views of homosexuality influenced by social norms and cultural values? ■

Bisexuality. Bisexuality is defined as a sexual orientation or attraction to both men and women. Many studies on bisexuality include homosexuals in their research samples, and this has made the understanding of bisexuality more difficult. Bisexuality can be viewed from different perspectives. Some people believe that it is a distinct sexual orientation, whereas others view bisexuality as a transition from one sexual orientation to another. Still others contend that bisexuality can be an individual's attempt to deny a true homosexual identity. Very few people actually identify themselves as being bisexual (Miracle, Miracle, and Baumeister, 2003).

Interest in the behavior and characteristics of bisexual men has increased in light of the acquired immunodeficiency syndrome (AIDS) epidemic and the need to design effective preventive interventions for HIV infection. One problem that has been identified with bisexual orientation is that the sexual risk behaviors of bisexual men are quite high. However, their lack of identification with and participation in the homosexual community make them unlikely to be reached by the gay community's safe sex and AIDS prevention programs.

Transvestism. Transvestism is defined as cross-dressing, or dressing in the clothes of the opposite sex. Most often the transvestite who seeks treatment is a male; very little is known about female transvestism. No reliable statistics concerning the incidence of transvestism are available, but many professionals believe it is more common than generally assumed.

Transvestites tend to be married men who report heterosexual behavior. Although they occasionally or frequently dress in female clothes, they do not want hormonal or surgical sex change. Many transvestites try to find willing partners, and typically their activities of cross-dressing do not prevent sexual relationships with others.

Transsexualism. The term *transsexual* simply implies going from one sex to another. Transsexualism is a condition in which one has a profound discomfort with his or her own sex and a strong and persistent identification with the opposite gender. A transsexual is an individual with a **gender identity disorder.** They experience a mismatch between their biological sex and their gender identity. This person lives as a member of the opposite sex either part- or full-time and may seek to change his or her sex through hormone therapy and sex reassignment surgery.

Many times the transsexual patient describes himself or herself as "feeling trapped in the wrong body." Transsexuals genuinely believe that they belong to the other sex. Many experience intense emotional turmoil because of stigma from society. No accurate estimates of the incidence of transsexualism are available; however, postoperative transsexuals in the United States now number in the thousands.

Transsexuality is different from homosexuality in that homosexuals are comfortable with their anatomical identity and do not want to change their sex. Many transsexuals are heterosexual and express distaste for homosexual activity. Transsexuals are essentially heterosexual, not homosexual, but are often mistaken by others or themselves as homosexual, as seen in this clinical example.

CLINICAL EXAMPLE

Mr. L is a 21-year-old biological male who was admitted to the psychiatric unit for evaluation after a serious suicide attempt. Mr. L told his nurse that he tried to kill himself because he has been "sexually mixed up for years" and is tired of feeling like a freak of nature. He said that his friends make fun of him and tell him he is a homosexual. Although he does feel sexually attracted to other men, he does not believe he is a homosexual. "I guess I don't feel like a man, I feel like a woman inside a man's body, and as a woman I am attracted to men."

Selected Nursing Diagnoses

- Ineffective sexual pattern related to conflicting sexual feelings, as evidenced by verbalizations of confusion and happiness
- Risk for self-directed violence related to sexual identity confusion, as evidenced by suicide attempt ■

Think of a patient you took care of last week. How would your care have been different if you knew this patient was a homosexual, bisexual, transvestite, or transsexual? ■

The Sexual Response Cycle. In addition to modes of sexual expression or sexual orientation, the physiological and psychological responses to sexual stimulation also can be described. The four stages of the sexual response cycle are **desire, excitement, orgasm,** and **resolution.** They are described in Box 26-1.

Sexual dysfunctions are more prevalent in women (43%) than men (31%) (Figure 26-3). They are highly associated with negative experiences in sexual relationships and overall well-being (Laumann, Paik, and Rosen, 1999). The most common problems for women are:

- **Lack of orgasm** caused by sexual inhibition, inexperience, lack of knowledge, or psychological factors such as anxiety or early sexual trauma.
- **Vaginismus** or painful, involuntary spasm of the muscles that surround the vaginal entrance, which interferes with sexual intercourse. It occurs in women who fear that penetration will be painful and may stem from previous traumatic or painful experiences.

The most common problems for men are:

- **Erectile dysfunction,** also known as **impotence,** which is an inability to achieve or maintain an erection for satisfactory sexual intercourse.
- **Ejaculatory disorders** in which ejaculation occurs before or soon after penetration (**premature**), ejacula-

tion does not occur (**inhibited**), or the ejaculate is forced back into the bladder (**retrograde**).

Impairment in sexual response may occur in any one of the phases of the sexual response cycle. For example, both men and women may experience low sexual desire. If the excitement phase is inhibited, it may produce erectile dysfunction in males and problems with arousal in females. If the orgasm stage of the cycle is disrupted, premature, inhibited, or retrograde ejaculation may occur in males, and females may experience vaginismus or pain. Although sexual dysfunction can occur when any phase is disrupted, resolution phase inhibition is rarely responsible for specific sexual dysfunctions.

The etiology of sexual dysfunction is varied and complex. Emotional and stress-related problems can increase the risk of sexual dysfunction in all phases of the sexual response cycle for both men and women. Sex therapists agree that many sexual dysfunctions are caused by psychological factors ranging from unresolved childhood conflicts to adult problems, such as performance anxiety, lack of knowledge, or failure to communicate with a partner.

Sexual dysfunction also can be caused by physiological factors. Medical problems such as circulatory, endocrine, or neurological disorders, as well as medication side effects, can contribute to sexual problems. The interaction between physiological illness and the psychosocial aspects of that illness also can lead to sexual problems in the adult.

Predisposing Factors

No one theory can adequately explain sexual development or predisposing factors of maladaptive sexual responses. Several theories have been proposed, however, and are briefly described here.

Biological. Biological factors are initially responsible for the development of gender, that is, whether a person is genetically male or female. Somatotype includes chromosomes, hormones, internal and external genitalia, and gonads. Sex differentiation is determined by the Y chromosome. Research in humans confirms the general rule that maleness and masculinity depend on fetal and perinatal androgens.

A biological female typically has XX chromosomes, with estrogen as the predominant hormone, appropriate internal

---

| BOX **26-1** | |

Stages of the Sexual Response Cycle

Stage 1: Desire
Sexual fantasies and the desire for sexual activity

Stage 2: Excitement
Subjective sense of sexual pleasure along with physiological changes, including penile erection in the male and vaginal lubrication in the female

Stage 3: Orgasm
Peaking of sexual pleasure and the release of sexual tension accompanied by rhythmic contractions of the perineal muscles and pelvic reproductive organs

Stage 4: Resolution
Sense of general relaxation, muscular relaxation, and well-being
     Females may be able to respond to additional stimulation almost immediately during this stage; however, most males need some time before they can be restimulated to orgasm.

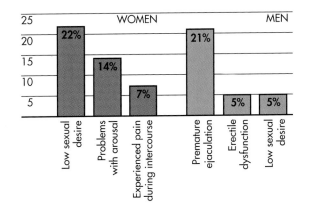

Figure 26-3   Sexual dysfunction in women and men. (From Patient page, *JAMA* 281(6), 1999.)

and external genitalia, and ovaries. A biological male typically has XY chromosomes, with androgen as the predominant hormone, appropriate internal and external genitalia, and testicles. However, each of these typical configurations may vary.

A person may have triple chromosomes, such as XXX, XXY, or XYY, or a single chromosome, XO. There is no YO chromosomal pattern. The triple pattern XXX and the single pattern XO (Turner's syndrome) result in a female body, whereas the triple patterns XXY (Klinefelter's syndrome) and XYY result in male bodies. Assuming no variation occurs, the biological factors result in a single, fully developed gender, either male or female.

Based on family studies and DNA samples of homosexual brothers, it has been suggested that a gene may be related to homosexuality. Early work in the field suggested that homosexuality may be inherited from the maternal side of the family through the X chromosome. Before such research is accepted as definitive, however, it will have to be validated by replication, and similar studies of lesbians have not yet been completed. In addition, such findings cannot account for all cases of homosexuality, but they do support a possible biological basis.

Psychoanalytical. Freud saw sexuality as one of the key forces of human life. In *Three Essays of the Theory of Sexuality* (1905) he proposed that sexuality began before puberty and that sexuality during infancy was central to personality development. He also believed that a person's choice of sexual expression depended on a mix of heredity, biology, and social factors.

The child, according to Freud, passes through a series of developmental stages in which a different erogenous zone is dominant. The first is the oral stage (birth to 12 or 18 months), in which the infant's chief sense of pleasure is derived from stimulation of the lips and mouth, that is, sucking. In the second, or anal, stage (ages 1 to 3 years), the child's attention is focused on elimination functions and control over body sphincters. The phallic stage follows (ages 3 to 5 years), in which the child's focus is on the genitals.

An important occurrence in this stage is the development of the Oedipus and Electra complexes. In the **Oedipus complex in boys** and the **Electra complex in girls,** the child experiences sexual feelings for the parent of the opposite sex and resents the parent of the same sex. According to Freud, the boy fears retaliation from his father for desiring the mother and fantasizes that the father will cut off his penis (castration anxiety). This fear is the impetus for the young boy's eventually giving up the resentment of the father and identifying with him and the male gender role. The girl, on the other hand, has no penis to fear losing. She believes that at one time she had a penis but it was cut off, and she blames her mother for this.

After the resolution of the Oedipus or Electra complex, the child enters a prolonged stage where sexual impulses are repressed (latency stage). This stage lasts until adolescence, when the child enters the genital stage and sexual urges

reawaken. The reemergence of Oedipal or Electra feelings and the need to assert themselves with parents also occur during this phase of development. The adolescent then makes the final transition into mature genital sexuality.

In recent years much criticism of Freud's theory of psychosexual development has been voiced. Feminists argue that psychoanalytical theory is male centered and views women as anatomically inferior to men (because they have no penis). Lack of scientific evidence is one of the major problems with Freud's theory. Other criticisms include that Freud was a victim of the Victorian era, a time of sexual repression, and that his thoughts and writings were bound by the period in which he lived. Finally, Freud's data were collected from observations of his patients, who were probably not representative of the total population because they were emotionally ill.

What impact has Freud's theory of psychosexual development had on society's view of women? ■

Behavioral. For the behaviorist, sexual reactions are the observable responses to overt, measurable stimuli. Behaviorists are not concerned with the intrapsychic process of early childhood and adolescence; rather, they view sexual behavior as a measurable physiological and psychological response to a learned stimulus or reinforcement event. Behaviorists consider the sexual behavior of adults who care for children as being important in the children's later sexual development. They are thus interested in sexual difficulties that result from sexual abuse in childhood.

A number of studies suggest that negative attitudes about sex and a variety of sexual dysfunctions may result from childhood sexual abuse. Although it is true that not all survivors of childhood sexual abuse experience sexual difficulties as adults, a large proportion do (Courtois, 2000).

Sexual difficulties can be seen in both men and women. A survey of 1410 men and 1749 women conducted to examine sexual behavior in the United States found that women who experience sexual victimization were more likely to have arousal disorders and men who were sexually victimized as children were 3 times as likely to experience erectile dysfunction and twice as likely to experience premature ejaculation and low sexual desire. Both men and women who were victims of unwanted sexual activity showed long-term effects on sexual functioning (Laumann, Paik, and Rosen, 1999). The care of people who have experienced abuse and violence is described in detail in Chapter 39.

Precipitating Stressors

Physical Illness and Injury. Physical illness may alter sexuality. Nurses often care for patients with sexual dysfunctions or altered sexuality patterns; they need to discuss and therapeutically intervene in patients' responses to these changes.

A person with rheumatoid arthritis may have body disfiguration and a change in body image caused by swollen areas around joints. The same patient may have decreased sexual interest because of joint pain during intercourse. People who have had a myocardial infarction may have decreased sexual interest because they fear sexual arousal may cause a heart attack. Vascular disease associated with diabetes might affect adequate arousal. Cardiovascular disease may inhibit intercourse secondary to dyspnea. Urinary incontinence may cause discomfort or embarrassment, leading to dysfunction or decreased sexual activity.

Gynecological conditions also can contribute to sexual difficulties. Hysterectomy, gynecological malignancies, and breast cancer present medical and mortality concerns and may alter perceptions of femininity that may result in decreased sexuality. Normal changes in a woman's reproductive life related to puberty, pregnancy, postpartum, and menopause can present unique problems. Puberty may lead to concerns regarding sexual identity. Pregnancy and the postpartum period are often associated with a decrease in sexual activity, desire, and satisfaction, which may be prolonged with lactation. The state of menopause may result in physical changes, as well as alterations in mood and a decline in desire, arousal, and frequency of intercourse (Phillips, 2000).

Psychiatric Illness. Psychiatric illness affects a person's sexuality as well as the sexual behavior and satisfaction of the person's partner (see A Family Speaks). Depression can be either the result or cause of sexual dysfunction. As many as

A FAMILY SPEAKS

Our daughter was diagnosed with schizophrenia 5 years ago when she was 17 years of age. Since that time we have received very good care for her. Although we understand that she may never be completely well, she has her illness under control and has even started taking some courses at the local community college. She has also met some people her age and seems to enjoy their company.

But ever since she began doing better, we have had the added concern about her sexual needs and activities. As involved parents, we raised this issue with the different health care providers who were managing her care over the years. In each case, almost without exception, we were told "Don't worry about such things; be grateful your daughter is as healthy as she is." Although their intentions may have been good, they didn't help resolve our questions or fears. But then our daughter was assigned to a nurse who we were told would be her case manager.

The first time they met, the nurse took a detailed history and asked our daughter the unthinkable: What sexual feelings did she have and how was she managing her sexual needs? It was as if the floodgate had opened for all of us, and that session marked the beginning of an ongoing discussion we would all have about the very topic we had been worrying so much about.

For that nurse asking just the right question, we will always be grateful, and if we could share one thought with future nurses in training, it would be to remember that patients are whole people and that sexuality is as important to those with psychiatric illness as it is to people everywhere.

70% of depressed patients have decreased sexual desire and decreased frequency of intercourse. Most often, depressed men engage in intercourse less often; depressed women may participate in sex but with less enjoyment. In contrast, hypersexuality may be the first symptom of a manic episode. People with bipolar illness have decreased sexual inhibitions, often impulsively choose sexual partners or begin extramarital affairs, display inappropriate sexual behavior, or act seductively or flirtatiously.

The sexual expression of patients with psychotic illnesses may be inappropriate and at times intrusive. Delusions and hallucinations may present with sexual content. Mental illness can interfere with one's ability to think coherently and express oneself in a clear and direct manner. Thus a patient's capacity for intimate relationships and sexual expression may be altered.

Although having a psychotic illness such as schizophrenia does not imply sexual dysfunction, sexual expression can be affected. The patient may not be able to understand or control sexual thoughts or impulses. For example, a patient may openly masturbate on an inpatient unit or inappropriately touch others. Thinking and judgment also may be impaired, resulting in sexual behavior that may be detrimental to the patient's health, such as unsafe sexual practices.

Questions also have been raised about the sexual lives of persons with serious and persistent mental illness who live in residential treatment facilities. It has been suggested that each facility and group of staff caring for residents need to identify ways to acknowledge and respect the normal sexual needs of these individuals and balance this with the need to keep the residents safe from sexually transmitted diseases, unwanted pregnancies, and nonconsensual sexual advances or assaults (Ford et al, 2003).

The nurse must therefore assess a psychiatric patient's sexual behavior carefully and intervene if inappropriate or dangerous sexual behavior is expressed. A study that examined the social function of a small group of patients with schizophrenia found that they wanted an intimate relationship but lacked the knowledge about how to attain one. They also reported that mental health staff did not talk with them about intimacy and sexual functioning (McDonald and Badger, 2002).

The nurse can help the patient identify and express needs related to sexuality. This includes helping the patient form healthy relationships with others, learn about safe sex practices, engage in healthy sexual expression, and decrease potentially dangerous sexual encounters.

Medications. Some medications contribute to sexual dysfunction, and nurses need to be knowledgeable about the medications they administer. The index of medications that can create sexual side effects continues to grow. These medications, which may include antihypertensives, antihistamines, anticholinergics, chemotherapeutic agents, and antiseizure drugs can cause diminished sexual desire and/or orgasmic disorders in both women and men. Some medications, especially antihypertensive agents, also can cause erectile difficulties in men.

The sexual side effects of psychiatric medications, including neuroleptics and benzodiazepines, are well documented (Wincze and Carey, 2001). A study of 636 patients with schizophrenia found that both atypical and conventional antipsychotics can cause sexual dysfunction in men and women, which may lead to noncompliance with taking the medication (Bobes et al, 2003).

Sexual dysfunctions are also a common side effect of the selective serotonin reuptake inhibitors (SSRIs). These antidepressants can cause problems in any phase of the sexual response cycle. Men commonly complain of anorgasmia or ejaculatory difficulties. The most common complaint in women is delayed or absent orgasm (Moore and Rothschild, 1999). Psychiatric medications and their side effects are described in detail in Chapter 27.

Nurses should be familiar with the sexual side effects of medications, educate their patients about them, and encourage patients to notify a health professional when these effects occur. For example, a man may not be aware that his medication can cause impotence, yet he may be embarrassed and hesitate to talk with the physician or nurse about the problem.

Often the medication itself or the dosage can be changed to correct the problem. Abuse of alcohol or nontherapeutic drugs also may have a debilitating effect on sexuality. Although many people believe alcohol is a sexual stimulant, prolonged use can cause erectile difficulty and other dysfunctions.

Consider two medications that you commonly administer to patients. Do you know whether they have sexual side effects, and have you talked about this possibility with your patients? ■

HIV/AIDS. Fear of contracting a sexually transmitted disease (STD) may create change in sexual behavior. The most frightening STD is acquired immune deficiency syndrome (AIDS), which is caused by the human immunodeficiency virus (HIV). HIV/AIDS is a leading worldwide health problem despite the attempts by health care professionals to educate society about safe sex practices. These practices include the following:

- Using condoms
- Reducing the number of sexual partners
- Promoting sexual behaviors that decrease the exchange of body fluids

Although in the United States the majority of those infected with HIV are men (82%), HIV is spreading rapidly among women. Heterosexual contact has surpassed intravenous (IV) drug use as the most common mode of transmission in women. The Centers for Disease Control and Prevention (CDC) estimated in 2001 that 65% of women with AIDS acquired it by heterosexual contact and 32% acquired it by IV drug use.

The number of young people with AIDS is also alarming. In 2001, 18% of persons diagnosed with HIV were under age 30 years. Although the number of young people with AIDS is beginning to decline, their represented proportion of all people with AIDS is significant. Of people with AIDS, 16% are in their twenties (CDC, 2001). Although the success of treatment for AIDS is promising, the effects of this illness have a significant impact on all aspects of society.

Many people infected with HIV also may have psychiatric and drug dependence problems. Nurses and other health care providers need to actively identify those at risk and work with policymakers to ensure the availability of appropriate testing, counseling, and treatment for these individuals (Bing et al, 2001; Lyon, 2001; Satriano, 2002; Essock et al, 2003).

The Aging Process. In the past researchers suggested that sexual activity decreased with aging. More recent studies indicate that patterns of sexual activity remain stable over middle and late adulthood years with only a small decline in later life. In 1999 the American Association of Retired Persons (AARP) conducted a sexual survey of 1384 adults over age 45 years. They found that overall 7 in 10 of those with partners reported engaging in intercourse at least once a month. In addition, the majority of respondents felt good about their lives now and felt that a satisfying sexual relationship was important to the quality of their lives (Jacoby, 1999).

There is nothing in the biology of aging that automatically shuts down sexual functioning; however, specific physiological changes do occur. In postmenopausal women, vaginal functioning changes in three ways. There is a reduced elasticity in the walls of the vagina and decreased vaginal lubrication. The decrease in vaginal lubrication is the result of decreased blood flow to the vagina, which is caused by low estrogen levels. The vagina also atrophies, both in width and length. In men several physiological changes occur in sexual response. Greater time and more direct stimulation is often needed for the penis to become erect, and erections tend to be less firm. The amount of semen is reduced, ejaculation is less intense, and the physical need to ejaculate is diminished. The refractory period also becomes greater with age (DeLamater and Friedrich, 2002; Zeiss and Kasl-Godley, 2001).

In Western culture the myth of the older adult as asexual still prevails. Therefore, when health professionals care for older people who express an interest in sex or are sexually active, the professional often judges the older adult to be an exception to the rule. Older adults themselves may accept society's false beliefs about sexuality and aging. Many deny sexual attractions and feelings because they have been socialized to believe that sexual behavior in older people is abnormal or perverted. Older adults are influenced by cultural values of Western society that prize youth and vitality and often disapprove of an elderly person doing anything other than sitting in a rocking chair.

One important variable affecting sexuality in older adults is the lack of knowledge about the normal changes that occur with the aging process. Often nurses and older adults mistake a side effect of a medication or a symptom of a chronic medical illness for an expected part of the aging process. It is important for the nurse to understand the normal changes that occur with aging so that he or she can teach patients about these changes. This allows patients to learn what to expect and how they might compensate for the normal changes related to aging and sexual behavior.

It is equally important for nurses to realize that organic illness can affect sexual functioning. Many of the disease states seen in the elderly can interfere with sexual expression. People with arthritis have limited range of motion capabilities. Persons with chronic obstructive pulmonary disease (COPD) can experience dyspnea on exertion. A stroke can cause problems with nerve pathways that can lead to erectile dysfunction in men and anorgasmy in women, and also can change one's body image leading to feelings of unattractiveness and worthlessness.

Medications taken by the elderly can lead to difficulties with sexual functioning as well. β-blockers and diabetes can contribute to impotence in men, and testosterone deficiency can create anorgasmy in women. These can be significant problems, and they often can be successfully treated.

Psychological factors, such as self-esteem, also can influence sexual activity in older adults. Older adults may be less inclined to be sexually active if they believe the physical changes that occur with aging make them unattractive. Marital status can influence sexuality. Because men die at younger ages than women, women are more likely to be widowed and live the last part of their lives alone. Because there are fewer men in the population, it is more difficult for older women to find partners than it is for older men.

Opportunities for sexual activity also may be limited for individuals who become dependent on others for their care. Older adults who must move in with their adult children or move to a personal care facility or a nursing home may find it difficult to engage in any form of sexual expression. Many nursing homes restrict physical activity, so residents lack privacy from staff, who tend to care for older adults in a parental way. Physical contact between nursing home residents is often discouraged by nursing home staff, and many residents may feel restricted in their sexual expression.

However, nurses are becoming more sensitive about the sexual needs of nursing home residents. By recognizing their sexual needs, nurses can act as advocates and help residents with sexual expression by encouraging discussion of sexual concerns, closing doors to ensure privacy, and allowing socialization with sexual partners.

While working in a long-term care facility you walk into a patient's room and see two patients engaged in sexual relations. How would you respond? ■

Appraisal of Stressors

Feelings of oneself as a sexual being change throughout the life cycle, and they are influenced by a person's appraisal of the stressful situation. Sexual identity cannot be separated from self-concept or body image. Therefore, when bodily or emotional changes occur, sexual responses change as well.

Coping Resources

It is important for the nurse to assess the patient's coping resources because these can have a significant impact on sexual health. Resources may include the person's knowledge about sexuality, positive sexual experiences the patient has had in the past, supportive people in the patient's environment, and social or cultural norms that encourage healthy sexual expression. It is also helpful to include the person's sexual partner whenever possible. This allows the nurse to evaluate the quality of this relationship and to frame all nursing interventions within the context of a supportive, loving partnership.

Coping Mechanisms

Coping mechanisms related to sexual response may be adaptive or maladaptive, depending on how and why they are being used. **Fantasy** is a coping mechanism used to enhance sexual experiences. Men and women may escape to erotic fantasies with unknown lovers during sex with their spouse. Although many people fear that fantasies about people other than their sexual partner indicate that they are unsatisfied or unattracted to their partner, this is typically not the case. Fantasies are often a creative way to increase sexual excitement and enjoyment and do not usually indicate dissatisfaction with a current partner. However, excessive fantasy can be maladaptive when used as a replacement for actual sexual expression or the development of intimate relationships with others.

Maladaptive coping mechanisms may result from problems with self-concept. Often one member of a sexually dysfunctional couple may use **projection** in blaming his or her partner for the total problem, absolving himself or herself from any responsibility: "I never had a sex problem with any of my previous lovers; I think you are the problem." Projection is also the coping mechanism used when a person's thoughts and feelings are unacceptable and anxiety producing. For example, a wife constantly accuses her husband of wanting to have an affair when actually the wife is contemplating an affair. Because her feelings are unacceptable to her, she projects them onto her husband and accuses him.

Denial and **rationalization** also are common coping mechanisms. Both allow the person to avoid dealing with sexual issues. The following are maladaptive examples:

- Denial: "I don't have a problem with sex" or "I never feel sexual."
- Rationalization: "I don't need sex; I'm fine without it. Besides, a good marriage is a lot more than just sex."

To cope with unacceptable feelings about becoming vulnerable and the resulting ambivalent feelings about intimacy, some people withdraw from any form of sexual behavior. Others may engage in increased sexual behavior with multiple partners to protect themselves from one intimate relationship.

◤ DIAGNOSIS

Nursing Diagnoses

When developing nursing diagnoses for variations in sexual response, the nurse should consider all the information gathered in the assessment phase and the components of the Stuart Stress Adaptation Model (Figure 26-4). The identified nursing diagnoses serve as a foundation for future problem solving.

There are two primary NANDA nursing diagnoses concerned with sexual response. The first is **ineffective sexuality**

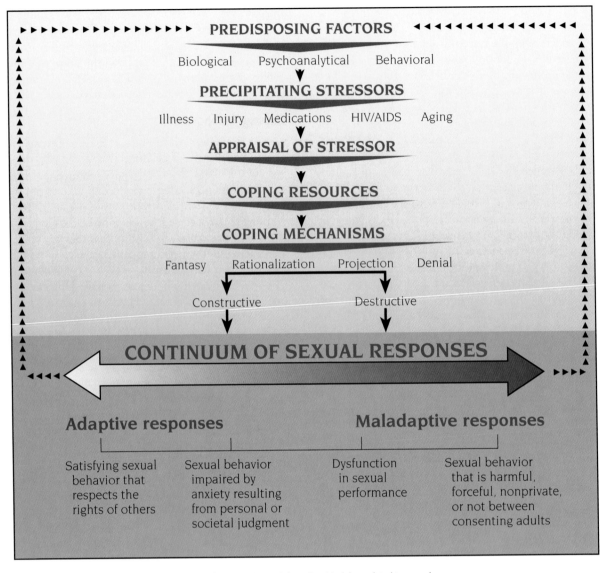

Figure 26-4   The Stuart Stress Adaptation Model as related to sexual responses.

pattern, which includes difficulties, limitations, or changes in sexual behaviors or activities. The second is **sexual dysfunction,** which includes lack of sexual satisfaction, alterations in perceived sex role, and conflicts involving values.

Other related nursing diagnoses that address additional behavioral problems also may need to be included. For example, a patient may be sexually functional but sexual identity may be unclear. Nursing diagnoses related to the range of possible maladaptive responses and related medical diagnoses are identified in the Medical and Nursing Diagnoses box (Box 26-2). The primary NANDA diagnoses and examples of expanded nursing diagnoses are presented in the Detailed Diagnoses table (Table 26-1).

Medical Diagnoses

Many people who have transient variations in sexual response do not have a medically diagnosed health problem. Those with more severe or persistent problems are classified into one of three categories of variations in sexual response according to the *DSM-IV-TR*: **sexual dysfunctions, para-**philias (sexual perversions or deviations), or **gender identity disorders** (American Psychiatric Association, 2000). The medical diagnoses and the essential features of each of these diagnostic classes according to the *DSM-IV-TR* are described in the Detailed Diagnoses table (see Table 26-1).

OUTCOME IDENTIFICATION

Goals must be formulated realistically, remembering the uniqueness of each person. The expected outcome for patients with maladaptive sexual responses is:

The patient will obtain the maximum level of adaptive sexual responses to enhance or maintain health.

This outcome can be made more specific through the use of short-term goals. These goals must be mutually identified with the patient, priorities must be established, and criteria used to measure progress toward the goals must be defined. Examples of short-term goals include the following:

- The patient will describe personal values and beliefs regarding sexuality and sexual expression.
- The patient will identify sexual questions and problems.

■ **BOX 26-2** *Medical and Nursing Diagnoses Related to* **Variations in Sexual Response**

RELATED MEDICAL DIAGNOSES (*DSM-IV-TR*)*	RELATED NURSING DIAGNOSES (NANDA)†
Sexual Dysfunctions Hypoactive sexual desire disorder Sexual aversion disorder Female sexual arousal disorder Male erectile disorder Female orgasmic disorder Male orgasmic disorder Premature ejaculation Dyspareunia Vaginismus Sexual dysfunction due to a general medical condition Substance-induced sexual dysfunction **Paraphilias** Exhibitionism Fetishism Frotteurism Pedophilia Sexual masochism Sexual sadism Transvestic fetishism Voyeurism **Gender Identity Disorders** Childhood, adolescence, or adulthood	Anxiety Body image, Disturbed Fear Grieving, Dysfunctional Health maintenance, Ineffective Pain, Acute or Chronic Personality identity, Disturbed Powerlessness Role performance, Ineffective Self esteem, Chronic or Situational low **Sexual dysfunction‡** **Sexuality pattern, Ineffective‡** Social interaction, Impaired Spiritual distress

*From American Psychiatric Association: *Diagnostic and statistical manual of mental disorders*, ed 4, text revision, Washington, DC, 2000, American Psychiatric Association.
†From North American Nursing Diagnosis Association: *NANDA nursing diagnoses: definitions and classification 2003-2004*, Philadelphia, 2003, The Association.
‡**Primary nursing diagnosis for variations in sexual response.**

- The patient will relate accurate information about sexual concerns.
- The patient will implement one new behavior to enhance sexual functioning.
- The patient will report decreased anxiety and greater satisfaction with sexual health.

After identifying goals in partnership with the patient, the nurse begins to implement the appropriate nursing interventions.

PLANNING

The nurse's level of expertise determines the degree of planning. The planning phase can simply involve reviewing assessment data, exploring options, and making referral sources known and available. This phase also can include sexual instruction for the patient or the patient and partner together. The nurse and patient can discuss a specific sexual issue and approaches that will provide the needed information.

IMPLEMENTATION

Health Education

Primary prevention strives to promote health and prevent problems through specific methods such as teaching and planning, described in Chapter 13. Before engaging in health education or counseling, however, nurses must examine their values and beliefs about sexual behavior. This can be facilitated by exploring commonly held myths regarding human sexuality. Table 26-2 lists some common sexual myths, the results of believing them, and the facts related to each one.

Education is the most common method of primary prevention of sexual problems. The content and methods of sex education have changed little over the past several decades. Many people receive most of their sex education from friends, who may not provide accurate information. Too few parents discuss sexual issues with their children, and school sex education programs, to avoid discussion of controversial subjects, often focus only on biological factors, which is insufficient for the needs of today's youth.

Recently, because of the epidemic rates of teenage pregnancies and abortions and the spread of AIDS, many experts are suggesting more comprehensive sex education programs, and some are suggesting that these programs begin as early as preschool and kindergarten. **Sex education is a lifelong process with the primary goal of promoting sexual health.** This includes helping people develop positive views of sexuality, gain information and skills about taking care of their sexual health, and acquire decision-making abilities regarding sexual issues.

Table 26-1	*Detailed Diagnoses Related to* **Sexual Responses**

NANDA DIAGNOSIS STEM	**EXAMPLES OF EXPANDED DIAGNOSIS**
Sexual dysfunction	Sexual dysfunction related to prenatal weight gain, as evidenced by verbal statements of physical discomfort with intercourse
	Sexual dysfunction related to joint pain, as evidenced by decreased sexual desire
Ineffective sexuality pattern	Ineffective sexuality pattern related to financial worries, as evidenced by inability to reach orgasm
	Ineffective sexuality pattern related to mastectomy, as evidenced by statements such as "My husband won't want to touch me" and "I don't feel like a woman"
	Ineffective sexuality pattern related to fear of pregnancy, as evidenced by stopping before penetration

***DSM-IV-TR* DIAGNOSIS**	**ESSENTIAL FEATURES***
Sexual Dysfunctions	
Hypoactive sexual desire disorder	Persistent or recurrent deficit or absence of sexual fantasies and desire for sexual activity
Sexual aversion disorder	Persistent or recurrent extreme aversion to and avoidance of genital sexual contact with a sexual partner
Female sexual arousal disorder	Persistent or recurrent inability to attain, or to maintain until completion of the sexual activity, an adequate lubrication-swelling response of sexual excitement
Male erectile disorder	Persistent or recurrent inability to attain, or to maintain until completion of the sexual activity, an adequate erection
Female orgasmic disorder	Persistent or recurrent delay in or absence of orgasm following a normal sexual excitement phase; diagnosis based on the clinician's judgment that the woman's orgasmic capacity is less than would be reasonable for her age, sexual experience, and the adequacy of sexual stimulation she receives
Male orgasmic disorder	Persistent or recurrent delay in or absence of orgasm following a normal sexual excitement phase during sexual activity that the clinician, taking into account the person's age, judges to be adequate in focus, intensity, and duration
Premature ejaculation	Persistent or recurrent ejaculation with minimal sexual stimulation before, on, or shortly after penetration, before the person wishes it
Dyspareunia	Recurrent or persistent genital pain before, during, or after sexual intercourse
Vaginismus	Recurrent or persistent involuntary spasm of the musculature of the outer third of the vagina that interferes with coitus
Sexual dysfunction due to a general medical condition	Clinically significant sexual dysfunction etiologically related to a general medical condition
Substance-induced sexual dysfunction	Clinically significant sexual dysfunction that developed during significant substance intoxication or withdrawal
Paraphilias	
Exhibitionism	A persistent association, lasting at least 6 months, between intense sexual arousal, desire, acts, or fantasies, and exposing one's genitals to an unsuspecting stranger
Fetishism	A persistent association, lasting at least 6 months, between intense sexual arousal, desire, acts, or fantasies, and nonliving objects (such as female undergarments)
Frotteurism	A persistent association, lasting at least 6 months, between intense sexual arousal, desire, acts, or fantasies, and rubbing against a nonconsenting person
Pedophilia	A persistent association, lasting at least 6 months, between intense sexual arousal, desire, acts, or fantasies, and one or more children, aged 13 years or younger
Sexual masochism	A persistent association, lasting at least 6 months, between intense sexual arousal, desire, acts, or fantasies, and being humiliated, beaten, bound, or otherwise being made to suffer (real or imagined)
Sexual sadism	A persistent association, lasting at least 6 months, between intense sexual arousal, desire, acts, or fantasies, and the affliction of real or simulated psychological or physical suffering (including humiliation)
Transvestic fetishism	A persistent association, lasting at least 6 months, between intense sexual arousal, desire, acts, or fantasies, and cross-dressing
Voyeurism	A persistent association, lasting at least 6 months, between intense sexual arousal, desire, acts, or fantasies, and observing unsuspecting people who are either naked, in the act of disrobing, or engaging in sexual activity
Gender Identity Disorders	
Childhood, adolescence, or adulthood	Persistent and intense distress about being a male or a female, with an intense desire to be the opposite sex, a preoccupation with the activities of the opposite sex, and a repudiation of one's own anatomical structures

*From American Psychiatric Association: *Diagnostic and statistical manual of mental disorders,* ed 4, text revision, Washington, DC, 2000, American Psychiatric Association.

Table 26-2	Ten Common Myths and Facts About Human Sexuality	
MYTH	RESULT OF MYTH	FACT
Patients become embarrassed when nurses bring up the subject of sexuality and would prefer that nurses not ask questions about sex.	If nurses believe this, they deny the patients the opportunity to ask questions and clarify concerns related to sexual issues.	Patients prefer that nurses initiate discussions of sexuality with them.
Excessive masturbation is harmful.	People often feel guilty or ashamed about masturbating; some people deny themselves this experience because of uncomfortable feelings perpetuated by society.	There is no evidence that masturbation causes physical problems. If masturbation leads to satisfaction and pleasure, it is unlikely to be a problem.
Sexual fantasies about having sex with a partner other than a lover or spouse indicate relationship difficulties.	People may become uncomfortable about having a fantasy with a different partner. They may feel guilty and view the fantasy as a sign of infidelity.	Imagining sex with a different partner is a common sexual fantasy and does not necessarily indicate a desire to act out the fantasy.
Sex during menstruation is unclean and harmful.	Women often view their bodies as unclean and even unfit or inferior during menstruation. Women use menstruation as an excuse to avoid intercourse rather than simply saying no without a "good reason."	Medically, menstrual flow is in no way harmful or dirty. If women desire, there is no reason to abstain from intercourse during menstrual flow.
Oral and anal intercourse is perverted and dangerous.	Many people refrain from these behaviors or indulge in them only to feel ashamed and guilty afterward.	Oral and anal intercourse is not harmful if certain precautions are taken when performing anal intercourse, such as avoiding contamination of the vaginal tract and wearing a condom to prevent the transmission of disease.
Most homosexuals molest children.	Known homosexuals are often fired from teaching jobs, and many parents do not allow their children to spend any time with anyone who is homosexual.	Research shows that the adult heterosexual male poses a far greater risk to the underage child than does the adult homosexual male.
Homosexuals are sick and cannot control their sexual behavior.	Homosexuals are denied jobs and are sometimes jailed for their homosexuality. Children may be taken away from homosexual parents by courts.	Most homosexuals' social and psychological adjustment is the same as the heterosexual majority, and objectionable sexual advances are far more likely to be made by a heterosexual (usually male to female) than by a homosexual.
Because of sex education programs, most adolescents and young adults are aware of the risks of getting sexually transmitted diseases and practice safe sex.	When health educators believe that young adults have adequate knowledge about sexually transmitted diseases, they may not take the time to assess, add to this knowledge, and correct any misperceptions.	A study of over 500 first-year students at a large university reported that of those who had multiple partners, fewer than 50% used condoms to lower the risk of disease.
Advancing age means the end of sex.	Many older adults become victims of this myth not because their bodies have lost the ability to perform, but because they believe that they have lost the ability to perform.	Sexually, men and women in good health can function effectively throughout their lives.
Alcohol ingestion reduces inhibitions and therefore enhances sexual enjoyment.	Many people use alcohol in the hope that it will increase their sexual pleasure and performance. Alcohol ingestion can also provide an excuse for engaging in sexual behaviors—"I would never have gone to bed with him if I hadn't had all that wine."	Data do not support the belief that alcohol ingestion reduces inhibitions and enhances sexual enjoyment.

Schools and communities develop their own curriculum for sexual education. These programs range from abstinence-only-until-marriage to comprehensive sexual education. Abstinence-only-until-marriage programs encourage abstinence from all sexual behaviors outside of marriage. They do include information about HIV prevention but do not include information about preventing pregnancy. Often they

support marriage as the only morally acceptable context for sexual behavior (SIECUS, 2001).

Comprehensive sex education programs include information about human development, building positive relationships, enhancing interpersonal skills, promoting responsible sexual behavior, maintaining sexual health and understanding societal and cultural influences on sexuality. Comprehensive sexuality programs have been found to be effective in both delaying sexual intercourse and teen pregnancy (SIECUS, 2001).

It is also clear that teaching information about sex and sexuality is not enough. For a sex education program to be effective, it must promote behavioral change. The most effective sex education programs are comprehensive and skill based. For example, it is not enough to teach individuals to say no to sex; they must be taught *how* to say no. This could be done by teaching decision-making and assertiveness skills and by role playing potentially difficult sexual situations.

Which sexual myth from Table 26-2 did you believe before reading this chapter? How will knowing the truth affect your nursing practice? ■

Sexual Responses Within the Nurse-Patient Relationship

Sexual Responses of Nurses to Patients. A clinical situation in which a nurse feels sexual attraction to a patient is a problem that has received little attention in the nursing literature. One reason for this is that nurses often deny sexual feelings for their patients. However, sexual attraction and sexual fantasies are part of the human experience. If these feelings are not examined, they can interfere with the quality of care by shifting the focus from the patient's needs to those of the nurse.

First, nurses must acknowledge their feelings without judging them. Often nurses try to ignore or deny these feelings because they are uncomfortable and frightening. They make judgments about themselves, such as

"What's wrong with me? I shouldn't feel this way about my patients. I must be really weird."

"I'm sure I'm the only nurse who ever had these feelings."

The nurse who admits these feelings without judging them is able to deal with them.

One of the best ways to begin to deal with these feelings is to seek consultation from a more experienced nurse. A nurse should not tell the patient about these feelings, because it will only further complicate the issue. It is not the patient's responsibility to respond to the nurse's feelings. Rather, **it is always the nurse's responsibility to preserve professional boundaries, even when a nurse feels sexually attracted to a patient.**

The nurse needs to be aware of behaviors exhibited by the patient. The nurse should avoid flirtatious gestures or sharing personal information during interactions. Finally, **it is never acceptable for a nurse to engage in sexual behavior of any kind with a patient.** Such activity is unethical and can lead to allegations of sexual misconduct and litigation (Wysoker, 2000).

Sexual Responses of Patients to Nurses. One of the most common sexual behaviors of hospitalized patients is seductive behavior toward the nurse. This includes making passes and sexual comments, inappropriate touching, asking for a phone number and requesting a date. Nurses are often extremely uncomfortable with such behaviors. One study ex-amining nurses' responses to sexual harassment by patients revealed that often the quality of care given to both the harassing patients and other patients was negatively affected. Many of the nurses in this study used avoidance as a defense mechanism (Lobell, 1999).

If a patient makes a sexual advance, the nurse should let the patient know that the behavior is unacceptable. The nurse needs to respond in a firm, matter-of-fact manner that clearly states what limits are being set, such as

"Mr. Moore, I am uncomfortable when you suggest that I get into bed with you. Please stop saying that."

"Mr. Dean, take your hand off my breast."

Nurses are sometimes embarrassed or afraid to confront patients and attempt to laugh it off or ignore it. Patients do not have the right to be verbally offensive or to touch nurses' bodies without permission. Nurses are taught to be accepting of patients' behavior, and this principle is difficult to dispute. However, when the behavior violates nurses' rights, limits must be set.

Nurses have a responsibility as professionals to attempt to understand sexual behaviors and analyze their possible meanings. Patients may show seductive behaviors for various reasons, which may not include a serious desire for sex with the nurse. Seductive behavior is often a way of getting the nurse's attention. Hospitalized patients also can feel unattractive or insecure about themselves sexually; thus seductive behaviors may be a request for reassurance.

Sometimes patients confuse their gratitude for and appreciation of the nurse with sexual attraction. These feelings may in turn generate thoughts such as, "Wouldn't my nurse make a wonderful wife? She's so giving and understanding all the time." In this case the patient views professional behavior and concern as self-sacrificing and altruistic.

Finally, patients may have difficulty understanding the difference between a professional and a social relationship. In many ways the nurse-patient relationship is idealized for the patient. The patient receives all the attention and caring and is not expected to give anything in return. It is easy to see how the patient could be confused about his or her relationship with the nurse. The clinical example that follows illustrates this point. Table 26-3 summarizes nursing considerations in sexual responses of patients to nurses.

▌ CLINICAL EXAMPLE

Mr. P has been hospitalized for an exacerbation of a chronic illness for the past 3 weeks. Ms. S has been his primary nurse during this hospitalization. The following is a conversation between the nurse and patient the day before his discharge.

Mr. P: I wish my wife were more like you, Ms. S.

Ms. S: Mr. P, I'm not sure I understand what you are saying.

Mr. P: Well, it's just that you are always so concerned about me. You always try to make me feel good and want to help me all the time. Sometimes my wife's a grouch; she's so wrapped up in her job and the kids she doesn't always pay as much attention to me as you do.

Ms. S: I'm glad you feel taken care of, but it's impossible to compare my role as your nurse with your wife's role.

Mr. P: I'm not sure I follow you.

Ms. S: They are very different types of relationships. It's nice to have someone take care of us when we can't take care of ourselves, but when we are healthy, we don't need someone to take care of us all the time. Your relationship with your wife is more of a sharing one with mutual benefits. You take care of her needs, and she takes care of your needs in return. If you feel that your relationship with your wife is not a satisfying one, perhaps you need to talk this over with her. ■

Maladaptive Sexual Responses

Resulting From Illness. Stress, physical and emotional illness, injury, and aging can lead to changes in sexuality and sexual functioning. These changes and related nursing interventions differ based on whether the illness is acute or chronic. It is important for the nurse to obtain complete information on the nature and course of the illness, the types of medications used in its treatment, the patient's appraisal of the impact of the illness, and any physical limitation imposed by the illness that affects the patient's sexual health.

Several nursing interventions can then be implemented to facilitate the patient's adaptive sexual responses. The first is for the nurse to act in a **supportive** way and to help the patient express feelings, fears, and problems. Open communication between the patient and partner also should be encouraged. The nurse can reinforce the positive attributes of the patient, prevent social isolation, mobilize coping resources, and support adaptive coping mechanisms that have helped the patient deal with stressors in the past.

The nurse also can offer **anticipatory guidance** and give accurate information about the illness or injury, including what the patient may expect from medical or psychiatric treatment and its impact on sexual health (see A Patient Speaks). The nurse can initiate **counseling** about sexuality and alternative means of sexual expression. Relaxation techniques, autoerotic activities, and variations in movement and positions may be suggested. The nurse should emphasize that pleasure can be obtained in a variety of ways and stress the importance of a loving relationship. If the problem is complex and of a long duration, the patient should be **referred** for psychotherapy or sex therapy from a qualified professional.

A Patient Education Plan for patients recovering from an organic illness is presented in Table 26-4.

Should sexual behavior be permitted among patients who are residents of a long-term psychiatric facility? If so, what issues must be addressed by staff? If not, how will the sexual needs of these patients be met? ■

Table 26-3   Summary of Nursing Considerations in Sexual Responses of Patients to Nurses

Goal: Maintain a professional nurse-patient relationship that will enable the nurse to provide therapeutic nursing care

PRINCIPLE	RATIONALE	NURSING CONSIDERATIONS
Establish a trusting relationship.	An atmosphere of trust allows for open, honest communication between patient and nurse; this enables the nurse to aid the patient in discovering the underlying issues related to sexual feelings and behavior.	Express nonsexual caring and concern for the patient. Be a responsive listener, especially to feelings and needs that the patient may not be able to express directly. Reinforce the purpose of the therapeutic nurse-patient relationship.
Gain awareness of nurse's own feelings and thoughts.	Being aware of his or her feelings and thoughts enables the nurse to understand how they influence his or her behavior; with increased self-awareness the nurse can increase the effectiveness of his or her interactions with patients.	Recognize own feelings and thoughts. Identify any specific patient interaction or behavior that influences the nurse's feelings and thoughts. Identify the influence of the nurse's feelings and thoughts on one's behavior in an attempt to increase the effectiveness of nursing interventions.
Decrease patient's inappropriate expressions of sexual feelings and behaviors.	If the nurse is able to help the patient see that his or her sexual interactions and behaviors are being expressed to an inappropriate partner (the nurse), the sexual acting out will usually decrease; this allows the nurse to help the patient begin to identify the reasons for his or her behavior.	Set limits on patient's sexual behavior. Use a calm, matter-of-fact approach without implying judgment. Reaffirm nonsexual caring for the patient. Explore the meaning of the patient's feelings and behaviors.
Expand patient's insight into sexual feelings and behaviors.	Once the patient begins to identify the reasons for his or her sexual feelings and behaviors, he or she can see that the nurse is not an appropriate outlet for these feelings and behaviors and can move toward a more appropriate and therapeutic relationship.	Clarify misconceptions regarding any feeling patient may have about the nurse as a possible sexual partner. Point out the futile nature of the patient's romantic or sexual interest in the nurse. Redirect patient's energies toward appropriate health care issues.

Difficulties with Sexual Orientation. Most heterosexuals, homosexuals, and bisexuals accept their sexual orientations, although some have difficulty and seek professional help. For example, it is possible that one's sexual behavior may not match one's sexual desire. Someone in a heterosexual relationship may wish to be in a homosexual one, or vice versa, and feel constrained to act because of personal, sociocultural, legal, economic, or religious reasons. This can create internal conflict and distress, and the person may seek counseling.

Homosexuality is not a disorder or mental illness. However, research has suggested that homosexuals, both gay and lesbian,

and bisexual youth are at increased risk for suicidal and self-harm behaviors and certain mental health problems (Fergusson, Horwood, and Beautrais, 1999; Lock and Steiner, 1999; Skegg et al, 2003). Although the reasons for this increased risk are complex, it is reasonable to assume that society's lack of acceptance of homosexuals is a contributing factor.

Negative attitudes expressed or felt by health care providers and society at large can greatly affect the health care received by homosexuals and other sexually diverse patients. Homophobia, which is an irrational fear of homosexuals accompanied by negative attitudes and hostility toward them, can significantly reduce the quality of care provided to these patients. Questions have been raised about the impact homophobia among nurses has on providing competent nursing care to homosexual patients (Wright and Anthony, 2002; Fields and Scout, 2001).

Another prevailing attitude among health care workers is that all patients are heterosexual. This assumption, also termed **heterosexism** may distance homosexual and bisexual patients from the care they require. Heterosexism is often most evident in health care assessments and sexual history forms (Fields and Scout, 2001). These concerns require serious self-analysis by every nurse (see Citing the Evidence).

Great sensitivity must be displayed by the nurse toward patients to show acknowledgement and acceptance of the fact that patients may display a range of sexual responses. Replacing the term **spouse** with **partner** when addressing patients is a good place to start. Committing to this one simple change is a daily reminder that not all patients are heterosexual. Other strategies that may increase the homosexual's comfort with health care providers are (1) allowing partners to be involved in decision making regarding patients' care, (2) ensuring confidentiality, and (3) gaining knowledge of the coming out process (Taylor, 1999). **Coming out** simply refers to the process of disclosing one's homosexual orientation. This process can be very stressful, even if the reactions from family and friends are positive (Gramling, Carr, and McCain 2000).

Because of the homosexual element of bisexuality, bisexuals often encounter many of the same difficulties stemming

---

A PATIENT SPEAKS

It's bad enough to be depressed, but how's a person supposed to feel when the people taking care of him don't give him all the information he needs? From what I can see from talking to other patients in my group, my story is not that unusual.

For about 6 months I felt myself slipping deeper and deeper into the black hole of depression. I saw some ads on television and decided that maybe I needed some outside help, since I clearly wasn't getting better by myself. So off I go to a nearby clinic where I see someone who diagnoses me with depression and gives me some pills to take. In the beginning the drugs made me kind of jittery, but gradually I got over it. In a couple of months I actually almost felt like my old self again (all except for sex, that is). In that one area of my life, I simply couldn't experience the satisfaction I used to have and didn't know what was going on. Well, it turns out that the pills I'm on limit my sexual performance, but nobody ever bothered to mention this to me. I guess they thought it wasn't important or something, but they were really wrong.

Now that I understand what's going on, I can work around it, since the drugs have helped me in almost every other way. But still, it would be nice if the people that you turn to for help could give you all the information you need and not just talk about the parts that they think are important or limit themselves to the topics they're comfortable talking about.

Table 26-4	PATIENT EDUCATION PLAN	Sexual Responses after an Organic Illness
CONTENT	**INSTRUCTIONAL ACTIVITIES**	**EVALUATION**
Describe the variety of human sexual response patterns.	Discuss the range of sexual desires, modes of expression, and techniques.	The patient identifies personal sexual orientation and typical level of sexual functioning.
Define the patient's primary organic problem.	Provide accurate information regarding the disruption caused by the organic impairment.	The patient understands the specific organic illness.
Clarify relationship between the organic problem and patient's level of sexual functioning.	Reframe distorted or confused perceptions regarding the impact of the illness on patient's sexual functioning.	The patient accurately describes the impact of the illness on sexual functioning.
Identify ways to enhance patient's sexual functioning and improve interpersonal communication.	Describe additional experiences that would add to the sexual satisfaction and the relationship between the patient and patient's partner.	The patient and partner report reduced anxiety and greater satisfaction with their sexual responses.

from societal attitudes as homosexuals. Another factor that may present a problem for the bisexual is isolation from a support group. Because bisexuals are often accused of fence-sitting, they can be rejected by heterosexuals and homosexuals. Bisexuals may lack social support, and friends and family may pressure them to decide on one sexual orientation (usually heterosexual) so that they will be accepted by society.

An important step in working with patients who are attempting to come to terms with their homosexuality or bisexuality is to help them explore their beliefs about sexually diverse lifestyles, where these came from, and whether they are based in fact or fiction. The patient may have internalized some of society's prejudices, such as "Homosexuality is a sick and abnormal behavior; because I am a homosexual, I am sick and abnormal and should not act on my sexual feelings because they are wrong." Responses can be varied and include denial, confusion, and sexual promiscuity, especially among those trying to prove to themselves that they are not gay.

It is helpful to have patients list their beliefs about homosexuality and bisexuality and to discuss each one. However, a review of beliefs about sexuality may not be sufficient. Encouraging the person to read about sexual diversity is also helpful. Throughout this process the patient will be extremely sensitive to the nurse's acceptance or rejection.

Confidentiality is also a central issue. It is helpful for the nurse to demonstrate an appreciation for patients' concerns

about unwanted exposure of their homosexuality to family members, friends, or co-workers. The nurse should not encourage or discourage the patient's disclosure of homosexual concerns but rather help the patient explore and process the choice of disclosure or lack of disclosure with others, as in the following clinical example.

CLINICAL EXAMPLE

Ms. A, a 25-year-old single female, came to the mental health clinic with the complaint of a "sexual problem." Her history revealed that she had been sexually inactive for the past 5 years. At the age of 20, Ms. A had a brief sexual encounter with a man she had been dating for 2 years. She ended the relationship shortly afterward because she had no interest in maintaining a sexual relationship with the man. Recently she became involved in a relationship with a woman that was very satisfying to her. She felt she had to end the relationship because she would not tolerate thinking of herself as a homosexual. During one of the initial counseling sessions, Ms. A told the nurse that she must end the relationship before "it" happens again.

Nurse: What are you afraid will happen?
Ms. A: I'm afraid I'll feel attracted to her again.
Nurse: What about that frightens you?
Ms. A: (becoming upset) That will mean I'm homosexual!
Nurse: What does being homosexual mean for you?
Ms. A: It means I'm sick. It's a sin. I couldn't go to church anymore.
Nurse: Are all homosexuals sick?
Ms. A: Yes.
Nurse: How do you know this?
Ms. A: Everybody knows that homosexuality is morally wrong. Homosexuals have a lot of emotional problems.
Nurse: Do you know any homosexual people?
Ms. A: Well, not exactly.
Nurse: What have you read about homosexuality?
Ms. A: Nothing.
Nurse: Then it looks to me like you are basing all of your conclusions on hearsay and not real knowledge. I think that you and I need to explore your beliefs in more detail, then you can do some reading to find out the facts.

Selected Nursing Diagnoses

• Ineffective sexuality pattern related to questions about sexual preference related to recent interpersonal relationship, as evidenced by current attraction to a woman
• Spiritual distress related to conflicting values, as evidenced by questions about religious beliefs ■

CITING THE EVIDENCE ON
Nursing Students' Comfort With Diverse Groups

BACKGROUND: A sample of 196 nursing students were asked to complete a questionnaire regarding their exposure to a variety of culturally diverse patients. They were further asked about their comfort levels when caring for these patients.

RESULTS: Students reported relatively little discomfort when asked to care for individuals from various racial and ethnic groups. However, this was not true when they were asked to care for people who were lesbian, gay, bisexual, or HIV positive. Specifically, 44% reported that they would be uncomfortable caring for lesbian patients; 43% were uncomfortable with bisexuals; 42% were uncomfortable with patients who were HIV positive; and 35% were uncomfortable with gay men. Students who had experience with a particular group of people were more likely to report feeling comfortable working with them.

IMPLICATIONS: Nursing curriculum can be designed to help students evaluate their fears and prejudices toward people with different sexual orientations. Strategies that can be helpful include panel discussions with gay, lesbian, and bisexual people; small group discussions regarding caring for people with different orientations; and role playing effective assessment and therapeutic interactions. Faculty also can role model appropriate behavior related to the range of sexual diversities. These changes will promote quality nursing care for all patients.

Eliason M, Raheim S: *J Nurs Educ* 39:161, 2002.

In the preceding clinical example, the nurse and Ms. A developed a plan often used in sexual counseling to explore homosexuality. Some of the interventions included the following:

• Ms. A described her beliefs about homosexuality and homosexuals.
• The nurse encouraged Ms. A to explore the literature on homosexuality and suggested readings to help dispel the myths.
• The nurse then discussed these with Ms. A and suggested that she attend a social gathering for gay people to test out her new knowledge. The nurse sug-

gested the social gathering because many people struggling with a homosexual identity are frightened to test out situations that would dispel the myths.

- Finally, the nurse helped Ms. A explore her responses to these activities and integrate them into a positive view of self.

Difficulties With Gender Identity. Gender identity is a person's perceptions of his or her maleness or femaleness. Gender identity disorder or gender dysphoria is a profound discomfort with one's sex and a strong and persistent identification with the opposite gender. It can be experienced along a continuum of responses, with transsexualism being the most severe form of this disorder.

Treatment of the transsexual person has been controversial. A comprehensive review of the literature found that the majority of people with gender identity disorder who chose to undergo gender reassignment surgery reported a variety of improvements (Carroll, 1999). The benefits included enhanced psychological, vocational, sexual, and social functioning.

Standards of care for gender identity disorders provide guidelines for health professionals who work with patients who have gender problems (Harry Benjamin International Gender Dysphoria Association [HBIGDA], 2001). These standards were developed because of the serious consequences of available treatments. Patients who believe they are transsexual and request surgical reassignment must meet these standards. They require that two therapists agree that the reassignment is appropriate; that the patient be of legal age; and that the patient live in the role of the preferred gender for at least 1 year. The standards also recommend that follow-up care be provided.

Professionals who care for transsexual patients must be educated in sexuality. The assessment phase of treatment is especially important. The patient and therapist must be certain that implementing the treatment plan is the best approach because the surgery is not reversible. When transgendered individuals follow the HBIGDA's standards of care, they are more likely to have improved psychosocial outcomes (Carroll, 1999).

Pedophilia. Pedophilia is the sexual attraction to prepubescent children. It is one of the paraphilias and is considered a maladaptive sexual response because it does not involve mutual adult consent (Krueger and Kaplan, 2001; Cohen and Galynker, 2002). Paraphilia describes a condition in which one experiences sexually arousing fantasies, sexual urges, or sexual acts involving nonhuman objects, the suffering or humiliation of one's partner, or children or other nonconsenting persons.

In a report by the United States Justice department of over 60,00 cases of reported sexual assault, over 67% of the victims were under the age of 18; 34% were under age 12; and 14% were under age 6. The vast majority of sexual offenders to a juvenile population were male (94%). However, when women were the offenders they were more likely to assault children under 6 years of age; 34% of offenders were family members.

Psychiatric nurses are in a position to care for either the victim or the offender. However, since **the act of sexual behavior with a child is a crime**, very few pedophiles seek treatment. Usually treatment is a compulsory term of their sentence following conviction (Farella, 2002; Krueger and Kaplan, 2002).

One of the primary problems in the treatment of pedophilia is the high rate of recidivism. It has been proposed that continued compliance with a comprehensive treatment program may reduce relapse. A comprehensive treatment program may involve individual or group therapy, stress management, cognitive restructuring, behavioral modification techniques, and the use of antiandrogenic medications to lower sexual desires (Krueger and Kaplan, 2002).

The effects of child sexual abuse are long lasting and therefore nurses must be equipped to care for both child and adult survivors. Abuse can influence health in four major ways. It can cause behavioral problems such as substance abuse, high-risk sexual behavior, and suicidality, and social problems may arise as well. Revictimization is a social problem that many survivors of sexual abuse encounter in that they also become victims of sexual violence at least once in an adult relationship.

Another way in which adult survivors are impacted by their past abuse is how they perceive their daily existence. For example, they may overestimate a situation's potential danger or perceive themselves as helpless in dealing with their environment. These thoughts can lead to increased levels of stress. A fourth way in which child sexual abuse can affect overall health is through negative emotions. These negative emotions can lead to depression or posttraumatic stress disorder (Courtois, 2000; Kendall-Tackett, 2002). Care for survivors of abuse and violence is discussed in detail in Chapter 39.

Nurses can begin to care for patients by incorporating questions pertaining to a history of sexual abuse into comprehensive nursing assessments. Once it has been determined that a patient does have a history of sexual abuse, the nurse can investigate whether current health problems are related. Referral can then be made to an advanced practice psychiatric nurse who specializes in helping victims of sexual abuse. Patients can be assisted in realizing that they are in control of their thoughts and behavior. They then can be taught methods to decrease anxiety, build trusting relationships, and decrease overall stress, thus improving health.

A Nursing Treatment Plan Summary for maladaptive sexual responses is presented in Table 26-5. **Empirically validated treatments** for paraphilias and sexual dysfunction are summarized in Box 26-3 (Nathan and Gorman, 2002).

What role do social institutions such as churches, schools, and health centers have in protecting youth from sexual improprieties? ∎

Table 26-5	NURSING TREATMENT PLAN SUMMARY	Maladaptive Sexual Responses

Nursing Diagnosis: Ineffective sexuality pattern
Expected Outcome: The patient will obtain the maximum level of adaptive sexual responses to enhance or maintain health.

SHORT-TERM GOAL	INTERVENTION	RATIONALE
The patient will describe values, beliefs, questions, and problems regarding sexuality.	Listen to sexual concerns implied and expressed. Communicate respect, acceptance, and openness to sexual concerns. Help the patient explore sexual beliefs, values, and questions. Encourage open communication between the patient and partner.	An accepting therapeutic relationship will allow patients to be free to question, grow, and seek help with sexual concerns.
The patient will relate accurate information about sexual concerns.	Clarify sexual misinformation. Dispel myths. Provide specific education about sexual health practices, behaviors, and problems. Give professional "permission" to continue sexual behavior that is not physically or emotionally harmful. Reinforce positive attitudes of the patient.	Accurate information is helpful in changing negative thoughts and attitudes about particular aspects of sexuality. It can also prevent or limit dysfunctional behavior. Giving permission allows the person to continue the behavior and alleviates anxiety about normalcy. It allows patients to incorporate sexual behavior into a positive and accepting self-concept.
The patient will implement one new behavior to enhance sexual response.	Set clear goals with the patient. Identify specific behaviors that can be carried out that focus on enhancing self-concept, role functioning, and sexuality. Encourage relaxation techniques, redirection of attention, positional changes, and alternative ways of sexual expression as appropriate. Become familiar with the sex therapy resources available in the community. Refer the patient to a qualified sex therapist as needed.	Giving a patient direct behavioral suggestions can help relieve a sexual problem or difficulty and is a useful intervention when the problem is of recent onset and short duration. Although all nurses need to screen for maladaptive sexual responses and provide basic nursing care, complex problems should be referred to qualified sex therapists for further treatment.

BOX 26-3	SUMMARIZING THE EVIDENCE ON Sexual Responses

Disorder	Paraphilias
Treatment	◆ Cognitive, behavioral, and cognitive-behavioral treatments lower rates of recidivism.
	◆ Somatic treatments, such as medroxy-progesterone and cyproterone acetate, that lower testosterone levels are also somewhat effective.
Disorder	Sexual dysfunction
Treatment	◆ Pharmacological therapies for erectile disorders (sildenafil) and rapid ejaculation (SSRIs: fluoxetine, sertraline, clomipramine, paroxetine) are successful in reversing sexual dysfunction. There is less efficacy for the sense of sexual satisfaction and couple interaction. The evidence concerning pharmacological treatment of female sexual disorder is very limited.

From Nathan P, Gorman J: *A guide to treatments that work*, ed 2, New York, 2002, Oxford University Press.

Dysfunctions of the Sexual Response Cycle

Both the advanced practice nurse and the nurse generalist should have a good knowledge base related to the causes of and treatment for sexual dysfunction (Mahan, 2003). Treating sexual dysfunctions is beyond the scope of the nurse generalist. However, the nurse should be aware of the principles involved and should know creditable sex therapists in the community for referral of patients. Two common models of sex therapy are briefly discussed here: the Masters and Johnson and the Helen Singer Kaplan models. They have been reported to be useful for several types of sexual dysfunction, and some long-term follow-up studies have shown the positive sustained effect of therapy on individuals' and couples' sense of sexual satisfaction.

Masters and Johnson Model. Masters and Johnson began their pioneering research in sexuality in the 1950s. Before their work, patients with problems in sexuality were generally referred to a psychiatrist for psychotherapy or psychoanalysis, because health professionals incorrectly assumed that anyone who had a problem with sexuality was emotionally disturbed. Masters and Johnson's (1970; Masters, Kolodny, and Johnson, 1986) treatment includes short-term education with step-by-step instructions regarding the physical aspects of sexual activity and supportive psychotherapy. They believe that attitudes and ignorance are responsible for most sexual dysfunctions.

Their approach to patients begins with obtaining a detailed sexual and background history. Then the couple is instructed to carry out a sensate focus exercise in which each partner instructs the other in specific ways of caressing for sensual pleasure without involving the breasts or genitals. The next day the exercise is repeated, including breasts and genital areas, but without coitus. The exercise's purpose is to alleviate performance anxiety and to enhance warm, comfortable feelings between partners. After the sensate focus exercises are completed, the therapy is directed to the sexual dysfunction. The Masters and Johnson model emphasizes education, communication, and cooperation between partners.

Helen Singer Kaplan Model. Kaplan's (1975, 1979) method of treating sexual dysfunctions combines specific tasks with psychodynamic insights, dream interpretations, and gestalt and transactional techniques. Treatment begins with an extensive evaluation, including marital, psychiatric, sexual, medical, and family history from both partners. If serious intrapsychic or interpersonal difficulties are found, the couple may be referred to individual or conjoint therapy and is not accepted for sex therapy at that time.

Like Masters and Johnson, Kaplan uses sensate focus exercises and variations, such as showering together, to begin sex therapy or to further evaluate a person's suitability for sex therapy. Therapy itself consists of erotic tasks performed at home plus weekly or semiweekly meetings with the therapist. Couples and the therapist explore feelings experienced during the erotic exercises. The exercises take into account the motivations and dynamics of the relationship. The role of the therapist includes education, clarification, and support. Both Kaplan and Masters and Johnson emphasize communication between partners and exploration of the relationship and emotional concerns.

Pharmacological Treatment. One of the greatest advances in treating men with erectile disorders has been in understanding its medical etiology and therefore being able to treat it with drugs, devices, or surgery. Sildenafil (Viagra) was the first oral medication used to treat this dysfunction. This drug acts by improving the effects of nitric oxide, which boosts relaxation of the smooth muscle in the penis allowing it to become erect.

Viagra is taken in pill form 1 hour before sex and requires sexual stimulation to be effective. Viagra has been effective for many men suffering from erectile dysfunction; however, sex therapists caution that although Viagra may eliminate a physical cause for erectile dysfunction, it is not a magic pill that will cure all. Relationship issues also must be addressed for satisfactory treatment of this dysfunction.

The use of Viagra is also being explored for treatment of female sexual dysfunction. In a preliminary study, sildenafil (Viagra) was given to women who complained of lowered sexual desire, which included decreased sensation, engorgement, and lubrication. Seventy seven percent had no history of childhood sexual abuse and 23% did. Fifty one percent reported an increase in vaginal lubrication. Seventy seven percent of the women reported an increase in sensation, and 68% reported that it was easier to achieve orgasm. Women without a history of childhood sexual abuse were twice as likely to report benefits of sildenafil treatment than women who were sexually abused as children. The researchers propose that ideal patients for medication are women who have a medical reason for their lowered sexual arousal. They also recommend treating female sexual dysfunction with both medication and psychotherapy.

Other medications to treat sexual dysfunction are Levitra and Cialis. These medications may be prescribed to treat the sexual side effects resulting from other medication treatments.

EVALUATION

In the evaluation phase, the nurse works with the patient to evaluate the effectiveness of the sexual counseling or intervention. Factors to consider include the following:

- **Sense of well-being.** How does the person feel about himself or herself? Have these feelings improved during the treatment?
- **Functioning ability.** If the person was dysfunctional, is functional ability restored? Somewhat improved? What about the person's ability to function within primary relations at work? With friends?
- **Satisfaction with treatment.** Does the patient believe that the treatment was helpful? Were the patient's goals adequately met?

Evaluation of any form of sexual counseling or intervention should be ongoing. The nurse and patient should work together on goals, problems, and alternatives.

A Clinical Exemplar of a Psychiatric Nurse
DONALD RIBELIN, RN, C

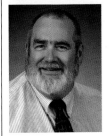

Having worked in nursing for over 20 years, I tend to have certain defined responses to almost any given situation. This works well until something comes along that doesn't fit into those preconceived notions of how things should be. I was working as evening charge nurse on an adult acute care psychiatric unit when one of the mental health assistants came to the desk to report that he had seen Mr. B and Ms. G sneaking into the solarium and that they appeared to be "getting it on." Almost every nurse has had to confront patients, visitors, or both in a sexual situation of one type or another. We'd had our share of such encounters in the past, but the staff reacted very differently this time.

To begin with, Mr. B was a 72-year-old "street" person who had been admitted with a diagnosis of rule-out dementia, and Ms. G was a lovely 70-year-old widow with a diagnosis of situational depression. Mr. B's apparent dementia had proven to be secondary to malnutrition and vitamin B_{12} deficiency. Once he had received treatment for these, we had found him to be a remarkable person whose ready sense of humor lightened many an evening group. Ms. G had been admitted with one of the flattest affects I had ever seen. Her family reported that she had been increasingly depressed since her husband's death 3 years ago. This depression increased dramatically around the anniversary of Mr. G's death, which was right around this time of the year. Over the past week, Ms. G's depression had lifted noticeably. She could be seen talking, laughing, and joking with Mr. B during any free moment. They seemed to always be together, sitting next to each other during groups or meals or walking side by side on outings. We had all commented on how much they had helped each other and what a nice couple they made. Suddenly Mr. B and Ms. G had stopped being a nice "old" couple and had become two psychiatric patients sneaking off to have "sex."

I found myself torn between several reactions to this news. The empathic nurse in me responded, "This is great: Two lonely people in the twilight years of their lives have found love and companionship." The analytical nurse in me wondered whether this relationship would really be therapeutic for Ms. G given Mr. B's background. The cautious nurse in me wondered whether Mr. B could simply be trying to ensure he had somewhere to stay after discharge. But the administrative nurse in me won out, thinking that I don't let other patients behave in this manner, so I have to intercede. Somewhat loudly I walked down the hall and into the solarium, taking a very long time fumbling for the light switch. The lights revealed Ms. G and Mr. B sitting side by side, holding hands and red faced. Ms. G's blouse was only partially buttoned, and she was ob-

viously upset. I apologized to them, explaining that I had planned to spend my break in the solarium and hadn't meant to startle them. As they quickly stood up and headed toward their rooms, I could see a look of sadness and possibly shame replacing the happy smile that we had been seeing the past few days on Ms. G's face. Mr. B also looked sad, and for a moment I thought I saw the return of the shuffling gait he had at admission. By doing the "right" thing, I now felt like I had done the very worst thing possible.

During my shift report, I gave the incident only brief comment. Talking more about the possible therapeutic benefits of the relationship, I didn't mention the sexual aspects at all. Guilt can be a great censor and rewriter of history, and I was obviously really feeling guilty. Well, time may heal all wounds, but it only gives rumors time to grow. I was very surprised when, upon returning to work the next evening, my nurse manager asked for the incident report on Mr. B and Ms. G having sex in the solarium. She also wanted to know why I hadn't documented the incident in my nursing notes. By the time I had explained the previous evening's happenings, what had started out as two people wanting to be together had become a major event. Damage control began with a meeting of all unit staff, where we discussed what had and had not happened. It didn't stop there. A psychiatric unit is often like a small town where there are no secrets. That evening, in group, the patients brought up our hapless couple's "making out." Again I found myself in a position where I felt anything I said could and probably would be wrong. After careful thought, I responded by first reminding them that this was a hospital and there were certain rules of conduct that had to be adhered to, even when we might personally disagree with them. Members of the group were asked to share their feelings about these rules and why they were or were not necessary. As the group proceeded, I kept a careful eye on Ms. G and Mr. B. They were sitting about as far from each other as possible and both were very quiet. As the patients talked, I kept trying to think of something to say or do to alleviate the obvious pain and embarrassment of our elderly, who were now the center of attention. Suddenly Mr. B stood up, smiled at the group, and said, "You know, I've been feeling real bad today. I felt like I had done something wrong and that I was just waiting for my punishment to come." Then he stated, "Yeah! I was feeling real bad until just a moment ago, when I remembered a button I saw once. It said, 'Old people need love, too,' and you know that's right because everyone needs to know that someone cares about them, needs them, and loves them. So it really doesn't matter what any of you think because I've found someone to love me and for me to love." I'll always remember that moment as a time that patients and staff clapped, cried, and laughed together. ∎

- Sexuality is defined as a desire for contact, warmth, tenderness, and love. Adaptive sexual behavior is consensual, free of force, performed in private, neither physically nor psychologically harmful, and mutually satisfying.
- The nurse's level of self-awareness is a critical component of discussions with patients regarding sexual issues. Developing self-awareness involves clarification of values regarding human sexuality and four phases of the nurse's growth: cognitive dissonance, anxiety, anger, and action.
- Patient behaviors related to sexual responses include heterosexuality, homosexuality, bisexuality, transvestism, and transsexual-

ism. The physiological and psychological responses to sexual stimulation consist of four stages: desire, excitement, orgasm, and resolution.
- Predisposing factors for variations in sexual response are described from biological, psychoanalytical, and behavioral perspectives.
- Precipitating stressors that may change sexuality include physical illness and injury, psychiatric illness, medications, and HIV/AIDS.
- Coping mechanisms used with expressions of sexuality include fantasy, projection, denial, and rationalization.
- Primary NANDA diagnoses are sexual dysfunction and ineffective sexuality pattern.

CHAPTER **FOCUS POINTS**—cont'd

- Primary *DSM-IV-TR* diagnoses are categorized as sexual dysfunctions, paraphilias, and gender identity disorders.
- The expected outcome of nursing care is that the patient will obtain the maximum level of adaptive sexual responses to enhance or maintain health.
- Education is the most common method of primary prevention of sexual problems. Sex education is a lifelong process with the primary goal of promoting sexual health.
- It is always the nurse's responsibility to preserve professional boundaries, even when a nurse feels sexually attracted to a patient. It is never acceptable for a nurse to engage in sexual behavior of any kind with a patient.
- If a patient makes a sexual advance, the nurse should let the patient know that the behavior is unacceptable. Nurses have a responsibility as professionals to attempt to understand sexual behaviors and analyze their possible meanings.
- Interventions in maladaptive sexual responses include providing support, anticipatory guidance, counseling, and referral.
- Negative attitudes by health care providers and society at large can affect the health care received by patients who are sexually diverse.
- Pedophilia, which is the sexual attraction to prepubescent children, is a crime.
- Dysfunctions of the sexual response cycle should be referred to sex therapists for treatment. Medications are also available to treat sexual dysfunctions.
- In evaluating nursing care the nurse and patient should consider the patient's sense of well-being, functional ability, and satisfaction with treatment.

KEY TERMS

bisexuality, 542
cognitive dissonance, 540
gender identity, 556
gender identity disorder, 556

heterosexuality, 542
homophobia, 554
homosexuality, 542
paraphilia, 556

pedophilia, 556
sexual orientation, 542
transsexualism, 542
transvestism, 542

CHAPTER REVIEW QUESTIONS

1. Match each term in Column A with the correct definition in Column B.

Column A
_____ Bisexuality
_____ Gender identity
_____ Gender role
_____ Genetic identity
_____ Heterosexuality
_____ Homophobia
_____ Homosexuality
_____ Orgasm
_____ Pedophilia
_____ Sexual orientation
_____ Transsexualism
_____ Transvestism

Column B
A. A person's chromosomal gender
B. A person's perception of his or her maleness or femaleness
C. Condition in which there is a profound discomfort with one's own sex and a strong and persistent identification with the opposite gender
D. Condition in which usually a male has a sexual obsession for or addiction to women's clothing
E. Peaking of sexual pleasure and the release of sexual tension accompanied by rhythmic contractions of the perineal muscles and pelvic reproductive organs
F. Irrational fear of homosexuals along with a negative attitude and hostility toward them
G. Sexual attraction to members of the opposite sex
H. Sexual attraction to members of the same sex
I. Sexual attraction to persons of both sexes
J. The cultural role attributes attributed to one's gender, such as expectations regarding behavior, cognitions, occupations, values, and emotional responses
K. The gender to which one is romantically attracted
L. Sexual attraction to prepubescent children

2. Fill in the blanks.

A. When a nurse holds two opposing beliefs at the same time, it is called _____.

B. A biological female typically has _____ chromosomes, whereas a biological male typically has _____ chromosomes.

C. According to Freud, in the _____ complex the child experiences sexual feelings for the parent of the opposite sex and resents the parent of the same sex.

D. Behaviorists believe that _____ may predispose one to sexual difficulties later in life.

E. _____ is the most common method of primary prevention of sexual problems.

F. The nurse's first step in working with a patient in relation to maladaptive sexual responses is to communicate _____.

3. Provide short responses for the following questions.

A. Identify five criteria for adaptive sexual behavior.
B. Design a sex education program for adolescents that includes a focus on safe sex practices.
C. Critique the assessment form used in your treatment center for its inclusion of information related to a patient's sexual responses.
D. Describe specific ways in which culture defines a society's view of "normal" sexual behavior.

Visit Evolve for additional resources related to the content of this chapter.
http://evolve.elsevier.com/Stuart/principles/

• Topical Course Outline • Student Workbook Exercises • Critical Thinking Questions and Activities • Case Studies • Research Topics
• Monthly Content Updates • WebLinks

Student Study CD-ROM

Access the accompanying CD-ROM for animations, interactive exercises, review questions for the NCLEX examination, and an audio glossary.

REFERENCES

Altemeyer B: Changes in attitudes toward homosexuals, *J Homosexuality* 42:63, 2001.

American Psychiatric Association: *Diagnostic and statistical manual of mental disorders,* ed 4, text revision, Washington, DC, 2000, American Psychiatric Association.

Bing EG et al: Psychiatric disorders and drug use among human immunodeficiency virus-infected adults in the United States, *Arch Gen Psychiatry* 58:721, 2001.

Bobes J et al: Frequency of sexual dysfunction and other reproductive side effects in patients with schizophrenia treated with rispiridone, olanzapine, quetiapine or haloperidol: the results of the EIRE study, *J Sex Marital Ther* 29:125, 2003.

Carroll RA: Outcomes of treatment for gender dysphoria, *J Sex Educ Ther* 24:128:1999.

Centers for Disease Control and Prevention: *HIV/AIDS surveillance report,* Atlanta, 2001, US Department of Health and Human Services.

Cohen LJ, Galynker II: Clinical features of pedophilia and implications for treatment, *J Psychiatr Prac* 8:276, 2002.

Courtois CA: The sexual after-effects of incest/child sexual abuse, *SIECUS Rep* 29:11, 2000.

DeLamater J, Friedrich WN: Human sexual development, *J Sex Res* 39:10, 2002.

Essock SM et al: Risk factors for HIV, hepatitis B, and hepatitis C among persons with severe mental illness, *Psychiatr Serv* 54:836, 2003.

Farella C: The unthinkable problem of pedophilia, *Nurs Spec* 3:36mw, 2002.

Fergusson DM, Horwood LJ, Beautrais AL: Is sexual orientation related to mental health problems and suicidality in young people? *Arch Gen Psychiatry* 56:876, 1999.

Fields CB, Scout BJ: Addressing the needs of lesbian patients, *J Sex Educ Ther* 26:182, 2001.

Foley T, Davies M: *Rape: nursing care of victims,* St Louis, 1983, Mosby.

Ford E et al: Managing sexual behavior on adult acute care inpatient psychiatric units, *Psychiatr Serv* 54:346, 2003.

Freud S: *Three essays of the theory of sexuality,* ed 3, London, 1962, Hogarth Press (originally published 1905).

Gramling LF, Carr RL, McCain NL: Family responses to disclosure of self-as-lesbian, *Issues Ment Health Nurs* 21:653, 2000.

Harry Benjamin International Gender Dysphoria Association: Standards of care for gender identity disorders (6th version), 2001, www.hbigda.org/soc.html [retrieved on 5/14/03].

Jacoby S: Great sex: what's age got to do with it? *Modern Maturity* 42R:43, 1999.

Kaplan HS: *The illustrated manual of sex therapy,* New York, 1975, New York Times Book Co.

Kaplan HS: *Disorders of sexual desire and other new concepts and techniques in sex therapy,* New York, 1979, Brunner/Mazel.

Kendall-Tackett K: The health effects of childhood abuse: four pathways by which abuse can influence health, *Child Abuse Negl* 26:715, 2002.

King BM: *Human sexuality today,* ed 3, Upper Saddle River, NJ, 1999, Prentice-Hall.

Kinsey A et al: *Sexual behavior in the human female,* Philadelphia, 1953, WB Saunders.

Krueger RB, Kaplan MS: The paraphilic and hypersexual disorders: an overview, *J Psychiatr Pract* 7:391, 2001.

Krueger RB, Kaplan MS: Behavioral and psychopharmacological treatment of the paraphilic and hypersexual disorders, *J Psychiatr Pract* 8:21, 2002.

Lamp J et al: Nurses' knowledge, attitudes and skills related to sexuality, *J Nurs Scholarsh* 32:391, 2000.

Laumann EO, Paik A, Rosen RC: Sexual dysfunction in the United States: prevalence and predictors, *JAMA* 281:537, 1999.

Lobell S: Registered nurses' responses to sexual harassment, *Pelican News* 55:14, 1999.

Lock J, Steiner H: Gay, lesbian, and bisexual youth risks for emotional, physical and social problems: results from a community-based survey, *J Am Acad Child Adolesc Psychiatry* 38:297, 1999.

Lyon DE: Human immunodeficiency virus (HIV) disease in persons with severe mental illnesses, *Issues Ment Health Nurs* 22:109, 2001.

Mahan V: Assessing and treating sexual dysfunction, *J Am Psychiatr Nurs Assoc* 9:90, 2003.

Masters W, Johnson V: *Human sexual inadequacy,* Boston, 1970, Little, Brown.

Masters WH, Kolodny RC, Johnson VE: *Masters and Johnson on sex and human loving,* Boston, 1986, Little, Brown.

Mc Donald J, Badger TA: Social function of persons with schizophrenia, *J Psychosoc Nurs* 40:42, 2002.

Miracle TS, Miracle AW, Baumeister RF: *Human sexuality: meeting your basic needs,* Upper Saddle River, NJ, 2003, Prentice Hall.

Moore BE, Rothschild AJ: Treatment of antidepressant induced sexual dysfunction, *Hosp Pract* 34:89, 1999.

Nathan P, Gorman J: *A guide to treatments that work,* ed 2, New York, 2002, Oxford University Press.

Phillips N: Female sexual dysfunction: evaluation and treatment, *Am Fam Physician* 62:141, 2000.

Satriano J: Routine HIV testing for the severely mentally ill: considerations and cautions, *J Psychiatr Pract* 8:143, 2002.

SIECUS Fact Sheet, Issues and answers: Fact sheet on sexuality education, *SIECUS Rep* 29:30, 2001.

Skegg K et al: Sexual orientation and self-harm in men and women, *Am J Psychiatry* 160:541, 2003.

Taylor B: 'Coming out' as a life transition: homosexual identity formation and its implications for health care practice, *J Adv Nurs* 30:520, 1999.

Wincze JP, Carey MP: *Sexual dysfunction: a guide for assessment and treatment,* ed 2, New York, 2001, Guilford Press.

Wright R, Anthony P: Lesbians and mental health: are we helping or hindering? *Ment Health Pract* 5:12, 2002.

Wysoker A: Sexual misconduct, *J Am Psychiatr Nurs Assoc* 6:131, 2000.

Zeiss AM, Kasl-Godley J: Sexuality in older adults' relationships, *Generations* 25:18, 2001.

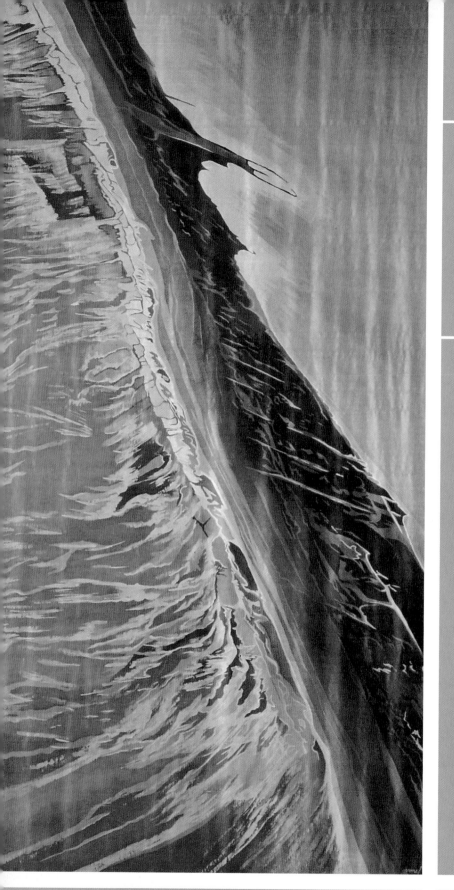

Unit Four

Fire Island (New York)
107" x 55" batik on silk 1995

Fire Island is my art addressing AIDS as a crisis. The burning diagonal represents a fiery issue in our country and holds a hieroglyphic message that has not yet been decoded to cure this disease. The waves to the left beat against the backbone of my now dead friend. The calm to the right is love and support of a spiritual nature.

Treatment Modalities

Maybe there have been times when you felt that the problems people experience are truly overwhelming and you wondered how you could ever really help. Sure you are a nurse, but how can one person reduce the world's stress, illness, and social injustice? Although it is true that societal problems are great, it is also true that the contribution of each person is like a ripple in a pool that can eventually turn the tide of life. One person can make a difference. But to be effective you need to have the right tools for the task, tools that will allow you to help people think about their own life situations and learn to change their behavior, tools that will help you work therapeutically with individuals, families, and groups.

In this unit you will be exposed to a wide range of treatment tools; do not think of these strategies as applying only to patients with psychiatric illnesses. Many people, not just psychiatric patients, take psychotropic medications, and nurses work with people who are struggling with issues of control, fear, agitation, and aggression in almost all clinical settings. Also, strategies intended to change negative thinking patterns and problematic behavior can apply to children and adults throughout their experiences with health and illness. And finally, are not groups an essential part of every health care delivery system? And do not all patients have families? As you can see, the skills you will learn in this unit will enhance your nursing practice regardless of the setting and patient population. So grab your highlighters and get ready to add to your growing repertoire of nursing skills and competencies, because you can and will make a difference.

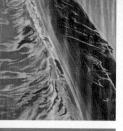

Medicines are nothing in themselves, if not properly used, but the very hands of the gods, if employed with reason and prudence.

HEROPHILUS

27 PSYCHOPHARMACOLOGY

Michele T. Laraia

evolve Visit Evolve for additional resources related to the content of this chapter.
http://evolve.elsevier.com/Stuart/principles/

This chapter introduces the nurse to psychopharmacology and describes important principles of drug therapy in the treatment of patients with neurobiological brain disorders, or mental illnesses. The pharmacological agents described in this chapter are all approved by the Food and Drug Administration (FDA), although not always for the indication described. Included in this chapter are discussions about drug augmentation and off-label uses of pharmacological agents. Dietary supplements, herbal preparations, and hormones used to treat the symptoms of mental illness are described in Chapter 29.

The theoretical framework for psychopharmacology in this chapter is one of integration in that drug therapy complements other evidence-based therapies, such as cognitive-behavioral, psychosocial, interpersonal, psychodynamic, and complementary and alternative interventions. Drug therapy is not viewed as a quick fix or miracle pill. Psychopharmacological agents treat specific symptoms of neurobiological illnesses with significant effectiveness, although side effects and adverse reactions of drug therapy require expertise and sound clinical judgment on the part of the nurse.

Psychopharmacology is the gold standard in the treatment of neurobiological illnesses, more and more of which are found to have genetic underpinnings. However, drugs alone do not treat the patient's personal, social, or environmental components of or responses to these illnesses. This underscores the need for an integrated and comprehensive approach to the treatment of persons with mental illness.

ROLE OF THE NURSE

Psychopharmacological treatment should be integrated with the principles of psychiatric nursing practice presented throughout this book. The psychiatric nurse has a wealth of knowledge and competencies that make the nursing care provided to people with psychiatric disorders unique in many ways. Following are some examples of the nurse's role in psychopharmacological treatment of persons with neurobiological illness.

Patient Assessment

Psychoactive drugs treat specific symptoms of neurobiological brain disorders. However, not all patient behaviors are treated by drug therapy, and not every identified personality trait is a symptom of illness targeted for treatment with drugs. It is essential that a thorough patient baseline assessment, including history, physical and laboratory examination (see Chapter 6), psychiatric evaluation (see Chapter 7), sociocultural assessment (see Chapter 8), and a medication history, be completed for each patient before any treatment interventions are initiated. This information helps distinguish aspects of the psychiatric illness from aspects of the patient's personality that were present before the onset of illness.

As a result of the baseline assessment, a diagnosis is made, psychiatric symptoms are identified as appropriate targets for drug treatment, and an integrated treatment plan is developed. Residual symptoms of the patient's illness may need

specific interventions to enhance treatment effectiveness, and dysfunctional personality characteristics not related to the psychiatric disorder can be addressed by nonpharmacological treatments if appropriate.

Drug side effects that emerge after treatment is begun should be identified and appropriately treated as they appear. Symptoms of organ system dysfunction, being either a component of an illness or a side effect of drug treatment, should be identified and treated. Current nonpsychiatric diagnoses and treatments also are documented at the baseline level, as well as documentation of use of over-the-counter remedies and complimentary and alternative treatments the patient may be taking. Finally, careful baseline assessment of each patient can help identify undiagnosed medical illnesses that are concurrent with the psychiatric illness or that may be causing the psychiatric symptoms. Box 27-1 provides a medication assessment tool to guide the nurse in taking a drug and substance history.

Coordination of Treatment Modalities

The nurse has an important role in designing a comprehensive treatment program. The most appropriate treatment choices should be individualized for each patient and reflected in the treatment plan. The coordination of treatment modalities is often the primary responsibility of the nurse who works with the patient in an ongoing therapeutic alliance as part of the health care team. The nurse is in a position to integrate drug treatments with the wide range of nonpharmacological treatments in a manner that is knowledgeable, safe, effective, and acceptable to the patient.

Psychopharmacological Drug Administration

No one on the health care team has a greater daily impact on the patient's experience with psychopharmacological agents than the nurse. In many inpatient, day treatment, home health, and other outpatient settings, the nurse administers the medication dose, works out a dosing schedule based on drug requirements and the patient's needs and preferences, and is continually alert for and treats drug effects. This role defines the nurse as a key professional in maximizing therapeutic effects of drug treatment and minimizing side effects in such a way that the patient is a true collaborator in managing the medication regimen.

Monitoring Drug Effects

The nurse has the important role of consistently monitoring the effects of psychopharmacological drugs. This includes making standardized measurements of drug effects on baseline target symptoms of illness, evaluating and minimizing side effects, treating adverse reactions, and noting the often subtle effects on the patient's self-concept and sense of trust.

A drug should be given within the recommended dose range and for the appropriate amount of time before it can be determined whether the drug has had an adequate therapeutic trial for a particular patient. Therapeutic drug monitoring is important because some drugs have a narrow therapeutic range (such as lithium), they can cause sudden serious ad-

BOX **27-1**

Medication Assessment Tool

For each of the following categories of drugs taken by the patient:
- Prescribed psychiatric medications ever taken
- Prescribed nonpsychiatric medication taken in the past 6 months or taken for major medical illnesses if more than 6 months ago
- Over-the-counter (OTC) medication taken in the past 6 months

Obtain the following information from the patient and other sources:
- Name of the drug
- Reason taken
- Dates started and stopped
- Highest daily dose
- Who prescribed it?
- Was it effective?
- Side effects or adverse reactions
- Was it taken as directed?
- If not, how was it taken?
- History of drug taken by first-degree relative
- Drugs taken prescribed by others
- Supplements, herbs, essential oils, and other complementary and alternative remedies either prescribed or OTC

For each of the following categories of drugs taken by the patient:
- Alcohol
- Tobacco
- Caffeine
- Street drugs

Obtain the following information from the patient and other sources:
- Name of substance
- Dates and schedule of use
- Summarize effects
- Adverse reactions/withdrawal symptoms
- Attempts to stop/treatments to stop
- Impact of substance on:
  - Quality of life
  - Relationships/spouse/children
  - Occupation/education
  - Health/productivity
  - Self-image
  - Expense

---

verse reactions (such as neuroleptic malignant syndrome), and drugs are often co-administered, thereby altering the drug metabolism and clearance rates.

Almost all drugs are metabolized by one of the many families of metabolic enzymes, or "cytochromes," usually referred to as the *CYP 450 system,* found predominantly in the liver. Some drugs, called **inducers,** speed up one or more of these systems, thus decreasing the blood level of drugs metabolized by that system, potentially causing a lack of effectiveness of those drugs. Other drugs, called **inhibitors,** slow down one or more systems, thus increasing blood levels of the drugs metabolized by that system, potentially causing increased side effects or even toxicity from those drugs. This is known as cytochrome P-450 inhibition. Additionally, some racial and ethnic groups have genetic predispositions toward deficiencies in some enzymes, making them at greater risk for CYP-450 problems.

It is the responsibility of the medication prescriber to anticipate these possibilities and prescribe accordingly. The nurse should be vigilant for signs of drug effects that seem inconsistent with the doses prescribed or that are adverse reactions.

Medication Education

The nurse is in a pivotal position to educate the patient and the family about medications. This includes teaching complex information to the patient so that it can be understood, discussed, and accepted. Patients should be well informed about each drug prescribed for them. They should be well educated about the expected benefits and potential risks, understand additional potential treatments for their condition, and know what to do and whom to contact if a question or problem arises. Medication education is an important key to the effective and safe use of psychotropic drugs, to patient collaboration in the treatment plan, and to patient adherence with drug treatment regimens.

Drug Maintenance Programs

For some patients the drug maintenance program may last many months and perhaps even a lifetime. The nurse can assume the important role of continuing a therapeutic alliance with a patient on drug maintenance. The nurse is often the contact for patients who may have ongoing questions about their current drug regimen, drug effects on lifestyle and concurrent illnesses, and new treatments as they become available. Advanced practice nurses may be the primary health care provider for patients during both acute and maintenance phases of treatment.

Clinical Research Drug Trials

As a member of the interdisciplinary research team, the nurse can contribute to the body of scientific knowledge, often adding a nursing perspective to team research efforts. The nurse can be included on many levels, from research data collector and principal investigator to funding agency monitor and consultant. The nurse's roles in interdisciplinary clinical research drug trials continue to evolve. Nurses involved in psychopharmacological **randomized controlled trials (RCTs)** can enhance the research experience for the patient, who will need significant information about informed consent, double-blind randomization, experimental treatments, placebo-controlled trials, and patient rights.

Prescriptive Authority

Legislation has been passed in almost every state in the United States authorizing advanced practice registered nurses (APRNs) to have at least some degree of authority to prescribe medications, and in some states APRNs have full autonomy in this role. Psychiatric mental health nurse practitioners, and in some states this includes clinical nurse specialists, who are qualified under their state nurse practice acts are thus able to prescribe pharmacological agents to treat the symptoms and improve the functional status of patients with psychiatric illnesses. Specific psychopharmacological agents can be prescribed by APRNs based on the state nurse practice act, state board of nursing regulations, diagnostic criteria, clinical practice guidelines, and medication prescribing protocols.

Thus the role of nurses in psychopharmacological treatments has been expanded to encompass medication prescriptive authority in order to capitalize on the expertise of APRNs and to increase patient access to quality and cost-effective health care. Collaborative relationships with one's supervisor, any other health care providers and agencies involved in the care of one's patients, and with one's peers are considered an important part of the nurse prescriber's role. The use of collective practical knowledge and wisdom by experienced APRN prescribers is a valuable learning tool in the education of nurses who have assumed this expanded role (Hale, 2002).

Does your state grant medication prescriptive authority to psychiatric–mental health APRNs? If so, what are the requirements for prescriptive practice? ■

■ PHARMACOLOGICAL PRINCIPLES

Pharmacokinetics

Pharmacokinetics is the study of how the body affects a drug. It answers the question: How does the body get drugs to and from their intended target? Body functions such as **absorption** (how the drug is moved into the blood stream from the site of administration), **distribution** (how much drug is moved into various body tissues), **metabolism** (how the drug is altered, usually by liver enzymes, into its active and inactive parts), and **elimination** (how much of the drug is removed from the body in a specific amount of time) are all pharmacokinetic properties.

The time course and location of drug concentrations in the body can be predicted, appropriate dosing schedules can be designed, side effects can be anticipated, and the time it takes a drug to become effective can be estimated by using pharmacokinetic models. Additional pharmacokinetic properties that assist in understanding the mechanisms of psychopharmacological agents and how the body affects a drug are described next.

Bioavailability (how much of the drug reaches systemic circulation unchanged) is an estimate used to compare various drug preparations, particularly if the same generic drug is made by several different manufacturers. In general, generic instead of trade name drugs are used when writing prescriptions to assure more accuracy of the bioavailability estimate, because trade name drugs can differ from one another. Using generic drug names also facilitates being able to take advantage of price differences among manufacturers and prevents possible confusion when a drug later becomes available as a generic (when the patent runs out and the drug can be made by any company, usually at a lower cost). Once a drug does become a generic, the patient should be instructed to continuously use the same company brand of a drug because the bioavailability of psychoactive drugs may vary significantly from one company to another, thus affecting drug dose and steady state. The patient can be taught to use one pharmacy regularly, and the pharmacist can be asked to use the same manufacturer every time when filling generic prescriptions of a particular drug, again to assure a constant bioavailability.

A drug's half-life is the time it takes for the dose amount of drug in the body to decrease by 50%. For example, the benzodiazepine alprazolam has a half-life of approximately 11 hours, so it takes about 2.5 days for nearly all traces of the drug to be eliminated from the body after taking a single dose.

Half-life determines how long it will take the body to achieve steady state. Steady state means that the plasma drug concentration remains relatively constant between doses because the amount of drug excreted equals the amount ingested, and this equilibrium occurs in approximately five half-lives of any given drug. Until steady state is reached, the drug level in the body continues to fluctuate, accounting for some acute side effects and preventing determination of the optimum dose for a particular patient. Assessing a blood level measurement is not an accurate method of determining a proper dose range; the daily dose may have to be divided in order to minimize the peak level of drug concentration after each ingestion.

Termination of drug treatment is also affected by half-life. The effects of drugs with a long half-life, or with active metabolites, can last a long time (sometimes weeks) after the last dose has been taken. Drugs with a shorter half-life usually must be tapered (discontinued gradually) over several days or weeks. In general, most psychoactive drugs should be tapered to avoid uncomfortable discontinuation symptoms. Drugs with addiction potential, such as benzodiazepines, must be tapered gradually to avoid serious withdrawal symptoms.

Drug interactions can be the result of pharmacokinetic properties. One drug may interfere with the absorption, metabolism, distribution, and elimination of another drug, thus raising or lowering the levels of that second drug in the blood and tissue. As noted above, some drugs inhibit and others induce the activity of liver drug-metabolizing enzymes, thereby affecting the liver's ability to keep levels of psychopharmacological drugs stable.

For example, most of the antidepressants (selective serotonin reuptake inhibitors [SSRIs] and nefazodone), some of the typical antipsychotics (haloperidol, perphenazine, and fluphenazine), the mood stabilizer topiramate, and even grapefruit juice can inhibit drug-metabolizing liver enzymes in the CYP-450 system, potentially causing toxic levels of other drugs (such as imipramine, which is metabolized by some of the affected enzymes). The mood stabilizer carbamazepine, St. John's wort, and even smoking cigarettes can markedly reduce many psychotropic drug levels, such as some antipsychotic drugs, rendering them ineffective (Boland and Keller, 2004).

Pharmacodynamics

Pharmacodynamics is the study of the effects of a drug on the body and, in particular, the interaction of a drug on the receptor that is its targeted site of action. Pharmacodynamics answers the question: What does a drug do once it gets where it's going? The time course and intensity of drug effects on the body can be determined, drug interactions can be better understood, and safety profiles can be developed that affect clinical decision making by using pharmacodynamic models. Several pharmacodynamic properties related to how drugs affect the body include those listed here.

Receptor Mechanisms. Receptors are channels sitting on cells that are the gatekeepers of brain communication. They recognize and respond to molecules (messengers) that affect their biological function. Thus receptors are targets for drugs acting as messengers, which modify the biological activity of the receptors, bringing a dysfunctional system back toward normal.

A drug modifies a receptor by attaching (binding) to one (like a key in a single lock) or many (like a master key for many locks) subtypes of receptors in several ways: A drug can stimulate the receptor to fully (in which case the drug is an agonist) or partially (partial agonist) open its channel; it can inhibit or block (antagonist) another chemical agonist from stimulating the receptor to open its channel; or it can directly close (inverse agonist) the receptor channel. For example, benzodiazepines are agonists for the gamma-aminobutyric acid (GABA) system (they enhance the activity of GABA, an inhibitory neurotransmitter), and most antipsychotic drugs are antagonists at dopamine (DA) receptors (they inhibit the activity of dopamine).

The Dose-Response Curve. If the concentration of the drug is plotted against the effects of the drug on a graph, the curve produced is a measure of drug potency. Potency is the amount of dose required to achieve certain effects. It answers the question: How much of this drug is needed to get these results? This concept is helpful when comparing the actions of one drug to another. For example, atypical antipsychotics differ in potency—risperidone is more potent than clozapine, therefore requiring lower doses to achieve a therapeutic effect.

The Therapeutic Index. The therapeutic index is a relative measure of the safety and toxicity of a drug. The ratio produced by measuring the amount of drug necessary for 50% of patients to experience a therapeutic effect (median effective dose) and the highest amount of drug at which a toxic effect is produced in 50% of patients (median toxic dose) is called the *therapeutic index*. It answers the question: What is the lowest dose of this drug needed to begin to produce a thera-

peutic effect, and what is the highest dose at which a toxic effect is produced in the average patient?

A **low therapeutic index** means that the difference between the amount of drug needed to achieve the desired effect and the amount that would cause toxic effects has a narrow range (like a window with a narrow opening). For example, the mood-stabilizer lithium has a low therapeutic index and requires frequent blood level checks and careful monitoring and stabilizing measures to ensure its safe use. On the other hand, the typical antipsychotic haloperidol has a **high therapeutic index** and thus is safely prescribed in a wide range of doses (like a window opened very wide). Individual patient differences such as age, gender, and race also can affect the therapeutic index of a specific drug.

The Development of Tolerance, Dependence, and Withdrawal Symptoms. Some patients become less responsive to the same dose of a particular drug over time which is called tolerance, requiring that higher doses of the drug be given over time to obtain the same initial therapeutic effect. The development of tolerance to some drugs like benzodiazepines (BZs) or opioids also may be associated with physical dependence on the drug, requiring tapering (gradual dose reduction) during discontinuation to avoid withdrawal symptoms. BZ withdrawal symptoms can be quite uncomfortable and, rarely, even fatal.

Drug Co-Administration

Once generally discouraged, the use of more than one psychopharmacological drug in the same patient at the same time is rapidly becoming standard clinical practice under specific circumstances. Patients who are prescribed multiple medications or are taking over-the-counter medications in addition to their prescribed medications can potentially receive benefits from these combinations, but also may be at risk for increased side effects, drug interactions, lack of clarity concerning which drug is causing which effect, complex dosing schedules, and higher costs of treatment.

Box 27-2 lists guidelines for drug co-administration. Box 27-3 alerts the nurse to which patients may be at higher risk for drug interactions. Table 27-1 is a reference list for the more common interactions of psychotropic drugs. The following drug co-administration principles will guide the nurse when multiple medications are prescribed.

Primary Medication. The medication used to treat the target symptoms of the patient's primary diagnosis is the primary medication in a drug treatment regimen. For example, antidepressants are the primary medications used in treatment of a primary diagnosis of major depression.

Combination Drug Therapy. Combination drug therapy refers to simultaneous use of two or more psychopharmacological drugs in the same class for long-term treatment. For example, in a patient who gains only partial relief from a mood stabilizer given for bipolar disorder, a second mood stabilizer may be added to the drug regimen to increase the treatment effect in long-term treatment.

BOX 27-2

Guidelines for Drug Co-Administration

- Identify specific target symptoms for each drug.
- If possible, start with one drug and evaluate effectiveness and side effects before adding a second drug.
- Be alert for adverse drug interactions.
- Consider the effects of a second drug on the absorption and metabolism of the first drug.
- Consider the possibility of additive side effects.
- Change the dose of only one drug at a time and evaluate results.
- Be aware of increased risk of medication errors.
- Be aware of increased cost of treatment.
- Be aware of decreased patient adherence when medication regimen is complex.
- In follow-up treatment, eliminate as many drugs as possible and establish the effective dose of the drugs used.
- Patient education programs regarding concomitant drug regimens must be particularly clear, organized, and effective.
- Patient follow-up contacts should be more frequent.
- If a patient has more than one prescriber, integration of care is required.

BOX 27-3

Increased Risk Factors for Development of Drug Interactions

- Drug co-administration
- High doses
- Geriatric patients
- Debilitated/dehydrated patients
- Concurrent illness
- Compromised organ system function
- Inadequate patient education
- History of nonadherence
- Failure to include patient in treatment planning

Why do you think patients often fail to report over-the-counter remedies when asked what medicines they are taking? How can you, as a nurse, be sure to obtain this information? ■

Special Populations

Although this chapter focuses on the adult patient, special populations such as children (see Chapters 36 and 37), the elderly (see Chapters 23 and 38), seriously medically ill patients (see Chapter 40), and cross-cultural members of various racially and ethnically diverse or disadvantaged groups are regularly given psychoactive drugs, even though these drugs are rarely adequately tested in randomized clinical trials on these populations. An understanding of relevant issues will help the nurse administer psychopharmacological agents safely to persons who are members of special populations.

Children. Few systematic studies of psychotropic drugs in children have been conducted, yet children and adolescents can experience quite severe psychiatric illnesses. Generally children metabolize drugs more rapidly than adults and therefore do not usually need lower doses than adults just because they may weigh less and have a smaller body size. Children and young adolescents exhibit a variable response to these drugs and thus need vigilant monitoring.

Geriatric Patients. Drug distribution, hepatic metabolism, and renal clearance are all affected by age. This often results in the elderly having slower metabolism and elimination of drugs and increased susceptibility to side effects. It is important to begin with a lower than recommended adult dose and titrate up at a rate slower than the usual recommended adult rate—or **"start low and go slow."** Geriatric patients often take multiple medications, so the nurse should be aware of the increased risk for drug interactions, complex dosing regimens, and cost.

Pregnant and Lactating Women. If a pregnant woman takes psychoactive drugs, the unborn infant may experience drug effects in utero and even withdrawal symptoms after birth. Because pregnant women are systematically excluded from randomized clinical trials, knowledge of drug reactions in animal studies and in human anecdotal reports is very use-

Augmentation or Adjunctive Therapy. Augmentation is the addition of another class of medication to supplement the effectiveness of the primary medication. It is becoming a widely accepted clinical practice. This is done when the primary medicine falls short of expectation and needs to have its effectiveness augmented, or boosted.

An example is the addition of one antidepressant (for example, fluoxetine) to the primary antidepressant drug (for example, paroxetine) to treat persistent depressive symptoms or to alleviate only partial remission of symptoms in a patient with major depression. This is also done when the primary drug treats target symptoms effectively, but other symptoms remain. For example, an antidepressant is added to the primary antipsychotic drug for persistent symptoms of depression in a patient with schizophrenia.

Concurrent Pharmacology. Some patients with more than one illness need drug treatments for each illness. An example is the diabetic patient taking insulin who also needs an antidepressant for a concurrent depression. Great effort must be employed to properly integrate the care of such a patient in order to optimize treatments and avoid incompatible therapies, complex dosing regimens, and high drug costs.

Polypharmacy. Polypharmacy is the use of multiple psychopharmacological medications for long-term treatment. It is considered to be outside the usual practice standards or clinical guidelines (although sometimes this term is mistakenly used to include all types of combined drug therapy).

An example of polypharmacy is maintaining a patient on two antipsychotics without having ever tried therapeutic doses of just a single antipsychotic.

Table 27-1	Interactions of Psychotropic Drugs and Other Substances
PSYCHOTROPIC CATEGORY	POSSIBLE INTERACTIONS

Antianxiety Agents

Benzodiazepines with:

Central nervous system (CNS) depressants (alcohol, barbiturates, antipsychotics, antihistamines, cimetidine)	Potential additive CNS effects, especially sedation and decreased daytime performance
Selective serotonin reuptake inhibitors (SSRIs), disulfiram, estrogens	Increased benzodiazepine effects
Antacids, tobacco	Decreased benzodiazepine effects

Sedative-hypnotics with:

CNS depressants (alcohol, antihistamines, antidepressants, narcotics, antipsychotics)	Enhancement of sedative effects; impairment of mental and physical performance; may result in lethargy, respiratory depression, coma, death
Anticoagulants (oral)*	Decreased coumarin plasma levels and effect; monitor and adjust dose of coumarin

Antidepressants

Tricyclics (TCAs) with:

Monoamine oxidase inhibitors (MAOIs)*	May cause hypertensive crisis
Alcohol and other CNS depressants	Additive CNS depression; decreased TCA effect
Antihypertensives* (guanethidine, methyldopa, clonidine)	Antagonism of antihypertensive effect
Antipsychotics and anti-parkinsonians	Increased TCA effect; confusion, delirium, ileus
Anticholinergics	Additive anticholinergic effects
Antiarrhythmics (quinidine, procainamide, propranolol)	Additive antiarrhythmic effects; myocardial depression
SSRIs*	Increased TCA serum level/toxicity through inhibition of cytochrome P-450 system
Anticonvulsants	Decreased TCA effect; seizures
Tobacco	Decreased TCA plasma levels

SSRIs with:

Clomipramine, maprotiline, bupropion, clozapine	Increased risk of seizures
MAOIs*	Serotonin syndrome
Barbiturates, benzodiazepines, narcotics	Increased CNS depression
Carbamazepine	Neurotoxicity: nausea, vomiting, vertigo, tinnitus, ataxia, lethargy, blurred vision
Aripiprazole	Fluoxetine and paroxetine lower levels
Risperidone	Fluoxetine and paroxetine may increase risperidone to toxic levels
Selegiline*	Hypertensive crisis; increased serotonergic effects; mania
St. John's wort, naratriptan, rizatriptan, sumatriptan, zolmitriptan, tramadol*	Serotonin syndrome
Haloperidol	Decreased effect of either drug
Calcium channel blockers	Neurotoxicity; dizziness, nausea, diplopia, headache
Valproate	Decreased valproate serum concentration
Cimetidine, erythromycin, isoniazid, fluconazole	Somnolence, lethargy, dizziness, blurred vision, ataxia, nausea; increased carbamazepine levels
Clozapine*	Avoid due to increased risk of agranulocytosis
Aripiprazole	Increased blood levels of aripiprazole
Rifampin	Decreased carbamazepine levels

Antipsychotics With:

Antacids, tea, coffee, milk, fruit juice	Decreased phenothiazine effect
CNS depressants (narcotics, antianxiety drugs, alcohol, antihistamines, barbiturates)	Additive CNS depression
Anticholinergic agents (levodopa)*	Additive atropine-like side effects and increased anti-Parkinson effects
SSRIs	Increased neuroleptic serum level and extrapyramidal side effects (EPS)

Antipsychotics

Clozapine with:

Carbamazepine*	Additive bone marrow suppression
Benzodiazepines*	Circulatory collapse, respiratory arrest
SSRIs*	Increased risk of seizures

*Potentially clinically significant.

ful information when prescribing for pregnant and lactating women, as is the FDA rating system for pregnancy risk of drugs (Millard, 2002). The FDA rates drug teratogenicity or its adverse effects on the fetus. The categories related to use during pregnancy are as follows:

- A—Controlled studies show no risk
- B—No evidence of risk in humans
- C—Risk cannot be ruled out
- D—Positive evidence of risk; however, potential benefits may outweigh potential risks
- X—Contraindicated in pregnancy

A careful risk-to-benefit analysis of the psychiatrically symptomatic mother should include these risks: inattention to prenatal care, poor maternal health, adverse effect on mother-infant bonding, increased stress levels on the fetus and infant, history of adverse drug effects on the fetus, and blood levels of a particular drug measured in breast milk. When the benefits outweigh the risks, some psychotropic drugs may be given during pregnancy and breast-feeding.

For example, the SSRIs (with the exception of fluoxetine because of its long half-life) are considered safe during pregnancy and breast-feeding (Carlat, 2003). Unless a bipolar woman is severely symptomatic, mood stabilizers are contraindicated during pregnancy and breast-feeding because of an increased risk for adverse effects on the fetus and infant. A number of psychotherapeutic drugs (including but not limited to alprazolam, lorazepam, amitriptyline, divalproex, and lithium) have an FDA pregnancy rating of category D. Low-potency typical antipsychotics, such as chlorpromazine, have been associated with increased congenital anomalies and infant sedation during breast-feeding, although high-potency drugs such as haloperidol have not. The atypical antipsychotics have not been systematically studied during human pregnancy and lactation.

Cross-Cultural Perspectives, Ethnopsychopharmacology, and Gender.

Various cultural groups can differ in the way in which its members seek help for illness, express symptoms of illness, relate to health care professionals of different backgrounds, and believe in the effectiveness of treatments. Cultural heritage can affect individual and family attitudes, beliefs, and practices regarding health and illness. This diversity can complicate the communication necessary for accurate diagnosis and successful treatment outcomes. The nurse should be knowledgeable about and sensitive to cross-cultural issues in patients and their families.

Race, ethnicity, and gender also can affect biological response to medications. Genetic differences can affect how psychotropic drugs can be used by an individual or a group with common genetic ancestry. Pharmacokinetic and pharmacodynamic processes that are biologically or biochemically mediated have the potential to exhibit differences between racial and ethnic groups.

Psychopharmacogenetics deals with genetic and environmental factors that control or influence psychotropic drug metabolizing enzymes, such as the CYP-450 metabolic enzyme system. Differences in the genetically determined structure of these enzymes can account for the ethnic variations that have been reported in drug responses (Ruiz, 2000). Although little systematic study of these issues has been done, they are becoming more important, and an emphasis on research in this area is increasing. This is because the population is becoming more diverse as a result of increasing geographical mobility and because more new psychopharmacological agents are becoming available.

In addition, provider bias toward racially and ethnically diverse or disadvantaged patients has been shown to effect treatment selection, thereby increasing disparities in health status associated with racial and ethnic populations. For example, studies have found that black patients with schizophrenia were more likely to be prescribed long-acting injectable antipsychotics, less likely to be prescribed the new generation atypical antipsychotic medications, less likely to be prescribed adjunctive medication to treat comorbid psychiatric illness, and less likely to have their antipsychotic medication side effects treated when compared to white patients (Kreyenbuhl et al, 2003; Mark et al, 2003).

Gender differences in pharmacokinetics and reproductive changes should be taken into account when psychotropic drugs are given to women. Compared with men, women receive more prescriptions and experience more side effects. Women are at higher risk for tardive dyskinesia from conventional antipsychotics and for activating side effects caused by antidepressants. Depressed premenopausal women respond better to SSRIs, and men respond better to tricyclic antidepressants.

The following issues should be considered when women, compared with men, take psychotropic drugs (Miller, 2000):

- Differences in pharmacokinetics in women: Gastric emptying is slower, gastric acidity is lower, blood volume is lower, renal clearance of drugs is decreased, and percent of body fat is higher. Thus women experience greater biological activity than men at a given dose of most psychotropic medicines.
- Dosage adjustment across the menstrual cycle and after menopause: Pharmacokinetics can differ significantly at different phases of a woman's menstrual cycle, necessitating dosage adjustment across the cycle for some drugs; women of reproductive age require lower doses of antipsychotic drugs; increased prolactin levels caused by some antipsychotic drugs can inhibit ovulation and cause menstrual cycle irregularity.
- Interactions between psychotropic agents and prescribed hormones: Oral contraceptives can magnify pharmacokinetic differences, necessitating dosage adjustments in some cases; drugs that induce hepatic enzymes, such as carbamazepine, can increase the metabolism of oral contraceptives, resulting in unwanted pregnancy; in women with bipolar disorder, hormone replacement therapy can trigger rapid cycling.
- Risks during pregnancy and breast-feeding: (See "Pregnant and Lactating Women" above).

Medically Ill Patients. Medically ill patients with concomitant psychiatric illness may have an increased sensitivity to the adverse effects of psychotropic drugs, changes in metabolism and excretion, and interactions with co-administered medications. Patients with liver disease are extremely sensitive to most psychoactive drugs, and patients with renal impairment are particularly sensitive to lithium.

It is important to collaborate with all the prescribers treating the patient to assure the compatibility of prescriptions. As with children and the elderly, good clinical practice for mentally ill patients involves beginning with lower doses and titrating up slowly while evaluating frequently for both clinical benefit and adverse effects.

Biological Basis for Psychopharmacology

All communication in the brain involves neurotransmission, or neurons "talking" to each other across synapses at receptors. Neurons are the basic functional unit of the brain structures of the nervous system, and the study of this communication process forms the basis of many of the neurosciences (see Chapter 6). The following description is a basic frame of reference from which to view the complexity of neuropharmacological mechanisms.

The synapse is a narrow gap separating two neurons: the presynaptic cell and the postsynaptic cell (Figure 27-1). Most receptors, organized into many subtypes, are three-dimensional

"gates" (channels) located on cells (neurons) that are targets for chemical first messengers (e.g., neurotransmitters, peptides, drugs). Depending on the message it receives, the receptor opens or closes its channel, allowing or stopping a flow of electrolytes (ions) into and out of the neuron, affecting the electrical nerve impulse of the neuron (stimulating or inhibiting its biological activity).

This process causes a cascade of activity by the chemical second messengers within the neuron, activating the neuron's genetic code (gene expression). Gene expression is what tells the neuron how to respond and continue the process of communication to the next neuron. This genetically determined communication within and between neurons controls how the brain functions and ultimately how the body responds and the person behaves.

Neurochemical messengers are synthesized (manufactured) from certain dietary amino acids (called *precursors*) by a chain of enzyme activity within the cell. These messengers are then stored in the presynaptic cell waiting to be released into the synapse. After neurotransmission takes place at a synapse, neurochemicals remaining in the synapse are either reabsorbed (reuptake) and stored by the presynaptic cell for later use or are metabolized (broken down) by enzymes, such as monoamine oxidase (MAO) and cholinesterase (ChE).

Many psychiatric disorders are thought to be caused by a **dysregulation** (imbalance) in the complex process of brain

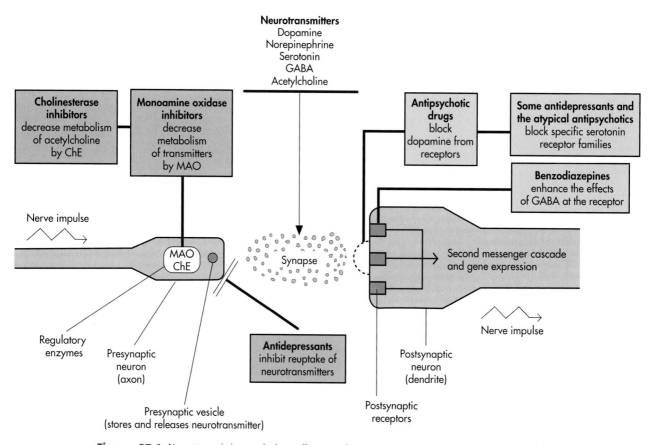

Figure 27-1 Neurotransmission and drug effects at the synapse. *GABA,* Gamma-aminobutyric; *MAO,* monoamine oxidase; *ChE,* cholinesterase.

structures communicating with each other through neurotransmission. For instance, psychosis is thought to involve excessive dopamine and serotonin dysregulation. Mood disorders are thought to result from disruption of normal patterns of neurotransmission of norepinephrine, serotonin, and other transmitters. Anxiety is thought to be a dysregulation of GABA and other transmitters. Alzheimer's disease is thought to result from a dysregulation of acetylcholine and other transmitters.

If a particular psychiatric illness is known to result from a dysregulation or imbalance of neurotransmission in a particular neurotransmitter system, and if the mechanism of action of psychiatric drugs is understood, then some order in the various pharmacological strategies used in psychiatric treatment can be recognized. This process of cell-to-cell communication at the synapse resulting in brain function can be affected by drugs in several important ways:

- **Release:** More neurotransmitter is released into the synapse from the storage vesicles in the presynaptic cell.
- **Blockade of postsynaptic receptors:** The neurotransmitter is prevented from binding to the target receptor.
- **Blockade of alpha-2 presynaptic autoreceptors:** This negative feedback system is prevented from turning off the release of norepinephrine into the synapse.
- **Receptor sensitivity changes:** The receptor becomes more or less responsive to the neurotransmitter.
- **Reuptake inhibition:** The presynaptic cell does not reabsorb the neurotransmitter well, leaving more neurotransmitter in the synapse and therefore enhancing or prolonging its action.
- **Interference with storage vesicles:** The neurotransmitter is either released again into the synapse (more neurotransmitter) or released to metabolizing enzymes (less neurotransmitter).
- **Precursor chain interference:** The process that makes the neurotransmitter is either facilitated (more is synthesized) or disrupted (less is synthesized).
- **Synaptic enzyme inhibition:** Less neurotransmitter is metabolized, so more remains available in the synapse and the presynaptic neuron.
- **Second messenger cascade:** A chemical chain reaction within the cell is initiated by neurochemical effects at the receptor during neurotransmission, activating genetically determined brain function.

Not all of these strategies have yielded clinically relevant treatments to date. Those that have are emphasized in this chapter (see Figure 27-1):

- **Antipsychotic** drugs block dopamine from the receptor site.
- **Antidepressants** block the reuptake of norepinephrine and/or serotonin and regulate the areas of the brain that manufacture these chemicals.
- **Monoamine oxidase inhibitors** (MAOIs) decrease enzymatic metabolism of norepinephrine and serotonin.
- **Cholinesterase (ChE) inhibitors** decrease the metabolism of acetylcholine (see Chapter 23).

- **Benzodiazepines** (BZs) potentiate (enhance the effects of) GABA.
- **Some antidepressants and atypical antipsychotics** block specific subtypes of serotonin receptors (thought to be responsible for serotonin side effects), thereby enhancing serotonin transmission at serotonin receptors implicated in depression.

Understanding synaptic and cellular functions has led to various treatment approaches in pharmacotherapy that attempt to modify one or more of the steps in neurotransmission. It has also led to research focused on developing drugs with more specificity (drugs that go to areas in the brain specifically targeted for their action, such as the brain regions implicated in mental illness, rather than also going to nonspecific or untargeted areas, causing drug side effects).

The future of psychopharmacology holds much promise as new discovery techniques, results of the Human Genome Project; changes in the way drugs are developed; and new theories are proven. Drug effects on gene expression and receptor function are most likely the bases of psychopharmacological efficacy in the treatment of psychiatric disorders. It is also likely that future diagnostic conceptualizations of the etiology of psychiatric disorders may be organized by neurotransmitter activity and dysregulation rather than the current *DSM-IV-TR* (American Psychiatric Association, 2000) symptom cluster approach.

ANTIANXIETY AND SEDATIVE-HYPNOTIC DRUGS

Anxiety is a normal emotion under circumstances of threat and is part of the fight-or-flight instinct necessary for survival. The diagnosis of anxiety (symptoms of anxiety that are disproportionate to the circumstances) is based on the patient's description, the nurse's observation of behaviors, and assessment of *DSM-IV-TR* diagnostic criteria, and the elimination of alternative diagnoses (see Chapter 16).

The possibility of a nonpsychiatric cause for anxiety symptoms also must be considered. Hyperthyroidism, hypoglycemia, cardiovascular illness, severe pulmonary disease, and a variety of medications and substances are often associated with high levels of anxiety. In addition to a careful physical assessment and a review of laboratory tests, the patient should be asked about the use of prescription and over-the-counter drugs, as well as "recreational" substances such as alcohol, caffeine, nicotine, and street drugs.

Anxiety also accompanies many psychiatric disorders. For example, depression and anxiety are often **comorbid** illnesses (existing together). In general, the primary disorder should be treated with the appropriate medication. For example, anxiety associated with a primary diagnosis of schizophrenia or major depression often goes away when the target symptoms for the primary disorder are treated successfully.

This section divides antianxiety and sedative-hypnotic drugs into two categories: the benzodiazepines and several nonbenzodiazepine antianxiety drugs. **The benzodiazepines are the most widely prescribed drugs in the world.** Their popularity is related to their effectiveness, prompt onset of action, and wide margin of safety. Concerns that are largely unfounded regarding physiological dependence, withdrawal, and abuse potential have limited their use somewhat.

Although benzodiazepines have almost entirely replaced barbiturates in the treatment of anxiety and sleep disorders, they recently have been considered to be second-line agents after the antidepressants in the long-term treatment of anxiety disorders such as panic disorder and social phobia. Antidepressants are discussed in detail in the next section.

What sociocultural factors may help explain why benzodiazepines are the most commonly prescribed medications in the United States? ■

Benzodiazepines

The BZs are thought to reduce anxiety because they are powerful potentiators (receptor agonists) of the inhibitory neurotransmitter GABA. A postsynaptic receptor site specific for the BZ molecule is located next to the GABA receptor. The BZ molecule and GABA bind to each other at the GABA receptor site. The result is an enhancement of the actions of GABA, resulting in an **inhibition** of neurotransmission (a decrease in the firing rate of neurons), resulting in a clinical decrease in the person's level of anxiety.

Clinical Use. The major indications for the use of BZs include anxiety and anxiety disorders, insomnia, alcohol withdrawal, anxiety associated with medical disease, skeletal muscle relaxation, seizure disorders, the anxiety and apprehension experienced before surgery, and substance-induced (except for amphetamines) and psychotic agitation in emergency rooms (Raj and Sheehan, 2004). Used in higher doses, the high-potency BZs alprazolam and clonazepam have been effective in the treatment of panic disorder and social phobia. The target symptoms for use of BZs are listed in Box 27-4.

Another clinical indication for the use of BZs is as a sedative-hypnotic to improve sleep. Insomnia includes difficulty falling asleep, difficulty staying asleep, or awakening too early with an inability to go back to sleep. It is a symptom with many causes and often responds to nonpharmacological strategies such as talking about problems, increased daytime exercise, elimination of stimulants such as caffeine, and incorporating physical comfort measures into the nighttime routine (see Chapter 17).

When used as hypnotics, the BZs should induce sleep rapidly, and their effect should be gone by morning. Any BZ can be an effective sedative-hypnotic when administered at bedtime, although the choice of drug should be tailored to the patient's complaints. For example, BZs with a short half-life are effective for patients who have trouble falling asleep, but they may wear off too soon to help patients with early morning awakening.

Because the BZs are in the same pharmacological class as alcohol, they can be used to suppress the alcohol withdrawal syndrome and are the treatment of choice for this indication (see Chapter 24). The ingestion of these two substances together is contraindicated, particularly for the patient using dangerous equipment or driving a car, because it can produce extreme sedation.

BOX 27-4

Target Symptoms for Antianxiety and Sedative-Hypnotic Benzodiazepines

Psychological
- Irritability, uneasiness, worry, fear
- Sense of impending doom or panic
- Insomnia

Physical
- Flushed skin
- Hot or cold flashes
- Sweating
- Dilated pupils
- Dry mouth
- Nausea or vomiting
- Diarrhea
- Tachycardia, palpitations
- Dizziness
- Shortness of breath
- Hyperventilation
- Paresthesias
- Tremor
- Restlessness
- Headache
- Urinary frequency

The BZs have no significant clinical advantages over each other, although **differences in half-life** (Table 27-2) can be clinically useful. For example, patients with persistent high levels of anxiety should take a drug with a long half-life. Patients with fluctuating anxiety might do better with either a short-acting drug or a drug with a sustained-release formulation (alprazolam, chlorazepate, diazepam, and adinazolam). Sustained-release BZs blunt the peaks of toxicity and the troughs of symptom breakthrough and are becoming a popular alternative to the original formulations.

In addition, the **lipid solubility** of each BZ determines the rapidity of onset and the intensity of effect, and this should be considered when selecting a BZ. For example, diazepam is more lipid soluble than lorazepam, thus it more readily moves into and then out of the central nervous system (CNS) and is more extensively distributed to peripheral sites, particularly to fat cells.

The **rate of absorption** of the different BZs from the gastrointestinal tract varies considerably, thus affecting the rapidity and intensity of onset of their acute effects. Antacids and food in the stomach slow down this process when these drugs are taken by mouth.

The injectable BZs (lorazepam and midazolam) have been proven reliable when administered in the deltoid muscle. Diazepam results in predictable and rapid rises in the blood level when used intravenously. Concentrations of BZs in the blood have not yet been firmly correlated to clinical effects, so blood level measurements are not clinically helpful.

Some patients may need to take antianxiety drugs for extended periods. Because of the potential disadvantages of BZs, they should always be used along with nonpharmacological treatments for the patient with chronic anxiety or insomnia. Psychotherapy, behavioral techniques, environmental changes, stress management, sleep hygiene, and an ongoing therapeutic relationship continue to be important in the treatment of anxiety disorders and insomnia.

In general, **treatment with benzodiazepines should be brief** and used during a time of specific stress or for a specific indication. The patient should be observed frequently during the early days of treatment to assess target symptom response

Table 27-2	Antianxiety and Sedative-Hypnotic Drugs: Benzodiazepines			
GENERIC NAME (TRADE NAME)	ACTIVE METABOLITES	APPROXIMATE HALF-LIFE (HR)	USUAL ADULT DOSAGE RANGE (MG/DAY)*	PREPARATION
Antianxiety Drugs				
Alprazolam (Xanax)	Yes (not significant)	14	1-4	PO
Chlordiazepoxide (Librium)	Yes	20-30	10-40	PO, IM
Clonazepam (Klonopin)	No	>20	0.5-10	PO, ODT
Clorazepate (Tranxene)	Yes	60	10-40	PO, SD
Diazepam (Valium)	Yes	10-60	2-40	PO, SR, IM, IV
Halazepam (Paxipam)	Yes	60	60-160	PO
Lorazepam (Ativan)	No	14	1-6	PO, IM, IV
Oxazepam (Serax)	No	9	15-120	PO
Prazepam (Centrax)	Yes	60	10-60	PO
Sedative-Hypnotic Drugs				
Estazolam (ProSom)	Yes	16	1-4 HS	PO
Flurazepam (Dalmane)	Yes	100	15-30 HS	PO
Temazepam (Restoril)	No	8	7.5-30 HS	PO
Triazolam (Halcion)	No	3	0.125-0.5 HS	PO
Quazepam (Doral)	Yes	39	7.5-15 HS	PO

*Dosage ranges are approximate and should be individualized for each patient.
PO, Oral tablet or capsule; *IM*, intramuscular; *ODT*, orally disintegrating tablet; *SD*, single dose; *SR*, oral slow-release tablet; *IV*, intravenous; *HS*, at bedtime.

Table 27-3	Benzodiazepine Side Effects and Nursing Considerations
SIDE EFFECTS	NURSING CONSIDERATIONS
Common	
Drowsiness, sedation	Activity helps; use caution when using machinery.
Ataxia, dizziness	Use caution with activity, prevent falls.
Feelings of detachment	Discourage social isolation.
Increased irritability or hostility	Observe, support, be alert for disinhibition.
Anterograde amnesia	Inability to recall events that occur while on drug.
Cognitive effects with long-term use	Interference with concentration and memory of new material.
Tolerance, dependency, rebound insomnia/anxiety	Short-term use; discontinue, using a slow taper; contraindicated with drug or alcohol abuse.
Rare	
Nausea	Dose with meals, decrease dose.
Headache	Usually responds to mild analgesic.
Confusion	Decrease dose.
Gross psychomotor impairment	Dose related, decrease dose.
Depression	Decrease dose; antidepressant treatment.
Paradoxical rage reaction	Discontinue drug.

BOX 27-5

Benzodiazepine Withdrawal Syndrome

- Agitation
- Anorexia
- Anxiety
- Autonomic arousal
- Dizziness
- Generalized seizures
- Hallucinations
- Headache
- Hyperactivity
- Insomnia
- Irritability
- Nausea and vomiting
- Sensitivity to light and sounds
- Tinnitus
- Tremulousness

harmless. Table 27-3 summarizes these reactions and nursing considerations.

The BZs generally do not live up to their reputation of being strongly addictive, especially if they are discontinued gradually, if they have been used for appropriate purposes, and if their use has not been complicated by other factors such as chronic use of other CNS depressants such as barbiturates or alcohol. Because of their calming effects, they have the reputation of being frequently misused.

Tolerance can develop to the sedative effects of BZs, which in some ways is an advantage, but it is unclear whether tolerance also develops to induced sleep or antianxiety effects. These drugs should be tapered to minimize withdrawal symptoms (Box 27-5) and rebound symptoms of insomnia or anxiety. If these symptoms occur, the dose should be raised until symptoms are gone and then tapering is resumed at a slower rate.

Because the BZs have a very high therapeutic index, overdoses of BZs alone almost never cause fatalities. The BZ antagonist, flumazenil (Romazicon), can reverse all BZ actions and is marketed as a treatment for BZ overdose.

and monitor side effects so that the dose can be adjusted as needed. Some patients, such as those with panic disorder, may require regular daily dosing and long-term BZ treatment.

Side Effects and Adverse Reactions. BZ side effects are common, dose related, usually short-term, and almost always

Elderly patients are more vulnerable to side effects because the aging brain is more sensitive to sedatives. Dosing ranges from one-half to one-third of the usual daily dose used for adults. The BZs with no active metabolites (see Table 27-2) are less affected by liver disease, the age of the patient, or drug interactions.

BZs have been used successfully in **children** to treat sleepwalking, in single doses to allay anticipatory anxiety, and to treat panic, generalized anxiety disorder (GAD), and avoidant personality disorder, but in general, they can increase anxiety and produce or aggravate behavior disorders, especially attention deficit/hyperactivity disorder (ADHD).

BZs during **pregnancy** have been associated rarely with palate malformations and intrauterine growth retardation, especially when used during the first trimester. When used late in pregnancy or during breast-feeding, these drugs have been associated with floppy infant syndrome, neonatal withdrawal symptoms, and poor sucking reflex. Thus they are not recommended.

Nonbenzodiazepine Antianxiety Agents

Buspirone, a nonbenzodiazepine anxiolytic drug, is a potent antianxiety agent with no addictive potential (Table 27-4) and has FDA approval for the treatment of generalized anxiety disorder. Buspirone does not exhibit muscle-relaxant or anticonvulsant activity, interaction with CNS depressants, or sedative-hypnotic properties. It is not effective in the management of drug or alcohol withdrawal or panic disorder. Generally it takes several weeks for its antianxiety effects to become apparent. It probably is most effective in patients who have never taken BZs and therefore are not expecting immediate effects from drug treatment.

Table 27-4	Nonbenzodiazepine Antianxiety and Sedative-Hypnotic Agents	
GENERIC NAME (TRADE NAME)	**DOSE (MG/DAY)**	**HALF-LIFE (HR)**
Antianxiety Agents		
Buspirone (BuSpar)	15-60	2-5
Propranolol (Inderal)	60-160	3
Clonidine (Catapres)	0.2-0.6	6-20
Sedative-Hypnotic Agents		
Zolpidem (Ambien)	5-10	1-2.5
Zaleplon (Sonata)	5-10	1-2.5
Antihistamines (also used for sleep)		
Diphenhydramine (Benadryl)	50	Unknown
Hydroxyzine (Atarax, Vistaril)	100-300	Unknown
Antidepressant		
Trazodone (Desyrel)	50-200	4

Propranolol (a β-blocker) and clonidine (an α₂ receptor agonist) have been used for the **off label** treatment of anxiety. These classes of drugs act by blocking peripheral or central noradrenergic (norepinephrine) activity and many of the manifestations of anxiety (e.g., tremor, palpitations, tachycardia, sweating). Propranolol is used in the treatment of performance anxiety found in some forms of social phobia and in panic disorder if rapid heart beat is a significant deterrent to the patient's ability to function.

Clonidine is also used to block physiological symptoms of opioid withdrawal and the tachycardia and excessive salivation seen with the atypical antipsychotic clozapine (Schatzberg, Cole, and DeBattista, 2003).

Once the atypical antipsychotic drugs were used to treat anxiety but have fallen out of use for this purpose because of their short- and long-term side effects. Recently low doses of the atypical antipsychotics for the treatment of anxiety or insomnia have begun to appear in the literature. It remains to be seen whether evidence for this use supports this practice.

Interestingly, many of the SSRIs and some of the newer antidepressants seem to be taking first line status in the treatment of specific anxiety disorders (although it is likely that most of the SSRIs are effective across the range of anxiety disorders) and have received FDA approval for these indications:

- Paroxetine for generalized anxiety disorder (GAD), posttraumatic stress disorder (PTSD), and social phobia
- Fluoxetine for obsessive-compulsive disorder (OCD), bulimia, and premenstrual dysphoric disorder (PMDD)
- Sertraline for OCD and PTSD
- Venlafaxine for GAD

Clomipramine is the only tricyclic antidepressant (TCA) shown to be effective in the treatment of OCD, and studies have shown that TCA imipramine and the MAOI phenelzine effectively treat panic disorder. The antidepressant drugs are discussed later in this chapter.

Nonbenzodiazepine Sedative-Hypnotic Agents

Zolpidem is the first of a new class of compounds for short-term treatment of insomnia. Structurally unrelated to BZs, it binds more selectively to neuronal receptors involved in inducing sleep (benzodiazepine-1 receptors on the BZ/GABA receptor complex) and has fewer of the BZ side effects. It is well tolerated and appears to have little antianxiety, anticonvulsant, or muscle-relaxant properties. Side effects can include daytime drowsiness, dizziness, and diarrhea. Zolpidem is a schedule IV controlled substance.

Zaleplon is another new nonbenzodiazepine sedative-hypnotic, similar to zolpidem in that it binds to the BZ-1 receptor, but has a half-life of only 1 hour. It has a very rapid onset of action, can be taken even if the patient has only 4 hours before he or she must awaken, and has no morning hangover effects. It also has sedative, anxiolytic, muscle-relaxing, and anticonvulsant properties, and is a schedule IV controlled substance.

Antihistamines are sometimes used as sedative-hypnotic agents for their sedating effects. They usually are not as effective as the BZs but do not cause physical dependence or abuse and are easily obtained by patients as over-the-counter drugs. A disadvantage of the antihistamines is that they lower the seizure threshold and cause anxiety and insomnia in some people.

Trazodone is an antidepressant with significant sedating effects and is the preferred antidepressant used for insomnia. It is not well studied for this use but is popular because it offers sedation with few cholinergic effects, has a much greater safety profile in overdose compared to tricyclic antidepressants, and shows no evidence of dependence or withdrawal. Side effects include orthostatic hypotension, anxiety, and a rare but very serious adverse effect, priapism (sustained and painful penile erection), which can occur with daily doses as low as 50 to 200 mg, the doses recommended for sleep.

Barbiturates and Older Antianxiety and Sedative-Hypnotic Drugs

Barbiturates (secobarbital and pentobarbital) and other older nonbenzodiazepine antianxiety and sedative-hypnotic agents (such as meprobamate, alcohols, and chloral hydrate) have many disadvantages that have led to their greatly decreased use. These include the following:

- Tolerance develops to their antianxiety and sedative effects.
- They are very addictive.
- They cause serious, even lethal, withdrawal reactions.
- They are dangerous in cases of overdose.
- They cause CNS depression.
- They can cause a variety of dangerous drug interactions, particularly when mixed with CNS depressants such as alcohol.

■ ANTIDEPRESSANT DRUGS

Research on the biology of depression has led to many new discoveries and even more hypotheses. It has been proposed that **serotonin, norepinephrine, and other neurochemicals are dysregulated in mood disorders**. The biological understanding of antidepressant drug actions supports this theory.

Antidepressants enhance the neurotransmission of these transmitters by several actions: they can block the reuptake of neurotransmitters at the presynaptic neuron, inhibit their metabolism and subsequent deactivation, and affect the activity of receptors on the postsynaptic neuron. Thus antidepressant drugs regulate neurotransmitter systems and their balance with each other. They enhance communication in brain structures responsible for mood and emotion, as well as many of the anxiety disorders, because the biochemical underpinnings of mood and anxiety are similar.

These actions at the synapse are immediate, but it takes several weeks for antidepressants to affect mood. This delay of clinical efficacy is the subject of considerable research. One proposal is that depression occurs when a depletion of neurotransmitters in the synapse causes the post-synaptic receptors for these transmitters to increase in number (up-regulation), as if they were adjusting to too little available transmitter. As the antidepressants make more transmitter available again in the synapse, it takes the receptors several weeks to return their numbers back to normal, allowing a normalization of synaptic activity. This time frame matches the several weeks it takes to see clinical improvement after initiation of antidepressant therapy.

The primary clinical indications and other suggested uses for antidepressant drugs are listed in Table 27-5. Table 27-6

Table 27-5	Indications for Antidepressant Drugs	
Primary Indications		
Major depression		Acute depression, maintenance treatment of depression and prevention of relapse, bipolar depression (when used with a mood stabilizer), atypical depression, and dysthymic disorder
Anxiety disorders		Panic disorder, obsessive-compulsive disorder (OCD), social phobia, generalized anxiety disorder, posttraumatic stress disorder
Evidence for Other Antidepressant Categories		
Selective serotonin reuptake inhibitors (SSRIs)	Strong evidence:	Bulimia, premenstrual dysphoric disorder (full- and half-cycle administration)
	Moderate evidence:	Obesity, substance abuse, impulsivity, and anger associated with personality disorders, pain syndromes
	Preliminary evidence:	Body dysmorphic disorder, hypochondriasis, anger attacks associated with depression, attention deficit/hyperactivity disorder (ADHD)
Other newer antidepressant agents	Moderate evidence:	Trazodone: Insomnia, dementia with agitation, minor sedative-hypnotic withdrawal
		Bupropion: ADHD, sexual side effects of antidepressants
Tricyclic antidepressants	Strong evidence:	Panic disorder (most), OCD (clomipramine), bulimia (imipramine, desipramine), enuresis (imipramine)
	Moderate evidence:	Separation anxiety, ADHD, phobias, generalized anxiety disorder (GAD), anorexia, headaches, diabetic neuropathy and other pain syndromes (amitriptyline, doxepin), sleep apnea (protriptyline), cocaine abuse (desipramine)
Monoamine oxidase inhibitors (MAOIs)	Strong evidence:	Panic disorder, bulimia
	Moderate evidence:	Other anxiety disorders, anorexia, body dysmorphic disorder

Data from Schatzberg AF, Nemeroff CB: *The American Psychiatric Publishing textbook of psychopharmacology*, ed 3, Washington DC, 2004, American Psychiatric Publishing.

presents antidepressant synaptic activity and receptor binding actions. Table 27-7 lists possible clinical effects of synaptic activity. Table 27-8 lists the antidepressant drugs. Box 27-6 lists the antidepressant drug target symptoms. Table 27-9 presents comparative side effect profiles of many of the antidepressant drugs.

Patients who respond to the initial course of treatment with an antidepressant should continue taking the drug at the same effective dosage for a **continuation phase of at least 6 to 9 months**. If they are symptom-free during that time, they can then be tapered off the medication and monitored for potential relapse.

Patients who have relapses after the continuation treatment is ended may require **maintenance phase medication of 1 or more years' duration** to prevent recurring depression. Patients who have had three or more episodes of major depression have a 90% chance of having another and are therefore potential candidates for long-term maintenance medication. Patients who have a history of suicide attempts, severe disability when depressed, or a history of depression in first-degree relatives also may be candidates for long-term antidepressant treatment. The long-term maintenance medication is generally given at the same dose that was effective in the acute phase of treatment.

When treating anxiety disorders with antidepressants, dose ranges are usually the same as those used for the treatment of depression, although the initial dose usually is lower, titration up to a therapeutic range may be slower, and for some patients, doses may have to be ultimately higher for the treatment of anxiety disorders such as obsessive-compulsive

Table 27-6 Antidepressant Drug Synaptic Activity

ANTIDEPRESSANT DRUG	PRIMARY SYNAPTIC ACTIVITY
All TCAs	Receptor blockade: H_1, ACh, alpha$_1$, 5-HT$_2$
Particularly tertiary amines	Reuptake inhibition: 5-HT
Particularly secondary amines	Reuptake inhibition: NE
MAOIs	Receptor blockade: ACh
	Enzymatic inhibition: MAO
SSRIs	Reuptake inhibition: 5-HT
Other Antidepressants	
Amoxapine	Reuptake inhibition: 5-HT and NE
	Receptor blockade: D_2, ACh, H_1
Bupropion	Reuptake inhibition: NE and DA
Maprotiline	Reuptake inhibition: NE
	Receptor blockade: H_1, ACh
Mirtazapine	Presynaptic autoreceptor inhibition: alpha$_2$
	Receptor blockade: 5-HT$_2$ and 5-HT$_3$
Nefazodone	Reuptake inhibition: 5-HT and NE
	Receptor blockade 5-HT$_2$, alpha$_1$
Reboxetine	Reuptake inhibition: NE
Trazodone	Reuptake inhibition: 5-HT
	Receptor blockade: 5-HT$_2$, H_1, alpha$_2$, alpha$_1$
Venlafaxine	Reuptake inhibition: 5-HT, NE, and DA

TCAs, Tricyclic antidepressant; H_1, histamine receptor; *ACh,* acetylcholine; *alpha$_1$* and *alpha$_2$,* norepinephrine receptors; *5-HT$_2$,* serotonin receptor; *5-HT,* serotonin; *NE,* norepinephrine; *MAOIs,* monoamine oxidase inhibitors; *SSRIs,* selective serotonin reuptake inhibitors; D_2, dopamine receptor; *DA,* dopamine.

BOX 27-6

Antidepressant Drug Target Symptoms

- Middle and terminal insomnia
- Appetite disturbances
- Anxiety and anxiety disorders
- Fatigue
- Poor motivation
- Somatic complaints
- Agitation
- Motor retardation
- Dysphoric mood
- Subjective depressive feelings (anhedonia, poor self-esteem, pessimism, hopelessness, self-reproach, guilt, helplessness, sadness)
- Suicidal thoughts

Table 27-7 Possible Clinical Effects of Synaptic Activity by Psychotropic Drugs

SYNAPTIC ACTIVITY	POSSIBLE CLINICAL EFFECTS
Serotonin (5-HT) reuptake inhibition	Reduced depression, antianxiety effects, gastrointestinal disturbances, sexual dysfunction
Norepinephrine (NE) reuptake inhibition	Reduced depression, tremors, tachycardia, erectile/ejaculatory dysfunction
Dopamine (DA) reuptake inhibition	Reduced depression, psychomotor activation, anti-parkinsonian effects
5-HT$_2$ receptor blockade	Reduced depression, reduced suicidal behavior, antipsychotic effects, hypotension, ejaculatory dysfunction
Dopamine D_2 receptor blockade	Extrapyramidal movement disorders
Muscarinic/cholinergic (ACh) receptor blockade	Anticholinergic side effects (blurred vision, dry mouth, constipation, sinus tachycardia, urinary retention, cognitive dysfunction)
Histamine (H_1) receptor blockade	Sedation/drowsiness, hypotension, weight gain
Alpha$_1$-adrenergic receptor blockade	Postural hypotension, dizziness, drowsiness, memory dysfunction, reflex tachycardia, potentiation of antihypertensive effect of prazosin and terazosin
Alpha$_2$-adrenergic receptor blockade	Priapism, blockade of the antihypertensive effects of clonidine and α-methyldopa

disorder and panic disorder. Patients who have recurrent severe depression, concurrent anxiety disorders, history of suicide attempts, and first-degree relatives with an anxiety disorder also may need long-term maintenance treatment with antidepressants.

> *Your patient who has been taking antidepressant medication for 2 months tells you that he feels better and wants to stop taking it. How would you respond?* ■

Antidepressants have no known long-term adverse effects, tolerance to therapeutic effects does not usually develop, and persistent side effects often can be minimized by a small de-

Table 27-8 Antidepressant Drugs

GENERIC NAME (TRADE NAME)	USUAL ADULT DAILY DOSE (MG/DAY)*	PREPARATIONS
Selective Serotonin Reuptake Inhibitors (SSRIs)		
Citalopram (Celexa)	20-40	PO, L
Escitalopram (Lexapro)	20-40	PO
Fluoxetine (Prozac)	20-60	PO, L
Fluvoxamine (Luvox)	100-200	PO
Paroxetine (Paxil)	20-50	PO, CR
Sertraline (Zoloft)	50-200	PO, L
Other New Antidepressant Drugs		
Amoxapine (Asendin)	200-300	PO
Bupropion (Wellbutrin)	150-450†	PO, SR
Maprotiline (Ludiomil)	50-200†	PO
Mirtazapine (Remeron)	15-45	PO
Serotonin antagonist and reuptake inhibitors (SARIs)		
Nefazodone (Serzone)	300-500	PO
Trazodone (Desyrel)	150-300	PO
Serotonin-norepinephrine reuptake inhibitor (SNRI)		
Venlafaxine (Effexor)	75-375	PO, XR
Tricyclic Antidepressant Drugs (TCAs)		
Tertiary (parent)		
Amitriptyline (Elavil)	150-300	PO, IM
Clomipramine (Anafranil)	100-250	PO
Doxepin (Sinequan)	150-300	PO, L
Imipramine (Tofranil)	150-300	PO
Trimipramine (Surmontil)	150-300	PO
Secondary (metabolite)		
Desipramine (Norpramin)	150-300	PO, L
Nortriptyline (Pamelor)	50-150	PO, L
Protriptyline (Vivactil)	15-60	PO
Tetracyclics		
Amoxapine (Asendin)	150-400	PO
Maprotiline (Ludiomil)	150-225	PO
Monoamine Oxidase Inhibitors (MAOIs)		
Isocarboxazid (Marplan)	20-60	PO
Phenelzine (Nardil)	45-90	PO
Selegiline (Eldepryl, Emsam)	20-50	PO, TS
Tranylcypromine (Parnate)	20-60	PO

*Dosage ranges are approximate; initiate at lower dose for most patients.
†Antidepressants with a ceiling dose due to dose-related seizures.
PO, Oral tablet/capsule; L, oral liquid; CR, controlled release; SR, sustained release; XR, extended release; IM, intramuscular; TS, transdermal system patch.

crease in dose without loss of effectiveness. **Because antidepressants do not cause physical addiction, psychological dependence, or euphoria, they have no abuse potential.** Their long half-life (24 hours or longer) allows most of them to be conveniently administered once a day after steady state is reached. If the patient experiences drowsiness, the drug should be taken at night. If the patient is activated after taking the drug, it should be taken in the daytime.

Patients with bipolar illness may be inadvertently switched into mania by antidepressants, thus they should be on concurrent mood stabilizers, and watched closely for increased activity, greater difficulty in concentrating and eating, and decreased sleeping patterns if an antidepressant is added to their drug regimen. Prescribers must be alert to CYP 450 problems when antidepressants are co-prescribed.

Selective Serotonin Reuptake Inhibitors

All the SSRIs inhibit the reuptake of serotonin at the **presynaptic** membrane. This results in an increase of available serotonin in the synapse and therefore at **post-synaptic** receptors, promoting serotonin neurotransmission. Although their actions and effectiveness are similar, they are structurally different from each other, accounting for some variation in their side effect profiles and some differences in effectiveness in some patients.

Many initial side effects are short term and tolerance may develop, although some may last for as long as the patient takes the drug. Thus if a patient cannot tolerate one of the SSRIs (due to side effects) or receives only minimal effectiveness (the patient is a SSRI partial responder or nonresponder), several choices can be considered.

For problems with SSRI side effects (Table 27-10), choices include lowering the dose, at least temporarily, to see whether side effects improve without a simultaneous loss of effectiveness; waiting for tolerance of the side effect to develop; using one of the nursing strategies to decrease side effects (Table 27-11); using drug co-administration strategies to treat the side effect (such as sildenafil for sexual dysfunction in men and women [Table 27-12]); and switching the patient to another antidepressant with a different side effect profile.

For SSRI nonresponders, choices include raising the dose to the limits of the therapeutic range (and the patient's tolerance); augmenting the primary antidepressant with another drug (such as another antidepressant, a stimulant, lithium, thyroxine, or buspirone) to increase effectiveness; and switching to another SSRI or other antidepressant). SSRIs can cause weight gain in some patients, thus making it necessary to watch the patient for this side effect and put the patient on weight reducing activities, or switch the patient to an antidepressant without this side effect.

The SSRIs have antidepressant effects comparable to those of the other classes of antidepressant drugs, yet without significant anticholinergic, cardiovascular, and sedative side effects. In addition, they are fairly **safe in overdose.** These properties have made them very popular, even though they cost more than the older tricyclic compounds.

Particular care must be taken when combining SSRIs with other serotonin drugs and with drugs that are metabolized by

Table 27-9	Comparative Side Effect Profiles of Some Antidepressant Medications						
	CENTRAL NERVOUS SYSTEM			**CARDIOVASCULAR**		**OTHER**	
	ANTICHOLINERGIC*	DROWSINESS	INSOMNIA/ AGITATION	POSTURAL HYPOTENSION	CARDIAC ARRHYTHMIA	GASTROINTESTINAL DISTRESS	WEIGHT GAIN (OVER 6 KG)
Amitriptyline	4+	4+	0	4+	3+	0	4+
Clomipramine	4+	4+	1+	3+	3+	1+	3+
Desipramine	1+	1+	1+	2+	2+	0	1+
Doxepin	3+	4+	0	2+	2+	0	3+
Imipramine	3+	3+	1+	4+	3+	1+	3+
Nortriptyline	1+	1+	0	2+	2+	0	1+
Protriptyline	2+	1+	1+	2+	2+	0	0
Trimipramine	1+	4+	0	2+	2+	0	3+
Amoxapine	2+	2+	2+	2+	3+	0	1+
Maprotiline	2+	4+	0	0	1+	0	2+
Mirtazapine	1+	4+	1+	2+	0	1+	2+
Nefazodone	1+	3+	1+	2+	0	3+	0
Venlafaxine	1+	1+	3+	0	0	3+	0
Trazodone	0	4+	0	1+	1+	1+	1+
Bupropion	0	0	2+	0	1+	1+	0
Fluoxetine	0	0	2+	0	0	3+	0
Paroxetine	0	0	2+	0	0	3+	0
Sertraline	0	0	2+	0	0	3+	0
Fluvoxamine	0	0	2+	0	0	3+	0
Citalopram	0	1+	2+	0	1+	3+	0
MAOIs	1+	1+	2+	2+	0	1+	2+

*Dry mouth, blurred vision, urinary hesitancy, constipation.
0, Absent or rare; 1+, 2+, in between; 3+, 4+, common.

liver enzymes that SSRIs may inhibit. For instance, combining serotonergic drugs can cause serotonin syndrome, a life-threatening crisis. See Table 27-11 for side effects of antidepressant drugs. Also, because the SSRIs may inhibit the cytochrome P-450 enzymes, which are responsible for the metabolism of many other drugs, care also has to be taken to monitor patients on multiple medications for signs of toxicity.

Other New Antidepressant Drugs

A growing number of new antidepressant drugs differ chemically from each other and from other classes of antidepressants and also differ significantly in their effects at the synapse. They therefore have varying side effect profiles, although their effectiveness is generally the same as that of other antidepressants, as is the length of time required for antidepressant or antianxiety effects to occur (several weeks at optimal dose). Like SSRIs, the other newer antidepressants are safer than TCAs and MAOIs in side effect profiles and overdose. Some of these drugs appear to have more specificity than many of the other antidepressants. These include the following:

- Bupropion is a norepinephrine and dopamine reuptake blocker (NDRI).
- Venlafaxine is a "dual" reuptake inhibitor because it inhibits both norepinephrine and serotonin reuptake (SNRI).
- Nefazodone and trazodone block (antagonize) a subtype of the serotonin 5-HT$_2$ postsynaptic receptor

that is thought to be associated with side effects and block serotonin reuptake (and norepinephrine to a lesser extent); thus they are serotonin antagonists and reuptake inhibitors (SARIs).
- Mirtazapine has several complex actions: it blocks presynaptic α_2 autoreceptors, increasing levels of norepinephrine (doing so ultimately increases serotonin) in the synapse; it serves as an agonist to the serotonin 5-HT$_1$ postsynaptic receptor, which is thought to be the serotonin receptor implicated in mood disorders; it antagonizes the 5-HT$_2$ receptor (thought to cause side effects); and it has fewer receptor actions in other neurotransmitter systems than some other antidepressants, so it is marketed as having a lower side effect profile (Schatzberg and Nemeroff, 2004).

Tricyclic Antidepressants

Although the TCAs as a class include some drugs that are structurally dissimilar, they are all quite similar in their clinical effects and adverse reactions (see Table 27-10). To varying degrees, TCAs all have the same primary actions, such as serotonin and norepinephrine reuptake inhibition (therapeutic effects), as well as blockade of three receptors not implicated in depression: muscarinic cholinergic receptors (anticholinergic side effects), histamine H$_1$ receptors (sedation and weight gain), and alpha$_1$ noradrenergic receptors (orthostatic hypotension and dizziness).

Table 27-10	Antidepressant Drug Side Effects	
	RECEPTORS/ NEUROTRANSMITTERS	SIDE EFFECTS
Antidepressants		
TCAs	H_1	Sedation/drowsiness, hypotension, weight gain
	ACh	Anticholinergic side effects: blurred vision, dry mouth, constipation, tachycardia, urinary retention, cognitive dysfunction
	$Alpha_1$	Postural hypotension, dizziness, tachycardia, memory dysfunction
	$5\text{-}HT_2$	Hypotension, ejaculatory dysfunction
	5-HT	Gastrointestinal (GI) disturbances (nausea, diarrhea), sexual dysfunction
	NE	Tremors, tachycardia, erectile/ejaculatory dysfunction
MAOIs	ACh	Anticholinergic side effects
SSRIs	5-HT	GI disturbances (nausea, diarrhea), sexual dysfunction
Other Antidepressants		
Amoxapine	NE	Tremors, tachycardia, erectile/ejaculatory dysfunction
	5-HT	GI disturbances (nausea, diarrhea), sexual dysfunction
	D_2	Extrapyramidal symptoms and tardive dyskinesia (rare)
	ACh	Anticholinergic effects
	H_1	Sedation/drowsiness, hypotension, weight gain
Bupropion	DA	Psychomotor activation
	NE	Tremors, tachycardia, erectile/ejaculatory dysfunction
Maprotiline	NE	Tremors, tachycardia, erectile/ejaculatory dysfunction
	H_1	Sedation, drowsiness, hypotension, weight gain
	ACh	Anticholinergic side effects
Mirtazapine	H_1	Sedation, drowsiness, hypotension, weight gain
	ACh	Anticholinergic effects
Nefazedone	5-HT	GI disturbances (nausea, diarrhea), sexual dysfunction
	NE	Tremors, tachycardia, erectile/ejaculatory dysfunction
	$5\text{-}HT_2$	Hypotension, ejaculatory dysfunction
	$Alpha_1$	Postural hypotension; dizziness, tachycardia, memory dysfunction
Trazedone	5-HT	GI disturbances (nausea, diarrhea), sexual dysfunction
	$5\text{-}HT_2$	Hypotension, ejaculatory dysfunction
	H_1	Sedation/drowsiness, hypotension, weight gain
	$Alpha_1$	Postural hypotension, dizziness, tachycardia, memory dysfunction
	$Alpha_2$	Priapism
	ACh	Dry mouth, constipation, tachycardia, urinary retention
Venlafaxine	NE	Tremors, tachycardia, erectile/ejaculatory dysfunction
	5-HT	GI disturbances (nausea, diarrhea), sexual dysfunction
	DA	Psychomotor activation

Additional side effects and adverse reactions of antidepressant drugs less clearly related to receptor/neurotransmitter effects:

TCAs	ECG changes, dizziness/lightheadedness
	TCA withdrawal syndrome (malaise, muscle aches, chills, nausea, dizziness, coryza), hallucinations, delusions, activation of schizophrenic or manic psychosis, excessive perspiration
MAOIs	Hypertensive crisis, lightheadedness, drowsiness, insomnia, weight gain, sexual dysfunction
SSRIs	Nervousness, activation, headache, cytochrome P-450 inhibition, serotonin syndrome, insomnia
Venlafaxine	Sweating, nausea, constipation, vomiting, somnolence, dry mouth, dizziness, anxiety, blurred vision, headache, hypertension, insomnia

TCAs, Tricyclic antidepressants; H_1; histamine receptor; *ACh,* acetylcholine; *alpha1,* norepinephrine receptor; $5\text{-}HT_2$, serotonin receptor; *5-HT,* serotonin; *NE,* norepinephrine; *MAOIs,* monoamine oxidase inhibitors; *SSRIs,* selective serotonin reuptake inhibitors; D_2, dopamine receptor; *ECG,* electrocardiogram.

TCAs also can have **dangerous cardiac side effects,** requiring electrocardiograms in adults over age 40 years, all children and young adolescents, and any patient with cardiac conduction problems. Because TCAs are **lethal in overdose,** careful baseline and ongoing suicide assessment is important. Elderly patients and patients with a medical illness may require lower doses of these drugs than healthy adults and careful assessments for side effects while they are taking the drugs.

The TCAs (except amoxapine and trimipramine) have clinically relevant blood levels, making monitoring therapeutic doses more precise if necessary. TCAs are as effective as the newer drugs, and because they have been on the market for many decades, many of them are much less expensive

Table 27-11 Nursing Considerations for Antidepressant Drug Side Effects

SIDE EFFECT	NURSING CARE AND TEACHING CONSIDERATIONS
Anticholinergic Side Effects	
Blurred vision	Temporary; avoid hazardous tasks.
Dry mouth	Encourage fluids, frequent rinses, sugar-free hard candy and gums; check for mouth sores.
Constipation	Increase fluids, dietary fiber and roughage, exercise; monitor bowel habits; use stool softeners and laxatives only if necessary.
Tachycardia	Temporary, usually not significant (except with coronary artery disease), but can be frightening; eliminate caffeine; β-blockers might help; supportive therapy.
Urinary retention	Encourage fluids and frequent voiding; monitor voiding patterns; bethanecol; catheterize.
Cognitive dysfunction	Temporary; avoid hazardous tasks, adjust lifestyle; supportive therapy.
Cytochrome P-450 inhibition*	SSRIs inhibit the liver isoenzyme cytochrome P-450, which is instrumental in the metabolism of a variety of drugs (TCAs, trazodone, barbiturates, most benzodiazepines, carbamazepine, narcotics, neuroleptics, phenytoin, valproate, verapamil). This effect can be potentially life-threatening because it increases serum concentrations as well as therapeutic and toxic effects of these drugs.
Dizziness/lightheadedness	Dangle feet; adequate hydration, elastic stockings; protect from falls.
ECG changes	Careful cardiac history; pretreatment ECG for patients over 40 and children; ST segment depression, T wave flattened or inverted, QRS prolongation; worsening of intraventricular conduction problems; do not use if recent myocardial infarction or bundle-branch block.
Ejaculatory dysfunction	Dose after sexual intercourse, not immediately before.
GI disturbances (nausea, diarrhea)	Take with meals or at HS; adjust diet if indicated.
Hallucinations, delusions, activation of schizophrenic or manic psychosis	Change to another antidepressant class of drug, initiate antipsychotics or mood stabilizers if appropriate.
Hypertensive crisis*	See Box 27-6.
Hypotension	Frequent BP; hydrate; elastic stockings; may need to change drug. For postural hypotension: lying and standing BP, gradual change of positions, protect from falls.
Insomnia	Dose as early in the day as possible; sleep hygiene, decrease evening activities; eliminate caffeine; relaxation techniques; sedative-hypnotic therapy.
Memory dysfunction	Temporary; encourage concentration, make lists, provide social support, adjust lifestyle.
Perspiration (excessive)	Frequent change of clothes, cotton/linen clothing, good hygiene; increase fluids.
Priapism	Change dose, change drug.
Psychomotor activation	Take drug in morning rather than HS, adjust lifestyle.
Sedation/drowsiness	Administer drug at HS, avoid hazardous tasks.
Serotonin syndrome (SS)*	SS is a life-threatening emergency resulting from excess central nervous system 5-HT caused by combining 5-HT-enhancing drugs or administering SSRIs too close to the discontinuation of MAOIs. Symptoms are confusion, disorientation, mania, restlessness/agitation, myoclonus, hyperreflexia, diaphoresis, shivering, tremor, diarrhea, nausea, ataxia, headache. Discontinue all serotonergic drugs immediately; anticonvulsants for seizures; serotonin antagonist drugs may help; clonazepam for myoclonus, lorazepam for restlessness/agitation, other symptomatic care as indicated; do not reintroduce serotonin drugs.
Sexual dysfunction	Dose after sexual intercourse, use lubricant if vaginal dryness is present; antidotes such as sildenifal, bupropion, or bethanecol.
Tachycardia	See anticholinergic side effects.
TCA withdrawal syndrome	Symptoms: malaise, muscle aches, chills, nausea, dizziness, coryza; when discontinuing drug, taper over several days or weeks.
Tremors	Temporary; adjust lifestyle if indicated.
Weight gain	Increase exercise; reduced calorie diet if indicated; may need to change class of drug.

NOTE: Always educate the patient and use the techniques in this table. Consider decreasing or dividing drug dose. Change drug only if necessary.
*Potentially life-threatening.
SSRIs, Selective serotonin reuptake inhibitors; *TCAs,* tricyclic antidepressants; *ECG,* electrocardiogram; *GI,* gastrointestinal; *HS,* at bedtime (hour of sleep); *BP,* blood pressure; *5-HT,* serotonin; *MAOIs,* monoamine oxidase inhibitors.

than most drugs used to treat depression and anxiety, so they may be a good choice for some patients.

Monoamine Oxidase Inhibitors

MAOIs are very effective antidepressant/antipanic/antiphobic drugs and were the first clinically effective antidepressants to be discovered in the 1950s. The MAOIs used in psychiatry are listed in Table 27-8. MAOIs inhibit both types of the enzyme (MAO A and MAO B) that metabolizes serotonin and norepinephrine. This inhibition is irreversible, lasting until the body is able to manufacture new MAO after the drug is discontinued, and is linked to the control of blood pressure because of its inhibition of norepinephrine.

BOX 27-7

Food Cautions for Patients Taking MAOIs

Foods to be Avoided
- Any cheeses *except* cottage and cream cheese
- Overripe (aged) fruit
- Fava beans
- Sausage, salami
- Sherry, liqueurs, red wine
- Sauerkraut
- Monosodium glutamate
- Pickled or smoked fish
- Brewer's yeast
- Beef and chicken liver
- Fermented products

Foods to be Eaten in Moderation and With Caution
- Alcohol, beer, white wines
- Caffeine-containing beverages
- Ripe avocado
- Yogurt
- Soy sauce
- Ripe bananas
- Chocolate
- Figs
- Meat tenderizers
- Raisins

MAOIs, Monoamine oxidase inhibitors.

BOX 27-8

Signs and Treatment of Hypertensive Crisis on MAOIs

Warning Signs
- Increased blood pressure
- Palpitations
- Headache

Symptoms of Hypertensive Crisis
- Sudden elevation of blood pressure
- Explosive occipital headache
- Head and face flushed and feel "full"
- Palpitations, chest pain
- Sweating, fever, nausea, vomiting
- Dilated pupils, photophobia

Treatment
- Hold MAOI doses
- Do not lie down (elevates blood pressure in head)
- IM chlorpromazine 100 mg, repeat if necessary (*mechanism of action:* blocks norepinephrine)
- IV phentolamine, administered slowly in doses of 5 mg (*mechanism of action:* binds with norepinephrine receptor sites, blocking norepinephrine)
- Manage fever by external cooling techniques
- Evaluate diet, adherence, and teaching

MAOIs, Monoamine oxidase inhibitors; *IM*, intramuscular administration; *IV*, intravenous administration.

Table 27-12	Adjunctive Agents for Antidepressant-Induced Sexual Dysfunction	
DRUG	**USUAL ADULT DOSE**
Buspirone	20-60 mg/day
Bupropion	75-150 mg/day
Sildenafil	50-100 mg/prn
Ginkgo biloba	60-240 mg/day
Amantadine	100-300 mg/day
Cyproheptadine	4-12 mg/prn
Yohimbine	5.4 mg/tid

Table 27-13	Drugs To Be Avoided in Combination With MAOIs	
DRUGS THAT MAY INTERACT WITH MAOIs	**NATURE OF DRUG INTERACTION**
Other MAOIs	Potentiation of side effects, seizures
SSRIs, fenfluramine, L-tryptophan	Serotonin syndrome
TCAs, carbamazepine, cyclobenzaprine	Severe side effects, hypertension, convulsions
Stimulants, buspirone, direct sympathomimetics, nasal and sinus decongestants, allergy and asthma remedies	Hypertension
Indirect sympathomimetics	Hypertensive crisis
Meperidine	Severe, potentially fatal interaction
Hypoglycemics (including insulin)	Worsening of hypoglycemia
Dextromethorphan	Reports of brief psychosis

MAOIs, Monoamine oxidase inhibitors; *SSRIs*, selective serotonin reuptake inhibitors; *TCAs*, tricyclic antidepressants.

A dangerous elevation in blood pressure can result from high levels of norepinephrine not metabolized by MAO. Thus patients taking these drugs must **avoid foods and drugs that are norepinephrine agonists** (Box 27-7 and Table 27-13) in order to avoid a **hypertensive crisis** (Box 27-8), which can cause intracerebral hemorrhage and death (Krishnan, 2004). Careful patient education is required with the use of these drugs.

MAO B is thought to convert some amines into toxins that may cause damage to neurons. Drugs that are selective inhibitors of MAO B have no antidepressant properties, have no risk of hypertension, and are used to prevent progression of neurodegenerative diseases such as Parkinson's disease.

A novel class of MAOI (not yet available in the United States) with antidepressant effectiveness comparable to that of other antidepressants is reversible and selective for inhibitors of MAO A, called *reverse inhibitors of monoamine oxidase A (RIMAs)* (moclobemide and brofaromine). Unlike the irreversible and nonselective MAOIs, RIMAs are short-acting drugs, allowing the recovery of enzyme activity in hours rather than weeks. Thus they have fewer side effects, (specifically the absence of severe hypertensive interaction) and do not require food and drug restrictions. RIMAs may prove to be valuable additions to the list of antidepressant drugs in the future.

BOX 27-9

Target Symptoms for Mood-Stabilizing Drug Therapy

Mania
- Irritability
- Expansiveness
- Euphoria
- Manipulativeness
- Lability with depression
- Sleep disturbance (decreased sleep)
- Pressured speech
- Flight of ideas
- Motor hyperactivity
- Assaultiveness/ threatening behavior
- Distractibility
- Hypergraphia
- Hypersexuality
- Persecutory and religious delusions
- Grandiosity
- Hallucinations
- Ideas of reference
- Catatonia

Depression
- Irritability
- Sadness
- Pessimism
- Anhedonia
- Self-reproach
- Guilt
- Hopelessness
- Somatic complaints
- Suicidal ideation
- Motor retardation
- Slowed thinking
- Poor concentration and memory
- Fatigue
- Constipation
- Decreased libido
- Anorexia or increased appetite
- Weight change
- Helplessness
- Sleep disturbance (insomnia or hypersomnia)

■ MOOD-STABILIZING DRUGS

Bipolar disorder is a common, recurrent, and often severe psychiatric illness associated with high rates of morbidity and mortality if left untreated (see Chapter 19). Yet treatment is sophisticated and complex. The goals of treatment are the same as for any chronic illness: rapid, complete remission of acute episodes, prevention of further episodes, suppression of symptoms that remain after the syndrome has been successfully treated (subsyndromal symptoms), and optimization of functional outcome and quality of life (Keck and McElroy, 2004).

It is important to develop a comprehensive treatment plan for the patient with bipolar disorder, including individual, family, and psychosocial therapies, and psychopharmacology is a critical component. Mood stabilizing drugs approved by the FDA for the treatment of bipolar disorder number just a few, but a range of other drugs are commonly used in clinical practice for this illness. The mood stabilizers include lithium, several types of anticonvulsants, atypical antipsychotics, benzodiazepines, and calcium channel blockers.

Box 27-9 lists the target symptoms of mania and of depression for mood-stabilizing drug therapy for patients with bipolar disorder. Table 27-14 lists the mood-stabilizing drugs. The nurse is advised to frequently refer to current adminis-

Table 27-14 Mood Stabilizing Drugs

DRUG CLASS GENERIC NAME (TRADE NAME)	HALF-LIFE (HR)	*USUAL ADULT DOSE (MG/DAY)	PREPARATIONS
Antimania			
Lithium (Eskalith, Lithobid)	18-36	600-2400	PO, CR, SR
Lithium citrate	18-36	600-2400	L/S
Anticonvulsants			
Valproic acid (Depakene); valproate (Depacon), divalproex (Depakote)	9-16	15-60 mg/kg/day	PO, L/S, ER, IM
Lamotrigine (Lamictal)	25-32	300-500	PO, Ch
Carbamazepine (Tegretol)	25-65	200-1600	PO, Ch
Gabapentin (Neurontin)	5-7	900-3600+	PO
Oxcarbazepine (Trileptal)	2-9	600-2400	PO, S
Topiramate (Topamax)	20-30	200-400	PO
Tiagabine (Gabatril)	7-9	4-32	PO
Atypical Antipsychotics See Table 27-15.			
Benzodiazepines See Table 27-2.			
Calcium Channel Blockers			
Verapamil (Calan)	3-7	240	PO
Nifedipine (Adalat, Procardia)	4	240	PO
Nimodipine (Nimotop)	2	60-120	PO

Data from Schatzberg AF, Nemeroff CB: *The American Psychiatric Publishing textbook of psychopharmacology*, ed 3, Washington, DC, 2004, American Psychiatric Publishing.
PO, Oral tablets or capsules; CR, controlled release; SR, slow release; L/S, liquid/syrup; ER, sustained release; IM, injection; Ch, chewable tablets; S, suspension.
* The dosage range is approximate and must be individualized for each patient.

tering and/or prescribing updates when treating patients on mood-stabilizing drugs.

Lithium

Lithium, a naturally occurring salt, is a first-line treatment for patients with acute mania and for the long-term prevention of recurrent episodes. Lithium also has a role in the treatment of recurrent bipolar depression, unipolar depression, aggressive behaviors, conduct disorder, and schizoaffective disorder. The exact mechanism of action of lithium is not fully understood, but many neurotransmitter functions are altered by the drug. It has been suggested that lithium may correct an ion exchange abnormality in the neuron, normalize synaptic neurotransmission of norepinephrine, serotonin, dopamine, and acetylcholine, and regulate second-messenger systems during neurotransmission (Freeman et al, 2004).

The use of lithium requires a comprehensive and vigilant approach. **Because lithium is excreted by the kidneys and can adversely affect the thyroid, and because it has a narrow therapeutic index and can quickly become fatal, initial and ongoing health assessment and laboratory monitoring is required** (Box 27-10). Also, health teaching of the patient, family, and support system is critical. The patient must be able to differentiate side effects from potentially life-threatening toxic effects (Box 27-11) and maintain a stable lithium level (Box 27-12). **Lithium toxicity is a medical emergency requiring rapid treatment** (Box 27-13).

Lithium may take weeks to months to significantly treat the symptoms of bipolar illness, and many patients may still continue to experience at least some symptoms of mood swings, anxiety, and psychosis. Therefore it is not uncommon to augment lithium with additional agents such as another mood stabilizer, an antidepressant, a benzodiazepine, or an atypical antipsychotic agent, depending on the target symptoms.

The nurse working with a patient on lithium needs a sophisticated understanding of the principles of lithium administration in order to keep lithium blood levels in the patient within the therapeutic range (between 0.6 and 1.4 mEq/L for

---

BOX 27-10

Prelithium Work-Up

Renal: Urinalysis, blood urea nitrogen (BUN), creatinine, electrolytes, 24-hour creatinine clearance; history of renal disease in self or family; diabetes mellitus, hypertension, diuretic use, analgesic abuse

Thyroid: Thyroid-stimulating hormone (TSH), T_4 (thyroxine), T_3 resin uptake, T_4 I (free thyroxine index); history of thyroid disease in self or family

Other: Complete physical, history, electrocardiogram (ECG), fasting blood sugar, complete blood count (CBC)

Maintenance Lithium Considerations

Every 3 months: Lithium level (for the first 6 months)
Every 6 months: Reassess renal status, lithium level, TSH
Every 12 months: Reassess thyroid function, ECG
Assess more often if patient is symptomatic

BOX 27-11

Lithium Side Effects and Toxicity

Body image: Weight gain (60% of patients)
Cardiac: Electrocardiogram (ECG) changes, usually not clinically significant
CNS: Fine hand tremor (50% of patients), fatigue, headache, mental dullness, lethargy
Dermatological: Acne, pruritic maculopapular rash
Endocrine: Thyroid dysfunction: Hypothyroidism (5% of patients); replacement hormone
Diabetes mellitus: Diet or insulin therapy
Gastrointestinal: Gastric irritation, anorexia, abdominal cramps, mild nausea, vomiting, diarrhea (dose with food or milk; further divide dose)
Renal: Polyuria (60% of patients), polydipsia, edema
Nephrogenic diabetes insipidus: Decrease dose; drink plenty of fluids; thiazide diuretics paradoxically reduce polyuria
Microscopic structural kidney changes (10% to 20% of patients on lithium for 1 year); does not cause clinical morbidity

Lithium Toxicity/Usually Dose Related

Prodrome of intoxication (lithium level ≥2.0 mEq/L): Anorexia, nausea, vomiting, diarrhea, coarse hand tremor, twitching, lethargy, dysarthria, hyperactive deep tendon reflexes, ataxia, tinnitus, vertigo, weakness, drowsiness
Lithium intoxication (lithium level ≥2.5 mEq/L): Fever, decreased urine output, decreased blood pressure, irregular pulse, ECG changes, impaired consciousness, seizures, coma, death

CNS, Central nervous system.

BOX 27-12

Stabilizing Lithium Levels

Common Causes for an Increase in Lithium Levels

- Decreased sodium intake
- Diuretic therapy
- Decreased renal functioning
- Fluid and electrolyte loss, sweating, diarrhea, dehydration, fever, vomiting
- Medical illness
- Overdose
- Nonsteroidal antiinflammatory drug therapy

Ways To Maintain a Stable Lithium Level

- Stabilize dosing schedule by dividing doses or use of sustained-release capsules.
- Ensure adequate dietary sodium and fluid intake (2 to 3 L/day).
- Replace fluid and electrolytes lost during exercise or gastrointestinal illness.
- Monitor signs and symptoms of lithium side effects and toxicity.
- If patient forgets a dose, a dose may be taken if less than 2 hours have elapsed; if longer than 2 hours, the dose should be skipped and the next dose taken as scheduled; never double up on doses.

BOX **27-13**

Management of Serious Lithium Toxicity

- Assess quickly; obtain rapid history of incident, especially dosing; offer support and explanations to patient.
- Hold all lithium doses.
- Check blood pressure, pulse, rectal temperature, respirations, and level of consciousness. Be prepared to initiate stabilization procedures, protect airway, and provide supplemental oxygen.
- Obtain lithium blood level immediately; obtain electrolytes, BUN, creatinine, urinalysis, CBC when possible.
- Electrocardiograph; monitor cardiac status.
- Limit lithium absorption; if acute overdose, provide an emetic; nasogastric suctioning.
- Vigorously hydrate: 5 to 6 L/day; balance electrolytes; IV line; indwelling urinary catheter.
- Patient will be bedridden: range of motion, frequent turning, pulmonary toilet.
- In moderately severe cases:
  - Implement osmotic diuresis with urea or mannitol.
  - Increase lithium clearance with aminophylline and alkalinize the urine with IV sodium lactate.
  - Ensure adequate intake of sodium chloride to promote excretion of lithium.
  - Implement peritoneal or hemodialysis in the most severe cases (serum levels between 2.0 and 4.0 mEq/L) with decreasing urinary output and deepening CNS depression.
- Ascertain reasons for lithium toxicity, increase health teaching efforts, mobilize postdischarge support system, arrange for more frequent clinical visits and blood level checks, assess for depression and suicidal intent.

BUN, Blood urea nitrogen; *CBC*, complete blood count; *CNS*, central nervous system.

adults), side effects minimized, quality of life maximized, and the bipolar patient adherent to the treatment regimen. Intensive medication management and ongoing patient education and psychotherapeutic support are the gold standard for the long-term treatment of the patient with bipolar illness. **Use of lithium during pregnancy is not recommended, particularly during the first trimester** (0.01% to 0.02% risk for cardiac anomalies: teratogenicity category D).

Your patient's wife calls you and is upset. Her husband says he enjoys his manic highs and does not want to take his medication, which dulls his enjoyment of life. How would you help this family? ■

Anticonvulsants

A variety of anticonvulsant drugs have beneficial effects in the treatment of bipolar disorder and several have FDA approval for this indication. It is thought that the anticonvulsant mood-stabilizing drugs work in bipolar disorder by enhancing the effects of the inhibitory neurotransmitter GABA and by desensitizing the "kindling" effect in bipolar illness.

Kindling occurs when the brain becomes neurochemically sensitized to events such as stress or trauma or the effects of street drugs and eventually seems to cause the brain to spontaneously respond in a dysfunctional manner even in the absence of these events (see Chapter 6). Kindling is a model used to theorize about the cause of cyclical illnesses such as bipolar illness and the intermittent symptoms of other illnesses such as panic attacks or the craving of substances of abuse. As with lithium, side effect profiles, adverse effects, and contraindications require a sophisticated clinical approach for the safe and effective use of anticonvulsant mood-stabilizing drugs in patients with bipolar illness.

Divalproex (Depakote), a derivative of valproic acid, has a superior therapeutic index, a better toxicity profile, and a wider range of effectiveness in subtypes of bipolar disorder (such as rapid cycling and mixed mood states) as compared with lithium. For these reasons it has surpassed lithium as the drug most commonly used to treat bipolar disorder in the United States. It is effective in both the manic and depressed phases of bipolar disorder and in schizoaffective disorder. Response usually occurs in 1 to 2 weeks, and it can be used in long-term maintenance alone or with other drugs such as lithium, antipsychotics, or antidepressants.

Divalproex is well tolerated in general; side effects include gastrointestinal complaints such as anorexia, nausea, vomiting, and diarrhea; neurological symptoms of tremor, sedation, headache, dizziness, and ataxia; and increased appetite and weight gain. Thrombocytopenia, with bruising, petechiae, hematoma, and bleeding, may necessitate a decrease in dose or discontinuation of the drug. Very rare but serious side effects include pancreatitis and severe hepatic dysfunction, thus comprehensive laboratory tests are conducted at baseline and are repeated every 1 to 4 weeks for the first 6 months and then every 3 to 6 months.

Divalproex is not recommended in patients during pregnancy (1% to 2% risk of neural tube defects, spina bifida: teratogenicity category D) or in those with hepatic disease, blood dyscrasias, organic brain disease, or renal function impairment. **It can be lethal in overdose**.

Lamotrigine (Lamictal), another anticonvulsant, with FDA approval as a mood stabilizer, is useful in delaying onset of mood episodes in patients receiving standard treatment for acute mood episodes in bipolar disorder. It appears to decrease glutamate release, modulate the reuptake of serotonin, and generally block the reuptake of monoamines, including dopamine. It is thought that these mechanisms may explain its mood stabilizing effects.

Lamotrigine is generally well tolerated. Common side effects include dizziness, headache, double vision, unsteadiness, sedation, and uncomplicated rash. Lamotrigine is started at 25 mg/day for the first week, and the dosage is increased by 25 to 50 mg every 2 weeks, with an upper dose target of 500 mg or more per day.

Lamotrigine increases the risk of serious skin reactions including Stevens-Johnson syndrome, which may be fatal (the risk is increased further by too rapid dose titration) to 1 in 1000 adults and 1 in 100 children (Schatzberg, Cole, and DeBattista, 2003). When used in conjunction with divalproex, doses of lamotrigine should be lowered because serum levels are increased. When used in conjunction with carbamazepine, higher doses of lamotrigine may be needed because serum levels are decreased. **Overdoses can be serious, and lamotrigine is a teratogenicity category C, thus is not recommended for use during pregnancy.**

Carbamazepine (Tegretol) is a third line agent behind divalproex and lithium, even though it does not have FDA approval for this indication. It has its peak effects within 10 days of administration and is used either alone or in combination with other drugs in the treatment of bipolar disorder. Side effects include drowsiness, dizziness, ataxia, double vision, blurred vision, nausea, and fatigue. Less common are gastrointestinal upset and a variety of skin reactions, occasionally requiring discontinuation of the drug. A temporary benign 25% decrease in the white blood cell count does not require discontinuation.

Because carbamazepine induces the CYP-450 liver enzyme system, it could cause a decrease in serum concentrations of other anticonvulsants, benzodiazepines, anticoagulants, and oral contraceptives, causing a decrease in effectiveness of these drugs. A rare but serious side effect is carbamazepine-induced agranulocytosis, a significant decrease in the white blood cell count that does not return to normal. Blood cell and platelet counts and hepatic and renal function tests are taken at baseline and intermittently throughout treatment. **Carbamazepine can be lethal in overdose, is not recommended during pregnancy, and should not be used in patients with a host of other medical illnesses, such as diabetes and bone marrow suppression.**

A related new compound, oxcarbazepine (Trileptal), does not appear to induce liver enzymes as much and is generally better tolerated. Although it is not being actively studied in large scale trials for the treatment of bipolar disorder, some practitioners have begun to use it for that purpose instead of carbamazepine. It remains to be seen whether evidence-based data eventually support this practice.

Several newer anticonvulsants also have become popular in the treatment of bipolar disorder. They are gabapentin (Neurontin), topiramate (Topamax), and tiagabine (Gabitril). Although very few systematic double-blind studies to date have assessed the safety and efficacy of these drugs in the treatment of bipolar disorder, they have been reportedly successful in treating mixed states and rapid cycling in people who have not received adequate benefit from or who are intolerant to lithium, carbamazepine, or valproic acid.

Gabapentin may be more effective in treating anxiety and agitation than carbamazepine and valproic acid. Topiramate is the only anticonvulsant mood stabilizer not associated with weight gain and in fact is associated with weight loss in up to 50% of patients. Tiagabine has mixed results thus far in open label studies. More controlled studies are needed to document the safety and efficacy profiles of these drugs in the treatment of bipolar disorder.

Atypical Antipsychotics

The atypical antipsychotic olanzapine has FDA approval for the treatment of acute mania. Evidence indicates that it has mild antidepressant properties as well. Data suggest that olanzapine will prove useful in preventing subsequent cycles of mania or depression as a maintenance treatment (Schatzberg, Cole, and DeBattista, 2003).

Numerous reports have indicated that the other atypical antipsychotic drugs are also effective in the treatment of bipolar disorder. The prescription of these drugs, particularly in combination with other mood stabilizers, is becoming common clinical practice. However, their precise mechanism of action for this disorder is unclear.

Benzodiazepines

BZs have been used as adjunctive treatment for anxiety in patients with bipolar disorder for many years, although they also have modest antimanic and antidepressant activity. Their use is limited because of their potential for abuse and risk for disinhibition. Additionally they may be used to treat insomnia, anxiety, or agitation during initiation of therapy with agents that are more effective in treating acute mania (Ketter et al, 2003).

Calcium Channel Blockers

Dysregulation of intracellular calcium may be involved in some affective disorders, and this has lead to the investigation of a class of drugs primarily used to treat hypertension, angina, and supraventricular arrhythmias. Calcium channel blockers (verapamil, nifedipine, and nimodipine) modulate mood by inhibiting calcium channels in the postsynaptic neuron, affecting the noradrenergic neurotransmitter system.

This action is similar to that of lithium, and these drugs have shown benefits similar to those of lithium in clinical use, and clinicians are beginning to use them for bipolar disorder in some patients. Patients who have not responded well to lithium or the anticonvulsants likely will not respond to these drugs either (Schatzberg and Nemeroff, 2004).

Calcium channel blockers may be best used in bipolar patients with hypertension or supraventricular arrhythmias, or for **pregnant bipolar patients** because the teratogenic risk is much lower than that in standard mood stabilizing agents. Side effects include dizziness, headache, and nausea. Serious but rare side effects include malignant arrhythmias, hepatotoxicity, severe hypotension, and syncope. More research is needed to determine what role this class of drugs will ultimately have in future bipolar treatment regimens.

■ ANTIPSYCHOTIC DRUGS

The original drugs from the 1950s used to treat psychosis are called "typical" or "conventional" antipsychotic drugs. They revolutionized the treatment of schizophrenia and other psychotic disorders. The newer or second generation antipsychotic drugs from the 1990s are called "atypical" or "novel" antipsychotic drugs and offer a different pharmacological mechanism of action, an expanded spectrum of therapeutic effectiveness, and a more acceptable side effect profile. Thus their development again revolutionized the treatment of psychosis, and they are considered first-line choices by many clinicians for the treatment of psychotic disorders.

The major uses for antipsychotic drugs are in the treatment of schizophrenia, schizoaffective disorder, organic brain syndrome with psychosis, and delusional disorder, in both acute and maintenance regimens (see Chapter 21). Several atypical drugs have been approved for the treatment of agitation associated with Alzheimer's disease and for bipolar disorder.

Their short-term use may be indicated in severe depression with psychotic features and in substance-induced psychosis. They also treat the aggressiveness and behavioral problems seen in patients with pervasive developmental disorders and in elderly patients with dementia and delirium with agitation and psychosis. They also decrease the vocal tics in Tourette's syndrome. The antipsychotic drugs are listed in Table 27-15.

The clinical symptoms of psychosis that are considered the major target symptoms for pharmacotherapy with the antipsychotic drugs are listed in Box 27-14. The initial nursing treatment plan should address target symptoms, selection of drug, dose, response, and observed side effects and their treatment, along with patient safety, education, and reassurance.

Although the relationship the nurse establishes with the patient who is very psychotic forms the basis for an ongoing therapeutic alliance, active nonpharmacological treatment of the residual symptoms of psychosis is more successful when the patient's behavior, mood, and thought processes begin to show improvement with pharmacotherapy.

Atypical Antipsychotics

All the atypical drugs exert blocking effects at the dopamine 2 (D_2) and serotonin 2 (5-HT_2) postsynaptic receptors. Thus they are DA and 5-HT antagonists. Aripiprazole is unique in that it is the first of a new generation of atypical antipsychotics, a dopamine-serotonin stabilizer. It is a partial agonist (enhancer) at D_2 and 5-HT_{1A} receptors and has antagonistic (blocking) activity at 5-HT_{2A} receptors.

Like the typical antipsychotics, the atypical antipsychotics improve the positive symptoms of schizophrenia, but unlike the typical drugs, they also improve the negative symptoms. Also, they rarely cause extrapyramidal syndrome (EPS) or tardive dyskinesia, side effects of the typical drugs implicated in patient nonadherence with drug regimens. Most importantly, atypical drugs also are reported to treat mood symptoms, hostility, violence, suicidal behavior, diffi-

Table 27-15 Atypical Antipsychotic and Typical Antipsychotic Drugs

Generic Name (Trade Name)	Therapeutic Equivalent (Potency, mg)	Half-Life (hr)	Usual Adult Daily Dose: Range (mg)*†	Preparations
Atypical Antipsychotic Drugs				
Clozapine (Clozaril)	50	8-12	100-900	PO
Risperidone (Risperdal, Consta)	0.5	3-24	2-8	PO, L, L-A
Olanzapine (Zyprexa, Zydis)	5	27	5-20	PO, ODT
Quetiapine (Seroquel)	50-100	7	150-750	PO
Ziprasidone (Geodon)	40	5	40-160	PO, IM, L
Aripiprazole (Abilify)	5	50-80	10-15	PO
Typical Antipsychotic Drugs				
Phenothiazines				
Chlorpromazine (Thorazine)	100	23-37	200-1000	PO, IM, L, Sup
Thioridazine (Mellaril)	100	24-36	200-800‡	PO, IM, L
Mesoridazine (Serentil)	50	24-42	75-300	PO, IM, L
Perphenazine (Trilafon)	10	9	8-32	PO, IM, L
Trifluoperazine (Stelazine)	5	24	5-20	PO, IM, L
Fluphenazine (Prolixin)	2	22	2-60	PO, IM, L, L-A
Fluphenazine decanoate (Prolixin D)	0.25 cc/month	q2-3 weeks	12.5-50 q 2-4 weeks	L-A
Thioxanthene				
Thiothixene (Navane)	4	34	5-30	PO, L, IM
Butyrophenone				
Haloperidol (Haldol)	2	24	2-20*	PO, IM, L
Haloperidol decanoate (Haldol D)	50-300	3 weeks	50-300 q 3-4 weeks	L-A
Dibenzoxazepine				
Loxapine (Loxitane)	10	4	20-100	PO, IM, L
Dihydroindolone				
Molindone (Moban)	10	1.5	50-225	PO, L
Diphenybutylpiperidine				
Pimozide (Orap)	2	55	2-6	PO

PO, Oral tablet, capsule; *L*, oral liquid, elixir; *L-A*, long-acting injectable preparation; *ODT*, orally disintegrating tablets; *IM*, intramuscular injection; *Sup*, suppository.
*Dose is for PO unless noted.
†Dose range varies by patient and should be individualized.
‡Upper limit to avoid retinopathy.

culty with socialization, and the cognitive impairment seen in schizophrenia.

Thus, although the treatment of schizophrenia with current antipsychotic drugs continues to be complex and research on more effective drugs continues, the atypical drugs provide new hope for patients with psychosis. The biggest disadvantage to the atypical drugs is the increase in cost over that of the typical agents. However, cost-benefit analyses show that the cost is outweighed by the improved effectiveness and quality of life experienced by patients on these drugs.

Although the atypical drugs are similar in their effectiveness compared with each other, they differ in side effects (Table 27-16) because of their different receptor-binding profiles (Woo et al, 2004):

- Risperidone tends to elevate serum prolactin levels and may cause EPS at higher doses.
- Weight gain and metabolic disturbances are common and problematic side effects of these drugs (with the probable exception of ziprasidone and aripiprazole). Olanzapine and clozapine seem to have the highest likelihood of causing these problems. Educational interventions can help patients minimize weight gain (see Citing the Evidence).
- Sedation is commonly observed in patients taking quetiapine, olanzapine, or clozapine.

- Because ziprasidone has been associated with Q-T interval (corrected for heart rate [QTc]) prolongation, it should not be given to patients with a current or past history of cardiac disease, and some clinicians have been slow to prescribe it for their patients in general.
- Clozapine is usually reserved for patients with treatment resistant illness because of its side effect of agranulocytosis, seizures, and myocarditis. Prescribers must follow a treatment protocol that includes entering patients in a national registry, monitoring white blood cell (WBC) count weekly for 6 months, then biweekly for as long as patients are taking the drug, and writing prescriptions for only 1 to 2 weeks at a time. For the refractory patient, however, clozapine may make a significant difference in treatment outcome.

Although these drugs offer some relief from many of the symptoms of schizophrenia, patients taking these medications still need help with other aspects of their psychosocial functioning because schizophrenia is still so debilitating, even with today's treatment. Psychoeducation, social skills training, group support, and other rehabilitative interventions are beneficial in improving their overall level of functioning and quality of life (see Chapter 15).

How would you help a family evaluate the risk/benefit ratio for clozapine treatment of their relative? ■

BOX 27-14

Antipsychotic Drug Target Symptoms

Typical and Atypical Antipsychotics
Positive symptoms: an excess or distortion of normal function*
Psychotic disorders of thinking
- Delusions (somatic, grandiose, religious, nihilistic, or persecutory themes)
- Hallucinations (auditory, visual, tactile, gustatory, olfactory)
Disorganization of speech and behavior
- Positive formal thought disorder (incoherence, derailment, illogicality)
- Bizarre behavior (catatonic motor behaviors, disorders of movement, deterioration of social behavior)

Atypical Antipsychotics
Negative symptoms: A diminution or loss of normal function†
- Affective flattening: Limited range and intensity of emotional expression
- Alogia: Restricted thought and speech
- Avolition/apathy: Lack of initiation of goal-directed behavior
- Anhedonia/asociality: Inability to experience pleasure or maintain social contacts
- Attentional impairment: Inability to mentally focus
Mood symptoms, cognitive impairment, and difficulty with socialization

*Responsive to traditional and atypical antipsychotics.
†Unresponsive to traditional antipsychotics, responsive to atypical antipsychotics.

CITING THE EVIDENCE ON
Antipsychotic Medication and Weight Gain

BACKGROUND: This study assessed the effect of an educational intervention on antipsychotic-induced weight gain among patients with schizophrenia. It used a quasi-experimental study design. Seventy patients with a DSM-IV diagnosis of schizophrenia or schizoaffective disorder entered this 6-month study conducted in the United States. All participants began receiving olanzapine treatment when they entered the study. The patients were then randomly assigned to an intervention group or a standard care group. Over the next 4 months, the intervention group participated in weekly psychoeducation classes focused on nutrition, exercise, and living a healthy lifestyle. Patients were followed for an additional 2 months to assess weight change.

RESULTS: A statistically significant difference in weight change between the two groups was observed posttreatment and at endpoint. At endpoint, the mean weight change of the intervention group was −0.6 pounds, whereas the mean weight change in the standard care group was 9.57 pounds. In both groups, men gained significantly more weight than did women.

IMPLICATIONS: The results indicate that a structured educational intervention can have a positive effect on antipsychotic-induced weight gain among patients with schizophrenia.

Littell KH et al: *J Nurs Scholarsh* 35:237, 2003.

Table 27-16   Comparison of Typical, Atypical, and Newest Antipsychotic Drugs

Clinical Efficacy	TYPICAL ANTIPSYCHOTICS	CLOZAPINE	RISPERIDONE	OLANZAPINE	QUETIAPINE	ZIPRASIDONE	ARIPIPRAZOLE
Dosage (mg/day)	Various	25-600+	2-8	5-20	150-750	80-160	10-15
Acute psychosis overall	+++	+++	+++	+++	+++	+++	+++
Acute positive symptoms	+++	+++	+++	+++	+++	+++	+++
Acute negative symptoms	+	+++	+++	+++	+++	+++	+++
Treatment-refractory psychosis	0	++	?	?	?	?	?

Side Effect Profile of Typical Antipsychotics

Agitation	+ to ++
Agranulocytosis	Rare
Anticholinergic effects	+ to +++
EPS	+ to +++
Dose-related increase in EPS	Yes
Nausea/dyspepsia	+
Orthostatic hypotension	+ to +++
Elevation of prolactin levels	+ to ++
Sedation	++ to +++
Seizures	+
Tardive dyskinesia	+++

Side Effect Profile of Atypical Antipsychotics

	SEDATION	EPS	WEIGHT GAIN
Clozapine	High	Low	High
Risperidone	Low	Low	Moderate
Olanzapine	Low	Moderate	High
Quetiapine	Low	Moderate	Moderate
Ziprasidone	Low	Moderate	Low
Aripiprazole	Low	Low	Low

Data from Schatzberg AF, Nemeroff CB: *The American Psychiatric Publishing textbook of psychopharmacology*, ed 3, Washington, DC, 2004, American Psychiatric Publishing.
Efficacy: + = mild, ++ = moderate, +++ = marked, +/− = minimal, ? = uncertain, 0 = none.
Side effects: + = mild, ++ = moderate, +++ = marked, +/− = minimal, ? = uncertain, 0 = none.
EPS, Extrapyramidal symptoms.

Typical Antipsychotics

The typical antipsychotic drugs are predominantly dopamine (DA) antagonists, thus they block postsynaptic D_2 receptors in several DA tracts in the brain, accounting for a decrease in positive symptoms of schizophrenia (listed in Box 27-14), as well as EPS. They have other synaptic effects in other transmitter systems, accounting for their broad side effect profile. Thus selection of a drug is determined by the extent, type, and severity of side effects.

For instance, a low-potency drug such as chlorpromazine can reduce the risk of EPS, and a high-potency drug such as haloperidol can minimize postural hypotension, sedation, and anticholinergic effects (Table 27-17). These drugs are equally effective in treating the positive symptoms, are equally less effective in treating the negative symptoms, and may even worsen those symptoms. In addition, they have not been particularly effective in treating cognitive impairment and mood symptoms, the other symptom dimensions of schizophrenia.

The side effects of typical antipsychotic drugs and treatment considerations are listed in Table 27-18. Side effects can range from merely uncomfortable and easily treated to a life-threatening emergency. Most EPS side effects are common and are often painful and disabling. They are also stigmatizing but usually can be prevented or minimized and effectively treated. Tardive dyskinesia is the exception because no effective treatment has been found to date. Drug strategies to treat EPS include lowering the dose of the drug, changing to a drug with a lower incidence of that side effect, or administering one of the drugs in Table 27-19.

A rare but potentially fatal (14% to 30% mortality) side effect of antipsychotic drugs is neuroleptic malignant syndrome (NMS). It is important for the nurse to assess for NMS and other serious drug side effects. Because many patients are taking more than one drug at a time, it can become confusing when symptoms of these side effects are similar. Table 27-20 compares the life-threatening side effects of serotonin syndrome with NMS.

It is important to minimize the patient's fears, decrease any sense of stigmatization, and enhance adherence to drug treatment through effective patient education and support and intensive and comprehensive medication management. Because of the importance in managing patients taking psychotropic medications and the problems they cause, medication-induced movement disorders are coded on Axis I of the *DSM-IV-TR* (American Psychiatric Association, 2000).

Table 27-17   Acute Side Effect Profile: Antipsychotic Drugs

DRUGS	SEDATION	EXTRAPYRAMIDAL SYMPTOMS	ANTICHOLINERGIC	POSTURAL HYPOTENSION
Low Potency				
Chlorpromazine	4	2	3	4
Thioridazine	4	1	4	4
Clozapine	4	1	4	3
Olanzapine	2	0	2	2
High Potency				
Trifluoperazine	2	3	2	2
Thiothixene	2	3	2	1
Loxapine	2	3	2	2
Molindone	2	3	2	2
Mesoridazine	3	2	3	3
Perphenazine	2	3	2	2
Fluphenazine	1	4	2	1
Haloperidol	1	4	1	1
Risperidone	2	1	1	2

1, Lowest incidence; *4*, highest incidence.

Table 27-18   Nursing Considerations for Antipsychotic Drug Side Effects

CNS SIDE EFFECTS	NURSING CARE AND TEACHING CONSIDERATIONS

Extrapyramidal symptoms (EPS)	General treatment principles:
	  Tolerance usually develops by the third month.
	  Decrease dose of drug.
	  Add a drug to treat EPS, then taper after 3 months on the antipsychotic.
	  Use a drug with a lower EPS profile.
	  Give patient education and support.

Acute dystonic reactions: oculogyric crisis, torticollis	Spasms of major muscle groups of neck, back, and eyes; occur suddenly; frightening; painful; medicate, parenteral works faster than PO; have respiratory support available; more common in children and young males, and with high potency drugs. Taper dose gradually when discontinuing antipsychotic drugs to avoid withdrawal dyskinesia.
Akathisia	Cannot remain still; pacing, inner restlessness, leg aches are relieved by movement; rule out anxiety or agitation; medicate.
Parkinson's syndrome: akinesia, cogwheel rigidity, fine tremor	More common in males and elderly; tolerance may not develop; medicate with DA agonist amantadine (must have good renal function).
Tardive dyskinesia (TD)	Can occur after use (usually long use) of conventional antipsychotics; stereotyped involuntary movements (tongue protrusion, lip smacking, chewing, blinking, grimacing, choreiform movements of limbs and trunk, foot tapping); if using typical antipsychotics, use preventive measures and assess often; consider changing to an atypical antipsychotic drug; there is no treatment at present for TD.
Neuroleptic malignant syndrome (NMS)*	Potentially fatal: Fever, tachycardia, sweating, muscle rigidity, tremor, incontinence, stupor, leukocytosis, elevated creatine phosphokinase (CPK), renal failure; more common with high-potency drugs and in dehydrated patients; discontinue all drugs; supportive symptomatic care (hydration, renal dialysis, ventilation, and fever reduction as appropriate); can treat with dantroline or bromocriptine; antipsychotic drugs can be cautiously reintroduced eventually.
Seizures*	Occur in approximately 1% of people taking these drugs; clozapine has a 5% rate (in patients on 600 to 900 mg/day); may have to discontinue clozapine.
Other Side Effects of Antipsychotic Drugs	
Agranulocytosis*	This is an emergency; it develops abruptly, with fever, malaise, ulcerative sore throat, leukopenia. High incidence (1% to 2%) is associated with clozapine; must do weekly CBC and prescribe only 1 week of drug at a time; discontinue drug immediately; may need reverse isolation and antibiotics.
Photosensitivity	Use sunscreen and sunglasses; cover body with clothing.
Anticholinergic effects	Symptoms: Constipation, dry mouth, blurred vision, orthostatic hypotension, tachycardia, urinary retention, nasal congestion; see Table 27-11 for nursing care.
Sedation, weight gain	See Table 27-11 for nursing care.

*Potentially life-threatening.
PO, Oral tablet/capsule; *DA*, dopamine; *CBC*, complete blood count.

Table 27-19	Drugs To Treat Extrapyramidal Side Effects	
Generic Name (Trade Name)	**Adult Dosage** Range (mg/day)	**Preparations**
Anticholinergics		
Benztropine (Cogentin)	2-6	PO, IM
Trihexyphenidyl (Artane)	4-15	PO, L
Biperiden (Akineton)	2-8	PO
Procyclidine (Kemadrin)	10-20	PO
Antihistamine		
Diphenhydramine (Benadryl)	50-300	PO, IM, L
Dopamine Agonist		
Amantadine (Symmetrel)	100-300	PO, L
Benzodiazepines		
Diazepam (Valium)	2-6	PO, IV
Lorazepam (Ativan)	0.5-2	PO, IM
Clonazepam (Klonopin)	1-4	PO

PO, Oral tablet/capsule; *IM*, intramuscular; *L*, oral liquid; *IV*, intravenously.

Table 27-20	Comparison of Serotonin Syndrome and Neuroleptic Malignant Syndrome	
Clinical Symptoms	**Serotonin Syndrome**	**Neuroleptic Malignant Syndrome**
Mental status	Confusion, disorientation, mania	Dazed mutism
Autonomic dysfunction*	50%-90%	>90%
Neuromuscular activity		
• Muscle rigidity	50%	90%
• Hyperreflexia	Common	Rare
• Myoclonic jerking	Common	Rare
• Ataxia	Common	Rare
• Extrapyramidal effects	Rare	Common
Hyperthermia	Mild-marked	Mild-marked
Leukocytosis	Rare	>80%
CPK elevation	Rare	Common
Acute renal failure	Possible	Possible

*Tachycardia, labile blood pressure, diaphoresis, tremor, incontinence, dyspnea, shivering, restlessness.
CPK, Creatine phosphokinase.

General Pharmacological Principles

Dosage requirements for individual patients vary considerably and must be adjusted as the target symptoms change and side effects are monitored. Some patients begin to respond to the sedating effects of the typical drugs in 2 to 3 days, and some take as long as 2 weeks. Full benefits may take 4 or more weeks.

The atypical drugs may begin to work in a week, but take several months to reach maximum efficacy. Thus the patient, family, and clinician must wait until the antipsychotic agent takes effect and not give in to the temptation to continue increasing the dose prematurely, because this strategy usually increases side effects and not effectiveness. A brief course of a benzodiazepine may help the patient maintain control during this time.

A patient who is unresponsive to an adequate antipsychotic trial often responds to another antipsychotic drug, so a second trial is given. Clozapine is usually considered only after a second trial failure (at this point the patient is considered treatment resistant), particularly if the patient failed to respond to the atypical drugs. When switching a patient from one antipsychotic to another, in order to avoid destabilizing the patient, one drug is gradually decreased while the new drug is gradually increased (**cross-titration**), usually by 25% each every for 2 to 4 days.

Several typical (e.g., haloperidol) and atypical (e.g., ziprasidone) antipsychotic drugs have a short-acting injectable preparation and can be administered by intramuscular routes for use in acutely agitated patients. This approach often provides relief for the acutely ill patient while the oral formulations begin to work, or until the acute crisis is resolved.

For maintenance treatment of the patient who is unable to adhere adequately to a daily dosing regimen, several long-acting injectable preparations (haloperidol decanoate, fluphenazine decanoate, and Risperdal Consta) of both the typical and atypical drugs are available (see Table 27-15). The patient's ability to tolerate these drugs should be tested by first administering the oral form for several days before administering an injection of a drug that may last for many weeks.

The antipsychotic drugs should be tapered slowly over several days to weeks to avoid dyskinetic reactions and some rebound side effects and because precipitous discontinuation is associated with increased risk for relapse (Woo et al, 2004). Antipsychotic drugs do not cause chemical dependency, and tolerance to their antipsychotic effects does not develop. They have a very low abuse potential, and they are relatively safe in overdose. The effects of antipsychotics on the fetus are inconclusive, although what is best for a psychotic pregnant mother must be carefully considered.

The nurse is encouraged to remain up to date with the treatment approaches for psychotic disorders, not only to provide the best care for these patients but also because over the next few years additional third and even fourth and fifth generation antipsychotic drugs are likely to be available, which will again revolutionize the treatment of psychosis. In the near future, as it becomes more feasible to accurately identify individuals who are vulnerable to schizophrenia, the currently controversial proposal of preventing psychosis in vulnerable individuals by pretreating them with atypical antipsychotic drugs may become common clinical practice.

■ FUTURE DEVELOPMENTS
New Psychopharmacological Agents

Currently just over 100 medicines for psychiatric illnesses are in development (Figure 27-2). It is important to evaluate new drugs very carefully as they come into clinical use. The nurse should determine the advantages and disadvantages of a new drug as compared with the standard drugs in that class and in re-

Table 27-21 New Drugs in Development for Mental Illness (2003)

PRODUCT NAME	INDICATION	DEVELOPMENT STATUS	MANUFACTURER
Aprepitant (substance P antagonist)	Affective disorders	Phase III	Merck
	Anxiety disorders		
Duloxetine (SNRI)	Depression	IND appl filed	Eli Lilly
DU 127090	Psychotic disorders	Phase III	Novartis/Titan
Escitalopram	GAD	Phase III	Forrest
	Panic disorder		
Gepirone (5-HT$_{1A}$ receptor agonist)	Depression	IND appl filed	Organon
Hoperidone	Psychotic disorders	Phase III	Novartis/Titan
Olanzapine/fluoxetine combination	Affective disorders	IND appl filed	Eli Lilly
	Treatment resistant depression		
	Bipolar depression		
Olanzapine IM	Psychotic disorders	IND appl filed	Eli Lilly
ORG 5222	Psychotic disorders	Phase III	Organon
ORG 24448	Psychotic disorders	Phase II	Organon
Osanetant	Psychotic disorders	Phase II	Sanofi-Synthelabo
NGD 91-3	Anxiety disorders	Phase II	Neutrogena/Pfizer
Pregabalin	Anxiety disorders	Phase III	Pfizer
Selegiline (TS)	Affective disorders	IND appl filed	Somerset
Methylphenidate (TS)	ADHD	IND appl filed	Noven

Modified from New medications in development, Washington, DC, 2003, PhARMA.
SNRI, Serotonin norepinephrine reuptake inhibitor; *IND appl*, investigational new drug application (filed with the FDA requesting drug approval); *TS*, transdermal system.

lation to the patient's reactions and preferences. The following list is a partial guide to help evaluate new drugs. Ask whether a new drug, compared with current drugs, has the following:

- A different mechanism of action that is more specific to the desired biological actions
- Quicker onset of action
- Fewer drug interactions
- A lower side effect profile
- No addictive or abuse potential
- No long-term adverse effects
- No suicide potential
- Permanent or curative effects on neurotransmitter regulation
- Several routes of administration
- A wide therapeutic index
- Fewer discontinuation problems
- Advantage in cost-effectiveness

Table 27-21 lists new drugs for which an investigational new drug (IND) application has been filed with the FDA or that are currently in phase II or III of the clinical trials. The drug development and approval process includes the following steps:

- Preclinical testing: Laboratory and animal studies to assess biological activity and safety
- Phase I: Safety and dosage studies of healthy volunteers
- Phase II: Small trials designed to evaluate effectiveness and look for side effects
- Phase III: Final phase of experimental drug testing designed to confirm effectiveness and monitor adverse reactions from long-term use
- IND application is filed: All study results are submitted to the FDA for drug approval
- Phase IV: Post marketing studies to support the indication and document safety of the drug over time.

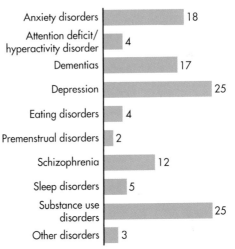

*Some medicines are in development for more than one disorder.

Figure 27-2 Medicines being developed for the treatment of mental illness. (From Pharmaceutical Research Manufacturers of America, Washington, DC, 2002.)

Several novel directions are being taken in the early trial phases of research involving antidepressants. For example, among the more promising areas are the use of anticortisol agents that impact the hypothalamic-pituitary-adrenal (HPA) axis and the use of glucocorticoid receptor antagonists that block the effects of cortisol, because severe depression is often characterized by elevated cortisol levels. Another line of antidepressant research involves the use of peptide hormonal antagonists, including substance-P, somatostatin, and cholecystokinin. The next decade should bring a variety of other new approaches to the pharmacological treatment of depression.

Genomics

The future of psychopharmacological research and drug discovery will be forever changed as a result of the findings of the Human Genome Project (see Chapter 6). With the complete decoding of all the genes that make up a human, researchers will have almost unlimited targets for drug development. This is particularly relevant to mental health because it is estimated that 5000 human genes code for brain-specific proteins, which creates the potential for 15,000 different classes of brain specific drugs (Preskorn, 2000).

In the coming era of genomic health care, new techniques of drug discovery will not only yield new targets for drug action but also help determine drug concentration relative to dose for each individual, thereby helping to determine why some patients respond to a given dose of a given drug, whereas others do not, and still others develop toxicity.

At some point in the foreseeable future, gene discovery (Figure 27-3) will make it possible to provide gene therapy that can prevent illness and diagnostic tests that can genetically identify persons at risk. Pharmacogenomics will make it possible to predict which drug will be most effective and produce the fewest side effects for any given individual, and new drugs will be developed that specifically target brain receptors for focused treatments (Collins, 2003).

■ PSYCHIATRIC NURSING PRACTICE

The psychiatric nurse should make use of competency documents and clinical guidelines and stay up to date on new, evidence-based theories and treatments for psychiatric illnesses. In addition, the safe practice of clinical psychopharmacology requires that nurses have competencies in diagnosis, biological assessment, knowledge of available drugs, and the design of medication regimens, as well as competence in prescriptive practice at the advanced level.

Important components of the psychiatric nurse's role are the ability to provide patient education regarding medications and the ability to identify side effects and then appropriately intervene to halt or lessen those side effects being experienced by patients as a result of their medication regimens. It is also important that nurses participate in activities that highlight psychiatric nursing and provide role models (e.g., to precept nursing students during their clinical rotations and to participate in community health fairs) to increase recruitment of qualified nurses into psychiatric nursing and to increase the visibility of nursing in the community as a whole.

Psychopharmacology Guidelines and Algorithms

Psychotropic medications are commonly used in the treatment of psychiatric disorders. It is therefore essential for psychiatric nurses to have a thorough understanding of psychopharmacol-

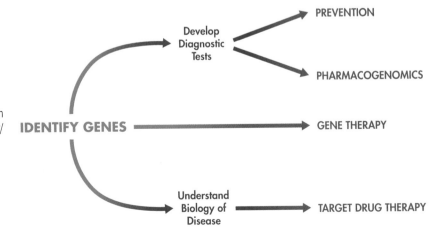

Figure 27-3 Gene discovery: new avenues to prevention and treatment. (From Collins F: *NAMI Advocate*, Summer/Fall, p 29, 2003.)

ogy. The American Nurses Association published a document (1994) that describes the skills and knowledge psychiatric nurses need to guide them in their work with psychopharmacological agents (Box 27-15). The document identifies specific areas that nurses can review to evaluate their ability to deliver competent nursing care.

Advanced practice psychiatric nurses are guided by these focal points of nursing and by various interdisciplinary treatment guidelines designed to inform medication prescribing for psychiatric disorders. In 2003, the National Organization of Nurse Practitioner Faculties (NONPF) published a comprehensive set of competencies defining the scope and practice of psychiatric mental health nurse practitioners (PMHNP). They are a continuation of a series of similar competencies for many nurse practitioner specialties (NONPF, 2003). An ex-

ample of a competency specific to medication prescribing for PMHNPs follows:

The PMHNP "prescribes psychotropic and related medications based on clinical indicators of a patient's status, including results of diagnostic and lab tests as appropriate, to treat symptoms of psychiatric disorders and improve functional health status."

In addition, various other professional organizations and groups have developed practice guidelines and psychopharmacology treatment algorithms (see Chapter 5). In particular, the Texas Medication Algorithm Project provides an evidence-based decision tree with information about how to make decisions regarding selection of medications, how and when to change medications, and how to augment medications. Figure 27-4 presents an algorithm showing

Step 1	**Patient with appropriate diagnosis and baseline psychiatric and medical history, physical, and evaluation.** Drug target symptoms Concomitant psychiatric and medical illnesses and treatments History of drug response in self and first-degree relatives Contraindications, allergies, lifestyle issues, and cost considerations Coordination of treatments among patient's providers Patient education and inclusion in treatment plan
Step 2	**Choose monotherapy from primary first line medications for indication.** Drug has positive efficacy/side effect profile for patient Patient education and consent Nonmedication therapy as appropriate
Step 3	**Wait appropriate time period to see response.** Side effects are minimized Dose is titrated/laboratory values as appropriate Target symptom rating is ongoing
Step 4	**Evaluate Response.** **(A) Good Response** *Is patient tolerating medication?* If yes, continue for appropriate time frame. If no, adjust dose; add adjunctive treatment; change primary medication. Repeat **Step 3**. - **(B) Partial Response** *Is dose adequate?* If no, adjust dose. Repeat **Step 3**. If yes, *is patient taking medication as prescribed?* If no, patient education and re-consent; initiate/increase nonmedication therapy; reevaluate patient's preference. If yes, *has illness exacerbated or is there a concomitant illness?* If yes, adjust dose or begin concomitant treatment; initiate/increase nonmedication therapy. Repeat **Step 3**. If no, *is diagnosis correct?* If no, repeat baseline diagnostic evaluation; consultation. If yes, consider: Augmentation; switch to another first line medication; switch to a second/third line medication; initiate/ increase nonmedication therapy; consultation. Repeat **Step 3**. - **(C) No Response** *Check:* Dose, patient adherence, diagnosis (see **B, Partial Response**). If diagnosis is correct, consider: Switch to another first line medication; switch to a second/third line medication; combination therapy with two agents with different mechanisms of action; triple medication combinations; other interventions as scientific data and clinical experience dictate. Repeat **Step 3**. Repeat **Step 4**. *Consider:* Referral.

Figure 27-4 Medication algorithm: overview. (Modified from Rush et al: *J Clin Psychiatry* 60:284, 1999.)

strategic recommendations for the use of psychopharmacological agents.

Documentation

In addition to routine documentation of pharmacological activities, the nurse may have special documentation considerations in the pharmacological treatment of mental illness. The following categories of information are particularly important to document when working with psychiatric patients:

- Drugs administered outside usual recommended levels
- Rationale for medication or dose changes
- Drugs used for indications other than those approved by the FDA
- Continued use of a drug that is causing clinically significant side effects
- Co-administration, augmentation, and polypharmacy rationale
- Patient and family knowledge, attitudes, and preferences

Patient Education

Patients taking psychotropic drugs must be knowledgeable about them. Serious consequences can result from not adhering to what may appear to the patient as minor changes in some of the instructions for drug use, such as skipping medication one day, eating cheese, or failing to recognize certain side effects.

Patients and their families need thorough and ongoing instruction on psychotropic drug treatment. Nursing programs focused on patient education need to address essential elements, such as missed medication doses, focus on self-management, and documenting effectiveness. Box 27-16 identifies specific nursing activities from the Nursing Interventions Classification (NIC) project related to teaching a patient how to take prescribed medications safely (Dochterman and Bulechek, 2004).

Many chronic mentally ill people have social workers as their case managers. What skills and knowledge would psychiatric nurses bring to this patient population that differ from those of social workers? ■

BOX 27-16

NIC Interventions for Teaching: Prescribed Medication

Definition
Preparing a patient to safely take prescribed medications and monitor for their effects.

Activities
Instruct the patient to recognize distinctive characteristics of the medication(s), as appropriate.
Inform the patient of both the generic and brand names of each medication.
Instruct the patient on the purpose and action of each medication.
Explain how health care providers choose the most appropriate medication.
Instruct the patient on the dosage, route, and duration of each medication.
Instruct the patient on the proper administration/application of each medication.
Review patient's knowledge of medications.
Acknowledge patient's knowledge of medications.
Evaluate the patient's ability to self-administer medications.
Instruct the patient to perform needed procedures before taking a medication (e.g., check pulse, glucose), as appropriate.
Inform the patient what to do if a dose of medication is missed.
Instruct the patient on which criteria to use when deciding to alter the medication dosage/schedule, as appropriate.
Inform the patient of consequences of not taking or abruptly discontinuing medication(s), as appropriate.
Instruct the patient on specific precautions to observe when taking medication(s) (e.g., no driving/using power tools), as appropriate.
Instruct the patient on possible adverse effects of each medication.
Instruct the patient how to relieve and/or prevent certain side effects, as appropriate.

Instruct the patient on appropriate actions to take if side effects occur.
Instruct the patient on the signs and symptoms of overdosage/underdosage.
Inform the patient of possible drug-food interactions, as appropriate.
Instruct the patient how to properly store the medication(s).
Instruct the patient on the proper care of devices used for administration.
Instruct the patient on proper disposal of needles and syringes at home, as appropriate, and where to dispose of the sharps container in his/her community.
Provide the patient with written information about the action, purpose, side effects, and so on, of medications.
Assist the patient to develop a written medication schedule.
Instruct the patient to carry documentation of his/her prescribed medication regimen.
Instruct the patient how to fill his/her prescription(s), as appropriate.
Inform the patient of possible changes in appearance and/or dosage when filling generic medication prescription(s).
Warn the patient of the risks associated with taking expired medication.
Caution the patient against giving prescribed medication to others.
Determine the patient's ability to obtain required medications.
Provide information on medication reimbursement, as appropriate.
Provide information on cost savings programs/organizations to obtain medications and devices, as appropriate.
Provide information on medication alert devices and how to obtain them.
Reinforce information provided by other health care team members, as appropriate.
Include the family/significant others, as appropriate.

From Dochterman JM, Bulechek GM, editors.: *Nursing interventions classification (NIC)*, ed 4, St Louis, 2004, Mosby.

Patient Assistance Programs

Because of limitations on health care coverage nationally for persons with psychiatric diagnoses and rising health care costs in general, including the increased expense of newer drugs and long-term maintenance therapy regimens, patients are finding it more difficult to afford their medications. Additionally, many psychiatric patients are unable to earn a living unless they are on successful treatment regimens, including psychopharmacology.

An important part of the nursing role, therefore, is to assist the patient with this problem by educating him or her about patient assistance programs (PAPs) offered by many pharmaceutical companies (Box 27-17). Although these programs are not available to all patients and do not offer assistance with the cost of all drugs, they can be helpful to many patients who have few other resources (Goldsmith, 2003).

Although each manufacturer has different requirements, most programs require an application either from the patient or the prescriber documenting the patient's financial status and need for the drug. Some patients who qualify for Medicaid, have private insurance, or exceed the income cap may be ineligible. More detailed information can be obtained by calling the drug manufacturer or by going to the Internet website.

Promoting Patient Adherence

Patients who do not take their medications as prescribed or who do not recognize warning signs of illness exacerbation or drug side effects are at risk for unsuccessful results and adverse reactions. Various research studies on medication adherence in psychiatric treatment identify patient nonadherence as a major problem (Dolder et al, 2002; Navon and Ozer, 2003). Poor adherence contributes to the economic costs of psychiatric illness (Thieda et al, 2003). Yet studies also note that nurses and other providers remain invested in patient adherence (Kemppainen et al, 2003).

The threats to patient adherence are many. Some of them come from the mental health team, others from the patient, and still others reflect a shared failure of the therapeutic alliance. Nurses and patients should work together to minimize misunderstandings and unnecessarily complex medication regimens.

However, too often clinicians blame patients for nonadherence without fully evaluating the treatment plan from the patient's perspective or understanding the patient's reasons for nonadherence (see Critical Thinking About Contemporary Issues). Pope and Scott (2003) compared clinician knowledge of reasons for nonadherence with patients' stated reasons for nonadherence and found that clinicians were not fully aware of the main reasons patients would stop medication treatment.

Risk factors for potential patient nonadherence are listed in Box 27-18. Understanding this issue from the patient's perspective will allow the nurse to anticipate problems and design nursing interventions that can target areas of potential difficulty.

Patients should be encouraged by the nurse to discuss their questions, fears, problems, and concerns about medication

---

BOX **27-17**

Patient Assistance Programs for Low-Income and Indigent Patients

These programs may be subject to change.

LillyCares
For indigent patients without any coverage: No fees
(800) 545-6962

LillyAnswers
For low income Medicare enrollees with no coverage:
   $12/month/script
(877) 795-4559
http://www.lillyanswers.com/

Pfizer for Living Share Card
For Medicare enrollees with no other coverage:
   $15/month/script
(800) 717-6005
http://www.pfizerforliving.com

Together Rx
For Medicare enrollees with no other coverage:
   20% to 40% discount on select drugs from Abbott,
   AstraZeneca, Aventis, Bristol-Myers-Squibb, GlaxoSmithKline,
   Johnson and Johnson, Novartis
(800) 865-7211
http://www.together-rx.com

Directory of Prescription Drug Patient Assistance Programs
From the Pharmaceutical Research and Manufacturers
   of America
http://www.phrma.org

AstraZeneca Foundation Patient Assistance Program
(800) 424-3727
http://www.astrazeneca-us.com/pap/pap.asp

GlaxoSmithKline: Bridges to Access
(866) 728-4368
http://bridgestoaccess.gsk.com/

Novartis Patient Assistance Program
(800) 277-2254
http://www.pharma.us.novartis.com/novartis/pap/pap.jsp

Critical Thinking *About* Contemporary Issues

Is Nonadherence a Patient Problem or a Nursing Problem?

Every nurse and many patients and their families have had the difficult experience of facing relapse in psychopharmacologically treated psychiatric illness. An obvious problem-solving approach includes an assessment of adherence—is the patient taking the drug as prescribed? In the absence of concomitant medical illness, differences in bioavailability among generic brands of a drug, and increases in life stressors, the nurse and family return to the issue of adherence and wonder why the patient deviated from a previously effective drug regimen. Even if patients deny nonadherence, they usually carry the burden of blame for relapse, and their future relationships with mental health care providers may be jeopardized.

The interactions of cultural belief systems and psychotropic drug effects are poorly understood. A relatively unacknowledged but well-documented fact is that the effects of pharmacoactive agents are not solely determined by their pharmacological properties. In the cultural context of care it must be recognized that psychotropic drugs affect diverse populations in diverse ways. Thus cultural differences must be considered in the patient and family medication education plan and in interactions with patients throughout the course of treatment.

The potential incompatibility between lay and professional values and between belief system and explanatory models of illness often determine patients' satisfaction with treatment, medication adherence, and clinical outcome (Ruiz, 2000; Navon and Ozer, 2003). The understanding, acceptance, and communication necessary to create a culturally competent and effective plan of care for the patient with mental illness rest with the nurse and the mental health care team. If treatment planning is individualized and is a mutual and shared responsibility between the nurse and patient, then patient adherence or nonadherence must be viewed as a shared outcome of that responsibility.

BOX **27-18**

Risk Factors for Patient Medication Nonadherence

- Failure to form a therapeutic alliance with the patient
- Devaluation of pharmacotherapy by treatment staff
- Inadequate patient and family education regarding treatment
- Poorly controlled side effects
- Insensitivity to patient beliefs, wishes, complaints, or opposition to the idea of taking medication
- Multiple daily dosing schedule
- Polypharmacy
- History of nonadherence
- Social isolation
- Expense of drugs
- Failure to appreciate patient's role in drug treatment plan
- Lack of continuity of care
- Increased restrictions on patient's lifestyle
- Unsupportive significant others
- Remission of target symptoms
- Increased suicidal ideation
- Increased suspiciousness
- Unrealistic expectations of drug effects
- Concurrent substance use
- Failure to target residual symptoms for nonpharmacological therapies
- Relapse or exacerbation of clinical syndrome
- Failure to alleviate intrafamilial and environmental stressors that precipitate symptoms
- Potential for stigmatization
- Bothered by the idea of chronic illness

before treatment is initiated, or altered. The nurse should realize that in addition to the quality of the nurse-patient relationship and the strength of the therapeutic alliance, understanding an individual patients' reasons for nonadherence plays an extremely important role in whether a patient will adhere to a pharmacological treatment plan and be successful in the recovery process.

COMPETENT CARING

A Clinical Exemplar of a Psychiatric Nurse
DIANA LAIKAM, MS, RN, CS

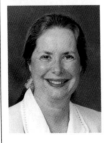

Henry David Thoreau wrote: "If one advances confidently in the direction of his dreams, and endeavors to lead the life which he imagined, he will meet with a success unexpected in common hours." Thirty years ago I confidently began my sojourn into the field of nursing. The journey has led to my role as a Psychiatric Clinical Nurse Specialist with prescriptive authority. When I began psychiatric nursing, hospital admissions lasted months instead of days. Lithium carbonate was still in clinical trials. Serotonin reuptake inhibitors were yet to be developed. And yet, from the beginning of my practice as a psychiatric nurse, I have known that working with the severely and persistently mentally ill was to be my life's work.

Psychotropic medications are the primary means of treating the symptoms of these illnesses. The medication treatment goals for my patients include management, reduction, and cessation of symptoms; establishment of an extended period of partial or complete remission; prevention of exacerbation or relapse symptoms; and prevention, identification, and treatment of side effects. I have learned over time that medication compliance is critical if the severely and persistently mentally ill patient is to avoid hospitalization. And I have had some success in this area.

One such success involved Mr. M, a 40-year-old man with a diagnosis of bipolar affective disorder, recurrent. Throughout his 20-year history of mood lability, he had been prescribed many antipsychotic and mood-stabilizing drugs. Most of his hospitalizations occurred as a result of medication noncompliance. He was referred to me on discharge from the inpatient psychiatric unit for medication monitoring, and I readily accepted the challenge.

My first glance at Mr. M was of him sitting in the waiting area before his appointment with me. He had a large, crumpled, brown paper bag at his feet. An anxious Mr. M brought the brown bag into my office. The bag contained 22 bottles of assorted medications. He told me that he was feeling much better but that his medications had all been changed while he was an inpatient. He was confused regarding the names of the medications, the dosages he should take, and the times that he should take the medications. Some of the medicines were for his medical illnesses and some for his psychiatric illness.

As the appointment progressed, it became clear to me that even with sorting out the medications and explaining how to take them that he was still feeling overwhelmed. With his involvement, a plan evolved. Prescriptions were rewritten with medica-

tion names he recognized (brand rather than generic) and, whenever possible, prescribed at times convenient to his lifestyle. Medication information was transferred to a sheet of paper so he could read which medication to take and when to take it. He found this particularly helpful because he could not read the small print on the bottles. A medication reminder was to be filled weekly with my assistance until he could manage his own medication.

A year has passed. Medication treatment goals have been met. Mr. M is quite proud that he now takes his medication in an organized manner without a medication reminder. He is acutely aware of subtle changes in his mental status and knows how to observe for side effects. Most importantly, he has not required hospitalization. So each day Mr. M's spirit rejuvenates me in a very real way as I proceed in the direction of my dreams—practicing the profession I love. ∎

CHAPTER FOCUS POINTS

- Psychopharmacology is the gold standard in the treatment of mental illness, and the psychiatric nurse makes a unique contribution to the implementation of this important modality.
- Various principles of psychopharmacology relate to pharmacokinetics, pharmacodynamics, drug co-administration, and the role of neurotransmitters in the development of psychiatric disorders.
- Benzodiazepines, the most widely prescribed class of drugs, have almost completely replaced the class of barbiturates as antianxiety and sedative-hypnotic agents. They are therapeutic and have a wide margin of safety in overdose. They can be addictive, especially when taken in high doses over a long time. Common side effects include drowsiness, dizziness, slurred speech, and blurred vision.
- Antidepressant drugs are effective and nonaddicting, but some can be lethal in overdose. Tricyclics, selective serotonin reuptake inhibitors, and newer drugs are more commonly used than monoamine oxidase inhibitors because they are safer in combination with other substances. Many of them are now first-line treatments for several anxiety disorders as well. Side effects of antidepressants are usually mild.
- The mood stabilizers include lithium, a range of anticonvulsants, atypical antipsychotics, and calcium channel blockers. These classes

of drugs are not addictive, but several of them can be toxic, which requires that patients be well educated concerning the effects of these drugs and that laboratory values be closely monitored.
- The various classes of typical antipsychotic drugs have similar therapeutic effects but are dissimilar in side effect profiles. Side effects are varied and can be disabling and life-threatening. The newer, atypical antipsychotic agents offer a different pharmacological mechanism of action, an expanded spectrum of therapeutic effectiveness, and a generally more acceptable side effect profile.
- New psychopharmacological agents are being tested in clinical drug trials throughout the United States. Many of them will be beneficial to patients with psychiatric illness.
- The findings from genomics research will change the future of drug discovery and psychopharmacology forever. With the complete decoding of all the genes that make up a human, researchers will have almost unlimited targets for drug development.
- Important issues related to psychopharmacology and psychiatric nursing practice include following psychopharmacology guidelines, documentation, patient education, patient assistance programs, and promoting patients' adherence to their pharmacological treatment plans.

KEY TERMS

CHAPTER REVIEW QUESTIONS

1. Match each term in Column A with the correct definition in Column B.

Column A
_____ Barbiturates
_____ Selective serotonin reuptake inhibitors
_____ Antianxiety drugs
_____ Cytochrome P-450 inhibition
_____ Anti-parkinsonian drugs
_____ Tricyclics
_____ Serotonin syndrome
_____ Sedative-hypnotics
_____ Atypical antipsychotics
_____ Hypertensive crisis
_____ Typical antipsychotics
_____ Mood stabilizers

Column B
A. SSRIs with MAOIs
B. Clozapine and risperidone
C. MAOIs with decongestants/cold remedies
D. Triazolam (Halcion) and flurazepam (Dalmane)
E. Imipramine (Tofranil) and amitriptyline (Elavil)
F. Lithium and divalproex (Depakote)
G. Chlorpromazine (Thorazine) and thiothixene (Navane)
H. Fluoxetine (Prozac) and sertraline (Zoloft)
I. Alprazolam (Xanax) and lorazepam (Ativan)
J. Secobarbital (Seconal) and pentobarbital (Nembutal)
K. SSRIs with various other drugs
L. Benztropine (Cogentin) and trihexyphenidyl (Artane)

2. Match the synaptic activity in Column A with the possible clinical effects in Column B.

Column A
_____ H$_1$ receptor blockade
_____ DA reuptake inhibition
_____ Alpha$_2$ receptor blockade
_____ NE reuptake inhibition
_____ ACh receptor blockade
_____ 5-HT reuptake inhibition
_____ Alpha$_1$ receptor blockade
_____ 5-HT$_2$ receptor blockade

Column B
A. Reduced depression, reduced suicidal behavior, antipsychotic effects, hypotension, sexual dysfunction
B. Sedation/drowsiness, hypotension, weight gain effects
C. Reduced depression, antianxiety effects, GI disturbances, sexual dysfunction
D. Postural hypotension, dizziness, tachycardia, memory dysfunction
E. Decreased depression, psychomotor activation, anti-parkinsonian effects
F. Priapism
G. Reduced depression, tremors, tachycardia, sexual dysfunction
H. Anticholinergic side effects

3. Fill in the blanks.

A. Patient assessment, coordination of treatment modalities, psychopharmacological drug administration and prescribing, medication education, monitoring and maintenance, and research are all within the _____.

B. Concurrent use of drugs, a frequently necessary and often complex practice in pharmacological interventions, is called

_____.

C. _____ is the term used when one drug affects the absorption, metabolism, distribution, and excretion of another drug.

D. Many of the psychiatric disorders are thought to be caused by problems in the regulation of communication in the brain, such as an overresponse or an underresponse somewhere along the complex process of neurotransmission. This hypothesis of mental illness is called the

_____.

E. The ANA Psychopharmacology Guidelines for Psychiatric Mental Health Nurses includes three broad categories that are essential content for nurses working with patients on psychotropic

drugs. These categories are _____,

_____ and _____.

4. Indicate whether the following statements are true (T) or false (F).

_____ A. Serotonin syndrome is the enhancement of action of combinations of antidepressant drugs for better efficacy in patients with depression.
_____ B. Neuroleptic malignant syndrome, a common side effect of antipsychotic drugs, responds well to increased doses of any of the psychotropic drugs used to treat mental illness.
_____ C. Hypertensive crisis, a result of MAOIs and tyramine-rich foods, is treated by holding the next dose of drug, elevating the patient's head, and administering a dose of chlorpromazine.
_____ D. Lithium toxicity occurs when blood levels of lithium are raised beyond the therapeutic window by fluid and electrolyte loss, decreased renal functioning, or overdose.
_____ E. Tricyclic antidepressants should be avoided if possible, or prescribed in amounts for 1 week at a time, in patients who are at risk for suicide.

5. Provide short answers for the following questions.

A. List the symptoms of schizophrenia, and note which respond better to atypical antipsychotics as compared with typical antipsychotics.
B. Briefly describe the difference between reuptake inhibition and receptor blockade. Identify a psychiatric disorder that might benefit from each of these strategies, and state why it is thought that this is so.
C. Discuss the reasons why suicide assessment should continue for several weeks after the depressed patient appears to be responding to antidepressants.

Visit Evolve for additional resources related to the content of this chapter.
http://evolve.elsevier.com/Stuart/principles/
• Topical Course Outline • Student Workbook Exercises • Critical Thinking Questions and Activities • Case Studies • Research Topics
• Monthly Content Updates • WebLinks

Student Study CD-ROM

Access the accompanying CD-ROM for animations, interactive exercises, review questions for the NCLEX examination, and an audio glossary.

REFERENCES

American Nurses Association: *Psychiatric mental health nursing psychopharmacology project: ANA task force on psychopharmacology,* Washington, DC, 1994, The Association.

American Psychiatric Association: *Diagnostic and statistical manual of mental disorders,* ed 4, text revision, Washington, DC, 2000, American Psychiatric Association.

Boland RT, Keller MB: Treatment of depression, Chapter 52. In Schatzberg AF, Nemeroff CB, editors: *The American Psychiatric Publishing textbook of psychopharmacology,* ed 3, Washington, DC, 2004, American Psychiatric Publishing.

Carlat D: Breast-feeding and antidepressants: an update, *The Carlat Report* 1:1, 2003.

Collins F: The genome era and mental illness, *NAMI Advocate,* Summer/Fall:29, 2003.

Dochterman JM, Bulechek GM: *Nursing interventions classification (NIC),* ed 4, St Louis, 2004, Mosby.

Dolder CR et al: Antipsychotic medication adherence: is there a difference between typical and atypical agents? *Am J Psychiatry* 159:103, 2002.

Freeman MP et al: Lithium, Chapter 35. In Schatzberg AF, Nemeroff CB, editors: *The American Psychiatric Publishing textbook of psychopharmacology,* ed 3, Washington, DC, 2004, American Psychiatric Publishing.

Goldsmith J: What's happened to American health care? *Am J Nurs* 103:21, 2003.

Hale A: Perspectives on prescribing: pioneers' narratives and advice, *Perspect Psychiatr Care* 38:79, 2002.

Keck PE, McElroy SL: Treatment of bipolar disorder, Chapter 53. In Schatzberg AF, Nemeroff CB, editors: *The American Psychiatric Publishing textbook of psychopharmacology,* ed 3, Washington, DC, 2004, American Psychiatric Publishing.

Kemppainen JK et al: Psychiatric nursing and medication adherence, *J Psychosoc Nurs Ment Health Serv* 41:38, 2003.

Ketter TA et al: The diverse roles of anticonvulsants in bipolar disorders, *Ann Clin Psychiatry* 15:95, 2003.

Kreyenbuhl J et al: Racial disparity in the pharmacological management of schizophrenia, *Schizophr Bul* 29:183, 2003.

Krishnan K: Monoamine oxidase inhibitors, Chapter 18. In Schatzberg AF, Nemeroff CB, editors: *The American Psychiatric Publishing textbook of psychopharmacology,* ed 3, Washington, DC, 2004, American Psychiatric Publishing.

Mark TL et al: Examination of treatment pattern differences by race, *Ment Health Serv Res* 5:241, 2003.

Millard M: Adverse drug reactions, Chapter 5. In Wynne AL, Woo TM, Millard M, editors: *Pharmacotherapeutics for nurse practitioner prescribers,* pp 49-57, Philadelphia, 2002, FA Davis.

Miller L: Psychopharmacology and women, *Behav Health Trends* 6, 2000.

National Organization of Nurse Practitioner Faculties (NONPF): Psychiatric mental health nurse practitioner competencies, Washington, DC:, 2003; National Panel for Psychiatric Mental Health NP Competencies, website: www.nonpf.com.

Navon L, Ozer N: Ordinary logic in unordinary lay theories: a key to understanding proneness to medication nonadherence in schizophrenia, *Arch Psychiatr Nurs* 17:108, 2003.

Pope M, Scott J: Do clinicians understand why individuals stop taking lithium? *J Affect Disord* 74:287, 2003.

Preskorn S: The Human Genome Project and modern drug development in psychiatry, *J Psychiatr Pract* Sept:272, 2000.

Raj A, Sheehan D: Benzodiazepines, Chapter 24. In Schatzberg AF, Nemeroff CB, editors: *The American Psychiatric Publishing textbook of psychopharmacology,* ed 3, Washington, DC, 2004, American Psychiatric Publishing.

Ruiz P: Ethnicity and psychopharmacology, *Rev Psychiatry* 19:4, 2000.

Schatzberg AF Cole J, DeBattista C: *Manual of clinical psychopharmacology,* ed 4, Washington, DC, 2003, American Psychiatric Publishing.

Schatzberg AF, Nemeroff CB, editors: *The American Psychiatric Publishing textbook of psychopharmacology,* ed 3, Washington, DC, 2004, American Psychiatric Publishing.

Thieda P et al: An economic review of compliance with medication therapy in the treatment of schizophrenia, *Psychiatr Serv* 54:508, 2003.

Woo T et al: Treatment of schizophrenia, Chapter 54. In Schatzberg AF, Nemeroff CB, editors: *The American Psychiatric Publishing textbook of psychopharmacology,* ed 3, Washington, DC, 2004, American Psychiatric Publishing.

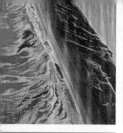

Canst thou not minister to a mind diseas'd,
Pluck from the memory rooted sorrow,
Raze out the written troubles of the brain,

And with some sweet oblivious antidote
Cleanse the stuff'd bosom of the perilous stuff
Which weights upon the heart?

WILLIAM SHAKESPEARE, *MACBETH*, ACT V

28 SOMATIC THERAPIES

Carol M. Burns

LEARNING OBJECTIVES

After studying this chapter, the student should be able to:

1. Analyze the use, indications, mechanism of action, and adverse effects of electroconvulsive therapy (ECT) as a treatment strategy for psychiatric illness (I).
2. Discuss the nursing care needs of the patient receiving ECT (II).
3. Analyze the use, indications, mechanism of action, and adverse effects of phototherapy as a treatment strategy for psychiatric illness (III).
4. Analyze the use, indications, mechanism of action, and adverse effects of sleep deprivation therapy as a treatment strategy for psychiatric illness (IV).
5. Analyze the use, indications, mechanism of action, and adverse effects of transcranial magnetic stimulation as a treatment strategy for psychiatric illness (V).
6. Analyze the use, indications, mechanism of action, and adverse effects of vagus nerve stimulation as a treatment strategy for psychiatric illness (VI).

TOPICAL OUTLINE

evolve   Visit Evolve for additional resources related to the content of this chapter.
http://evolve.elsevier.com/Stuart/principles/

With the emergence of biological psychiatry and the growing knowledge bases in the neurosciences, interest has increased in somatic therapies for psychiatric illness. The limitations of psychotropic medications, increase in treatment-resistant psychiatric disorders, and refinement in treatment techniques have placed greater emphasis on evaluating the indications for and efficacy of somatic therapeutic interventions.

Psychiatric nurses are commonly involved in caring for patients who are receiving a somatic therapy. Thus it is essential that all nurses understand how these treatment modalities work and understand what nursing care enhances their effectiveness. This chapter discusses contemporary somatic therapies used for psychiatric illnesses: electroconvul-

sive therapy, phototherapy, sleep deprivation therapy, transcranial magnetic stimulation, and vagal nerve stimulation.

ELECTROCONVULSIVE THERAPY

Electroconvulsive therapy (ECT) was first described by Cerletti and Bini in 1938 as a treatment for schizophrenia. At that time it was believed that epileptics were rarely schizophrenic and therefore hypothesized that convulsions would cure schizophrenia. Later research did not support this hypothesis. Further experience with ECT showed that it is much more effective as a treatment for affective disturbances than it is for schizophrenia. It also has been noted that epilepsy and schizophrenia sometimes occur together.

Electroconvulsive therapy is a treatment in which a grand mal seizure is artificially induced in an anesthetized patient by passing an electrical current through electrodes applied to the patient's head. Traditionally the electrodes have been applied **bilaterally**. Alternative electrode placements are now routinely used, including **unilateral** and **bifrontal**. It has been reported that patients have fewer cognitive side effects with these alternative placements, including less disorientation and fewer disturbances of verbal and nonverbal memory (Lisanby et al, 2000; Weiner, 2000).

However, unilateral ECT, under many conditions, may not be as reliably effective as bilateral ECT (Krystal et al, 2000;

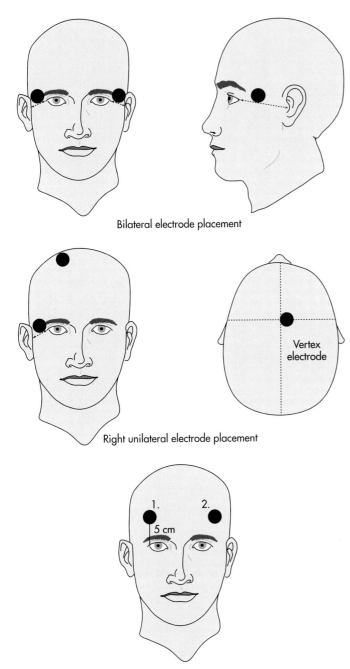

Bilateral electrode placement

Right unilateral electrode placement

Vertex electrode

Bifrontal electrode placement

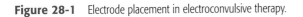

Figure 28-1   Electrode placement in electroconvulsive therapy.

McCall et al, 2000; Sackeim et al, 2000). Bifrontal placement combines the efficacy of bilateral with the cognitive profile of unilateral (Bailine et al, 2000). Further studies in this area are ongoing. Figure 28-1 illustrates the different electrode placements.

Current clinical wisdom notes that for ECT to be effective, a **grand mal seizure** must occur. The electrical stimulus is generally adjusted to the minimum level of energy that will produce a seizure. The number of treatments in a series varies according to the patient's therapeutic response. **A usual course is 6 to 12 treatments given two to three times a week.** Patients with schizophrenia may require more.

ECT is an effective treatment and is generally well-tolerated by patients (Brodaty et al, 2003; UK ECT Review Group, 2003) (see Citing the Evidence). In some cases, after a successful initial treatment episode, continuation of outpatient ECT combined with antidepressant medication may be recommended: weekly treatments for the first month after remission, gradually tapering to monthly treatments (Gagne et al, 2000; Sackeim et al, 2001a).

ECT is sometimes called "shock therapy." Describe how use of this term stigmatizes mental illness and its treatment. ■

Indications

The primary indication for ECT is major depression. ECT's response rate of 80% or more for most patients is better than response rates associated with antidepressant medications. It can be useful for people in most age-groups who cannot tolerate or fail to respond to treatment with medication (Hermann et al, 1999; Rabheru, 2001). Box 28-1 lists the primary and secondary criteria for the use of ECT as determined by the American Psychiatric Association (APA) Task Force on Electroconvulsive Therapy (2000).

CITING THE EVIDENCE ON
Improvement Following Electroconvulsive Therapy

BACKGROUND: From the perspective of the consumer, improvement is important in the assessment of treatment outcome. To gain a better understanding of health related factors that are meaningful to service recipients, patients who had been hospitalized for electroconvulsive therapy were surveyed following discharge to the community.

RESULTS: Nearly 80% of the patients reported improvement at 3 to 37 months after inpatient electroconvulsive therapy (ECT) treatment. More than 60% reported "much" or "very much" improved. Self-reported improvement was related to frequency of social contact and being able to engage in useful work. The receipt of aftercare was not related to the degree of patient self-reported improvement.

IMPLICATIONS: It is important to ask patients about their perception of improvement following mental health care, as well as about those factors that contributed to their recovery. For this group of patients, ECT was an effective treatment choice.

Rohland B: *Admin Policy Ment Health* 28:193, 2001.

BOX **28-1**

Criteria for the Use of Electroconvulsive Therapy

Primary Use
Situations in which electroconvulsive therapy (ECT) may be used before a trial of psychotropic medications include, but are not limited to, the following:
- Need for rapid, definitive response owing to the severity of a psychiatric or medical condition
- Risks of other treatments outweigh the risks of ECT
- History of poor medication response or good ECT response in one or more previous episodes of the illness
- Patient preference

Secondary Use
In other situations, a trial of an alternative therapy should be considered before referral for ECT. Subsequent referral for ECT should be based on at least one of the following:
- Treatment resistance (taking into account issues such as choice of medication, dosage, duration of trial, and compliance)
- Intolerance or adverse effects with pharmacotherapy that are deemed less likely or less severe with ECT
- Deterioration of the patient's psychiatric or medical condition that creates a need for a rapid, definitive response

From American Psychiatric Association: *The practice of electroconvulsive therapy: recommendations for treatment, training, and privileging,* ed 2, Washington DC, 2000, The Association.

Primary criteria in which ECT may play a life-saving role involve patients who are extremely depressed and suicidal or, alternatively, are so hyperactive that they are in grave danger of self-harm, such as in those with acute mania and those with affective disorders with psychosis. On occasion, ECT may be used for conditions other than affective disorders, such as Parkinson's disease (Gaylord, 2003). ECT is considered appropriate for patients with schizophrenia in a few situations, including when a psychosis is exacerbated, when psychotic symptoms have an abrupt or recent onset, when the duration of illness is short, when catatonia is present, or when the patient has responded well to ECT in the past.

Finally, ECT should be considered as an initial intervention when its anticipated side effects are considered less harmful than those associated with drug therapy in populations such as the elderly, patients with heart block, and women who are pregnant (Rabheru, 2001; Flint and Gagnon, 2002). The potential effectiveness of ECT is reduced in those with personality disorders (Sareen, Enns, and Guertin, 2000). Box 28-2 summarizes behaviors for which ECT is and is not effective.

Why would ECT be particularly indicated for depressed patients with heart block? ■

Mechanism of Action

Despite much research, the precise mechanism of action of ECT is still not known. Most theories about the mode of action of ECT focus on its efficacy with depressed patients and include the following:

BOX **28-2**

Target Behaviors for Electroconvulsive Therapy

Electroconvulsive Therapy Effective
Hyperemotionality
Hypermotility
Catatonia
Severe psychosis with acute onset
Life-threatening psychiatric conditions
Rigidity of parkinsonism or neuroleptic malignant syndrome

Electroconvulsive Therapy Ineffective
Severe character pathology
Substance abuse and dependence
Sexual identification disorders
Psychoneurosis
Chronic illness without obvious psychopathology

- **Neurotransmitter theory** suggests that ECT acts like tricyclic antidepressants by enhancing deficient neurotransmission in monoaminergic systems. Specifically, it is thought to improve dopaminergic, serotonergic, and adrenergic neurotransmission.
- **Neuroendocrine theory** suggests that ECT releases hypothalamic or pituitary hormones or both, which results in its antidepressant effects. ECT releases prolactin, thyroid-stimulating hormone, adrenocorticotropic hormone, and endorphins; but the specific hormones responsible for the therapeutic effect are not known.
- **Anticonvulsant theory** suggests that ECT treatment exerts a profound anticonvulsant effect on the brain that results in an antidepressant effect. Some support for this theory is based on the fact that a person's seizure threshold rises over the course of ECT and that some patients with epilepsy have fewer seizures after receiving ECT.

Adverse Effects

The mortality rate associated with ECT is estimated to be the same as that associated with general anesthesia in minor surgery (approximately 1 death per 10,000 patients). Mortality and morbidity are believed to be lower with ECT than with the administration of antidepressant medications despite the frequent use of ECT in patients with medical complications and in the elderly (American Psychiatric Association, 2000; Shiwach, Reid, and Carmody, 2001).

Medical adverse effects can, to some extent, be anticipated and prevented. Patients with preexisting cardiac illness, compromised pulmonary status, a history of central nervous system problems, or medical complications after anesthesia are likely to be at increased risk. Thus the workup preceding ECT should include a thorough review of the patient's history, and may include a complete blood count, serum chemistry profile, chest and spinal radiographs, electrocardiography, and computed tomography scan of the head.

Adverse effects can potentially occur in the following categories:

- **Cardiovascular effects**. Transient cardiovascular changes are expected in ECT. Routine ECGs should be performed to rule out baseline pathology, with further workup as indicated.
- **Systemic effects**. Headaches, nausea, muscle soreness, and drowsiness may occur after ECT, but they usually respond to supportive management and nursing intervention.
- **Cognitive effects**. ECT is associated with a range of cognitive side effects including a period of confusion immediately after the seizure and memory disturbance during the treatment course, although a few patients report persistent deficits. The onset of cognitive side effects varies considerably among patients (Lisanby et al, 2000; Weiner, 2000). It is believed that patients with preexisting cognitive impairment, neuropathological conditions, and those receiving psychotropic medication during ECT are at increased risk of developing more side effects. No evidence has been found to indicate that ECT causes brain damage (Ende et al, 2000; Madsen et al, 2000; Zachrisson et al, 2000).

NURSING CARE IN ELECTROCONVULSIVE THERAPY

Psychiatric nurses have always had a role in assisting with the ECT procedure. This role has evolved to include independent and collaborative nursing actions.

Emotional Support and Education

Nursing care begins as soon as the patient and family are presented with ECT as a treatment option. An essential role of the nurse is to allow the patient an opportunity to **express feelings,** including concerns associated with myths or fantasies involving ECT. Patients may describe fears of pain, dying of electrocution, suffering permanent memory loss, or experiencing impaired intellectual functioning. As the patient reveals these fears and concerns, the nurse can clarify misconceptions and emphasize the therapeutic value of the procedure. Supporting the patient and family is an essential part of nursing care before, during, and after treatment.

After the patient has had an opportunity to express feelings, the nurse can begin the important role of **teaching,** taking into consideration the patient's anxiety, readiness to learn, and ability to comprehend. Family teaching may occur at the same time as patient teaching, and the amount of information to be shared should be individualized. The nurse should review with the family and patient the information they have received from the physician and respond to any questions they might have.

During this assessment process, the nurse also should attempt to define specific patient behaviors the family associates with the patient's illness and determine whether the patient or family member has received ECT in the past. Any information about the family's previous experiences with ECT helps the nurse identify familial beliefs about the patient's illness, ECT treatment, and expected prognosis.

Open-ended questions may give the nurse the opportunity to identify and correct misinformation and address specific concerns the patient or family has about the procedure. Nursing actions may facilitate the family's ability to provide support to the patient during the treatment course and thus further alleviate the patient's anxiety (Harrison and Kaarsemaker, 2000).

Various media may be used to teach the patient and family about ECT, including written materials and videotape presentations. These should be individualized for each patient. A tour of the treatment suite itself may help familiarize the patient with the area and equipment. Encouraging the patient to talk with another patient who has benefited from ECT may be worthwhile.

Finally, facilitating flexibility in family visiting arrangements, particularly during the patient's first few treatments, may be helpful in allaying the family's anxieties and concerns about the treatment while encouraging the family to support the patient. If the family cannot or does not want to visit, the nurse should contact the family after treatments to provide information. The nurse also should encourage the family throughout the course of treatment to discuss changes they observe in the patient or concerns that arise.

There are many misconceptions regarding ECT. Many of these are perpetuated by movies. Observe ECT in person, then watch the movies One Flew Over the Cuckoo's Nest, Frances, *and* Ordinary People, *and critique the way in which ECT is presented.* ■

Informed Consent for Electroconvulsive Therapy

Before ECT treatment begins, an informed consent form must be signed by the patient or, if the patient does not have the capacity to give consent, by a legally designated person (see Chapter 10). This consent acknowledges the patient's rights to obtain or refuse treatment. Although it is the physician's ultimate responsibility to explain the procedure when obtaining consent, the nurse plays an important part in the consent process.

Informed consent is a dynamic process that is not completed with the signing of a formal document; rather, the process continues throughout the course of treatment. As such, it suggests a number of nursing activities.

First, it is helpful if a nurse is present when the treatment for which consent is required is discussed with the patient, preferably a nurse who already has established a trusting and therapeutic relationship with the patient. The presence of this nurse may enable the patient to feel comfortable asking questions of the physician. The nurse also can ensure that the patient has understood fully the explanation of the treatment, including its nature, purpose, and implications, and that the patient has the option to withdraw consent at any time, before the patient signs the form. After the consent form has been signed, but before the beginning of treatment, the nurse should again thoroughly review the information and discuss the treatment with the patient in an open and direct manner.

Certain patients pose particular challenges to the nurse when obtaining informed consent. If a patient is unable to make independent judgments and meaningful decisions about care and treatment, the nurse is responsible for acting as a patient advocate. For example, concentration is often impaired in depressed patients, so they are less likely to comprehend and retain new information. For these patients it is essential that the nurse repeat the information at regular intervals because new knowledge is seldom fully absorbed after only one explanation. Then, throughout the patient's treatment course, the nurse should reinforce the relevant information, remind the patient of anything that may have been forgotten, and answer any new questions.

Pretreatment Nursing Care

Providing optimal nursing care for the patient undergoing ECT includes evaluating the pretreatment protocol to ensure that it has been followed according to hospital policy. This involves **reviewing recommended consultations, noting that any abnormalities in laboratory tests have been addressed, and checking that equipment and supplies are adequate and functional**.

The treatment nurse is responsible for ensuring proper preparation of the treatment suite. Box 28-3 provides a list of standard equipment needed to provide optimal patient care, as designated by the APA Task Force on ECT. A crash cart with defibrillator should be readily available for emergency use.

Patient preparation for ECT is similar to that for any **brief surgical procedure**. General anesthesia is required, so fluids

---

Equipment for Electroconvulsive Therapy

- Treatment device and supplies, including electrode paste and gel, gauze pads, alcohol preps, saline, electroencephalogram (EEG) electrodes, and chart paper
- Monitoring equipment, including electrocardiogram and EEG electrodes
- Blood pressure cuffs (two), peripheral nerve stimulator, and pulse oximeter
- Stethoscope
- Reflex hammer
- Intravenous and venipuncture supplies
- Bite blocks with individual containers
- Stretchers with firm mattress and siderails and with the capability of elevating the head and feet
- Suction device
- Ventilation equipment, including tubing, masks, Ambu bags, oral airways, and intubation equipment with an oxygen delivery system capable of providing positive-pressure oxygen
- Emergency and other medications as recommended by anesthesia staff
- Miscellaneous medications not supplied by the anesthesia staff for medical management during electroconvulsive therapy such as labetalol, esmolol, glycopyrrolate, caffeine, curare, midazolam, diazepam, thiopental sodium (Pentothal), methohexital sodium (Brevital), and succinylcholine

---

should be withheld from the patient for 6 to 8 hours before treatment to prevent the potential for aspiration. The exception to this nothing-by-mouth (NPO) status is in the case of patients who routinely receive cardiac medications, antihypertensive agents, or H_2 blockers. These drugs should be administered several hours before treatment with a small sip of water.

The patient should be encouraged to wear comfortable clothing, which can include loose-fitting street clothes, pajamas, or a hospital gown, preferably clothing that can be opened in the front to facilitate the placement of monitoring equipment. The patient also should be reminded to remove prostheses before coming to the treatment area to prevent loss or damage. This may include dentures, glasses, contact lenses, and hearing aids. The patient's hair should be clean and dry to facilitate optimal electrode contact.

The patient should void immediately before receiving ECT to help prevent incontinence during the procedure and to minimize the potential for bladder distention or damage.

Nursing Care During the Procedure

The patient should be brought to the treatment suite either ambulatory or by wheelchair, accompanied by a nurse with whom the patient feels at ease. If possible, **the nurse should remain with the patient throughout the treatment** to provide support. On arrival, the patient should be introduced to each member of the treatment team and given a brief explanation of everyone's role in the ECT procedure.

The patient should then be assisted onto a stretcher and asked to remove shoes and socks. This allows for the placement of a blood pressure cuff on an ankle and clear observation of the patient's extremities during the treatment. Once the patient is positioned comfortably on the stretcher, a member of the anesthesia staff inserts a peripheral intravenous line while the treatment nurse and other members of the treatment team place leads for various monitors. One member of the treatment team should explain the procedure while it is occurring.

EEG monitoring consists of two electrodes, one on the forehead and one on the left mastoid (Figure 28-2). A set of three-lead ECGs, connected to the oscilloscope, is placed on

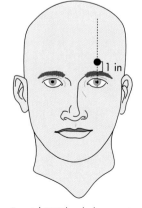
Frontal EEG lead placement

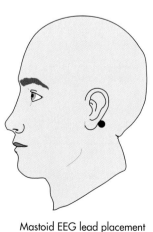
Mastoid EEG lead placement

Figure 28-2 Electroencephalogram (EEG) electrode placement.

the patient's chest. A pulse oximeter is clipped to the patient's finger to monitor oxygen saturation. Blood pressure monitoring throughout the treatment is accomplished by either a manual or automatic cuff. A peripheral nerve stimulator, preferably placed on the ankle over the posterior tibial nerve, serves to determine muscle relaxation.

The treating psychiatrist or nurse cleans areas of the patient's head with mild soap at the sites of electrode contact. This cleansing process facilitates optimal stimulus electrode contact during treatment, thus eliminating the potential for skin burns and minimizing the amount of electrical stimulus needed for the treatment. The areas being cleaned will be either the forehead, if bilateral or bifrontal electrode placement is to be used, or the right temple and top of the head 1 inch to the right of the midline, if unilateral placement is used.

Once the preparation is completed, an anticholinergic agent, such as glycopyrrolate (0.1 to 0.4 mg) or atropine (0.3 to 0.6 mg) may be administered intravenously to decrease oral secretions and minimize cardiac bradyarrhythmias in response to the electrical stimulus. Next, an anesthetic, usually methohexital or propofol (usual dose approximately 1 mg/kg), is administered. When the patient is asleep, the blood pressure cuff on the ankle is inflated, allowing it to serve as a tourniquet.

A muscle relaxant, succinylcholine (usual dose approximately 0.75 mg/kg), is then administered to minimize the patient's motor response to the ECT treatment. Because the tourniquet is in place on one ankle, the succinylcholine is not effective in that extremity. This is a desired effect because it is used in detecting a motor response of the seizure. Progressive muscle relaxation is monitored by the nerve stimulator, as well as by observing the patient for the cessation of fasciculations. As the muscle relaxant takes effect, the anesthesiologist provides oxygen by mask to the patient through positive pressure ventilation.

Although most muscles become completely relaxed, the patient's jaw muscles are stimulated directly by the ECT, causing the patient's teeth to clench. This creates the need for a protective device, or bite block, to be inserted in the patient's mouth by the treatment nurse before the electrical stimulus. This disposable or autoclavable device prevents tooth damage and tongue or gum laceration during the stimulus. The bite block is placed between the upper and lower teeth. The patient's chin is firmly supported against the bite block during delivery of the brief electrical stimulus. After delivery of the stimulus, the bite block may be removed.

The electrical stimulus causes a brief generalized seizure, the motor manifestations of which can be observed in the cuffed foot. Characteristic EEG changes also may be observed. One member of the treatment team records the time elapsed during the seizure. A motor seizure lasting 20 seconds is generally considered adequate to produce a therapeutic effect, and seizures lasting longer than 2 minutes should be terminated to prevent a prolonged post-ictal state. The seizure may be terminated by using a benzodiazepine, such as diazepam, thiopental sodium (Pentothal), or additional anesthetic, given at half the induction dose.

Anesthesia staff continuously ventilate the patient with oxygen during the procedure until the patient is able to breathe spontaneously. Vital signs should be monitored by the nurse both before and after the ECT treatment. Once the patient is stabilized, the anesthesiologist clears the patient for transfer to the recovery area.

Posttreatment Nursing Care

The recovery area should be adjacent to the treatment area to provide accessibility for anesthesia staff in case of an emergency. The area should contain **oxygen, suction, pulse oximeter, vital sign monitoring,** and **emergency equipment.** The area should be appropriately staffed and provide a minimal amount of sensory stimulation.

Once in the recovery area with pulse oximeter in place, the patient should be unobtrusively observed by a staff member in close proximity until the patient awakens. At this time, the staff should be aware of the potential for falls from the stretcher that could be caused by patient restlessness and should maintain patient safety.

When the patient awakens, a nurse should discuss the treatment and check vital signs. Most patients do not remember receiving the treatment and may be confused and disoriented, similar to patients recovering from anesthesia. The nurse should provide frequent reassurance and reorientation and repeat this information at regular intervals until the patient retains it. Being postictal, the patient may have somewhat concrete thinking. Providing brief, distinct direction is most beneficial.

When the patient awakens and appears ready to return to the hospital room, the nurse verifies that the patient's vital signs and mental status have returned to an acceptable level of functioning and that a continuous oxygen saturation level is being maintained at 90% or above. Then the nurse should help move the patient from the stretcher to a wheelchair for transport from the recovery area; the seatbelt should be securely fastened. If functioning well enough, the patient may be allowed to ambulate if desired.

The ECT treatment nurse then conveys information regarding the patient to the unit nursing staff. The most beneficial information includes medications that have been given to the patient and may be evidenced in the patient's behavior or vital signs and any change in the procedure or the patient's response to treatment that may affect the patient's behavior on return to the unit. Table 28-1 identifies some common problems patients may have and the related nursing interventions.

Assessing the patient's condition is an important nursing function needed to determine the level of observation required. If desired, the patient may return to bed and sleep, but the nurse should encourage eating breakfast and resuming normal activities as soon as possible. If the patient chooses to return to bed, the siderails should be in an upright position.

The patient should be observed at least once every 15 minutes. If the patient is agitated, confused, or restless, one-to-one observation may be required until the patient's condition has stabilized. Level of orientation should be assessed every 30 minutes, if the patient is awake, until mental status

Table 28-1 Common Patient Problems and Nursing Interventions Related to Electroconvulsive Therapy

PATIENT PROBLEM	NURSING INTERVENTIONS
Pretreatment with β-blockers may cause a decrease in blood pressure, pulse, or both.	Vital signs should be monitored frequently until they return to normal.
Lengthy seizures (more than 2 minutes) may increase the duration of disorientation or confusion.	Reorientation may need to be repeated for longer periods than usual.
If given a barbiturate or benzodiazepine to terminate the seizure, the patient may be more drowsy than usual.	Patient may need more time to rest after treatment.
After-effects may increase potential for falls.	Increase intensity of observation to prevent falls.
Nausea/vomiting creates potential for aspiration.	Extended stay in the recovery area may be necessary to provide access to suctioning equipment.
Headache creates alteration in comfort.	After assessment for gag reflex return, an analgesic may be administered. If headache is a recurrent problem, a standing order for analgesia to be given as soon as possible after each treatment may be obtained. Change in activity schedule and environment to provide a darkened room or quiet area may be necessary.

Table 28-2 Nursing Interventions for the Patient Receiving Electroconvulsive Therapy

PRINCIPLE	RATIONALE	NURSING INTERVENTION
Informed participation in the procedure	A patient who understands the treatment plan will be more cooperative and have less stress than one who does not; an informed family is able to provide the patient with emotional support.	Educate regarding ECT, including the procedure and expected effects. Teach family about the treatment. Encourage expression of feelings by patient and family. Reinforce teaching after each treatment.
Biological integrity	General anesthesia and an electrically induced seizure are physiological stressors and require supportive nursing care.	Check emergency equipment before procedure. Maintain NPO status several hours before treatment. Remove potentially harmful objects, such as jewelry and dentures. Check vital signs. Maintain patent airway. Assist to ambulate. Offer analgesia or antiemetic as needed.
Dignity and self-esteem	Patients are usually fearful before ECT treatment; amnesia and confusion may lead to anxiety and distress; patient will need help to function appropriately.	Remain with the patient and offer support before and during treatment. Maintain the patient's privacy during and after treatment. Reorient the patient. Help family members understand behavior related to amnesia and confusion.

ECT, Electroconvulsive therapy; NPO, nothing by mouth.

returns to baseline. If sleeping, the patient should remain undisturbed unless additional nursing intervention is warranted. Sleeping may help the patient return to baseline values more quickly.

After assessing the return of the gag reflex, medications and breakfast may be offered. When fully awake, the patient should be observed when getting out of bed for the first time to ensure complete return of muscle functioning after administration of muscle relaxants. Throughout the posttreatment interval, the nurse provides support and reassurance to the patient to eliminate distress that may result from posttreatment amnesia.

Any confusion or disorientation is likely to be of short duration. The patient may respond well to restricted environmental stimulation, and frequent nursing contacts will serve to remind the patient that he or she has received ECT treatment and will provide reorientation. Memory loss affects primarily material that has been recently learned and any information acquired during the time of the ECT treatments.

Memory loss is distressing for the patient, so the nurse should reiterate often that most memory difficulties will pass within several weeks; a minimal amount of difficulty may last up to 6 months. However, some information cannot be retrieved, including the experience of the treatment itself and events that occurred just before the procedure, such as IV placement. In addition, events that occurred during treatment may be unclear. A summary of nursing interventions for patients receiving ECT is presented in Table 28-2.

What kind of post-ECT environment do you think would be most conducive to the patient's recovery? ■

Interdisciplinary Collaboration

The nurse is part of an interdisciplinary treatment team that not only administers the treatments but also collaborates to evaluate the effectiveness of ECT and recommend changes in the patient's treatment plan as appropriate. Within the team, the nurse identifies patterns of patient behavior and evaluates their implications as related to treatment. These include behaviors indicative of a positive treatment response, such as improvement in activities of daily living; adaptive changes in social interactions with others; increases in energy, appetite, and weight; or other positive changes in target symptoms.

The nurse also would report any adverse behaviors associated with ECT, including prolonged periods of confusion or disorientation, recurrent nausea or headaches, elevation in blood pressure that does not resolve within several hours after treatment, or an increase in the intensity or occurrence of target symptoms.

With these clinical observations and judgments, the nurse becomes an active participant in treatment planning. Together the team evaluates issues such as the length of the ECT treatment course, the need for alternative management strategies and adjustments in the frequency of treatments, considerations for maintenance ECT, indications for additional consultations, and other possible modifications in the treatment plan.

Give specific examples of ways in which the psychiatric nurse's role in ECT has evolved from the dependent function of implementing physicians' orders to more independent and interdependent areas of psychiatric nursing practice. How have patients benefited from this change? ■

Nursing Staff Education

Despite recent increases in the use of ECT and its effectiveness in the treatment of certain psychiatric illnesses, the procedure continues to elicit emotional responses from the public as well as the medical and nursing communities. Some of these responses may be positive, but many people react negatively to ECT based on outdated ideas and procedures (see Critical Thinking About Contemporary Issues).

It is essential that, when a patient is referred for ECT, **the patient and family should be presented with information regarding treatment options in a balanced and unbiased manner**. If a nurse has ambivalent or negative feelings about ECT, these feelings will probably be communicated to the patient and render the treatment course less effective. To function as patient advocates, nurses need to examine their attitudes and have as much information about the procedure as possible (Wysoker, 2003).

Educational efforts should be directed toward nurses who work on units where ECT is implemented as a treatment strategy. Programs should be developed that address both cognitive and attitudinal content because the more knowledge and clinical experience mental health professionals have with ECT, the more positive their attitude will be toward it.

Such programs might be initiated by asking staff to discuss their beliefs and feelings about ECT, including its potential

Critical Thinking *About* Contemporary Issues

Is Electroconvulsive Therapy a Therapeutic Treatment or a Primitive Punishment?

Electroconvulsive therapy (ECT) is still controversial. The controversy is not about its efficacy or safety, because these have been well established in numerous studies. Rather, it is about its presumed effects on the brain, public fears of the procedure, and health care professionals' lack of education concerning its beneficial effects. Some people regard ECT as a punishment, believing that it is inhumane. Still others are concerned that permanent brain damage could result.

The opposing view holds that it is more inhumane to allow a person to suffer from a severe emotional disorder when ECT can provide prompt relief. They believe that the stigmatization related to ECT does considerably more harm than the treatment itself. Part of the stigma associated with ECT stems from the fact that mental illness is seen as social deviance rather than a medical disorder. As a result, the treatment of mental illness is seen as a stigmatizing punishment.

The second major reason for the stigmatization of ECT is that few people understand the current administration of the procedure. Properly administered, ECT induces far less discomfort and medical complications than most surgical and many psychopharmacological treatments.

The third reason rests in the language used to describe the treatment. The fact that it used to be called "shock therapy" conjures up the image of pain that further stigmatizes this treatment option.

It is up to each professional to reach a personal resolution on this issue. This decision should be based on objective data, observation of the treatment, and personal experiences in working with patients who have and have not received ECT.

therapeutic value, perceived risks, nature of the procedure itself, and ethical and legal issues concerning its use. The content can then progress to a discussion of factual material about ECT, including the rationale for the treatment, possible mechanisms of action, its efficacy relative to other treatment options, risks and side effects resulting from ECT, and current research on its indications and benefits.

Time should be spent discussing the way in which the procedure has changed over the years, and all nurses should be encouraged to observe the ECT procedure as performed in their institution.

These discussions could be supplemented with written handouts, reference articles, and teaching videotapes on the topic of ECT. This information can be incorporated into the unit's daily nursing care by the establishment of nursing standards of care for patients receiving ECT and a standardized nursing care plan that identifies appropriate nursing diagnoses, goals, and interventions.

In addition to informing nurses who routinely care for patients undergoing ECT, the nursing community at large needs more information about ECT. Psychiatric nurses who work with ECT can provide inservice instruction to nurses in other clinical settings, such as geriatrics, neurology, or medicine, to dispel myths, clarify misconceptions, and provide current, accurate information.

> *What stereotypical views did you have about ECT before reading this chapter? How have they changed, and how might this experience help you educate patients and colleagues about this treatment procedure?* ■

■ PHOTOTHERAPY

Phototherapy, or light therapy, consists of exposing a patient to artificial therapeutic lighting about 5 to 20 times brighter than indoor lighting. Patients usually sit, with eyes open, about 3 feet away from and at eye level with a set of broad-spectrum fluorescent bulbs designed to produce the intensity and color composition of outdoor daylight. They then can engage in their usual activities, such as reading, writing, or eating (Figure 28-3). Light boxes currently cost between $180 and $500.

The most recently developed light therapy device is the light visor, a device shaped like a baseball cap and worn on the head, with the light contained in a visor portion suspended above and in front of the eyes. The obvious advantage to such a device is that it allows the person to move about while receiving treatments. However, the results of studies testing the device show great variability in effectiveness (Meesters et al, 1999).

The timing and dosage of the light vary from person to person. Most literature indicates that light treatment administered in the morning is most effective (Terman et al, 2001). The amount of light to which a person is exposed depends on the intensity of the light source and the duration of exposure. The brighter the light, the more effective the treatment per unit of time (Lee and Chan, 1999). For example, 2 hours of treatment with 2500 lux/day appears to have an antidepressant effect equal to that of 30 minutes/day at 10,000 lux (Figure 28-4).

Light therapy appears to have important positive effects. Treatment is rapid and can be repeated. **Most patients feel relief after 3 to 5 days; however, they relapse equally rapidly if light treatment is stopped.** Therefore patients should continue treatment throughout the winter and discontinue use only during the summer months (George and Kozel, 2002).

Treatment can be received at home, and it need not disrupt daily routine; however, initial therapy sessions should be supervised by a professional with experience and training. The long-term efficacy of light therapy has not yet been fully evaluated.

Indications

Phototherapy has a 60% to 90% response rate in patients with well-documented, nonpsychotic winter depression or seasonal affective disorder (SAD) (Lee and Chan, 1999). SAD is a cyclical mood disorder characterized by periods of depression that begin in October and subside in April (see Chapter 19 for a full discussion of mood disorders).

Although people in all latitudes can suffer from SAD, the prevalence of the disorder increases in the northernmost parts of the country. About 6% of the adult population in the United States, or 15 million people, suffer from the symptoms of SAD, which include sadness, irritability, increased appetite, carbohydrate craving, weight gain, hypersomnia, and decreased energy. In addition, 14% of Americans experience a more mild condition called "winter blues."

In a study examining predictors of response to light treatment, responders were characterized by atypical symptoms, especially hypersomnia, afternoon and evening slump, reverse diurnal variation (evenings worse), and carbohydrate craving. In contrast, nonresponders were characterized mainly by melancholic symptoms including retardation, sui-

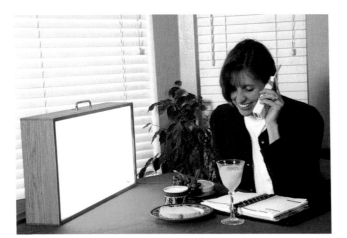

Figure 28-3   Broad-spectrum fluorescent lamps like this one are used in daily therapy sessions from autumn until spring for people with seasonal affective disorder (SAD), who report feeling less depressed within 3 to 7 days after treatment begins. (Courtesy Apollo Light Systems.)

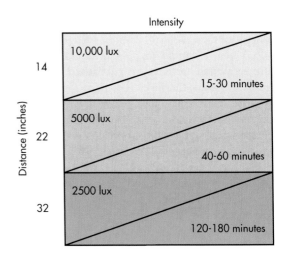

Figure 28-4   Timing, dosage, and exposure to light. All times are average durations and may vary with each person. *Lux,* Luminous flux density (unit of illuminance).

cidality, depersonalization, typical diurnal variation (mornings worse), anxiety, early and late insomnia, appetite loss, and feelings of guilt.

Light therapy is a safe and satisfactory treatment for many, but may be insufficient for more severely ill patients (Lee and Chan, 1999). Light therapy is a less conventional treatment that may be of value to patients who do not respond to drug therapy or prefer nonpharmacological treatments, or it may be used as an adjunct to drug treatments.

Mechanism of Action

Phototherapy is based on biological rhythms, particularly those related to light and darkness (see Chapter 6). However, despite much investigation, the exact etiology of SAD and the mechanism of action of phototherapy remain unclear. The therapeutic effect appears to be mediated primarily by the eyes, not the skin. It appears that certain people may have a neurochemical vulnerability, related to melatonin, that causes them to develop SAD in the absence of adequate exposure to environmental light (Wehr et al, 2001).

Do you think that people who experience common disturbances in body rhythms such as jet lag and shift work can be helped by phototherapy? ■

Adverse Effects

Side effects, when they occur, are generally mild. The most common adverse effects of phototherapy are eyestrain and headache. Patients with a history of mania or hypomania should use light therapy with caution because it may precipitate those conditions. Other adverse effects include irritability, insomnia, fatigue, nausea, and dryness of the eyes, nasal passages, and sinuses. These usually can be managed by decreasing the duration of therapy or increasing the patient's distance from the light.

The long-term effects of phototherapy, if any, are currently unknown. Light therapy should be used with caution in those with specific ophthalmic conditions.

■ SLEEP DEPRIVATION THERAPY

It has been reported that as many as 60% of depressed patients improve immediately after one night of total sleep deprivation (Colombo et al, 1999). Unipolar and bipolar patients appear to do equally well. Although these findings have been reported in the literature, few randomized controlled clinical studies have been conducted on sleep deprivation therapy. Thus these findings should be considered with caution.

Unfortunately, **many patients who respond to this therapy become depressed again when they resume sleeping even as little as 2 hours a night.** This disadvantage has tended to discourage the use of sleep deprivation in clinical practice. However, there is some suggestion that improvement can be maintained if the sleep manipulation can be used repeatedly over time, such as by initially shifting the timing of sleep to earlier in the night and then gradually ad-

vancing the time of sleep toward a more acceptable schedule. For example, the patient can initially go to sleep at 5 PM and arise at 2 AM and then gradually shift the hours of sleep to 11 PM to 6 AM.

In addition, medications or light therapy may help prevent relapse after sleep deprivation therapy. It is interesting to note that some antidepressants, especially the monoamine oxidase inhibitors, often interfere with sleep (see Chapter 27). This has led some researchers to wonder whether part of the efficacy of these drugs is a result of their ability to induce partial sleep deprivation.

How can a patient's expectations of a treatment influence its effectiveness? Can you think of a placebo treatment for sleep deprivation that would control this problem? ■

Indications

Evidence suggests that depressed patients with symptoms of marked diurnal variation are the ones most likely to improve after sleep deprivation. Patients who respond favorably to sleep deprivation also appear to have abnormally elevated nighttime body temperatures. Some evidence also indicates that patients with SAD respond positively to sleep deprivation.

Mechanism of Action

The biological mechanisms of the antidepressant effects of sleep deprivation have not been identified. It has been hypothesized that sleep deprivation works by interrupting rapid eye movement (REM) sleep. Another theory proposes that neuroendocrine changes accompanying sleep deprivation account for its antidepressant effects.

Adverse Effects

Unfortunately, sleep deprivation appears to induce mania in some patients with bipolar disorder. Thus sleep deprivation, as with some antidepressant medications, should be used with caution in patients who are susceptible to mania or have a family history of bipolar illness (Colombo et al, 2000).

On the other hand, the knowledge that sleep deprivation may induce mania can have important preventive applications. For example, people who are biologically vulnerable to bipolar illness may want to monitor disruptions to their sleep caused by work schedules, travel, drugs, or other life events, thus preventing sleep loss at times of stress to possibly prevent the occurrence of mania.

■ TRANSCRANIAL MAGNETIC STIMULATION

Transcranial magnetic stimulation (TMS) is a noninvasive procedure in which a changing magnetic field is introduced into the brain to influence the brain's activity. The field is generated by passing a large electric current through a wire stimulation coil over a brief period.

The insulated coil is placed on or close to a specific area of the patient's head, allowing the magnetic field to pass through the skull and into target areas of the brain (Figure 28-5). The shape of the coil determines the properties and size of the magnetic field. A figure-of-8 shape is frequently used, because that shape makes it possible to create a well-focused field (Hasey, 2001).

When the magnetic stimulus is administered as a train of multiple stimuli per second, it is called **repetitive transcranial magnetic stimulation (rTMS)**. Initially used to study various functions within the brain, such as attention, memory, and language, rTMS also was noted to change activity within the neurons. Therefore, in recent years, the technique has been studied as a potentially therapeutic device for some neurological and psychiatric illnesses (Kozel and George 2002). When used for these indications, rTMS is administered at daily sessions. The number of sessions vary, depending on patient response.

Although now accepted as a standard clinical treatment in Europe and Canada, rTMS is still considered experimental in the United States. Work is progressing in an effort to determine its efficacy and safety. Studies to determine optimal treatment conditions also are underway. These include num-

ber of treatment sessions, most effective number of stimuli per second (i.e., "fast" [20 Hz] vs. "slow" [5 Hz]), and modification of coil placement (i.e., left vs. right) for the treatment of specific conditions.

Another form of TMS, called magnetic seizure therapy (MST), has been developed most recently based upon the ECT model. MST uses a magnetic stimulus to produce a seizure. This new and more powerful form of magnetic stimulation has shown promising results in preliminary studies (Lisanby, 2002).

Indications

TMS has been studied for a number of indications. The most frequently cited indication for this therapy in psychiatry has been in the treatment of **mood disorders** (Fitzgerald, Brown, and Daskalakis, 2002; Gershon, Dannon, and Grunhaus, 2003). Imaging studies have found that depressed patients have reduced perfusion in the prefrontal cortex area of the brain, especially on the left side. The results of numerous

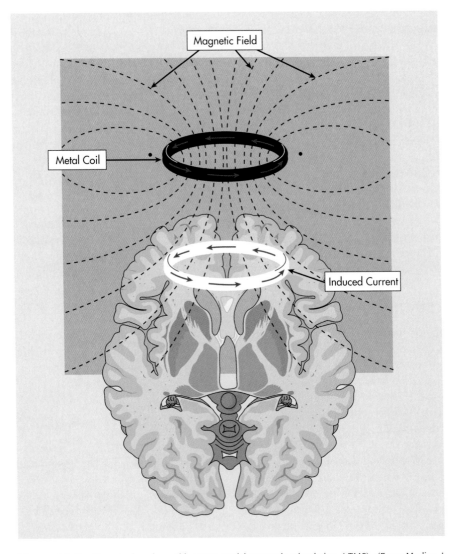

Figure 28-5 The physics of repetitive transcranial magnetic stimulation (rTMS). (From Medina J: *Psychiatric Times,* August 2001.)

small studies have suggested that rTMS, when administered at the left prefrontal cortex, may be an effective treatment for nonpsychotic depression (Janicak et al, 2002; Grunhaus et al, 2003), although not all studies agree with these results (Loo et al, 2003).

Conversely, some data suggest that rTMS, administered at the right prefrontal cortex, can be helpful for those with mania. Additionally a few small studies have suggested that rTMS may be helpful for other psychiatric disorders such as obsessive-compulsive disorder, and posttraumatic stress disorder. It has not been found to be helpful in those with schizophrenia (Nahas et al, 2000; McNamara et al, 2001).

At the present time studies describing the duration of improvement with rTMS are ongoing; however, it appears that daily sessions extending over 3 weeks or more may be required for optimal response (George and Kozel, 2002).

Mechanism of Action

The mechanism of action of TMS is based on the principle of *Faraday induction*. According to this principle, when an electric current is passed through a coil, a magnetic field is generated. If another conductive material, such as a neuron in the brain, is exposed to a changing magnetic field, a second electrical field is activated within that material. This activation may result in neurochemical changes based on alterations in gene expression, such as an increase in some receptor binding.

Therefore, unlike ECT, **with TMS the brain is directly stimulated** to produce neurochemical changes. However, as with ECT, the exact changes that make the treatment effective are still under investigation.

Adverse Effects

The biggest concern when using rTMS is the potential for **inducing seizures**, even in patients with no preexisting epilepsy. Seven such cases have been described worldwide (Kozel and George, 2002). Most occurred during early studies designed to test rTMS safety, and they appeared to be related to higher frequency pulses. Recommendations for treatment parameters have now been made, which should avoid further occurrences.

The potential for tinnitus or even transient hearing loss caused by the high frequency noise produced by the treatment apparatus has prompted the routine use of ear plugs for both patient and investigator, thereby minimizing the occurrence of this adverse effect. The most common reported adverse effect from rTMS is the occurrence of headaches. The etiology appears to be contraction of scalp muscles during the stimulation. In most cases this discomfort resolves with standard analgesics. Mild, transient cognitive disturbances during the stimulation sessions also have been reported.

As a result of the strong (1 to 2 Tesla) magnetic fields involved in this treatment, some patients may not be candidates. These patients include those with metal objects such as screws, plates, or shrapnel anywhere in the body, unless it is known that the object will not create a problem.

Patients with pacemakers or other implants that might create a low-resistance current path should not be considered for rTMS. Patients with heart disease would be at increased risk (Frei and Osorio, 2001), as would those with increased intracranial pressure because of the increased risk in the event of a seizure. Although one case of safe administration of rTMS in a pregnant woman has been reported (Nahas et al, 1999), in general, rTMS is not generally indicated in this group. Patients at increased risk for seizures should be considered with caution.

How would you explain to patients who have metal in their bodies why TMS is contraindicated for them? ■

■ VAGUS NERVE STIMULATION

Vagus nerve stimulation (VNS) is another somatic therapy currently under investigation. VNS was first studied in animals during the 1980s, when it was discovered that intermittent stimulation of the vagus nerve could be helpful in the treatment of seizures.

In the 1990s some epileptic patients receiving VNS via an implanted device reported improved mood. These reports stimulated interest in VNS as a treatment for depression. Results from a multicenter study, showing a 40% to 50% reduction in depressive symptoms among patients receiving VNS, validates its potential as a promising somatic therapy in psychiatry (Rush et al, 2000).

VNS involves surgically implanting a small (pocket watch–sized) generator (Figure 28-6) into the patient's chest.

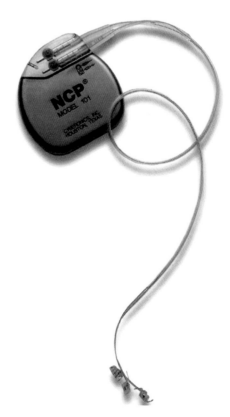

Figure 28-6 Vagus nerve stimulation (VNS) generator. (Courtesy Cyberonics, Inc.)

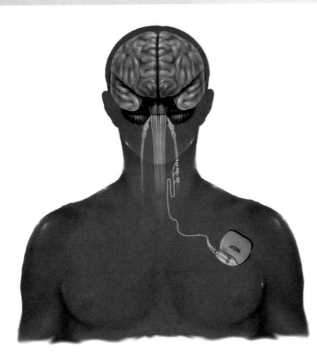

Figure 28-7 Vagus nerve stimulation (VNS) implantation. (Courtesy Cyberonics, Inc.)

An electrode is threaded subcutaneously from the generator to the vagus nerve on the left side of the patient's neck. The end of the electrode is wrapped around the nerve (Figure 28-7). Once implanted, the generator is programmed via computer for the frequency and intensity of the stimulus.

Indications

At the present time, VNS is approved only for clinical use in the treatment of epilepsy in the United States. The most compelling use in psychiatry is in the treatment of affective disorders, particularly depression. Given the multiple functions of the vagus nerve, VNS merits study in the treatment of other conditions including anxiety disorders, obesity, chronic pain syndromes, addictions, and sleep disorders (George et al, 2000).

One pilot study suggests that VNS may improve cognition in patients with Alzheimer's disease (Sjogren et al, 2002). Clinical trials examining the efficacy of VNS with treatment-resistant, depressed patients found that VNS was most effective for patients with low to moderate antidepressant resistance, but not effective for more severely ill patients (Sackeim et al, 2001b).

Mechanism of Action

As with other somatic therapies, the exact mechanism of action of VNS is unknown, but thought to work via the neurotransmitter system. The vagus nerve has many functions; however, in this instance, the left vagus is chosen because it is composed of mostly afferent sensory fibers. These fibers connect to brainstem and deep brain structures that are thought to be involved in epilepsy and some psychiatric disorders. Stimulation of these fibers is thought to cause changes in the function of some of these structures and also affects the concentration of some neurotransmitters, such as γ-aminobutyric acid (GABA) and glutamate.

Adverse Effects

In general, reported adverse effects of VNS have been mild and tolerable. The most frequently reported adverse effect is hoarseness, which is most likely related to the stimulation. Other reported stimulation-related effects include throat pain, neck pain, headache, and shortness of breath. A few incidences of infection at the incision sites, coughing, voice alteration, vocal cord paralysis, lower facial muscle paresis, changes in heart rate, and an accumulation of fluid over the generator have been reported (Ben-Menachen, 2001; Frei and Osorio, 2001).

A patient with a history of chronic, severe depression asks you if she would be a good candidate for a new treatment she learned of on the Internet called vagus nerve stimulation. How would you respond? ■

COMPETENT CARING **A Clinical Exemplar of a Psychiatric Nurse**
Dean Olivet, RN, MS, C

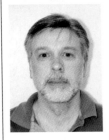

On this particular morning, I arrived at work as usual and performed all the morning rituals that a nurse does before venturing out on the clinical floor. After having been off for several days, I learned from reading reports and from listening to my coworkers that the acuity on the unit was high. Not only was the unit psychiatrically tense, but several geriatric patients had been admitted for evaluation and electroconvulsive therapy (ECT) treatment. On a general psychiatric unit, such patients often elicit a variety of feelings from the staff, ranging from mild anxiety to downright fear. Therefore, I opted to take a few of the older, acute patients, including Mr. J, who was 80 years old.

Mr. J was newly admitted for evaluation of medications and a possible course of ECT. The staff who had contact with him described him as needy, confused, and wanting constant reassurance. At my first contact, Mr. J was asleep in his bed. He was disheveled, as was his room. When he awoke, I introduced myself to him and found out immediately why he seemed to have caused the staff to be anxious. He grabbed my arm and spoke to me in a high-pitched whine that anyone would want to avoid. My initial reaction was a flight response. To resist this, I began to assess his level of independence, and it soon became clear that he was unable to make any choices with regard to planning his morning. In organizing my care, I decided to outline the morning routine for him in small time increments and assess his ability to make decisions with regard to his basic needs.

We began with his activities of daily living. Mr. J needed help to meet these physiological needs, and his anxiety level made it necessary for me to maximize his safety and security. He told me that his daughter and son had helped him the night before. He assured me that I was too busy and they would help him the next time they visited as well. My nursing pride was somewhat injured, and I was puzzled about the necessity for his family to perform what seemed to be a nursing responsibility. Nonetheless, I carried on with my care and convinced him to bathe while I cleaned up his room and made his bed. Implementing this minor intervention made me feel more comfortable in his room, and he didn't seem quite as overwhelmed.

Because his anxiety was still moderately high, I consulted with the nurse who was giving his medications and reviewed his chart. Here I learned that this was his second hospitalization, with many preceding years being free of symptoms of depression. During his first hospital stay, he had received a course of ECT that was very successful in helping him get well. I also learned that he was being cared for by his wife and daughter. Their treatment of choice was to medicate him until he slept. Learning this, I sensed the need to evaluate the quality of his experience with his last course of ECT, as well as the current need for possible ECT and medication education for the family. These two educational needs became an ongoing process dependent on his and his family's readiness to learn.

My plan of care was quite simple. I would make sure that his activities of daily living were completed each morning, his environment kept orderly, and his introduction to the milieu made in short intervals. This was necessary to keep him safe from patients with less impulse control and to avoid overwhelming him or the other patients. Mr. J needed some peer contact as well, and I introduced him to other patients as appropriate.

That afternoon his family came to visit, and I met with them to assess their need for information and their readiness to learn. I outlined Mr. J's day and apologized for his insistence that they perform his activities of daily living. I thought that perhaps they might be annoyed about this issue and was relieved when they expressed their appreciation for my interest in him. They explained to me that I was the first person they had had substantial contact with since he was admitted. In fact, they were quite upset with his condition the night before, and were considering raising the issue with the staff. After listening to their concerns, I outlined my plan of care for Mr. J and explained that in my absence, the rest of the nursing staff would use the care plan to meet his daily needs. At this point, the family became an ally to the total hospital experience, and I became a resource for the patient and the family. This brought comfort to the family, which in turn allowed Mr. J to meet his basic needs and have the security necessary for him to meet the challenge of recovering from his illness.

The family members were satisfied with my interventions, and a possibly problematic hospital experience was averted. As nurses, we all can relate to experiences in which we have cared for patients only to have family members complain about the care or lack of care their significant other received. We also can describe occasions when it was very rewarding to have a patient respond to our care and to have the family recognize this nursing effort. Given this dichotomy, which do you prefer? The answer really reflects the crux of good psychiatric nursing practice. ∎

CHAPTER **FOCUS POINTS**

- Electroconvulsive therapy (ECT) is an effective treatment for major depression, with an efficacy rate of 80% or more, which is equal to or better than response rates to antidepressant medications. It is particularly useful for people who cannot tolerate or fail to respond to treatment with medication.

- Nursing care in ECT involves providing emotional and educational support to the patient and family; assessing the pretreatment protocol and the patient's behavior, memory, and functional ability before ECT; preparing and monitoring the patient during the actual ECT procedure; and observing and interpreting patient responses to ECT, with recommendations for changes in the treatment plan as appropriate.

- Phototherapy, or light therapy, consists of exposing patients to bright, artificial lighting for a specified period each day. It is a treatment option for patients with nonpsychotic winter depression or seasonal affective disorder (SAD).

- Sleep deprivation therapy has been reported to be effective with depressed patients; however, many become depressed again when they resume sleeping even as little as 2 hours a night.

- Transcranial magnetic stimulation (TMS) consists of using a magnetic field to produce changes in brain chemistry. It is a promising new treatment for mood disorders, especially depression, and has a relatively low side effect profile.

- Vagus nerve stimulation (VNS) involves surgically implanting a nerve stimulator into the patient's chest. An electrode is threaded from the generator to the vagus nerve on the left side of the patient's neck. Early studies have found this stimulation effective in relieving depressive symptoms.

KEY TERMS

electroconvulsive therapy, 603
magnetic seizure therapy (MST), 612

phototherapy, 610
sleep deprivation therapy, 611

transcranial magnetic stimulation (TMS), 611
vagus nerve stimulation (VNS), 613

CHAPTER REVIEW QUESTIONS

1. Indicate whether the following statements are true (T) or false (F).

_____ A. For ECT to be effective, a grand mal seizure must occur.

_____ B. ECT cannot be followed by antidepressant medications because adverse reactions will occur.

_____ C. Evidence indicates that ECT causes brain damage and permanent memory loss.

_____ D. A seizure lasting 30 to 60 seconds is generally considered adequate for producing a therapeutic effect.

_____ E. The timing and dosage of light therapy vary from person to person.

_____ F. Substantial research documents the long-term effectiveness of light therapy.

_____ G. Light therapy is particularly effective as a treatment for more severely ill patients.

_____ H. Many patients who respond to sleep deprivation therapy become depressed again when they resume sleeping at night.

_____ I. TMS is an invasive procedure that directly impacts the brain structures.

2. Fill in the blanks.

A. For affective disorders, _____ to

_____ ECT treatments are normally
administered.

B. For schizophrenia, as many as _____

to _____ ECT treatments may be
administered.

C. The primary indication for ECT is _____.

D. ECT's response rate of _____ or more
is equal to or better than response rates to antidepressant
medications.

E. Preparation for ECT is similar to that implemented for any

brief _____ procedure.

F. Potential side effects that may occur immediately after ECT that

may be treated symptomatically include _____,

_____, and _____.

G. Phototherapy has a _____% to _____%
response rate in patients with winter depression or SAD.

H. Sleep deprivation appears to produce _____
in some patients with bipolar illness.

I. TMS is most frequently used for the treatment of

_____ disorders.

J. _____ is the newest somatic therapy
currently under investigation.

3. Provide short answers for the following questions.

A. You're talking with a nursing colleague and he asks you,
"What exactly is ECT?" How would you respond?

B. ECT is often recommended for women with severe depression who are in their first trimester of pregnancy. Why do
you think this is?

C. Obtain the informed consent form used for ECT by your
treatment facility. Review it for the elements described in
this chapter. Try explaining the procedure to a friend or
family member.

D. Review the incidence of depression among people geographically distributed in some of the most northern and
southern states in the United States. Make a case for the
impact of light and seasonal affective disorder among
these populations.

Visit Evolve for additional resources related to the content of this chapter.

http://evolve.elsevier.com/Stuart/principles/

• Topical Course Outline • Student Workbook Exercises • Critical Thinking Questions and Activities • Case Studies • Research Topics
• Monthly Content Updates • WebLinks

Student Study CD-ROM

Access the accompanying CD-ROM for animations, interactive exercises, review questions for the NCLEX
examination, and an audio glossary.

REFERENCES

American Psychiatric Association: *The practice of electroconvulsive therapy: recommendations for treatment, training, and privileging,* ed 2, Washington, DC, 2000, The Association.

Bailine SH et al: Comparison of bifrontal and bitemporal ECT for major depression, *Am J Psychiatry* 157:121, 2000.

Ben-Menachem E: Vagus nerve stimulation, side effects, and long term safety, *J Clin Neurophysiol* 18:415, 2001.

Brodaty H et al: Perceptions of outcome from electroconvulsive therapy by depressed patients and psychiatrists, *Aust N Z J Psychiatry* 37:196, 2003.

Colombo C et al: Rate of switch from depression into mania after therapeutic sleep deprivation in bipolar depression, *Psychiatry Res* 86:267, 1999.

Colombo C et al: Total sleep deprivation combined with lithium and light therapy in the treatment of bipolar depression: replication of main effects and interaction, *Psychiatry Res* 95:43, 2000.

Ende G et al: The hippocampus in patients treated with electroconvulsive therapy: a proton magnetic resonance spectroscopic imaging study, *Arch Gen Psychiatry* 57:937, 2000.

Fitzgerald PB, Brown TL, Daskalakis ZJ: The application of transcranial magnetic stimulation in psychiatry and neurosciences research, *Acta Psychiatr Scand* 105:324, 2002.

Flint AJ, Gagnon N: Effective use of electroconvulsive therapy in late-life depression, *Can J Psychiatry* 47:734, 2002.

Frei MG, Osorio I: Left vagus nerve stimulation with the neurocybernetic prosthesis has complex effects on heart rate and on its variability in humans, *Epilepsia* 42:1007, 2001.

Gagne GG Jr et al: Efficacy of continuation ECT and antidepressant drugs compared to long-term antidepressants alone in depressed patients, *Am J Psychiatry* 157:1960, 2000.

Gaylord K: Parkinson's disease and electroconvulsive therapy: a nursing perspective, *J Am Psychiatr Nurs Assoc* 9:9, 2003.

George MS: Vagus nerve stimulation: a new tool for brain research and therapy, *Biol Psychiatry* 47:287, 2000.

George M, Kozel FA: Other antidepressant therapies: light therapy, ECT, TMS, VNS. In Thase M, Potokar J, editors: *Advances in the management and treatment of depression,* London, 2002, Martin and Dunitz, Ltd.

Gershon AA, Dannon PN, Grunhaus L: Transcranial magnetic stimulation in the treatment of depression, *Am J Psychiatry* 160:835, 2003.

Grunhaus L et al: A randomized controlled comparison of electroconvulsive therapy and repetitive transcranial magnetic stimulation in severe and resistant nonpsychotic major depression, *Biol Psychiatry* 53:324, 2003.

Harrison B, Kaarsemaker B: Continuous quality improvement to an electroconvulsive therapy delivery system, *J Psychosoc Nurs Ment Health Serv* 38:27, 2000.

Hasey G: Transcranial magnetic stimulation in the treatment of mood disorders: a review and comparison with electroconvulsive therapy, *Can J Psychiatry* 46:720, 2001.

Hermann RC et al: Diagnoses of patients treated with ECT: a comparison of evidence-based standards with reported use, *Psychiatr Serv* 50:1059, 1999.

Janicak PG et al: Repetitive transcranial magnetic stimulation versus electroconvulsive therapy for major depression: preliminary results of a randomized trial, *Biol Psychiatry* 51:659, 2002.

Kozel F, George M: Meta-analysis of left prefrontal repetitive transcranial magnetic stimulation (rTMS) to treat depression, *J Psychiatr Pract* 8: 270, 2002.

Krystal AD et al: ECT stimulus intensity: are present ECT devices too limited? *Am J Psychiatry* 157:963, 2000.

Lee TM, Chan CC: Dose-response relationship of phototherapy for seasonal affective disorder: a meta-analysis, *Acta Psychiatr Scand* 99:315, 1999.

Lisanby SH et al: The effects of electroconvulsive therapy on memory of autobiographical and public events, *Arch Gen Psychiatry* 57:581, 2000.

Lisanby SH: Update on magnetic seizure therapy: a novel form of convulsive therapy, *J ECT* 18:182, 2002.

Loo CK et al: Double-blind controlled investigation of bilateral prefrontal transcranial magnetic stimulation of the treatment of resistant major depression, *Psychol Med* 33:33, 2003.

Madsen TM et al: Increased neurogenesis in a model of electroconvulsive therapy, *Biol Psychiatry* 47:1043, 2000.

McCall WV et al: Titrated moderately suprathreshold vs fixed high dose right unilateral electroconvulsive therapy: acute antidepressant and cognitive effects, *Arch Gen Psychiatry* 57:438, 2000.

McNamara B et al: Transcranial magnetic stimulation for depression and other psychiatric disorders, *Psychol Med* 31:1141, 2001.

Meesters Y et al: Prophylactic treatment of seasonal affective disorder (SAD) by using light visors: bright white or infrared light? *Biol Psychiatry* 46:239, 1999.

Nahas Z et al: Safety and feasibility of repetitive transcranial magnetic stimulation in the treatment of anxious depression in pregnancy: a case report, *J Clin Psychiatry* 60:50, 1999.

Nahas Z et al: TMS in schizophrenia. In George MS, Belmaker RH, editors: *Transcranial Magnetic Stimulation in Neuropsychiatry*, Washington, DC, 2000, American Psychiatric Press.

Rabheru K: The use of electroconvulsive therapy in special patient populations, *Can J Psychiatry* 46:710, 2001.

Rush AJ et al: Vagus nerve stimulation (VNS) for treatment-resistant depressions: a multicenter study, *Biol Psychiatry* 47:276, 2000.

Sackeim HA et al: A prospective, randomized, double-blind comparison of bilateral and right unilateral electroconvulsive therapy at different stimulus intensities, *Arch Gen Psychiatry* 57:425, 2000.

Sackeim HA et al: Continuation pharmacotherapy in the prevention of relapse following electroconvulsive therapy: A randomized controlled trial, *JAMA* 285:1299, 2001a.

Sackeim H et al: Vagus nerve stimulation (VNS) for treatment-resistant depression: efficacy, side-effects, and predictors of outcome, *Neuropsychopharmacology* 25:713, 2001b.

Sareen J, Enns MW, Guertin JE: The impact of clinically diagnosed personality disorders on acute and one-year outcomes of electroconvulsive therapy, *J ECT* 16:43, 2000.

Shiwach RS, Reid WH, Carmody TJ: An analysis of reported deaths following electroconvulsive therapy in Texas, 1993-1998, *Psychiatr Serv* 52:1095, 2001.

Sjogren MJ et al: Cognition-enhancing effect of vagus nerve stimulation in patients with Alzheimers disease: a pilot study, *J Clin Psychiatry* 63:972, 2002.

Terman JS et al: Circadian time of morning light administration and therapeutic response in winter depression, *Arch Gen Psychiatry* 58:69, 2001.

UK ECT Review Group: Efficacy and safety of electroconvulsive therapy in depressive disorders: a systematic review and meta-analysis, *Lancet* 361:799, 2003.

Wehr TA et al: A circadian signal of change of season in patients with seasonal affective disorder, *Arch Gen Psychiatry* 58:1108, 2001.

Weiner RD: Retrograde amnesia with electroconvulsive therapy: characteristics and implications, *Arch Gen Psychiatry* 57:591, 2000.

Wysoker A: Electroconvulsive therapy, *J Am Psychiatr Nurs Assoc* 9:103, 2003.

Zachrisson O et al: No evident neuronal damage after electroconvulsive therapy, *Psychiatry Res* 96:157, 2000.

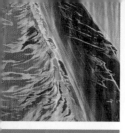

Through the like, disease is produced, and through the application of the like it is cured.
HIPPOCRATES, FOURTH CENTURY BC

29 | COMPLEMENTARY AND ALTERNATIVE THERAPIES

Therese K. Killeen

LEARNING OBJECTIVES

After studying this chapter, the student should be able to:
1. Evaluate the evidence base and ethical issues related to complementary and alternative therapies (**I**).
2. Analyze complementary and alternative therapies used to treat depression, anxiety, substance use disorders, eating disorders, attention deficit hyperactivity disorder, and dementias (**II, III, IV, V, VI, VII**).
3. Discuss nursing implications for the use of complementary and alternative therapies in psychiatric care (**VIII**).

TOPICAL OUTLINE

 Visit Evolve for additional resources related to the content of this chapter.
http://evolve.elsevier.com/Stuart/principles/

Complementary and alternative medicine (CAM) is the term commonly used to describe a broad range of healing philosophies, approaches, and therapies that focus on the whole person, including biopsychosocial and spiritual aspects. CAM therapies are often used alone (referred to as **alternative**), in combination with other CAM therapies, or in combination with other conventional therapies (referred to as **complementary**). Some therapies are consistent with principles of Western medicine, and others involve healing systems with a different origin. Some therapies are outside the realm of accepted Western medical practice, others are becoming established in mainstream health care.

■ OVERVIEW OF CAM

People in the United States are increasingly utilizing and paying out of pocket for CAM therapies. Enhanced public health education has heightened health care awareness and concern, prompting people to become more active in their health care and more willing to make lifestyle changes. CAM therapies often seem to be more available, accessible, and therefore more appealing to the health care consumer. In addition, the benefits of CAM therapies may outweigh the barriers that are associated with conventional therapies. For example, people identify many **benefits** of CAM therapy that include less cost, more convenience, fewer side effects, more individualized care, and more contact with practitioners.

Patients are more often disclosing their use of CAM to their primary health care providers, and providers are including more questions about the use of CAM in their routine assessments. Since the development of the National Center for Complementary and Alternative Medicine (NCCAM), more research on the efficacy and safety of CAM has emerged. This has enabled practitioners to approve and recommend certain complementary therapies that may be of benefit to their patients. In contrast, CAM without empirically based efficacy may be harmful to patients or delay their seeking conventional empirically based medical care.

Some patients turn to CAM after the failure of their conventional therapy, particularly patients with severe stress and pain. CAM is more often used in combination with conventional therapies than used alone (Consumer Reports, 2000; Kessler et al, 2001; Unutzer et al, 2000). Given the high use of CAM by depressed and anxious patients, it is especially important for all mental health practitioners to be aware of available CAM therapies and document any that their patients may be using (see Citing the Evidence).

Recent research findings have alerted the public to the **potential dangers of certain CAM therapies, particularly some herbal medicines**. Serious medical events attributed to the use of ephedra, an over-the-counter stimulant, have prompted the Food and Drug Administration (FDA) to intervene by implementing restrictions on ephedra products. Problems with other herbal products such as kava (*Piper methysticum*), L-tryptophan, comfrey (*Symphytum officinale*), and yohimbe (*Pausinystalia johimbe*) also have been identified. In addition, more information is known now about possible serious drug interactions that can occur when combining herbal products and medications (Fontanarosa, Rennie, and DeAngelis, 2003).

Nurses must inform themselves on a continuing basis of research findings related to CAM because nurses play an important role in educating consumers about the evidence supporting these new therapies, as well as about the dangers involved in using some of them. Evidence-based outcomes provide more information about efficacy, tolerability, dosage, safety, and interactions with other treatments.

NCCAM has developed a classification system of five major domains of CAM (USDHHS, 2000). Table 29-1 lists the five domains and gives a description of each along with specific examples of CAM therapies that fall under each classification.

Many CAM therapies use energy and system theories to support a rational approach to treatment. A proper balance

CITING THE EVIDENCE ON
CAM Therapies for Anxiety and Depression

BACKGROUND: This interview was conducted to identify CAM therapies utilized by individuals with anxiety and depression. A total of 2055 individuals completed the interview.

RESULTS: In all, 57% of respondents reporting anxiety attacks and 54% of respondents reporting severe depression used CAM therapies for these conditions in the last 12 months. Relaxation techniques, spiritual healing by others, imagery, self-help groups, energy healing, and massage were the therapies most often used.

IMPLICATIONS: Individuals with anxiety and depression use CAM therapies more often than they use conventional mental health treatments. Given the emerging research on safety and efficacy of certain CAM therapies, conventional mental health practitioners need to be kept informed regarding the CAM therapies of their patients.

Kessler RC: *Am J Psychiatry* 158:289, 2001.

Table 29-1	Major Domains of Complementary and Alternative Medicine	
DOMAIN	**DEFINITION**	**CAM THERAPY**
Alternative medical systems	Complete systems of theory and practice that have evolved independently of, and often prior to, the conventional biomedical approach	Traditional oriental medicine, Ayurveda, homeopathy, naturopathy
Mind-body interventions	Employ a variety of techniques designed to facilitate the mind's capacity to affect bodily function and symptoms	Meditation; hypnosis; prayer; art, music, and dance therapy
Biologically based therapies	Natural and biologically based practices, interventions, and products, many of which overlap with conventional medicine's use of dietary supplements	Herbal, special dietary, orthomolecular, and individual biological therapies
Manipulative and body-based methods	Methods based on manipulation and/or movement of the body	Chiropractic, massage and body work, reflexology
Energy therapies	Focus on either energy fields believed to originate within the body (biofields) or those emanating from other sources (electromagnetic fields)	Qi gong, Reiki, therapeutic touch, electromagnets

From US Department of Health and Human Services: Expanding horizons of healthcare: five-year strategic plan, 2001-2005, NCCAM (SuDoc HE 20.3002: H 78), Washington, DC, 2000, USDHHS.
CAM, Complementary and alternative medicine.

of energy within the biopsychosocial and spiritual systems must be maintained. The individual is an open system and exchanges energy with the environment to maintain balance and prevent illness. Illness is associated with an imbalance of energy, either deficiency or excess. The environment, as well as the needs of individuals, are constantly changing throughout life; thus adaptation is synonymous with health.

Evidence-Based Practice

Research in CAM continues to increase, and studies have become more rigorous in the scientific methodology being employed (see Critical Thinking About Contemporary Issues). Currently more studies are using double-blind placebo-control designs. **Few CAM therapies claim to cure diseases; rather they propose to have therapeutic benefits related to the reduction or relief of symptoms and the promotion of well-being.**

However, controversy among CAM researchers continues in regard to subjecting their research to the same empirical

---

Critical Thinking *About* Contemporary Issues

Does Science Play a Role in Complementary and Alternative Health Care?

Critics of complementary and alternative medicine (CAM) claim that no scientific evidence indicates that these therapeutic approaches work. This controversy is at an important juncture because it involves the potential acceptance or rejection of certain "healing" therapies by both health care professionals and consumers. Many patients and providers have divergent opinions on whether these unproven treatments can or ever will be cost-effective, accessible, and medically useful and safe. Yet in recent years, such criticism has become somewhat outdated as research into these treatment modalities has increased in the United States. In addition, much research on CAM therapies has been published in other countries, although often the results have been discounted or ignored by the U.S. medical community.

It is important to differentiate between complementary approaches that truly represent alternatives and those that are simply unusual. From a cultural historical perspective, it seems reasonable to assume that approaches that had no value probably would have died out a long time ago. Conversely, approaches deemed to be quite unusual tend to have no cultural traditions associated with them. Typically, such approaches are instead associated with just a few people who are unwilling or unable to scientifically replicate the results of their therapy. To date, complementary approaches that have been validated by contemporary science are generally those with long cultural histories.

Finally, one of the most important ways in which CAM may become accepted and integrated into conventional medicine is by the use of an evidence-based approach. This process assumes (1) that an adequate scientific methodology is in place, (2) that any treatment effects are measured and are clinically meaningful, and (3) that some application of the therapy can be made to clinical practice. Evidence to enlighten and inform clinical practice is the starting point and ending point of this engaging controversy.

---

standards required in Western medicine. Practitioners of CAM often develop individualized treatment plans, and thus different people receive different treatments for similar symptoms. This makes it difficult to determine what would be considered a specific intervention for an experimental or treatment group.

Other methodological criticisms of CAM research include the small number of participants, high drop-out rates, self-report social response bias, maturation bias, selection bias, nonrandomization, use of nonclinical populations, and the possibility that placebo CAM therapies also produce some beneficial outcomes. Better methods of diagnosing and describing clinical characteristics of participants also are needed.

Only a modest number of well-designed CAM research studies involve mental health. With the exception of certain herbal treatments, such as St. John's wort for depression and kava-kava for anxiety, few high-quality studies of the main CAM treatments (such as acupuncture, homeopathy, other herbal products, meditation, yoga, exercise, and biofeedback) are available for any of the major mental illnesses. Even when mental health outcomes are assessed, most research has not examined the psychiatrically ill. For example, although many trials show a decrease in patient anxiety scores after massage, most of the trials have studied acute anxiety associated with cancer, intensive care, or surgery, not with mental illness.

This creates a barrier that hampers the transition of CAM outcome findings into psychiatric clinical practice. Considering that CAM interventions use mind-body approaches, it is surprising that research in this area is not being explored more aggressively. For example, it has been reported that 43% of survey participants used an alternative therapy to treat anxiety and 40% used an alternative therapy to treat depression. Aside from neck and back problems, more respondents used alternative therapies for depression and anxiety than for any other condition (Eisenberger et al, 1998). In another study that looked at the rates of psychiatric disorders in patients receiving complementary medical care, 69% met criteria for at least one lifetime *DSM-IV-TR* Axis I disorder, with major depression being the most common diagnosis (Davidson et al, 1998).

With the increased usage of these therapies by the public and the establishment of NCCAM, more attention has been given and more money made available to study the effectiveness of CAM therapies. Future research should continue to investigate and replicate promising CAM therapies using well-designed methodology.

Many advocates of CAM therapies dispute the value of randomized, controlled clinical trials and will not participate in such studies. How does this affect their being accepted by the larger community of health care providers? ■

Ethical Issues

Ethical concerns about CAM therapies include issues of **safety** and **effectiveness,** as well as the **expertise and qualifications of the practitioner**. Of equal importance is the **com-**

munication between CAM and traditional health care providers. This is particularly important in regard to recent findings of adverse drug and herb interactions.

Care must be taken to monitor medications being combined with herbal products. For example, ginkgo biloba may interact with aspirin or warfarin to prolong bleeding times, thus potentially placing the patient with bleeding disorders in jeopardy. Also it has been shown that the herbal product St. John's wort lowers blood levels of protease inhibitors, thereby decreasing their effectiveness by an average of 57%. This increases the chances that HIV-positive patients who are taking protease inhibitors would not respond to that treatment if they were also taking St. John's wort (Piscitelli et al, 2000).

The possibility always exists that symptoms relieved by CAM therapies may mask signs of serious illnesses, thereby causing delays in seeking conventional, evidence-based treatment. Other concerns are related to effective symptom management, possible side effects, and the lack of regulation of herbal products for purity and potency. Because herbal products are unregulated, the consumer has no guarantee of the ingredients in the herbal products. This increases the potential for adverse effects and drug interactions.

Given these concerns, the nurse who refers a patient to a CAM practitioner needs to explore the options, as well as the health risk-benefit ratios. Local and state regulatory boards, other health regulatory agencies, and consumer affairs departments also can provide information about practitioner qualifications such as licensure, education, accreditations, and complaints that may have been filed.

Box 29-1 provides information health consumers should consider when trying to decide whether to use a complementary or alternative therapy. In addition, the website www.consumerlab.com provides testing results of the authenticity of ingredients on product labels. The FDA website www.fda.gov provides consumer reports on dietary supplements.

The following sections describe the most common **evidence-based CAM therapies** that have been used for some of the **major psychiatric disorders**.

■ DEPRESSION

Depression is one of the most common conditions for which people use alternative therapies. A review of the most beneficial CAM therapies for depression found evidence to support the use of exercise, herbal therapy (St. John's wort), self-help or bibliotherapy, and light therapy for seasonal depression. Other therapies with some supportive evidence include massage, acupuncture, light therapy for nonseasonal depression, relaxation, S-adenosyl-L-methionine (SAMe), folate, and yoga (Jorm et al, 2002).

Herbal Products

One of the most widely researched herbal products is **hypericum (St. John's wort)**. It is currently used throughout Europe and the United States to treat mild to moderate depression, anxiety, seasonal affective disorder, and sleep disorders.

The herb's mechanism of action may involve serotonin, dopamine, gamma-aminobutyric acid (GABA), and norepinephrine reuptake inhibition. Other reported effects of St. John's wort include anti-inflammatory, antiviral, antimicrobial, antiulcerogenic, and astringent activity (Barnes et al, 2001).

The herb is available in tea, capsule, or tincture form, usually standardized to contain 0.3% hypericin. Most recent findings show that the hyperforin (0.05% to 5%) constituent may contribute more to the antidepressant effects than the hypericin constituent. The standard dose is 300 mg 3 times a day. Side effects are minimal and include dry mouth, dizziness, gastrointestinal symptoms, and photosensitivity.

BOX 29-1

Patient Guidelines for Considering Complementary and Alternative Therapies

- Ask a health care provider about the safety and effectiveness of the desired therapy or treatment. Information also can be found in current publications and on the National Center for Complementary and Alternative Medicine (NCCAM) website.

- Contact a state or local regulatory agency with authority over practitioners who practice the therapy or treatment being sought. Complementary and alternative medicine (CAM) usually is not as regulated as is the practice of conventional medicine; but licensing, accreditation, and regulatory laws are increasingly being implemented. Check to see whether the practitioner is licensed to deliver the identified services.

- Talk with those who have had experience with the practitioner you are considering, both health care providers and other patients. Find out about the confidence and competence of the practitioner and whether patients have lodged any complaints.

- Talk with the practitioner in person. Ask about education, additional training, licenses, and certifications, both conventional and unconventional. Find out how open the practitioner is to communicating with patients about technical aspects of methods, possible side effects, and potential problems.

- Visit the practitioner's office, clinic, or hospital. Ask how many patients are typically seen in a day or week, and how much time is spent with each patient. Look at the conditions of the office or clinic. The primary issue here is whether the service delivery adheres to regulated standards for medical safety and care.

- Find out what several practitioners charge for the same treatment to get a better idea about the appropriateness of costs. Regulatory agencies and professional associations also may provide cost information.

- Most important, discuss all issues regarding therapies and treatments with your usual health care provider, whether a practitioner of conventional or alternative medicine. Competent health care management requires knowledge of both conventional and alternative therapies for the provider to have a complete picture of your treatment plan.

Hypericum interferes with the metabolism of many medications and should not be taken with post transplant antirejection drugs, oral contraceptives, statin anticholesterol drugs, protease inhibitors, antineoplastics, antiretrovirals, anticonvulsants, digoxin, theophylline, triptans, serotonin reuptake inhibitors (SSRIs), and anticoagulants (FDA, 2000). A 2-week wash-out period is recommended before initiating another antidepressant.

A number of well-designed placebo-controlled studies have been conducted to determine the efficacy of hypericum for depression. Several studies have compared hypericum to either placebo or other antidepressants, namely tricyclics and SSRIs, in patients with mild to moderate depression and have found comparable efficacy (Brenner et al, 2000; Philipp, Kohnen, and Hiller, 1999; Schrader, 2000; Lecrubier et al, 2002). These studies show a much lower side effect profile for hypericum compared with tricyclics and SSRIs. However, as dosage of hypericum is increased, the side effect profile becomes more similar to that of the SSRIs.

In contrast, studies comparing hypericum to placebo in patients with major depression have found no differences for depression scores (Shelton et al, 2001; Hypericum Depression Trial Study Group, 2002). **Thus the evidence suggests that although St. John's wort may have some efficacy in mild to moderate depression, it is not an evidence-based treatment for major depression**. Although the methodology of these studies have improved, they are still criticized for using various strengths of the hypericum constituents, not using therapeutic doses of comparative antidepressants, and not doing longer follow-ups (Brown and Gerberg, 2001).

Other herbal products and dietary supplements have been used successfully to promote sleep in patients with depressive disorders. **Melatonin**, a hormone secreted by the pineal gland, works by synchronizing circadian rhythms. In a small, double-blind, randomized controlled trial, improvement in sleep using slow-release melatonin (2.5 to 10 mg) plus antidepressant therapy (fluoxetine, 20 mg) was shown to be superior to antidepressant therapy plus placebo (Dolberg, Hirschmann, and Grunhaus, 1998). Several studies found melatonin to be effective for improving sleep in elderly depressed patients. This population is at a higher risk for suffering the adverse effects associated with use of benzodiazepines (Brown and Gerberg, 2001). Melatonin also may be effective in patients who are discontinuing benzodiazepines. One study showed that patients who received melatonin (2 mg) were more successful at discontinuing benzodiazepines at 6 weeks and reported more improved sleep quality than patients who received placebo (Garfinkel et al, 1999).

Although research is scant, **valerian** may have a mild sedative effect by virtue of its action on GABA receptors. Specifically, valerian may improve slow wave (stages 3 and 4) restorative sleep. The dosages used are 300 to 1200 mg at bedtime or 2 to 3 g of the dried root 3 times a day. Side effects are possible potentiation of other central nervous system depressants, blurred vision, headache, nausea, and excitability. Valerian has not been shown to produce the adverse effects commonly seen after taking benzodiazepines (McEnany, 2000).

SAMe, a dietary supplement, has been used for the treatment of mild to moderate depression and attention deficit/hyperactivity disorder (ADHD). SAMe is a naturally occurring substance found in living cells and is involved in many biochemical reactions. Transmethylation, one reaction that effects neurotransmitter levels, is most likely responsible for the antidepressant action (Keller, 2001). Several randomized, double-blind, placebo-controlled studies using SAMe concluded that SAMe was more effective than placebo and as effective as several tricyclic antidepressants for the treatment of mild to moderate depression (Brown and Gerberg, 2001). Some anecdotal evidence even suggests that SAMe may have efficacy in treatment-resistant depression when used as an adjunct to antidepressant therapy.

The usual oral dose of SAMe for the treatment of depressive symptoms is 800 to 1000 mg twice a day. Because of the instability of the substance, it is recommended that an enteric-coated formulation be used. SAMe has additional benefits over other antidepressants in that it is well-tolerated, particularly in medically ill patients. The side effect profile is equivalent to that for placebo. SAMe should not be combined with other psychotropic medications unless medically supervised and should not be taken by patients with bipolar or manic disorders.

Omega-3 fatty acids, a supplement found mostly in fish oils, may have some efficacy in patients with affective disorders. Some evidence indicates that mood disorders are associated with low omega-3 fatty acid levels. In a small randomized, double-blind study, eicosapentaenoic acid (E-EPA), a specific omega fatty acid, or placebo was added to antidepressant therapy. The dosage of E-EPA was 1 g twice a day. The mean reduction in depression scores from baseline to 4 weeks was significantly lower in the E-EPA group than in the placebo group (Nemets, Stahl, and Belmaker, 2002). In another study involving 30 women with borderline personality disorder, E-EPA 500 mg twice a day was more efficacious than placebo in improving depression and aggression scores at 8 weeks (Zanarini and Frankenburg, 2003).

Conduct an informal survey of your friends and family. How many of them have taken St. John's wort? Were they aware that in a Los Angeles Times survey, 3 out of 10 brands of St. John's wort had no more than half the potency listed on the labels? As a nurse, how would you advise them? ■

Acupuncture

Acupuncture involves the insertion of needles into acupoints located along the body's meridians (energy channels that run throughout the body) for the purpose of restoring energy balance. It is believed that acupuncture may stimulate the synthesis and release of endorphins, serotonin, and norepinephrine. In several randomized control trials, electroacupuncture was as effective in reducing depression as the tricyclic antidepressant, amitriptyline (Ernst and Pittler, 2002; Luo et al, 1998). Specifically, electroacupuncture produced significantly better changes in anxiety, somatization, cognitive processing, and reactive depression. In addition, electroacupuncture had a lower side effect profile. Another study using a double-blind procedure found that the group receiving specific or real acupuncture had significantly less depression after 8 weeks than the control groups given nonspecific acupuncture or no treatment (Allen, 1999). At a 6-month follow-up study, the antidepressant effects of acupuncture persisted (Gallagher et al, 2001).

Acupuncture also has been used as an adjunct to antidepressant therapy. In one study specific and nonspecific acupuncture added to the antidepressant mianserin had comparable outcomes on depressive symptoms at 8 weeks, and both acupuncture groups had depression improvement that was better than the mianserin alone group. The effects of acupuncture in this study did not appear to be site-specific, suggesting effects may be attributed to the attention provided by the acupuncture intervention (Roschke et al, 2000). No studies currently exist comparing acupuncture to the newer antidepressants.

Exercise

Exercise has been investigated over the years for its positive benefits on mood. **Physical exercise in the form of muscular strength training, flexibility training, and cardiovascular aerobic endurance has been associated not only with positive medical benefits but with improvement in mood and self-esteem, decreased tension, and a feeling of accomplishment and renewed energy.** Numerous studies suggest that levels of depression are lower in exercise groups compared with control groups, with some showing equivalent outcomes when compared with psychotherapy and antidepressants (Lawlor and Hopker, 2001; Manber, Allen, and Morris, 2002).

One study randomized older depressed patients to a group aerobic exercise program 3 times a week, the antidepressant sertraline, or both exercise program and sertraline for 16 weeks. Sixty to 70% of patients no longer met criteria for major depression at the end of the study period, with no differences shown between the three groups. However, the sertraline group took less time to respond and the exercise group had lower relapse rates at 10-month follow-up (Babyak et al, 2000). Another randomized study compared exercise with health education classes for 10 weeks in 86 older depressed patients to determine whether the effects of exercise were attributed to socialization. Significantly more participants in the exercise group had a positive response than those in the health education group (Mather et al, 2002).

Massage

Only a few controlled studies have evaluated the effects of massage therapy for the treatment of depression. These studies have shown that participants receiving massage therapy report improvements in mood and well being. However, these effects were short term and the clinical relevance is questionable (Manber, Allen, and Morris, 2002). None of these studies compared massage with established medication or psychotherapy treatments.

What physiological changes are stimulated by massage therapy? How might these relate to one's thoughts and emotions? ■

Light Therapy

Exposure to bright light, or phototherapy, has been shown to be effective for the treatment of seasonal affective disorder (SAD). Phase delayed sleep brought on by the reduced sunlight in winter disrupts circadian rhythms. It has been suggested that the onset of melatonin level and minimum body temperature, which peak at specific times during the sleeping hours, are delayed in SAD. Individuals with SAD sit in front of a light box with 10,000 lux illumination upon awakening in the morning (see Chapter 28). However, cost and inconvenience have made this approach less practical.

Another form of light therapy, **dawn stimulation**, involves exposure to a gradually increasing low level light (maximum 400 lux) in the early morning hours while the individual is still asleep. In a well-designed double-blind, placebo-controlled study, 95 individuals who met DSM-IV criteria for SAD were randomized to either bright light (10,000 lux) for 30 minutes upon awakening at 6 AM, dawn stimulation (peaking to 250 lux) while asleep from 4:30 to 6:00 AM, or placebo dawn stimulation (peaking at 0.5 lux) while asleep from 4:30 to 6:00 AM. At the end of 6 weeks, the dawn stimulation group had significantly greater response and remission rates compared with the bright light and placebo groups (Avery, 2001).

Meditation and Yoga

Meditation and yoga exercises have been associated with antidepressant effects and stress reduction. These interventions involve focusing attention and self-regulation. One type of meditation, Sudarshan Kriya Yoga (SKY) uses different breathing rhythms to induce a tranquil state. In one study, 45 depressed patients were randomized to receive SKY for 45 minutes 6 days a week, electroconvulsive therapy (ECT), or imipramine 150 mg daily for 4 weeks. Remission rates were 67% for the group receiving SKY, 93% for the ECT group, and 73% for the imipramine group. The SKY and imipramine groups had comparable responses (Janakiramaiah et al, 2000).

Another type of meditation, mindfulness-based stress reduction, involves development of skills to learn to acquire an attitude of "living in the moment" and acceptance. This intervention may hold promise in preventing relapse to depression but may require too much concentration effort in acutely depressed patients (Bishop, 2002).

■ ANXIETY

Anxiety disorders are one of the major reasons people use CAM therapies. Anxiety disorders that have been investigated using CAM therapies include generalized anxiety disorders, social and specific phobias, panic disorder, obsessive-compulsive disorder (OCD), and posttraumatic stress disorder (PTSD). Because anxiety and depressive disorders often co-occur, many of the therapies that are used for depressive disorders are also used for anxiety disorders.

Relaxation

Relaxation techniques are an accepted therapeutic strategy and often are used in psychotherapy, particularly in patients with anxiety disorders (see Chapter 31). Progressive muscle relaxation (PMR) uses a process of tensing and releasing groups of muscles starting from facial muscles and moving down the body to the muscles in the feet. Individuals learn the systematic technique and gain control over anxiety-provoking thoughts and muscle tension.

PMR also has been used in conjunction with imagery, breathing retraining, autogenic training, and biofeedback. In a randomized, controlled study using PMR on medicated and nonmedicated individuals with insomnia, those receiving PMR experienced a significant improvement in anxiety and sleep efficiency and quality and reduced their use of sleep medication by 80% (Lichstein et al, 1999).

Mindfulness meditation also has been suggested as being beneficial for those with generalized anxiety and panic disorders. As a technique for gaining control over emotions, mindfulness meditation involves an intentional suspended awareness of the present-moment experience that excludes reaction, judgment, or partiality. Overall, however, little research has explored the efficacy of meditation in psychiatric populations.

Therapeutic Touch

Although not investigated in psychiatric populations, therapeutic touch has been explored for possible stress reduction in nonpsychiatric populations. Therapeutic touch involves the intentional exchange of energy between the practitioner and patient to promote healing and well-being. The use of the hands is the conduit for the energy exchange. This intervention is proposed to work by eliciting the relaxation response.

Therapeutic touch has been embraced by nursing in all areas of practice and is probably one of the most widely researched interventions in the nursing literature. One study found alterations in immunoglobulin levels and a decreased percentage of suppressor T cells with the use of therapeutic touch (Clark, 1999). Another study found lowered pulse amplitude indicating peripheral vasoconstriction in participants receiving therapeutic touch compared with placebo therapeutic touch. This finding is contrary to the expected vasodilatation response, which is characteristic of the relaxation response (Engle and Graney, 2000). The literature on therapeutic touch, however, has been criticized for only emphasizing positive findings (O'Mathuna, 2000).

Why do you think that therapeutic touch has been relatively unexplored as a treatment for psychiatric patients? ■

Yoga

Several types of yoga have been used for stress and anxiety disorders. Yoga is a physical and emotional conditioning of the body produced by engaging in a series of postures, stretching exercises, breath control, and meditation. A randomized study using one type of yoga, Kundalini Yoga (KY), was found to have efficacy in treating obsessive-compulsive disorder (OCD). This intervention consisted of eight primary and three nonmandatory KY techniques. One technique, requir-

ing participants to perform left nostril breathing, was suggested to be specific for OCD. At the end of 3 months, participants in the KY group had a significant improvement (38% reduction) in their symptoms compared with a control group receiving relaxation response and mindfulness meditation (14% reduction). When the groups were merged at 3 months and all participants received KY, a 15-month follow-up study showed a 71% reduction in obsessive-compulsive symptoms for all participants. Specifically, after receiving KY, the original control group had a 44% reduction. The investigators also noted that these improvements were superior to several placebo-controlled, double-blind medication trials (Shannahoff-Khalsa et al, 1999).

Herbal Products

Several herbs are marketed for the relief of anxiety, but few have been empirically studied. **Kava-kava**, a plant found in the South Pacific, is proposed to have anxiolytic, sedative, and muscle relaxant properties. A kava product standardized for 70% kava pyrone content (proposed active ingredient) was used in a randomized, placebo-controlled 25-week outpatient trial with 101 outpatients suffering various anxiety disorders. Statistically significant improvements in anxiety were seen in the kava group versus the control group at all follow-up assessments starting at 8 weeks. The only possibly related side effect reported was "stomach upset." Thus kava may be better tolerated than other pharmacological agents presently used for anxiety disorders. The dosage used in this study was 90 to 110 mg of the 70% kava pyrone extract given 3 times a day (Volz and Kieser, 1997).

In a review of the research exploring the efficacy of kava, seven high quality studies revealed that kava was superior to placebo in reducing anxiety (Pittler and Ernst, 2002). However, in Canada and several European countries, kava has been associated with liver damage and toxicity. Investigators have not been able to determine which individuals may be at most risk for kava liver toxicity. Chronic overuse of kava, combined with alcohol or other drugs and preexisting liver conditions may be contributing factors (Grossman, 2002).

The FDA Consumer Advisory and Consumer Reports medical experts have cautioned against the use of kava (Consumer Reports, 2003). Use of kava combined with other central nervous system medications can be harmful, and kava may have addictive properties with long-term use. Other medications used in combination with kava that have reported adverse drug interactions include levodopa, dopamine agonists, benzodiazepines, cimetidine, and terazosin (Ayd, 2001).

Another herbal product, **valerian**, has been used for insomnia, a symptom common to many anxiety disorders. The active constituent, valepotriate, may act on GABA receptor binding. Several small studies have shown valerian to improve sleep latency and sleep quality in mild to moderate insomnia (Ernst and Pittler, 2002). Valerian may potentiate the effects of other central nervous system depressants and hypnotics.

Eye Movement Desensitization and Reprocessing

Eye movement desensitization and reprocessing (EMDR) is an intervention that requires the patient to generate a number of rapid lateral eye movements while engaging in imagery recall of significant aspects of a particular traumatic memory or feared stimuli. This therapy is based on the observations that spontaneous multiple eye movements combined with a number of traditional cognitive behavioral and exposure procedures are associated with attempts to diffuse negative emotions and cognitions.

In a meta-analysis, Davidson and Parker (2001) evaluated 34 EMDR studies. When compared to no treatment (wait list) or nonexposure treatments (i.e., relaxation), EMDR had better outcomes with regard to PTSD symptoms, psychophysiological measures, and other more global psychiatric symptoms. The effects of EMDR were similar in comparison to exposure therapies. A few reports have supported the efficacy of EMDR for panic disorders and phobias.

It remains unclear, however, whether the eye movements are integral to the treatment. For example, it has been suggested that the eye movements are necessary because they simulate rapid eye movement (REM) sleep, a stage of sleep when normal consolidation and integration of memories occurs (Shapiro and Maxfield, 2002). Other studies have shown that the effectiveness of EMDR may be related to correcting cognitive intrusions (Lee et al, 2002; Lytle, Hazlett-Stevens, and Borkovec, 2002).

■ SUBSTANCE USE DISORDERS

Acupuncture

One of the most widely researched CAM therapies used to treat addiction is acupuncture. **Many chemical dependency programs in the United States use auricular acupuncture as an additional therapy.** The National Acupuncture Detoxification Association (NADA) has trained thousands of individuals on the standard 4- to 5-point auricular acupuncture procedure (Figure 29-1). This procedure has been used with reported success in one New York clinic since 1975. In 1997 a consensus panel for the National Institutes of Health and Medicine stated that there was sufficient evidence to support the possibility that acupuncture may be effective for the treatment of addictions.

A qualitative study with eight substance-abusing participants receiving auricular acupuncture revealed several prevailing themes. Mood elevation, relaxation, and improved sleep were among the beneficial effects experienced by participants (Berstein, 2000). Recent quantitative studies with better methodologies have questioned the efficacy of site-specific acupuncture. In a large multisite randomized control study, 620 cocaine-addicted participants were randomized to receive NADA addiction acupuncture, placebo acupuncture, or a relaxation control condition for 8 weeks with posttreatment, 3-month and 6-month follow-up assessments. At all follow-ups no significant differences were noted between groups in the percentage of positive urine drug screens or treatment retention (Margolin et al, 2002). One drawback to this study was the low number of counseling sessions attended by participants in all three groups.

Auricular acupuncture is not meant to be a stand-alone treatment. An earlier smaller study with a similar design that included only cocaine-dependent methadone-maintained patients found that participants in the NADA auricular acupuncture group had more cocaine-negative urine drug screens than the placebo acupuncture group or the relaxation control group throughout the 8-week treatment (Avants et al, 2000). Killeen and colleagues (2002) found no differences in cue-elicited cocaine craving between participants after receiving one session of NADA acupuncture or sham acupuncture. Both groups reported a reduction in craving measures. Thus replication of well-designed studies is needed to provide empirical support for the use of auricular acupuncture for the treatment of cocaine addiction.

Auricular acupuncture also has been explored for use with smoking cessation programs. One hundred forty-one patients were randomized to receive NADA addiction acupuncture alone, NADA addiction acupuncture plus education, or sham acupuncture plus education for 5 weeks. At the end of treatment and follow-up, participants in the addiction acupuncture plus education group had significantly better cessation rates and had a greater percentage of decrease in cigarette consumption than participants in the other two groups (Bier et al, 2002).

Yoga

Only one study has compared hatha yoga with psychodynamic therapy. The interventions were delivered for 5 months in a group setting to methadone-maintained patients. Both groups showed reduction in both drug use and criminal activity (Shaffer, La Salvia, and Stein, 1997).

Biofeedback

Some small studies have investigated the use of biofeedback for the treatment of addictions and other psychiatric disorders. Biofeedback is an intervention in which physiological responses such as heart rate, skin conductance, skin temperature, and muscle activity are monitored for the purpose of teaching the patient to consciously regulate these processes. Often patients engage in relaxation exercises or other cogni-

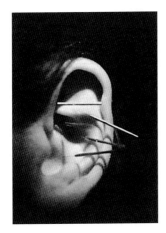

Figure 29-1   Auricular acupuncture points.

tive behavioral techniques to decrease arousal and activation of these physiological responses (Patrick, 2002).

Neurotherapy or neurofeedback is a specific biofeedback that transmits electroencephalogram (EEG) signals and provides information about neuronal activity in the cerebral cortex. One study randomized patients to receive transcendental meditation (TM), electromyographic biofeedback (BF), neurotherapy (NT), or routine therapy alone (RT) for the treatment of alcoholism. The NT and RT groups were the control groups. Outcome results 18 months after treatment showed significant increases in the number of nondrinking days for the TM and BF groups but not for the NT or RT groups (Taub et al, 1994).

■ EATING DISORDERS

Bulimia nervosa is a disorder of affect and anxiety dysregulation and an inability to self-soothe. In a group of 50 patients who met criteria for bulimia nervosa, guided imagery interventions were significantly more effective in reducing binge and purge frequencies and eating disorder psychopathology and improved ability to self-soothe at the end of 6 weeks of treatment (Esplen et al, 1998). More research is needed in this area.

■ ATTENTION DEFICIT/HYPERACTIVITY DISORDER

Neurofeedback, previously described in the addiction section, has been explored for the management of attention deficit/hyperactivity disorder (ADHD) symptoms. Several small studies show children exhibiting neurofeedback display improvements in attention, impulse control, and information processing (Brue and Oakland, 2002).

■ DEMENTIAS

Gingko biloba, an extract obtained from the leaves of the maidenhair tree in China, is another herbal product that has been studied in psychiatric populations for its cognitive enhancing effects, specifically in those with Alzheimer's disease. It may act by dilating blood vessels and increasing blood supply, reducing blood viscosity, decreasing free radicals, and altering neurotransmitter levels (McEnany, 2000).

In a meta-analysis, gingko was shown to be superior to placebo for improving cognitive function, activities of daily living, and measures of mood and emotional function at doses between 120 and 240 mg/day at 12, 24, and 52 weeks. No differences were found in adverse events between the gingko and placebo groups. Gingko was also just as efficacious as four cholinesterase inhibitors for enhancing cognition in patients with mild to moderate Alzheimer's (Birks et al, 2002). Reports have indicated that gingko may interact with anticoagulants and aspirin to increase the risk of bleeding.

■ NURSING IMPLICATIONS

CAM therapies can have an important impact on psychiatric nursing practice. They are beneficial, safe, cost-effective, and easily implemented throughout psychiatric settings. Nurses on psychiatric inpatient units using CAM therapies report better patient compliance, as well as a more relaxed, manageable milieu (Gurevich et al, 1996).

Most CAM therapies can be prescribed and implemented by nurses. Nurses should continue to follow the research literature to track the emerging evidence regarding the effectiveness of these therapies. Another valuable resource is the Cochrane Collaboration, which has an ongoing registry of randomized clinical trials related to CAM that can be accessed over the Internet.

With its holistic framework, nursing is in an ideal position to gain ownership of many CAM therapies for the management of symptoms experienced by psychiatric populations. In addition, CAM therapies that empower the patient can play an important part in strengthening the nurse-patient partnership.

COMPETENT CARING

A Clinical Exemplar of a Psychiatric Nurse
PAULA E. JOHNSON, MSN, RN, CS

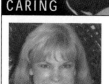

As a psychiatric nurse who has spent 15 years working in academic medical centers and 5 years in private psychotherapy practice, I have had the opportunity to study, personally experience, and offer to my patients many therapeutic modalities that are not commonly found in traditional or conventional health care settings. I have come to appreciate the value and power of these practices commonly known as "alternative" therapies. I rarely use the term alternative therapy, however, because I do not see my work as precluding other forms of therapy. I believe that the most effective therapy incorporates an alternative perspective and includes rather than excludes the use of appropriate conventional treatments.

Early in my own personal quest for physical and mental wellness, I was drawn to the practices of yoga, meditation, and conscious breathing. Later in nursing school, I was given the opportunity to experience and investigate other holistic approaches to health care including therapeutic touch and guided imagery. After graduation, my interest and excitement in alternatives continued to grow. I pursued certification in reflexology, Reiki, transformational breathing, and the self-inquiry work of Byron Katie. With each of these alternative therapies, I first experience and apply it in my own life. Eventually I bring those techniques that have a positive impact on my own health and wellness to my patients, the majority of whom enjoy similar results.

For example, after years of meditation practice, I began to incorporate the use of conscious breathing and mindfulness into my time with my patients. My intention is to pass on to them the healing effects of calmness, presence, and relaxation that I have experienced. In simple and clear ways, I talk with them about the power of conscious awareness and instruct them in how to use the breath to consciously bring themselves into the present moment and to increase their realization of what they are experiencing within their bodies. I have observed that when patients grow in their personal awareness of their internal experience, they are better able to express their feelings, are more likely to pay attention to early symptoms of distress and take appropriate action, and eventually are more comfortable in their bodies.

I recently worked with a woman who was experiencing marital and job-related stress and severe anxiety. I noticed that every sentence she spoke contained within it some projection into the future. "I won't be able to stand it if he doesn't change." "My boss will never appreciate what I do for him and the company." When I asked how she feels when she has these thoughts, she said she felt tremendous fear. I suggested some homework in between sessions. I simply asked her to check in with herself throughout the day, notice her breathing, and for a few minutes practice being totally present in the moment. The following week she told me that she had never before realized just how little of her time is spent fully aware in the present moment. I observed her growing attention and even excitement as she learned to acknowledge and report her internal experiences. As she continued to apply this practice more and more in her everyday life, she reported that her husband seemed to be changing, she had started to ask her boss for what she wants, and she was feeling more in control of her own life.

Through this and many similarly powerful experiences with alternative modalities, I came to see that these practices to which I seemed to have been drawn were in fact not alternative to me but rather more closely resonating with my own nature than many of the conventional approaches. I am now able to distinguish more clearly between what is normal and what is natural and to assist my patients in making that distinction for themselves.

More and more I find myself choosing to offer those alternative therapies that self-empower and give patients responsibility for their own healing and wellness. Through the practice of alternative therapies with my patients, I have come to know the tremendous benefits of shared common experience. Many of the patients I work with in private practice speak to me of the pain and suffering of anxiety, depression, mood swings, and addiction—all responses to life situations that I can find within myself. When I am able to recognize and acknowledge our common human condition, I no longer feel separate from them. This recognition never compromises our nurse-patient relationship. In fact, it actually creates an opening in which we can truly communicate, perhaps for the first time.

Alternative therapies offer an approach to creating and maintaining health that is often not available in a conventional health care setting. Yet this growing field of practices is perhaps nothing more than the manifestation of our growing conscious awareness of ourselves and how we exist in the universe. As I see it, the greatest benefit for patient and therapist is the opportunity to experience a relationship that honors and respects, listens and hears, and is open to all possibilities.

As nurses we can begin by looking within ourselves for the answers. To believe that we have reached the pinnacle of development in health care, that the physical world is all there is, or that we are separate from each other is to live in a myth. Whether it is an alternative therapy or a more conventional one, our full presence in the here and now makes the difference. This is where true healing begins. ∎

CHAPTER **FOCUS POINTS**

- Complementary and alternative medicine (CAM) is the term used to describe a broad range of nontraditional healing philosophies, approaches, and therapies. CAM can be delivered alone or in combination with conventional therapies.
- Well-designed CAM research studies in mental health and psychiatric disorders are beginning to provide empirical evidence for practice. Nurses must continue to inform themselves of research findings related to CAM because nurses play an important role in educating consumers about the evidence supporting these new therapies, as well as the dangers involved in using some of them.

- Ethical concerns include issues of safety and effectiveness, the expertise and qualifications of the practitioner, and communicating the use of CAM therapies to the traditional health care provider.
- Evidence-based CAM therapies for various psychiatric disorders include herbal products, acupuncture, exercise, massage, light therapy, meditation, therapeutic touch, yoga, eye movement desensitization and reprocessing, and biofeedback.
- CAM therapies can be used by psychiatric nurses and potentially can have a significant impact on their practice.

KEY TERMS

acupuncture, 622
biofeedback, 625
complementary and alternative
  medicine (CAM), 618

eye movement desensitization and
  reprocessing (EMDR), 625
mindfulness meditation, 624
phototherapy, 623

progressive muscle relaxation (PMR),
  623
therapeutic touch, 624
yoga, 624

CHAPTER REVIEW QUESTIONS

1. Indicate whether the following statements are true (T) or false (F).

_____ A. In the United States fewer people are using CAM therapies because of concerns from traditional health care providers.

_____ B. Relatively few scientific studies of CAM in patients with major psychiatric illnesses have been conducted.

_____ C. Herbal products are not regulated for purity and potency.

_____ D. St. John's wort can be safely taken with other antidepressants.

_____ E. Mindfulness meditation has been found to be beneficial in those with generalized anxiety and panic disorders.

_____ F. Acupuncture has been found to be effective in treating cocaine and other substance use disorders.

2. Fill in the blanks.

A. _____ is the term used to describe a broad range of healing philosophies, approaches, and therapies that focus on the whole person.

B. _____ is the most common herbal alternative therapy used for depression.

C. A hormone secreted by the pineal gland that works by synchronizing circadian rhythms is called _____.

D. The process of tensing and releasing groups of muscles in the body is called _____.

E. _____ involves the intentional exchange of energy between the practitioner and patient to promote healing and well-being.

F. The herbal product most commonly used for anxiety is

_____.

G. _____ is an herbal product that has been studied in psychiatric populations for its cognitive enhancing effects.

3. Provide short answers for the following questions.

A. Give three reasons why CAM therapies are seen as desirable by many people.

B. Identify four ethical concerns related to CAM therapies.

C. Describe the proposed mechanism of action of acupuncture.

Visit Evolve for additional resources related to the content of this chapter.

  http://evolve.elsevier.com/Stuart/principles/
• Topical Course Outline • Student Workbook Exercises • Critical Thinking Questions and Activities • Case Studies • Research Topics
• Monthly Content Updates • WebLinks

Student Study CD-ROM

Access the accompanying CD-ROM for animations, interactive exercises, review questions for the NCLEX examination, and an audio glossary.

REFERENCES

Allen J: Innovative study shows acupuncture promising as depression treatment, *Psychiatric News*, August 6, 1999.

Avants SK et al: A randomized controlled trial of auricular acupuncture for cocaine dependence, *Arch Intern Med* 160:2305, 2000.

Avery DH: Dawn stimulation and bright light in the treatment of SAD: a controlled study, *Biol Psychiatry* 50:205, 2001.

Ayd F: Interactions between prescription drugs and natural remedies, *Psychiatric Times*: 64, August 2001.

Babyak M et al: Exercise treatment for major depression: maintenance of therapeutic benefit at 10 months, *Psychosom Med* 62:633, 2000.

Barnes J et al: St. John's wort (Hypericum perforatum L.): a review of its chemistry, pharmacology and clinical properties, *J Pharm Pharmacology* 53:583, 2001.

Bernstein KS: The experience of acupuncture for treatment of substance dependence, *J Nurs Scholarsh* 32:267, 2000.

Bier ID et al: Auricular acupuncture, education, and smoking cessation: a randomized, sham-controlled trial, *Am J Public Health* 92:1642, 2002.

Birks J et al: Gingko biloba for cognitive impairment and dementia, *The Cochrane Library of Systemic Review* 4:CD003120, 2002.

Bishop SR: What do we really know about mindfulness based stress reduction? *Psychosom Med* 64:71, 2002. (Erratum in *Psychosom Med* 64:449, 2002.)

Brenner R et al: Comparison of an extract of hypericum (LI 160) and sertraline in the treatment of depression: a double-blind, randomized pilot study, *Clin Ther* 22:411, 2000.

Brown R, Gerbarg P: Herbs and nutrients in the treatment of depression, anxiety, insomnia, migraine and obesity, *J Psychiatr Pract* 7:75, 2001.

Brue AW, Oakland TD: Alternative treatments for attention-deficit/hyperactivity disorder: does evidence support their use? *Altern Ther Health Med* 8:68, 2002.

Clark C: Concepts and issues. In Clark CC, editor: *Encyclopedia of complementary health practice*, New York, 1999, Springer.

Consumer Reports: *Kava: a supplement to avoid*, 68:8, 2003.

Consumer Reports: *The mainstreaming of alternative medicine*, p 17, May 2000.

Davidson P, Parker K: Eye movement desensitization and reprocessing: a meta analysis, *J Consult Clin Psychol* 67:305, 2001.

Davidson JR et al: Psychiatric disorders in primary care patients receiving complementary medical treatments, *Compr Psychiatry* 39:16, 1998.

Dolberg OT, Hirschmann S, Grunhaus L: Melatonin for the treatment of sleep disturbances in major depressive disorder, *Am J Psychiatry* 155:1119, 1998.

Eisenberg DM et al: Trends in alternative medicine use in the United States, 1990-1997: results of a follow-up national survey, *JAMA* 280:1569, 1998.

Engle VF, Graney MJ: Biobehavioral effects of therapeutic touch, *J Nurs Scholarsh* 32:287, 2000.

Ernst E, Pittler MH: Herbal medicine, *Med Clin North Am* 86:149, 2002.

Esplen MJ et al: A randomized controlled trial of guided imagery in bulimia nervosa, *Psychol Med* 28:1347, 1998.

Fontanarosa PB, Rennie D, DeAngelis CD: The need for regulation of dietary supplements—lessons from ephedra, JAMA 289:1568, 2003.

Food and Drug Administration (FDA): Risk of drug interactions with St John's wort, JAMA 283:1679, 2000.

Gallagher SM et al: Six-month depression relapse rates among women treated with acupuncture, *Complement Ther Med* 9:216, 2001.

Garfinkel D et al: Facilitation of benzodiazepine discontinuation by melatonin: a new clinical approach, *Arch Intern Med* 159: 2456, 1999.

Grossman L: The curious case of kava, *Time*, p 58, April 8, 2002.

Gurevich MI et al: Is auricular acupuncture beneficial in the inpatient treatment of substance-abusing patients? *J Subst Abuse Treat* 13:165, 1996.

Hypericum Depression Trial Study Group: Effect of *Hypericum perforatum* (St. John's wort) in major depressive disorder: a randomized controlled trial, JAMA 287:1807, 2002.

Janakiramaiah N et al: Antidepressant efficacy of Sudarshan Kriya Yoga (SKY) in melancholia: a randomized comparison with electroconvulsant therapy (ECT) and imipramine, *J Affect Disord* 57:255, 2000.

Jorm AF et al: Effectiveness of complementary and self-help treatments for depression, *Med J Aust* 176 Suppl:S84-96, 2002.

Keller K: SAM-e: more research, more uses, *Adv Nurs*, p 36, October 15, 2001.

Kessler RC et al: The use of complementary and alternative therapies to treat anxiety and depression in the United States, *Am J Psychiatry* 158:289, 2001.

Killeen TK et al: The effect of auricular acupuncture on psychophysiological measures of cocaine craving, *Issues Ment Health Nurs* 23:445, 2002.

Lawlor DA, Hopker SW: The effectiveness of exercise as an intervention in the management of depression: systemic review and meta-regression analysis of randomized control trials, *BMJ* 322:763, 2001.

Lecrubier Y et al: Efficacy of St. John's wort extract Ws 5570 in major depression: a double-blind, placebo-controlled trial, *Am J Psychiatry* 159:1361, 2002.

Lee C et al: Treatment of PTSD: stress inoculation training with prolonged exposure compared to EMDR, *J Clin Psychol* 58:1071, 2002.

Lichstein KL et al: Relaxation to assist sleep medication withdrawal, *Behav Modif* 23:379, 1999.

Luo H et al: Clinical research on the therapeutic effects of the electroacupuncture treatment in patients with depression, *Psychiatry Clin Neurosci* 52(suppl):S338, 1998.

Lytle RA, Hazlett-Stevens H, Borkovec TD: Efficacy of Eye Movement Desensitization in the treatment of cognitive intrusions related to a past stressful event, *J Anxiety Disord* 16:273, 2002.

Manber R, Allen JJ, Morris MM: Alternative treatments for depression: empirical support and relevance to women, *J Clin Psychiatry* 63:628, 2002.

Margolin A et al: Acupuncture for the treatment of cocaine addiction: a randomized controlled trial, JAMA 287:55, 2002.

Mather AS et al: Effects of exercise on depressive symptoms in older adults with poorly responsive depressive disorder: randomized control trial, *Br J Psychiatry* 180:411, 2002.

McEnany G: Herbal psychotropics. Part 4: Focus on gingko biloba, L-carnitine, lactobacillus acidophilus, and ginger root, *J Am Psychiatr Nurs Assoc* 7:22, 2000.

Nemets B, Stahl Z, Belmaker RH: Addition of omega-3 fatty acid to maintenance medication for recurrent unipolar depressive disorder, *Am J Psychiatry* 159:477, 2002.

O'Mathuna DP: Evidenced-based practice and reviews of therapeutic touch, *J Nurs Scholarsh* 32:279, 2000.

Patrick G: Biofeedback applications for psychiatric nursing, *J Am Psychiatr Nurs Assoc* 8:109, 2002.

Philipp M, Kohnen R, Hiller KO: Hypericum extract was better than placebo and equivalent to imipramine for moderate depression, *BMJ* 319:1534, 1999. (Erratum in *BMJ* 320:361, 2000.)

Piscitelli S et al: Indinavir concentrations and St. John's wort, *Lancet* 355:547, 2000.

Pittler M, Ernst E: Kava extract for treating anxiety, *The Cochrane Library for Systemic Review* 4:1, 2002.

Roschke J et al: The benefit from whole body acupuncture in major depression, *J Affect Disord* 57:73, 2000.

SAMe for depression, *Med Lett* 41:107, 2000.

Schrader E: Equivalence of St. John's wort extract (Ze 117) and fluoxetine: a randomized, controlled study in mild-moderate depression, *Int Clin Psychopharmacol* 15:61, 2000.

Shaffer HJ, La Salvia TA, Stein JP: Comparing Hatha yoga with dynamic group psychotherapy for enhancing methadone maintenance treatment: a randomized clinical trial, *Altern Ther Health Med* 3:57, 1997.

Shannahoff-Khalsa D et al: Randomized controlled trial of yogic meditation techniques for patients with obsessive-compulsive disorder, *CNS Spectrums* 4:34, 1999.

Shapiro F, Maxifield L: Eye Movement Desensitization and Reprocessing (EMDR): information processing in the treatment of trauma, *J Clin Psychol* 58:933, 2002.

Shelton RC et al: Effectiveness of St. John's wort in major depression: a randomized controlled trial, JAMA 285:1978, 2001.

Taub E et al: Effectiveness of broad-spectrum approaches to relapse prevention in severe alcoholism: a long-term randomized, controlled trial of transcendental meditation, EMG biofeedback and electronic neurotherapy, *Alcohol Treat Q* 11:187, 1994.

US Department of Health and Human Services (USDHHS): Expanding horizons of healthcare: five-year strategic plan, 2001-2005, NCCAM (SuDoc HE 20.3002: H 78), Washington, DC, 2000, USDHHS.

Unutzer J et al: Mental disorders and the use of alternative medicine: results from a national survey, *Am J Psychiatry* 157:1851, 2000.

Volz HP, Kieser M: Kava-kava Extract WS 1490 versus placebo in anxiety disorders—a randomized placebo-controlled 25-week outpatient trial, *Pharmacopsychiatry* 30:1, 1997.

Zanarini MC, Frankenburg FR: Omega-3 fatty acid treatment of women with borderline personality disorder: a double-blind, placebo-controlled pilot study, *Am J Psychiatry* 160:167, 2003.

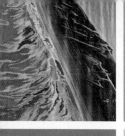

Healthy children raised in decent conditions among loving people in a gentle and just society where freedom and equality are valued will rarely commit violent acts toward others.

RAMSAY CLARK, *A FEW MODEST PROPOSALS TO REDUCE INDIVIDUAL VIOLENCE IN AMERICA*

30 PREVENTING AND MANAGING AGGRESSIVE BEHAVIOR

Christine Diane Hamolia

LEARNING OBJECTIVES

After studying this chapter, the student should be able to:

1. Discuss the prevalence of aggressive behavior among psychiatric patients and reasons for its increase (**I**).
2. Compare passive, assertive, and aggressive behavioral responses (**II**).
3. Describe theories on the development of aggressive behavior (**III**).
4. Identify factors useful in predicting aggressive behavior among psychiatric patients (**IV**).
5. Assess patients for aggressive behavioral responses (**V**).
6. Analyze nursing interventions for preventing and managing aggressive behavior (**VI**).
7. Develop a patient education plan to promote patients' appropriate expression of anger (**VI**).
8. Describe the implementation of crisis management techniques (**VII**).
9. Evaluate prevention strategies related to educating staff, working with staff who have been assaulted, and understanding legal implications (**VIII**).

evolve Visit Evolve for additional resources related to the content of this chapter.
http://evolve.elsevier.com/Stuart/principles/

Nurses provide care for patients with many types of problems. People who enter the health care system are often in great distress and may exhibit maladaptive coping responses. Nurses who work in settings such as emergency rooms, critical care areas, and trauma centers often care for people who respond to events with angry and aggressive behavior that can pose a significant risk to themselves, other patients, and health care providers (Anderson, 2002). Thus preventing and managing aggressive behavior are important skills for all nurses to have.

Psychiatric nurses in particular work with patients who have inadequate coping mechanisms for dealing with stress. Patients admitted to an inpatient psychiatric unit are usually in crisis, so their coping skills are even less effective. During these times of stress, acts of physical aggression or violence can occur. It is also true that nursing staff spend more time with patients on an inpatient unit than do nurses in other disciplines. Thus they are more likely to be involved in preventing and managing aggressive behavior and are more at risk for being victims of acts of violence by patients. For these reasons, it is critical that psychiatric nurses be able to assess patients at risk for violence and intervene effectively with patients before, during, and after an aggressive episode.

■ DIMENSIONS OF THE PROBLEM

High rates of assaultive behavior have been reported in a variety of health care settings including outpatient clinics, nursing homes, and emergency departments. By far the highest rates of assault occur in psychiatric settings. Studies

630

have found that as many as 75% of all psychiatric nursing staff have been assaulted at least once in their careers. Although most assaults occur in inpatient settings, nurses in outpatient mental health settings are also at high risk for violence. Injury rates from violence in public sector psychiatric settings are alarmingly high across nursing employment categories.

Many explanations have been offered for the increasing incidence of violent behavior in psychiatric settings. As more emphasis is placed on outpatient and partial hospital treatment programs in the community, an increasing number of patients referred for inpatient care are hospitalized because they display aggressive or dangerous behavior. Before patients can be committed to the hospital, most states require evidence that patients are dangerous to themselves or others (see Chapter 10). This results in a larger proportion of aggressive and violent patients on inpatient units.

The nature of the inpatient milieu also has changed because of increasing patient acuity and shortened lengths of stay. Economic constraints have resulted in fewer nurses being assigned to inpatient units. Finally, evolving legal directives and perplexing ethical issues challenge the use of chemical and mechanical restraints and raise questions regarding patients' rights to refuse treatment and the nature of the least restrictive environment. This often results in a delicate balance between patient rights and the safety of others.

Members of different disciplines sometimes have different views on how to manage aggressive behavior. Talk with nurses and physicians who care for psychiatric patients about their personal experiences and clinical judgments regarding this problem. ∎

∎ BEHAVIORAL RESPONSES

Within each person lies the capacity for passive, assertive, and aggressive behavior. When in a threatening situation, the choices are to be (1) **passive** and fearful and flee, (2) **aggressive** and angry and fight, or (3) **assertive** and self-confident and to confront the situation directly. The situation and the characteristics of the people involved determine the appropriate response.

Passive Behavior

Passive people subordinate their own rights to their perception of the rights of others. When passive people become angry, they try to hide it, thereby increasing their own tension. If other people notice the anger by observing nonverbal cues, passive people are unable to confront the issue. This also can increase their tension. This pattern of interaction can seriously impair interpersonal growth. The following clinical example illustrates passive behavior.

⟨ CLINICAL EXAMPLE

Ms. J was a staff nurse on a busy surgical unit. She enjoyed her work and liked the patients. She also placed a high value on getting along with her co-workers. Other staff members always spoke positively of her. Ms. C, the head nurse, valued Ms. J as an employee, stating particularly, "She's not like the rest of them. She never complains."

Ms. J made it a practice never to refuse a request made by a patient or another staff member. If a patient who was assigned to another nurse asked her to explain his diet or straighten his bed, she would do so, even if she was then behind in her own work. She never asked for help from others because she felt that her assignment was her responsibility. If a co-worker asked to change days off with her, Ms. J always agreed, even if she had plans, rationalizing that the other person probably had more important plans.

Ms. C began to sense a tenseness when she was around Ms. J. Because she could not think of any problem at work, she assumed that Ms. J must have been having a problem at home. She was concerned and asked Ms. J if she could help. To her amazement, Ms. J recited a long list of angry feelings related to the work situation. Ms. C then felt guilty when she realized that she and the other staff members had been taking advantage of Ms. J. ∎

Although Ms. J thought that she was acting in a healthy way, she was actually negating her own needs and diminishing her self-respect. Her co-workers, who superficially liked her, in reality felt uncomfortable with her because they were never allowed to reciprocate her acts of kindness. Ms. C's guilty response quickly changed to anger when she realized that she had been a victim of Ms. J's passivity. If Ms. J had informed Ms. C of her feelings, she would have treated her more equitably.

Passivity is also expressed nonverbally. The person may speak softly, often in a childlike manner, and make little eye contact. The person may be slouched in posture, with arms held close to the body.

Sarcasm is another indirect expression of anger. This usually provokes anger in the person who is the target. It is different from assertive behavior because it usually infringes on the rights of the other. A sarcastic remark generally conveys the message "You are not worthy of my respect." Sarcasm may be disguised as humor. Confrontation may then be responded to with a disclaimer such as "Can't you take a joke?" Humor that derogates another person is hostile and is indulged in for the purpose of self-enhancement. It tends to backfire because the joker is revealed as insecure.

Assertive Behavior

Assertiveness is at the midpoint of a continuum that runs from passive to aggressive behavior. **Assertive behavior conveys a sense of self-assurance but also communicates respect for the other person.** Assertive people speak clearly and distinctly. They observe the norms of personal space appropriate to the situation. Eye contact is direct but not intrusive. Gestures emphasize speech but are not distracting or threatening. Posture is erect and relaxed. The overall impression is that the person is strong, but not threatening.

Assertive people feel free to refuse an unreasonable request. However, they will share their rationale with the other person. They will also base the judgment about the reasonableness of the request on their own priorities. On the other hand, assertive people do not hesitate to make a request of others, assuming that they will inform them if their request is unreasonable. If the other person is unable to refuse, assertive people will not feel guilty about making the request.

Assertiveness also implies communicating feelings directly to others. As a result, anger is not allowed to build up, and the expression of feeling is more likely to be in proportion to the situation. If dissatisfaction is verbalized, the reason for the feeling is included. Assertive people also remember to express love to those to whom they are close. Compliments are given when deserved. Assertion also involves acceptance of positive input from others.

Aggressive Behavior

At the opposite end of the continuum from passivity is aggression. **Aggressive people ignore the rights of others. They assume that they must fight for their own interests, and they expect the same behavior from others.** For them, life is a battle. An aggressive approach to life may lead to physical or verbal violence. The aggressive behavior often covers a basic lack of self-confidence. Aggressive people enhance their self-esteem by overpowering others and thereby proving their superiority to themselves. The next clinical example describes aggressive behavior.

⎰ CLINICAL EXAMPLE

Suzy was a 9-year-old girl brought to the child psychiatric clinic by her mother on referral from the school nurse. She was described as a tomboy who loved active play and hated school. She was the first girl to make the neighborhood Little League baseball team and had proved her right to be there by beating up several male team members. Suzy was sent to the clinic after the teacher caught her forcing younger children to give her their lunch money.

When Suzy came to the clinic, she presented a facade of toughness. She did not deny her behavior and explained it by saying that the "little kids don't need much to eat anyway. I let them keep some of the money." Suzy was saving money for a new baseball glove. When she was asked about school, she said angrily, "I'm not dumb. I could learn that junk, but who needs it? I just want to play ball."

Psychological testing revealed that Suzy's IQ was slightly below average. She attended school with a group of upper-middle-class college-bound children. Even in fourth grade she was feeling insecure and unable to compete. She masked her insecurity with her bullying behavior, striving for acceptance in sports, where she did have ability. The medical diagnosis was conduct disorder, undersocialized, aggressive. When Suzy's problem was explained to

her parents and the school, some of the pressure for academic achievement was alleviated. Her parents spent extra time helping her with her homework. Also, she was given genuine recognition for her athletic ability, demonstrated by the gift of a new baseball glove. Suzy gradually responded to the positive input from others by developing a sense of positive regard for herself. As she did so, she no longer needed to bully other children and began to grow into some real friendships. ■

Aggressive adults are not unlike Suzy. They try to cover up their insecurities and vulnerabilities by acting aggressive. The behavior is self-defeating because it drives people away, thus reinforcing the low self-esteem and vulnerability to rejection.

Aggressive behavior is also communicated nonverbally. Aggressive people may invade personal space. They may speak loudly and with great emphasis. They usually maintain eye contact over a prolonged period of time so that the other person experiences it as intrusive. Gestures may be emphatic and often seem threatening (for example, they may point their finger, shake their fists, stamp their feet, or make slashing motions with their hands). Posture is erect, and often aggressive people lean forward slightly toward the other person. The overall impression is one of power and dominance. Table 30-1 summarizes the major characteristics of passive, assertive, and aggressive behaviors.

Do you use passive, assertive, or aggressive behaviors most often in your personal life? How does this compare with your behavior in your professional life as a nursing student? ▪

■ THEORIES ON AGGRESSION

It is useful for nurses to view aggressive and violent behavior along a continuum with verbal aggression at one end and physical violence at the other. **Violence is the result of extreme anger (rage) or fear (panic).** Specific reasons for aggressive behavior vary from person to person. Nurses need to communicate with patients to understand the events that they perceive as anger-provoking.

In general, anger occurs in response to a perceived threat. This may be a threat of physical injury or, more often, a threat to the self-concept. When the self is threatened, peo-

Table 30-1	Comparison of Passive, Assertive, and Aggressive Behaviors		
	PASSIVE	**ASSERTIVE**	**AGGRESSIVE**
Content of speech	Negative	Positive	Exaggerated
	Self-derogatory	Self-enhancing	Other-derogatory
	"Can I?" "Will you?"	"I can," "I will"	"You always," "You never"
Tone of voice	Quiet, weak, whining	Modulated	Loud, demanding
Posture	Drooping, bowed head	Erect, relaxed	Tense, leaning forward
Personal space	Allows invasion of space by others	Maintains a comfortable distance; claims right to own space	Invades space of others
Gestures	Minimal, weak gesturing, fidgeting	Demonstrative gestures	Threatening, expansive gestures
Eye contact	Little or none	Intermittent, appropriate to relationship	Constant stare

ple may not be entirely aware of the source of their anger. In this case, the nurse and patient need to work together to identify the nature of the threat.

A threat may be external or internal. Examples of external stressors are physical attack, loss of a significant relationship, and criticism from others. Internal stressors might include a sense of failure at work, perceived loss of love, and fear of physical illness.

Anger is only one of the possible emotional responses to these stressors. Some people might respond with depression or withdrawal. However, those reactions are usually accompanied by anger, which may be difficult for the person to express directly. Depression is sometimes viewed as anger directed toward the self, and withdrawal also may be a passive expression of anger.

Anger often seems out of proportion to the event. An insignificant stressor may be "the last straw" and result in the release of a flood of feelings that have been stored up over time. Nurses need to be aware of this and not personalize anger expressed by a patient. The nurse may seem to be a safer target than significant others with whom the patient also may be angry.

A number of theories on the development of aggressive behavior have influenced the treatment of violent patients. They can be categorized as psychological, sociocultural, and biological. Current thinking in the field suggests that aggressive behavior is the result of the interaction among all three and that each of these factors must be considered when determining nursing care.

Psychological

One psychological view of aggressive behavior suggests the importance of predisposing developmental or life experiences that limit the person's capacity to select nonviolent coping mechanisms. Some of these experiences are listed in Box 30-1. They may limit a person's ability to use supportive relationships, leave the person very self-centered, or make the person particularly vulnerable to a sense of injury that can easily be provoked into rage.

It also has been suggested that a disruption in the mother-infant bonding process can lead to the development of poor interpersonal behavior that may increase the likelihood of vi-

olent behavior. When combined with neurological deficits, the risk of violent behavior is increased.

Figure 30-1 shows how these factors can contribute to an intergenerational transmission of violent behavior. Box 30-2 presents background information about the patient that also may be associated with violence.

Social learning theory proposes that aggressive behavior is learned through the socialization process as a result of internal and external learning. Internal learning occurs through the personal reinforcement received when enacting aggressive behavior. This may be the result of achieving a desired goal or experiencing feelings of importance, power, and control. For example, 4-year-old Johnny wants a cookie just before dinner. When his mother refuses, Johnny has a temper tantrum. If his mother then gives him a cookie, Johnny has learned that an aggressive outburst will be rewarded and he will get what he wants. If similar situations also elicit the desired response, Johnny will continue to use an aggressive approach.

External learning occurs through the observation of role models such as parents, peers, siblings, and sports and entertainment figures. Sociocultural patterns that lead to the imitation of aggressive behavior suggest that violence is an acceptable way of solving problems and achieving social status. According to this view, activities such as violent crime, aggressive sports, and other forms of violence depicted through the media or witnessed in person reinforce aggressive behavior and desensitize the viewers to the consequence of violence (Anderson and Dill, 2000; Miller, 2001).

Sociocultural

Social and cultural factors also may influence aggressive behavior. Cultural norms help define acceptable and unacceptable means of expressing aggressive feelings. Sanctions are applied to violators of the norms through the legal system. By this means, society controls violent behavior and attempts to maintain a safe existence for its members.

Unfortunately, this prohibition against violent behavior also may be extended to include any expression of anger. This can inhibit people from the healthy expression of angry feelings and lead to other maladaptive responses. A cultural

---

BOX 30-1

Developmental Factors Limiting Use of Nonviolent Coping Techniques

- Organic brain damage, mental retardation, or learning disability, which may impair capacity to deal effectively with frustration
- Severe emotional deprivation or overt rejection in childhood, or parental seduction, which may contribute to defects in trust and self-esteem
- Exposure to violence in formative years, either as a victim of child abuse or as an observer of family violence, which may instill a pattern of using violence as a way to cope

---

BOX 30-2

Background Information Associated With Violent Behavior

- Childhood cruelty to animals or other children
- Fire setting or similar dangerous actions
- Recent violent behavior toward self or others
- Recent accidents, threats, or poor judgment in potentially dangerous situations
- Altered states of consciousness
- Escalating irritability, sensitivity, or hostility
- Fear of losing control
- Efforts to obtain help
- Bothering family, neighbors, or police
- History of abuse of alcohol or other disinhibiting substances

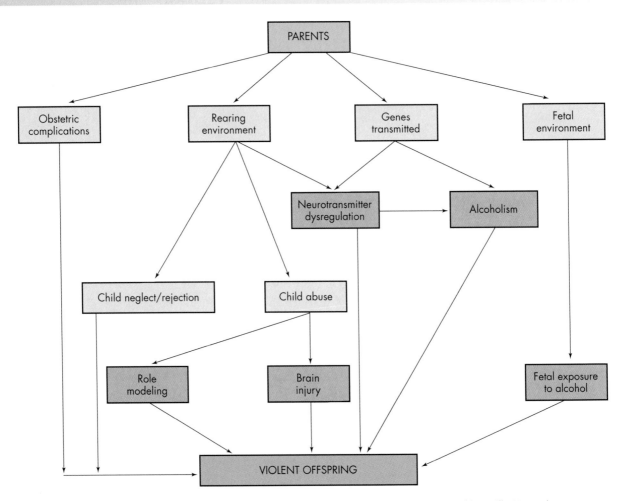

Figure 30-1 Intergenerational transmission of violence. (From Volavka J: *J Neuropsychiatry Clin Neurosci* 2:307, 1999.)

norm that supports verbally assertive expressions of anger will help people deal with anger in a healthy manner. A norm that reinforces violent behavior will result in physical expression of anger in destructive ways.

Finally, a number of studies have attempted to explore the influences of race, culture, economics, and environmental factors on violent behavior. Physical crowding and heat appear to be related to violent behavior. Other social determinants of violence are linked in a cycle and include the following:
- Poverty and the inability to have basic necessities of life
- Disruption of marriages
- Production of single-parent families
- Unemployment
- Difficulty in maintaining interpersonal ties, family structure, and social control

Biological

Current neurobiological research has focused on three areas of the brain believed to be involved in aggression: the limbic system, the frontal lobes, and the hypothalamus (Figure 30-2). Neurotransmitters also have been suggested as having a role in the expression or suppression of aggressive behavior (Niehoff, 2002; Hoptman, 2003). Each of these areas is described in detail in Chapter 6.

The **limbic system** is associated with the mediation of basic drives and the expression of human emotions and behaviors such as eating, aggression, and sexual response. It is also involved in the processing of information and memory. Synthesis of information to and from other areas in the brain influences emotional experience and behavior. Alterations in functioning of the limbic system may result in an increase or decrease in the potential for aggressive behavior. In particular, the amygdala, part of the limbic system, mediates the expression of rage and fear. The surgical removal of this region makes aggressive wild rhesus monkeys docile and lethargic, unable to respond to threats to their safety. Perhaps in those prone to violence, the amygdala may be overresponsive, perceiving threats where there are none.

The **frontal lobes** play an important role in mediating purposeful behavior and rational thinking. They are the part of the brain where reason and emotion interact. Damage to the frontal lobes can result in impaired judgment, personality changes, problems in decision making, inappropriate conduct, and aggressive outbursts.

The **hypothalamus**, at the base of the brain, is the brain's alarm system. Stress raises the level of steroids, the hormones secreted by the adrenal glands. Nerve receptors for these hormones become less sensitive in an attempt to compensate,

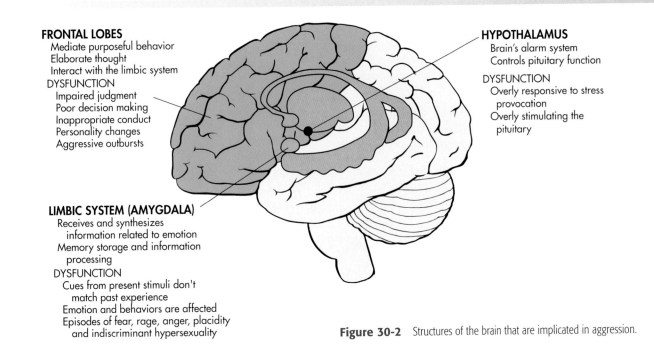

FRONTAL LOBES
  Mediate purposeful behavior
  Elaborate thought
  Interact with the limbic system
DYSFUNCTION
  Impaired judgment
  Poor decision making
  Inappropriate conduct
  Personality changes
  Aggressive outbursts

HYPOTHALAMUS
  Brain's alarm system
  Controls pituitary function
DYSFUNCTION
  Overly responsive to stress
    provocation
  Overly stimulating the
    pituitary

LIMBIC SYSTEM (AMYGDALA)
  Receives and synthesizes
    information related to emotion
  Memory storage and information
    processing
DYSFUNCTION
  Cues from present stimuli don't
    match past experience
  Emotion and behaviors are affected
  Episodes of fear, rage, anger, placidity
    and indiscriminant hypersexuality

Figure 30-2   Structures of the brain that are implicated in aggression.

and the hypothalamus tells the pituitary gland to release more steroids. After repeated stimulation, the system may respond more vigorously to all provocations. That may be one reason why traumatic stress in childhood may permanently enhance one's potential for violence.

Neurotransmitters are brain chemicals that are transmitted to and from neurons across synapses, resulting in communication between brain structures. An increase or decrease in these substances can influence behavior. Changes in the balance of these compounds can aggravate or inhibit aggression.

It has been suggested that low levels of the neurotransmitter serotonin are associated with irritability, hypersensitivity to provocation, and rage. People who commit impulsive arson, suicide, and homicide have lower than average levels of 5-HIAA, the breakdown product of serotonin, in their spinal fluid.

Other neurotransmitters often associated with aggressive behaviors are dopamine, norepinephrine, and acetylcholine, and the amino acid γ-aminobutyric acid (GABA). For example, animal studies indicate that increasing brain dopamine and norepinephrine activity significantly enhances the likelihood that the animal will respond to the environment in an impulsively violent manner.

The prefrontal cortex also may play an important role in inhibiting aggressive behavior. The specific area of the prefrontal cortex known as the orbitofrontal region appears to inhibit aggressive behavior. Stimulation of this area leads to inhibition of anger and aggression whereas lesions lead to impulsive behavior. In a study using mental imagery of aggressive behavior, PET scans revealed a decrease in regional cerebral blood flow in the medial orbitofrontal cortex of violent murderers compared to nonviolent subjects, providing further evidence that this area may play a role in the control of aggression (Pietrini et al, 2000).

Findings related to a gene associated with violent behavior are inconclusive. The evidence on whether men with high testosterone levels are more aggressive or prone to violence than those with moderate levels of testosterone is conflicting. Current understanding of the neurobiology of aggressive behavior is just the beginning; more research is needed on the delicate balance of neurotransmitters and the influence of environmental forces on neurochemistry and brain function.

■ PREDICTING AGGRESSIVE BEHAVIOR

Researchers have tried to determine which patients are more likely to become violent (Swanson et al, 2002). Demographic variables such as age, sex, race, marital status, education, and socioeconomic level have not been useful in predicting violent behavior. In contrast, psychiatric diagnosis has often been correlated with assaultiveness. However, the ability of this variable to predict violence is complicated by the fact that many patients have more than one diagnosis.

In addition, patients may have different clinical symptoms depending on the severity and acuity of their illness. Thus a patient's diagnosis is suggestive of future behavior at best. In general, research indicates that two populations of patients are at increased risk of violence (Soliman and Reza, 2001; Nolan et al, 2003):

- Patients with **active psychotic symptoms.** In particular, those patients who have symptoms related to a perceived threat or an overriding of internal controls, such as delusions of thought control, are at increased risk of committing violence.
- Patients with **substance abuse disorders**. The prevalence of violence is 12 times greater for those with alcohol abuse or dependence and 16 times greater for those with other drug dependence compared with those who have no psychiatric diagnosis. Comorbid substance abuse has an added effect in increasing the risk of violence for people with major psychiatric disorders.

The best single predictor of violence is a history of violence. Research also suggests that perhaps mental illness is not a risk factor for violence at all, and that mentally ill persons who commit acts of violence do so for the same reasons

CITING THE EVIDENCE ON
Patient and Staff Perceptions of Aggression

BACKGROUND: This study examined the views of patients and staff involved in incidents of aggression to help understand emotions experienced, perceptions of causes, and recommendations for ways of reducing the frequency of aggression.

RESULTS: Significant differences were found between staff and patient perceptions of the causes of aggression and ways to reduce it. Many staff members perceived the patient's illness as being the cause of the aggression and believed that, to manage aggression, changes in medication were largely indicated. In contrast, patients perceived illness, interpersonal factors, and environmental factors as being almost equally responsible for their aggression, and nearly all patients emphasized the need for improved staff-patient communication and more flexible unit rules in helping to reduce aggression. Patients and staff were generally satisfied with the way the aggressive incidents were handled, but more staff than patients had an opportunity to debrief.

IMPLICATIONS: Staff and patients had different perceptions of causes of aggression and ways to reduce it. Staff supervision and training should highlight the need for understanding patients' perspectives.

Ilkiw-Lavalle O, Grenyer B: *Psychiatr Serv* 54:389, 2003.

as persons without mental illness who become violent (Stuart and Arboleda-Florez, 2001). In fact, psychopathic and antisocial personality traits are proving to be more predictive of violent behavior than mental illness (Nestor, 2002).

Situational and **environmental factors** also can be important in escalating patient behavior from dangerous to violent. These factors include aspects of the physical facilities and the presence of staff and other patients. Several studies have found that the number of violent incidents is greater when patients move or gather in groups, are overcrowded, lack privacy, or are inactive (Ng et al, 2001).

Clinicians also may intentionally or inadvertently precipitate an outbreak of violence because staff attitudes and actions have a powerful impact on patient behavior (Fagan-Pryor et al, 2003). Inexperienced staff, provocation by staff, poor milieu management, understaffing, close physical encounters, inconsistent limit setting, and a norm of violence may all negatively affect the inpatient environment.

Finally, a patient's **appraisal of a situation** and level of **perceived environmental, cognitive, and communication stress** also affect one's response (see Citing the Evidence). When an environment is interpreted as hostile, the response is likely to be hostile in return. Those suffering from psychiatric illness, substance abuse, past traumatic experiences, or brain damage may have distorted perceptions that can lead to aggressive responses. A model for the development of aggression in inpatient settings that incorporates these various factors is presented in Figure 30-3.

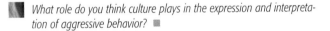

What role do you think culture plays in the expression and interpretation of aggressive behavior? ■

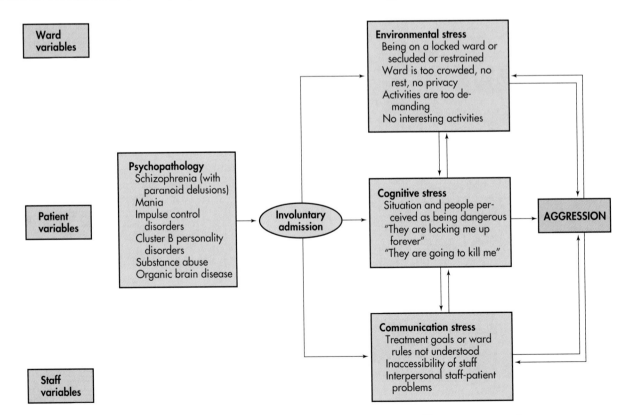

Figure 30-3 Model of inpatient aggression. (From Nijman H et al: *Psychiatr Serv* 50:832, 1999.)

■ NURSING ASSESSMENT

Accurate prediction of patient violence is not possible. For this reason, it is important for psychiatric nurses to be alert for symptoms of increasing agitation that could lead to violent behavior (Box 30-3).

Using a hierarchy of aggressive behaviors (Figure 30-4) in which lower levels of aggression may lead to more violent behavior may be helpful in evaluating patients. Some of these early behaviors include **motor agitation** such as pacing, inability to sit still, clenching or pounding fists, and tightening of jaw or facial muscles. **Verbal clues** also may be present, such as threats to real or imagined objects or intrusive demands for attention. Speech may be loud and pressured, and posture may become threatening.

Another critical factor in the assessment of a potentially violent patient is the **affect** associated with escalating behaviors. Anger often is seen in patients who are imminently violent. Inappropriate euphoria, irritability, and lability in affect may indicate that a patient is having difficulty in maintaining control. **Changes in level of consciousness**, including confusion, disorientation, and memory impairment, also may be an indication of future violent behavior.

In summary, psychiatric nurses should carefully assess all patients for their potential for violence. A screening or assessment tool such as the one presented in Figure 30-5 can be useful. Once completed, a violence assessment tool can help the nurse:

- Establish a therapeutic alliance with the patient.
- Assess a patient's potential for violence.
- Develop a plan of care.
- Implement the plan of care.
- Prevent aggression and violence in the milieu.

Following the assessment, if the patient is believed to be potentially violent, the nurse should:

- Implement the appropriate clinical protocol to provide for patient and staff safety.
- Notify co-workers.
- Obtain additional security if needed.
- Assess the environment and make necessary changes.
- Notify the physician and assess the need for prn medications.

BOX **30-3**

Behaviors Associated With Aggression

Motor Agitation
Pacing
Inability to sit still
Clenching or pounding fists
Jaw tightening
Increased respirations
Sudden cessation of motor activity (catatonia)

Verbalizations
Verbal threats toward real or imagined objects
Intrusive demands for attention
Loud, pressured speech
Evidence of delusional or paranoid thought content

Affect
Anger
Hostility
Extreme anxiety
Irritability
Inappropriate or excessive euphoria
Affect lability

Level of Consciousness
Confusion
Sudden change in mental status
Disorientation
Memory impairment
Inability to be redirected

■ NURSING INTERVENTIONS

The nurse can implement a variety of interventions to prevent and manage aggressive behavior. These interventions can be thought of as existing on a continuum (Figure 30-6). They range from **preventive strategies** such as self-awareness, patient education, and assertiveness training to **anticipatory strategies** such as verbal and nonverbal communication, environmental changes, behavioral interventions, and the use of medications. If the patient's aggressive behavior escalates despite these actions, the nurse may need to implement crisis management techniques and **containment strategies** such as seclusion or restraints.

Self-Awareness

The most valuable resource of a nurse is the ability to use one's self to help others. To ensure the most effective use of self, it is important to be aware of personal stress that can interfere with one's ability to communicate therapeutically with patients. If the nurse is tired, anxious, angry, or apa-

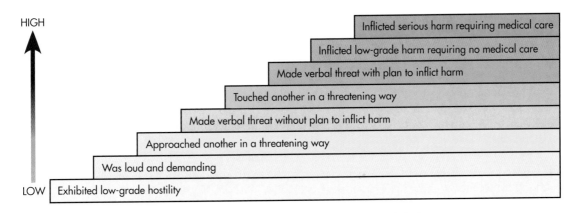

Figure 30-4 Hierarchy of aggressive and violent patient behaviors.

ASSAULT AND VIOLENCE ASSESSMENT TOOL

Description: This tool is used if a patient
                 a. Has a history of violence
                 b. Is currently threatening violence
                 c. Was threatening violence at the time of the referral

Directions: a. Assess each key factor.
                 b. Circle one (of three) descriptor for each factor that best describes the patient.
                 c. Add the points for each circled item to obtain the total score.

Key Factors	High Risk	Moderate Risk	No Precautions
History of Violence	Any single episode of violence with injury to others while hospitalized -OR- Multiple assaults with injury while outside hospital 2	Destruction of property without injury to others while in hospital -OR- A single assault outside the hospital resulting in injury -OR- Multiple assaults outside the hospital not resulting in injury 1	Violence only when using drugs or alcohol -OR- Destruction of property outside hospital -OR- No history of violence 0
History of Recent Aggression	Physically threatening at time of referral/admission 2	Verbally threatening at time of referral/admission 1	Nonthreatening at time of referral/admission 0
History of Aggression in Family of Origin	Victim or perpetrator of physical or sexual abuse 2	Witness of physical or sexual abuse 1	Witness or victim of verbal aggression -OR- No history of aggression in family 0
Substance Abuse Status	Recent alcohol/substance abuse actively detoxing -OR- Currently under the influence of alcohol or drugs 2	Recent substance/alcohol abuse with absence of withdrawal symptoms 1	Rehabilitated abuser -OR- No history of alcohol/substance abuse -OR- Past history (>3 months ago) alcohol/substance abuse with no rehabilitation 0
Paranoia/Hostility	Paranoia or hostility generalized to people in the immediate environment 2	Paranoia or hostility generalized toward inaccessible people 1	No apparent paranoia No apparent hostility 0
Impulsivity	Physically impulsive 2	Verbally impulsive -OR- History of physical impulsivity 1	No apparent impulsivity 0
Agitation	Psychomotor agitation with constant pressured physical activity 2	Psychomotor agitation with intermittent bursts of hyperactivity 1	No apparent psychomotor agitation 0
Sensorium	Disoriented with impaired memory 2	Oriented with impaired memory 1	Oriented with intact memory 0

Scoring Key   9 or more   =   High-risk precautions

                 3-8   =   Moderate-risk precautions

                 0-2   =   No precautions

Total Score: _____

Assessed by (RN): _____

Date: _____

Time: _____

Figure 30-5   Assault and violence assessment tool.

thetic, it will be difficult to convey an interest in the concerns and fears of the patient. If the nurse is overwhelmed with personal or work problems, the energy available for patients is greatly reduced.

When dealing with potentially aggressive patients, it is important to be able to assess the situation objectively despite the positive or negative countertransference that might be present. **Countertransference** is an emotional reaction of the nurse to some aspect or behavior of the patient (see Chapter 2). Negative countertransference reactions may lead to nontherapeutic responses on the part of the staff (Rossberg and Friis, 2003). Ongoing self-awareness and supervision can assist the nurse in ensuring that patient needs, rather than personal needs, are addressed.

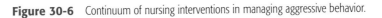

Preventive Strategies   **Anticipatory Strategies**   **Containment Strategies**

Self-awareness   Communication   Crisis management
Patient education   Environmental change   Seclusion
Assertiveness training   Behavioral actions   Restraints
                                Psychopharmacology

Figure 30-6   Continuum of nursing interventions in managing aggressive behavior.

Table 30-2   PATIENT EDUCATION PLAN   Appropriate Expression of Anger

CONTENT	INSTRUCTIONAL ACTIVITIES	EVALUATION
Help the patient identify anger.	Focus on nonverbal behavior. Role play nonverbal expression of anger. Label the feeling using the patient's preferred words.	Patient demonstrates an angry body posture and facial expression.
Give permission for angry feelings.	Describe situations in which it is normal to feel angry.	Patient describes a situation in which anger would be an appropriate response.
Practice the expression of anger.	Role play fantasized situations in which anger is an appropriate response.	Patient participates in role play and identifies behaviors associated with expression of anger.
Apply the expression of anger to a real situation.	Help identify a real situation that makes the patient angry. Role play a confrontation with the object of the anger. Provide positive feedback for successful expression of anger.	Patient identifies a real situation that results in anger. Patient is able to role play expression of anger.
Identify alternative ways to express anger.	List several ways to express anger, with and without direct confrontation. Role play alternative behaviors. Discuss situations in which alternatives would be appropriate.	Patient participates in identifying alternatives and plans when each might be useful.
Confrontation with a person who is a source of anger.	Provide support during confrontation if needed. Discuss experience after confrontation takes place.	Patient identifies the feeling of anger and appropriately confronts the object of the anger.

Patient Education

Teaching patients about communication and the appropriate way to express anger can be one of the most successful interventions in preventing aggressive behavior (see Patient Education Plan, Table 30-2). Many patients have difficulty identifying their feelings, needs, and desires and even more difficulty communicating these to others. Thus teaching health anger management skills is an important area of nursing intervention (Thomas, 2001; Chan et al, 2003).

Teaching patients that feelings are not right or wrong or good or bad can allow them to explore feelings that may have been bottled up, ignored, or repressed. The nurse can then work with patients on ways to express their feelings and eval-uate whether the responses they select are adaptive or maladaptive. Providing patients with available choices in managing anger, such as those listed in Box 30-4, may be effective in reducing more restrictive interventions.

Assertiveness Training

Teaching assertive communication skills is an important nursing intervention (see Chapter 31). Interpersonal frustrations often escalate to aggressive behavior because patients have not mastered the assertive behaviors. Assertive behavior is a basic interpersonal skill that includes the following:

- Communicating directly with another person
- Saying no to unreasonable requests

BOX 30-4

Ways To Manage Anger

- Positive self-talk
- Change of environment
- Writing about your feelings
- Thinking of the consequences
- Listening to music
- Watching television
- Deep breathing exercises
- Taking a walk

- Counting to 50
- Comfort wrap with a blanket
- Relaxation exercises
- Talking about your feelings
- Using adaptive coping skills
- Reading
- Being alone
- Medication

- Being able to state complaints
- Expressing appreciation as appropriate

Patients with few assertive skills can learn them by participating in structured groups and programs. In these settings patients can watch staff demonstrate specific skills and then role play the skills themselves. Staff can provide feedback to patients on the appropriateness and effectiveness of their responses. Homework also can be assigned to patients to help them generalize these skills outside the group milieu. Aggressive behaviors may diminish as the patient learns new and more effective social skills.

How can a nurse who has difficulty being assertive with peers and interdisciplinary colleagues effectively teach assertiveness skills to patients? ■

Communication Strategies

The psychiatric nurse often can prevent a crisis situation through the use of early verbal and nonverbal intervention. This is sometimes called "talking the patient down." Because it is much less dangerous to prevent a crisis than to respond to one, every effort should be made to carefully monitor patients who are at risk for violent behavior and intervene at the first possible sign of increasing agitation.

It is important for nurses to notice the early verbal and behavioral signs indicating that a patient is becoming increasingly agitated. By understanding where a patient may be on the continuum of escalation and the meaning of the patient's behavior, they can assess the potential danger and provide the necessary intervention to assist the patient to deescalate (Johnson and Hauser, 2001; Chabora, Judge-Gorny, and Grogan, 2003). Strengthening the therapeutic alliance is an important part of this process.

Speaking in a calm, low voice can help decrease a patient's agitation. Agitated patients often speak loudly and use profanity. It is important that nurses not raise their voices in response because this can be perceived as competition and further escalate the volatile situation. The nurse should use short, simple sentences and avoid laughing or smiling inappropriately.

The nurse also can help reduce a rising level of agitation by acknowledging the patient's feelings and reassuring the patient that the staff is there to help. The importance of allowing the patient to communicate his or her concerns without

interruption and engaging the patient's participation in treatment decisions cannot be overemphasized.

In a survey of 59 mental health consumers, the importance of being treated with respect by staff members, being listened to, and being included in treatment decisions was strongly emphasized. Of these patients, 74% stated that they would like to complete an advance directive if given the opportunity (Allen et al, 2003).

Psychiatric advance directives can provide staff with strategies to assist a patient in the event that he or she becomes unable to participate in treatment decisions (see Chapter 10). Whenever possible, collaboration with patients is important not only to minimize further trauma to the patient but also to decrease the chances that the patient may respond in an angry or aggressive manner.

It is also important that the nurse communicate expected behavior in a way that encourages the patient to maintain control of any violent impulses. At this early stage some patients, with encouragement, may be willing to remove themselves from an overstimulating environment, thus facilitating their self-control.

The specific nonverbal communication used by the nurse also can greatly affect the outcome of the intervention. A calm and relaxed posture that does not tower over the patient is much less intimidating than a posture in which hands are placed on the hips and the nurse looms over the patient. Crossing the arms across the chest is another posture that communicates emotional distance and an unwillingness to help.

The nurse's hands should be kept open and out of pockets. Threatening, nervous, and sudden gestures should be avoided. Altering position so that the nurse's eyes are at the same level as those of the patient allows the patient to communicate from an equal rather than inferior position.

The nurse should assume a supportive stance that is at least one leg length or 3 feet from the patient. It is helpful if the nurse remains at an angle to the patient and the patient's need for personal space is respected. It has been noted that violence-prone people need 4 times more personal space than nonviolence-prone people. Intrusion into a patient's personal space can be perceived as a threat and provoke aggression.

Finally, when approaching potentially violent patients, nurses should carefully observe their behavior. Clenched fists, tightening of the facial muscles, and movement away from the nurse may suggest that the patient is feeling threatened. The nurse should respond by giving the patient as much distance as possible. These communication strategies are summarized in Box 30-5.

Why do you think that standing at an angle to the patient is less threatening than facing the patient full face? Try the two stances with a friend and describe your feelings about each one. ■

Environmental Strategies

Violent behavior is more likely to occur in a poorly structured milieu with undefined program rules and a great deal of unscheduled time for patients. Inpatient units that provide many productive activities reduce the chance of inappropriate patient behavior and increase adaptive social and leisure functioning. Both the unit norms and the rewards associated with such activities may reduce the amount of disorganized patient behavior and the number of aggressive acts.

In contrast, units that are overly structured with too much stimulation and little regard for the privacy needs of patients may increase aggressive behavior. For example, some psychiatric hospitals have patients eat in dining rooms that are crowded during mealtimes. Other hospital units restrict patients to a central day room to allow for better observation by staff and minimize patient isolation. In such situations, often only one television is provided and sometimes only one patient telephone is available. For patients who lose much of their privacy when they are admitted to a psychiatric unit, the lack of personal privacy and loss of control over their lives can foster anger and hostility when their ability to cope is already challenged.

Aggressive behavior may be more effectively managed by allowing those at risk to spend time in their rooms away from the hectic day room rather than encouraging them to interact with others in a crowded milieu. The environment that may have been therapeutic in the days of extended hospital stays may no longer be suitable for patients who are hospitalized on short-term, acute inpatient units where the acuity of the patients is extremely high. Inpatient units should adapt the environment to best meet the needs of the patients they treat. The impact of the environment is seen in the following clinical example.

CLINICAL EXAMPLE

Mr. T was a 36-year-old man who was admitted for the third time to an acute care unit at a state psychiatric hospital. His medical diagnosis was bipolar disorder, manic. The nursing staff was apprehensive because the patient had a history of assaultive behavior on earlier admissions. At the time of this admission, the unit atmosphere was tense because one of the other patients had made a suicide attempt requiring emergency room treatment.

Mr. I was Mr. T's primary nurse from his previous admission. He was working when the patient arrived on the unit. During the nursing assessment, Mr. I discussed the nursing interventions that had seemed to be helpful in the past. He validated with Mr. T that he was usually able to maintain control of his behavior by participating in a structured physical activity when he was feeling upset. In addition, he recalled that the patient would begin to pace rapidly and sing when he was losing control. Mr. T agreed with these observations.

Mr. T responded very quickly to the tension on the unit. He began to pace up and down the hall and sing in a moderately loud tone of voice. Other patients also began to show signs of increased agitation. The nursing staff held a brief consultation. They decided that the charge nurse would gather the patients for a community meeting to discuss their feelings about the suicide attempt. Meanwhile, Mr. I would take Mr. T for a walk with one of the other staff.

The interventions were successful. More intensive nursing actions were not needed. ■

Room Program. In an inpatient setting, the use of a structured room program is an effective tool for the management

BOX 30-5

Communication Strategies Used To Prevent Aggressive Behavior

- Present a calm appearance.
- Speak softly.
- Speak in a nonprovocative and nonjudgmental manner.
- Speak in a neutral and concrete way.
- Put space between yourself and the patient.
- Show respect for the patient.
- Avoid intense direct eye contact.
- Demonstrate control over the situation without assuming an overly authoritarian stance.
- Facilitate the patient's talking.
- Listen to the patient.
- Avoid early interpretations.
- Do not make promises you cannot keep.

of agitated patients. A room program limits the amount of time patients are allowed in the unit milieu. For example, patients initially may be asked to stay in their rooms for a certain length of time, or conversely be allowed out of their rooms for a specific amount of time every hour. The amount of time in the milieu may then be increased by increments of 15 minutes as patients tolerate the environment.

Another way of implementing a room program is to allow patients to come out of their rooms during certain designated hours, such as when the unit is quiet or when other patients are off the unit. Such a structured program allows patients time away from situations that may increase agitation and provides a way to regulate the amount of stimulation patients receive. Its purpose is the prevention of a crisis that could result in more serious patient complications.

Cathartic Activities. Many clinicians support the use of cathartic activities as a way of helping patients deal with their anger and agitation. These can be of two types: physically cathartic and emotionally cathartic.

The first type is based on the assumption that some physical activity can be useful in releasing aggression and can prevent more explosive or destructive forms of aggression or violence. However, research suggests that aggressive behavior exists on a continuum and that minor manifestations of aggression can lead to further aggressive behavior (Bushman, Baumeister, and Stack, 1999).

Thus the evidence challenges the effectiveness of physically cathartic activities and calls into question some traditional nursing interventions, such as encouraging patients to release tension through the use of exercise equipment or allowing patients to pace the halls in the expectation that their tension will decrease. Because these strategies are not supported by research and may increase the patient's potential for aggressive behavior, they are not recommended nursing actions. This is also an excellent example of the way in which nursing evidence can challenge traditional nursing interventions and help psychiatric nurses base their practice on empirical data rather than commonly held but untested assumptions.

In contrast, there is support for emotionally cathartic activities. Having patients write about their feelings, do deep breathing or relaxation exercise, or talk about their emotions with a supportive person can help the patient regain control and lower feelings of tension and agitation.

Behavioral Strategies

Nursing interventions include applying principles of behavior management to the aggressive patient. These are described in detail in Chapter 31. Effective limit setting is one of the most basic interventions in this area.

Limit Setting. Limit setting is a nonpunitive, nonmanipulative act in which the patient is told what behavior is acceptable, what is not acceptable, and the consequences of behaving unacceptably. By explaining the rationale for the limit and communicating to the patient in a calm and respectful manner, potentially aggressive behavior can be avoided. When nursing staff communicate in an authoritarian, parental, controlling, or disrespectful way, patients are more likely to respond in an angry, aggressive manner.

The nurse does not assume responsibility for the patient's behavior, adaptive or maladaptive. It is recognized that the patient has the right to choose a behavior and understands its consequences. Limits should be clarified before negative consequences are applied.

Once a limit has been identified, the consequences must take place if the behavior occurs. Every staff member must be aware of the plan and carry it out consistently. If staff do not do so, the patient is likely to manipulate staff by acting out and then pointing out areas of inconsistent limit setting. Clear, firm, and nonpunitive enforcement of limits is the goal.

It is also important for nurses to understand that when limit setting is implemented, the maladaptive behavior will not immediately decrease; in fact, it may briefly increase. This is consistent with behavioral principles and testing behavior. If staff understand the dynamics of this intervention, they will be able to implement this strategy effectively and understand that patient behavior will eventually change.

Behavioral Contracts. If a patient uses violence to win control and make personal gains, the nursing care must be planned to eliminate the rewards the patient receives while still allowing the patient to assume as much control as possible. Once the rewards are understood, nursing care can be planned that does not reinforce aggressive and violent behavior. Behavioral contracts with the patient can be helpful in this regard. For example, head-injured patients with low impulse control can be told that staff will take them for a walk if they can refrain from using profanity for 4 hours.

To be effective, contracts require detailed information about the following:

- Unacceptable behaviors
- Acceptable behaviors
- Consequences for breaking the contract
- The nurse's contribution to care

Patients also should have input into the development of the contract to increase their sense of self-control. This negotiated process increases the mutuality of the therapeutic alliance and reduces the possibility of aggressive behavior.

Time-Out. In an inpatient setting, the use of time-out can be an effective tool for the management of agitated patients. It is a strategy that can decrease the need for seclusion and restraint. Time-out from reinforcement is a behavioral technique in which socially inappropriate behaviors can be decreased by short-term removal of the patient from overstimulating and sometimes reinforcing situations.

Patients who appear to be escalating are prompted to enter time-out, which is usually a quiet, low-traffic area of the unit or the patients' room. They remain there until they have been nonaggressive for a couple of minutes. Time-out allows the patient time away from a stimulating environment to regain control of himself or herself. Time-out may be initiated by the patient or by the staff. It is not considered to be seclusion and therefore is not subject to the regulations required for seclusion.

In time-out the patient is allowed out of the time-out area when he or she is able to remain calm. Patients determine their own readiness to leave the time-out area. If the patient is prevented from leaving the area for any reason, this intervention then becomes seclusion and is subject to the monitoring, documentation, and evaluation required of seclusion.

Token Economy. Another effective behavioral strategy is the implementation of a token economy. In this intervention, identified interpersonal skills and self-care behaviors are rewarded with tokens that can be used by the patient to buy items or receive rewards or privileges.

Behaviors to be targeted are specific to each patient. Guidelines should clearly specify desired behaviors required to receive tokens, the number of tokens to be received for each behavior, and the length of time a desired behavior must be exhibited to receive tokens. In a token economy, undesired behaviors can result in the loss of tokens.

Research has shown that inpatient units that have implemented token economies have significantly fewer aggressive episodes than more traditional settings (LePage, 1999). This strategy for managing aggressive behavior is particularly useful with chronic lower-functioning patient populations. The following clinical example describes the use of this intervention.

CLINICAL EXAMPLE

A regressed patient, Ms. S, refused to get out of bed in the morning. She would not shower, dress, or wash her clothes. When encouraged to do these things, Ms. S became agitated, swore, and threatened to hit anyone who tried to help her. A token store was set up with the number of tokens required to purchase each item. Under her contract, Ms. S would receive two tokens for each of the following behaviors:

- Getting out of bed by 7:30 AM
- Showering before 8:00 AM
- Dressing before 8:00 AM

- Being at the breakfast table by 8:15 AM
- Eating 100% of the food on her breakfast tray by 8:45 AM
- Arriving at the community meeting by 9:00 AM

Her contract also included the following penalty:

- An episode of swearing will result in the loss of 4 tokens. ■

Psychopharmacology

Pharmacological interventions have proven effective in the management of aggressive behavior (Allen et al, 2003). They include a variety of therapeutic agents, all of which are discussed in greater detail in Chapter 27.

Patients should be given the option of an oral medication whenever possible. Liquid formulations are preferred because of their more rapid onset and increased ability to verify that the patient did indeed swallow the medication. Intramuscular injections may increase the risk of side effects as well as trauma to the patient.

Antianxiety and Sedative-Hypnotics. These drugs are effective in the management of acute agitation. Benzodiazepines such as lorazepam are often used during psychiatric emergencies to sedate combative patients. Lorazepam in particular is frequently used because of its quick onset and because it can be administered either orally or intramuscularly.

Antianxiety medications are not recommended for long-term use because they can result in confusion and dependency and may worsen depressive symptoms. Most importantly, some patients experience a disinhibiting effect from benzodiazepines that can result in increased impulsive and aggressive behavior.

Buspirone, an antianxiety drug that may be effective in the management of aggressive behavior associated with anxiety and depression, also has een shown to decrease aggression and agitation in patients with head injuries, dementia, and developmental disabilities.

Antidepressants. The selective serotonin reuptake inhibitors (SSRIs) appear to reduce the risk of violence associated with posttraumatic stress.

Mood Stabilizers. Valproate is effective in the treatment of aggression resulting from mania. Lithium is also useful in decreasing aggression resulting from mania and other disorders such as mental retardation, head injuries, schizophrenia, and personality disorders, and in children with conduct disorder. In patients with temporal lobe epilepsy, lithium may actually increase the frequency of aggressive acts. Carbamazepine has been shown to be effective in managing aggressive behavior in patients with abnormal electroencephalograms (EEGs). Some evidence also indicates that carbamazepine may be effective in managing agitated behavior associated with dementia.

Antipsychotics. These drugs are often used for the treatment of aggression. The most common medication strategy for managing violent patients in a psychiatric emergency is the high potency typical antipsychotic haloperidol, in combination with the benzodiazepine lorazepam. Both medications are considered effective for decreasing agitation and both can be given by injection with a quick onset of action. Droperidol is also highly effective in decreasing agitation. It acts quickly and effectively to calm violent patients.

Patients given typical antipsychotics should be assessed for the occurrence of acute neuroleptic-induced akathisia, which can appear as worsening of agitation and acute dystonic reaction. This complication can be frightening and uncomfortable for patients.

Atypical antipsychotics are also used often to manage potentially violent behavior. They are less likely to cause extrapyramidal side effects. Recent data show that the liquid concentrate of risperidone plus lorazepam may be just as effective as intramuscular (IM) haloperidol plus lorazepam. In addition, the atypical antipsychotics olanzapine and ziprasidone are available in IM formulations. Finally, the atypical antipsychotics clozapine and risperidone may be effective not only for patients with schizophrenia but also for people with dementia, brain injuries, and mental retardation.

Other Medications. Several case reports have suggested that naltrexone, an opiate antagonist, may reduce self-injurious behavior. This effect is particularly notable in patients with developmental disabilities.

β-blockers such as propranolol also have been shown to decrease aggressive behavior in children and adults and particularly in patients with organic mental disorder. Nurses should be aware of the side effects of β-blockers including hypotension, bradycardia, and in some cases depression.

Psychostimulants are used to treat aggressive behavior in children with attention deficit/hyperactivity disorder (ADHD). Lithium and the atypical antipsychotics are more effective than stimulants in the treatment of aggression in children and adolescents with conduct disorders.

How do the strategies for managing aggressive behavior relate to the theories of aggression described earlier in this chapter? ■

■ CRISIS MANAGEMENT TECHNIQUES

At times early interventions are unsuccessful and more active intervention is necessary. Experience and wisdom are needed to determine when verbal and other less restrictive interventions may be unsuccessful. Nonviolent physical control and restraint should be used only as a last resort. Like medical emergencies, psychiatric emergencies require immediate action.

Team Response

Effective crisis management must be organized and should be directed by one clearly identified crisis leader (Box 30-6). Because psychiatric nurses are responsible for the management of patient care 24 hours a day, it is most appropriate that the crisis leader be a nurse. The leader may be the charge nurse, the primary nurse, nurse manager, or a staff nurse; however, the person designated as the leader should be chosen in advance. Other staff members, including physicians, nurses, and counselors, can provide support. The crisis leader must decide the intervention necessary to ensure the safety of both patients and staff. The decision can be a difficult one to make, especially when the acuity of the situation does not always allow adequate time to discuss all possible strategies with the entire treatment team.

Once the decision to intervene has been made, the crisis leader must obtain assistance to manage the crisis. All members of the crisis team should be trained in crisis management and have experience working as a cohesive group. The staff should be prepared to intervene under the direction of the crisis leader.

In many inpatient facilities, hospital security personnel are also notified when assistance is needed. It is the responsibility of the crisis leader to be acquainted with the security officers, give them a brief description of the situation, describe the intervention, and identify the role of security personnel in managing the crisis. Because security officers are not mental health professionals, their assistance should be used only when the patient cannot be physically managed by the nursing staff. Often there is little time for planning, and the leader must balance the need to act quickly with the need to be organized so that the safety of the patients and staff is not jeopardized.

The leader is also responsible for ensuring the safety of the other patients during a crisis. This can be accomplished by assigning a staff member to remove the other patients from the area. Quite often other patients become more acutely distressed in response to a psychiatric emergency on the unit and require extra nursing attention both during and after the crisis. After the crisis has passed, allowing patients to verbalize their anxiety and concern about the crisis and processing it with them can be helpful. It is not appropriate to encourage this activity during a crisis intervention.

A room without furniture should always be readily available for an emergency. If restraints are necessary, they must be obtained from an easily accessible place. To protect the patient and staff, the leader must assess the situation quickly and devise a plan. This plan should include a brief explanation to the staff of the patient's behavior and the intervention necessary.

Staff members who will be directly involved in the intervention should each be assigned to secure one of the patient's limbs when directed to do so. The leader must also explain to the team what will be said to the patient and on what signal the staff should secure the patient's limbs. As the group approaches within 6 to 8 feet of the patient, the leader should express concern for the patient's safety and the behavior demonstrated that has caused such concern. The patient should then be escorted to the appropriate room and informed of the necessary intervention. It should be emphasized that the intervention is not a punishment but is being provided to help ensure the safety of the patient and the rest of the unit.

If restraints are to be used, the patient should be asked to lie on the bed with arms at his or her side. Quite often the presence of several staff is enough to enlist the patient's cooperation. If the patient is unable to cooperate, the patient should be told that the staff will be assisting. Patients often hesitate at this point in their attempt to remain in control. If patients cannot cooperate within several seconds, they may be unable to cooperate at all, and the leader must then direct the staff to restrain the patient as planned. This can be very frightening for patients, and they may need several reminders that they will not be hurt but that the staff will protect them from their impulses.

During this time it is critically important that the leader relate to the patient in a calm, steady voice and manner. Any anxiety or ambivalence will be conveyed to the patient and contribute to a feeling of insecurity. A leader who is anxious will be unable to think clearly about the situation. Many patients are afraid of losing control, and they become assaultive not because they want to frighten people but because they themselves are frightened.

If the staff shows control of the situation, the patient's agitation is often defused. When the crisis team is overwhelmed by their own fears of the patient, they cannot be effective in reducing the patient's fear. Consistency is also important so that the patient cannot bargain with or manipulate staff members. If the leader is indecisive, inconsistent, or easily manipulated, the patient will not be assured that the staff can guarantee safety by controlling the situation.

After the crisis is over, the team should discuss any concerns they may have had during the crisis because this type of intervention can be stressful for both staff and patients. The patient's behavior may have evoked feelings of guilt, anger, or aggression in the staff. These issues should be discussed as a team so that care is consistent, interventions are therapeutic, and staff do not become discouraged, negative, or burned out. Ongoing reevaluation of the patient's status and gradual reintegration of the patient into the milieu is important as soon as the patient is no longer a danger to self or others.

BOX **30-6**

Procedure for Managing Psychiatric Emergencies

- Identify crisis leader.
- Assemble crisis team.
- Notify security officers if necessary.
- Remove all other patients from area.
- Obtain restraints if appropriate.
- Devise a plan to manage crisis and inform team.
- Assign securing of patient limbs to crisis team members.
- Explain necessity of intervention to patient and attempt to enlist cooperation.
- Restrain patient when directed by crisis leader.
- Administer medication if ordered.
- Maintain calm, consistent approach to patient.
- Review crisis management interventions with crisis team.
- Process events with other patients and staff as appropriate.
- Process event with the patient.
- Gradually reintegrate patient into milieu.

Seclusion and Restraints

Seclusion is the involuntary confining of a person alone in a room from which the person is physically prevented from leaving (Brown, 2000). It is one of the most restrictive interventions used in psychiatric facilities and is viewed as a negative experience by most patients.

Although numerous articles have been written on the subject of seclusion and restraints, no evidence has shown that seclusion has therapeutic value other than as a last resort to ensure safety (Sailas and Fenton, 2002; Horsfall and Cleary, 2003). The evidence does suggest, however, that seclusion and restraints may actually cause further trauma and harm to patients who have often suffered significant physical and psychological trauma in the past (Cusack et al, 2003; Oberleitner, 2000; Mohr and Mohr, 2000; Finke, 2001).

Physical restraints are any manual method or physical or mechanical device attached to or adjacent to the patient's body that he or she cannot easily remove and that restricts freedom of movement or normal access to one's body, material, or equipment (Brown, 2000). Chemical restraints are medications used to restrict the patient's freedom of movement or for emergency control of behavior, but it is not a standard treatment for the patient's medical or psychiatric condition (Murphy, 2002). Medications are often considered to be a less invasive alternative to the use of physical restraints, but both are practices that must be implemented with caution (see Critical Thinking About Contemporary Issues).

Critical Thinking *About* Contemporary Issues

Are Chemical Restraints Less "Restraining" Than Physical Restraints?

Although there is some lack of agreement about what constitutes "chemical restraint," the concern regarding the use of forced or involuntary medications in psychiatric practice is clear. No national data exists related to the frequency with which chemical restraint is used in psychiatric emergencies, but it is believed to be a widespread occurrence (Currier, 2003). Similarly, little literature about the topic is available to assist health care workers with clinical decision making. Some even believe that any medication that is taken orally is a voluntary form of treatment, regardless of the amount of influence exerted by the staff.

Recent federal regulations, however, equate chemical and physical restraint and treat them in the same way. Concerning the use of medications, the main focus of these regulations involves the distinction between whether they are used as treatments or as chemical restraints. This distinction hinges on whether the medications are given as part of a documented plan of care or are used solely to control behavior. These regulations emphasize that restraints of any kind can be used only after less restrictive interventions have been ineffective. They may not be used as a coercive measure for a patient refusing treatment because it is within the rights of a competent patient to refuse treatment (see Chapter 10). Given the frequency with which forced medication occurs, more research is needed to understand the use and abuse of this intervention.

Because seclusion and restraints represent restriction of patient freedom and can result in harm to both the patient and the staff who implement them, they should be used only as an emergency intervention to ensure the safety of the patient or others and only when other less restrictive interventions have been ineffective. They are a violation of patient rights if used as a means of coercion, discipline, or convenience of staff (Brown, 2000).

The use of seclusion and restraints received national attention in October 1998 after a series of articles published in the Hartford Courant newspaper documented 142 deaths related to the use of seclusion and restraints in psychiatric units, group homes, and residential facilities. Consumer advocacy groups, members of Congress, and professional organizations became active in the debate about the need for regulation or legislation regarding the use of restraints and seclusion.

In 1999 the Centers for Medicare and Medicaid Services (CMS), formerly the Health Care Financing Administration (HCFA), implemented the new Patients' Rights Condition of Participation regulations for hospitals that treat Medicare patients. Under the new Patients' Rights Condition of Participation, all hospital staff who have direct contact with patients are required to have ongoing education and training in the proper use of seclusion and restraints and alternative interventions to avoid the use of seclusion and restraints.

CMS also requires that a physician or other licensed independent practitioner evaluate the patient's need for seclusion and restraints within 1 hour after the initiation of this intervention. Under the new condition, restraints can be ordered for a maximum of 4 hours for adults, 2 hours for adolescents ages 9 to 17, and 1 hour for children under age 9. Orders may be renewed for 24 hours before another face to face evaluation is necessary by a physician or licensed independent practitioner.

In addition, the new condition requires continual assessment, monitoring, and reevaluation of patients in restraints or seclusion. For patients who are both restrained and secluded, the condition requires that the patient be constantly monitored face to face or by both audio and video equipment.

It also states that patients must be released from seclusion or restraints as soon as possible. The Joint Commission on Accreditation of Healthcare Organizations (JCAHO), the organization which monitors hospitals that voluntarily request their review, also developed standards regarding the use of seclusion and restraints (JCAHO, 1996). In order to ensure that hospitals continue to decrease the use of seclusion and restraints, the JCAHO requires that seclusion and restraint be included as a performance improvement priority (Kozub and Skidmore, 2001).

It has been noted that nonclinical factors, such as cultural biases, staff role perceptions, and the attitude of hospital administration, have a great influence on rates of seclusion and restraint. Facilities that have been successful in decreasing the use of seclusion and restraint have included top-level administrative support, involvement from consumers of mental health services, and a change in culture, staff education, data analysis, and individualized treatment (American Psychiatric Nurses Association, 2003; Donat, 2003; Fisher, 2003).

Seclusion. Degrees of seclusion vary. They include confining a patient in a room with a closed but unlocked door or placing a patient in a locked room with a mattress but no linens and with limited opportunity for communication. Patients may be dressed in their clothes or in hospital clothing. A mattress and sheet or blanket are the minimally acceptable conditions for seclusion.

The rationale for the use of seclusion is based on three therapeutic principles:

- Containment
- Isolation
- Decrease in sensory input

Using the principle of **containment**, patients are restricted to a place where they are safe from harming themselves and other patients. **Isolation** addresses the need for patients to distance themselves from relationships that, because of the illness, are pathologically intense. Some patients, particularly those with paranoia, distort the meaning of the interactions around them. Their distortions create such psychic pain that seclusion may provide some relief and may be the only place they feel safe from their "persecutors." The third principle is that seclusion provides a **decrease in sensory input** for patients whose illness results in a heightened sensitivity to external stimulation. The quiet atmosphere and monotony of a seclusion room may provide some relief from the sensory overload.

Legal requirements for the care of the secluded patient vary from state to state. Good nursing care includes optimum fulfillment of basic human needs and concern for personal dignity. The nurse must help the patient meet biological needs by providing food and fluids, a comfortable environment, and the opportunity for use of the bathroom. Frequent observation and monitoring is essential. The room must be constructed so the patient can be observed without being unnecessarily exposed to those who are not involved in his or her care.

Staff should be able to communicate with the patient. Careful records should include all nursing care and observation of the isolated patient. The need for continued isolation should be assessed on a regular basis. It may be necessary for the nurse to initiate this review of the patient's condition with other health team members. Box 30-7 identifies nursing interventions related to seclusion from the Nursing Interventions Classification (NIC) project (Dochterman and Bulechek, 2004).

One of the best ways to understand patients' points of view is to "walk in their shoes." Arrange to spend 15 minutes alone in the seclusion room on a psychiatric unit. Dare you try on the restraints? Describe your thoughts and feelings. ■

BOX 30-7

NIC Interventions Related to Seclusion

Definition
Solitary containment in a fully protective environment with close surveillance by nursing staff for purposes of safety or behavior management

Activities
Obtain a physician's order, if required by institutional policy, to use a physically restrictive intervention.
Designate one nursing staff member to communicate with the patient and to direct other staff.
Identify for patient and significant others those behaviors that necessitated the intervention.
Explain procedure, purpose, and time period of the intervention to patient and significant others in understandable and non-punitive terms.
Explain to patient and significant others the behaviors necessary for termination of the intervention.
Contract with patient (as patient is able) to maintain control of behavior.
Instruct on self-control methods, as appropriate.
Assist in dressing in clothing that is safe and in removing jewelry and eyeglasses.
Remove all items from seclusion area that patient might use to harm self or nursing staff.

Assist with needs related to nutrition, elimination, hydration, and personal hygiene.
Provide food and fluids in nonbreakable containers.
Provide appropriate level of supervision/surveillance to monitor patient and to allow for therapeutic actions, as needed.
Acknowledge your presence to patient periodically.
Administer prn medications for anxiety or agitation.
Provide for patient's psychological comfort, as needed.
Monitor seclusion area for temperature, cleanliness, and safety.
Arrange for routine cleaning of seclusion area.
Evaluate, at regular intervals, patient's need for continued restrictive intervention.
Involve patient, when appropriate, in making decisions to move toward a more/less restrictive intervention.
Determine patient's need for continued seclusion.
Document rationale for restrictive intervention, patient's response to intervention, patient's physical condition, nursing care provided throughout intervention, and rationale for terminating the intervention.
Process with the patient and staff, on termination of the restrictive intervention, the circumstances that led to the use of the intervention, as well as any patient concerns about the intervention itself.
Provide the next appropriate level of restrictive intervention (e.g., physical restraint or area restriction), as needed.

From Dochterman JM, Bulechek GM, editors.: *Nursing interventions classification (NIC)*, ed 4, St. Louis, 2004, Mosby.

Restraints. The patient in physical or mechanical restraints may be confused or delirious and will probably be frightened at the limitation of movement. The nurse should not assume that the patient understands the need for restraints. Support and reassurance are essential.

Restraints should be applied efficiently and with care not to injure a combative patient. Adequate personnel must be assembled before the patient is approached. Each staff member should be assigned responsibility for controlling specific body parts. Restraints should be available and in working order. Padding of cuff restraints helps to prevent skin breakdown. For the same reason, the patient should be positioned in anatomical alignment.

Privacy is important. If visitors are allowed, the nurse should explain the reason for restraints or seclusion before they see the patient. This may help them accept the situation. Physical needs must be included in the nursing care plan. Vital signs should be checked, and regular observation of circulation in the extremities is necessary. Fluids should be offered regularly and opportunities for elimination provided. Skin care is also essential. Restraints should be released at least every 2 hours to allow exercise of the extremities. Nursing interventions related to the use of physical restraints from the Nursing Interventions Classification (NIC) project are presented in Box 30-8 (Dochterman and Bulechek, 2004).

Terminating the Intervention

Patients should be removed from seclusion or restraints as soon as they meet criteria for release. It is important to review with the patient the behavior that precipitated the interven-

---

BOX 30-8

NIC Interventions Related to Physical Restraint

Definition

Application, monitoring, and removal of mechanical restraining devices or manual restraints that are used to limit physical mobility of patient

Activities

Obtain a physician's order, if required by institutional policy, to use a physically restrictive intervention or to reduce use.

Provide patient with a private, yet adequately supervised, environment in situations in which a patient's sense of dignity may be diminished by the use of physical restraints.

Provide sufficient staff to assist with safe application of physical restraining devices or manual restraints.

Designate one nursing staff member to direct staff and communicate with the patient during the application of physical restraints.

Use appropriate hold when manually restraining patient in emergency situations or during transport.

Identify for patient and significant others those behaviors that necessitated the intervention.

Explain procedure, purpose, and time period of the intervention to patient and significant others in understandable and non-punitive terms.

Explain to patient and significant others the behaviors necessary for termination of the intervention.

Monitor the patient's response to procedure.

Avoid tying restraints to side rails of bed.

Secure restraints out of patient's reach.

Provide appropriate level of supervision/surveillance to monitor patient and to allow for therapeutic actions, as needed.

Provide for patient's psychological comfort, as needed.

Provide diversional activities, (e.g., television, reading to patient, visitors, mobiles), when appropriate, to facilitate patient cooperation with the intervention.

Administer prn medications for anxiety or agitation.

Monitor skin condition at restraint site(s).

Monitor color, temperature, and sensation frequently in restrained extremities.

Provide for movement and exercise, according to patient's level of self-control, condition, and abilities.

Position patient to facilitate comfort and prevent aspiration and skin breakdown.

Provide for movement of extremities in patient with multiple restraints by rotating the removal/reapplication of one restraint at a time (as safety permits).

Assist with periodic changes in body position.

Provide the dependent patient with a means of summoning help (e.g., bell or call light) when caregiver is not present.

Assist with needs related to nutrition, elimination, hydration, and personal hygiene.

Evaluate, at regular intervals, patient's need for continued restrictive intervention.

Involve patient in activities to improve strength, coordination, judgment, and orientation.

Involve patient, when appropriate, in making decisions to move toward a more/less restrictive form of intervention.

Remove restraints gradually (i.e., one at a time if in four-point restraints), as self-control increases.

Monitor patient's response to removal of restraints.

Process with the patient and staff, on termination of the restrictive intervention, the circumstances that led to the use of the intervention, as well as any patient concerns about the intervention itself.

Provide the next appropriate level of restrictive action (e.g., area restriction or seclusion), as needed.

Implement alternatives to restraints, such as sitting in chair with table over lap, self-releasing waist belt, geri-chair without tray table, or close observation, as appropriate.

Teach family the risks and benefits of restraints and restraint reduction.

Document the rationale for use of restrictive intervention, patient's response to the intervention, patient's physical condition, nursing care provided throughout the intervention, and rationale for terminating the intervention.

From Dochterman JM, Bulechek GM, editors.: *Nursing interventions classification (NIC)*, ed 4, St Louis, 2004, Mosby.

tion and the patient's current capacity to exercise control over his or her behavior. Patients should be told which behaviors they need to exhibit and which behaviors or impulses they need to control before the intervention can be discontinued. Communication and careful documentation are critical in making an accurate assessment of a patient's level of control.

Debriefing is an important part of terminating the use of seclusion or restraints. Debriefing is a therapeutic intervention that includes reviewing the facts related to an event and processing the response to them. It provides staff and patients with an opportunity to clarify the rationale for the seclusion, offer mutual feedback, and identify alternative methods of coping that might help the patient avoid seclusion in the future (Petti et al, 2001).

Debriefing can be used after any stressful event. Describe how talking with your friends after an examination can be seen as a kind of debriefing. ∎

∎ PREVENTION

Employers have a duty to provide a work environment that is free from hazards that may cause death or serious physical harm to employees. Workplace violence is a recognized hazard for psychiatric nurses. For this reason, health care facilities are required by law to develop a plan to decrease the risk to nursing staff who are frequently the targets of violent patients.

Workplace Guidelines

In 1998 violence prevention guidelines were published to assist health care and social service employers provide an environment that reduces exposure of employees to violence in the workplace (U.S. Department of Labor, OSHA, 1998). The guidelines include the following:
- Management commitment and employee involvement
- Worksite analysis
- Prevention and control
- Safety and health training

For a workplace violence prevention program to be successful, administrators and managers must be willing to commit energy and resources to this initiative. The guidelines state that the goals and objectives related to the prevention of workplace violence be established by each facility and that a policy of zero-tolerance for workplace violence be communicated.

The guidelines also recommend that a worksite analysis be completed to identify areas of potential vulnerability for workplace violence. The analysis should include the review of procedures and operations as well as prior incidents to identify trends. Input from employees is an important aspect of this analysis. Quantifying the frequency and severity of incidents is also needed so that improvement can be measured over time. The items in Box 30-9 can assist in an analysis of the worksite.

Once potential hazards are identified, physical changes may be needed to decrease the risk of violence. The installation of alarm systems or other security devices such as panic

---

BOX 30-9

Items To Consider in a Violence Prevention Worksite Analysis

- Analyze incidents, including the characteristics of assailants and victims, an account of what happened before and during the incident, and the relevant details of the situation and its outcome. When possible, obtain police reports and recommendations.
- Identify jobs or locations with the greatest risk of violence and processes and procedures that put employees at risk of assault, including how often and when.
- Note high-risk factors such as types of clients or patients (e.g., psychiatric conditions or patients disoriented by drugs, alcohol, or stress); physical risk factors of the building; isolated locations/job activities; lighting problems; lack of phones and other communication devices, areas of easy, unsecured access; and areas with previous security problems.
- Evaluate the effectiveness of existing security measures, including engineering control measures. Determine whether risk factors have been reduced or eliminated, and take appropriate action.

---

buttons can be crucial in enlisting necessary assistance in the event of a psychiatric emergency. Also changes in procedures and practices can be implemented to minimize the risk of danger to staff who provide care for potentially violent patients. Box 30-10 outlines practices and procedures that can decrease the risk of workplace violence.

Staff Development

Effective management of potentially dangerous patients requires highly skilled staff and attention to environmental and workplace factors. Nurses, physicians, and other support staff, including security personnel, must be trained in emergency psychiatric care and crisis management techniques. This includes training in early detection of behaviors that can lead to violence, strategies to verbally intervene with agitated patients, the use of alternative interventions that can avoid seclusion and restraint and seclusion, nonviolent self defense skills, and crisis management techniques.

The JCAHO Standards (1996) on Restraint and Seclusion and the Center for Medicare and Medicaid Services Patients' Rights Condition of Participation requirements also should be an essential part of a staff education program. Education should focus on assessment of the patient, particularly mental status, motor behavior, affect, and speech. Verbal intervention should be stressed as a way of defusing agitation, and helpful and non-helpful responses should be reviewed.

All nursing interventions should be grounded in theory and current research, and crisis intervention in psychiatric emergencies is no exception. The theoretical basis and supporting research for various intervention strategies should be discussed as part of the training. Pharmacological interventions should be reviewed, with particular attention given to the choice of medication, its purpose, and its potential ad-

BOX 30-10

Practices To Decrease the Risk of Workplace Violence

- State clearly to patients, clients, and employees that violence is not permitted or tolerated.
- Establish liaison with local police and state prosecutors. Report all incidents of violence.
- Provide police with physical layouts of facilities to expedite investigations.
- Require employees to report all assaults or threats to a supervisor or manager (e.g., can be confidential interview).
- Keep log books and reports of such incidents to help in determining any necessary actions to prevent further occurrences.
- Advise and assist employees, if needed, of company procedures for requesting police assistance or filing charges when assaulted.
- Provide management support during emergencies.
- Respond promptly to all complaints.
- Set up a trained response team to respond to emergencies.
- Use properly trained security officers, when necessary, to deal with aggressive behavior.
- Follow written security procedures.
- Ensure adequate and properly trained staff for restraining patients or clients.
- Provide sensitive and timely information to persons waiting in line or in waiting rooms.
- Adopt measures to decrease waiting time.
- Ensure adequate and qualified staff coverage at all times. Times of greatest risk occur during patient transfers, emergency responses, meal times, and at night. Locales with the greatest risk include admission units and crisis or acute care units. Other risks include admission of patients with a history of violent behavior or gang activity.
- Institute a sign-in procedure with passes for visitors. Enforce visitor hours and procedures.
- Establish a list of "restricted visitors" for patients with a history of violence. Copies should be available at security checkpoints, nurses' stations, and visitor sign-in areas.
- Review and revise visitor check systems, when necessary.
- Limit information given to outsiders on hospitalized victims of violence.
- Supervise the movement of psychiatric clients and patients throughout the facility.
- Control access to facilities other than waiting rooms, particularly drug storage or pharmacy areas.
- Prohibit employees from working alone in emergency areas or walk-in clinics, particularly at night or when assistance is unavailable.
- Employees should never enter seclusion rooms alone.
- Establish policies and procedures for secured areas, and emergency evacuations, and for monitoring high-risk patients at night (e.g., open versus locked seclusion).

- Ascertain the behavioral history of new and transferred patients to learn about any past violent or assaultive behaviors.
- Establish a system such as chart tags, log books, or verbal census reports to identify patients and clients with assaultive behavior problems, keeping in mind patient confidentiality and worker safety issues. Update as needed.
- Treat and/or interview aggressive or agitated clients in relatively open areas that still maintain privacy and confidentiality (e.g., rooms with removable partitions).
- Use case management conferences with co-workers and supervisors to discuss ways to effectively treat potentially violent patients.
- Prepare contingency plans to treat clients who are "acting out" or making verbal or physical attacks or threats.
- Transfer assaultive clients to "acute care units," "criminal units," or other more restrictive settings.
- Make sure that nurses and physicians are not alone when performing intimate physical examinations of patients.
- Discourage employees from wearing jewelry to help prevent possible strangulation in confrontational situations.
- Periodically survey the facility to remove tools or possessions left by visitors or maintenance staff which could be used inappropriately by patients.
- Provide staff with identification badges, preferably without last names, to readily verify employment.
- Discourage employees from carrying keys, pens, or other items that could be used as weapons.
- Provide staff members with security escorts to parking areas during evening or late night hours.
- Parking areas should be highly visible, well-lighted, and safely accessible to the building.
- Use the "buddy system," especially when personal safety may be threatened.
- Encourage home health care providers, social service workers, and others to avoid threatening situations.
- Staff should exercise extra care in elevators, stairwells, and unfamiliar residences; immediately leave premises if there is a hazardous situation; or request police escort if needed.
- Develop policies and procedures covering home health care providers, such as contracts on how visits will be conducted, the presence of others in the home during the visits, and the refusal to provide services in a clearly hazardous situation.
- Establish a daily work plan for field staff to keep a designated contact person informed about workers' whereabouts throughout the workday. If an employee does not report in, the contact person should follow-up.
- Conduct a comprehensive post-incident evaluation, including psychological and medical treatment, for employees who have been subjected to abusive behavior.

verse effects. And finally the program should be evaluated for its effectiveness as related to the knowledge, attitude, and behavioral interventions used by the staff (Calabro, Mackey, and Williams, 2002; Taxis, 2002; Morrison et al, 2002; Morrison and Carney Love, 2003).

Ongoing practice sessions in crisis management should be required of all staff. These sessions should include basic self-protection maneuvers and strategies for restraining assaultive patients. Each member of the staff should be able to function as a leader in the event of a crisis, and the staff as a whole must be able to function smoothly as a cohesive emergency team. The nursing and medical care of these patients should be reviewed, as should the impact of countertransference issues.

The guidelines for preventing workplace violence also recommend the following as part of staff education:

- The workplace violence prevention policy
- Risk factors that cause or contribute to assaults
- Early recognition of escalating behavior or recognition of warning signs or situations that may lead to assaults
- Ways of preventing or diffusing volatile situations or aggressive behavior, managing anger, and appropriately using medications as chemical restraints
- Information on multicultural diversity to develop sensitivity to racial and ethnic issues and differences
- A standard response action plan for violent situations, including availability of assistance, response to alarm systems, and communication procedures
- How to deal with hostile persons other than patients and clients, such as relatives and visitors
- Progressive behavior control methods and safe methods of restraint application or escape
- The location and operation of safety devices such as alarms systems, along with the required maintenance schedules and procedures
- Ways to protect oneself and co-workers, including use of the "buddy system"
- Policies and procedures for reporting and record-keeping
- Policies and procedures for obtaining medical care, counseling, workers' compensation, or legal assistance after a violent episode or injury

Staff Support

Unfortunately, nurses are sometimes assaulted by patients. It is impossible to predict and prevent all episodes of violent behavior in a psychiatric setting. If a staff member is assaulted, the support and assistance of colleagues are needed.

Nurses who have been assaulted may experience symptoms such as anger, anxiety, helplessness, irritability, hyper-alertness, depression, shock, or disbelief that the assault occurred. It is not unusual for nurses to blame themselves for the assault or to question their competence in managing potentially violent patients.

Nurses can be supported by allowing adequate time off from work to address their physical and emotional needs. Discussing the event in a nonblaming manner also can be helpful. Validation from others that assaults occur despite clinical competence and appropriate interventions can help the assaulted nurse in healing.

Acknowledging the nurse's right to take legal action against the patient also can be helpful. In fact, many argue that it is therapeutic to bring criminal charges against assaultive patients. Legal action can help patients take responsibility for their behavior, and perhaps decrease future violent episodes. For the assaulted nurse, taking legal action articulates a position that the personal trauma of being physically assaulted should not be an accepted consequence of caring for others.

Another way of helping nursing staff members who have been assaulted is through a peer support group, which legitimizes staff responses and allows for the expression of feelings in a supportive setting. Developing a staff action program made up of volunteers who work with staff in critical incident debriefing, run support groups, and offer specialized services such as family and community meetings is another effective strategy (Erdos and Hughes, 2001).

A final suggestion is the implementation of a nursing consultation support service that responds to the needs of assault victims and sets the tone for institutional attitudes of nonblaming concern. All of these programs have merit, and each organization should select the best way to deal with the problem of staff assault based on the environment, group process, and institutional resources.

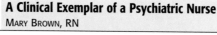

COMPETENT CARING   **A Clinical Exemplar of a Psychiatric Nurse**
Mary Brown, RN

When I think about aggressive behavior, I think back to an incident that could have ended badly, but instead resulted in the people involved receiving the help needed. I was working as a case manager for an agency that provided intensive case management for chronically mentally ill people. The event took place on a weekend. Office hours were 9 AM to 5 PM during the week, and a person was assigned to be on call after working hours and on all weekends.

I was the person on call this particular weekend. One of the agency's patients had been hospitalized and was now ready for discharge. This patient was deaf, and I was to pick him up from the hospital and see that he got settled in his home. After I left the hospital with the patient, my beeper went off indicating I needed to call the answering service. I was close to the office, so I stopped there to use the phone. The building has two stories, and I had access only to the top floor. I climbed the stairs, the discharged deaf patient behind me, unlocked the door, walked in, and then turned around to shut the door, but a large hand kept me from doing so.

The hand belonged to a man who was over 6 feet tall, weighed approximately 250 pounds, and appeared to be psychotic. He forced his way into the building with the patient and me. I was terrified at this point. He stated, "I came to get my money," in an angry and loud tone of voice.

I then recognized him as a patient I had worked with before and could see the changes in him, which made me feel unsafe to be alone with him. I tried very hard not to let him know how frightened I was of him. I told him the office was closed and he needed to come back Monday, when the appropriate people could help him. He shouted, "I want my money now!" I became increasingly frightened. There was no panic button to push for help. There were no other staff to distract him to allow me to get my deaf patient and myself to safety. I was the one who needed to protect us.

In a calm voice, I told him I couldn't help him get his money. I told him I would need to go to the staff room (he was aware that patients were not allowed in this room) to call someone to help him. He followed me into the room. I firmly told him that he was not allowed in the room and to please leave. He sat down anyway. I told him I was only at the office to return an emergency call. I called the service and the doctor who paged me was checking to see whether everything went okay with the discharged patient. I told him about the intrusion from the angry and irrational man who was insisting on staying until he got his money. The doctor said he would call the police. While waiting for the police, I kept trying to get the patient to leave the room. He repeatedly refused. He sat at one end of the table and I sat at the other end. The deaf patient was watching our interaction intensely.

The angry patient appeared to be responding to internal stimuli. He was looking at me and began to laugh. He stopped laughing and said, "Why won't you go out with me?" as he proceeded to my end of the table. I told him firmly that this behavior was not appropriate. I reinforced that I was his nurse and again I asked him to leave the room. He stopped, looked at me inexplicably, and said, "I'll be back on Monday to get my money."

When I heard the door slam, I quickly locked the door. The doctor called back to say that the police were on their way and asked whether everything was okay. While shivering, I managed to say, "yes." The police picked the angry patient up downstairs and found that he was carrying a screwdriver. He told them that he was at the office before I arrived and intended to break into the office to take his money. The deaf patient who was watching all this communicated with me by writing on a piece of paper, "Are you all right? I could tell you were afraid of him." I was amazed. Nonverbal communication can be deciphered by a lay person as well as a skilled observer.

As a nurse, I am trained to evaluate what is not being said and make a determination. I realized that the deaf patient also was able to look at my nonverbal communication and make a determination. I also was reminded of the value of setting firm limits and giving clear, consistent, and nonthreatening messages at all times when managing aggressive behavior. ∎

CHAPTER **FOCUS POINTS**

- High rates of assaultive behavior have been reported in a variety of health care settings including outpatient clinics, nursing homes, and emergency departments. By far the highest rates of assault occur in psychiatric settings.
- Within each person lies the capacity for passive, assertive, or aggressive behavior. The situation and the characteristics of the person define the most appropriate response.
- Theories on the development of aggressive behavior include psychological, sociocultural, and biological factors.
- Two populations of patients are at increased risk of violence: patients with active psychotic symptoms and patients with substance abuse disorders.
- The best single predictor of violence is a history of violence.
- Nurses need to assess all patients for their potential for violence including their motor agitation, verbalizations, affect, and level of consciousness. A formal screening tool may be useful in this process.

- Many nursing interventions may be helpful in dealing with aggressive behavior, including self-awareness, patient education, assertiveness training, communication strategies, environmental strategies, behavioral strategies, and psychopharmacology.
- Effective crisis management must be organized and clearly directed by one team leader.
- Seclusion and restraints should be used only as a last resort.
- Employers have a duty to provide a work environment that is free from hazards that may cause death or serious physical harm to employees. Health care facilities are required by law to develop a plan to decrease the risk to nursing staff who are often the targets of violent patients.
- Staff development issues include educating staff in crisis management techniques, working with staff who have been assaulted, and understanding the implications of possible legal action.

◀ KEY TERMS

assertiveness, 631	limit setting, 642	seclusion, 645
chemical restraints, 645	physical restraints, 645	time-out, 642
debriefing, 648	room program, 641	token economy, 642

CHAPTER REVIEW QUESTIONS

1. Match each term in Column A with the correct definition in Column B.

Column A

_____ Assertive behavior

_____ Debriefing

_____ Limit-setting

_____ Passive behavior

_____ Restraint

_____ Seclusion

_____ Token economy

Column B

A. Acting in a way that conveys a sense of self-assurance but also communicates respect for the other person by using nonpunitive, nonmanipulative behavior in which someone is told what is acceptable, what is not acceptable, and the consequences of behaving in an unacceptable way

B. Positive reinforcement in which patients are rewarded for performing desired targeted behaviors

C. Separating a patient from others and placing him or her in a safe, contained environment

D. Subordinating one's own rights to the perception of the rights of others

E. Therapeutic intervention that includes reviewing the facts related to an event and processing the response to them

F. Use of mechanical or manual devices to limit the physical mobility of the patient

G. A nonpunitive, nonmanipulative act in which the patient is to told what behavior is acceptable, what is not acceptable, and the consequences of behaving unacceptably

2. Indicate whether the following statements are true (T) or false (F).

_____ A. Patients who are mildly aggressive should be allowed to pace the halls to decrease tension.

_____ B. Overly crowded and stimulated environments may increase aggressive behavior.

_____ C. A patient's diagnosis is a good predictor of future violent behavior.

_____ D. A minority of psychiatric patients are responsible for a majority of the violent incidents.

_____ E. Failing to set effective limits with patients can lead to provocation and assault.

3. Provide short answers for the following questions.

A. Identify the three areas of the brain that are believed to be involved in aggression.

B. Identify two preventive strategies, two anticipatory strategies, and two containment strategies for managing aggressive behavior.

C. A patient who appears agitated and potentially threatening approaches you. How should you physically position yourself when interacting with this patient?

D. Do you think that physical restraints are more or less restrictive than the use of chemical restraints with the aggressive patient? Defend your position.

Visit Evolve for additional resources related to the content of this chapter.

http://evolve.elsevier.com/Stuart/principles/

• Topical Course Outline • Student Workbook Exercises • Critical Thinking Questions and Activities • Case Studies • Research Topics • Monthly Content Updates • WebLinks

Student Study CD-ROM

Access the accompanying CD-ROM for animations, interactive exercises, review questions for the NCLEX examination, and an audio glossary.

REFERENCES

Allen MH et al: Treatment of behavioral emergencies: a summary of the expert consensus guidelines, *J Psychiatr Pract* 9:16, 2003.

Allen MH et al: What do consumers say they want and need during a psychiatric emergency? *J Psychiatr Pract* 9:39, 2003.

American Psychiatric Nurses Association: *Learning from each other: successful stories and ideas for reducing restrain/seclusion in behavioral health*, Washington, DC, 2003, APNA.

Anderson C: Workplace violence: are some nurses more vulnerable? *Issues Ment Health Nurs* 23:351, 2002.

Anderson CA, Dill KE: Video games and aggressive thoughts, feelings and behavior in the laboratory and in life, *J Pers Soc Psychol* 78:772, 2000.

Bushman BJ, Baumeister RF, Stack AD: Catharsis, aggression, and persuasive influence: self-fulfilling or self-defeating prophecies? *J Pers Soc Psychol* 76:367, 1999.

Brown J: Restraints and Seclusion State Policies for Psychiatric Hospitals, pp 1-21, 2000, Department of Health and Human Services Office of Inspector General.

Calabro K, Mackey TA, Williams S: Evaluation of training designed to prevent and manage patient violence, *Issues Ment Health Nurs* 23:3, 2002.

Chabora N, Judge-Gorny M, Grogan K: The Four S Model in action for de-escalation: an innovative state hospital-university collaborative endeavor, *J Psychosoc Nurs Ment Health Serv* 41:22, 2003.

Chan HY et al: Effectiveness of the anger-control program in reducing anger expression in patients with schizophrenia, *Arch Psychiatr Nurs* 17:88, 2003.

Currier GW: The controversy over "chemical restraint" in acute care psychiatry, *J Psychiatr Pract* 9:59, 2003.

Cusack KJ et al: Trauma within the psychiatric setting: a preliminary empirical report, *Adm Policy Ment Health* 30:453, 2003.

Dochterman JM, Bulechek GM, editors: *Nursing interventions classification (NIC)*, ed 4, St Louis, 2004, Mosby.

Donat DC: An analysis of successful efforts to reduce the use of seclusion and restraint at a public psychiatric hospital, *Psychiatr Serv* 54:1119, 2003.

Erdos BZ, Hughes DH: Emergency psychiatry: a review of assaults by patients against staff at psychiatric emergency centers, *Psychiatr Serv* 52:1175, 2001.

Fagan-Pryor EC et al: Patients' views of causes of aggression by patients and effective interventions, *Psychiatr Serv* 54:549, 2003.

Finke L: The use of seclusion is not evidence-based practice, *J Child Adolesc Psychiatr Nurs* 14:186, 2001.

Fisher WA: Elements of successful restraint and seclusion reduction programs and their application in a large, urban, state psychiatric hospital, *J Psychiatr Pract* 9:7, 2003.

Hoptman MJ: Neuroimaging studies of violence and antisocial behavior, *J Psychiatr Pract* 9:265, 2003.

Horsfall J, Cleary M: Patient concerns about seclusion: developing a leaflet, *Issues Ment Health Nurs* 24:575, 2003.

Johnson ME, Hauser PM: The practices of expert psychiatric nurses: accompanying the patient to a calmer personal space, *Issues Ment Health Nurs* 22:651, 2001.

Joint Commission on Accreditation of Healthcare Organizations (JCAHO): *Revised standards and scoring guidelines for restraint and seclusion*, Oakbrook Terrace, 1996, JCAHO.

Kozub ML, Skidmore R: Seclusion and restraint: understanding recent changes, *J Psychosoc Nurs Ment Health Serv* 39:24, 2001.

LePage J: The impact of a token economy on injuries and negative events on an acute psychiatric unit, *Psychiatr Serv* 50:941, 1999.

Miller M: Does violence in the media cause violent behavior? *Harvard Ment Health Lett* September 5, 2001.

Mohr WK, Mohr BD: Mechanisms of injury and death proximal to restraint use, *Arch Psychiatr Nurs* 14:285, 2000.

Morrison EF, Carney Love C: An evaluation of four programs for the management of aggression in psychiatric settings, *Arch Psychiatr Nurs* 17:146, 2003.

Morrison E et al: Reducing staff injuries and violence in a forensic psychiatric setting, *Arch Psychiatr Nurs* 16:108, 2002.

Murphy M: The agitated psychotic patient: guidelines to ensure staff and patient safety, *J Am Psychiatr Nurs Assoc* 8:S2, 2002.

Nestor PG: Mental disorder and violence: personality dimensions and clinical features, *Am J Psychiatry* 159:1973, 2002.

Ng B et al: Ward crowding and incidents of violence on an acute psychiatric inpatient unit, *Psychiatr Serv* 52:521, 2001.

Niehoff D: *The biology of violence*, New York, 2002, Free Press.

Nolan KA et al: Characteristics of assaultive behavior among psychiatric inpatients, *Psychiatr Serv* 54:1012, 2003.

Oberleitner LL: Aversiveness of traditional patient restriction, *Arch Psychiatr Nurs* 14:93, 2000.

Petti TA et al: Perceptions of seclusion and restraint by patients and staff in an intermediate-term care facility, *J Child Adolesc Psychiatr Nurs* 14:115, 2001.

Pietrini P et al: Neural correlates of imaginal aggressive behavior assessed by positron emission tomography in healthy subjects. *Am J Psychiatry* 157:1772, 2000.

Rossberg JI, Friis S: Staff members' emotional reactions to aggressive and suicidal behavior of inpatients, *Psychiatr Serv* 54:1388, 2003.

Sailas E, Fenton M: Seclusion and restraint for people with serious mental illness, *Cochrane Library*, Issue 3, 2002.

Soliman AE, Reza H: Risk factors and correlates of violence among acutely ill adult psychiatric patients, *Psychiatr Serv* 52:75, 2001.

Stuart HL, Arboleda-Florez JE: A public health perspective on violent offenses among persons with mental illness, *Psychiatr Serv* 52:654, 2001.

Swanson JW et al: The social-environmental context of violent behavior in persons treated for severe mental illness, *Am J Public Health* 92:1523, 2002.

Taxis JC: Ethics and praxis: alternative strategies to physical restraint and seclusion in a psychiatric setting, *Issues Ment Health Nurs* 23:157, 2002.

Thomas S: Teaching healthy anger management, *Perspect Psychiatr Care* 37:41, 2001.

U.S. Department of Labor, OSHA: Guidelines for preventing workplace violence for healthcare and social service workers. www.osha.gov/ safety and health topics/workplace violence/Guidelines for preventing workplace violence for healthcare and social service workers, 1998.

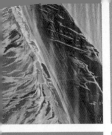

> *But humanism stands for the whole person, the whole individual striving to become as conscious and responsible as possible about everything in the universe.*
>
> DORIS LESSING, *THE GOLDEN NOTEBOOK*

31 COGNITIVE BEHAVIORAL TREATMENT STRATEGIES

Gail W. Stuart

evolve Visit Evolve for additional resources related to the content of this chapter.
http://evolve.elsevier.com/Stuart/principles/

Cognitive behavioral treatment strategies apply learning theories to problems of living, with the aim of helping people overcome difficulties in everyday life. These difficulties often occur along with a medical or psychiatric disorder. The techniques of cognitive behavioral therapy can be applied to school, work, home, family, and leisure activities. In these situations cognitive behavioral treatment strategies help people achieve personal growth by expanding their coping skills. They can be used by nurses with any background and in any health care setting to promote healthy coping responses and to change maladaptive behavior.

Cognitive behavioral therapy is problem focused, goal oriented, and deals with here-and-now issues. It views the individual as the primary decision maker regarding goals and issues to be dealt with during treatment. This chapter reviews the key concepts of cognitive behavioral therapy, the treatment process, and specific strategies that can be used in nursing practice.

DEFINITION OF BEHAVIOR

Behavior is any observable, recordable, and measurable act, movement, or response. A behavior must be accurately described before it can be measured, and this is done in different ways. For example, the behavior of eating can be broken down into parts such as selecting the food items, preparing the meal, setting the table, eating the meal, and cleaning the dishes after the food is eaten. In contrast, this behavior can be more globally described as simply eating dinner.

This example shows that there can be several different and accurate definitions for what appears to be a single, simple behavior. It also points to the need to begin by describing what is seen or heard and then clarifying this information until the participants agree with the description.

A behavior is what is observed—not the conclusion, inferences, or interpretations drawn from the observation. For example, hyperactivity is not a behavior but is a conclusion drawn from observing a set of behaviors. Hyperactivity cannot be measured. What can be measured is the number of times a child gets out of his or her seat, interrupts a conversation, drops a book, or completes required homework assignments. Thus treatment for the child should focus not on hyperactivity but on the specific behaviors that interfere with the child's adjustment to school, home, or the community.

Other examples of inferences rather than behaviors are psychiatric diagnoses and the labeling of patients as uncooperative, aggressive, difficult, noncompliant, or hostile. These adjectives globally describe a person but do not reflect the specific behavior that led to such conclusions.

Similarly, when formulating a nursing diagnosis, it is essential that the nurse identify the specific defining characteristics of the nursing diagnosis that apply to the patient. In this way, the nurse will have recorded specific behaviors that can be measured over time. These can then be used to evaluate the patient's progress toward expected outcomes.

A clear definition of a behavior minimizes subjective interpretations. It is **measurable, not subject to interpretation,** and **states what the person does**.

> *Think about your experiences in psychiatric–mental health nursing. In your view, how much treatment is based on inference rather than on behavior? What impact does this have on patient adherence to treatment plans?* ■

■ CLASSICAL CONDITIONING

Classical conditioning focuses on the process by which **involuntary behavior** is learned. It is derived from Pavlov's (1927) famous work in which he taught dogs to salivate at the sound of a bell by associating the bell with meat presented at the same time. The explanation is that when two stimuli are repeatedly paired (presented to the subject at the same time), the response that is produced can be elicited later by either stimulus alone. Other examples of classical conditioning include the following:

- Blinking in response to a puff of air directed toward someone's eye
- Salivating at the aroma of cookies baking
- Automatically raising the leg when the patellar tendon is struck

A clinical example is that of a person who has become conditioned to feel fear in neutral situations that have become associated with anxiety, such as fear of heights or of traveling by way of public transportation (e.g., by bus or airplane). Inconsistent pairings of the two stimuli lead to less reliable learning, and the response gradually disappears if the pairings are discontinued.

■ OPERANT CONDITIONING

Operant conditioning has been credited to the work of B.F. Skinner (1953) and his colleagues. It is concerned with the relationship between **voluntary behavior** and the environment. Operant behaviors are those that are influenced by the consequences of an action, and they are regarded as a more complex form of learning. Examples include correcting a spelling mistake when writing a letter or studying class notes before an examination.

The basic idea is that behaviors are influenced by their consequences and that operant behaviors are cued by environmental stimuli. Behaviors that have a positive consequence will be stronger and are likely to be repeated. In contrast, behaviors that result in negative consequences will be weakened and are less likely to occur.

For example, if a person tells a joke and everyone who is listening to it laughs heartily, the person will probably repeat that joke in another social setting. However, if the person tells the joke and everyone stares blankly or appears quiet and embarrassed, the person will probably not repeat that joke in the future.

Unlike classical conditioning, operant conditioning is strengthened rather than weakened by inconsistent pairings of the behaviors and consequences. That is, a certain behavior is more likely to recur when it is followed unpredictably by positive or negative consequences.

Many of the techniques used in operant conditioning fall under the heading of behavior modification. They are based on the assumption that a high-frequency, preferred activity can be used to reinforce a low-frequency, nonpreferred activity. For example, if a boy enjoys playing with toy racing cars, this high-frequency preferred activity can be used to reinforce the low-frequency, nonpreferred activity of tidying his room. The terms **reinforcement** and **punishment** do not have the same meaning when used in operant conditioning as when used by most laypeople.

> *Give an example of classical and operant conditioning from your work in a psychiatric setting related to either patient or staff behavior.* ■

Increasing Behavior

Reinforcers are anything that increases the frequency of a behavior. By far the most commonly used form of reinforcement is positive reinforcement, or rewarding stimuli. An example is a teacher praising students for remaining in their assigned seats. Because of the praise, the students are likely to remain seated more often.

However, what is regarded as a positive reward can be quite subjective, and many times people intending to decrease a behavior actually wind up reinforcing it. For example, when a father yells at his son for fighting with his sibling, the yelling may represent to the son a form of desired parental attention and thus may be interpreted as positive reinforcement. As a consequence, the son is likely to continue fighting with his sibling.

Negative reinforcement also increases the frequency of a behavior by reinforcing the power of the behavior to control an aversive, rather than a rewarding, stimulus. An example is putting on sunglasses in glaring sunlight. The sunlight is an aversive stimulus; putting on the sunglasses is the behavior; and escaping the sun's glare is the negative reinforcer. It is negative because it removes or subtracts something from the environment (sunlight), resulting in an increase in the desired behavior (wearing sunglasses). Other examples of negative reinforcement include the following:

- A child who is being scolded by his mother goes up to her and kisses her, and her scolding stops.
- An adolescent who is having trouble in school runs away from home, thus avoiding her parents' displeasure.
- Drivers maintain the speed limit to avoid receiving a traffic ticket.

Decreasing Behavior

Three techniques are used to reduce the frequency of behavior: punishment, response cost, and extinction. Punishment is an aversive stimulus that occurs after the behavior and decreases its future occurrence. An example is a child who must stay in from recess because he or she disrupted the class.

Table 31-1 Operant Conditioning Procedures

PROCEDURE	DEFINITION	EXAMPLE
Increasing Behavior		
Positive reinforcement	Adding a rewarding stimulus as a consequence of a behavior, thus increasing the probability that it will occur again	Behavior → Rewarding stimulus → Behavior ↑
Negative reinforcement	Removing an aversive stimulus as a consequence of a behavior, thus increasing the probability that it will occur again	Aversive stimulus → Behavior → Aversive stimulus removed → Behavior ↑
Decreasing Behavior		
Punishment	Presentation of an aversive stimulus as a consequence of a behavior, thus decreasing the probability that it will occur again	Behavior → Aversive stimulus → Behavior ↓
Response cost	Loss or withdrawal of a reinforcer as a consequence of a behavior, thus decreasing the probability that it will occur again	Behavior → Loss of reinforcer → Behavior ↓
Extinction	Withholding a reinforcer as a consequence of a behavior, thus decreasing the probability that it will occur again	Behavior → Reinforcement → Behavior → No reinforcement → Behavior ↓

Response cost decreases behavior through the experience of a loss or penalty following a behavior. Examples include paying a fine for overdue library books, losing an allowance for not keeping a clean room, or not being able to attend the next school dance as a result of coming home after curfew.

Extinction is the process of eliminating a behavior by ignoring it or not rewarding it. For example, a child who has frequent temper tantrums is sent to summer camp. On the first day at camp, the child has a tantrum because he or she is not allowed to sleep in a specific bunk. The counselor ignores the child and continues to interact with the other campers. In the next 2 days the child has three more tantrums, and the counselor continues to ignore the outbursts. After the fourth day the child has no more temper tantrums.

The procedures of operant conditioning are summarized in Table 31-1. These procedures are incorporated into many cognitive behavioral treatment strategies, and they can be used by nurses in all areas of practice to help patients overcome a wide range of problems and then resume productive lives.

▨ *Do you think the procedures of operant conditioning can be used by nurses working in medical-surgical settings? Give an example from your experience.* ▨

▍ROLE OF COGNITION

Cognition is the act or process of knowing. Cognitive therapy proposes that it is not the events themselves that cause anxiety and maladaptive responses but rather people's expectations, appraisals, and interpretations of these events. It suggests that maladaptive behaviors can be altered by dealing directly with a person's thoughts and beliefs (Beck, 1976; Beck, 1995).

Specifically, cognitive therapists believe that maladaptive responses arise from cognitive distortions. Such distortions might include errors of logic, mistakes in reasoning, or individualized views of the world that do not reflect reality. The distortions may be either positive or negative.

For example, someone may consistently view life in an unrealistically positive way and thus take dangerous chances, such as denying health problems and claiming to be "too young and healthy for a heart attack." Cognitive distortions also may be negative, such as those expressed by a person who interprets all unfortunate life situations as proof of a complete lack of self-worth. Common cognitive distortions are listed in Table 31-2.

The goal of cognitive therapy is to change irrational beliefs, faulty reasoning, and negative self-statements that underlie behavioral problems. Research has shown that cognitive therapy is an effective intervention for a wide range of clinical problems, particularly depression, anxiety, eating disorders, personality disorders, and schizophrenia (Wright and Beck, 2000). It can be used in inpatient, outpatient, and psychosocial rehabilitation treatment programs. Therefore interventions that include principles of cognitive therapy have much to contribute to psychiatric nursing practice.

▨ *Give an example from your personal experiences of each cognitive distortion listed in Table 31-2. What was the consequence of each distortion, if any?* ▨

▍COGNITIVE BEHAVIORAL THERAPY AND THE NURSING PROCESS

There are many misperceptions about cognitive behavioral therapy. One misperception is that it involves controlling the patient. Another misperception is that relationship factors are neglected in the treatment process. Neither of these perceptions is true. The major characteristics of cognitive behavioral therapy are listed in Box 31-1.

Cognitive behavioral therapy is totally **patient centered**. It views the person as a unique individual who has a problem of living rather than a psychopathological condition. Maladaptive behaviors, as well as adaptive coping responses, are believed to be acquired through the process of learning. Thus emphasis is placed on behavioral monitoring and on the completion of homework by the patient to reinforce the skills

Table 31-2	Cognitive Distortions	
DISTORTION	**DEFINITION**	**EXAMPLE**
Overgeneralization	Draws conclusions about a wide variety of things on the basis of a single event	A student who has failed an examination thinks, "I'll never pass any of my other exams this term and I'll flunk out of school."
Personalization	Relates external events to oneself when it is not justified	"My boss said our company's productivity was down this year, but I know he was really talking about me."
Dichotomous thinking	Thinking in extremes—that things are either all good or all bad	"If my husband leaves me I might as well be dead."
Catastrophizing	Thinking the worst about people and events	"I'd better not apply for that promotion at work because I won't get it and then I'll feel terrible."
Selective abstraction	Focusing on details but not on other relevant information	A wife believes her husband doesn't love her because he works late, but she ignores his affection, the gifts he brings her, and the special vacation they are planning together.
Arbitrary inference	Drawing a negative conclusion without supporting evidence	A young woman concludes "my friend no longer likes me" because she did not receive a birthday card.
Mind reading	Believing that one knows the thoughts of another without validation	"They probably think I'm fat and lazy."
Magnification/minimization	Exaggerating or trivializing the importance of events	"I've burned the dinner, which goes to show just how incompetent I am."
Perfectionism	Needing to do everything perfectly to feel good about oneself	"I'll be a failure if I don't get an A on all my exams."
Externalization of self-worth	Determining one's value based on the approval of others	"I have to look nice all the time or my friends won't want to have me around."

learned in therapy and to promote their use in real life. Rather than trying to remove problems by changing subconscious dynamics, the cognitive behavioral therapist works with the patient to plan experiences that encourage the development of new skills.

Another important characteristic is the high degree of **mutuality** in the treatment process. Cognitive behavioral therapists collaborate with the patient in defining the problem, identifying goals, formulating treatment strategies, and evaluating progress.

Because the focus is on the patient's self-control, cognitive behavioral therapy is seen as **educational and skill building** rather than curative, with the therapist taking a facilitative role. The therapeutic relationship and the responsive dimensions of genuineness, warmth, and empathy are all critically important, and full recognition is given to their significance in influencing the effectiveness of treatment.

From this overview it is evident that cognitive behavioral therapy has many things in common with the nursing process. The steps of the nursing process closely resemble the steps involved in cognitive behavioral therapy. Similarly, both approaches are patient centered and strongly emphasize mutuality.

Cognitive behavioral therapy also places a strong emphasis on an objective assessment process. Specifically, it uses standardized measurement tools, bases treatment strategies on research evidence, and values ongoing evaluation of patient progress.

These characteristics suggest that cognitive behavioral treatment strategies can make a significant contribution to the therapeutic effectiveness of nursing care. Therefore they have relevance for psychiatric nurses practicing in any setting and with any patient population.

BOX 31-1

Characteristics of Cognitive Behavioral Therapy

Empirically based. Extensive evidence supports cognitive behavioral methods for the treatment of many clinical problems.

Goal oriented. Explicit treatment goals are identified by the patient and therapist. They are then used to evaluate the patient's progress and treatment outcome.

Practical. The patient and therapist focus on defining and solving current problems of living. They discuss the here and now, not the history of the patient.

Collaborative. Collaboration with the patient and active participation by the patient in the treatment process are the norm. Cognitive behavioral therapy helps people change.

Open. The therapeutic process is open and explicit. The patient and the therapist share an understanding of what is going on in treatment.

Homework. The patient is often given homework assignments for data collecting, skill practice, and reinforcement of new responses.

Measurements. Baseline measurements of the problem behavior are made during the assessment process. These measurements are repeated at regular intervals during and at the completion of treatment. Thus the treatment process is rigorously monitored.

Active. Change and progress in treatment must be meaningful to the patient and have a positive impact on the quality of the patient's life. Both the patient and the therapist are active in therapy. The therapist serves as a teacher and coach, and the patient practices the strategies learned in therapy.

Short term. Cognitive behavior therapy is a short-term treatment that usually lasts 6 to 20 sessions.

■ COGNITIVE BEHAVIORAL ASSESSMENT

Cognitive behavioral therapy places great importance on assessment. Cognitive behavioral therapists assess the patient's **actions, thoughts,** and **feelings** in particular situations. Assessment includes collecting information, identifying problems from the data, defining the problem behavior, deciding how to measure the problem behavior, and identifying environmental variables that influence the problem behavior. It also includes a review of the patient's strengths and deficits and minimizes the use of assumptions and unvalidated inferences.

Nurses form conclusions about the physiological problems of patients after using a variety of tools and tests to collect objective evidence. Why do you think nurses dealing with psychosocial problems often forget to use the scientific approach and instead frequently base their care on unsubstantiated inferences? ■

It is important that the patient's problem be defined as clearly as possible. Initially the nurse addresses the following questions:

- What is the problem?
- Where does the problem occur?
- When does the problem occur?
- Who or what makes the problem occur?
- What is the feared consequence related to the problem?

The nurse can then assess the frequency, intensity, and duration of the problem.

The next step is to find out more about the patient's experience with the problem by using a behavioral analysis (Figure 31-1). This analysis consists of three parts **(the ABCs of behavior):**

- Antecedent: The stimulus or cue that occurs before the behavior and leads to its manifestation
- Behavior: What the person does or does not say or do
- Consequence: What type of effect (positive, negative, or neutral) the person thinks results from the behavior

Antecedents can include the physical environment, the social environment, or the person's behavior, feelings, or thoughts. Behaviors can be broken down into discrete actions or a series of steps. Consequences can be viewed as powerful rewards or punishments of a person's actions. Thus each is a critical element of the assessment. An example of a behavioral analysis is as follows:

- **Problem** = Anxiety
- **Feared consequence** = Fear of losing control or dying
- **Antecedent** = Leaving the house
- **Behavior** = Avoiding stores, restaurants, and public places
- **Consequence** = Restriction of daily activities

Another way to assess a person's experiences is to consider the three systems **(the ABCs of treatment)** that are interrelated in this treatment framework:

- **Affective:** Emotional or feeling responses
- **Behavioral:** Outward manifestations and actions
- **Cognitive:** Thoughts about the situation

Figure 31-2 shows that these three elements are interrelated in explaining human behavior because:

- **Feelings influence thinking.**
- **Thinking influences actions.**
- **Actions influence feelings.**

An assessment of each one of these areas has important implications for understanding the problem and treating it effectively.

Another aspect to be considered in the assessment process is whether the problem is expressed as an observable behavior and whether this behavior is current and predictable. Mutually agreed upon treatment goals and strategies can then be determined. Finally, throughout the treatment process, cognitive behavioral therapists use various methods to measure problem severity, including standardized rating scales.

In your mental health setting, are standardized rating scales used by staff members who work with patients? If so, how are they used? If not, how could their use influence patient care? ■

■ TREATMENT STRATEGIES

Cognitive behavioral therapy is the most heavily researched form of psychotherapy and has a strong evidence base in the treatment of a wide variety of clinical problems. It is useful in working with children, adolescents, adults, elderly, and families and may be implemented both individually and in groups (see Citing the Evidence). In general, cognitive behavioral treatment strategies are aimed at the following:

- **Increasing activity**
- **Reducing unwanted behavior**

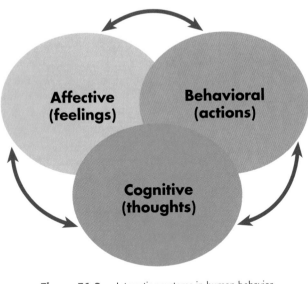

Figure 31-2   Interacting systems in human behavior.

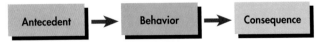

Figure 31-1   Phases of behavior.

- **Increasing pleasure**
- **Enhancing social skills**

The three groups of cognitive behavioral treatment strategies are listed in Box 31-2. These techniques may be used alone or in combination. They also require practical skills and efforts from both the nurse and the patient. This may include activities outside the clinical setting, such as taking a bus ride, riding an elevator, or going to a supermarket with a patient.

Anxiety Reduction

Relaxation Training. As a therapeutic tool, relaxation training effectively decreases tension and anxiety. It can be used alone, in combination with other cognitive behavioral techniques, or in addition to supportive or insight therapy. The basic premise is that muscle tension is related to anxiety. If tense muscles can be made to relax, anxiety will be reduced.

All relaxation procedures involve rhythmic breathing, reduced muscle tension, and an altered state of consciousness. Clinical experience suggests that there are individual differences in the experience of relaxation. Not everyone demonstrates all of the characteristics of a relaxed physiological state. The physiological, cognitive, and behavioral manifestations of relaxation are listed in Box 31-3.

Systematic relaxation training involves tensing and relaxing voluntary muscles in an orderly sequence until the body, as a whole, is relaxed. For this technique, the patient should be seated in a comfortable chair. Soft music or pleasant visual cues may be present. Before beginning the exercises, a brief explanation should be given about how anxiety is related to muscle tension. The relaxation procedure also should be described.

The patient begins by taking a deep breath and exhaling slowly. This is followed by a sequence of tension-relaxation exercises beginning with the hands and ending with the feet. The patient is instructed to tense each muscle group for approximately 10 seconds while the nurse describes how tense and uncomfortable this body part feels. The nurse then asks the patient to relax this muscle group as the nurse comments, "Notice how all the hardness and tension is draining from your hands. Now notice how they feel—warm, soft, and calm. Compare this feeling to when they were tense and see how much better they feel now." The patient should be reminded to tense only the muscle group named. The patient then proceeds to the next muscle group in the sequence listed in Box 31-4.

The final exercise asks the patient to become completely relaxed, beginning with the toes and moving up through the body to the eyes and forehead. Once the patient has learned the procedure, these exercises can be performed only for the

---

■ CITING THE EVIDENCE ON
Cognitive Behavioral Therapy for Schizophrenia

BACKGROUND: Despite advances in psychopharmacology, many patients with schizophrenia continue to experience persistent delusions and hallucinations, which result in increased anxiety and depression, disability, and risk of suicide. The aim of this study was to test whether the clinical benefits of cognitive behavioral therapy (CBT) and supportive counseling (SC) observed at posttreatment and 1 year are maintained 2 years after the end of treatment. Patients were randomly assigned to CBT plus routine care, SC and routine care, or routine care alone. Treatment took place over 3 months, and follow-up was made 12 and 24 months after treatment finished.

RESULTS: Patients who received only routine care did worse at 2 years for positive and negative symptoms, relapse, and rehospitalization.

IMPLICATIONS: Adjunct psychological treatments, including CBT, can have long-lasting benefits in the treatment of patients with chronic schizophrenia.

Tarrier N et al: *J Consult Clin Psychol* 68:917, 2000.

BOX 31-2

Cognitive Behavioral Treatment Strategies

Anxiety Reduction
Relaxation training
Biofeedback
Systematic desensitization
Interoceptive exposure
Flooding
Vestibular desensitization training
Response prevention
Eye movement desensitization and reprocessing

Cognitive Restructuring
Monitoring thoughts and feelings

Questioning the evidence
Examining alternatives
Decatastrophizing
Reframing
Thought stopping

Learning New Behavior
Modeling
Shaping
Token economy
Role playing
Social skills training
Aversive therapy
Contingency contracting

BOX 31-3

Manifestations of Relaxation

Physiological
Decreased pulse
Decreased blood pressure
Decreased respirations
Decreased oxygen consumption
Decreased metabolic rate
Pupil constriction
Peripheral vasodilation
Increased peripheral temperature

Cognitive
Altered state of consciousness

Heightened concentration on single mental image
Receptivity to positive suggestion

Behavioral
Lack of attention to and concern for environmental stimuli
No verbal interaction
No voluntary change of position
Passive movement easy

BOX 31-4

Sequence of Progressive Muscle Relaxation

Hands. First the fists are tensed and relaxed, then the fingers are extended and relaxed.

Biceps and triceps. These are tensed and relaxed.

Shoulders. They are pulled back and relaxed and then pushed forward and relaxed.

Neck. The head is turned slowly as far to the right as possible and relaxed, then turned to the left and relaxed. It is then brought forward until the chin touches the chest and relaxed.

Mouth. The mouth is opened as wide as possible and then relaxed. The lips form a pout and then relax. The tongue is extended out as far as possible and then relaxed, then retracted into the throat and then relaxed. It is pressed hard into the roof of the mouth and relaxed, then pressed hard into the floor of the mouth and relaxed.

Eyes. They are opened as wide as possible and relaxed, then closed as hard as possible and relaxed.

Breathing. The patient inhales as deeply as possible and relaxes, then exhales as much as possible and relaxes.

Back. The trunk of the body is pushed forward so that the entire back is arched, then relaxed.

Midsection. The buttocks muscles are tensed and then relaxed.

Thighs. The legs are extended and raised approximately 6 inches off the floor and then relaxed. The backs of the feet are pressed into the floor and relaxed.

Stomach. It is pulled in as much as possible and relaxed, then extended and relaxed.

Calves and feet. With legs supported, the feet are bent with the toes pointing toward the head and then relaxed. Feet are then bent in the opposite direction and relaxed.

Toes. The toes are pressed into the bottom of the shoes and relaxed. They are then bent to touch the top inside of the shoes and relaxed.

---

muscles that usually become tense. This is different for each person and may include the shoulders, forehead, back, or neck. Patients may also eliminate the tensing exercises and perform only the relaxation ones.

Meditation also may be used to evoke the relaxation response (LaTorre, 2001). It may follow or replace systematic relaxation. The basic components for meditation include the following:

- A quiet environment
- A passive attitude
- A comfortable position
- A word or scene to focus on

The first three components are necessary for any relaxation procedure. The fourth component refers to **visualization**—the process in which the patient selects a cue word or scene with pleasant connotations. The nurse then instructs the patient to close both eyes, relax each of the major muscle groups, and begin repeating the word silently at each exhalation.

Other relaxation techniques include guided imagery, centering, mindful meditation, and focusing. Although each of these approaches varies slightly, the intent of all of them is to use the mind to get in touch with the inner self. As such, they have been found to promote relaxation, enhance sleep, reduce pain, and increase creativity.

 Name four clinical settings in which nurses can use relaxation training with patients. Identify whether such training would be a primary, secondary, or tertiary prevention activity in each setting. ■

Biofeedback. Biofeedback uses a machine to reduce anxiety and modify behavioral responses. Small electrodes connected to the biofeedback equipment are attached to the patient's forehead. Brain waves, muscle tension, body temperature, heart rate, and blood pressure can then be monitored for small changes. These changes are communicated to the patient by auditory and visual means. The more relaxed the patient becomes, the more pleasant are the sounds or sights presented. These pleasant sights and sounds stop when the patient stops relaxing, and they resume when the patient reachieves the relaxed state. After developing the ability to relax, the patient is encouraged to apply the technique during stressful situations (Patrick, 2002).

Systematic Desensitization. Systematic desensitization was designed to decrease the avoidance behavior linked to a specific stimulus (e.g., heights, airplane travel). The goal of systematic desensitization is to help the patient change his or her response to a threatening stimulus (Kormos, 2003). It involves combining deep muscle relaxation with imagined scenes of situations that cause anxiety. The assumption is that relaxation is incompatible with anxiety. Therefore if the person is taught to relax while imagining such scenes, the real-life situation depicted by the scene will cause much less anxiety.

With systematic desensitization, the patient must first be able to relax the muscles. Next, a hierarchy of the anxiety-provoking or feared situations is constructed. These situations are ranked from 1 to 10 in order of difficulty, with 1 evoking little or no anxiety and 10 evoking intense or severe anxiety. Box 31-5 presents a sample hierarchy of a patient with agoraphobia.

With **in vitro**, or imagined, desensitization, the patient proceeds with the imagined pairing of the hierarchy items with the relaxed state, progressing from the least anxiety-provoking item to the most anxiety-provoking item. **In vivo** desensitization exposes the patient to real rather than imagined life situations. In vivo exposure is widely considered to be the treatment of choice for simple and social phobias and for obsessive-compulsive disorders.

This technique works through a combination of positive reinforcement for confronting anxiety-provoking stimuli and the extinction of maladaptive behavior that occurs when it is realized that the feared negative consequences never occurred. It is helpful for the nurse to share the following thoughts with the patient during exposure therapy:

- Anxiety is unpleasant but is not dangerous; that is, the patient will not die or lose control.

- Anxiety does eventually decrease and does not continue indefinitely.
- Practice makes perfect; the more the patient repeats a particular exposure exercise, the easier it becomes.

For example, a boy may have a fear of spiders. His daily schedule may then include a series of planned activities involving reading about spiders. He may then begin gradual exposure to pictures and photographs of spiders, followed by looking at real spiders in his yard. Thus the exposure gradually leads to anxiety reduction and more adaptive behaviors.

Interoceptive Exposure. Interoceptive exposure is a technique used to desensitize a patient to catastrophic interpretations of internal bodily cues such as tachycardia, blurred vision, and shortness of breath. A hierarchy is made of the specific symptoms that increase the patient's anxiety. The patient is then asked to do the things that cause these symptoms in a gradually increasing, repetitive manner in order to desensitize him or her to these cues. Patients can be asked to jump in place, run up a flight of stairs, or spin in circles. This technique is especially helpful for patients who do not have agoraphobia but have spontaneous, unprovoked panic attacks that cause them increased worry and anxiety.

Flooding. Flooding is another form of exposure therapy in which the patient is immediately exposed to the most anxiety-provoking stimulus instead of being exposed gradually or systematically to a hierarchy of feared stimuli. If this technique uses an imaginary event instead of a real life event, it is called **implosion**.

Vestibular Desensitization Training. Vestibular desensitization training is an exposure therapy for patients whose panic attacks are provoked by environmental cues that cause them to have symptoms of motion sickness (e.g., dizziness, imbalance, vertigo, nausea, tinnitus, blurred vision, or headache). These environmental cues can include suddenly changing position, walking on floors with patterns, walking down a grocery store aisle that is stacked high with products on both sides, or riding in a car on a hilly road.

A desensitization hierarchy is created to include activities that cause these symptoms, such as getting up suddenly from a prone position, making sudden head movements, or making sudden stop-and-go movements. Patients who get motion sickness when standing in a wide open space with no object to break the horizon are taught to turn in a full circle while keeping their eyes on a selected object for orientation, much like ballet dancers do when they turn repetitively.

Response Prevention. In response prevention the patient is encouraged to face a particular fear or situation without engaging in the accompanying behavior. This technique is based on the concept that repeated exposure to an anxiety-producing stimulus without the presence of the anxiety-reducing response will lead to anxiety reduction because the feared consequence does not occur.

> ### BOX 31-5
>
> #### Sample Patient Hierarchy for Phobias
>
> A hierarchy of phobias is a list of your fears and avoidances in order of severity. Your greatest phobia should be at the top of the list and your smallest fear at the bottom. In between, rank your other fears and phobias in order of severity. Try to list 10 but not more than 20 phobias. These activities should be convenient to do, because you will be doing them from several times a day to at least several times per week.
>
> For example, think of yourself standing at the end of a football field marked off in 10-yard lines. Closest to you, at the 0-yard line, is something you are mildly fearful of or avoid doing sometimes but not always; the farthest end of the field is your biggest fear; at the 50-yard line is a medium fear; and on the 10-yard line is a minor fear but one that is stronger than at the 0-yard line.
>
> Remember that everyone's hierarchy will be different. There are no "right" or "wrong" hierarchies. Your hierarchy is a tool to help you approach feared situations in a systematic and controlled way.
>
> **Sample Hierarchy**
>
> | | |
> |---|---|
> | 100 | Driving alone across a high bridge in the rain |
> | 90 | Driving alone on the interstate far from home |
> | 80 | Driving alone on side streets that are unfamiliar |
> | 70 | Speaking in front of groups of people |
> | 60 | Using elevators alone |
> | 50 | Eating in restaurants alone |
> | 40 | Going to large public gatherings with safe people |
> | 30 | Eating with friends or family in familiar restaurants |
> | 20 | Driving more than several miles from home with a passenger in the car |
> | 10 | Going shopping with a safe person in big stores and malls |
> | 0 | Going shopping with a safe person in small stores near home |

For example, a patient may fear using a public restroom and engage in hand washing up to 20 times a day. With response prevention treatment, the patient's daily schedule would include using a public restroom, turning on the water faucets, and washing hands for only 30 seconds. Over time, the maladaptive behaviors would be reduced because the feared consequence of germs and illness did not occur.

Eye Movement Desensitization and Reprocessing. Eye movement desensitization and reprocessing (EMDR) is based on specific and repetitive rapid eye movements similar to those experienced naturally in rapid eye movement (REM) sleep. The principle behind this treatment is that the brain lays down biological memory tracks during early traumatic experiences. These memory tracks are provoked later during seemingly unrelated events, causing anxiety and perhaps depression.

With EMDR, the patient is asked to think about past traumatic events while the therapist moves his or her hand back and forth in front of the patient's face; the patient's eyes follow the therapist's hands. In this way, the neural tracks are hypothesized to become reprogrammed and less sensitized to anxiety-provoking experiences (Shapiro and Forrest, 1997).

EMDR is being used to treat a variety of psychological problems, including anxiety, stress, phobias, recurrent nightmares, substance abuse, and posttraumatic stress disorder (Lee, Beaton, and Ensign, 2003). However, meta-analyses of existing research studies do not show clear evidence of its effectiveness (Davidson and Parker, 2001; Shepherd, Stein, and Milne, 2000). What appears to be useful with EMDR is the behavioral desensitization aspect of the treatment, which is not new. Furthermore the same effect may be achieved with other forms of rhythmic stimulation, such as finger tapping or musical tones.

> *Do you think a highly anxious nurse can effectively implement anxiety-reduction strategies with patients? Why or why not?* ■

Cognitive Restructuring

Monitoring Thoughts and Feelings. Changing cognitions begins with identifying what is reinforcing and maintaining the patient's dysfunctional thinking and maladaptive behavior. An important first step is for patients to become more aware of and monitor their own thinking and feeling. Patients can be helped to do this through the use of the Daily Record of Dysfunctional Thoughts Form (Figure 31-3).

The patient uses this form by recording information in each of five columns, beginning with a brief description of a particular situation or event in the first column. The patient writes down his or her feelings or emotions, as well as the automatic thoughts in response to the situation. The strength of each is also rated by the patient. The patient is then encouraged to think of a more rational response to the situation and record that in the fourth column. Finally, in the last column, the patient reevaluates his or her level of belief in the automatic thought and subsequent emotions.

By using such a form, patients are taught to distinguish between thoughts and feelings and to identify more adaptive responses to problematic situations. They also begin to recognize the connection between certain thoughts and maladaptive emotions and behaviors.

Questioning the Evidence. The next step is for the patient and therapist to examine the evidence that is used to support a certain belief. Questioning the evidence also involves examining the source of the data. Patients with distorted thinking often give equal weight to all sources of information or ignore all data except those that support their distorted thinking. Having patients question their evidence with staff, family, and other members of their social support network can clarify misinformation and result

	Situation	Emotion(s)	Automatic Thought(s)	Rational Response	Outcome
Date	Describe: 1. Actual event leading to unpleasant emotion, or 2. Stream of thoughts, daydream, or recollection, leading to unpleasant emotion	1. Specify sad, anxious, angry, etc. 2. Rate degree of emotion, 1-100.	1. Write automatic thought(s) that preceded emotion(s). 2. Rate belief in automatic thought(s) 0-100%.	1. Write rational response to automatic thought(s). 2. Rate belief in rational response 0-100%.	1. Rerate belief in automatic thought(s), 0-100%. 2. Specify and rate subsequent emotions, 0-100.
10/9/04	1. Event- My boyfriend was supposed to call me tonight to discuss our plans but he never did. 2. He must be too busy for me. Maybe he's seeing someone else and wants to break it off with me.	1. Anxious - 90 2. Sad - 50 3. Angry - 10	1a. I'll never be able to keep a boyfriend - 60% 1b. I am not a "good enough" date or girlfriend - 70%	1. Lots of men at school seem to enjoy talking and spending time with me - 80% 2. I'll have plenty of time in the future to meet more men and develop relationships - 50%	1a. I'll never be able to keep a boyfriend - 30% 1b. I am not a "good enough" date or girlfriend - 40% 2. Anxious - 20 Sad - 5 Angry - 30

Explanation: When you experience an unpleasant emotion, note the situation that seemed to stimulate the emotion. (If the emotion occurred while you were thinking, daydreaming, etc., please note this.) Then note the automatic thought associated with the emotion. Record the degree to which you believe this thought: 0%, not at all; 100%, completely. In rating degree of emotion: 1, a trace; 100, the most intense possible.

Figure 31-3 Daily Record of Dysfunctional Thoughts form. (Modified from Beck A et al: *Cognitive therapy of depression*, New York, 1979, Guilford.)

in more realistic and appropriate interpretations of the evidence.

Examining Alternatives. Many patients see themselves as having lost all options. This type of thinking is particularly evident in suicidal patients. Examining alternatives involves working with patients to generate additional options based on their strengths and coping resources.

Decatastrophizing. Decatastrophizing is also called the "what-if" technique. It involves helping patients evaluate whether they are overestimating the catastrophic nature of a situation. Questions that the nurse can ask include, "What is the worst thing that can happen?" "Would it be so terrible if that really took place?" "How would other people cope with such an event?" The goal of this intervention is to help the patient see that the consequences of life's actions are generally not "all or nothing" and thus are less catastrophic.

Reframing. Reframing is a strategy that changes a patient's perception of a situation or behavior. It involves focusing on other aspects of the problem or encouraging a patient to see the issue from a different perspective.

Patients who dichotomize events may see only one side of a situation. Weighing the advantages and disadvantages of maintaining a particular belief or behavior can help patients gain balance and develop a new perspective. By understanding both the positive and negative consequences of an issue, the patient can attain a broader perspective of it. For example, suggesting that a mother's overinvolvement with her son is actually a sign of her loving concern may help a family see the situation in a new light.

This strategy also creates an opportunity to help challenge the meaning of a problem or behavior; once the meaning of a behavior changes, the person's response will also change. For example, this strategy might involve helping a patient see an adversity as a potentially positive event. The loss of a job may be perceived as a stressor, but it also can be viewed as an opportunity for pursuing a new job or career.

> *Think of a problem you encountered in the past year. How might you have used the technique of cognitive reframing to see the situation in a more positive way?* ■

Thought Stopping. Dysfunctional thinking often can have a snowball effect on patients. What begins as a small or insignificant problem can, over time, gather importance and momentum that can be difficult to stop. The technique of thought stopping is best used when the dysfunctional thought first begins. The patient can picture a stop sign, imagine a bell going off, or envision a brick wall to stop the progression of the dysfunctional thought.

To begin, the patient identifies the problematic thought and talks about it as the problem scene is imagined. The nurse interrupts the patient's thoughts by shouting "STOP." Thereafter the patient learns to interrupt thoughts in a similar way. Finally, the patient converts the "stop" into an in-audible phrase or image and thus learns to use the technique quietly in everyday situations.

Learning New Behavior

Modeling. Modeling is a strategy used to form new behavior patterns, increase existing skills, or reduce avoidance behavior. The target behavior is broken down into a series of separate stages that are ranked in order of difficulty or distress, with the first stage being the least anxiety provoking. The patient observes a person modeling the behavior in a controlled environment. The patient then imitates the model's behavior. In participant modeling, the model and patient perform the behavior together before the patient performs it alone. For the treatment to be most effective, it is particularly important that the model selected for this treatment be credible to the patient.

Shaping. Shaping induces new behaviors by reinforcing behaviors that approximate the desired behavior. Each successive approximation of the behavior is reinforced until the desired behavior is attained. Skillful use of the technique requires that the nurse carefully look, wait, and reinforce. The nurse needs to look for the desired behavior, wait until it occurs, and then reinforce it when it does occur. An example of this strategy is the nurse noticing that an aggressive child is playing cooperatively with a peer and then praising the child for this behavior.

Token Economy. A token economy is a form of positive reinforcement used most often on a group basis with children or patients in a psychiatric hospital. It consists of rewarding the person in various ways (e.g., tokens, passes, or points) for performing desired target behaviors. These target behaviors might include performing hygienic grooming, attending classes, or verbally expressing frustration rather than striking out at others. Tokens also may be lost for inappropriate behaviors. If tokens or points are used, they may be cashed in periodically for rewards such as free time, off-unit outings, games, or nutritious snacks.

Role Playing. Role playing allows patients to rehearse problematic issues and obtain feedback about their behavior. It can provide practice for decision making and exploring consequences. A related practice is role reversal, in which the patient switches roles with someone else and thus experiences the difficult situation from another point of view.

Social Skills Training. Smooth social functioning is central to most human activity, and social skills problems exist in many psychiatrically ill patients. Social skills training is based on the belief that skills are learned and therefore can be taught to those who do not have them. The principles of skill acquisition include the following:

- **Guidance**
- **Demonstration**
- **Practice**
- **Feedback**

These principles must be included in implementing an effective social skills training program, which is often a component of psychiatric rehabilitation programs (see Chapter 15). Guidance and demonstration are usually used early in the treatment, followed by practice and feedback. Treatment typically follows four stages:

1. **Describing** the new behavior to be learned
2. **Learning** the new behavior through the use of guidance and demonstration
3. **Practicing** the new behavior with feedback
4. **Transferring** the new behavior to the natural environment

The types of behaviors that are often taught in these programs include asking questions, giving compliments, making positive changes, maintaining eye contact, asking others for specific behavior changes, speaking in a clear tone of voice, and avoiding fidgeting and self-criticism. This treatment strategy is most often used with patients who lack social skills, assertiveness (assertiveness training), or impulse control (anger management), as well as with patients who exhibit antisocial behavior.

Aversion Therapy. Aversion therapy helps reduce unwanted but persistent maladaptive behaviors. Aversive conditioning applies an aversive or noxious stimulus when a maladaptive behavior occurs. An example is for a patient to snap a rubber band on the wrist when being bothered by an intrusive thought. Covert sensitization is an aversive technique in which patients imagine scenes that pair the undesired behavior with an unpleasant consequence. By imagining aversive consequences for a behavior such as overeating, the patient gains control by providing a form of punishment for his or her own behavior.

> *Aversion therapy has sometimes been criticized as unethical and detrimental to patients' well-being. Do you agree? If not, what conditions should be present before implementing aversive therapy with patients?* ■

Contingency Contracting. Contingency contracting involves a formal contract between the patient and the therapist, defining what behaviors are to be changed and what consequences follow the performance of these behaviors. Included are positive consequences for desirable behaviors and negative consequences for undesirable behaviors.

■ ROLE OF THE NURSE

Much of the early history of behavioral therapy took place in the United States. The first report of nurses functioning as behavioral therapists came from Ayllon and Michael (1959), who taught nurses to use operant skills in modifying the behavior of patients in long-term psychiatric institutions. It was believed that nurses were a natural choice because they made up the majority of the staff caring for the patients. Since that time, the practice of cognitive behavioral therapy nursing has been more dominant in Britain than in the United States.

In 1975 Isaac Marks, a psychiatrist and researcher in London, established the first program to prepare nurses to be cog-

nitive behavioral therapists. This program continues today at the Institute of Psychiatry at Maudsley in London. The clinical outcomes these nurses achieved were at least as good as those obtained by other professionals.

Marks also calculated the cost-benefit ratio of employing nurses as therapists. He found that people treated by nurses used fewer health care resources after treatment than before, resulting in a significant savings of resources (Ginsberg and Marks, 1977). These were impressive findings, and cognitive behavioral therapy became an increasingly important component of the nurse's role in England and Scotland in the years that followed.

In contrast, cognitive behavioral therapy has been integrated into the role of the psychiatric nurse much less in the United States (see Critical Thinking About Contemporary Issues). This needs to change because nurses are the front-

---

■ **Critical Thinking** *About* **Contemporary Issues**

Does Humanistic Nursing Care Embrace Cognitive Behavioral Treatment Strategies?

Humanistic care is highly valued in nursing. However, the definition and boundaries of such care are often vague and unspecified. Many believe in the primacy of psychodynamic psychotherapy, yet relatively little research specifies the clinical conditions and disorders for which it is effective. In comparison, the evidence is overwhelmingly in support of the effectiveness of cognitive behavioral therapy in treating a variety of psychiatric illnesses. This leads one to wonder why cognitive behavioral therapy is not incorporated to a greater degree into the practice of psychiatric nurses.

In fact, too few nurses are skilled in the principles and techniques of cognitive behavioral therapy. There are several possible reasons for this. First, nurses may have little formal exposure to cognitive behavioral treatment strategies in the course of their education. Second, nurses have been traditionally reinforced for their unconditional nurturance of patients and their compliance with physicians' orders. In contrast, cognitive behavioral therapy requires the use of independent judgment, limit setting, reframing, and the selective use of rewards, skills that nurses may not be encouraged to use in clinical settings. Third, nurses place great emphasis on the therapeutic use of self, and this approach to nursing has sometimes created confusion between the concepts of caring and treatment. It incorrectly suggests that these are different events, with nurses being responsible for caring and physicians being responsible for treating. Fourth, myths continue to surround the field of cognitive behavioral therapy, and nurses have been slow to acknowledge the facts about this treatment modality.

Current changes in the scope and functions of contemporary psychiatric nursing practice underscore the need for all nurses to learn cognitive behavioral therapy skills. Contemporary psychiatric nursing practice includes both caring and treating activities. The reality is that nurses have always been involved with helping patients reduce anxiety, change cognitions, and learn new behaviors. As influential agents of behavioral change, nurses need to be aware of their ability to promote adaptive or maladaptive responses and increase their skills and knowledge in effective treatment strategies.

line providers of care. They are the group called on most often to carry out selective reinforcement, modeling, extinction, skills training, shaping, and role playing. Because of their direct patient contact, nurses are best able to observe patients, assess problem areas, and recommend targets for cognitive behavioral intervention.

There are three basic roles for nurses involved in cognitive behavioral therapy. Each of these roles can be performed by all nurses at various levels of expertise—from novice through generalist and specialist:

1. Providing direct patient care
2. Planning treatment programs
3. Teaching others the use of cognitive behavioral techniques

Psychiatric nurses provide direct patient care in both inpatient and community settings, and the value of cognitive behavioral therapy is evident throughout the continuum of care. Most treatments are ideally suited to community settings, and they can include interventions across the continuum of coping responses—from promoting health, to intervening in acute illness, to fostering rehabilitation.

Nurses also may function as planners and coordinators of complex treatment programs, consultants, and teachers of other nurses, professionals, patients, and their families. It is clear that with the current emphasis on cost-effective treatment and documented outcomes of care, cognitive behavioral therapy will be a growing area of expertise for all psychiatric nurses in the next decade.

COMPETENT CARING
A Clinical Exemplar of a Psychiatric Nurse
DARCY O'NEILL, RN

I first met A, a 13-year-old girl, when she was admitted by her mother to our combined child and adolescent psychiatric unit. Her mother reported that A was becoming increasingly oppositional, refusing to attend school, having sexual relations with multiple partners, running away from home for long periods, and exhibiting destructive outbursts when confronted. A was admitted to our unit following a 3-day runaway. She appeared tired and disheveled, somewhat older than her chronological age, and was extremely angry about hospitalization. However, despite her angry demeanor, it was rapidly apparent that A was a very bright and charming young girl. I was intrigued.

During this hospitalization A continued to have unpredictable violent outbursts. At times the most benign redirection would result in verbal threats, screaming, and cursing, which would often escalate into physical attacks on staff. At other times, a similar or more emphatic directive would be calmly accepted and performed. I was puzzled and rather frustrated by trying to balance this child's need to express some deeply felt anger while maintaining the safety of the milieu.

Our unit uses a token economy as part of a patient's treatment. Depending on the age and cognitive abilities, patients earn points or stickers for attending activities and participating in treatment. Points are earned as rewards and may be exchanged for special privileges. Although we specialize in short-term assessment and evaluation, many children quickly engage in this token economy and are able to address behavioral issues in a direct and timely fashion. Unfortunately, A was not one of these children. Her participation in the point system was as unpredictable and sporadic as her behavior.

The team began to discuss the therapeutic effectiveness of an individually designed behavioral program for A. As a new graduate nurse who knew little about the use of behavioral therapies, I balked. I felt that what A needed was more one-to-one time to process the strong emotions underlying her behavior. A and I were beginning to have regular but brief interactions in which she began to share some of her feelings. I feared that by making a more concrete program, obviously different from the program her peers experienced, we risked alienating a child who already had great difficulties with trust. I also

feared that from a position of frustration we were falling into a punitive stance. Unfortunately, A was discharged to an outpatient program before the formulation of a new behavioral program. It seemed that many of my questions concerning the therapeutic value of special behavioral programs would remain unanswered.

After I had been on the unit for 6 months, A was readmitted. At this admission her mother reported an increase in the severity and frequency of the behaviors that had precipitated A's first admission. In the time that had passed since her first admission, I had had quite a few opportunities to work with individually designed behavioral programs. I had begun to appreciate this therapeutic approach and to understand that for many children these programs provided a sense of security and an opportunity to address their problem behaviors more concretely.

What I had not understood at the time of A's first admission was that these programs increase the amount of one-to-one while helping children take more control of their own behavior. I had discovered that behavioral programs provided the framework for increased teaching and learning.

From the outset of her second admission, A was increasingly difficult to reach. She had become more physically and verbally threatening. I continued to try to engage her in the point system and had moderate success.

A was even more unpredictable. At one minute she was willing to discuss her emotions and was open to nurturance and support, and at the next she was isolated and violent, with no tolerance of any perceived frustration. I was quickly exasperated. I truly liked this charming, bright young girl who showed me through her behavior that she was in a great deal of pain. Many times after a violent or threatening outburst she would cry inconsolably, curled in the fetal position, appearing much younger than her 13 years. I agonized along with the team members on how to help this child out of a self-destructive, downward spiral.

The team quickly returned to the discussion of a special behavioral program. Almost as quickly the staff became divided on how to best design and implement this program. Individual philosophies, differing levels of appreciation for behavioral therapies, and personal limits and tolerances were shared in numerous discussions.

With A's full participation and tenuous acceptance, a preliminary program was designed and implemented. Within 3 days some minor improvements were noted, but they were buried in continually violent and impulsive behavior. It took a great deal of painstaking discussion for staff to identify the positive behavior changes and suggest appropriate modifications in the behavior plan in an effort to increase these positive behaviors. Unfortunately, this was not effective for A, and within the next few days she needed seclusion to remain safe.

Again, the team reassessed the program and decided to adopt a more concrete contract with A. A could earn immediate rewards by either exhibiting new positive behaviors or by refraining from old negative behavior. The hope was to extinguish dangerous, self-destructive behaviors while replacing them with new coping strategies. Again, the changes were subtle and erratic and were surrounded by what appeared to be setbacks. This program necessitated hypervigilance on the part of staff to be aware of any positive change, no matter how slight.

I recall one time I was attempting to process with A after she was placed in open seclusion after threatening staff. I found myself desperately searching for positive feedback to offer her. All I could immediately identify was total frustration with her behavior and the program, in addition to my own feelings of inadequacy.

Yet with a little reflection, I was able to see a number of significant changes as I reviewed her behavioral contract. She had walked to seclusion independently; she needed only one directive to go to the seclusion room; and she was able to sit there without swearing at or threatening me. As soon as I realized all the changes I was witnessing, I became elated. Although she was still unable to talk with me, I continued to state how impressed I was by her ability to eliminate these behaviors. I made a point of sharing this information with passing staff, loud enough for A to hear. In time she was able to process what had happened and reintegrate into the milieu.

Through this trying, challenging experience I believe I was able to grow professionally and personally. I learned in a very deep way the therapeutic necessity of a fully functioning interdisciplinary team, as well as my integral role on that team. More important, I gained a new respect for behavioral programs and the opportunities they offer not only for patients but also for nurses. A well-designed behavioral program provides numerous opportunities for teaching, one-to-one relationship building, and a framework for continual assessment, planning, and evaluation.

Although the desired outcomes may be slow in coming and the process difficult, I readily look forward to the next opportunity to use my skills creatively in designing and implementing a behavioral treatment program. ∎

CHAPTER FOCUS POINTS

- Cognitive behavioral treatment strategies are aimed at helping people overcome difficulties in any area of human experience. They are problem focused and goal oriented, and they deal with here-and-now issues.
- Behavior is any observable, recordable, and measurable act, movement, or response. It is what is observed—not the conclusions drawn from the observation.
- Classical conditioning focuses on the processes by which involuntary behavior is learned.
- Operant conditioning focuses on the processes by which voluntary behavior is learned, including increasing and decreasing behavior.
- Increasing behavior occurs through reinforcers. Positive reinforcement increases the frequency of behavior by supplying rewarding stimuli. Negative reinforcement also increases the frequency of behavior by reinforcing the power of the behavior to control an aversive, rather than rewarding, stimuli.
- Decreasing behavior occurs through implementing punishment, response cost, and extinction.
- Cognitive therapists believe that maladaptive responses arise from cognitive distortions, and the goal of therapy is to change irrational beliefs, faulty reasoning, and negative self-statements that underlie behavioral problems.
- Cognitive behavioral therapy is similar to the nursing process in that both are patient centered, emphasize mutuality, and place a strong emphasis on the measurement of progress and evaluation.
- Cognitive behavioral assessment includes collecting information, identifying problems, defining the problem, deciding how to measure the problem, and identifying environmental variables that influence the problem behavior.
- The ABCs of behavior are antecedent, behavior, and consequence.
- The ABCs of treatment are affective, behavioral, and cognitive.
- Cognitive behavioral treatment strategies are aimed at increasing activity, reducing unwanted behavior, increasing pleasure, and enhancing social skills.
- A variety of cognitive behavioral treatment strategies may be used alone or in combination. They focus on anxiety reduction, cognitive restructuring, and learning new behavior.
- Three basic roles for nurses involved in cognitive behavioral therapy are (1) providing direct patient care, (2) planning treatment programs, and (3) teaching others the use of behavioral techniques. These roles may be enacted by all nurses in various practice settings.

KEY TERMS

antecedent, 658
aversion therapy, 664
behavior, 654, 658
biofeedback, 660
classical conditioning, 655
cognition, 656
cognitive distortions, 656
consequence, 658
contingency contracting, 664
decatastrophizing, 663
extinction, 656

eye movement desensitization and reprocessing (EMDR), 661
flooding, 661
interoceptive exposure, 661
modeling, 663
negative reinforcement, 655
operant conditioning, 655
positive reinforcement, 655
punishment, 655
relaxation training, 659

response cost, 656
response prevention, 661
role playing, 663
shaping, 663
social skills training, 663
systematic desensitization, 660
thought stopping, 663
token economy, 663
vestibular desensitization training, 661

CHAPTER REVIEW QUESTIONS

1. Match each term item in Column A with the correct definition in Column B.

Column A

_____ Behavior
_____ Biofeedback
_____ Contingency contracting
_____ Extinction
_____ Flooding
_____ Punishment
_____ Shaping
_____ Social skills training
_____ Systematic desensitization
_____ Reframing

Column B

A. An aversive stimulus that decreases behavior
B. Any observable, recordable, measurable act or response
C. Combines deep muscle relaxation with imagined scenes of situations that cause anxiety
D. Immediate exposure to one's most anxiety-provoking stimulus
E. Induces new behaviors by reinforcing behaviors that approximate the desired behavior
F. Involves a formal contract between the patient and the therapist, defining behaviors to be changed and the consequences
G. Monitors brain waves and body activities, allowing a patient to modify behavioral responses
H. Process of eliminating a behavior by ignoring it or not rewarding it
I. Strategy used to modify or change a person's perception of a situation or behavior
J. Technique for learning new behavior; consists of guidance, demonstration, practice, and feedback

2. Fill in the blanks.

A. A person's pupil constricting when exposed to bright sunlight is an example of _____.
B. Putting on sunscreen lotion to avoid a sunburn is an example of _____.
C. The three operant conditioning techniques used to decrease behavior are _____, _____, and _____.
D. Cognitive therapy proposes that it is not the event itself but a person's _____ of the event that causes adaptive or maladaptive responses.
E. A list of a person's fears, avoidances, or maladaptive responses in order of severity is called a _____.
F. The three roles for nurses involving cognitive behavioral therapy are _____, _____, and _____.
G. In cognitive behavioral therapy, emphasis is placed on behavioral monitoring and the completion of _____ by the patient.

3. Provide short answers for the following questions.

A. Analyze the nursing assessment form you use in your clinical work from the perspective of a cognitive behavioral therapist. What changes would you make from this perspective?
B. Describe the ABCs of behavior and the ABCs of cognitive behavioral treatment.
C. For 2 days use the daily record of dysfunctional thoughts and evaluate its value for your work with patients.
D. Try the steps of relaxation training on yourself. Note your thoughts, feelings, and behaviors during the process.

Visit Evolve for additional resources related to the content of this chapter.

http://evolve.elsevier.com/Stuart/principles/
• Topical Course Outline • Student Workbook Exercises • Critical Thinking Questions and Activities • Case Studies • Research Topics
• Monthly Content Updates • WebLinks

Student Study CD-ROM

Access the accompanying CD-ROM for animations, interactive exercises, review questions for the NCLEX examination, and an audio glossary.

REFERENCES

Ayllon T, Michael J: The psychiatric nurse as a behavioral engineer, *J Exp Anal Behav* 2:323, 1959.

Beck AT: *Cognitive therapy and the emotional disorders,* Philadelphia, 1976, Center for Cognitive Therapy.

Beck J: *Cognitive therapy: basics and beyond,* New York, 1995, Guilford.

Davidson PR, Parker KC: Eye movement desensitization and reprocessing (EMDR): a meta-analysis, *J Consult Clin Psychol* 69:305, 2001.

Ginsberg G, Marks I: Costs and benefits of behavioral psychotherapy: a pilot study of neurotics treated by nurse therapists, *Psychol Med* 7:685, 1977.

Kormos T: Behavioral treatment for fear of flying, *J Am Psychiatr Nurs Assoc* 9:145, 2003.

LaTorre M: Meditation and psychotherapy: an effective combination, *Perspect Psychiatr Care* 37:103, 2001.

Lee GK, Beaton RD, Ensign J: Eye movement desensitization and reprocessing: a brief and effective treatment for stress, *J Psychosoc Nurs Ment Health Serv* 41:22, 2003.

Patrick G: Biofeedback applications for psychiatric nursing, *J Am Psychiatr Nurs Assoc* 8:109, 2002.

Pavlov I: *Conditioned reflexes,* London, 1927, Oxford University Press.

Shapiro F, Forrest M: *EMDR: the breakthrough therapy for overcoming anxiety, stress and trauma,* New York, 1997, Basic Books.

Shepherd J, Stein K, Milne R: Eye movement desensitization and reprocessing in the treatment of post-traumatic stress disorder: a review of emerging therapy, *Psychol Med* 30:863, 2000.

Skinner BF: *Science and human behavior,* New York, 1953, Free Press.

Wright J, Beck A: Cognitive therapy. In Hales RE et al, editors: *American Psychiatric Press Textbook of Psychiatry,* ed 3, Washington, DC, 2000, American Psychiatric Press.

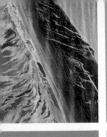

Self and world are correlated, and so are individualization and participation.... Participation means: being a part of something from which one is, at the same time, separated.

PAUL TILLICH, *THE COURAGE TO BE*

32 THERAPEUTIC GROUPS

Paula M. LaSalle ■ *Arthur J. LaSalle*

LEARNING OBJECTIVES

After studying this chapter, the student should be able to:

1. Define a group (**I**).
2. Describe the components of a small group (**II**).
3. Compare the stages of group development (**III**).
4. Analyze small-group evaluation factors (**IV**).
5. Examine the responsibilities and qualities of nurses as group leaders and the types of groups they lead (**V**).

TOPICAL OUTLINE

 Visit Evolve for additional resources related to the content of this chapter.
http://evolve.elsevier.com/Stuart/principles/

Groups provide nurses with wonderful opportunities to facilitate therapeutic growth in patients. They offer members a variety of relationships as they interact with each other and with the group leader. Since group members come from many backgrounds, they have the opportunity to learn to deal with the likes, dislikes, similarities, and dissimilarities of others outside their usual social circle. They are confronted with envy, timidity, anger, aggression, fear, joy, generosity, attraction, competitiveness, and the many other emotions and motives presented by others (Yalom, 1995). All of this takes place in the context of the dynamics of the group process in which, with careful leadership, members give and receive feedback about the meaning and effect of their various interactions with each other.

Groups can be formed to support those of many different populations and can be conducted in a variety of settings, including inpatient units, community and university health centers, schools, churches, and places of employment. Groups may be formed to address the needs of the families of people with serious mental illness for the purpose of receiving instruction, assistance with coping, mutual support, and crisis intervention. School nurses may

lead groups for children who share developmental milestones or life problems, such as parental divorce or death. In each of these situations the format, setting, and goal of the group varies. Thus facilitating group work is an important skill for all nurses to master, regardless of their practice setting or specialty area.

Think of some specific patient situations in which a group approach would be more effective than an individual nurse-patient encounter. Discuss the reasons for this. Describe other situations in which a group format would be less helpful. ■

■ DEFINITION

A group is a collection of people who have a relationship with one another, are interdependent, and may have common norms. Therapeutic groups have a shared purpose. For example, a group's purpose might be to help members who consistently engage in destructive relationships identify and change their maladaptive behaviors. Each group has its own structure and identity. The power of the group lies in the contributions made by each member and the leader to the shared purpose of the group. These contributions are both content and process oriented.

Content functions of the group are met when members share their experiences in an effort to help another. They tell their stories, relate their problems and what they did that worked or did not work to solve those problems. They tell the group their own history as it relates to the themes of the group. When members share all of these elements, they are addressing the group's content functions.

Process functions allow an individual to receive feedback from other members and the leader concerning how the member interacts and is perceived within the group. The group can be viewed as a laboratory or arena in which to observe, experiment, and define relationships and behaviors. For example, a member who complains that his wife is always accusing him of being domineering may receive feedback from the group as to whether others see him acting in a similarly domineering way. Then he has the opportunity to work on changing his behavior in the group setting before risking the change in the outside world.

The group has primary and secondary tasks. The primary task is necessary for the group's survival or existence; secondary tasks may enhance the group but are not basic to its survival. An example of a primary task for a group of mothers might be that of improving mothering skills; a secondary task might be to add to the mothers' social network. Relationships in the group may limit or enhance their willingness to share concerns about mothering.

■ COMPONENTS OF SMALL GROUPS

For one to be effective in therapeutic group work, it is necessary to understand the complex processes that occur and to be able to use various approaches to increase the therapeutic potential of the group for its members. The components of small groups are summarized in Table 32-1.

Group Structure

Group structure is the group's underlying order. It describes the boundaries, communication and decision-making processes, and authority relationships within the group. The structure offers the group stability and helps regulate behavioral and interactional patterns. Examples of group structure include set meeting times and place, rules regarding attendance, and rules for behavior in the group, for example, no smoking while interacting with the group.

Group Size

The preferred size of an interpersonally oriented group is 7 to 10 members. The group must have enough people to give members the opportunity to receive consensual validation and hear the expression of different viewpoints. If the group has too many people, not all members will be given enough time to speak and some will feel excluded. Also the available time will be insufficient to analyze and discuss interactions. If the group has too few members, too little sharing and interaction may occur.

Length of Sessions

The optimum length of a session is 20 to 40 minutes for lower-functioning groups and 60 to 120 minutes for higher-functioning ones. For the latter groups, a few minutes are spent warming up to the task of working, then most of the session is spent on group work, and finally the last few minutes are used to summarize and take care of any unfinished business that relates to that session. Some groups end with the assigning of "homework," such as practicing saying "No" three times to various requests before the next group session.

Communication

One of the group leader's primary tasks is to observe and analyze the communication patterns within the group. Using feedback, the leader helps members become aware of the group dynamics and communication patterns so that they may realize the significance of these patterns for the group and for themselves. The group or individual members may then experiment and change these patterns if they choose.

Observable verbal and nonverbal elements of the group's communication include the following:
- Spatial and seating arrangements
- Common themes expressed by the group
- How often and to whom members communicate
- How members are listened to in the group
- What problem-solving processes occur in the group

Table 32-1	Components of Small Groups
COMPONENTS	CHARACTERISTICS
Group structure	The group's underlying order; includes boundaries, communication, and decision-making processes, as well as authority relationships; offers stability and helps regulate behavior and interactional patterns.
Group size	Preferred size is 7 to 10 members.
Length of sessions	Optimum length of a session is 20 to 40 minutes for lower-functioning groups and 60 to 120 minutes for higher-functioning groups (divided into time for a brief warm-up, work time, and a brief wrap-up).
Communication	Feedback is used to help members identify group dynamics and communication patterns.
Roles	Determined by behavior and responsibilities assumed by the members of the group.
Power	Ability to influence the group and other members.
Norms	Standards of behavior in the group; influence communication and behavior; communicated overtly or covertly.
Cohesion	The strength of the members' desire to work together toward common goals; related to group's attraction and member satisfaction.

- Facial and/or hand gestures that might indicate emotional content

These behaviors help the leader assess the following: resistance within the group; interpersonal conflict; the roles assumed by some of the members; the level of competition; and how well the members understand and are working on the task.

Group Roles

In studying groups it is important to observe the roles that members assume in the group. Each role has certain expected behaviors and responsibilities.

The role a member takes can be determined by observing communication and behavioral patterns. The following factors influence role selection: the member's personality, the interaction in the group, and the member's position in the group. Three types of roles people can play in groups are (Benne and Sheats, 1948) as follows:

- **Maintenance roles,** which involve group processes and functions
- **Task roles,** which deal with completing the group's task
- **Individual roles,** which are not related to the group's tasks or maintenance; they may be self-centered and distracting for the group

Table 32-2   Group Roles and Functions

ROLE	FUNCTION
Maintenance Roles	
Encourager	To be a positive influence on the group
Harmonizer	To make/keep peace
Compromiser	To minimize conflict by seeking alternatives
Gatekeeper	To determine level of group acceptance of individual members
Follower	To serve as an interested audience
Rule maker	To set standards for group behaviors (such as time and dress)
Problem solver	To solve problems to allow group to continue its work
Task Roles	
Leader	To set direction
Questioner	To clarify issues and information
Facilitator	To keep the group focused
Summarizer	To state current position of the group
Evaluator	To assess performance of the group
Initiator	To begin group discussion
Individual Roles	
Victim	To deflect responsibility from self
Monopolizer	To actively seek control by incessant talking
Seducer	To maintain distance and gain personal attention
Mute	To seek control passively through silence
Complainer	To discourage positive work and vent anger
Truant/latecomer	To invalidate significance of the group
Moralist	To serve as judge of right and wrong

Modified from Benne KD, Sheats P: *J Soc Issues* 4:41, 1948.

These roles are summarized in Table 32-2. A person who acts as a harmonizer and peacemaker would be taking a maintenance role. A person in the task role of questioner might clarify and seek new information.

Members may experience a conflict when there is a difference between the role they seek or assume and the role given to them by the group. For example, a member may be expected to be a peacemaker because of having performed that role previously. Now, however, this member may be under additional stress or feel angry with someone in the group and may choose to start rather than resolve conflict. Often the group will be confused and upset by the person assuming this new role.

Consider the last group of which you were a member. Identify the roles that were taken by each group member. Which helped and which interfered with task accomplishment? Give an example of the behavior that was associated with each role. ■

Power

Power is the member's ability to influence the group as a whole and its other members individually. The power structure in the group is usually resolved in its initial stages. To determine the power of various members, it is helpful to assess which members receive the most attention, which are listened to most, and which make decisions for the group. Power may be granted or assumed based on any number of factors including gender, age, previous experience, length of time in the group, or willingness to speak in the group.

Resolution of the power struggle does not necessarily mean that everyone will be satisfied with the arrangement. Sometimes a continual struggle for power occurs. This may be functional if the members are trying to gain new leadership that will contribute to their therapeutic goals. The power struggle can be dysfunctional when it takes the group's energy and attention away from other tasks.

Norms

Norms are standards of behavior. They are expectations of how the group will act in the future based on its past and present experiences. It is important to understand norms because they influence the quality of communication and interaction within the group.

The observance of norms results in conforming behavior by group members. Any member who does not follow the norms of the group may be considered rebellious or resistant by the other group members. Conforming to group norms is essential to being a fully accepted member. For example, if the group norm is to start meetings on time, a member who is always late to meetings is not conforming to group norms. The group will decide to what extent it will tolerate nonconforming behavior.

Norms are created to do the following:

- Facilitate accomplishment of the group's goals or tasks
- Control interpersonal conflict
- Interpret social reality
- Foster group interdependence

Norms may be communicated overtly or covertly. Overt expression of norms may be written or clearly stated. For example, members may tell a new member that smoking is not allowed in the group. Covert expression of norms may be implied through members' behavior. For example, a member who uses foul language may be ignored by the other members.

A highly cohesive group may have appropriate or inappropriate norms. For example, a group of patients may unite to help a patient sneak a cigarette when such behavior is contraindicated because of that patient's health problems. The group also may unite to do what it can to prevent that patient from smoking.

One concern that is vitally important for a group to address is **confidentiality**. For a group to be most effective, members need to feel free to talk about issues that may be painful, embarrassing, or disturbing. The group members need to agree that whatever is discussed in the group belongs to the group and that group content will not be discussed outside of the group unless it is specifically discussed beforehand and agreed to by all members. This norm should be communicated overtly. Some groups may even want members to sign an agreement of confidentiality.

Identify and describe group norms that you have observed in a selected clinical setting and in the classroom. Did anyone deviate from a norm? How did the group respond? How did the leader respond? ■

Cohesion

Cohesion is the strength of the members' desire to work together toward common goals. It influences members to remain in the group. It is related to each member's attraction to and satisfaction received from the group.

Cohesion is a basic fiber of any group because it affects its life span and success. Many factors contribute to the level of cohesion, including agreement of members on group goals, interpersonal attractiveness between the members, degree to which the group satisfies individual needs, similarities among members, and satisfaction of members with the leadership style.

Cohesion is such an important dimension that some group leader interventions are aimed specifically toward promoting it. These may include encouraging members to talk directly with each other, discussing the group in "we" terms, and encouraging all members to sit within the space reserved for the group. A leader also can promote cohesion by pointing out similarities among group members, helping members listen to each other, and encouraging cooperation among the members.

The group leader continually monitors the level of cohesion in the group. Group leaders might observe how much members express interest in each other and recognize each other for their individuality. Another way to measure cohesion is to find out whether members identify with the group and whether they want to remain in the group.

■ GROUP DEVELOPMENT

Groups, like individuals, have the capacity for growth and development. Likewise, they have the ability to regress and resist working effectively. Every group develops according to a series of three interpersonal stages:

1. Inclusion—Being in or out
2. Control—Being top or bottom
3. Affection—Being near or far

Each stage is characterized by members expressing various aspects of the same interpersonal issue or conflict.

In group development, phases may overlap, or a group may regress to a previous phase. For example, group regression can occur when a new member is added. Phases of group development can be thought of as a path that a group takes to form and accomplish its objectives. The leader's task is to understand and assist the group as it moves along its growth path.

Pregroup Phase

An important factor to consider when starting a group is what will be its **goals**. The group's purpose will greatly influence many of the leader's behaviors. The group may have more than one goal; if so, the primary goal should be clearly stated. To guarantee success, the group's goals must be understood by all people involved, including the members and sponsoring agencies. It is the leader's role to clarify the task and help the group achieve it.

Once the purpose is established, the leader must be sure that the group has **administrative permission**. A written group proposal is one effective way to request this. Box 32-1 lists information to include in a group proposal. To avoid possible problems, the leader should explore any administrative limitations. For example, an agency may not permit a group to meet outside of its own physical facilities or may prefer

---

BOX **32-1**

Group Proposal Guideline

List the group goals, primary and secondary.
List group leaders and their related expertise.
List theoretical frameworks used by the leaders to meet the group goals.
List criteria for membership.
Describe the referral and screening process.
Describe the structure of the group.
  Meeting place
  Meeting time
  Length of each meeting
  Number of members
  Duration of the group
  Expected member behaviors
  Expected leader behaviors
Describe the evaluation process for members and the group.
Describe resources needed for the group, such as coffee, a movie projector, or audiovisual equipment.
If pertinent, describe the expected cost and financial benefits incurred by the group.

that the leader not use certain techniques in the group. Also, any potential cost to the agency should be clearly identified.

The leader is also responsible for finding **physical space** in which the group can meet. The leader identifies the room requirements of the group. For example, in a patient education group, resources such as flipcharts or a DVD player may be needed. A psychotherapy group may need space for comfortable chairs to be placed in a circle without a table. In a group that plans to use human relations exercises, a more spacious room will probably be needed. In all cases the group room should be comfortable, private, and quiet. The same room should be used for each meeting. Leaders often have to adapt inadequate space to fit the needs of the group. The session itself is more important than where it is conducted.

The next responsibility of the group leader is to **select members**. The selection is based on the purposes of the group, referrals to the group, and interviews with potential members. The leader or the agencies must provide information about the group to potential sources of referrals. All information should clearly identify the group's purpose and state the criteria for membership eligibility and the time, place, and duration. The leaders' names and professional credentials should be provided.

Membership will greatly influence the group's outcome. In selecting members the leader should consider group cohesion and therapeutic problem solving. Selection criteria include problem areas, motivation, age, sex, cultural factors, educational level, socioeconomic level, ability to communicate, intelligence, and coping and defensive styles. Homogeneous groups will share preselected criteria (e.g., all members will be women who suffered incest as children). Heterogeneous groups will include a mixture of people, such as a group for men and women who want to build their self-esteem.

If possible, the leader should decide whether the membership of the group will be closed or open before screening members. In a **closed group**, no new members are added once the group is started. In an **open group**, members leave and new members are added throughout the duration of the group. Open groups may retain their initial purpose for the duration of the group but experience both a change of members and leaders.. Such groups usually continue indefinitely with no termination date. The closed group offers the advantage of consistency of leadership, norms, and expectations. The open group, on the other hand, continually brings fresh ideas and opportunities for learning to its members.

The primary purpose of the screening interview is to determine the appropriateness of the potential member to the group. Secondary purposes accomplished during the screening interview include the following:

- Beginning to develop a relationship between the leader and the member
- Determining the motivation of the possible member
- Determining whether the candidate's goals are in agreement with the group goals
- Educating the candidate about the nature of the group
- Determining the type of group experience the person has had in the past

- If appropriate, beginning to review the group contract with the candidate

In addition to or instead of the screening interview, some clinicians use group intake meetings. Several new members meet in a group to learn about the group process and identify some possible treatment goals. This approach is less costly and has the same objectives as the screening interview.

As soon as possible a decision should be made about group membership. Candidates not selected should be referred to other treatment options. The reasons for not being selected should be explained to the candidate and, if appropriate, to the person who made the referral.

You are asked to develop a group treatment program for victims of discrimination. What membership characteristics will you list as necessary for inclusion in the group? What will you say to the patients who are not selected for inclusion in your group? ◼

Initial Phase

The initial phase includes meetings in which the group's members begin to settle down to work. This phase is characterized by anxiety about being accepted by the group, the setting of norms, and the casting of various roles. This phase has been subdivided into three stages by Yalom (1995): the **orientation, conflict,** and **cohesive** stages. These stages correspond to Tuckman's (1965) first three phases of group development: **forming, storming,** and **norming.** Table 32-3 summarizes Tuckman's and Yalom's stages of group development.

Orientation Stage. This stage corresponds to Tuckman's **forming** stage. The leader is more directive and active than in other stages. The leader orients the group to its primary task and helps the group arrive at a group contract. Some common factors that may be included in the group contract are goals, confidentiality, meeting times, honesty, structure, and communication rules (for example, only one person may talk at a time).

Because an important part of this phase is norm setting, the leader should ensure that the norms will help the group achieve its goals. Another task of the leader in this stage is to foster a sense of belonging or cohesion among the members. To accomplish this, the leader encourages interaction among members and maintains the group at a working level of anxiety. For example, the leader could refer to the group as "our" group and suggest how members can help each other. Members could be encouraged to state what they hope to learn from the group. The leader would then reinforce realistic expectations and give examples of how the group might meet them.

During the first stage the members are evaluating each other, the group, and the leader. They are deciding whether they are going to be a part of the group and how much they will participate. Some common conscious or unconscious concerns of members during this stage are fear of being rejected, fear of self-disclosure, and fear of not being seen as an individual. Social behaviors are important, and the members are attempting to develop their social roles. The roles members assume during this stage are often renegotiated during other stages.

Table 32-3	**Developmental Phases in Small Groups**			
YALOM PHASE	TUCKMAN PHASE	DEFINITION	TASK ACTIVITY	INTERPERSONAL ACTIVITY
Orientation	Forming	Group members concerned with orientation	To identify task and boundaries regarding it	Relationships tested; interpersonal boundaries identified; dependent relationship with leaders, other group members, or preexisting standards established
Conflict	Storming	Group members are resistive to task and group influence	To respond emotionally to task	Intergroup conflict
Cohesive	Norming	Resistance to group overcome by members	To express intimate personal opinions about task	New roles adopted; new standards evolved in group feelings; cohesiveness developed
Working	Performing	Creative problem solving engaged; solutions emerge	To direct group energy toward completion of task	Interpersonal structure of group becomes a tool to achieve its task; roles become flexible and functional

Members of groups will often test out their dependency needs and wishes on the leader. They look to the leader for structure, approval, and acceptance and may try to please the leader with reward-seeking behaviors. The leader is not responsible for meeting all the dependency wishes of the members but must encourage them to interact more with one another. This supports members in becoming more interdependent and less dependent on the leader. The dependency issue between the leader and the members may lead the group into conflict and thus into the second stage.

Conflict Stage. This stage of the group corresponds to Tuckman's **storming** stage of group development. Issues related to control, power, and authority become primary. Members are concerned about the pecking order or deciding who is top or bottom in control and decision making. The dependency conflict may be openly or covertly expressed, with members being polarized between independent and dependent issues.

This stage reflects a struggle between the counterdependent and dependent members, with the counterdependent members wanting to assume the leader's role. For example, a group may be divided over the issue of whether members can telephone each other. Some members may want the leader to decide, whereas others may think that the leader's statements are irrelevant.

During this phase the counterdependent members might usurp the leader's position and let the leader know that his or her directions have been unsuccessful or unheard. The dependent members might ask the leader for more directions. Other members who are neutral (neither dependent nor counterdependent) eventually may help the group resolve this conflict.

Subgroups usually form within the group, and hostility may be expressed. Often the hostility is directed toward the leader, but it also may be expressed toward other members. The leader's tasks are to allow expression of both negative and positive feelings, help the group understand the underlying conflict, and prevent or examine nonproductive behaviors such as scapegoating. This phase is usually the most difficult for a new leader because some members may try to convince the leader to believe that he or she has failed the group by not living up to its unrealistic expectations.

The leader must be careful not to avoid or suppress the group members' anxiety and, at times, should encourage the expression of hostility. If hostility toward the leader is expressed indirectly, such as anger toward other authority figures (staff members, teachers, or parents), the leader should help the group express its anger more directly. A useful technique is for the leader to give the group permission to discuss its anger by acknowledging that the group may be disappointed or angry at the leader.

By the end of the conflict stage, the leader may be dethroned, and his or her omnipotent role, with its "magical" solutions, may be discarded. Slowly the leader becomes humanized. Members learn that responsibilities for the group are shared. Members also may learn that expressions of anger and disappointment do not destroy the leader and may help the group assess its resources and limitations more accurately. The group's resources can then be used to achieve its tasks. Members may realize that conflicts need not be avoided; instead, through discussion, open conflicts may increase the group's maturity and usefulness.

Cohesive Stage. Tuckman's **norming** phase is closely related to the cohesive stage. Group members, after resolving the second stage, feel a strong attraction toward one another and a strong attachment to the group. Positive feelings toward one another and the group are often expressed, but negative feelings usually are not shared.

At this stage, members feel free to give self-disclosing information and share more intimate concerns. However, the group's problem-solving ability is restricted because negative communication is usually avoided in order to maintain the high group morale.

The leader's task is to make a connection between the members' disclosures and the group's primary task. The leader should not interfere with the group's basic cohesion but should encourage the group to use its problem-solving ability.

The leader shows how a group member can have individual concerns and values and still be productive within the group. In other words, the leader demonstrates that differing and opposite opinions may not necessarily destroy the group identity.

At the resolution of this stage, members may learn that self-discoveries and differences should not be feared. They also learn that similarities and differences between the members may help the group achieve its tasks. At the end of the cohesive stage, the group begins to see task achievement as a reality. The members gain a more realistic and honest view of their ability to work together and accomplish their primary and secondary tasks.

Compare behaviors that would indicate that a group is in the orientation stage, the conflict stage, and the cohesive stage. Give specific examples. What leader interventions would be appropriate at each stage?

Working Phase

The working phase of a group can be compared with Tuckman's **performing** stage of group development. During this stage the group becomes a team. It directs its energy mainly toward completing its tasks. Although they are hard at work, this phase is enjoyable for both the leader and the members. Responsibility for the group is more equally shared, anxiety is usually decreased and tolerated better, and the group is more stable and realistic.

Therapeutic forces occur in group therapy. Eleven of these therapeutic or curative factors are presented in Table 32-4 (Yalom and Vinogradov, 1989). Although these factors were identified in relationship to therapy groups, they apply to experiences in all types of groups (Bender and Ewashen, 2000). Other therapeutic factors important in promoting positive change in short-term groups include self-responsibility and self-understanding.

The leader's major role is to help the group complete its tasks by maximizing effective use of its curative properties. Because the members are fully participating in the group's work, the leader's activity level decreases. The leader now acts more as a consultant to the group. The leader helps keep the group goal-directed and tries to decrease the impact of anything that may regress or retard the group.

Because this phase is the group's creative problem-solving and resolution phase, there are few, if any, specific guidelines for the leader. The leader's interventions are based primarily on theoretical frameworks, experiences, personality, and intuition, as well as the needs of the group and its members.

In addition to fostering group cohesion, maintaining its boundaries, and encouraging the group to work on its tasks, the leader may help the group solve specific problems. Because these problems are unique to the group, many are not predictable. Some of the more common problems are the formation of subgroups, the management of conflict, determining the optimum level of self-disclosure, and dealing with resistance.

Subgroups that conflict with the group's goals and are not acknowledged by the group can restrict its work. Other members may feel excluded, and loyalties will be divided between the subgroup and the whole group. For example, in a women's group, two of the members may become close friends, keeping secrets from the group and engaging in private conversations during the session. Other members may feel excluded from this pair and be ineffective in working with them. To decrease the negative impact of a subgroup, its consequences and the group's reactions should be openly discussed.

Conflict is unavoidable but can be used to foster growth. However, expression of conflict may need to be controlled so that the intensity does not exceed the group's tolerance. Examples of conflict are competition among members for the leader's attention and a disagreement between two members. A leader may manage conflicts by identifying the conflict, explaining that conflicts are natural and can lead to growth, and encouraging members to discuss the reasons for the conflict. Successful conflict resolution is related to the amount of group cohesion, trust, and acceptance among the members.

Self-disclosure in the group is usually related to the amount of acceptance and trust the member feels. Self-disclosure is always risky. If people give private information

Table 32-4	Yalom's Curative Factors	
FACTOR	**DEFINITION**
Imparting information	Receiving didactic information and advice
Instillation of hope	Increasing hopefulness of group members
Universality	Realization that others experience similar thoughts, feelings, and problems
Altruism	Experience of sharing part of oneself to help another
Corrective reenactment	Ability of members to alter learning experience previously obtained from primary family group in their families
Development of social interaction techniques	Opportunity to increase awareness of social interactions and develop social skills
Imitative behaviors	Opportunities to increase skills by imitating behaviors of others in group
Interpersonal learning	Ability to engage in wider range of interpersonal exchanges, thereby increasing each member's understanding of responsibility and complexity of interpersonal relationships and decreasing members' interpersonal distortions
Existential factors	Ability of group to help members deal with meaning of their own existence
Catharsis	Opportunity to express feelings previously unexpressed
Group cohesion	Attraction of member for group and other members

Modified from Yalom ID, Vinogradov S: *Group psychotherapy*, Washington, DC, 1989, American Psychiatric Press.

too quickly, they will feel vulnerable. On the other hand, if people disclose too little during the working phase they may not be able to form supportive interpersonal relationships. Their growth potential in the group may be decreased.

Resistance, or holding back the therapeutic process, can be expected in therapy groups. Resistance to working on the therapeutic goal can occur at both an individual and a group level. Group work can initially be anxiety producing because working through interpersonal issues can be personally threatening and emotionally painful. The leader must actively structure the group to make it as nonthreatening as possible and to allow for some early successes for patients.

It is one matter to agree on goals and another to work on obtaining the actual therapeutic outcomes. Resistance by individual members may take many forms, such as avoiding discussion of a conflict, frequent or prolonged silences, attempting to become an assistant leader, absence from the group, pairing between two members, and prolonged or unusually intense expression of hostility. Resistance by the group or a majority of its members may be expressed in ways similar to those used by individuals. Other examples of group resistance include shared silence among the members, unusual amounts of dependency on the leader, scapegoating, subgroup formations, and the wish for magical solutions to resolve group conflict.

Resistance to group psychotherapeutic efforts can have a demoralizing effect on the therapist. With experience, handling resistance will become less threatening. The nurse should realize that resistance is a signal that treatment is progressing, that the therapist and the group members are getting close to crucial issues. Resistance also may occur because of increased anxiety related to conflict or change.

The management of resistance depends on the type of group, the group contract, and the therapist's theoretical framework. Some methods of decreasing resistance are to establish trust, make observations regarding the group process or individual behaviors, offer interpretations, counteract the resistant behavior, and demonstrate more adaptive behavioral patterns.

By the end of the second phase, members have made significant progress toward goal achievement. They have a sense of their own productivity and accomplishments. The need for the group or their involvement in the group is less apparent. The group must then begin to deal more actively with its final task: separation.

Termination Phase

The work of termination begins during the first phase of the group. However, as the group or individual members approach termination, certain processes are more likely to occur. The termination phase is not always discussed as a definite phase in the literature. It is discussed as a separate phase here because of the significance it may have for the members.

There are two types of termination: termination of the group as a whole and termination of individual members. A closed group usually terminates as an entire group; in an open group, members (and perhaps the leader) terminate separately. Members and groups may terminate prematurely, unsuccessfully, or successfully.

Termination is a highly individual process. Members and groups will terminate in unique ways. If the group has been successful, termination may be painful and involve grieving or a sense of loss. It may cause the group to experience increased anxiety, regression, and a feeling of accomplishment. Permitting members to avoid discussing termination would deprive them of a possible growth experience. Leadership behaviors include encouraging an evaluation of the group or its terminating members, reminiscing about important events that occurred in the group, and encouraging members to give each other feedback.

Evaluation usually focuses on the degree to which the group's or individual's goals have been met. Leaders must be careful not to collude with members in denying termination; rather, they should encourage full discussion. Termination should be talked about several sessions before the final session to allow members time to work through issues that may surface. Termination may lead to discussion of many related topics, such as other separations, death, aging, and the use and passage of time. If terminated successfully, members may feel a sense of resolution about the group experience and use these experiences in many other life situations.

Premature termination means that the group ends before its tasks are completed or a member leaves the group before his or her work is finished. Premature termination may occur for appropriate and inappropriate reasons. Appropriate reasons include moving to another city before the group is terminated. Inappropriate reasons might include a member's unwillingness to discuss an issue central to the group but painful to that person.

As a staff nurse you are given the responsibility for developing a transition group for patients who are to be discharged from a day treatment program. Outline the points you will need to consider and the steps you would take to establish the group. ■

■ EVALUATION OF THE GROUP

Evaluation of the group and the group members' progress is an ongoing process that begins in the selection interview. Notes detailing the group sessions should be descriptive to help identify goal achievement. To make record keeping easy, it is usually helpful to have a group notebook. In this notebook leaders can write pertinent data on individual members such as their goals, their telephone numbers, their addresses, the screening note, any individual comments, and a termination summary note. In another section of the group notebook the leader can describe each group meeting.

One format for quickly recording each group meeting is provided in Box 32-2. In most agencies summary notes are also included in individual members' clinical records.

In addition, it is helpful to determine each member's goal attainment periodically during the course of the group. This can be done using subjective ratings by the group leader and by obtaining individual members' perceptions on how they

---

BOX 32-2

Group Session Note Outline

Date _____   Group Meeting No. _____
Membership:
    List members attending (state whether new member).
    List members who were late.
    List absent members.
List individual members' pertinent issues or behaviors discussed in the group.
List group themes.
Identify important group process issues (such as developmental stage, roles, and norms).
Identify any critical leadership strategy used.
List proposed future leadership strategies.
Predict member and group responses for the next session.

---

are meeting their goals. For a slightly more objective evaluation, members are asked to rate their goal achievement on a Likert scale (one that allows members to rate their response along a continuum, with 1 being low, 5 being high, for example). Members' goal achievement should always be evaluated at termination.

In addition, before, during, and at the end of the group the clinician should use **behavioral rating scales** to assess progress toward expected outcomes. The scales selected should be related to the expected changes in the group. For example, an anxiety scale should be administered to members attending a group whose major goal is to reduce anxiety.

It is also essential to identify specific **outcomes** so that the impact and validity of nursing group interventions can be communicated to consumers and health care organizations. For example, possible short-term outcome measures for nurse-led groups could include increased knowledge of coping skills and increased insight into the members' own effective and ineffective coping behaviors. Long-term outcomes may be related to a decrease in specific symptoms, such as anxiety or depression, as measured by specific behavioral rating scales.

In contrast, a nursing staff support group might have as measurable outcomes the use of a problem-solving approach, the development of a unit communication tool, or the identification of strategies to negotiate staff conflict, seek assistance from each other when stressed, decrease patient complaints, or reduce staff turnover.

■ NURSES AS GROUP LEADERS

Nurses who are group leaders must be concerned about the many previously discussed factors regarding the group. The group leader must be able to study the group and participate in it at the same time. The leader must constantly monitor the group and, whenever necessary, help the group achieve its goals.

The qualities of an effective nurse leader are the same qualities that are important in the therapeutic relationship

Critical Thinking *About* **Contemporary Issues**

Do Computer Networks Provide a New Way for Nurses to Interact with Groups of Patients?

Interactions through computer networks and online groups are growing in popularity. Nurses have begun to identify opportunities to establish patient groups using this technology and have reported on the potential effectiveness of computer network groups and telecommunication in providing information and support (Cudney and Weinert, 2000). Advantages to the members include convenience, ability to relate to a variety of people in similar situations, and ready access to peer support. This approach also offers the option of anonymity to group members.

Psychiatric nurses also need to consider the possible disadvantages of therapeutic groups online (Finfgeld, 2000). The inability to perceive nonverbal communication removes an important dimension from the communication process. Because interaction may not be simultaneous, time gaps can occur between interventions and the responses of various members. Spontaneity also may be lost. The development of trust among group members could proceed differently than in traditional groups. Confidentiality may be even more of a concern to members than it is in face-to-face groups.

Identifying and exploring the dimensions of computer network groups offer a challenge to psychiatric nurses. Nurses who lead groups need to adapt their skills to enhance the advantages of the technology and minimize the disadvantages. As more people become computer-literate and accustomed to online relationships, the potential for this new form of group support will evolve.

(see Chapter 2). In particular, these include the responsive and active dimensions of empathy, genuineness, and confrontation. In addition, creativity and opportunism are helpful qualities for leaders to possess. While they are listening to members' words, leaders also need to be aware of the group process. They must be alert to opportunities for the group to use themes and behaviors and see how these are related to individual issues.

Leaders may be compared to an orchestra conductor who seeks to focus on the sound of a particular instrument for the appreciation and reaction of the total orchestra. The leader may encourage examination of the music from different perspectives and look for possible variations that would create a new piece of music. Opportunities for creativity also may lead to the development of innovative group techniques (see Critical Thinking About Contemporary Issues).

Group leaders must make it safe for members to challenge their authority. In examining the interplay between the leader and the members, opportunities can be found to practice conflict management, confrontation, and assertive communication. The leader needs to accept confrontation without taking it personally.

Leaders also need to have assertive communication skills so that they can foster independence in the group but also help the group focus on reaching its goals. Achieving this balance requires a blend of skills and judgment, which can be gained by

CITING THE EVIDENCE ON

Self-Help Groups

BACKGROUND: The purpose of this study was to examine the efficacy of using an online, interactive group to support young widows. A survey instrument was constructed, and grounded theory was used to analyze the data.

RESULTS: The findings indicated the self-help group was helpful in reducing young widows' sense of isolation and helping them cope with their losses. It also allowed members a means of keeping in touch with others and obtaining needed information.

IMPLICATIONS: Although technology is often associated with creating distance between people, interactive, Internet-based support groups can, in fact, result in empathic support for those unable or unwilling to attend an in vivo group. Nurses knowledge of online resources and their comfort level in working with the Internet can provide a useful therapeutic modality for patients.

Bacon E et al: *J Psychosoc Nurs* 38:7, 2000.

practicing in group leadership, by being supervised by an experienced group facilitator, and by studying the group process.

It is also critical for leaders to be able to organize a great deal of information and to identify themes for the session. Novice leaders usually need to review the group experience with a supervisor after the session so that they can identify and analyze the important events.

Finally, a nurse leader also needs a sense of humor. Laughter helps reveal truth and enables participants to share and empathize when serious matters are being discussed; laughter can lessen the high levels of tension that often accompany such discussions. For example, in a women's co-dependent group, humor and laughter were used regularly. The group adopted this technique to talk about their "rescuing" and controlling behaviors. This group was composed of fragile women who grew up in abusive families. They worked hard at seeing, understanding, and changing their contributions to the destructive relationships they had developed. The members came to the weekly group sessions prepared to share examples of their "setting themselves up" behavior and laughed as they were able to find humor in recognizing behavior that was similar to their own. The humor also allowed the members to give feedback in a less confrontational manner.

Groups With Co-Leaders

For some groups, the presence of co-leaders may have advantages and disadvantages. When two clinicians share the leadership, the breadth of observation and the choice of interventions are greater than with just one leader. For example, a male and female team of leaders may represent the family and offer the group members an opportunity to deal with issues related to parents or other significant male and female figures.

A male-female team also offers group members opportunities to observe a man and a woman working together with mutual respect and without exploiting, sexualizing, or patronizing each other. When experienced co-leaders work together in learning and resolving problems, they are role-modeling adaptive behavior for the group. This can contribute significantly to the group's openness and power.

Disadvantages of the leadership team are often related to difficulties between the leaders themselves. When there is competition, a major philosophical difference, or great variance in strategy or style, the group will not work effectively. Differences in levels of experience can be handled successfully if both are comfortable with their roles of apprentice and senior leader. Conflict between co-leaders could lead to the splitting of the group or to the group developing an alliance with only one of the leaders, which could be very damaging. If the group becomes divided, or split, this dynamic must be openly interpreted in the group and dealt with by the group members and leaders.

Nurse-Led Groups

Nurses lead groups in a variety of health care settings. Some types of groups that may be led by nurses are task groups, self-help groups, teaching groups, supportive/therapy groups, psychotherapy groups, and peer support groups. The type of group intervention provided by an individual nurse is determined by the needs and goals of the patients and by the education and experience of the nurse.

Task Groups. Task groups are designed to accomplish a particular task. Nursing care planning meetings and committees are examples of task groups. The emphasis of these groups is on decision making and problem solving. They often have specific goals to accomplish and a deadline for completion of the work.

Self-Help Groups. Groups organized around a common experience are labeled **self-help groups** (see Citing the Evidence). Some examples include smoking cessation groups, Overeaters Anonymous, Alcoholics Anonymous, Parents and Friends of Lesbians and Gays, Parents Without Partners, and numerous groups related to specific health problems. They may not receive consultation from a health care provider, such as a professional nurse.

Although some self-help groups are established and organized by professionals, the groups are run by the members alone and often do not have a designated leader. Leadership evolves within the group depending on the need that arises. Nurses can support self-help groups by referring members and by offering advice and assistance if it is requested. They also can promote links between the self-help group and the health care system. Self-help groups are discussed in Chapter 13.

Educational Groups. The goal of teaching groups is to provide information. Examples are childbirth preparation, parent education groups, medication groups, and psychoeducation groups (Rindner, 2000). Inservice education groups for staff are also included in this category. The nurse leader is able to educate more people more efficiently using a group format. The members themselves often become co-teachers as they share their information and experiences (Webster and Austin, 1999). Psychoeducation groups are designed to teach symptom identification, symptom management, and recovery planning skills. They are discussed in Chapter 15.

Supportive Therapy Groups. The primary goal of supportive therapy groups is to help the members cope with

---

BOX 32-3

Planning Checklist for Time-Limited Psychotherapy Groups

Check for the following planning factors:

_____ **Clear administrative mandate:** Establish achievable annual goals for the number of therapy groups and the number of patients seen in these groups in a particular setting.

_____ **Clinical group coordinator:** Determine need for groups and guidelines for referrals, identify group therapists, conduct staff training, market the group, and establish pregroup and postgroup tests and outcome evaluations.

_____ **Population-based approach:** Identify the main diagnostic categories to be included and the needs of the target population that could be met by group therapy.

_____ **Group screening:** Pregroup orientation and screening ensure that patients understand how the group will operate and that the patient's needs will be addressed.

_____ **Clear referral criteria:** Clearly written referral guidelines help reduce clinician resistance to making referrals, promote effective use of the group, and increase patients' acceptance of the referral.

_____ **Regular status reports:** A weekly status report reminds referrers of the availability of groups. It should include the dates and times when groups meet, the types of groups, openings in groups, and the contact person.

_____ **Testing and evaluation:** Pretesting and posttesting help clarify the patient's response to treatment and allow for assessment of the effectiveness of the group.

_____ **Treatment models:** Use of a variety of group models (psychoeducational, social skills training, relapse prevention, crisis intervention, cognitive-behavioral, and so on) matches patients with their presenting problems and increases patient receptivity.

_____ **Training:** A group therapy apprenticeship (clinicians observe and assist the group and are observed themselves by experienced therapists) increases clinician effectiveness, acceptance of group modality, and appropriateness of referrals.

_____ **Adequate resources:** A reasonable fee schedule, adequate clinician time to develop and conduct groups, and appropriate physical space are essential for the group's success.

Modified from Crosby G, Sabin JE: *Psychiatr Serv* 47:25, 1996.

---

life stress. The focus is on dysfunctional thoughts, feelings, and behaviors. Supportive therapy groups have value for patients of all ages and with both medical and psychiatric diagnoses (Bonhote, Romano-Egan, and Cornwell, 1999; Washington and Moxley, 2001). Supportive therapy is discussed in Chapter 3.

Psychotherapy Groups. The goal of a psychotherapy group is the treatment of emotional, cognitive, or behavioral dysfunction. Group techniques and processes are used to help members learn about their behavior with other people and how it relates to core personality traits. The intent is for the members to change their behavior, not just understand or seek support for it (Diefenbeck, 2003; Dugas et al, 2003). Members also learn that they have responsibilities to others and can help other members achieve their goals.

Brief Therapy Groups. Many managed care organizations are placing a new emphasis on group therapy as a cost-effective alternative to individual therapy. Most recently, the focus on cost containment and outcome evaluation in the treatment of health-related problems has been a major influence on the increasing importance of time-limited or brief therapy groups that are linked to individual treatment plans.

The purpose of brief therapy groups is to focus on the actions participants can take to improve their current situation. Far less importance is given to the causes of the patient's problems or the accompanying emotional reactions. These groups target what can be done now to change a patient's problem-solving approach and help the patient implement more adaptive coping skills. The establishment of a recognized and self-sustaining group program is greatly facilitated by advanced planning, well-thought-out structure, and clearly stated goals. A planning checklist for establishing time-limited psychotherapy groups is included in Box 32-3.

Intensive Problem-Solving Groups. Intensive problem-solving groups are designed for 6 to 10 patients, each working on the identification and resolution of specific target problems, goals, and problem-solving strategies related to an individual treatment plan. They are based on cognitive, behavioral, and interpersonal therapy models implemented in a structured problem-solving format.

The goal is to identify and clarify the problem, explore alternative solutions, and get action-oriented commitments for change. The therapist acts as a leader, teacher, and coach, whose purpose is to teach group members the interpersonal skills needed to solve the problems identified in their treatment plans.

Multidisciplinary Teams. Nurses often are members of multidisciplinary teams consisting of psychiatrists, psychologists, social workers, rehabilitation counselors, occupational therapists, and so forth. The pooling of all of these resources allows for efficient use of available resources for the benefit of the patient (Melrose, 2000). However, one of the drawbacks of these groups is the tension that can be manifested between the different professional disciplines because of status issues; role conflict related to who is responsible for what part of the patient's care; communication issues resulting from team members working from different perspectives; and leadership issues resulting from conflict over who is, or should be, the leader of such a multidisciplinary team (Whyte and Brooker, 2001).

Activity Groups. Activity group therapy is designed to enhance the psychological and emotional well-being of psychiatric patients. Tasks can include drawing, exercising to music, baking, community trips, arts and crafts, and reviewing current events. The benefits that have been reported from the participation of psychiatric patients in such activity groups include the expression of positive and negative feelings and the greater acceptance of oneself (Gagner-Tjellesen, Yurkovich, and Gragert, 2001). As mental health care continues to move away from the more costly inpatient setting toward community-based programs for the seriously mentally ill, nurses are in a good position to care for these patients with creative and effective interventions.

Peer Support Groups. Finally, peer support groups are an effective way for professionals to share the stresses and problems related to their work. An example of a peer support group is a group of advanced practice psychiatric nurses who meet monthly. Group purposes may include case consultation, sharing information about educational opportunities, providing information about management skills, and decreasing professional isolation. Another example is a group of nurses who work with people who have HIV/AIDS. They meet regularly for nursing consultation and support in coping with the continual loss associated with this disease.

As a head nurse, you decide to form a staff support group. How would this differ from a therapeutic group? Discuss in terms of the roles of the leader and the members. Would there be any similarities? ■

COMPETENT CARING

A Clinical Exemplar of a Psychiatric Nurse
PAULA M. LASALLE, CS, RNP, LCPC

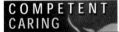

As a psychiatric clinical nurse specialist, I ran a community-based group for people living with HIV/AIDS. The purpose of the group was to support the members by providing a safe, confidential, nonjudgmental, consistent forum to help them cope with the emotional aspects of having HIV/AIDS. It was also a place where they could access medical, social services, educational, and legal resources.

The group was open, and membership changed from week to week in number and personalities. Some people came weekly for years, others came for a period after the initial diagnosis, and others came at crisis times. Members were gay, straight, old, young, and of diverse cultures and socioeconomic backgrounds. There were lawyers, prisoners, military personnel, parents, and people from other countries. The meetings were held in a room in a nonprofit agency that served families and children. As the leader I was the gatekeeper who interviewed potential members briefly on the phone. There was agreement in the group that new members could bring along a friend or family member for the first couple of meetings to enable anxious members to feel supported and encouraged in the joining process. With time it became evident that a family and significant others group was also needed, and thus one was begun.

M was a mother of three school-age children whose husband and brother-in-law had both died of AIDS. Her husband had attended a few meetings before he died. Her greatest fears involved what would happen to her children when she died. She came every week and especially appreciated the group when she was in a physical crisis. She was generous and nurtured other members in a sweet and gentle way that members could accept.

J was a nurse who had to deal with this disease in both his professional and personal life. His lover had died quickly from a rapidly progressing infection. He came to the group to grieve his loss and was eventually able to get tested and found himself to be HIV positive. He was a great resource regarding the newest regimens available to treat HIV. He taught the other members about the medical system and how to navigate it.

B was a single mother of three children who was a master at researching and learning all of the social and medical systems to gain access to funds and social services. She was politically active and a strong advocate for herself and others, especially when she believed there were issues of discrimination.

It was the longest running group of its kind in the state. They trusted one another and me and were passionate in their efforts to live as well as possible with HIV/AIDS. The group continues to meet and receive community support.

Leading the group was rewarding and difficult. When a member would become terminally ill, he or she would frequently come to group to do "life review." Although the member would be frightened, the group would do their best to be there to offer support and love. It was difficult to share the experiences of members who had been rejected by their families and friends. Some could no longer work due to illness. Others had to do battle with the legal system regarding the survivor benefits for their partners. I was allowed to share in the lives of many brave and strong people who managed their illness as best they could while continuing to raise families, earn a living, cope with recurrent bouts of illness, and sometimes prepare for their death.

The group taught me to respect and trust in the group. I was the consistent person who turned on the lights. I facilitated, not controlled, the content and process of the group. This group cried, laughed, ate, sang, and prayed together, depending on their needs. At its best, it served to offer a solid footing from which the members could cope and step out into their lives. ■

CHAPTER FOCUS POINTS

- A group is a collection of people who are interrelated and interdependent and may share common purposes and norms.
- Components of a small group include structure, size, length of sessions, communication, roles of members, norms, and cohesion.
- The phases of group development are pregroup, initial phase with orientation, conflict and cohesion stages, working phase, and termination.
- Small group evaluation is based on accomplishment of individual goals and expected group outcomes.

- Careful documentation of each group session is required.
- The responsibilities and qualities of nurse group leaders include empathy, nurturance, genuineness, creativity, acceptance of confrontation, assertive communication skills, organization, and a sense of humor.
- Types of nurse-led groups include task, self-help, educational, supportive therapy, psychotherapy, brief therapy, intensive problem solving, multidisciplinary teams, activity, and peer support groups.

KEY TERMS

cohesion, 671
group, 668

norms, 670
power, 670

CHAPTER REVIEW QUESTIONS

1. Match each term in Column A with the correct definition in Column B.

Column A

_____ Follower
_____ Moralist
_____ Truant
_____ Gatekeeper
_____ Encourager
_____ Questioner
_____ Facilitator
_____ Leader
_____ Complainer
_____ Summarizer

Column B

A. Decides who gets into the group and who does not
B. Keeps the group focused
C. Serves as judge of right and wrong
D. States current position of the group
E. Serves as an interested audience
F. Discourages positive work and vents anger
G. Clarifies issues and information
H. Invalidates significance of the group
I. Sets direction
J. Acts as a positive influence on the group

2. Fill in the blanks.

A. _____ is the member's ability to influence the group and its other members.
B. The stage of group development in which the leader is more directive and active than in other stages is the

_____ stage.

C. The optimum length of a session is _____ for higher-functioning groups and _____ for lower-functioning groups.
D. The four phases of a group's development identified by

Tuckman are _____, _____,

_____, and _____.
E. According to Yalom, the realization that others experience the same thoughts, feelings, and problems is called

_____, and the experience of sharing part of oneself to help another is called _____.

3. Provide short answers for the following questions.

A. Define a group and list eight components of small groups as described in this chapter.
B. Compare psychoeducational, intensive problem-solving, and activity groups.
C. Describe four functions that group norms serve.
D. Assess your own level of comfort working in groups. What roles do you usually assume?
E. What additional skills would you need to be an effective group leader?

Visit Evolve for additional resources related to the content of this chapter.
http://evolve.elsevier.com/Stuart/principles/
• Topical Course Outline • Student Workbook Exercises • Critical Thinking Questions and Activities • Case Studies • Research Topics
• Monthly Content Updates • WebLinks

Student Study CD-ROM

Access the accompanying CD-ROM for animations, interactive exercises, review questions for the NCLEX examination, and an audio glossary.

REFERENCES

Bender A, Ewashen C: Group work is political work: a feminist perspective of interpersonal group psychotherapy, *Issues Ment Health Nurs* 21:297, 2000.

Benne KD, Sheats P: Functional roles and group members, *J Soc Issues* 4:41, 1948.

Bonhote K, Romano-Egan J, Cornwell C: Altruism and creative expression in a long-term older adult psychotherapy group, *Issues Ment Health Nurs* 20:603, 1999.

Cudney SA, Weinert C: Computer-based support groups: nursing in cyberspace, *Comput Nurse* 18:35, 2000.

Diefenbeck CA: Group therapy for male batterers: comparison of cognitive behavioral and object relations approaches, *J Psychosoc Nurs Ment Health Serv* 41:18, 2003.

Dugas MJ et al: Group cognitive-behavioral therapy for generalized anxiety disorder: treatment outcome and long-term follow-up, *J Consult Clin Psychol* 71:821, 2003.

Finfgeld D: Therapeutic groups online: the good, the bad, and the unknown, *Issues Ment Health Nurs* 21:241, 2000.

Gagner-Tjellesen D, Yurkovich EE, Gragert M: Use of music therapy and other ITNI's in acute care, *J Psychosoc Nurs Ment Health Serv* 39:26, 2001.

Melrose CE: Facilitating a multidisciplinary parent support and education group guided by Allen's developmental health nursing model, *J Psycho Nurs Ment Health Serv* 38:18, 2000.

Rindner EC: Combined group process-psychoeducation model for psychiatric clients and their families, *J Psychosoc Nurs Ment Health Serv* 38:36, 2000.

Tuckman BW: Developmental sequence in small groups, *Psychol Bull* 63:384, 1965.

Washington OG, Moxley DP: A model of group treatment to facilitate recovery from chemical dependence, *J Psychosoc Nurs Ment Health Serv* 39:30, 2001.

Webster C, Austin W: Health-related hardiness and the effect of a psychoeducational group on clients' symptoms, *J Psychiatr Ment Health Nurs* 6:241, 1999.

Whyte L, Brooker C: Working with a multi-disciplinary team in secure psychiatric environments, *J Psychosoc Nurs Ment Health Serv* 39:26, 2001.

Yalom I, Vinogradov S: *Group psychotherapy*, Washington, DC, 1989, American Psychiatric Press.

Yalom I: *The theory and practice of group psychotherapy*, ed 4, New York, 1995, Basic Books.

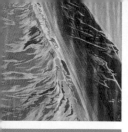

33 | FAMILY INTERVENTIONS

Janet A. Grossman

evolve Visit Evolve for additional resources related to the content of this chapter.
http://evolve.elsevier.com/Stuart/principles/

America is concerned about the health of families and the impact of family stress on our developing youth. Over the past two decades, the research on families and the development of family interventions has dramatically expanded. Nursing has played an important role in the development of family intervention science and the promotion of family health.

The term *family therapy* has both a specific meaning and a broader meaning. Family therapy is used to refer to both specific family interventions and a broader conceptual framework for intervention that includes family-centered treatment, family/couples psychotherapy, family skills building, multiple family groups, and in-home support.

The field of family therapy dates back to the early 1900s and the Child Guidance Movement when typically a psychiatrist provided treatment for the child, a social worker counseled the parents, and nurses provided milieu therapy. More recently the field of family interventions has been defined by federal initiatives, such as the 1999 Strengthening American Families Project to identify science-based interventions with evidence of effectiveness (DHHS, 1999; Institute of Medicine, 1994). Nursing curricula need to shift from traditional family approaches not supported by research to evidence-based family interventions.

■ THE CONTEXT OF FAMILY INTERVENTIONS
The Family Movement

The family movement in mental health started in the seventies and has since grown tremendously. Two motivating forces were behind the family movement: the deinstitutionalization of the mentally ill, which left families unprepared to care for their family member with a mental illness, and the tendency for health professionals and others to blame parents for mental illness in the family.

Several recent policy reports have served to educate professionals, policy makers, and lay persons about the needs of persons with mental illness and their families and about the problems of the mental health delivery system (see Chapter 9). Organizations also have been formed to serve families of the mentally ill. Three primary organizations that are committed to family support, advocacy, research, and public awareness include the National Alliance for the Mentally Ill (NAMI), the Federation for Families for Children's Mental

Advocacy

Elsie Weyrauch is a retired psychiatric nurse. Her husband Jerry is a retired navy officer. Elsie and Jerry lost their daughter Terri Ann, a physician, to suicide. Since that event they have worked tirelessly for suicide prevention. They founded Suicide Prevention Advocacy Network, Inc. (SPAN), a grassroots advocacy organization, in 1996 in Marietta, Georgia.

SPAN links the energy of those bereaved by suicide with the expertise of leaders in education, religion, science, business, government, and public service to significantly reduce suicide. It is a nonprofit organization dedicated to the creation and implementation of national, state, and local suicide prevention strategies. SPAN USA includes survivors left behind by suicide victims, suicide attempt survivors, and community activists. SPAN activities have included holding awareness events, visiting and writing letters to legislators, advocating for the passage of congressional resolutions related to suicide, participating in public hearings, hosting suicide awareness events in Washington, DC, cosponsoring a national suicide prevention strategy meeting, and sitting in federal advisory groups.

The story of SPAN is an inspiring testimonial to the role of consumers as advocates and the nurse consumer as champion. Despite the tremendous progress that has been made by this organization, the Weyrauchs continue to urge local, state, federal, and international communities to *never let up*. Now in their 70s, they exclaim, "We can't wait. We're too old."

Health, and the National Mental Health Association (NMHA). These groups offer rich resources for nurses working with families. Because of the efforts of these organizations, one of the most significant shifts in mental health service delivery in recent years has been the emergence of family involvement in decision making as it relates to their children.

Family advocacy refers to the mutual support, time, energy, and resources needed to advocate for improved services and opportunities for family members with psychiatric illness. Family advocacy is effective in raising awareness among service providers, legislators and the public (Reinhard, Grossman, and Piren, 2004). Box 33-1 illustrates the power of consumer grassroots activity.

Talk to a family member of someone who is mentally ill. Ask about that person's perception of the mental health delivery system. ■

Cultural Competence

Cultural competence is critical in family interventions. One multicultural framework uses the following set of beliefs in the treatment of families (Bruenlin, Schwartz, and Kune-Karrer, 1992):

- A matrix of sociocultual contexts of membership that contribute to value formation and interaction with therapist's values
- Ways to use these contexts in assessing opportunities and barriers for the family

- Therapeutic guidelines that consider the patient and therapist's multicultural contexts

Specific multicultural contexts include immigration status, economics, education, ethnicity, religion, gender, age, role, minority-majority status, and geography. The goodness of fit is the congruence of sociocultural background between the family and community and between the family and therapist.

Nurses need to examine their own sociocultural contexts, recognize similarities and differences with those of patients and families, be curious about and validate the sociocultural context of the patient and family, and include sociocultural considerations in the assessment and planning of care for the family (see Chapter 8). The following are examples of relevant and ethnically sensitive treatments provided by psychiatric nurses (Scott et al, 1999; Coatsworth et al, 1997).

An Advanced Practice Registered Nurse in Psychiatric–Mental Health (APRN-PMH) developed a health promotion clinic for recovering women in a therapeutic family drug court located in an urban area. Recognizing that a majority of the women were Hispanic, the advanced practice nurse recruited a bilingual nurse practitioner, who had previously practiced in a Hispanic country, to provide culturally sensitive health promotion based on a Hispanic cultural context and the women's language of preference. The nurse practitioner was cognizant of the variety of Hispanic heritages and the variability in the women's health beliefs.

In the same urban area (also with a majority Hispanic population), brief strategic family therapy with Hispanic youth was implemented that incorporated a cultural understanding of strong family cohesion and parental control, communication issues related to intergenerational and cultural conflicts, and knowledge of cultural barriers to participation. This family intervention with Cuban families was an early model that has since been replicated in other Hispanic populations.

Family Functioning

It is important for the family therapist to be able to differentiate adaptive from maladaptive family functioning in order to appropriately identify target symptoms that will be the focus for change. Characteristics of functional families are described in Chapter 11. At the opposite end of the continuum are dysfunctional families. Some of the more common dysfunctional family patterns (conceptualized as "symptoms" within a pathology paradigm and maladaptive coping within the empowerment model) include the following:

- The acting out adolescent who is a symptom bearer and whose symptoms bring the family to treatment
- The overprotective mother and distant father (distant through work, alcohol, or physical absence)
- The overfunctioning "superwife" or "superhusband" and the underfunctioning passive, dependent, and compliant spouse
- The spouse who maintains peace at any price and denies difficulties in the marriage but suddenly feels wronged and self-righteous when the mate is discovered to be in legal trouble or having an affair

- The child who exhibits evidence of poor peer relationships at school while attempting to parent younger siblings to compensate for ineffective or emotionally overwhelmed parents
- The overly close three generations of grandparent, parent, and grandchild in which lines of authority and generational identity are poorly defined and the child acts out because of a lack of effective limit setting by an agreed-on parental figure
- The family with a substance-abusing member
- The family subjected to physical, emotional, or sexual abuse by one of its members
- The child who is scapegoated by the family to diffuse marital conflict

Family Relational Diagnoses

Although no formal family diagnostic system exists, the nurse may find it useful to examine the **family relational problems** in terms of the categories described in the *Diagnostic and Statistical Manual of Mental Disorders* (*DSM-IV-TR*) (American Psychiatric Association, 2000). The *DSM-IV-TR* lists five relational categories (Table 33-1) under "Other Conditions That May Be a Focus of Clinical Attention." Relational problems often necessitate clinical attention in order to avoid further family deterioration, individual symptoms, and decreased quality of life of family members.

Many insurance and managed care companies may require a *DSM-IV-TR* psychiatric diagnosis (other than a family relational diagnosis), before authorizing family therapy treatment that they will reimburse. Many family interventions, such as family skills building (a parenting intervention), are yet to be reimbursed because third party payers are poorly informed about the impact of such programs in preventing dysfunctional behavior in children and families.

Training in Family Therapy

Clinical training programs in family therapy are open to psychiatric nurses and other health care professionals across the United States. They vary in duration, theoretical framework used, and the level of knowledge and credentials required for participation. Usually they are limited to clinicians with graduate degrees in mental health.

Although the nurse generalist needs knowledge of family systems in one's daily clinical work with patients, the nurse family therapist should have a master's degree with didactic content and clinical seminars focused on formal family work and individual or group counseling related to awareness of one's family of origin. The nurse also should be supervised on either an individual or group basis when doing family therapy to facilitate his or her refinement of clinical skills and deepening of theoretical understanding of family systems and interventions.

The American Association of Marriage and Family Therapy has defined what should constitute the education, training, and certification for family therapists, supervisors, and teachers. Licensing is also available through this organization. Students can be trained in family psychotherapy by acting as co-therapists with experienced therapists or being supervised by means of recorded sessions or live observation.

What are the qualifications of the person providing family therapy in your psychiatric clinical setting? ■

■ FAMILY THEORETICAL APPROACHES

Much of the original family therapy work was defined by specific schools, approaches, or models of family therapy. These approaches or frameworks include cognitive-behavioral, family systems, experiential, humanistic, integrative, brief therapy, systemic, narrative, psychodynamic, psychoanalytical, psychoeducational, solution-focused, strategic, structural, transgenerational, developmental, gender, organizational, cultural, functional, conflict, and ecological (Bruenlin, Schwartz, and Kune-Karrer, 1992; McFarlane, 2001; Sadock and Sadock, 2003; Wright and Leahy, 2000; White and Klein, 2002). Many of these family approaches have clinical evidence of effectiveness but not research evidence.

Currently, no unified system of family functioning has been established (Liddle et al, 2002). However, recent family approaches are more integrative than those used in the past and draw upon several theories. Commonly used contemporary family frameworks include systems, gender, developmental, cultural, conflict, and structural theories. Thus a family with an adolescent with an eating disorder could be viewed from different frameworks or theories, such as the following:

Table 33-1	Categories of Family Relational Problems in *DSM-IV-TR*
PROBLEM	ESSENTIAL FEATURES
Relational problem related to a mental disorder or general medical condition	Focus of clinical attention is a pattern of impaired family interaction in the presence of a mental disorder or a medical condition in a family member
Parent-child relational problem	Impairment includes faulty communication, overprotection, or inadequate discipline
	Clinically significant impairment or symptoms are present in an individual, in family functioning, or both
Partner relational problems	Pattern of interaction characterized by negative or distorted communication or noncommunication associated with clinically significant impairment in one or both partners
Sibling relational problems	Patterns of interactions associated with clinically significant impairment in individual or family members or the development of symptoms in one or more siblings
Relational problem not otherwise specified	Includes extra-family relational problems and difficulty with others, such as co-workers

From American Psychiatric Association: *Diagnostic and statistical manual of mental disorders*, ed 4, text revision, Washington, DC, 2000, American Psychiatric Association.

- **Systems**—How does the adolescent's eating disorder impact the parents' marital relationship?
- **Gender**—What are the roles of females in this family?
- **Developmental**—How does the family's stage of development affect individuation for this child?
- **Cultural**—How does the family interact at mealtimes?
- **Conflict**—How is disagreement between generations resolved?
- **Structural**—How is nurturing of the children expressed?

The **risk and protective factors model** also is used to prevent specific psychiatric disorders and suicide attempts (see Chapter 13). For example, certain family-centered preventive interventions, such as family skills building, reduce risk factors and increase protective factors that decrease the likelihood of substance abuse or other problem behaviors (DHHS, 1999).

Risk and protective factors can be biological, behavioral, personality, family, and environmental. Examples of family risk factors include a siblings' drug use or a lack of consistent discipline by parents. Family protective factors can include parental supervision and cohesion and attachment or bonding between parents and children. The risk and protective factors model is consistent with predisposing factors, precipitating stressors, and appraisal of stressors in the Stuart Stress Adaptation Model (see Chapter 4).

Box 33-2 lists risk and protective factors for children and adolescents. The Center for Substance Abuse Prevention

---

Risk and Protective Factors for Children and Adolescents

Individual Child Factors of Biology, Behavior, and Personality
Risk factors
- Antisocial and other problem behaviors such as stealing, vandalism, conduct disorder, attention deficit/hyperactivity disorder (ADHD), rebelliousness, and aggressiveness—particularly in boys
- Alienation
- High tolerance for deviance and strong need for independence
- Psychopathology
- Attitudes favorable to drug use
- High-risk personality factors such as sensation seeking, low harm avoidance, and poor impulse control

Protective factors
- Positive temperament
- Social coping skills
- Belief in one's own ability to exert control over what happens (self-efficacy) and in one's ability to adapt to changing circumstances
- Positive social orientation

Family Factors
Risk factors
- Family behavior concerning substance abuse:
  - Parental substance use and drug use modeling
  - Perceived parental permissiveness of youth's substance use
  - Siblings' drug use, particularly that of older brothers
- Poor family management and parenting practices:
  - Overinvolvement of one parent and distancing by the other
  - Low parental aspirations for children's educational achievement
  - Unclear or unrealistic parental expectations for children's behavior, especially as they relate to the child's developmental level
  - Poor disciplinary techniques, such as lack of or inconsistent discipline and extremely harsh punishment
- Poor maternal-child relationships:
  - Lack of maternal involvement in children's activities
  - Cold, unresponsive, underprotective mother
  - Low maternal attachment
  - Maternal use of guilt to control children's behavior

- Family conflict (a strong predictor of delinquency and antisocial behavior, including substance abuse)
- Physical abuse (the earlier the age of experience, the greater its negative effects)

Protective factors
- Cohesion, warmth, and attachment or bonding between parents and children during childhood
- Parental supervision
- Interaction and communication between and among parents, parents and children, and siblings

Environmental Factors
Risk factors
- Peer influence—rejection or low acceptance, particularly in early school years
- Deficient cultural and social norms and laws, such as poor enforcement of minimum purchase age for alcohol and tobacco products, social norms condoning use, and proliferation of tobacco and alcohol product advertisements
- Extreme poverty, for children with behavior problems and other risk factors
- Neighborhood disorganization that reduces the sense of community, increases experiences with crime, and creates high mobility and transience
- Failure to achieve in school, especially in the late elementary grades, regardless of whether it is due to behavior problems, truancy, learning disabilities, poor school environment, or other causes

Protective factors
- Sources of positive emotional support outside the family, such as close friends (one or several), neighbors, extended family, peers, and elders
- Formal and informal supports and resources available to the family
- Community and school norms, beliefs, and behavioral standards against substance abuse
- Successful school performance and strong commitment to school

From Substance Abuse and Mental Health Services Administration: *Preventing substance abuse among children and adolescents: family-centered approaches: a practitioner's guide*, DHHS Publication No. 3224 - FY98, Washington, DC, 1998, DDHS.

BOX 33-3

How Can Practitioners Have the Greatest Impact?

In addressing the various risk and protective factors around which family-centered approaches are built, practitioners should keep in mind the following principles:

1. Select prevention approaches according to the risk level of the targeted families:
   a. Families not yet known to have any risk factors (universal)
   b. Families with children who belong to subgroups that have risk factors but who currently have no problems (selective)
   c. Families with children who have risk factors and current problems (indicated)
2. Focus on families with young, school-aged children (before negative behaviors and family problems become entrenched).
3. Reduce exposure to risks.
4. Enhance protective factors.
5. Choose strategies that are developmentally and gender appropriate.
6. Develop interventions in multiple contexts and settings, such as schools, cultural life, religious institutions, neighborhoods, and communities.
7. Address multiple risk factors simultaneously, such as by working to reduce domestic conflict and children's antisocial behavior while improving parenting skills and school performance.
8. Build on families' strengths, preserve their integrity and encourage their leadership in the growth process.

From Department of Health and Human Services: *Family-centered approaches to prevent substance abuse among children and adolescents: a guideline*, Prevention Enhancement Protocol System (PEPS) (No. 277-92-1011), Washington, DC, 1999, US Government Printing Office.

also has identified principles practitioners (including nurses with all levels of preparation) should follow in addressing risk and protective factors in prevention approaches with families (DHHS, 1999). Box 33-3 lists these principles.

Think about your own family. Identify two risk and two protective factors related to your own upbringing. ∎

Family Therapy

Family therapy has two essential principles that distinguish it from individual or group therapy and from other types of family interventions, such as skills building.

- **The family is conceptualized as a behavior system with unique properties rather than as the sum of the characteristics of its individual members.**
- **It is assumed that a close relationship exists between the way a family functions as a group and the emotional adaptation of its individual members.**

Family therapy has evolved from these principles in order to link the disorders of family living to the disorders of individual members of a family within one therapeutic approach. This approach assumes that individual emotional differences stem from disturbances in the overall interaction of the natural biopsychosocial unit, the family (Sadock and Sadock, 2003). **The purposes of family therapy are to improve interpersonal skills, communication, behavior, and functioning.**

Deciding when family therapy is appropriate or indicated over individual or group therapy is not always easy. Resource availability is a factor; many settings do not have anyone trained in family therapy, and reimbursement issues have to be addressed. When the resources are available, the therapist's bias may have an influence on this decision. Some family therapists conceptualize all emotional problems within the family framework. Others recommend certain guidelines in determining which problems should be treated in family therapy. They suggest that family therapy is indicated in the following situations:

- The presenting problem appears in system terms, such as marital conflicts, severe sibling conflicts, or cross-generational conflicts (parents versus offspring, parents versus grandparents).
- Various types of difficulty and conflict arise between the identified patient and other family members.
- The family is experiencing a transitional stage of the family life cycle, such as beginning a family, marriage, birth of the first child, entrance of children into adolescence, the first child leaving home, retirement, or the death of a spouse or other family member.
- Individual therapy with one family member has resulted in symptoms developing in another family member.
- No improvement occurs with adequate individual psychotherapy. Enlarging the conceptual field to include the family in psychotherapy may produce therapeutic movement.
- The person in treatment seems unable to use individual psychotherapy for personal understanding and change, but rather uses therapy sessions primarily to talk about or complain about another member.

Another important component of family therapy, as in all treatments, is to be clear about the targets for therapeutic change. A target list will help determine the type of family therapy interventions that might be most effective and will keep the sessions focused on the goals and expected outcomes of treatment. To produce an appropriate target list, the nurse should be current on his or her knowledge of research findings that affect practice and be familiar with family rating scales.

Family Assessment

The goals of a family assessment and subsequent intervention are appraisal, reduction of psychiatric symptoms, increase in family resourcefulness or skills, improvement in individual psychological needs and family interactions, enhanced family awareness of how family patterns affect the health and satisfaction of their members, and the selection, implementation, and evaluation of treatment (Messer and Reiss, 2000).

Many methods of family assessment have been identified, including measures of relationships, family history, family

APGAR, family relational diagnoses, self-report inventories, and genograms (see Chapter 11). One example of a systems model for assessing families examines five levels including individuals, dyads, nuclear families, extended family, and community and cultural systems. The systems are assessed in the overlapping domains of cognition, affect, communication, interpersonal, structural, developmental, control, and sanctions (Snyder, Cozzi, and Mangrum, 2002). Multiple assessment strategies are then used to assess across domains including formal and informal self-report and observational techniques.

It is useful to consider the following guidelines when completing a family assessment:

- When the presenting problem is with a child, the therapist may meet with the whole family or just the parents.
- Children are usually involved in the sessions because they are relevant to the targeted problems.
- Younger children may be disruptive in the sessions so they should be excluded, although sometimes there may be a reason to include them. For example, when intervening with a family in which the mother is having a postpartum episode, it may be important to observe the mother's interaction with the infant and the husband's response to her interaction.
- Family genograms are constructed to capture history, structure, and genetics related to psychiatric disorders and health.

Review family genograms from Chapter 11. Construct a genogram for your own family. ∎

Family Interventions

Family interventions are aimed at engaging families and encouraging them to be active participants in treatment and rehabilitation, thereby increasing their knowledge and improving coping skills in both patients and their families (Kopelowicz, Liberman, and Zarare, 2002). The indications for family interventions are supported by research that suggests that stressful family environments predict the course of illnesses, such as mood disorders and schizophrenia (Simoneau et al, 1999).

Family interventions are delivered in a variety of settings, such as schools, homes, outpatient programs, offices, inpatient units, residential treatment programs, hospitals, courts, child development centers, churches, and other community settings. Nurses, psychiatrists, psychologists, and social workers can provide family interventions, as can licensed marriage and family counselors. However, the delivery of family and couples therapy requires advanced training and supervision.

Many family education, support, and skills building programs can be delivered by consumers and other community-based leaders trained in the intervention. For example, survivors of suicide can be trained as leaders of support groups for family and friend survivors of a loved one who died by suicide. This often enhances culturally competent programs. Nurse experts in family intervention can provide training,

supervision, and support and can play an important role in program development, preparation of funding applications, and dissemination of evidence-based family interventions in the community.

Family Outcome Measures

Outcomes of family interventions include not only individual change but also changes in interactions relevant to problem behaviors or social systems (Kumpfer, 1999; Liddle et al, 2002; Messer and Reiss, 2000). Instruments, such as the Family Burden Scale, are widely used by clinicians and researchers to examine the impact of medical and psychiatric disorders on the family. It is important for nurses to note that satisfaction is not a priority outcome, thus self-report of family satisfaction has limited value in measuring the impact of family interventions.

In selecting an instrument for family intervention one should use the best known, standardized, briefest, and most valid and reliable instruments. The instruments should be pilot tested. Interviews should begin with positive measures, should address the most sensitive measures half way through the interview, and should save the least important measures for the end of the interview. It is helpful to ask the questions using as few words as possible, and consideration should be given to developmental, culturally appropriate, and gender sensitive issues. Direct observation should be used to assess changes in parent/child interactions. Finally, distal or long-term changes in family dynamics or risk factors should be part of outcome evaluation.

Compare and contrast the usefulness of self-report, interview, and observation formats in working with families. ∎

∎ RESEARCH ON FAMILY INTERVENTIONS

Studies of family therapy effectiveness are new; they have been conducted in just the last two decades. They are based on family functioning theories and clinical practice. Research on families can include basic family research, family intervention research, and family-related research. In each of these areas of research, the conceptualization, measurement, and analysis aspects view the family as a unit or system and thus contribute to the knowledge of family functioning. For family-related research, the responses of individual family members or concepts related to families or family members are examined.

Family intervention research has included interventions for persons with mood disorders, schizophrenia, substance abuse, personality disorders, conduct disorders, developmental disorders, children of substance abusers, and those who are suicidal (see Citing the Evidence). Additional research is needed in areas such as family responses to illnesses, the suitability of assessments and interventions across cultural groups, methods useful for analyzing family data, and methods used to recruit and retain family members from a variety of cultural groups (Liddle et al, 2002). A sample of family interventions supported by research are described here.

CITING THE EVIDENCE ON
Family Interventions for Schizophrenia

BACKGROUND: Although a growing body of evidence on the efficacy of psychological interventions for schizophrenia now exists, this meta-analysis improves on previous systematic and meta-analytical reviews by including a wider range of randomized controlled trials and providing comparisons against both standard care and other active interventions. Literature searches identified randomized controlled trials of four types of psychological interventions: family intervention, cognitive-behavioral therapy (CBT), social skills training, and cognitive remediation.

RESULTS: Family therapy, in particular single family therapy, had clear preventive effects on the outcomes of psychotic relapse and readmission, in addition to benefits in medication compliance. CBT produced higher rates of 'important improvement' in mental state and demonstrated positive effects on continuous measures of mental state at follow-up. CBT also seems to be associated with low drop-out rates.

IMPLICATIONS: Family intervention should be offered to people with schizophrenia. CBT may be useful for those with treatment resistant symptoms. Both treatments, in particular CBT, should be further investigated in large trials across a variety of patients, in various settings, and in regard to factors that mediate treatment success.

Pilling S et al: *Psychol Med* 32:763, 2002.

Youth

In 1999 the Office of Juvenile Justice and Delinquency, in collaboration with the Center for Substance Abuse Prevention (CSAP), searched for "best practice" family-strengthening programs, specifically family programs that have proven to be effective in the prevention of youth substance abuse and other dysfunctional behavior (Alvarado et al, 2000). Interventions were evaluated using criteria for clinical and research evidence developed by the Institute of Medicine (1994) including the following categories: strong level of evidence, medium level of evidence, suggestive but insufficient evidence, and substantial evidence of ineffectiveness. Interventions were rated as Exemplary I and II, Model, and Promising.

A guideline was developed, known as the Prevention Enhancement Protocol System (PEPS), and titled "Preventing Substance Abuse Among Children and Adolescents: Family-Centered Approaches" (DHHS, 1999). PEPS is a systematic and analytical process that synthesizes a body of knowledge on specific prevention topics. This PEPS document is based on the belief that the family is the first line of defense and that there is a need to know which family interventions are effective in preventing substance abuse.

Three family-centered approaches with clinical and research evidence to support their efficacy were identified in PEPS: parent and family skills building, family in-home support, and family therapy. All three evidence-based programs target families with multiple risk factors or a high level of ex-

posure to one risk factor, such as divorce, parental substance abuse, or juvenile legal involvement.

As an intervention with youth, multisystemic family therapy is considered Exemplary I (meeting the highest level of research evidence for effectiveness). Multisystemic therapy (MST) is a family- and community-based treatment to prevent youth out-of-home placements, such as incarceration and psychiatric hospitalization (Henggler, 1999). MST has produced long-term outcomes and is cost effective for youth with serious problems.

A key feature of MST is the integration of empirically based approaches, such as structural family therapy, cognitive behavior therapy, and psychopharmacological treatment, to address a variety of risk factors across the family, peer, school, and community levels. Treatment principles are clearly identified, and the home-based therapists are actively supervised. MST has been the focus of federally funded projects with multiple replications, revisions, and adaptations, and it is included in policy recommendations for juvenile offenders.

Functional family therapy is another exemplary program. Functional family therapy (FFT) is an approach that integrates systems, behavioral, and cognitive views of dysfunction (Alexander, Holtzworth-Monroe, and Jameson, 1994). The treatment goal of FFT is to modify interaction and communication patterns to foster more adaptive family functioning.

This intervention has been used with families of juvenile offenders. These families manifest high rates of defensiveness in parent-parent and child-parent communication, negative attitudes, blaming, and low rates of mutual support as compared with families of nonoffenders (Kazdin, 2002). Although only a few studies of FFT have been conducted, the evidence thus far indicates that FFT decreases conduct problems in juvenile offenders, even $2\frac{1}{2}$ years after treatment completion.

A few family interventions have been designed specifically for families of suicidal youth. Successful Negotiation Acting Positively (SNAP) is a brief standardized cognitive-behavioral therapy program with the goal of reducing subsequent youth suicide attempts (Rotheram-Borus et al, 1994). SNAP is a six-session outpatient intervention, consisting of structured activities designed to create a positive family atmosphere, teach active problem-solving skills, and shift the family's view of problems from difficult family members to troublesome situations. Based on social learning theory, the experiences include structured role plays, therapist modeling, written case vignettes, and psychoeducation.

Family dysfunction also has been implicated as a risk factor in anorexia nervosa among youth. Family therapy has been used to treat adolescent and adult patients with anorexia nervosa. Minuchin's (Minuchin and Fishman, 1981) structural family therapy is often combined with individual therapy and nutritional counseling; however, studies of family therapy in eating disorders are limited. Some studies suggest the outcomes of family therapy are comparable or slightly better than those of individual therapy (Robin, Siegel, and Moye, 1995).

Finally, suicidal youth often present in the emergency department (ED). A few family-centered interventions have been developed that may improve treatment adherence and decrease the risk of a subsequent suicide attempt. An urban ED adherence program targeting Hispanic adolescent attempters included an orientation video for families, an on-call bilingual crisis therapist/crisis manager, and an interdisciplinary training program for ED personnel (Rotheram-Borus et al, 1994).

Another youth suicide prevention program trained ED staff to deliver a means restriction intervention to parents of youth at risk for suicide. Means restriction is intended to restrict access to firearms, medications, and other means of suicide. When this intervention was delivered, the parents were significantly more likely to lock up guns and medications (Kruesi et al, 1999). Although mental health professionals may be reluctant to discuss firearms with parents, nurses are well trained and well positioned to deliver this intervention.

Do you think nursing staff in emergency rooms are prepared to care for suicidal patients? What additional training do you think they would need to enhance the care they now provide to this group of patients? ■

Couples Therapy

Another area of research focuses on the relationships of couples. An example is Wallerstein and Blakeslee's (1995) qualitative work with functional couples in which they identified nine tasks of building a good marriage:

- To separate emotionally from the family of one's childhood so as to invest fully in the marriage and, at the same time, to redefine the lines of connection with both families of origin.
- To build togetherness by creating the intimacy that supports it while carving out each partner's autonomy.
- To embrace the daunting roles of being parents and to absorb the impact of a baby's dramatic entrance while working to protect their own privacy.
- To comfort and master the inevitable crises of life, maintaining the strength of the bond in the face of adversity.
- To create a safe haven for the expression of differences, anger, and conflict.
- To establish a rich and pleasurable sexual relationship and protect it from the incursions of the workplace and family obligations.
- To use laughter and humor to keep things in perspective and to avoid boredom by sharing fun, interests, and friends.
- To provide nurturance and comfort to each other, satisfying each partner's needs for dependency and offering continuing encouragement and support.
- To keep alive the early romantic, idealized images of falling in love while facing the sober realities of the change wrought by time.

The variability in the types of happy marriages is diverse. Persons in healthy marriages have better health, healthier lifestyles, and deal better with stress (Gollan and Jacobsen, 2002). Marital distress also increases the risk for developing psychiatric disorders and health problems, due in part to immunological suppression.

Marital therapy is the treatment of the distress in a committed relationship, or the education of a couple in regard to what makes healthy relationships, such as good communication skills. This modality has been used in the treatment of depression, substance abuse, sexual dysfunction, divorce, step-family conflict, and trauma. There is strong clinical evidence for the effectiveness of this intervention.

Typically this therapy is brief (12 to 20 sessions) and is contract-oriented. The therapy activities include enhancing communication skills, increasing caring activities, and linking current family issues to family of origin experiences. Contraindications for marital therapy include marital affairs, intense anxiety, a potential for violence, a lack of commitment to the relationship, and an inexperienced therapist.

Evidence exists for the effectiveness of six types of martial therapy including behavioral, emotion-focused, cognitive-behavioral, strategic, and insight-oriented. Behavioral marital therapy is a very successful and well-researched approach, based on the premise that distress in a couple results from efforts to get positive reinforcement that fails.

Family Psychoeducation

Psychoeducation for families that include persons with severe disorders, such as schizophrenia, major depression, and bipolar disorder, is typically combined with pharmacotherapy (Craighead et al, 2002a and b; Nathan and Gorman, 2003; Miklowitz et al, 2003). Programs often blend psychoeducation, communication enhancement training, and problem-solving skills training with information modules on symptoms, diagnosis, etiology, prognosis, interactions of stress and vulnerability, risk and protective factors, trajectory of the disorder, treatment, and strategies for relapse prevention (see Chapter 13). Skills building may include relapse prevention drills and disorder-related conflicts skills.

Evidence exists for the effectiveness of family psychoeducation for families of adults with bipolar disorder as compared with individually focused treatment on crisis management, relapse, depression, rehospitalization, and positive communication (Goldstein, Rea, and Miklowitz, 1996; Miklowitz et al, 2003; Simoneau et al, 1999). Similarly, family psychoeducation for families of persons with mood disorders, schizophrenia, and other psychiatric disorders improved global and symptomatic functioning and family rejection and burden. Marital psychoeducation of patients with bipolar disorder resulted in improved medication adherence and global functioning (Clarkin et al, 1998).

There is much overlap between psychoeducation and family and marital therapy for families with members who have schizophrenia and mood disorders. Psychoeducation is often combined with marital and family therapy. Both psychoeducation and psychotherapy focus on problem solving and communication therapy. Outcomes of these interventions have demonstrated decreases in feelings of rejection by family members and decreases in patient relapse and rehospitalization and improved family communication and patient functioning, recovery, and medication adherence.

The need for these approaches is indicated by the difficult family communication that can occur when a person is experiencing a psychiatric episode and by the impact of stressful environments, including those labeled as highly expressed

Critical Thinking *About* Contemporary Issues

Is Expressed Emotion a Concept that Perpetuates Family Blame?

Does the concept of expressed emotion (EE) perpetuate blaming families for the mental illness of their families? There are many views of this concept, and views have changed over time. The original research on this concept was developed in the 1970s in England. Relapse and rehospitalizations of persons with mental illness were found to correlate with high EE, particularly negative emotion, of family members. The researchers came to the conclusion that these patients were particularly sensitive to overstimulating environments and would fare better in more structured, nondemanding, and less stimulating environments.

On the other hand, the National Alliance for the Mentally Ill (NAMI), believes that EE studies and the resulting conclusions (family emotional characteristics contributing to psychiatric episodes) perpetuate family blaming. As an alternative explanation, NAMI suggests that when families cope with unusual behavior in a member with mental illness, the family may develop unique patterns of behavior.

In the eighties, as new models of psychoeducation developed, clinicians saw this as an opportunity to decrease family blaming and lower emotional expression through family education. This approach was based on the stress-diathesis model in which some people have a predisposition that make them decompensate under stress. Ironically, in the nineties, with the focus on biological psychiatry, family members complained that many psychiatrists were ignoring families.

This concept of EE has relevance to the psychiatric–mental health nurse in terms of planning and managing milieus and in providing psychoeducation to families. Different families relate to different explanations of etiology, such as focusing more on biology or more on the interaction of risk factors. Nurses need to respect these differences. Nurses can help families normalize their experiences in coping with their mentally ill member and learn new coping styles to use when responding to problems and crises. There is no simple answer to this question, and much remains to be learned about "what works" as nurses continue to partner with their patients and their families.

emotion, on relapse (see Critical Thinking About Contemporary Issues). These approaches have been used in inpatient and outpatient settings, in crisis programs, and with home-based interventions and multiple family groups.

Family Bereavement

A variety of programs have been developed for families of persons who died by suicide, homicide, or terrorism. Nurses at all levels of practice can be trained as group leaders in these programs. An example is the **Loving Outreach to Survivors of Suicide (LOSS) Program**, a family bereavement program that included concurrent groups for prepubertal children whose fathers had died by suicide and their mothers (Grossman, 1990). The curriculum included mother-child activities outside the group. For example, the mothers assisted their children in selecting and framing photographs of their fathers. Each child was given an opportunity to share

the picture with the group and then decided where to keep the photograph at home.

Another example is the **Families' Going On After Loss (GOALS) Project** developed by a group of mental health professionals that provides a range of services in the New Jersey–New York metropolitan area in response to the events of September 11, 2001. Through a two-part series of psychoeducational support groups, six sessions in length, these groups have addressed family losses while highlighting family resiliencies and strengths (Underwood et al, 2004).

Family and Parent Skills Building

The purposes of family and parent skills building are to (1) provide parents with new skills that they can use to nurture and protect their children, (2) train parents to deal with challenging children, and (3) help children develop prosocial skills. The level of evidence for the effectiveness of these programs is strong. The Kumpfer **Strengthening Families Program (SFP)** is an Exemplary I family skills building program. Like MST, the SFP has had over 15 years of implementation, replication, revisions, development of adaptations for specific groups, and federally funded evaluation (http://www.strengtheningfamilies.org).

Three components are involved in the 14-week SFP program: concurrent parent and child skills building groups, family dinner, and family skills building (Kumpfer and Tait, 2000). The parent skills building focuses on topics such as communication, problem solving, limit setting, behavioral programs, and the impact of alcohol and drugs on families. The child skills building and the family skills building activities are consistent with the parent topics for that week. The program is delivered through a manualized protocol. Advanced practice nurses have provided leadership in the dissemination of the Kumpfer SFP in family drug courts in several cities (Haack et al, 1999; Scott et al, 1999).

Another family skills building program is the **Effective Black Parenting Program (EBPP),** a cognitive-behavioral program designed to meet the specific needs of African-American families. Thousands of leaders have been trained to deliver child management skills using African American linguistic forms and emphasizing African-American achievement and competence. Evaluation of the program demonstrated significant decrease in parental rejection, increase in the quality of family relationships, and improvement in child behavior outcomes (Alvarado et al, 2000).

You need a license to drive a car, fish, and hunt but not to be a parent. Do you think a parenting skills building program should be required of all new parents? ■

■ THE ROLE OF NURSES

Family nurse researchers are well trained to engage families in research, ensure compliance with the research protocol over time, and search for families who have lost contact with the study group that could benefit from these. Several programs of interdisciplinary family research being led by nurse scientists have received extramural funding and are positively impacting health policy. Some examples include Deatrick, Knafl, and Murphy-Moore's (1999) studies of family management styles and normalization in families of children with health problems, Webster-Stratton's (Webster-Stratton, Hollingsworth, and Kolpacoff, 1989) studies of family-based interventions designed to prevent youth conduct disorders, McCubbin's (1993) studies of families responding to normative and nonnormative transitions and other family stresses, Gross's (Gross et al, 2003) studies of depressed mothers of preschoolers, and Eggert and Thompson's (Eggert et al, 1995) studies of school and family interventions with youth at risk for school dropout and suicide. Eggert and Thompson's interventions have been recognized as exemplary youth suicide prevention programs in several policy documents prepared by the Surgeon General and the Institute of Medicine.

Nurses are well prepared to enhance family functioning in traditional clinical settings and nontraditional settings. In addition, the knowledge, skills, and creativity of nurses enhance family compliance and improve the likelihood of completion of family interventions. Nurses at generalist and specialist levels of preparation can contribute to the implementation of family interventions, research, and education. However, these endeavors must be based on the available evidence, not on tradition, rich as it is.

Nurses need to integrate family-based theory and interventions into clinical programs, disseminate family intervention science, and advocate for family and third-party reimbursement for family interventions. Such proactive strategies will have a significant impact on strengthening families and helping people become competent adults.

COMPETENT CARING

A Clinical Exemplar of a Psychiatric Nurse
JULIE CARBRAY, DNSc, APN, BC

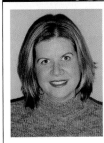

One of the pleasures of being a psychiatric nurse is that of enjoying the positive transformation of families that can occur through your guidance. I participated in such a transformation with a family I saw professionally in our outpatient child psychiatry setting. J was a 9-year-old white male, oldest son of two professional parents, who had been hospitalized for a suicidal gesture. During a family conflict, he had threatened to take his life in a letter he wrote to his parents. After he was stabilized in the hospital and started on antidepressant medication, he was discharged with a referral to my care for his medication management and family therapy.

In a preliminary family session, it became clear that each family member was stressed and that the family had a pattern of highly expressed emotion that typically fueled their conflicts. The mother, father, patient, and his younger sister each felt victimized by the anger in the home, and all agreed that the family did more criticizing than supporting. We discussed J's illness and how his own symptoms—irritability, low self-esteem, and aggression—always were preceded by one of these high conflict states at home.

The parents were educated about how depression manifests in children, that it was almost as if he were more sensitive because of the depression and that the conflict prompted him to respond or to withdraw. His aggression and suicidality were frequently the result of his feeling unable to control the situation at home. The family had a strong extended family history of mood disorders and alcoholism, and both parents were raised in families where conflict and expressed emotion were high. As children they had done their best to avoid these situations or "grew tough skin" to protect themselves. Their son's extreme sensitivity and reactivity appeared out of proportion to what they had experienced in their own childhood.

As part of the treatment plan, the parents agreed to try to empathize with their son because his hurting himself would be one of the worst scenarios they could imagine. His mother started by noting how she felt a need to nag others at home to help out more because she felt things should be orderly and because this behavior took care of "my control issues." The father shared his own struggles and the frustration he felt because of not having time with his wife, feeling as if everything he did was not enough for her, and that the family did very little together. These feelings contributed to a sense of isolation he felt at home, and so he frequently attempted to rescue his children from his wife when she was disciplining them. They had grown accustomed to a good guy–bad guy style of parenting that resulted in more conflict rather than less.

The family also was encouraged to discuss similarities and strengths. They all enjoyed joking with one another, enjoyed sports, and liked watching movies together. I used their sense of humor as a means of bringing them together and getting them to talk about difficult issues while at the same time reinforcing their affection for one another.

Yes, as a result of therapy this family did transform from one of high conflict and tension to one of support and shared responsibilities. This is why I became a psychiatric nurse...and this is why I remain one. ■

CHAPTER FOCUS POINTS

- Family advocacy refers to the mutual support, time, energy, and resources needed to advocate for improved services and opportunities for family members with psychiatric illness. It is effective in raising awareness among service providers, legislators, and the public.
- Commonly used contemporary family therapy frameworks include systems, gender, developmental, cultural, conflict, and structural theories.
- The goals of a family assessment and subsequent intervention are appraisal, reduction of psychiatric symptoms, increase in

family resourcefulness or skills, improvement in individual psychological needs and family interactions, enhanced family awareness of how family patterns affect the health and satisfaction of their members, and the selection, implementation, and evaluation of treatment.
- Family interventions supported by research exist in the areas of youth, couples therapy, family psychoeducation, family bereavement, and parent and family skills building.

◀ KEY TERMS

▶ CHAPTER REVIEW QUESTIONS

1. Indicate whether the following statements are true (T) or false (F).

_____ A. Family therapy is a term used to refer to both family interventions and a conceptual framework for family interventions.

_____ B. Family therapy is a role of the nurse generalist.

_____ C. There is one unified family theory.

_____ D. Family skills building targets families whose children are likely to be placed outside the home.

2. Fill in the blanks.

A. Two motivating forces behind the family movement are

_____ and _____.

B. A self-help and consumer advocacy group in the United

States is _____.

C. The *DSM-IV-TR* includes _____ under "Other Conditions That May Be a Focus of Clinical Attention."

D. Multisystemic family therapy is a family intervention focused

on _____.

E. Means restriction is an intervention used with parents to

restrict access to _____.

F. _____ is an Exemplary I family skills program.

3. Provide short answers for the following questions.

A. Critique the adaptive and maladaptive family functioning portrayed in family movies such as *Happy Meals, Terms of Endearment,* and *On Golden Pond.*

B. Discuss the relationship between a functional marital relationship and depression in a spouse.

C. Describe one type of family research conducted by nurse researchers.

Visit Evolve for additional resources related to the content of this chapter.
http://evolve.elsevier.com/Stuart/principles/
• Topical Course Outline • Student Workbook Exercises • Critical Thinking Questions and Activities • Case Studies • Research Topics
• Monthly Content Updates • WebLinks

Student Study CD-ROM

Access the accompanying CD-ROM for animations, interactive exercises, review questions for the NCLEX examination, and an audio glossary.

REFERENCES

Alexander J, Holtzworth-Monroe A, Jameson P: The process and outcome of marital and family therapy: review and evaluation. In Bergin A, Garfield S, editors: *Handbook of psychotherapy and behavior change*, ed 4, New York, 1994, Wiley.

Alvarado R et al: *Strengthening America's families*, University of Utah, 2000, Department of Health Promotion and Education.

American Psychiatric Association: *Diagnostic and statistical manual mental disorders*, ed 4, text revision, Washington, DC, 2000, American Psychiatric Association.

Bruenlin D, Schwartz R, Kune-Karrer B: *Metaframeworks: transcending the models of family therapy*, San Francisco, 1992, Jossey-Bass.

Clarkin J et al: Effect of psychoeducational intervention for married patients with bipolar disorder and their spouses, *Psychiatr Serv* 49:531, 1998.

Coatsworth J et al: Culturally competent psychosocial interventions with antisocial problem behavior in Hispanic youths. In Stoff D, Breiling J, Maser J, editors: *Handbook of antisocial behavior*, New York, 1997, Wiley.

Craighead W et al: Psychosocial treatments for major depressive disorder. In Nathan P, Gorman, J, editors: *A guide to treatment that works*, New York, 2002a, Oxford University Press.

Craighead W et al: Psychosocial treatments for bipolar disorder. In Nathan P, Gorman J, editors: *A guide to treatment that works*, New York, 2002b, Oxford University Press.

Deatrick JA, Knafl KA, Murphy-Moore C: Clarifying the concept of normalization, *Image J Nurs Sch* 31:209, 1999.

Department of Health and Human Services (DHHS): *Family-centered approaches to prevent substance abuse among children and adolescents: a guideline*, Prevention Enhancement Protocol System (PEPS) (No. 277-92-1011), Washington, DC, 1999, US Government Printing Office.

Eggert L et al: Reducing suicide potential among high-risk youth: tests of a school-based prevention program, *Suicide Life-Threatening Behav* 25:22, 1995.

Goldstein, M, Rea M, Miklowitz D: Family factors related to course and outcome of bipolar disorder. In Mundt C et al, editors: *Interpersonal factors in the origin and course of affective disorders*, London, 1996, Gaskell Books.

Gollan J, Jacobsen N: Developments in couple therapy research. In Liddle H et al, editors, *Family psychology: science-based interventions*, Washington, DC, 2002, American Psychological Association.

Gross D et al: Parent training of toddlers in day care in low-income urban communities, *J Consult Clin Psychol*, 71:261, 2003. Erratum in *J Consult Clin Psychol* 71:442, 2003

Grossman J: Child and parent bereavement program post paternal suicide, Unpublished Manual, Chicago, Illinois, 1990, College of Nursing, Rush University.

Haack M et al: *Strengthening African American families*, Washington, DC, 1999, Substance Abuse and Mental Health Services Administrative Department of Health and Human Services.

Henggler S: Multisystemic therapy: An overview of clinical procedures, outcomes, and policy implications, *Child Psychol Psychiatry Rev* 4:2, 1999.

Institute of Medicine: *Reducing risks for mental disorders: frontiers for preventive intervention research*, Washington, DC, 1994, National Academy Press.

Kazdin A: Psychosocial treatments for conduct disorders. In Nathan P, Gorman J, editors: *A guide to treatment that works*, New York, 2002, Oxford University Press.

Kopelowicz A, Liberman, P, Zarare R: Psychosocial treatments for schizophrenia. In Nathan P, Gorman J, editors: *A guide to treatment that works*, New York, 2002, Oxford University Press.

Kruesi M et al: Suicide and violence prevention: parent education in the emergency department, *J Am Acad Child Adolesc Psychiatry* 38:250,1999.

Kumpfer K: Outcome measures of interventions in the study of children of substance-abusing parents, *Pediatrics* 103:1128, 1999.

Kumpfer K, Tait C: Family skills training for parents and children, *Juvenile Justice Bulletin*, April, p 1, 2000.

Liddle H et al: *Family psychology: science-based interventions*, Washington, DC, 2002, American Psychological Association.

McCubbin M: Family stress theory and the development of nursing adaptation about family adaptation. In Feetham S et al, editors: *The nursing of families*, Newbury Park, Calif, 1993, Sage.

McFarlane M: *Family therapy and mental health: innovations in theory and practice*, Binghamton, NY, 2001, Haworth Clinical Practice.

Messer S, Reiss D: Family and relational issues measures. In *Handbook of psychiatric measures*, Washington, DC, 2000, American Psychiatric Association.

Miklowitz DJ et al: A randomized study of family-focused psychoeducation and pharmacotherapy in the outpatient management of bipolar disorder, *Arch Gen Psychiatry* 60:904, 2003.

Minuchin S, Fishman H: *Family therapy techniques*, Cambridge, Mass, 1981, Harvard University Press.

Nathan P, Gorman J: *A guide to treatment that works*, New York, 2002, Oxford University Press.

Reinhard S, Grossman J, Piren K: Advocacy. In Joel L, editor: *Advanced practice nursing*, Philadelphia, 2004, FA Davis.

Robin AL, Siegel PT, Moye A: Family versus individual therapy for anorexia: impact on family conflict, *Int J Eat Disord* 17:313, 1995.

Rotheram-Borus MJ et al: Brief cognitive-behavioral treatment for adolescent suicide attempters and their families, *J Am Acad Child Adolesc Psychiatry* 33:508:517, 1994.

Sadock B, Sadock V: *Kaplan & Sadock's synopsis of psychiatry*, ed 7, Philadelphia, 2003, Lippincott Williams & Wilkins.

Scott K et al: *Strengthening families through community partnerships*, Washington, DC, 1999, Substance Abuse and Mental Health Services Administration, Department of Health and Human Services.

Simoneau TL et al: Bipolar disorder and family communication: effects of a psychoeducational treatment program, *J Abnorm Psychol* 108:588, 1999.

Snyder D, Cozzi J, Mangrum L: Conceptual issues in assessing couples and families. In Liddle H et al, editors: *Family psychology: science-based interventions*, Washington, DC, 2002, American Psychological Association.

Underwood M et al: *The Families GOALS Project (Going On After Loss)*, NJ, 2004, NJ Mental Health Association.

Wallerstein J, Blakeslee S: *The good marriage: how and why love lasts*, New York, 1995, Warner Books.

Webster-Stratton C, Hollingsworth T, Kolpacoff M: The long-term effectiveness and clinical significance of three cost-effective training programs for families with conduct-problem children, *J Consult Clin Psychol* 57:550, 1989.

White J, Klein D: *Family theories*, Thousands Oaks, Calif, 2002, Sage.

Wright L, Leahey M: *Nurses and families: a guide to family assessment and intervention*, ed 3, Philadelphia, 2000, Davis.

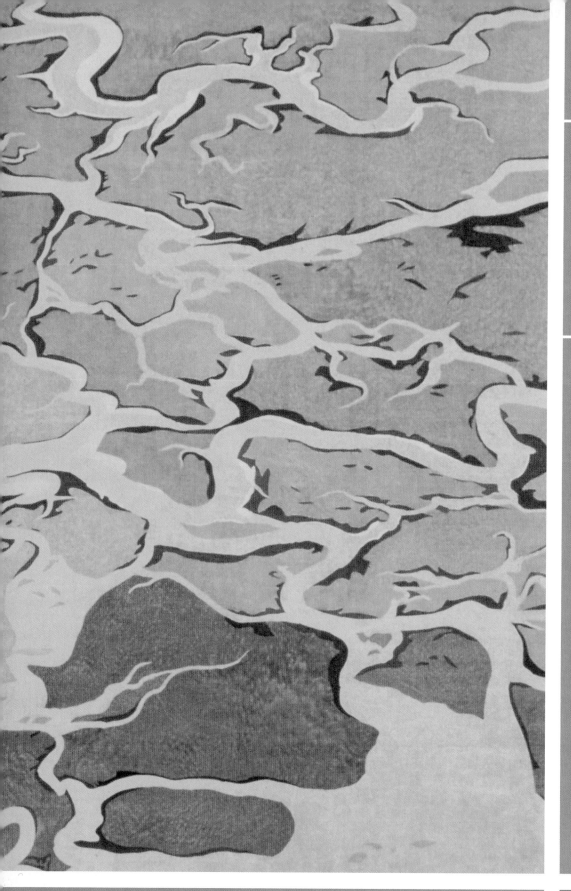

Unit Five

Salt Beds (San Francisco)
50" x 33" batik on silk 1991

Artist's Note: Every location is different from the air, and the flight over the salt beds in 1986 were foreign to me as an East Coast artist. The environment required a different approach—a lower, tighter angle through the lens. Salt has been thrown on the silk to disperse the dyes. The black edges create tension.

Treatment Settings

You may think that most people with emotional and psychiatric problems spend many days of their lives in an acute or long-term psychiatric hospital being cared for by specially trained staff. Years ago you would have been correct, but today most people with such problems live in the community and receive their mental health care in outpatient settings. These are the people you pass on the street, see at the mall, and laugh with at the movies. Today we no longer try to separate and isolate the mentally ill in large, impersonal institutions. Rather, we ask our caregivers to reach out to these people and their families in the neighborhoods in which they live, love, and learn.

In this unit you will discover how contemporary psychiatric hospitals take care of patients. You will read how inpatient psychiatric nurses protect and stabilize people in crisis and then turn their care over to a variety of community-based mental health care providers. As psychiatric treatment grows in the community, new and expanded roles are opening up for psychiatric nurses in such areas as home and forensic psychiatric care. These tap into nurses' spirit of innovation, creativity, and resourcefulness. So step up, step out, and step into the current practice settings of psychiatric care.

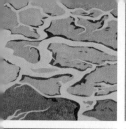

"We're all mad here. I'm mad. You're mad." "How do you know I'm mad?," said Alice. "You must be," said the Cat, "or you wouldn't have come here." Alice didn't think that proved it at all.

LEWIS CARROLL, *ALICE'S ADVENTURES IN WONDERLAND*

34 HOSPITAL-BASED PSYCHIATRIC NURSING CARE

ELIZABETH G. MAREE

 Visit Evolve for additional resources related to the content of this chapter.
http://evolve.elsevier.com/Stuart/principles/

The treatment of the mentally ill has always reflected social values and public policy. Before World War II, effective medications were largely unavailable, and the mentally ill were separated from the community and housed in institutions for the protection of patients as well as society. Nursing care for these patients was primarily custodial.

With changing social perspectives and the move toward more humane treatment, the psychiatric hospital came to be seen as a possibly powerful force that could influence patient behavior and help people recover from mental illness. More recently, scientific advances have led to the use of effective medications and somatic therapies to treat symptoms of psychiatric illness. These, used in conjunction with therapeutic principles and management strategies of the treatment milieu, offer hospital-based psychiatric nurses valuable tools for the care of the mentally ill.

■ INPATIENT PSYCHIATRIC CARE IN TRANSITION

Economic pressures are transforming all health care services in the United States. These forces are dramatically influencing inpatient psychiatric care facilities. All inpatient programs compete for limited resources and must generate revenues and manage expenses effectively in order to maintain their mission (Goldberg, 2001).

Psychiatric nurses must have a broad understanding of the challenges associated with the delivery of psychiatric care in an inpatient setting. **Lack of parity in funding for psychiatric treatment, stigma, limited use of evidence-based interventions, and a shortage of specialized mental health personnel, especially nurses, are a few of the major issues impacting inpatient psychiatric care** (Halter, 2002; Mechanic, 2002).

These concerns increase barriers to acute care treatment, resulting in stress on hospitals and community systems as they try to address unmet needs. Yet news headlines constantly remind society of the real need for psychiatric intervention and the danger of ignoring behaviors associated with mental illness.

Inpatient Programs

In recent years the focus of psychiatric care has moved away from extended care in predominantly inpatient settings and toward shorter lengths of inpatient stays and a wider choice among the continuum of care options. For example, in 1989 the average length of stay for acute psychiatric inpatient treatment was about 24 days, as compared with 7.6 days in 2001 (Figure 34-1). Most inpatient psychiatric settings now have an average length of stay of 5 to 10 days, and crisis stabilization inpatient programs may involve only a 2- or 3-day length of stay.

The major psychiatric diagnoses of patients admitted to inpatient and partial hospital programs are listed in Table 34-1. In previous years most patients with maladaptive coping responses entered the psychiatric hospital in the **acute treatment stage** and were able to stay in the hospital until the goal of symptom **remission** was attained. Today, however, the majority of patients are admitted to hospitals in the **crisis stage,** with the treatment goal of **stabilization** rather than symptom remission.

The indications for inpatient hospital use have become more focused in recent years and include the following:

- Prevention of harm to self or others
- Stabilization to allow treatment at a less restrictive level of care
- Initiation of a treatment process for patients with safety risks that must be monitored by specially trained personnel
- Management of severe symptoms resulting in significant confusion, disorganization, and inability to care for self
- Need for a rapid, multidisciplinary diagnostic evaluation that requires frequent observation by specially trained personnel

As the goals of hospitalization have shifted, treatment objectives also have become more focused and include the following:

- Rapid evaluation and diagnosis
- Decreasing behavior that is dangerous to self or others
- Preparing the patient and significant caregivers to manage the patient's care in a less restrictive setting

- Arranging for effective aftercare to facilitate continued improvement in the patient's condition and functional level

Specific treatment interventions include detoxification from substances, intervening in the family/significant other systems, initiation or modification of pharmacological treatment, and follow-up planning (Glick, Carter, and Tandon, 2003).

The Role of the State Hospital

The history of mental health services reveals a debate over the best location for treatment. This "institution vs. community" controversy has driven policy and legal reforms for the past 50 years (Geller, 2000). A large part of this debate is the concern over **institutionalism**, which is described as a pat-

Table 34-1	Major Diagnoses of Patients Admitted to Inpatient Programs and Less Than 24-Hour Care	
	DIAGNOSIS	PERCENTAGE
	Inpatient Programs	
	Affective disorders	40
	Schizophrenia	20
	Substance use disorders	12
	Adjustment disorders	5
	Organic mental disorders	4
	Personality disorders	2
	Less Than 24-Hour Care	
	Schizophrenia/affective	37
	Disruptive behavior	16
	Developmental disability	10
	Substance abuse	9
	Personality	2
	Other	1

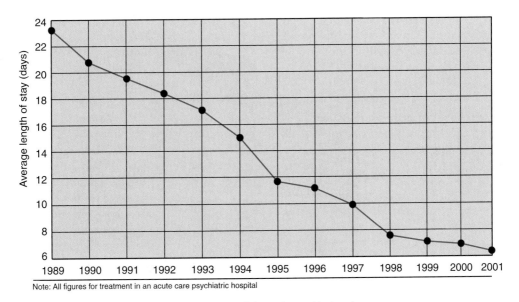

Note: All figures for treatment in an acute care psychiatric hospital

Figure 34-1 Hospital stays for psychiatric patients.

tern of passive dependent behavior observed among psychiatric inpatients that is characterized by hospital attachment and resistance to discharge (Wirt, 1999). The prevention of this condition and the belief in the superiority of community treatment that would allow for the integration of family and social living lead to an advocacy movement that discouraged the state hospital concept.

The philosophy of deinstitutionalization, changing health care economics, and advances in the treatment of mental illness, especially psychopharmacology developments, significantly influenced the transformation of state mental hospitals. These were major factors in the downsizing and increasingly frequent closure of these facilities. Fifty-four state psychiatric hospitals closed between 1940 and 1999 (Ross, 1999/2000). Only 14 of these closures occurred before 1990 (Figure 34-2). The period from 1970 to 1999 was a time of major downsizing, with the total number of state and county psychiatric beds decreasing by 50% (NASMHPD, 2000).

The downsizing and closing of psychiatric hospitals by state mental health agencies occurred as allocation of funds shifted from hospital to community-based services. In 1993, for the first time, states spent more on community-based services than on state psychiatric hospitals. By 1998, community mental health spending was about $9 billion, far exceeding the $6.6 billion spent on state psychiatric hospitals (Ross, 1999/2000).

What will be the role for state psychiatric hospitals in the next decade? Some advocates continue to seek resources for developing alternative settings and services in the community (Fisher et al, 2001). Others consider state mental health hospitals to be a component of the continuum of mental health services (Flannelly, Flannelly, and Cox, 2001). Although a majority of patients transitioning from state hospitals have been maintained in community services, concern for the population of persons with severe mental illness has been rising.

Despite advancements, some patients continue to require long-term, highly structured care on a 24-hour basis. Safety of the patient and society, inconsistent availability of appropriate and accessible services in the community, and preventing the mentally ill from becoming homeless or incarcerated are

a few of the concerns and challenges that must be dealt with in trying to meet the needs of the most severely mentally ill.

Some professionals argue that the debate over location of services has overshadowed the more important issue of how best to deliver quality, humane, and effective care (Geller, 2000). For a small number of patients with severe and persistent mental illness, the long-term care function of state hospitals may continue to provide the most appropriate care—making these hospitals an essential niche in the system of care (Fisher et al, 2001). Extremely disruptive or dangerous patient behaviors, staffing demands, discharge complications, and lack of funding all contribute to the difficulty of providing community services to this population.

The nursing role in the state psychiatric hospital is extremely challenging. From the outset nurses are confronted with the stigma of the population and the very real safety concerns, both of which contribute to the stressful environment of these hospitals. A host of other concerns are inherent in this care setting. Clinical decision making is often hampered by inadequate or incorrect patient information. Nurses also face multiple simultaneous demands and high noise levels. Other challenges include controlling the number and mix of patients on a unit, an inability to impact changes in the personnel system, the burden of paperwork, and the inflexibility of shift scheduling. Maintaining professional standards and navigating through the blurred role boundaries between nurses and paraprofessional staff is yet another challenge (Thomas et al, 1999a).

Still despite these challenges, there are also rewards for nurses working in state psychiatric hospitals. They have the opportunity to develop quality relationships with their patients; they can take pride in their ability to cope with the challenging circumstances; and they can derive gratification from the positive impact they have on patients' lives. Nurses' coping abilities can be enhanced further through opportunities to validate their experiences and expertise with others (Thomas et al, 1999b).

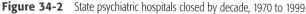 *Some say that state psychiatric hospitals have created a two-tiered (insured and indigent) system of mental health care that does not exist in general health care settings. How would you respond to this allegation?* ■

Crisis Beds

Crisis beds have been developed as an alternative to traditional inpatient hospitalization. The crisis bed concept was designed to decrease reliance on inpatient services, decrease costs, and improve the clinical outcomes of patients for whom this kind of care is appropriate. As the name implies, the focus is on assisting the patient through a brief crisis period lasting **72 hours or less**. After this brief but intensive intervention phase, patients usually can be discharged back to the community. For those who do not stabilize in that timeframe, transfer to inpatient hospitalization may be necessary.

The exact nature of the crisis bed concept depends on the structure of the behavioral health system in which it operates. Regardless of the structure, common goals underlie the devel-

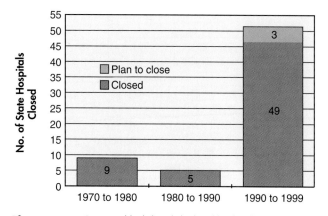

Figure 34-2   State psychiatric hospitals closed by decade, 1970 to 1999.

opment of a crisis program that are distinct from those for inpatient services. These goals include a focus on issues of suicidality, homicidality, and violence; clinical assessment; a rapid resolution of the crisis; decreased dependency on the hospital; prevention of regressive behaviors; and improved functioning of the inpatient environment (Ash and Galletly, 1997).

Residential crisis (RC) programs are delivered in community-based homes, not as a component of a short-stay inpatient admission. This alternative approach to crisis management of an acute exacerbation of serious mental illness in a voluntary patient has been demonstrated to extend care at less cost with comparable effectiveness (Fenton et al, 2002).

Crisis beds require a differentiated role in the continuum of care to be successful. Defined admission and discharge criteria and expert coordination of all levels of care ensure appropriate utilization. Communications within the service, a structured environment, and staff trained in crisis intervention are all necessary components. When these conditions are present, crisis beds become an important addition to a behavioral health continuum of care. The ability to offer safety and continuity while minimizing costs and improving clinical outcomes is crucial in the development of mental health care delivery systems.

Does your community have any crisis beds? If so, how often are they used and by what type of patient? ■

Partial Hospital Programs

Partial hospital or day treatment programs also have become an important part of the continuum of care for those needing mental health and chemical dependency treatment. Partial hospital programs are medically oriented, with a focus on providing specific treatments such as medication and individual, group, and family therapy in a highly organized, structured program. These programs are similar to inpatient programs without the room and board provided by hospitals.

Partial hospital programs are designed to perform the two major functions of crisis stabilization and intermediate-term treatment (Scheifler and Lefkovitz, 2003):

- **Crisis stabilization** is used to avert psychiatric hospitalization or to offer transitional treatment back to the community in order to shorten an episode of acute inpatient care.
- **Intermediate-term treatment** provides more extended, daily, goal-directed service for patients at high risk for hospitalization or readmission because of the serious and persistent nature of their disorder.

Indications for the use of partial hospitalization are very similar to those for inpatient admission; the primary differences are related to the stability and supportiveness of the patient's living environment that are necessary to maintain safety during treatment. Length of stay is determined by the treatment team, in collaboration with the patient.

Typically, the patient is in treatment all day, every day for the first 1 or 2 weeks. As the crisis stabilizes and the level of functioning improves, there is a reduction in the number of days per week the patient attends is reduced. This allows the patient to gradually make the transition back to work, home, or school.

The partial hospital psychiatric team is multidisciplinary and generally includes a psychiatrist, psychiatric nurse, social worker, activity therapist, and vocational counselor. Each member of the team has discipline-specific functions and some functions that overlap. For example, group therapy is an important component of most partial hospital programs, and psychiatric nurses, social workers, and activity therapists all may function as group psychotherapists or lead activity groups.

Unlike inpatient settings where the psychiatrist is expected to see patients daily, in most partial hospital programs the patient is usually seen weekly. The psychiatric nurse in most partial hospital programs assumes primary responsibility for assessing and identifying medical issues that may be contributing to the patient's psychiatric condition.

Studies combining inpatient care with an active, treatment-intensive partial hospital program can reduce symptoms and improve social functioning. A meta-analysis of 40 years of research examining partial versus full hospitalization for adults in psychiatric distress found similar outcomes among partial and full hospitalization patients (Horvitz-Lennon et al, 2001).

How do you think the changes in hospital-based psychiatric care affect the families and support systems of the mentally ill? How can nurses help them with the problems they face? ■

Today the majority of psychiatric nurses work in inpatient and partial hospital psychiatric settings. Hospital-based psychiatric nursing practice is rich in history and tradition. Psychiatric nurses are the only group of mental health professionals who are responsible for meeting the needs of inpatients 24 hours a day, 365 days a year. In partial hospital programs, it is not uncommon for psychiatric nurses to be in contact with patients throughout the full day of treatment, whereas clinicians in other disciplines move in and out of the program to provide specific treatments.

To deliver cost-effective, high-quality inpatient or partial hospital care, psychiatric nurses must manage the one-to-one nurse-patient relationship within a complex social and organizational environment. The scope of contemporary psychiatric nursing practice requires knowledge and expertise in three broad areas:

1. Managing the therapeutic milieu
2. Implementing caregiving activities
3. Integrating and coordinating care delivery

By incorporating these three components, psychiatric nurses can improve a patient's overall treatment outcome.

All psychiatric nurses, regardless of education or experience, engage in these activities every day. To do so requires that the nurse be aware of and value the full range of psychiatric nursing activities (see Chapter 1) and know about the changing mental health care delivery system (see Chapter 9). This chapter is organized around these three areas of functioning because they represent both the structure and the process of hospital-based psychiatric nursing care.

■ MANAGING THE THERAPEUTIC MILIEU

The basic difference between inpatient, crisis bed, partial hospital, and outpatient psychiatric care is the controlled environment, or milieu, in which it occurs. Hospital-based treatment facilities generally provide a milieu that physically shelters patients from what they perceive to be painful and frightening stressors.

This respite, although brief, provides patients with an opportunity to begin to stabilize while being protected from factors that would interfere with their treatment progress. Similarly, partial hospital treatment provides structure and respite for part of the day and intensive support and intervention to promote a home environment that supports positive therapeutic outcomes.

Understanding the concepts of the therapeutic milieu is an essential part of effective psychiatric nursing care. The aim of the therapeutic milieu is to provide patients with a stable and coherent social environment that facilitates the development and implementation of an individualized treatment plan. Many people have studied different aspects of the inpatient psychiatric environment and identified structures and principles that help in treating the mentally ill.

The Therapeutic Community

Maxwell Jones (1953) first described the inpatient environment as a **therapeutic community** with cultural norms for behaviors, values, and activity. He saw patients' social interactions with peers and health care workers as treatment opportunities. For example, he believed that interpersonal difficulties between patients provided fertile material for psycho-dynamic intervention. He also believed that the clinical staff should share community governance with the patient group on an equal basis. He further emphasized the benefit of mutual participation of patients in each others' treatment, predominantly through sharing of intimate information and giving feedback in group settings such as the community meeting.

Since its introduction, the concept of the therapeutic community seems to have lost some of its credibility and popularity (Delaney, Pitula, and Perraud, 2000). One reason for this is that its philosophy of democracy and egalitarianism among patients and clinical staff is not compatible with the medical model. Others point out that the concept of the therapeutic community was developed when patients spent months and even years in the hospital. This is in sharp contrast to the short-term nature of most current inpatient psychiatric hospitalizations.

The therapeutic community is an example of the social model of psychiatric care described in Chapter 3. Discuss how it differs from the medical model in the roles of patient and therapist and the therapeutic process. ■

The Therapeutic Milieu

More than a decade later, the idea of the therapeutic milieu was introduced (Abroms, 1969). It serves two main purposes:

1. **Sets limits on disturbing and maladaptive behavior**
2. **Teaches psychosocial skills**

Five categories of disturbing behaviors and interventions that would help patients keep maladaptive behaviors under control and allow treatment to progress are listed in Table 34-2.

Table 34-2	Managing Disturbing Behaviors in the Milieu	
DISTURBING BEHAVIOR	**DEFINITION**	**INTERVENTION**
Destructiveness	Physically destructive behavior—it is a response to a variety of feelings, such as fear or anger.	In working with destructive behavior, the goal is to control or set limits on the maladaptive response but support the feeling underlying the behavior. Validation is essential to help the patient recognize the feeling and ultimately regain control of maladaptive behavior.
Disorganization	Distorted or unusual behavior a psychotic patient may exhibit as symptomatic of the illness—it may be triggered by elevated anxiety, profound depression, or organic dysfunctions.	Reassure and help the patient while reducing the degree to which these behaviors inhibit therapeutic processes.
Deviancy	Behaviors often described as acting out—they are the result of the patient expressing conflicts overtly in the environment. It is often difficult to determine precisely what acting out behavior is, as well as what is justifiable or even tolerable, because much of it may be influenced by sociocultural factors.	The therapeutic goal in working with deviancy is to analyze how the behavior affects the milieu and how it inhibits the patient's progress. Examining the behavior with the patient and identifying consequences and alternatives are useful approaches.
Dysphoria	Patients with mood alterations may be dysphoric, which is evident in maladaptive responses such as withdrawal from the environment, obsessional behaviors, intrusiveness, or hyperreligiosity.	Establishing a therapeutic alliance is the first task. From there, the nurse and patient can explore feelings and dysfunctional thoughts and begin to modify behavioral responses.
Dependence	Evidenced by patients who do not identify and meet their own needs despite being able to do so—the avoidant nature of dependency interferes with therapeutic progress.	The initial therapeutic goal is to work with the patient to draw on any remaining areas of independence and strength. Then, situations can be identified in which the patient can apply these independent behaviors successfully.

Once maladaptive behaviors are limited, the therapeutic milieu can be used to foster the development of four important psychosocial skills in mentally ill patients, as follows.

- **Orientation.** All patients could achieve a greater level of orientation and reality awareness. Orientation is the patient's knowledge and understanding of time, place, person, and purpose. Awareness of these elements can be reinforced through all patient interactions and activities. For example, introducing oneself, one's role, and the rationale for an interaction helps disoriented patients attend to their surroundings. Another intervention would be a "current events" group conducted with patients.
- **Assertion.** The ability to express oneself appropriately can be modeled and exercised in a variety of ways in the treatment setting. Supporting patients in expressing themselves effectively and in a socially acceptable manner on a specific topic or issue is the overall goal. Some sample interventions include assertiveness training groups, focus groups for lower-functioning patients, or any facilitated, interactive patient group.
- **Occupation.** Patients can feel a sense of confidence and accomplishment through industrious activity. Many therapeutic opportunities are provided through completion of individual or group hands-on activities. Spending time working with patients on something as simple as a jigsaw puzzle can provide purposeful activity, physical skill development, and the added benefit of practiced social interaction.
- **Recreation.** The ability to engage in and enjoy constructive leisure activity is a beneficial outlet for pleasure and relaxation. Providing a variety of recreational opportunities helps patients apply many of the skills they have learned, including orientation, assertion, social interaction, and physical dexterity. Some examples include informal games such as cards, charades, or bingo and brief walks outdoors.

These are useful and practical ideas related to the therapeutic environment that continue to have value in both inpatient and partial hospital settings today. They support the use of some of the different therapies patients receive in structured settings, such as recreation therapy, occupational therapy, and art therapy. However, their appropriateness in short-term inpatient settings is being reevaluated given the acute nature of contemporary inpatient psychiatric care in many settings.

Perhaps the most important contribution to the concept of the therapeutic milieu came when Gunderson (1978) described five specific components of a therapeutic milieu: **containment, support, structure, involvement,** and **validation**. These functions are often used to measure the therapeutic effectiveness of the treatment environment.

How would you respond to a patient's wife who asks you why her husband is spending time in a fitness program and attending a current events discussion group when he has only 5 days of insurance to pay for his hospitalization for severe depression? ■

Containment. Containment provides for the physical well-being of patients. It includes providing food, shelter, and medical attention, as well as taking the steps necessary to prevent the patient from harming self or others. Thus it includes a continuum of interventions, with the use of seclusion and restraints being the most extreme. It is intended to reinforce temporarily the internal controls of patients.

Containment is necessary to provide safety and foster trust. Therapeutic use of containment communicates to patients that the nurse will impose external controls as necessary to keep them and the environment safe. Appropriate and consistent limit setting is essential to meeting this goal. Nursing examples of therapeutic containment include the use of time-outs, room programs, specified observation periods, and seclusion (see Chapter 30).

Planning for containment in partial hospital settings poses additional challenges. The nurse must not only attend to the structured therapeutic milieu of the treatment program but also plan how containment can be enacted in the patient's living environment outside program hours.

The nurse must assess the patient's home environment, both physical and interpersonal, to identify supports and potential problems. This assessment may be based on data collected from interviews with the patient and family members or living companions or may be based on data collected by direct observation during a home visit.

The knowledge gained from the home assessment can then be analyzed along with knowledge about the patient's triggers for disturbing behaviors and productive coping mechanisms that work best for the patient. In collaboration with the patient and others from the home environment, the nurse can develop an effective plan for reducing the triggers as much as possible and defining coping mechanisms for use in avoiding or managing disturbing behaviors.

Support. Support includes the staff's conscious efforts to help patients feel better and enhance their self-esteem. It is the unconditional acceptance of the patient, whatever his or her circumstances. The function of support is to help patients feel comfortable and secure and reduce their anxiety. It may take many forms, but it falls under the general heading of paying attention to the patient.

Support can be communicated through empathy, being available, appropriately offering encouragement and reassurance, giving helpful direction, offering food or beverages, and engaging patients in activities that they are reluctant to do. Other nursing examples include giving direction, suggestions, and education; promoting reality testing; and modeling healthy relationships and interactions.

To best accomplish this task, nursing staff activity must be coordinated, cohesive, and consistent with the patient's treatment goals. Supportive nurturance enhances self-esteem. Milieus that offer support also provide nurturance and encourage patients to become engaged in other therapeutic efforts.

In both inpatient and partial hospital programs, it is essential to coordinate support with others in the home so that they understand the behavioral changes the patient is attempting, how difficult it is to make such changes, the improbability of complete success in initial attempts, and the importance of recognition and support for all attempts.

Structure. Structure refers to all aspects of a milieu that provide a predictable organization of time, place, and person. This dependability in activity, staff, and environment helps the patient feel safe. Having a predictable timetable of meetings, group sessions, and other activities is one feature of structure. Other nursing examples include the setting of limits and the use of contracts, token economies, and required meetings.

The more these uses of structure are planned with the patient according to shared ideas of what is adaptive and maladaptive, the more the structure becomes therapeutic in itself. For partial hospital programs this also involves planning with the patient how he or she will structure his or her activities while outside the hospital.

The patient can then begin to accept responsibility for behavior and its consequences. Providing structure helps the patient control maladaptive behaviors. The nurse uses appropriate consequences if the patient is unable, for whatever reason, to impose or honor effective limits. As natural consequences are consistently applied, the patient learns to delay impulsive and inappropriate responses through consistent expectations and behavioral responses.

Involvement. Involvement is a part of the structure that goes beyond compliance with rules and activities. It refers to processes that help patients actively attend to their social environment and interact with it. The purpose is to strengthen a patient's ego and modify maladaptive interpersonal patterns. Interpersonal communication and shared activity provide patients with opportunities to interact with others in their community.

Nursing examples of involvement include the use of open doors and open rounds and facilitating patient-led groups, activities, and self-assertive experiences. Programs that emphasize involvement encourage the use of cooperation, compromise, and confrontation.

In addition, patients' patterns of involvement and interaction in their social environment can be identified. Progressively demanding opportunities for practicing these skills can then be planned and the results evaluated to help the patient build the skills necessary to develop the level of social involvement needed to support continued therapeutic progress.

Through this involvement, patients learn appropriate interaction patterns and experience the consequences of unacceptable behaviors. For example, a patient who displays anger or offensive behavior that distances others can participate in activities that will help in verbalizing feelings, working out differences, and receiving feedback. This supportive experience strengthens the patient's sense of self, behavioral control, and social interactive skills. Thus encouraging involvement provides corrective experiences for the patient.

Validation. Validation means that the individuality of each patient is recognized. It is the act of affirming a person's unique worldview. Validation can help patients develop a greater capacity for closeness and a more consolidated identity. The psychiatric nurse communicates this through individual attention, empathy, and nonjudgmental acceptance of the patient's thoughts, feelings, and perspective. Other nursing examples of validation include individualized treatment planning, showing respect for a patient's rights, and providing opportunities for the patient to fail as well as succeed.

Therapeutic listening and acknowledging the feelings underlying the patient's personal experience reinforce individuality. Clarification of these feelings helps the patient understand and accept his or her own unique experience. This strengthens the patient's sense of individuality and encourages the integration of pleasant and unpleasant aspects of personal experience.

Visit an inpatient psychiatric unit. Which of the five components of a therapeutic milieu did you observe? Which ones were missing? What barriers prevented the unit from fully implementing this concept? ■

Nursing Implications

One of the earliest advocates of the importance of the environment for nursing care was Florence Nightingale. She believed that the essential responsibilities of nursing included the provision of pure air and water, efficient drainage, cleanliness, and light. In addition, the "prudent" nurse prevented unnecessary noise and attended to the aesthetics and nutritional value of food and the comfort of bedding (Nightingale, 1960).

Since Nightingale's time, the inpatient environment and the therapeutic management of the milieu have continued to be important aspects of the role of all nurses, and this has now been expanded to provide direction for nurses working in partial hospital settings.

Managing the therapeutic milieu remains the domain of the psychiatric nurse. It is essential that psychiatric nurses working in structured settings realize the potential impact that the environment can have on the patient and consciously use it for the patient's benefit (see Critical Thinking About Contemporary Issues). The challenge is for psychiatric nurses to adapt to changes in the patient population and the mental health delivery system by evolving new approaches to managing the milieu as needed (Echternacht, 2001; Thomas, Shattell, and Martin, 2002; Tucker et al, 2001).

Milieu management is a deliberate decision-making process. The psychiatric nurse should first identify what each patient needs from the therapeutic milieu, while keeping in mind the needs of the larger patient group. Weighing individual needs against group needs can be difficult, but it is essential for the successful implementation of a therapeutic milieu. The nurse can then engage aspects of the therapeutic milieu to meet the patient's needs by providing the following:

- **Limits and controls (containment)**
- **Education about the patient's illness and treatment plan (support)**
- **Therapeutic and predictable activity schedules (structure)**
- **Opportunities for social interaction (involvement)**
- **Acknowledgment of the patient's feelings (validation)**

Activities related to each part of the therapeutic milieu can be incorporated into the nursing plan of care, thus maximizing the therapeutic effect of the environment.

Critical Thinking *About* Contemporary Issues

Can Inpatient Psychiatric Nurses Develop Creative, Dynamic Units?

Many conditions operate to stagnate the role of the inpatient psychiatric nurse and decrease the profession's contribution to the hospital-based psychiatric treatment setting (Delaney, 2002). These conditions include the following:

- Lack of studies by nursing researchers that focus on evidence-based interventions for inpatient practice
- Inability to articulate the unique contribution of nurses to the inpatient psychiatric setting
- Maintenance of traditional inpatient nursing practice through oral communications that depend on the availability of experienced nurses to transfer this knowledge
- Reliance on treatment models that have not been adequately researched to provide consistent frameworks for the organization of practice
- Advanced practice psychiatric nurses following a career path that takes them out of the hospital setting
- Lack of continuing education opportunities that address inpatient issues
- Medical model hierarchy that inhibits collaborative care
- Work processes that focus nurses' attention away from patient care

It is important that psychiatric nurses reflect on what they can do to overcome these conditions and improve their ability to positively impact care and outcomes in the inpatient psychiatric setting. Three suggestions for how nurses can direct their efforts toward changing these conditions are as follows:

1. Use the current focus on restraint reduction to examine the work of expert nurses, the impact of organizational factors on treatment, and the role culture plays in igniting discussions concerning unit redesign for patient-centered care.
2. Participate in the development of staffing level indicators that address the rationale for nurse:patient ratios, the skill mix of health care providers, and patient outcomes that are affected by staffing.
3. Become active in professional associations to build peer and collaborative partnerships and access a larger forum for discussing the issues unique to psychiatric nursing.

Clearly, these are just a few of the ways nurses could promote improvements in inpatient psychiatric treatment; however, all would require advocacy, assertiveness, and proactive actions by psychiatric nurses at all levels of education and experience. Psychiatric inpatient nurses are key players. They, perhaps more than any other group, understand the frustration of the mental health system and the human suffering that is caused by mental disorders (Benson and Briscoe, 2003). The need for competent care is great, and the time to act is now. The answer for psychiatric inpatients is high quality psychiatric nursing care.

Nurses have been challenged to better articulate the nursing component of the inpatient treatment program and what specifically they contribute to improving patient outcomes. The key processes of care should be centered on outcomes related to the stabilization of acute symptoms, the restoration of functioning, the establishment of a system of support and the formulation of a plan for symptom management.

To that end, it has been suggested that inpatient nursing interventions be developed in regard to four clinical functions: **safety, structure, support,** and **symptom management** (Delaney, Pitula, and Perraud, 2000). Three of these are core functions identified by Gunderson, but an important fourth function, that of symptom management, has been added. This Four S model has been suggested to help nurses organize inpatient practice because it combines interventions that operate at both the individual and environmental levels of care. Table 34-3 outlines how a nurse might think about outcomes of inpatient care in relation to nursing process and these four clinical functions.

Compare the components of the therapeutic milieu with the responsive and action dimensions of the therapeutic nurse-patient relationship described in Chapter 2. ■

■ IMPLEMENTING CAREGIVING ACTIVITIES

Hospital-based psychiatric nurses must have clinical knowledge and skills and apply them for the benefit of patients and their families. The atmosphere created by the psychiatric nurse strives to provide patients with activities and interactions carefully designed to meet their needs. This includes both direct and indirect psychiatric nursing care functions as well as dependent, independent, and interdependent aspects of psychiatric nursing practice. A few of these caregiving activities in the hospital-based setting merit special discussion.

Assessing and Intervening To Reduce Potential Risks

One of the most important aspects of psychiatric nursing practice is physical safety for the patient and others. This process begins with a thorough assessment of risks at the time of admission and throughout the course of treatment. Common areas of risk for psychiatric patients include potential for aggression or violence, suicide attempts, elopement, seizures, falls, allergic reactions, and communicable diseases.

Based on assessment findings, the nurse is responsible for selecting and implementing the appropriate safety precautions or treatment protocols. Implementation includes not only enacting the prescribed nursing care but also explaining the assessed risk and nursing care plan to the patient, as well as notifying other members of the nursing staff and treatment team of the identified risk.

Patient and Family Education

Education of patients and significant others is essential for sustained therapeutic progress. The process of education must begin with an assessment of the patient's barriers to learning. Such barriers may include lack of insight or denial related to the illness, illiteracy, sensory deficits such as visual or hearing

Table 34-3	Six Processes and Outcomes of Inpatient Psychiatric Treatment	
OUTCOME	**BASIC PROCESS LABEL**	**CLINICAL FUNCTION**
Resolve crisis	Increase patient's perception of control	Support, safety, and symptom management
	Increase supports to patient's system	
	Decrease patient's symptom acuity	
Normalize	Restore sleep pattern	Structure
	Re-engage in socialization	
Thorough assessment	Comprehensive battery of diagnostic interviews and testing completed in a timely manner	Symptom management
Mutual goal setting	Ascertaining patient's goals	Support
	Reaching understanding of what inpatient treatment can provide	
	Assessing patient's attributions of illness and treatment	
Client understands presumed efficacy of medication cognitive/behavioral techniques and rationale for referrals	Outpatient treatment planning	Symptom management
	Guide patient and family through logic of basic cognitive/behavioral approaches	
	Pharmacological recommendations and potentials of service agency referrals	
Do no harm	Provide physical and psychologically safe milieu	Safety structure
	Handle milieu tensions proactively	
	Use least restrictive methods in handling dyscontrol	
	Demonstrate persistent effort to develop collaborative relationship with patient	
	Adequately train staff to maintain safety, sustain structure, affect-attune with client, and understand symptom management techniques	

From Delaney K et al: *J Psychosoc Nurs Ment Health Serv* 38:7, 2000.

impairments, limited concentration and attention span, confusion, or impaired memory.

Once barriers have been identified, particular strategies can be incorporated into the teaching plan to help the patient retain and use the information. As with any learner, repetition of information, presenting information in ways that engage multiple sensory avenues, and providing opportunities for practice and feedback promote learning for psychiatric patients. Common topics for education include symptom recognition and management, desired effects and potential side effects of medication, relapse prevention, and importance of and plans for aftercare.

Almost every interaction provides an opportunity for informal education. For example, meal selection provides an opportunity to learn about nutrition and also to practice decision making and communication skills. Conflicts between patients provide opportunities to learn about and practice problem solving, anger management, negotiation, cooperation, and assertive communication. In addition to such impromptu opportunities for learning, more formal educational activities may be structured into patient care.

Given that patients are admitted to psychiatric units in acute distress, how should a nurse structure his or her own approach to facilitate patients' participation in and retention of educational information presented to them?

Activities, Groups, and Programs

Therapeutic nursing activities, groups, and programs provide a wide variety of opportunities for the nurse to influence the patient's progress toward treatment goals. In providing these corrective experiences, the psychiatric nurse must be clear on the purpose of these activities.

They should be designed to accomplish specific nursing and patient goals in a constructive, efficient, and supportive way. The nurse's challenge is to plan these events in a way that integrates the desired patient outcomes, the interests of the patients, and the ability of the patients to participate and derive feelings of pleasure and accomplishment.

Structured activities can accomplish several goals of the nursing process at the same time. For example, encouraging a cognitively impaired patient to play a common table game, such as cards, allows the nurse to assess the patient's concentration, orientation, memory, and abstract thinking. Based on these observations, the nurse can better understand the patient's learning needs and incorporate them into the plan of care. This same activity can help the socially withdrawn patient try out newly learned interactive skills, experience the role modeling of the nurse, and receive supportive feedback. In addition, the nurse can use these activities to evaluate the effect of nursing, somatic, and psychopharmacological treatments.

Therapeutic nursing groups and programs provide a cost-effective way to implement psychiatric nursing care. Nursing interventions applied in a group setting allow one or two nurses to work with many patients at the same time. Such interventions are productive not only in hospital-based settings but also across the continuum of care. For example, day treatment patients may join inpatients in the same groups or programs. This heterogeneity adds breadth of experience and perspective to the group. Each patient may accomplish a different goal within the same group or program, and such offerings can provide valuable structure to the therapeutic mi-

BOX 34-1

Examples of Psychiatric Nursing Groups or Programs

Medication Education Group

In this group, basic concepts related to medication can be discussed. Providing general information about taking medications, such as the influence of slight dosage or schedule changes, serum levels, the therapeutic window, or how some medication potentiates the effect of other medications, can help the patient and family understand the specifics of the prescribed regimen. Common problems encountered by patients taking psychotropic medication can be discussed, and strategies for dealing with these potential barriers can be shared.

Community Resource Groups

These can be ongoing groups with rotating topics. Topics should be selected based on the learning needs of the group members and their ability to share knowledge about and experiences with varied community resources. For example, a pertinent topic might be the public transportation system of the city. Using maps and information from the local transit authority, exercises can be constructed in which patients go from destination to destination as they practice navigating around the geographic area independently. Another topic may be how to use the newspaper, library, or telephone book to learn about and contact nonprofit, social service, health care, or philanthropic agencies, thus teaching the patient how to mobilize resources after discharge.

Nutrition Groups

Nutrition groups can help teach patients the importance of balanced diets and how to recognize and prepare healthful and appetizing meals for themselves. Food ingredients also provide excellent topics for discussion with psychiatric patients. For example, caffeine can be discussed, pointing out its subtle but pervasive effects on the body and its ability to interfere with the effectiveness of some medications. Other topics can include the basic food groups, shopping strategies, and the role of exercise in promoting health and balanced body weight.

Sleep Improvement Programs

How to improve sleep habits is knowledge often needed by psychiatric patients. Relaxation techniques such as simple yoga positioning, progressive muscle relaxation, and deep breathing may be helpful for some patients. The importance of a healthy sleep-wake cycle can be discussed. Group members can be encouraged to share their sleep-inducing secrets. Commonly used strategies for encouraging sleep can be shared with the group, such as spending time in a soothing bath, sipping warm milk, or reading with a soft light. Behaviors and influences that inhibit sleep may be discussed as well. Group members can be encouraged to try out the ideas and report back to the group on their effectiveness.

---

lieu. Some examples of psychiatric nursing groups are described in Box 34-1.

With the focus of psychiatric care shifting away from extended inpatient stays, opportunities for activity, group, and program development by psychiatric nurses are great. Nursing programs in social skills development, assertiveness, community-based support, crisis intervention, family preservation, and general health teaching are growing areas of psychiatric nursing responsibility.

Equally important are the nursing activities directed toward involving the family in the treatment plan as soon as possible (see Chapter 11). Shorter lengths of inpatient stays have increased caregiver burden and challenges. Patient/family education programs provide the necessary preparation to assume these additional often complex responsibilities (DesRoches et al, 2002). Although this may present challenges to those working in inpatient settings, promoting family involvement needs to be a priority of every treatment setting.

Ask an inpatient psychiatric nurse whether you can "shadow" him or her for a day. Group the nursing functions you see performed as direct or indirect and as dependent, independent, or interdependent. Did this experience change your perception of the inpatient psychiatric nursing role? ■

Meeting Physical Needs

Studies have documented the prevalence of physical illness among psychiatric patients in both inpatient and outpatient treatment settings (Roy-Byrne, 2002). Yet too often, physical illness goes undetected in this patient population. Physical illness may:

- Be the causative factor in a patient's presumed psychiatric illness.
- Exacerbate a psychiatric illness.
- Have no direct relationship to the psychiatric illness but still require medical and nursing intervention for the patient's well-being.

The increase in medical and psychiatric comorbidity among psychiatric patients emphasizes the need for psychiatric nurses to stay current with their physical assessment and medical-surgical nursing skills. It is not uncommon for patients in psychiatric programs to need dialysis, hyperalimentation, intravenous therapy, or dressing changes. Thus completing a physical assessment on admission and monitoring the patient's physical and psychological status throughout the hospitalization are essential functions of the psychiatric nurse.

Discharge Planning

The most obvious goal for inpatient or partial hospital care is to discharge the patient to outpatient status. Therefore a critical focus of the inpatient stay should be establishing the involvement of family members, significant other, and follow-up providers in discharge planning that increases the potential for ongoing care (Boyer et al, 2000).

The nurse must be knowledgeable about the patient's environment. Potential needs and resources should be identified on admission. Once the nurse has decided what knowledge, skills, and behaviors will help the patient adapt to the discharge environment, creative and purposeful activities can be planned to provide the needed resources.

Information regarding supportive resources and medications should be provided to patients and their families to encourage functional independence and decrease the chances of relapse once discharged. This can significantly influence patients' abilities to maintain adaptive coping responses.

Psychiatric discharge planning can be considered part of the psychiatric rehabilitation model that addresses biopsychosocial needs in a manner similar to the physical rehabilitation process. A discharge checklist can be used as an interdisciplinary tool to review the patient's discharge needs and include the patient in the planning process. Areas pertinent to discharge planning that should be included are medications, activities of daily living, mental health aftercare, residence, and physical health care. Special education and the need for financial assistance also should be reviewed with the patient and family.

Transitional care services for mentally ill patients leaving the hospital are often inadequate. Strong communication linkages between hospital-based and community-based providers are essential in order to ensure continuity of care, maximize the value of hospital-based services, and minimize future admissions (see Citing the Evidence). Some of the caregiving activities of hospital-based nursing practice can be seen in the following clinical example.

CLINICAL EXAMPLE

Ms. R was a 17-year-old single high school student who was admitted to an inpatient psychiatric unit with the diagnosis of bipolar disorder. She was admitted because of uncontrollable behavior (sexual promiscuity, running away from home, hyperverbalization, and extreme irritability).

The initial nursing assessment provided a data base that revealed a chaotic family system with a long history of mental illness on both sides of the family, a social and cultural environment in which drug and alcohol abuse were prevalent, and a community that, because of its low socioeconomic status, had limited mental health resources. However, the patient was very bright and cooperative and was motivated to benefit from her hospitalization.

The initial nursing actions were to administer the prescribed medications. The nurse assessed that there was an immediate need to protect the patient from her impulsive, uncontrollable behavior. The patient was placed under close nursing observation at all times until she was able to control her own behavior.

Once the patient's mood had stabilized, her case was presented in nursing rounds. During this time the patient was able to identify a great need for the nurse to teach her and her family about bipolar disorder and the importance of continued medication. The patient and staff agreed that a home visit would make it possible to explore the pressures that the family placed on the patient to function as a surrogate mother to her eight siblings. The patient also believed that it was important that her illness not be viewed in exactly the same manner as that of her sister, who was diagnosed with schizophrenia. The patient viewed her intellectual ability and the love that existed in her family system as her best resources. She thought that, with the help of the nursing staff, she and her family could develop more understanding of her illness and decrease the chaos within the family. After discharge the patient was followed up in outpatient therapy by her primary nurse. ■

■ INTEGRATING CARE DELIVERY

The integrative function of the hospital-based psychiatric nurse is very important, although it is often overlooked or taken for granted. It includes all activities involved in the coordination of patient care such as managing nursing resources, balancing costs and outcomes in decision making, evaluating nursing care delivery modalities, ensuring compliance with professional and regulatory standards, and encouraging communication, participative problem solving, and conflict resolution among mental health team members. In addition, the clinical practice of the nurse involves ongoing implementation of new ideas and approaches for improving quality and decreasing costs.

Teamwork and Coordinated Care

Almost all programs use a multidisciplinary team to deliver treatment. To integrate and coordinate patient care the psychiatric nurse must collaborate with professionals from other disciplines and manage a group of nursing care providers. If therapeutic outcomes are to be optimized, team members must work together to address targeted behaviors and treatment goals. To achieve this level of coordination, team communication must be open and active.

Nursing can enhance continuity of care by organizing the rich clinical data obtained from 24-hour patient involvement. Nursing shift reports should be focused and include updates on nursing assessments, medical information, specific

CITING THE EVIDENCE ON
Risk Factors and Key Strategies in Linkage to Outpatient Psychiatric Care

BACKGROUND: The purpose of the study was to identify patient characteristics resulting in nonadherence to outpatient follow-up after discharge and to identify inpatient interventions that significantly improved the linkage to continued care.

RESULTS: Sixty-five percent of the patients in the study failed to meet the first follow-up appointment after discharge from inpatient hospitalization. Risk factors for failure to link to outpatient treatment included the following: involuntary status at admission, longer length of stay, persistent mental illness, and lack of prior experience with public hospitalization. Three successful interventions were identified: (1) family involvement while the patient was hospitalized, (2) discussion of discharge plans with patient providers, and (3) beginning outpatient linkage before discharge.

IMPLICATIONS: Continuity of care between inpatient and outpatient modalities can be enhanced with successful bridging strategies. Interpersonal components of discharge planning should be prioritized during the inpatient stay in order to prevent gaps in service and improve outcome of care.

Boyer C et al: *Am J Psychiatry* 157:1592, 2000.

nursing interventions, and the short- and long-term goals of treatment. Nurses must be aware of the power of communication and construct reports that are "descriptive, objective, and future oriented" (Priest and Holmberg, 2000).

The degree of cooperation and cohesion among disciplines may vary widely. Interdisciplinary problems have been identified that could interfere with the quality of psychiatric care. Problems between providers may involve poor communication, professional self-doubt, role confusion, and conflict, all of which may be increased by work-related stress.

Whenever multiple people, each with a unique perspective, are working together, the potential for conflict exists. Handling conflict productively is an ongoing challenge for the psychiatric nurse. When poorly handled or avoided, conflict can interfere with the continuity of patient care and the management of a therapeutic milieu. However, effective management of conflict can facilitate stronger professional working relationships, model positive communication skills for patients, and contribute to the nurse's professional development.

Observe a multidisciplinary treatment team in the inpatient psychiatric setting. Did you see any areas of team conflict, role blurring, or turf struggles? If so, how did the team handle these issues? ■

Resource Allocation

Psychiatric nurses must be able to justify the type and level of nursing personnel needed to provide high-quality nursing care (Delaney, 2002). Inpatient unit staffing decisions should be based on accurate information regarding requirements for quality treatment and not solely on staffing ratios (Coleman and Paul, 2001). Thus attention to the most appropriate and efficient use of personnel and other resources is an important part of the psychiatric nurse's role.

The assignment of nursing resources must be based on identified patient care needs, clinical competencies, and available resources. This requires that all nurses become actively involved in examining patient needs, identifying realistic outcomes of care, and assessing the strengths and weaknesses of available nursing personnel.

You report to work one evening and discover that you and only one other staff member have been assigned to cover the 20-bed psychiatric unit. You know that the hospital has been reducing costs, but you believe that this assignment amounts to unsafe staffing. How would you present your case for more staff to nursing and hospital administration? ■

Professional, Regulatory, and Accreditation Standards

Professional standards of the American Nurses Association (ANA) for psychiatric–mental health clinical practice provide a basis for evaluating nursing care. In addition to the Standards of Care and Professional Performance Standards (see Chapter 12), other ANA standards are available to guide nursing activities in administrative and educational areas.

Regulatory and accreditation standards also must be considered by the hospital-based psychiatric nurse. These include the state laws and regulations governing nursing practice and facility licensure, the laws and regulations determining the payment of federal and state insurance funds (Medicaid and Medicare), and standards set forth by accrediting bodies. A health care facility may be required to show how any of these standards are met, including those pertaining to the condition of the physical facility, credentialing of employees, or the documentation of patient care. Requirements vary depending on the type of facility, state regulations, and types of services offered.

The Joint Commission on Accreditation of Healthcare Organizations (JCAHO) has become a leading accrediting agency for many different types of health care facilities. Their standards have served as a benchmark for many other regulatory agencies. JCAHO standards are a helpful and comprehensive guide for all aspects of health care delivery in this country.

The Centers for Medicare and Medicaid Services (CMS) is the federal agency that oversees the spending of Medicare and Medicaid funds. Each state has an identified agency that implements CMS policies locally. Often, in order for the care and treatment delivered by health care agencies to be reimbursed by Medicare or Medicaid, CMS consultants or representatives of the state agency first must conduct surveys of the facility. They may review patient records, inspect the physical plant, interview staff, and evaluate programs to ensure that their specific regulations are being met. Once the facility has shown that all required standards are met, it is eligible to receive payment for treating patients insured by Medicaid and Medicare. These standards are often similar to those of other regulatory and credentialing bodies and focus mainly on the sanitation and safety of the facility, competency of the personnel, and the adequacy and pertinence of the care delivered and documented.

Determine the bed charge for 1 day of care in your psychiatric inpatient unit. How does that compare with the bed charge in a medical-surgical unit? How much of that charge do you think is related to nursing services? ■

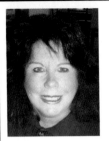

COMPETENT CARING

A Clinical Exemplar of a Psychiatric Nurse

SIMMY PALECKO, MSN, RN

One of the true rewards of psychiatric nursing is that many patients get better and return to functional lives in which they can again experience pleasure and increased self-esteem. It is unbelievably fulfilling to see patients regain a sense of independence and renewed control over their own destinies.

Ms. M is an example of how an intensive short-term psychiatric hospitalization can remarkably improve the quality of a patient's life. She was a 72-year-old woman who was admitted to our adult unit with electrolyte imbalance. She was psychotic and delusional, refusing to eat or drink, not sleeping, highly anxious, and refusing to perform her activities of daily living (ADLs). She believed that her body was rotting away. She was also extremely paranoid, insisting that the clients in the boarding home where she lived were plotting to kill her and that the staff were laughing and talking about her outside her door during the night. She complained of auditory hallucinations and how she felt tortured. Ms. M was extremely irritable and argumentative, as well as physically and verbally threatening. She refused to get out of bed and even ambulate. She insisted that we leave her alone so that she could die.

Ms. M was a recurrent patient on our unit. Her diagnoses were Axis I, bipolar affective disorder; Axis III, colon cancer status postresection, hypertension, degenerative joint disease, peptic ulcer disease, neurogenic bladder, and recurrent urinary tract infections. She was a particular challenge to the nursing staff that we were more than willing to undertake. We were able to use our medical-surgical skills while drawing blood repeatedly, placing IVs, doing ECGs and urinary catheterizations for residual volumes, making accurate intake and output calculations, and carrying out range-of-motion activities. Safety and emotional support were also a major focus of our patient care. Ms. M was placed on fall precautions with continued teaching and reinforcement, even though she was minimally receptive.

Within a few days of admission, her physical condition stabilized and she was scheduled for electroconvulsive therapy (ECT), which had been successful for her in the past. The staff impatiently waited for Ms. M's mood to improve, her appetite to increase, her nighttime sleeping to improve, her interest in her ADLs to increase, and her auditory hallucinations, negativism, and anxiety to decrease. After the fourth ECT treatment, the staff began to see Ms. M's return to her baseline. She was smiling more and her humor was returning. She no longer stated that her body was rotting. She even began to joke with the nursing staff.

Ms. M was discharged to the boarding home approximately 10 days after her admission. The change in the patient's mental and physical condition was remarkable, and I was again reminded of the intrinsic rewards of psychiatric nursing. ■

CHAPTER **FOCUS POINTS**

- The treatment goals, processes, expected outcomes, and length of stay related to hospital-based psychiatric care are changing. The majority of psychiatric nurses currently work in inpatient or partial hospital settings, but they must be ready and able to provide their services throughout the continuum of care.
- Crisis beds have been developed as an alternative to traditional inpatient hospitalization. Residential crisis programs are delivered in community-based homes instead of a short-stay inpatient admission.
- Partial hospital programs are medically oriented, with a focus on providing specific treatments such as medication and individual, group, and family therapy in a highly organized, structured program. They are similar to inpatient programs but without the room and board provided by hospitals.
- The aim of the therapeutic milieu is to provide patients with a stable and coherent social environment that facilitates the development and implementation of an individualized treatment plan.

- Components of the therapeutic milieu include containment, support, structure, involvement, and validation.
- Inpatient psychiatric nursing interventions should be developed along four clinical functions: safety, structure, support, and symptom management.
- Important nursing activities include assessing and intervening in potential risks, providing patient and family education, implementing activities, groups, and programs, meeting patients' physical needs, and planning discharge.
- The integrative function of the hospital-based psychiatric nurse includes all activities involved in the coordination of patient care such as those related to facilitating teamwork and coordinating care, managing nursing resources, and ensuring compliance with professional and regulatory standards.

▌ KEY TERMS

therapeutic milieu, 700

▌ CHAPTER REVIEW QUESTIONS

1. Match each example in Column A with the correct component of the therapeutic milieu in Column B.

Column A

_____ Allows for predictable organization of time, place, and person

_____ Affirming the patient's worldview

_____ Offering education and encouragement

_____ Promoting the patient's attention and interaction with the social environment

Column B

A. Containment
B. Involvement
C. Structure
D. Support
E. Validation

_____ Provision of food, shelter, medical care, and safety from harm

_____ Unconditional acceptance, nurturance, and promotion of self-esteem

_____ Use of contracts, token economies, and required meetings

_____ Use of individualized treatment plans and showing respect for patients' rights

_____ Use of open doors, open rounds, and patient-led groups

_____ Use of time-outs and room programs

2. Fill in the blanks.

A. Today the majority of patients admitted to psychiatric hospitals are in the _____ stage, with the treatment goal of _____.

B. A syndrome characterized by dependency on the hospital and resistance to discharge is known as _____.

C. The partial hospital psychiatric team is _____ in nature.

D. Maxwell Jones first described the inpatient environment as a _____ with cultural norms for behaviors, values, and activity.

E. One of the earliest advocates of the importance of the environment for nursing care was _____.

F. _____ is the leading accreditation agency for hospital-based facilities.

3. Provide short answers for the following questions.

A. What are the two major functions of partial hospitalization programs?

B. Discuss characteristics of crisis bed programs.

C. Analyze the need for state psychiatric hospitals in the current mental health care delivery system.

D. Describe how patient teaching would need to be modified in an inpatient setting in which patients were in the most acute stages of their illnesses.

E. In many hospital-based facilities, psychiatric nurses rotate between inpatient and partial hospital programs. Discuss how this can benefit both patients and the nursing staff.

Visit Evolve for additional resources related to the content of this chapter.

 evolve

http://evolve.elsevier.com/Stuart/principles/
• Topical Course Outline • Student Workbook Exercises • Critical Thinking Questions and Activities • Case Studies • Research Topics • Monthly Content Updates • WebLinks

---

Student Study CD-ROM

Access the accompanying CD-ROM for animations, interactive exercises, review questions for the NCLEX examination, and an audio glossary.

REFERENCES

Abroms GM: Defining milieu therapy, *Arch Gen Psychiatry* 21:553, 1969.

Ash D, Galletly C: Crisis beds: the interface between the hospital and the community, *Int J Soc Psychiatry* 43:193, 1997.

Benson WD, Briscoe L: Jumping the hurdles of mental health care wearing cement shoes: where does the inpatient psychiatric nurse fit in? *J Am Psychiatr Nurs Assoc* 9:123, 2003.

Boyer CA et al: Identifying risk factors and key strategies in linkage to outpatient psychiatric care, *Am J Psychiatry* 157:1592, 2000.

Coleman JC, Paul GL: Relationship between staffing ratios and effectiveness of inpatient psychiatric units, *Psychiatr Serv* 52:1374, 2001.

Delaney K: Inpatient psychiatric nursing: set up to stagnate? *J Am Psychiatr Nurs Assoc* 8:130, 2002.

Delaney KR, Pitula CR, Perraud S: Psychiatric hospitalization and process description: what will nursing add? *J Psychosoc Nurs Ment Health Serv* 38:7, 2000.

DesRoches C et al: Caregiving in the post-hospitalization period: findings from a national survey, *Nurs Econ* 20:216, 2002.

Echternacht M: Fluid group: concept and clinical application to the therapeutic milieu, *J Am Psychiatr Nurs Assoc* 7:39, 2001.

Fenton WS et al: Cost and cost-effectiveness of hospital vs residential crisis care for patients who have serious mental illness, *Arch Gen Psychiatry* 59:357, 2002.

Fisher WH et al: Long-stay patients in state psychiatric hospitals at the end of the 20th century, *Psychiatr Ser* 52:1051, 2001.

Flannelly LT, Flannelly KJ, Cox BA: Evaluating improvements in nursing staff at a state psychiatric hospital, *Issues Ment Health Nurs* 22:621, 2001.

Geller JL: The last half-century of psychiatric services as reflected in *Psychiatric Services, Psychiatr Serv* 51:41, 2000.

Glick I, Carter WG, Tandon R: A paradigm for treatment of inpatient psychiatric disorders: from asylum to intensive care, *J Psychiatr Pract* 9:395, 2003.

Goldberg RJ: Financial management challenges for general hospital psychiatry 2001, *Gen Hosp Psychiatry* 23:67, 2001.

Gunderson JG: Defining the therapeutic processes in psychiatric milieus, *Psychiatry* 41:327, 1978.

Halter MJ: Stigma in psychiatric nursing, *Perspect Psychiatr Care* 38:23, 2002.

Horvitz-Lennon M et al: Partial versus full hospitalization for adults in psychiatric distress: a systematic review of the published literature (1957-1997), *Am J Psychiatry* 158:676, 2001.

Jones M: *The therapeutic community*, New York, 1953, Basic Books.

McIntyre JS: A new subspeciality, *Am J Psychiatry* 159:1961, 2002.

Mechanic D: Removing barriers to care among persons with psychiatric symptoms, *Health Aff* 21:137, 2002.

NASMHPD: *State profile highlight: closing and reorganizing state psychiatric hospitals: 2000* (Contract No. 280-96-0003), Alexandria, Va, 2000, NASMHPD Research Institute, Inc.

Nightingale F: *Notes on nursing: what it is and what it is not*, New York, 1960, Dover.

Priest CS, Holmberg SK: A new model for the mental health nursing change of shift report, *J Psychosoc Nurs Ment Health Serv* 38:37, 2000.

Ross C: Role of state psychiatric hospitals as next century approaches, *NAMI Advocate* 11(Dec 1999/Jan 2000):2, 1999/2000.

Roy-Byrne P: Untreated medical comorbidity is high in patients with serious mental illness, *Journal Watch* 1:4, 2002.

Scheifler P, Lefkovitz P: *Standards and guidelines for partial hospitalization adult programs*, Fairfax, Va, 2003, AABH Publications.

Sharfstein S: The American Psychiatric Publishing Textbook of Consultation-Liaison Psychiatry: Psychiatry in the Medically Ill, ed 2, *Am J Psychiatry* 159:1796, 2002.

Thomas MD et al: Meanings of state hospital nursing. I: Facing challenges, *Arch Psychiatr Nurs* 13:48, 1999a.

Thomas MD et al: Meanings of state hospital nursing. II: Coping and making meaning, *Arch Psychiatr Nurs* 13:55, 1999b.

Thomas SP, Shattell M, Martin T: What's therapeutic about the therapeutic milieu? *Arch Psychiatr Nurs* 16:99, 2002.

Tucker S et al: Exploring the relationship between brief inpatient treatment intensity and treatment outcomes for mood and anxiety disorders, *J Am Psychiatr Nurs Assoc* 7:86, 2001.

Wirt GL: Causes of institutionalism: patient and staff perspectives, *Issues Ment Health Nurs* 20:259, 1999.

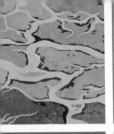

What life have you if you have not life together? There is no life that is not in community.

T. S. ELIOT, CHORUSES FROM "THE ROCK"

35 COMMUNITY-BASED PSYCHIATRIC NURSING CARE

Gail W. Stuart

LEARNING OBJECTIVES

After studying this chapter, the student should be able to:

1. Relate historical perspectives on community-based psychiatric care (I).
2. Describe a systems model of community-based psychiatric care that includes case management (II).
3. Assess the needs of vulnerable psychiatric populations living in the community (III).
4. Analyze evidence-based community interventions for patients and families experiencing psychiatric illness (IV).
5. Discuss the role of the nurse in psychiatric home care (V).
6. Discuss the role of the nurse in forensic psychiatric care (VI).

TOPICAL OUTLINE

 Visit Evolve for additional resources related to the content of this chapter.
http://evolve.elsevier.com/Stuart/principles/

The goal of the mental health delivery system is to allow the individual to achieve the promise of community living and to assure that consumers and families have access to timely and accurate information that promotes learning, self-monitoring, and accountability. The report from the New Freedom Commission on Mental Health, *Achieving the Promise: Transforming Mental Health Care in America*, (NFCMH, 2003) stated that successfully transforming the mental health service delivery system rests on two principles:

1. **Services and treatments must be consumer and family centered.**
2. **Care must focus on increasing consumers' ability to successfully cope with life's challenges, on facilitating recovery, and on building resilience.**

The report goes on to say that evidence shows that offering a full range of community-based alternatives is more effective than hospitalization and emergency room treatment. Thus giving consumers access to a range of effective, community-based treatment options is critical to achieving their full community participation. To ensure this access, the report recommends that the array of community-based treat-ment options be expanded. This is the challenge currently facing contemporary psychiatric care.

What factors do you think influence whether psychiatric nurses work in hospital-based or community-based psychiatric programs? ■

HISTORICAL PERSPECTIVES

The Community Mental Health Centers Act of 1963 marked the beginning of a major federal effort to provide comprehensive community-based mental health services to all people in need regardless of income. Each community mental health center was mandated by law to provide five essential mental health services.

Four of these services—**inpatient, emergency, partial hospitalization,** and **outpatient**—were to provide psychiatric care in the community to reduce the number of admissions to state hospitals (secondary and tertiary prevention). The goal of the fifth service, **consultation and education,** was to provide information about mental health principles to other community agencies, reduce the number of people at risk for mental illness, and increase community awareness of mental health practices through education (primary prevention). The large scope of this mission, care of those with diagnosed mental illness and prevention of mental illness, led to controversy in defining the purpose and function of community mental health that continues to the present day (Coddington, 2001).

By the mid 1970s many centers faced the end of federal funding, and state governments were unable or unwilling to take on the burden of funding them. The centers then had to rely heavily on third-party reimbursement through fee-for-service mechanisms, which were typically physician directed and illness oriented. These factors led to major amendments of the Community Mental Health Centers Act in 1975, requiring centers to offer services for people with serious mental illness who had been discharged from the state hospitals. These services included screening admissions to inpatient services, aftercare services, and transitional housing.

Because centers were not allowed to reduce the five original essential services and were not given sufficient funds to add these new services, decisions about priorities had to be made. Political and social pressures were mounting; the community was demanding that care be provided to those who were being discharged from the hospital into the community in large numbers. As a result, most community mental health centers reluctantly decreased their preventive efforts and focused more resources on the care of people with diagnosed mental illness.

Deinstitutionalization

At the patient level, deinstitutionalization refers to the transfer of a patient hospitalized for extended periods of time to a community setting. At the mental health care system level, it refers to a shift in the focus of care from long-term institution to the community, accompanied by discharging long-term patients and avoiding unnecessary admissions.

Between 1965 and 1995 nearly 700,000 patients were either discharged or diverted from state hospitals to care in the community. It was hoped that psychiatric treatment in community centers, combined with living arrangements provided by family or board and care homes, would allow these people to live more humane lives in their own communities.

However, it rapidly became clear that policymakers had seriously miscalculated both the service needs of this population and the ability of communities to accommodate the large numbers of people with mental illness who had been discharged from the state. Often, these former patients had to be readmitted to state hospitals. Others who could not meet the increasingly strict admission criteria of hospitalization drifted into the criminal justice system or into homelessness. Many who were elderly were admitted to nursing homes.

In reviewing the failures of this early attempt to move patients into community care, mental health experts agree that the following problems contributed to the lack of success:

- Poor coordination between state hospitals and community mental health centers
- Underestimation of the support systems needed to enable people with mental illness to live in the community

- Lack of knowledge about psychiatric rehabilitation
- Shortage of professionals trained to work with this population in the community
- Reimbursement systems that rewarded hospitalization
- Underestimation of community resistance to deinstitutionalization

How would you and your family feel about a group home for people with mental illness being built in your neighborhood? ■

Among the lessons learned from deinstitutionalization are that (Lamb and Bachrach, 2001):

1. Successful deinstitutionalization involves more than simply changing the locus of care.
2. Service planning must be tailored to the needs of each individual.
3. Hospital care must be available for those who need it.
4. Services must be culturally relevant.
5. Severely mentally ill persons must be involved in their service planning.
6. Service systems must not be restricted by preconceived ideology.
7. Continuity of care must be achieved.

In the 1999 *Olmstead v. L. C.* decision, the U.S. Supreme Court held that the unnecessary institutionalization of people with disabilities is discrimination under the Americans with Disabilities Act (see Chapter 10). The Court found that "confinement in an institution severely diminishes the everyday life activities of individuals, including family relations, social contacts, work options, economic independence, educational achievement, and cultural enrichment" (Olmstead, 1999). Nonetheless, today many adults and children remain in institutions instead of being in more appropriate community-based settings.

Do you think that people recovering from psychiatric illness are better off living independently, with their families, in group homes, or in psychiatric hospitals? ■

■ A SYSTEMS MODEL OF CARE

A systems model of community mental health operates on the philosophy that all aspects of a person's life need to be cared for—basic human needs, physical health needs, and needs for psychiatric treatment and rehabilitation—if a person is to live successfully in the community. The focus is on developing a comprehensive system of care and coordinating needed services into an integrated package for persons with severe and disabling mental illnesses.

A special federal initiative was launched to help states and communities develop comprehensive services for the psychiatric population. This initiative was led by the National Institute of Mental Health (NIMH), which began to fund demonstration programs for community support systems in all states. Community mental health centers were given primary responsibility for the development and implementation of community support systems for people in their service areas.

Case Management

In implementing these systems, case management became the primary means for ensuring that the components were available to every person with a chronic mental illness who needed them. Components of a community support system include **client identification and outreach, mental health treatment, crisis response services, health and dental care, housing, income support and entitlement, peer support, family and community support, rehabilitation services,** and **protection and advocacy** (Figure 35-1).

Case management involves linking the service system to the consumer and coordinating the service components so that he or she can achieve successful community living. It focuses on problem solving to provide continuity of services and overcome problems of rigid systems, fragmented services, poor use of resources, and problems of inaccessibility. The six activities of case management are as follows:

1. **Identification and outreach**
2. **Assessment**
3. **Service planning**
4. **Linkage with needed services**
5. **Monitoring service delivery**
6. **Advocacy**

In addition, core aspects and specific interventions related to clinical case management are listed in Table 35-1.

Which interventions of clinical case management listed in Table 35-1 do you think should be provided by a mental health professional and which ones, if any, can be carried out by a lay person? ■

At present, case management is an ambiguous concept without a clear base in any one professional discipline. Early definitions stressed the linking, brokering, and advocacy functions of the role. These roles evolved into a more clinically oriented definition. Furthermore, there are various models or types of case management, including full service, broker, therapist, intensive, social support, collaborative, community advocate, and problem-focused—each with its

own structure, purpose, and team composition (Schaedle and Epstein, 2000). Questions about the effectiveness of the different types of case management (Samele et al, 2002) and the recommended caseload of case managers remain unresolved (King, Le Bas, and Spooner, 2000).

The work of the case manager is very complex, covering a broad array of activities. With the advent of managed care, case management has come to reflect two basic but seemingly contradictory goals: increasing access to services and limiting costs. In the public sector, case management is intended to increase access to care and make more services available to those eligible and underserved. In the private sector, case management has become synonymous with utilization review, where the emphasis is placed on cost control and limitation of resource use.

Clearly, functions resembling case management will be an increasingly prominent part of mental health care in the fu-

Table 35-1	Aspects and Interventions of Clinical Case Management
ASPECT	**INTERVENTION**
Initial phase	Engagement
	Assessment
	Planning
Environmental interventions	Linkages with community resources
	Consultation with families and caregivers
	Maintenance and expansion of social networks
	Collaboration with physicians and hospitals
	Advocacy
Patient interventions	Individual psychotherapy
	Training in independent living skills
	Psychoeducation
Patient-environment intervention	Crisis intervention
	Monitoring

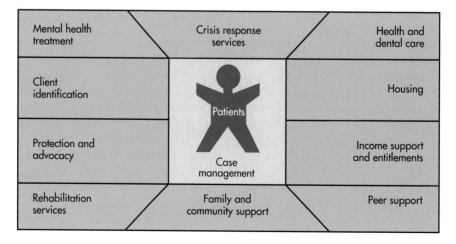

Figure 35-1 Components of a community support system. (Department of Health and Human Services: *Toward a model plan for a comprehensive community-based mental health system,* October 1987.)

ture as attempts are made to balance cost, access, and effectiveness. Resources of patients, families, providers, and society must be managed in order to carry out these complex goals. However, important questions such as the following remain: What are the tasks of case managers? Who should be doing case management (what personal qualities, education, and training are needed)? To whom is the case manager accountable? How should the work of case management be organized and evaluated (Bedell, Cohen, and Sullivan, 2000)? These are no small questions for the mental health delivery system to answer.

CLINICAL EXAMPLE

Jane M is single, 33 years old, and has a history of multiple psychiatric admissions. She was referred to the community mental health center case management unit on discharge from a 6-month stay at the state hospital. She had a diagnosis of undifferentiated schizophrenia in remission and was discharged to the care of her family on risperidone 4 mg daily. Jane has occasional auditory hallucinations, is somewhat suspicious, and has a long history of disruptive family relationships and noncompliance with medications.

The psychiatric nurse case manager volunteered to take the case and made an appointment with the family for a home visit. When she arrived, the family was visibly upset and related that in the week since Jane had been home, she slept much of the day and roamed around the house during the night, taking long showers, slamming kitchen cabinet doors, and playing loud rock music. When she was awake during the day, she would disappear for hours at a time, causing great anxiety for the family. The mother was tearful and wringing her hands in an agitated manner while the father sat on the sofa with his head bowed. Jane sprawled in a chair and intermittently swore at her mother as the mother described these events.

The nurse recognized that Jane's illness dominated the household, essentially putting her in control of the rest of the family. The nurse worked intensely with this family to restore generational boundaries by supporting the parents in making mutually agreed upon rules about behavior that would be tolerated in their household. She helped the family identify ways to support Jane while setting limits that would promote adaptive family functioning. The family found this exchange to be very helpful, and they called on the nurse to validate their ideas and provide them with ongoing information on Jane's illness. The nurse also evaluated the impact of the medication on Jane's behavior and her compliance with taking it.

Over the next few weeks, Jane began to sleep at night. With continued support from the nurse, the parents became skilled and comfortable at presenting a united front. Although Jane initially resisted, she adapted rather quickly to the new norms in the house, and a family crisis that might have resulted in Jane's readmission to the hospital was averted. ∎

VULNERABLE POPULATIONS IN THE COMMUNITY

Homeless People With Mental Illness

Homeless people are an inescapable presence in American society, where they live in subway tunnels and on steam grates and die in cardboard boxes on windswept corners in communities throughout the country. To most Americans, homelessness seems neither invisible nor insurmountable (Box 35-1).

People who are mentally ill and homeless reflect the tension between a mental health system that views housing as a social welfare problem and public housing agencies that believe that this population needs specialized residential programs provided by mental health agencies. Thus the needs of this population are underserved because services are fragmented and inaccessible (Box 35-2).

It has been estimated that one-third of the estimated 600,000 homeless people in the United States have a severe mental illness. However, only one in 20 persons with a severe mental illness is homeless. Among homeless persons with a mental illness, as few as 5% to 7% need to be institutionalized. Most can live in the community with appropriate, supportive housing.

Research has shown that when homeless people with mental illness are given the opportunity to participate in treatment programs that address their needs for services in areas such as housing, health care, substance abuse, and income support, many can be helped to find homes and achieve substantial improvements in their lives (Gelberg, Anderson, and Leake, 2000; Lam and Rosenheck, 2000). Thus mental health professionals have begun to explore the use of new approaches to providing treatment, rehabilitation services, and housing to homeless people with men-

---

BOX 35-1

What Americans Say About the Homeless

A national survey conducted for *Parade* magazine found the following:

- 70% saw homeless people in their own communities.
- 76% said something should be done to reduce homelessness in America.
- 36% can imagine a situation in which they might become homeless.
- 84% thought that at least half of the homeless could be helped enough to reenter society.
- 82% said the homeless should not be prohibited from public places.
- 77% thought homeless people are not adequately helped by the government.
- 69% did not want a legal procedure that would forcibly remove homeless people from the street.
- 7% thought homeless people were violent, but 60% said the homeless contribute to the rising crime rate.
- 56% thought homeless people were not responsible for the situation they were in.
- 30% said a homeless person who is nonviolent but has a diagnosed mental illness should be institutionalized against his or her will.
- 16% said they would go out of their way to avoid homeless people.

BOX 35-2

Reflecting on Homelessness

by Tyrone Garrett, Chair, Staten Island Consumer Committee

As I once again gazed upon the formidable, almost timeless building located on the perimeter of the hospital complex, I found myself filled with contradictory emotions of elation and dread. On the one hand, I was elated because I no longer was an occasional occupant of this homeless shelter. On the other hand, I felt dread because the memories of living there were so devastating. But I was glad that I'd returned to this place, the 30th Street Bellevue Men's shelter, for the October 2, 2002 march and rally for New York/New York III Housing.

I, along with numerous other consumers of mental health services, and various mental health provider agencies, joined together at this site to peacefully and publicly demand that our elected officials recognize not only our plea but also the plight of so many of our peers by providing 9000 new units of housing for the homeless mentally ill.

Looking back upon the twisted journey of my life, I am aware of how my history of homelessness was probably one of the main reasons that I'd languished so long outside mainstream society. I remember being shuttled from facility to facility with little access to effective services. The daily uncertainty of matters such as where I was going to eat and sleep contributed to my deteriorating psychiatric condition. Unable to form healthy relationships or achieve healthy pursuits, many of us homeless at times feel a little less than human.

We gathered outside the Bellevue shelter and as we marched through Manhattan, I considered the people passing in their mobile cocoons of comfort and luxury, who gazed at us with expressions of curiosity, wonder, and sometimes sympathy. I wondered if these citizens could even imagine what it was like to have nowhere to call your own.

The only place I had to store my belongings was a flimsy 3' × 5' locker. I was told when and where to sleep, and I usually stood in a long, sometimes fragrant line for an insufficient meal of questionable quality.

Most of the real world has no knowledge of the subculture of homeless people. The violence and degradation of the overpopulated circles of hell were the labyrinthine shelters of the 80s. They are no longer as visible, but these conditions and experiences do continue, although on a smaller and less obvious scale.

Recovery from mental illness is a difficult undertaking, especially since it requires people to act contrary to what may seem natural when they are sick. Being suspicious of people who are trying to help may seem natural to a sick person, but it is an obstacle to recovery, which requires honesty and trusting relationships.

If we, as a society, have the knowledge and means to remove homelessness as an obstacle to recovery, then we have a moral obligation to do so. If we stood tall in the face of 9/11, why can't we provide homes for our unfortunates during normally distressing times?

*(**New York City Voices** Editor's note: Tyrone Garrett has stayed at over seven homeless shelters throughout New York City. He is the current program supervisor and senior peer advocate of Baltic Street Mental Health Board's Staten Island Peer Advocacy Center, an advocacy and empowerment program.)*

From *New York City Voices*, vol VII, No. 4, September-October 2002.

---

tal illness—a population who often avoid contact with traditional mental health programs because of past difficulty in gaining access to care, demands from clinicians for treatment compliance, or past involuntary hospitalization (Rosenheck, 2000; Jones et al, 2003).

Key components of this focused treatment approach include the following:

- Frequent and consistent staff contact through assertive outreach
- Meeting the client where he or she is, both geographically and interpersonally
- Help with immediate survival needs such as food, emergency shelter, and clothing
- Gradual treatment through the development of trust
- An emphasis on client strengths
- Client choice of services and the right to refuse treatment
- The delivery of comprehensive services including mental health and substance abuse treatment, medical care, housing, social and vocational services, and help in obtaining entitlements

CLINICAL EXAMPLE

Neighbors reported that an unkempt, dirty, and bedraggled woman had taken to sleeping in a local park. She appeared to be physically unwell, with a cough and severe sunburn, and was scavenging food from garbage cans. She appeared frightened when approached and was refusing help. Several complaints had been made about her by a nearby school.

A variety of health services were contacted, and it appeared that she had been diagnosed 5 years previously with paranoid schizophrenia, had come from another state, and had taken to traveling around the area. She had a history of trauma and abuse, was noncompliant with treatment, and consistently eloped from hospitals if admitted.

A psychiatric nurse from the local community mental health center did a brief psychosocial assessment of the woman in the park. She was interviewed from about 10 feet away, which was as close as she would allow. Food, soap and towels, a small amount of money, and a warm blanket were left with her. She appeared frightened, thought disordered, and underweight. She did agree to the nurse visiting her on a regular basis to provide food. She was seen most days for 2 weeks during which she became more comfortable with the nurse. One day she allowed the nurse to briefly examine her in the park toilets. Soon thereafter she agreed to a 1-week hospital admission on a voluntary basis. ■

ACCESS Program. One particularly innovative program was the Access to Community Care and Effective Services and Supports (ACCESS) program. It was initiated in 1993 by the U.S. Department of Health and Human Services as part of a national agenda to end homelessness among people with serious mental illness. Demonstration projects developed integrated systems of care for this population. The purpose of the ACCESS program was to determine whether integration initiatives implemented at the program, policy, and organizational levels improve outcomes for the homeless people with mental illness beyond those obtained by integration at the direct service delivery level—that is, by case management (Randolph et al, 2002).

Data from studies show the project was successful in terms of service integration but not overall system integration. Furthermore there was little direct effect on clients (Goldman et al, 2002; Morrissey et al, 2002; Rosenheck et al, 2002). These findings are disappointing and underscore the need for resources for outreach and intensive clinical care as well as housing and rental subsidies to impact homelessness. They clearly reflect the complexity of problems facing the homeless mentally ill and the need for a transformed system of mental health care to bring about desired change.

Should people be allowed to choose to be homeless if they are not dangerous to themselves or others? ■

Rural Mentally Ill

Rural America makes up 90% of our Nation's landmass and is home to 25% of the population. Although the incidence and prevalence of mental illness among adults and serious emotional disturbances in children are similar in rural and urban areas, the issues related to the rural mentally ill are different in important ways.

Particularly in the more remote "frontier" areas that exist in 25 states and represent 45% of the land mass of the United States, barriers to mental health care are significant. They include insufficient access to crisis services, mental health and general medical clinics, hospitals, and innovative treatments (Rost et al, 2002). Rural residents also may face greater social stigma in regard to seeking mental health care, and basic community services such as transportation, electricity, water, and telephones that are important to providing health care may not be available.

Rural residents are at significant risk for substance use disorders and mental illness. Symptoms related to mood and anxiety disorders, trauma, and cognitive, developmental, and psychotic disorders appear to be as common among rural residents as among city dwellers, and rural suicide rates have surpassed urban suicide rates over the past 20 years. For these reasons, mental health issues are among the most prominent health concerns being faced in rural areas, and as a result, residents with mental health needs:

- Enter care later in the course of their disease than their urban peers.
- Enter care with more serious, persistent, and disabling symptoms.

- Require more expensive and intensive treatment response.

Two additional issues are problematic. The first is the lack of mental health professionals, including culturally competent or bilingual providers in these medically underserved areas (NACRH, 2002). The second is the fact that rural Americans have lower family incomes and are less likely to have health insurance benefits for mental health care. Thus rural residents have longer periods without insurance and are less likely to seek mental health care for which they cannot pay.

Finally, many ethical dilemmas arise when practicing in the community (see Critical Thinking About Contemporary Issues), and some of these are unique to the rural setting. When numbers of providers in isolated settings are limited, problems may arise because of overlapping social and professional relationships, altered therapeutic boundaries, challenges in protecting patient confidentiality, and differing cultural dimensions of mental health care. Ways to combat these dilemmas include the development of clinical support networks through electronic communications, attention to clinical ethics, and regular peer supervision or consultation.

What role do you think alternative and complementary therapies play in rural health care settings? ■

Critical Thinking *About* Contemporary Issues

What Ethical Issues Challenge Community Psychiatric Care?

Community psychiatric care is unique in three ways. First, the patients are some of the sickest, poorest, and overall least well-off members of the community. Second, community mental health care delivery systems tend to be structured in ways that emphasize a multisystem, multidisciplinary approach to patient care. Third, the community mental health care settings typically are underfunded and suffer from insufficient resources. One might question, therefore, whether these factors create unique ethical dilemmas as well.

Four general categories of ethical conflicts in community psychiatric care have been identified. The first relates to the patient's ability to give valid informed consent or refusal of treatment, particularly when circumstances are complex and many parties may be involved. The second is related to paternalism in which there is a conflict between meeting a patient's *needs* versus respecting a patient's *rights* to self-determination. Issues here include forced medication, coerced outpatient treatment, and involuntary commitment (see Chapter 10). The third issue is that of resource allocation, as providers frequently find themselves in positions of deciding *who* receives *what* resources *when* and *how frequently*. Given the scarce resources, these are often difficult decisions to make. The final problem arises around organizational relationships because the more systems that are involved in care, the greater the likelihood of differing treatment philosophies and priorities.

Unfortunately, the unique ethical conflicts in community psychiatric care have received little attention. Thus clinicians have little guidance in this area. More dialogue and study is needed to inform the field and assure quality, ethical community psychiatric care.

Mentally Ill People in Jail

In the United States about 80,000 patients are in psychiatric hospitals. In contrast, almost 1 in 5 inmates in the nation's state prisons and local jails and 1 in 14 federal inmates—or nearly 370,000 persons altogether—have reported a mental illness or spent at least one night in a psychiatric hospital at some time (Table 35-2). This is four and a half times the number of people in psychiatric hospitals throughout the country. Stated another way, **the rate of serious mental illness in the incarcerated population is about 3 to 4 times that of the general U.S. population.**

One in six persons in the community on probation gave similar histories. One in five reported being homeless in the year before being arrested, compared with 1 in 11 of the other inmates. Mentally ill inmates of both sexes reported higher rates of prior physical and sexual abuse than other inmates, were more likely to have a history of substance abuse, and had higher unemployment prior to incarceration.

In facilities housing state prison inmates, 70% report screening inmates at admission; 65% conduct psychiatric assessments; 51% provide 24-hour mental health care; and 73% distribute psychotropic medications (Beck and Maruschak, 2001). Six in 10 mentally ill persons in state and federal prisons and 4 in 10 persons in jails received some form of mental health care, most commonly prescription medication. Of all mentally ill populations, white female inmates were the most likely to receive care. They also related the highest rates of mental illness. Nearly 40% of white female inmates aged 24 and under reported being mentally ill.

Clearly, the presence of severely mentally ill persons in jails and prisons is an urgent problem (Diamond et al, 2001). These individuals are often poor, uninsured, dispro-portionately members of minority groups, and living with co-occurring substance abuse and mental disorders.

Some programs are attempting to deal with this problem in various parts of the United States. A community model for services (Figure 35-2) has been proposed that includes methods for preventing incarceration of people with mental illness and intervening effectively when such a person is jailed. This model is based on the formation of a community board and includes both preventive and post-release interventions.

So too, mental health courts are being created across the country to divert those individuals away from jails and into the mental health system to receive appropriate care (see Chapter 10). Additional approaches will be needed, however, to fully address this growing problem and meet the needs of this vulnerable population.

Have jails become today's substitute for yesterday's state hospitals for people with mental illness? If so, what should be done to address this problem? ∎

∎ EVIDENCE-BASED INTERVENTIONS
Assertive Community Treatment

Assertive Community Treatment (ACT) was developed in Wisconsin in the early 1970s as a program originally called Training in Community Living (TCL). It was created as a way of organizing outpatient mental health services for patients who were leaving large state mental hospitals and were at risk for rehospitalization.

Table 35-2	State Inmates and Jail Inmates Identified as Mentally Ill: By Sex, Race/Origin, and Age	
OFFENDER CHARACTERISTIC	PERCENT OF STATE INMATES IDENTIFIED AS MENTALLY ILL	PERCENT OF JAIL INMATES IDENTIFIED AS MENTALLY ILL
Gender		
Female	23.6	22.7
Male	15.8	15.6
Race/Origin		
White*	22.6	21.7
Black*	13.5	13.7
Hispanic	11.0	11.1
Age		
24 or younger	14.4	13.3
25-34	14.8	15.7
35-44	18.4	19.3
45-54	19.7	22.7
55 or older	15.6	20.4

From Ditton, Paula M: *Mental health and treatment of inmates and probationers,* Bureau of Justice Statistics Special Report, July 1999, NCJ 174463.
*Excludes Hispanics.

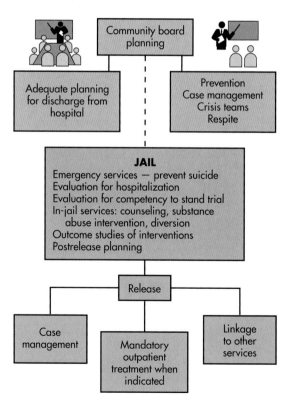

Figure 35-2   Community model for services. (From Laben J, Blum J: Persons with mental illness in jail. In Worley N, editor: *Mental health nursing in the community,* St Louis, 1997, Mosby.)

The original TCL model has been replicated in thousands of communities under names such as Continuous Treatment Teams (CTTs), Programs for Assertive Community Treatment (PACT), and Intensive Case Management (ICM). This model program provides a full range of medical, psychosocial, and rehabilitative services. The 10 principles of ACT are listed in Box 35-3.

ACT uses an interdisciplinary team-oriented approach that typically includes up to 10 staff members (nurses, psychiatrists, social workers, activity therapists) who meet regularly to plan individualized care for a shared caseload of about 120 patients. More than 75% of staff time is spent in the field providing direct treatment and rehabilitation. The services provided by ACT treatment team members are listed in Box 35-4.

Psychiatric nurses are typically an integral member of the ACT treatment team (see Citing the Evidence). These teams function as continuous care teams who work with patients with serious mental illness and their families over time to improve their quality of life. In effect, these programs function as a community-based "hospital without walls," providing a high-intensity program of clinical support and treatment.

BOX 35-3

Ten Principles of Assertive Community Treatment

1. Services are targeted to a specified group of individuals with severe mental illness.
2. Rather than brokering services, treatment, support, and rehabilitation services are provided directly by the assertive community treatment team.
3. Team members share responsibility for the individuals served by the team.
4. The staff-to-consumer ratio is small (approximately 1 to 10).
5. The range of treatment and services is comprehensive and flexible.
6. Interventions are carried out at the locations where problems occur and support is needed rather than in hospital or clinic settings.
7. There is no arbitrary time limit on receiving services.
8. Treatment and support services are individualized.
9. Services are available on a 24-hour basis.
10. The team is assertive in engaging individuals in treatment and monitoring their progress.

From Phillips S et al: *Psychiatr Serv* 52:771, 2001.

BOX 35-4

Services Provided by Assertive Community Treatment Team Members

Rehabilitative Approach to Daily Living Skills
Grocery shopping and cooking
Purchase and care of clothing
Use of transportation
Help with social and family relationships

Family Involvement
Crisis management
Counseling and psychoeducation with family and extended family
Coordination with family service agencies

Work Opportunities
Help to find volunteer and vocational opportunities
Provide liaison with and educate employers
Serve as job coach for consumers

Entitlements
Assist with documentation
Accompany consumers to entitlement offices
Manage food stamps
Assist with redetermination of benefits

Health Promotion
Provide preventive health education
Conduct medical screening
Schedule maintenance visits
Provide liaison for acute medical care
Provide reproductive counseling and sex education

Medication Support
Order medications from pharmacy
Deliver medications to consumers
Provide education about medication
Monitor medication compliance and side effects

Housing Assistance
Find suitable shelter
Secure leases and pay rent
Purchase and repair household items
Develop relationships with landlords
Improve housekeeping skills

Financial Management
Plan budget
Troubleshoot financial problems (for example, disability payments)
Assist with bills
Increase independence in money management

Counseling
Use problem-oriented approach
Integrate counseling into continuous work
Ensure that goals are addressed by all team members
Promote communication skills development
Provide counseling as part of comprehensive rehabilitative approach

From Phillips S et al: *Psychiatr Serv* 52:771, 2001.

CITING THE EVIDENCE ON

Nurses and ACT Teams

BACKGROUND: The investigators sought to identify case managers' perspectives on the critical ingredients, therapeutic mechanisms of action, and gaps in implementation of the critical ingredients of Assertive Community Treatment (ACT). The degree to which 16 clinical activities were beneficial to clients was rated by 73 ACT teams; the teams also rated the importance of 27 possible critical ingredients of the ideal team.

RESULTS: Having a full-time nurse on the team was rated as the most beneficial clinical activity. Critical elements that the teams reported as being the most underimplemented included the presence of a full-time substance abuse specialist, a psychiatrist's involvement on the team, team involvement with hospital discharge, and working with client support systems.

IMPLICATIONS: Case managers strongly endorsed the team approach and also endorse having a nurse as an essential member of the team. Despite broad consensus on critical ingredients of the ideal ACT team, several of them appear to be implemented inconsistently.

McGrew J, Pescocolido B, Wright E: *Psychiatr Serv* 54:370, 2003.

BOX 35-5

Nine Basic Principles of Multisystem Therapy

1. The primary purpose of assessment is to understand the fit between the identified problems and their systemic context.
2. Therapeutic contact should emphasize the positive, and interventions should use systemic strengths as leverage for change.
3. Interventions should promote responsible behavior and decrease irresponsible behavior.
4. Interventions should be present focused and action oriented, targeting specific and well-defined problems.
5. Interventions should target sequences of behavior within and among systems.
6. Interventions should be developmentally appropriate and fit the developmental needs of the young person.
7. Interventions should be designed to require daily or weekly effort by family members.
8. Intervention efficacy should be continuously evaluated from different perspectives.
9. Interventions should promote treatment generalization and long-term maintenance of therapeutic change.

Modified from Henggeler SW et al: *Treatment manual for family preservation using multisystemic therapy*, Charleston, 1994, South Carolina Health and Human Services Finance Commission.

Numerous controlled clinical trials of ACT have been conducted with a wide range of people with severe mental illness, including patients with schizophrenia, veterans, dually diagnosed patients, and homeless people. These studies report that patients spent less time in hospitals and more in independent community housing. Their symptoms were reduced, their treatment compliance was increased, and ACT costs were usually lower (Marshall and Lockwood, 2002; Schaedle et al, 2002; Calsyn et al, 2002; Ziguras and Stuart, 2000; Rowe et al, 2002).

The Program of Assertive Community Treatment (PACT) is recognized by the National Alliance of the Mentally Ill (NAMI) as the most effective service delivery model for community treatment of severe mental illness. As such, NAMI has launched a national grassroots effort called PACT Across America to educate people about PACT and to offer training, monitoring, certification, and management services to those mental health agencies wishing to implement the PACT model.

Why might the role of the psychiatric nurse on an interdisciplinary mental health care team be more difficult to define in community settings? ■

Multisystemic Therapy

Multisystemic therapy (MST) is a highly flexible treatment approach that addresses the multiple, interrelated needs of youths with serious behavioral and emotional problems and their families. It is usually delivered through the family preservation model of service delivery to provide interventions in home, school, and neighborhood settings.

The primary goal of family preservation has been to prevent out-of-home placement by providing home-based, intensive, and time-limited services to families whose children are at immediate risk of such placement. The goal of MST is to develop parent skills and resources needed to address the difficulties of raising teenagers and to teach youths to cope with family, peer, school, and neighborhood problems. At the peer or school level, a goal of treatment is to decrease the youth's involvement with deviant peers and to increase involvement with prosocial peers.

MST uses pragmatic, goal-oriented treatment strategies, and interventions are guided by nine principles (Box 35-5). MST is usually delivered by master's-level clinicians with caseload ratios of one staff to four to six families. Service duration usually ranges from 3 to 5 months, with an average of 40 to 60 hours of direct clinical contact over the course of treatment. Staff are available 24 hours a day, 7 days a week during the active treatment phase.

Controlled clinical trials have provided strong support for MST as a viable approach to adolescents and their families who have traditionally been regarded as unresponsive to treatment. It also has been shown to improve communication in families of juvenile offenders and parent-child interaction in abusive or neglecting families. Other reported outcomes include improved family relations and peer relations and the prevention of expensive out-of-home placements (Henggeler et al, 2002, 2003; Schoenwald et al, 2000).

ACT and MST programs are evidence-based models of psychiatric care. Determine whether they are being used in your community and the impact they may be having on vulnerable populations where you live. ■

Table 35-3	Differences Between Traditional Mental Health Care Systems, Assertive Community Treatment, and Multisystemic Therapy		
SERVICE ELEMENT	TRADITIONAL SYSTEM	ASSERTIVE COMMUNITY TREATMENT	MULTISYSTEMIC THERAPY
Primary locus of care	Hospital, residential programs, day programs, offices	In the field (community, home, neighborhood, workplace)	In the field (community, home, neighborhood, school)
Provider of care	Individual clinician for individual outpatients, multidisciplinary teams for inpatients; treatment time highly variable; outpatient caseloads high, inpatient caseloads low; fragmented continuity of care across loci of care	Generalist teams share fixed case load; ratio of staff to patients = 1:10-15; treatment time unlimited; direct services continuously available	Generalist teams share temporary case load; treatment time averages 4 months; ratio of staff to patients = 1:6; continuous services and emergency response available around the clock for treatment period
Treatment approach	Specific individual or group psychosocial therapies and biological treatments provided mostly in a health care facility; providers not held directly accountable for outcomes	Medication monitoring and social support (help with housing, health, basic needs) in natural community environment; providers held accountable for outcomes	Pragmatic approach addresses problems identified in the child, family, peer, school, and neighborhood; family taught to sustain benefits, providers held directly accountable for outcomes

From Santos A et al: *Am J Psychiatry* 152:1111, 1995.

Therapeutic Elements

ACT, used for adults with severe mental illness, and MST, used for adolescents with serious emotional disorders, share common elements that differ from traditional systems and that have important implications for mental health policy (Table 35-3). They both use a **social-ecological model** of behavior applied to mental health patients. In addition, therapeutic principles emphasizing **pragmatic, outcome-oriented treatment approaches, home-based interventions,** and **individualized treatment goals** are key elements of their success. Most importantly, both systems embody a therapeutic philosophy demanding **therapist accountability,** in which staff are rewarded for clinical outcomes and therapeutic innovation rather than for following a prescribed plan.

Being evidence-based approaches tested in multiple clinical trials using sound experimental designs, both ACT and MST provide a strong scientific foundation for continued mental health care innovation. They also illustrate the critical elements needed in designing new community treatments for behavioral as well as medical conditions.

Describe an innovative psychiatric nursing service that you could provide to people with mental illness in your community. ■

■ HOME PSYCHIATRIC NURSING CARE

Psychiatric home care is available to a broad segment of the population. Factors contributing to the development of this treatment setting include the following:

- Continued trend of deinstitutionalization
- Growth of managed care, which focuses on cost, outcomes, and earlier hospital discharges
- Advocacy by consumer groups to find less restrictive and more humane ways of delivering care to people with mental illness

Psychiatric home care programs are changing rapidly in response to the increased number of people with psychiatric illnesses living in the community and the competitive health care market. Although changes in Medicare home health reimbursement have limited the growth of psychiatric home care, these programs have proven to be effective in meeting the needs of the psychiatric patient in a cost-effective manner. Psychiatric home care is a natural "fit" for the psychiatric nurse (Fagin, 2001).

Perhaps the best reason to advocate for psychiatric home care is that it is a humane and compassionate way to deliver health care and supportive services. Home care reinforces and supplements the care provided by family members and friends and maintains the recipient's dignity and independence—qualities that are all too often lost in even the best institutions.

Psychiatric home care ranges from serving as an alternative to hospitalization to functioning as a single home visit for the purposes of evaluating a specific issue. Psychiatric home care programs receive and refer patients from the entire community's general medical and mental health care services (Box 35-6). The advantages of home care in relation to inpatient treatment involve its ability to serve as:

- An alternative to hospitalization by maintaining a patient in the community.
- A facilitator of an impending hospital admission through preadmission assessment.
- An enhancement of inpatient treatment through integration of home issues in the inpatient treatment plan.
- A way to shorten inpatient stays while keeping the patient engaged in active treatment.
- A part of the discharge planning process by assessing potential problems and issues.

Examples of other gains obtained by psychiatric home care include its outreach capacity and emphasis on patient participation, responsibility, autonomy, and satisfaction.

BOX **35-6**

Who Can Benefit From In-Home Psychiatric Nursing Services?

- Patients with repeated inpatient or crisis unit admissions
- Patients with a history of medication or treatment plan non-compliance or lack of follow-through with aftercare plans
- Patients with combined diagnoses of a medical and psychiatric nature (e.g., elderly or HIV-positive patients)
- Patients with combined substance abuse and psychiatric diagnoses
- Patients receiving injectable medications who are homebound or do not follow through with scheduled outpatient appointments
- Patients in need of laboratory monitoring who are homebound or do not follow through with outpatient laboratory appointments
- Patients who are depressed and neglect self-care
- Patients who suffer from anxiety or panic and have difficulty leaving the home

What specific kind of patients do you think would benefit most from psychiatric home care? ■

Reimbursement Issues

Reimbursement for psychiatric home care is largely provided by Medicare, Medicaid, managed care companies, and private insurance. Each payer has requirements for services covered and some require advance authorization for psychiatric nursing services in the home. The majority of psychiatric home care is paid for by Medicare. The second largest source is out-of-pocket payments.

The Medicare population with mental illnesses falls into two broad categories. One group is patients over 65 who may have a history of mental illness or a newly diagnosed mental illness, usually depression. The second group is composed of people under 65 who qualify for Medicare because of their disability. The most common diagnosis in this group is schizophrenia.

Medicare guidelines do not provide very specific information on psychiatric nursing services that are covered on home visits (Box 35-7). They do require that the patient:

- **Be homebound.**
- **Have a diagnosed psychiatric disorder.**
- **Require the skills of a psychiatric nurse.**

It is largely left up to the home care agencies to interpret the Medicare guidelines and apply them to psychiatric home care. This has created many problems in the field, and psychiatric home care programs continue to struggle with this reimbursement issue.

Psychiatric homebound status is qualitatively different from medical homebound status. In determining psychiatric homebound status, a useful definition is a patient who is unable to independently and consistently access psychiatric follow-up. This definition is broad enough to include a person who is physically healthy and mobile, but too depressed to get out of bed. It also includes patients with agoraphobia,

BOX **35-7**

Medicare Guidelines for Psychiatric Home Care Nursing

Psychiatric Evaluation, Therapy, and Teaching

The evaluation, psychotherapy, and teaching activities needed by a patient with a diagnosed psychiatric disorder that requires active treatment by a psychiatrically trained nurse, as well as the costs of the psychiatric nurse's services, may be covered as a skilled nursing service. Psychiatrically trained nurses are nurses who have special training and/or experience beyond the standard curriculum required for a registered nurse. The services of the psychiatric nurse are to be provided under a plan of care established and reviewed by a physician.

Modified from Health Care Financing Administration, Publication 11, Washington, DC, 1996.

BOX **35-8**

Conditions That Might Make a Patient Psychiatrically Homebound

- Confusion, disorientation, poor judgment
- Immobilizing depression
- Severe anxiety that interferes with independence
- Agoraphobia with or without panic attacks
- Vulnerability in the community
- Psychosis or paranoid delusions that interfere with safety
- Need for 24-hour supervision

as well as patients with psychotic thinking processes who are vulnerable in the community. Medicare considers a person to be homebound if:

- The condition restricts his or her ability to leave home without an assistive device or another person.
- The effort required to leave the home is considerable and taxing.
- It is medically contraindicated to leave the home.
- The patient leaves home very infrequently and the absences are of short duration, or attributable to the need to receive treatment.

Each patient is individually evaluated with regard to homebound status. Box 35-8 lists some conditions that might make a patient psychiatrically homebound.

Medicare is a retrospective payer; records are reviewed by fiscal intermediaries to determine the necessity and appropriateness of psychiatric nursing care. It is important for the psychiatric home care nurse to concentrate on Medicare-recognized reimbursable skilled nursing services such as teaching, assessment, skilled management of the care plan, and direct care activities when planning and delivering service.

As managed care companies control an increasing share of the market, psychiatric home care programs are beginning to develop specific programs for these companies. Some examples are in-home substance abuse programs, crisis intervention programs, and hospitalization prevention programs. Managed

BOX **35-9**

BOX **35-9**

Medicare Requirements for Psychiatric Nurses in Home Care*

- A registered nurse with a master's degree in psychiatric or community mental health nursing
- A registered nurse with a bachelor's of science in nursing (BSN) degree and 1 year of related work experience in an active treatment program for adult or geriatric patients in a psychiatric health care setting
- A registered nurse with a diploma or associate degree and 2 years of related work experience in an active treatment program for adult or geriatric patients in a psychiatric health care setting
- American Nurses Association (ANA) certification in psychiatric or community health nursing

*Other qualifications may be considered on an individual basis.

care companies' requirements for psychiatric home care services vary and preauthorization for services is the norm.

Psychiatric home care is a subspecialty that calls for a nurse with certain kinds of skills, education, and experience. Box 35-9 outlines Medicare requirements for psychiatric nurses practicing in the home setting.

Any nurse can be hired to work in an inpatient psychiatric unit, but Medicare has specific requirements for a psychiatric home care nurse. Discuss the implications of this from the point of view of the patient, the nurse, and the employing health care organization. ■

Context of Home Care

Psychiatric home care nursing provides unique challenges and opportunities to the nurse. In an inpatient clinic or office setting, the provider has the control and power that come with ownership. The patient is a guest and the nurse is the host. In the home setting the nurse is the guest and the patient sets the rules. This raises four key issues for the nurse: cultural competence, flexibility in boundary setting, trust, and safety.

Cultural Competence. Awareness of the patient's ethnic and cultural background is critical to effective care in all settings but nowhere is it more obvious to the attentive eye and more critical to treatment outcome than in the home care setting. The nurse is exposed to the patient's culture, and the patient will observe the nurse's reaction in these surroundings.

Ways of addressing members of the family, views of health and mental illness, the role of the nurse and health care providers in general, and the importance of alternative therapies are just a few of the issues that vary across cultures. All of these differences must be considered by the nurse planning care with the patient in the home. Recognition and use of the patient's cultural beliefs in delivery of nursing care can positively influence the patient's participation in recovery.

It is important that the nurse also have an understanding of one's own cultural background and the prejudices related

to socioeconomic status, gender, family structure, and ways of dealing with emotion emanating from that background. Self-awareness gives the nurse the ability to step back from a judgmental stance and ask whether a certain behavior, opinion, or way of coping stands in the way of the patient's ultimate health.

Imagine yourself providing psychiatric home care to an individual with a cultural background very different from your own. How would this effect your assessment of the patient's biopsychosocial needs and your related nursing interventions? What resources would you draw on to provide culturally competent nursing care? ■

Boundary Issues. Closely related to cultural issues are the differences in boundary issues. In the home setting it may be appropriate for the nurse to sit and share a cup of tea with the patient or eat a piece of cake. If the patient's culture is one that sees hospitality as connected closely to the sharing of food and refusal of food is thought of as an affront, then being willing to share in this ritual can build trust in the relationship between the nurse and patient. Although differing opinions exist regarding boundary issues in psychiatric home care, the experienced psychiatric home care nurse knows that nursing care must be adapted to the needs and environment of each patient and family.

Trust. The psychiatric home care nurse must consider many different factors when planning and implementing nursing care. Unlike nursing practice in the hospital or outpatient mental health center, psychiatric home care nurses have little control over their patients' environments. It is therefore essential to establish trust in the initial evaluation home visit. Trust then becomes a vital part of the nurse-patient relationship as the patient and nurse work together to solve problems and achieve goals. For example, the nurse trusts the patient to be home at scheduled visits, take medications, and participate fully in all aspects of the plan of care. The patient trusts the nurse to be reliable, clinically knowledgeable, competent, and caring.

Safety. In general, psychiatric home care patients are not at greater risk for violence than the general home care patient population. However, the assessment of the environment should include issues of safety for the patient and the nurse. Strategies must be identified for dealing with suicidal or aggressive behavior. In this way, home health nursing does have its limitations. The nurse and patient must work together to achieve an acceptable plan, given the reality of having intermittent visits. If the situation becomes unsafe, the nurse must leave the home. Patients' families, caregivers, and other community resources should be urged to notify the police or take the patient to the hospital for an evaluation if the patient becomes dangerous.

Nursing Activities

Nursing interventions in the home include assessment, teaching, medication management, administration of parenteral injections, venipuncture for laboratory analysis, and skilled management of the care plan. All of these interventions are recognized as reimbursable skilled nursing services by Medicare. Psychiatric home care nurses provide many other skilled nursing services. They act as case managers, coordinating an array of services including physical therapy, occupational therapy, social work, and community services such as home-delivered meals, home visitors, and home health aides. They collaborate with all of the patient's health care providers and often facilitate communication among members of the multidisciplinary team.

CLINICAL EXAMPLE

Sonia, a 49-year-old woman, was referred by a managed care company to psychiatric home care after a 2-week inpatient stay at a local psychiatric hospital. She had a long history of psychiatric admissions for stabilization of her schizophrenia. Most hospitalizations were preceded by the patient's noncompliance with her medication schedule and follow-up care at the mental health center.

Sonia lived with her sister and elderly mother in a small row house in the Hispanic section of a large city. The family's native language was Spanish; they spoke English as a second language and understood some written English. Sonia's sister was the family's caregiver. She cared for their bedridden mother and helped with Sonia's care. Sonia's sister could not understand why Sonia would be all right for long periods and then become "crazy" and not listen. Sonia agreed to psychiatric nursing visits but initially would not agree to treatment at the mental health center. Paranoia was a major component of her illness. Other barriers were financial concerns, a lack of knowledge about her illness, and cultural and language issues.

The psychiatric nurse's plan of care included educating the patient and her sister on the disease process, signs and symptoms of relapse, the importance of continued medical care, medication actions and side effects, and correct administration of the prescribed medication. As her care progressed and Sonia became stable, the nurse helped the patient and her sister make and attend a follow-up appointment at the mental health center. Sonia was discharged from home care and agreed to go to the mental health clinic for her follow-up medical care. ■

Psychiatric home care nurses make appropriate referrals to community agencies and help their patients access community resources independently. They educate families and patients, provide supportive counseling and brief psychotherapy, promote health and prevent illness, and above all, document everything in precise detail so that their agency can be reimbursed for the services they provide.

Documentation is one of the most challenging requirements of psychiatric home care. If the nurse's documentation does not reflect the skilled service given, the payment for that service can be denied by Medicare or other payers. Few guidelines are available for documentation of psychiatric home care, although standardized coding and classification systems are preferred. The psychiatric home care nurse must be very organized and detail oriented to successfully manage the extensive and precise paperwork.

How might the use of a laptop computer facilitate more concise and timely documentation in the home health setting? ■

■ FORENSIC PSYCHIATRIC NURSING CARE

A frontier for nurses working in the community is the specialized area of forensic nursing. Forensic nursing is defined as a subspecialty of nursing that has as its objective assisting the mental health and legal systems in serving individuals who have come to the attention of both (Love and Morrison, 2002).

Forensic nursing has two very different and sometimes conflicting goals. There is the goal of providing individualized patient care, and the goal of providing custody and protection for the community. The forensic focus for nursing is the therapeutic targeting of any aspect of the patient's behavior that links his offending activity and psychiatric symptomatology. As such, the forensic nurse functions as a patient advocate, a trusted counselor, an agent of control, and a provider of primary, secondary, and tertiary health care interventions to this incarcerated population. Interventions include crisis intervention, rehabilitation, suicide prevention, behavior management, sex-offender treatment, substance abuse treatment, and discharge planning.

Settings and Roles

Most forensic psychiatric nurses work in the public sector under state departments of mental health or in psychiatric units in jails, prisons, and juvenile detention centers. However, forensic nurses are also found working in the following areas (IAFN, 2003):

- Interpersonal violence
- Public health and safety
- Emergency/trauma nursing
- Patient care facilities
- Police and corrections, including custody and abuse

The scope of responsibility of forensic nurses can be quite broad, depending on the area of practice. Forensic nurses can practice in the emergency room, critical care setting, coroner's office, or correctional facility. One specific role is that of the Sexual Assault Nurse Examiner (SANE). This is a nurse who has received special training to provide care to the victim of sexual assault.

Nursing is the backbone of correctional health care, and nurses are the major providers of health services. Yet forensic nursing has to date received limited professional recognition (Love and Morrison, 2002). Although advanced education is desirable, it is not widely available in this specialized role. Curriculum for this nursing specialty should be based on the public health approach with coursework covering medicolegal issues, criminal justice and psychopathology, family issues involving violence, and investigational techniques (Goldkuhle, 1999; Love and Morrison, 2002). Forensic nurses also must have intact ego boundaries, hardiness, insight, receptivity to feedback, self-confidence, and a commitment to ongoing professional development.

Given the growing interest in forensic psychiatry, additional examination is needed related to the roles, functions, preparation, and work perceptions of forensic nurses (Hammer, 2000; Evans and Wells, 2001). With the need for improved mental health services and health outcomes, this role merits further exploration and development.

COMPETENT CARING

A Clinical Exemplar of a Psychiatric Nurse
SUZANNE SMITH, MSN, RN, CS

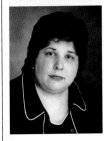

An experience I'll always remember involved a patient who was being discharged from the state psychiatric hospital; I had previously interviewed this patient for admission into an intensive case management program. R had been in and out of the state hospital for 3 years with the diagnosis of chronic schizophrenia. His frequent readmissions were related to the system's inability to place him in the community, which was due in part to his history of setting fires. Before this admission, he had burned down his residence during a psychotic episode. However, his psychosis had resolved quickly after he was admitted to the hospital and started on a regimen of neuroleptics.

R was admitted into the intensive case management program, and his first 6 months had been very busy. He had been placed in an apartment with a roommate and became responsible for managing the apartment, cooking his own food, balancing his checkbook, and paying his bills. His adjustment to life in the community was progressing well. I was able to work with R on almost a daily basis, and all was going well.

On this specific day, I had called R to let him know that I would be coming to take him to the bank. We discussed in detail his checking account balance and financial obligations for that month. When I arrived at his home, R's roommate informed me that R had gone to the store to get a cup of coffee. While waiting, I walked into the hallway to check on a problem thermostat. As I glanced into R's room, I noticed that something was amiss. There were several cigarette burns in the carpet. On the bed there were a number of cigarette lighters. Propped on the pillows were cover photos from several women's magazines. The mouths on the models had been enlarged and a cigarette had been placed through the hole. In the bedside table I found several more cigarette lighters. I noted all of these things, as well as the fact that R did not smoke.

On his return, we discussed some problems R was having with his roommate and banking affairs. His conversation was calm and rational. I then talked with him about what I had seen in his bedroom. Initially he was silent and refused to discuss the matter. I realized that one of his greatest fears was returning to the state hospital, so I assured him that if something was wrong and he needed to go back to the hospital, it would be for a short-term hospitalization. At that point he began to explain that he had not taken his medication in a week and that recently he drank a six-pack of beer with several other patients in the program. Since then, he had been hearing messages from God in which she told him to smoke cigarettes because carbon monoxide was needed to clear all the pollution on the earth.

After a consultation phone call, I told R that I thought he was becoming ill again and needed some time in the hospital. He agreed and we left in my car for an admission assessment at a local hospital. On the way, we stopped at the bank and R completed his banking business. When we arrived, several of my peers were surprised that I had let R ride in my car and go to the bank when he was obviously experiencing psychotic symptoms. They exclaimed that they would have certainly called for backup from the office or the mobile crisis unit. I explained to them that I had assessed R and felt that this decision would not endanger him or me. My decision was based on my skills as a psychiatric nurse, my experience in working with psychotic patients for a number of years, and my evaluation of R, with whom I had worked closely for 6 months.

When I think back to this experience, I realize that it captured some of the critical essence of psychiatric nursing decision making. I believe that it is calculated thinking woven into a fabric of clinical experience that guides psychiatric nursing practice. For R it was also a nursing act that expressed both caring for and caring about. After 5 days in the hospital, R was stabilized once more and returned to the life he so wanted to live. ■

CHAPTER FOCUS POINTS

- Transforming the mental health service delivery system rests on two principles: services and treatments must be consumer and family centered, and care must focus on increasing consumers' ability to successfully cope with life's challenges, on facilitating recovery, and on building resilience.

- The Community Mental Health Centers Act of 1963 marked the beginning of a major federal effort to provide comprehensive community-based mental health services to all people in need regardless of income.

- Between 1965 and 1995 nearly 700,000 patients were either discharged or diverted from state hospitals to care in the community in the movement known as deinstitutionalization. However, both the service needs of this population and the ability of communities to accommodate the large numbers of people with mental illness who had been discharged from the state were seriously miscalculated.

- Components of a community support system include client identification and outreach, mental health treatment, crisis response services, health and dental care, housing, income support and entitlement, peer support, family and community support, rehabilitation services, and protection and advocacy.

- The activities of case management are identification and outreach, assessment, service planning, linkage with needed services, monitoring service delivery, and advocacy. Questions exist about what the tasks of case managers are, who should be doing case management, to whom the case manager is accountable, and how the work of case management should be organized and evaluated.

- About one third of the estimated 600,000 homeless people in the United States have a severe mental illness, although as few as 5% to 7% of these need to be institutionalized. Most can live in the community with appropriate, supportive housing.

- Mental health issues are among the most prominent health concerns faced in rural areas. Residents with mental health needs enter care later in the course of their disease than their urban peers; enter care with more serious, persistent, and disabling symptoms; and require more expensive and intensive treatment response.

- The rate of serious mental illness in the incarcerated population is about 3 to 4 times that of the general U.S. population. Additional approaches are needed to fully address this growing problem of the mentally ill in jails.

- Assertive Community Treatment (ACT) is an evidence-based program that provides a full range of medical, psychosocial, and rehabilitative services for those with severe mental illness.

- Multisystemic therapy (MST) is a flexible treatment approach that addresses the multiple, interrelated needs of youths with serious

Continued

CHAPTER FOCUS POINTS—cont'd

behavioral and emotional problems and their families. It is usually delivered through the family preservation model of service delivery to provide interventions in home, school, and neighborhood settings.

- Psychiatric home care ranges from serving as an alternative to hospitalization to functioning as a single home visit for the purposes of evaluating a specific issue. Four key issues for the psychiatric home

care nurse are cultural competence, flexibility in boundary setting, trust, and safety.

- Forensic nursing is defined as a subspecialty of nursing that has as its objective to assist the mental health and legal systems in serving individuals who have come to the attention of both. Forensic nurses work in interpersonal violence, public health and safety, emergency/trauma nursing, patient care facilities, and police and corrections.

KEY TERMS

case management, 712
community support system, 712
deinstitutionalization, 711

forensic nursing, 722
multisystemic therapy (MST), 718

CHAPTER REVIEW QUESTIONS

1. Indicate whether the following statements are true (T) or false (F).

_____ A. The deinstitutionalization movement in the United States was successful in transitioning patients into the community.

_____ B. The Supreme Court's *Olmstead v. L. C.* decision furthered the movement toward community psychiatric care.

_____ C. Advocacy is one of the six core activities of case management.

_____ D. Most homeless people with mental illness need to be institutionalized.

_____ E. The rate of serious mental illness in the prison population is about the same as in the general population.

2. Fill in the blanks.

A. The five essential services community mental health centers were mandated to provide were _____,

_____, _____,

_____, and _____.

B. _____ is a type of program that functions as a community-based hospital without walls to provide intensive clinical support and treatment.

C. A treatment approach that addresses the needs of youth with behavioral and emotional problems and their families

is called _____.

D. A relatively new specialty of nursing caring for the mentally ill

in correctional facilities is called _____ nursing.

E. The majority of psychiatric home care is paid for by

_____.

3. Provide short answers for the following questions.

A. Describe common elements of ACT and MST programs.

B. What groups are at high risk for developing mental illness in your community? How many resources are devoted to prevention activities with these groups? How can you help to better match community needs with community resources?

C. Most case managers in this country are social workers. Describe how you as a nurse and a social worker might differ in implementing the case manager role.

D. What new roles that you read about in this chapter appeal to you as a potential career option?

Visit Evolve for additional resources related to the content of this chapter.

http://evolve.elsevier.com/Stuart/principles/
- Topical Course Outline • Student Workbook Exercises • Critical Thinking Questions and Activities • Case Studies • Research Topics
- Monthly Content Updates • WebLinks

Student Study CD-ROM

Access the accompanying CD-ROM for animations, interactive exercises, review questions for the NCLEX examination, and an audio glossary.

REFERENCES

Beck A, Maruschak L: Mental health treatment in state prisons, 2000, *Bureau of Justice Statistics, Special Report*, July 2001.

Bedell JR, Cohen NL, Sullivan A: Case management: the current best practices and the next generation of innovation, *Community Ment Health J* 36:179, 2000.

Calsyn RJ et al: Moderators and mediators of client satisfaction in case management programs for clients with severe mental illness, *Ment Health Serv Res* 4:267, 2002.

Coddington DG: Impact of political, societal, and local influences on mental health center service providers, *Adm Policy Men Health* 29:81, 2001.

Diamond PM et al: The prevalence of mental illness in prison, *Adm Policy Ment Health* 29:21, 2001.

Evans AM, Wells D: Scope of practice in forensic nursing, *J Psychosoc Nurs Ment Health Serv* 39:38, 2001.

Fagin C: Revisiting treatment in the home, *Arch Psychiatr Nurs* 15:3, 2001.

Gelberg L, Anderson RM, Leake BD: The Behavioral Model for Vulnerable Populations: application to medical care use and outcomes for homeless people, *Health Serv Res* 34:1273, 2000.

Goldkuhle U: Professional education for correctional nurses: a community-based partnership model, *J Psychsoc Nurs Ment Health Serv* 37:38, 1999.

Goldman HH et al: Lessons from the evaluation of the ACCESS program: Access to Community Care and Effective Services, *Psychiatr Serv* 53:967, 2002.

Hammer R: Caring in forensic nursing: expanding the holistic model, *J Psychosoc Nurs Ment Health Serv* 38:18, 2000.

Henggeler SW et al: Four-year follow-up of multisystemic therapy with substance-abusing and substance-dependent juvenile offenders, *J Am Acad Child Adolesc Psychiatry* 41:868, 2002.

Henggeler SW et al: One-year follow-up of multisystemic therapy as an alternative to the hospitalization of youths in psychiatric crisis, *J Am Acad Child Adolesc Psychiatry* 42:543, 2003.

International Association of Forensic Nurses (IAFN): About IAFN: at work, www.forensicnurse.org/about/work.html, January 2003.

Jones K et al: Cost-effectiveness of critical time intervention to reduce homelessness among persons with mental illness, *Psychiatr Serv* 54:884, 2003.

King R, Le Bas J, Spooner D: The impact of caseload on the personal efficacy of mental health case managers, *Psychiatr Serv* 51:364, 2000.

Lam JA, Rosenheck RA: Correlates of improvement in quality of life among homeless persons with serious mental illness, *Psychiatr Serv* 51:116, 2000.

Lamb HR, Bachrach LL: Some perspectives on deinstitutionalization, *Psychiatr Serv* 52:1039, 2001.

Love C, Morrison E: Forensic psychiatric nursing: struggling to happen, failing to thrive, www.forensicnursemag.com, 1:24, 2002.

Marshall M, Lockwood A: Assertive community treatment for people with severe mental disorders, *Cochrane Library*, 3, 2002, Oxford: Update Software.

Marshall M, Lockwood A, Green R: Case management for people with severe mental disorders, Cochrane Library, 3, 2002, Oxford: Update Software.

Morrissey JP et al: Integration of service systems for homeless persons with serious mental illness through the ACCESS program: Access to Community Care and Effective Services and Supports, *Psychiatr Serv* 53:949, 2002.

National Advisory Committee on Rural Health (NACRH): *A targeted look at the rural health care safety net*, Washington, DC, 2002.

New Freedom Commission on Mental Health (NFCMH): *Achieving the promise: transforming mental health care in America, final report*, DHHS Pub. No. SMA-03-3832, Rockville, Maryland, 2003, DHHS.

Olmstead v. L. C., 527 U. S. 581 (1999).

Randolph F et al: Overview of the ACCESS program: Access to Community Care and Effective Services and Supports, *Psychiatr Serv* 53:945, 2002.

Rosenheck RA: Cost-effectiveness of services for mentally ill homeless people: the application of research to policy and practice, *Am J Psychiatry* 157:1563, 2000.

Rosenheck RA et al: Service systems integration and outcomes for mentally ill homeless persons in the ACCESS program: Access to Community Care and Effective Services and Supports, *Psychiatr Serv* 53:958, 2002.

Rost K et al: Use, quality, and outcomes of care for mental health: the rural perspective, *Med Care Res Rev* 59:231, 2002.

Rowe M et al: Engaging persons with substance use disorders: lessons from homeless outreach, *Adm Policy Ment Health* 29:263, 2002.

Samele C et al: Patients' perceptions of intensive case management, *Psychiatr Serv* 53:1432, 2002.

Schaedle RW, Epstein I: Specifying intensive case management: a multiple perspective approach, *Ment Health Serv Res* 2:95, 2000.

Schaedle R et al: A comparison of experts' perspectives on assertive community treatment and intensive case management, *Psychiatr Ser* 53:207, 2002.

Schoenwald SK et al: Multisystemic therapy versus hospitalization for crisis stabilization of youth: placement outcomes 4 months postreferral, *Ment Health Serv Res* 2:3, 2000.

Ziguras SJ, Stuart GW: A meta-analysis of the effectiveness of mental health case management over 20 years, *Psychiatr Serv* 51:1410, 2000.

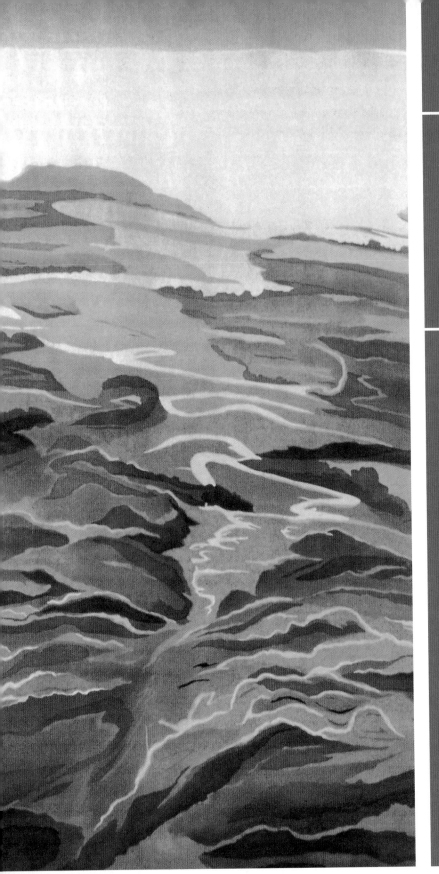

Unit Six

Fog on the Chesapeake
(Virginia)
59" × 35" batik on silk 1996

Artist's Note: When my brother and I were flying the Chesapeake, we could not get to the north shore because of the fog. As we made our way back up the bay, we could barely decipher the land on the other side. On crossing, we came to this scene. At many times in our lives we must explore options to find a solution.

Special Populations in Psychiatry

Life is unfair. It is unfair that many people who are very young or very old may have to suffer for reasons they are unable to control. But that is a reality of life that nurses, more than many others, need to understand and incorporate into their practice. It has been said that a society can be judged by how it treats its most vulnerable populations. Given that criterion, how would you rank American society? What level of compassion, protection, and caring is needed to make a society humane? What resources are given to health care providers to educate, empower, and help heal these vulnerable groups? These are questions you may wrestle with the remainder of your professional life.

In this unit you will enter the world of children, adolescents, and adults who are vulnerable to developing or being disabled by psychiatric illness. You will learn about their special needs and begin to search your heart and mind for ways in which you can reach out to help them. In that sense, you have come to the end of your journey in this textbook. Your next passage as a professional nurse will be in other pages of your life. Good luck and Godspeed.

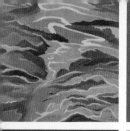

Youth's love
Embracingly integrates
Successfully frustrates
And holds together,

Often unwittingly,
All that hate, fear, and selfishness
Attempt to disintegrate.

R. BUCKMINSTER FULLER, *AND IT CAME TO PASS—NOT TO STAY*

36 CHILD PSYCHIATRIC NURSING

Sally Raphel ▪ Carole F. Bennett

LEARNING OBJECTIVES

After studying this chapter, the student should be able to:
1. Discuss issues related to psychiatric illness in children, including a framework for child psychiatric nursing practice (**I, II**).
2. Identify the major clinical areas and ego competency skills that should be included when assessing children (**III**).
3. Analyze medical and nursing diagnoses and plan interventions related to psychiatric illness in children (**IV, V**).
4. Implement therapeutic treatment modalities with children and evaluate their effectiveness (**VI, VII**).

evolve Visit Evolve for additional resources related to the content of this chapter.
http://evolve.elsevier.com/Stuart/principles/

In any given year **9%** to **13%** of children suffer from clinically significant psychiatric disorders that should be treated. Among children ages 1 to 14 years of age, suicide is the tenth leading cause of death. However, only 25% to 36% of children with mental disorders currently receive any form of treatment. The Global Burden of Disease Study indicates that by the year 2020, childhood neuropsychiatric disorders will increase by more that 50% internationally to become one of the five most common causes of morbidity, mortality, and disability among children in the world (Murray and Lopez, 1996).

There is also evidence that alcohol and drug use begins by age 8 years in some children and can be a significant problem by age 12 years. Studies have found that 50% of 8th graders have used alcohol more than once, that marijuana has been smoked by 2% of 8th graders, and that increasing numbers of children are inhaling butane, glue, and gasoline (Finke et al,

2002). These statistics concerning psychiatric problems among children are alarming. Adding to this concern is the increase in school-related shootings and other violent behavior displayed by young children in family and community settings.

Another disturbing issue is the prognosis of a child who has been diagnosed with a psychiatric illness. Mental illness that develops before age 6 can interfere with critical aspects of a child's emotional, cognitive, and physical development. For example, there is an association between conduct disorder in a child and the development of antisocial personality disorder later in life. So, too, prior anxiety, behavior, and mood disorders all increase the likelihood of the child having psychiatric problems as an adult.

Thus childhood disorders appear to set in motion a chain of maladaptive behaviors and environmental responses that foster more persistent psychopathology over time. These findings emphasize the importance of early identification and treatment of these children in order to reduce the risk for psychiatric disorders reaching into their adult lives.

Although the number of children receiving care has doubled in the last decade, the extent of unmet needs is still great (Pottick, 2002). It is well established that without treatment, psychological problems disrupt the child's social, academic, and emotional development and result in family turmoil.

■ CHILD PSYCHIATRIC CARE IN PERSPECTIVE

The earliest evidence of child or adolescent treatment for psychiatric disorders in the history of medical care was in 1799 when Jean Stard built residential schools for young people with mental retardation in Massachusetts and New York. These were to be educational institutions rather than asylums. The assumption was that after assistance, the youth would be able to function at home. By the end of the 19th century, the "state schools for idiots" as they were called, were primarily custodial and few of the children returned home.

In the early days of psychiatry, children were not seen as patients. An example is that Freud published his *Theory of Infantile Sexuality* in 1905, but it was 3 years before he saw any child professionally. When he treated "Little Hans" in 1909, it was through visits with his father, not Hans himself.

Current child psychiatric therapy began with Melanie Klein in 1932. She was a student of Freud who, along with Anna Freud, applied Freud's approach to children. Both clinicians substituted play therapy for adult free association, used drawing and dreams techniques. At this same time, child guidance clinics were being established. By 1930, 500 of these clinics had been established in the United States.

Child intelligence testing was begun by Alfred Binet in the early 20th century. This resulted in learning the extent to which a child differed from established norms in cognitive ability. Behaviorism was developed by John B. Watson in 1913, followed by special education training for teachers in 1914, and B.F. Skinner's operant conditioning in 1938. Behavioral modification based on operant conditioning theory (see Chapter 31) was not actually practiced with children until the mid 1960s to mid 1970s. It was first used on a consistent basis in child residential settings, regular and special education classrooms, and outpatient settings with children.

More recently in 1999, the Surgeon General of the United States released the landmark policy document *Mental Health: A Report of the Surgeon General* with a major section dedicated to children and adolescents (USDHHS, 1999). The national focus on vulnerable children was maintained by a number of subsequent reports including: *Report of the Surgeon General's Conference on Children's Mental Health: A National Action Agenda* (USDHHS, 2000b; Raphel, 2001), *A National Strategy for Suicide Prevention: Goals and Objectives for Action* (USDHHS, 2001a), and *Youth Violence: A Report of the Surgeon General* (USDHHS, 2001b).

Although a national dialogue about evidence-based practice and empirically validated treatments for children has

---

BOX 36-1

Events Affecting Child Psychiatric Nursing

1909-1930	Child guidance movement began. Nurses did not have formalized role in treatment of children.
1953	American Academy of Child Psychiatry formed to provide national forum for child psychiatrists.
1954	Boston University offered first graduate program for child psychiatric nurses. Other universities soon developed programs.
1959	Child psychiatry became an official subspecialty of psychiatry.
1971	Advocates for Child Psychiatric Nursing formed the first national nursing organization for nurses working in child and adolescent psychiatry.
1972	Claire Fagin published the classic text *Nursing in Child Psychiatry*.
1975	International Year of the Child declared.
1985	*Standards of Child and Adolescent Psychiatric and Mental Health Nursing Practice* published by the American Nurses Association. Claire Fagin became president of American Orthopsychiatric Association.
1988	*Journal of Child and Adolescent Psychiatric and Mental Health Nursing* began publication.
1999	*Mental Health: a Report of the Surgeon General* published with a major section dedicated to children and adolescents.
2000	*Children's Mental Health: a National Action Plan* published.
2001	*National Strategy for Suicide Prevention* and *Youth Violence: A Report of the Surgeon General* released.

---

been ongoing for some time now, youth and families continue to suffer because of missed opportunities for prevention of psychiatric disorders and early interventions in behavioral problems. A timeline of events affecting child psychiatric nurses is presented in Box 36-1.

Etiological Factors

Both **genetic factors (nature)** and **childhood experiences (nurture)** are recognized as predisposing and precipitating causes for the development of a psychiatric illness. With the current understanding of the roles of neurotransmitters and brain development, the effect of experience combined with genetic predisposition begins to explain the complexity of the development of child psychiatric illness.

For example, **traumatic events** are known to have a profound impact on children. The symptoms that are characteristic of posttraumatic stress disorder (PTSD) in children are those of increased arousal, including hypervigilance, irritability, anxiety, physiological hyperactivity, impulsivity, and sleep difficulty. These symptoms often are also diagnosed as attention deficit/hyperactivity disorder (ADHD), conduct disorder, anxiety disorder, and mood disorder.

It is now also recognized that the particular constellation of symptoms a child experiences are often related to the **family history**. Specifically, if a family member has a history of anxiety disorder, the child may experience symptoms that are more anxious in appearance. However, if family members have a strong history of alcoholism and sociopathy, symptoms may pertain more to conduct disorder. Thus it is believed that a genetic predisposition to certain symptoms is inherent and that these symptoms can be stimulated as a response to an event in the environment.

After traumatic events, many factors are important in the development of the intensity of symptoms, including the nature of the trauma, the degree to which body integrity is threatened, the threat posed by the event to the child's self-system and security, and the nature of the family support system.

The **neurophysiology** activated during acute stress is usually rapid and reversible. The brain has mechanisms that down-regulate the stress reaction after the threat has passed, returning the brain to its prior level of functioning. However, if the stress is prolonged, severe, or repetitive, the resulting increases in neurotransmitter activity are often not reversible.

This process has a significant impact on the development of the child's brain. A trauma-induced brain response would probably result in abnormal patterns, time, and intensity of catecholamine activity in the developing brain. Young children who are exposed to a high rate of stress-induced trauma are at risk for developing permanent changes in neuronal organization, making it more difficult for them to learn and to control their behavior.

Other psychiatric illnesses, such as ADHD, also illustrate the interplay of genetics and environment. Children with ADHD usually exhibit excessive activity and have difficulty paying attention. These behaviors are often tolerated by a family. However, when these children begin school, they are identified as problematic because these behaviors interfere with the child's academic performance and peer relationships. As in PTSD, children with ADHD often have a range of symptoms, including symptoms that overlap with anxiety disorders, oppositional defiant disorder, and conduct disorder.

Although the precise etiology of ADHD remains unclear, it is believed that environmental factors such as lead ingestion, prenatal and perinatal complications, socioeconomic factors, genetic factors, and brain dysfunction resulting from brain damage may contribute to the development of the illness. No one finding has adequately explained this complex disorder, but there is agreement that it has a neurobiological basis.

By the time a child and family seek treatment, the child may have developed secondary mental health problems such as **low self-esteem** and **poor socialization**. Thus the effect of this illness on the child is significantly mediated by its severity, the ability of the family to cope with the illness, and the secondary symptoms that result.

As these two examples show, psychiatric illness in children is complex and can be debilitating for both the child and the family. **Treatment usually involves the combination of medication to improve brain function, social skills training to improve socialization, behavior management to learn impulse control, cognitive therapy to practice problem solving and communication, and parent education to integrate the new behaviors and skills into the child's life.**

What influence did your social and physical environment have on your outlook on life today? ■

Resilience

A child's individual characteristics and early life experiences, as well as protective factors in their social and physical environment, contribute to resilience, their ability to withstand stress (Mandleco and Peery, 2000; Paris, 2000). Resilient children are active, affectionate, and good-natured. They are also humorous, confident and competent, realistic, flexible, and assured of their own inner resources and support from outside sources. They have a strong sense of personal control, take age appropriate responsibility, and exercise self-discipline. When faced with stressors, they show capacity to recover quickly from temporary collapse and attempt to master stress rather than retreat or defend against problems.

Although developmental consequences of living in chronic violence can be devastating for some children, not all children experience harm or develop psychiatric disorders. It has been estimated that 80% of children exposed to powerful stressors do not sustain developmental damage. Researchers find that children from similar family and community environments can be touched by the same negative experience (e.g., poverty, parental psychiatric and substance abuse disorders, war, dislocation) but not experience the same degree of emotional and physical problems (Werner and Johnson, 2000).

So what makes some children more resilient than others? Specific protective or resiliency factors of children have been identified (Mylant et al, 2002). A **sense of autonomy** is one resiliency factor. Another factor is **adaptive distancing**, which occurs when a child is able to distance oneself from too close involvement with a dysfunctional family, transcend a difficult past, not identify with troubled family members, and select healthy alternatives as they become available.

Other protective factors include the following:
- Cognitive competence
- Experiences of self-efficacy resulting in self-confidence
- Temperament characteristics that elicit positive responses from others
- Parenting that fosters competence
- Positive self-esteem
- Supportive adults who foster trust and act as gatekeepers
- Opportunities in major life transitions that allow competencies to be reinforced and rewarded

Issues related to the development of a positive self-concept and high self-esteem are discussed in Chapter 18.

A study of resourcefulness in school-aged children determined that coping and resiliency are learned throughout life in the context of an individual's situation. High maternal resourcefulness added to the child's own resourcefulness were predictors for positive outcomes (Zauszniewski et al, 2002). Resilient children have parents who are models of resilience and are available to them with reassurance and encouragement during times of trouble. These support persons help children understand and process stress and trauma.

Studies also show that a child can overcome emotional stress and physical disruption such as that caused by war or chronic violence if they remain with a parent or caretaker and are taken care of in a routine, stable way. The most important point is that the resilient child has the ability to make sense of threatening situations and can understand clearly what is occurring in their environment, which then helps them master stress.

Resiliency is fostered by the child having a supportive and caring adult in his or her life. How can nurses facilitate access to community support persons for young people? ■

■ A FRAMEWORK FOR NURSING PRACTICE

To be effective in the psychiatric nursing care of children, one must be well grounded in knowledge of child growth and development. The works of Piaget (1952), Erikson (1968), Kohlberg (1999), and Brazelton (1984) are very relevant to nursing practice. In addition, nursing interventions should be based on meeting the child where he or she is developmentally and not on parental, societal, or academic standards. This is critical to success in establishing trust with the child and implementing planned interventions.

Nurses are challenged to derive realistic, well-defined goals, respond to the complex social needs of the child, understand and advocate for the child, and develop a comprehensive treatment plan that identifies and integrates the child's needs and family resources. All of this must be done with the realization that the behavior of children is largely culturally based and must be viewed from a sociocultural perspective.

Organizing child psychiatric nursing care around **ego competency skills** is an effective and culturally sensitive way of planning and implementing nursing interventions for children regardless of psychiatric diagnosis or setting. The nine skills that all children need to become competent adults include the following (Strayhorn, 1989):

- Establishing closeness and trusting relationships
- Handling separation and independent decision making
- Negotiating joint decisions and interpersonal conflict
- Dealing with frustration and unfavorable events
- Celebrating good feelings and experiencing pleasure
- Working for delayed gratification
- Relaxing and playing
- Cognitive processing through words, symbols, and images
- Establishing an adaptive sense of direction and purpose

Communication

The first goal of the nurse is to establish a therapeutic alliance with the child and the parents. If the child's verbal communications are vague or unclear, the nurse needs to ask for additional explanation. Often a child will not respond to a problem-centered line of communication. In this case the nurse should start with discussing more general aspects of the child's life such as family members, school, or friends. Strategies for communicating with children are identified in Box 36-2.

Children with internalizing disorders such as depression or anxiety are often the best informants about their affective states. Children with externalizing disorders of ADHD or conduct disorder are typically poor informants and generally less cooperative in interview. They tend to blame others, thereby requiring reports from parents, teachers, day care, or school personnel to obtain information about problems and progress.

As a novice working with children, how can you establish trust? What would indicate to you that a child trusts you? ■

Cultural Competence

Nowhere is the importance of culturally competent care greater than in the delivery of mental health services to children and their families. Cultural issues and communication between the child, family members, and clinician are a critical part of the service and success of the child's outcomes.

BOX 36-2

Strategies for Communicating With Children

- Develop an understanding of age-related norms of development.
- Convey respect and authenticity.
- Assess and use familiar vocabulary at the child's level of understanding.
- Assess the child's needs in relation to the immediate situation.
- Assess the child's capacity to cope successfully with change.
- Use nonverbal communication and alternatives to verbalization (e.g., eye contact, reassuring facial expressions).
- Work to develop trust through honesty and consistency.
- Interpret the child's nonverbal cues back to him or her verbally.
- Use humor and active listening to foster the relationship.
- Increase coping skills by providing opportunities for creative, unstructured play.
- Use indirect age-appropriate communication techniques (e.g., storytelling, picture drawing, and creative writing).
- Use alternative, supplementary communication devices for children with specialized needs (e.g., sign language, computer-enhanced communication programs).

Adapted from Arnold EA, Boggs KU: *Interpersonal relationships: professional communication skills for nurses*, ed 4, St Louis, 2003, WB Saunders.

Child psychiatric nurses, family members, and other mental health professionals have identified culturally relevant clinical standards and implementation guidelines (USDHHS, 2000a). These are intended to fill the gap for mental health professionals working with African Americans, Hispanics, Native Americans/Alaska Natives, and Asian/Pacific Island Americans.

To ensure cultural competence, the nurse must understand the child's background, communicate effectively across cultures, and formulate treatment plans in partnership with the child and family. The nurse must develop knowledge, understanding, skills, and informed attitudes about differences related to the following:

- Symptom expression
- Attributions of mental illness (religious, supernatural)
- Role and manifestation of spiritual tradition, values, and practice beliefs
- Perceptions of stigma
- Thresholds of psychiatric and emotional distress
- Verbal and non-verbal language, speech patterns, and degree of English literacy
- Culturally acceptable help-seeking behavior for children
- Culturally related side effects of medications

A guideline for transcultural nursing care with children is presented in Table 36-1.

Legal and Ethical Issues

Much progress has been made related to legal and ethical issues affecting children with psychiatric disorders. However, challenges remain for advocacy by nurses for ethical issues impacting child psychiatric care (ACAPN, 2001). For example, the right to privacy and confidentiality is rarely granted to a child apart from his or her parents.

Confidentiality of patient information is an ethical and legal responsibility of every nurse. In mental health care, the provider is sometimes required to balance the child's wishes and interests against the parent's request for information. Clear exceptions are when a child reports a plan for self-harm or harm to others or relates information about child sexual or physical abuse, which must be reported to authorities as required by the court.

Inconsistency is found in statutory and case law regarding a child's status, capacity, competence, and liabilities. Minors are protected and deemed lacking the capacity to enter into contracts, but they are considered to be emancipated or free from parental authority if they are married, serving in the military, parenting a child, living separate from parents, or are self-supporting. In these cases the youth can contract for health services, give informed consent, and may be seen as an adult by law. Most states do not allow minors (under legal age 18) to obtain psychiatric care without parental consent.

■ ASSESSING THE CHILD

Assessment of the child requires a biopsychosocial approach with attention given to the contribution of biological development, medical illness, cognitive and personality characteristics, cultural context, and the child's family, school, and social environment. The goal of assessment is to determine the child's emotional, cognitive, social, and linguistic development, and to identify the nature of relationships with family, school, and social milieu (Delaney and Belmonte-Mann, 2001).

The components of a psychiatric assessment are shown in Box 36-3. Multiple sources of information can be accessed when forming one's assessment, including family (parents, caregivers), school and day care personnel (teachers, parents, counselors, principals), sitters, after school program staff, athletic coaches, scout leaders, and bus drivers. An understanding of the child's competencies related to his or her stage of development is critical to forming a well-grounded diagnosis.

Key Areas

Establishing a therapeutic alliance with the child begins during assessment and should move toward a working partnership (Morrison and Anders, 1999). Playing with or watching the child play with age-appropriate toys or games is an effective

---

BOX 36-3

Child Assessment Components

Family Interview
Define the problem(s), developmental and family history (genogram), parental mental and physical health, family interactions (see Chapter 33)

Interview With the Child
Mental state: Does he or she have a problem? School experiences, friendship, play, and teasing. Worries, fears, mood (including tears and suicidal ideas), expression of anger, sleep and appetite, habits and obsessions, and (when indicated) inquire about sexual/physical abuse, auditory hallucinations, and delusional ideas
Development of conscience and values, interests, hobbies, talents
Supplement the interview by play and drawing (ask the child to draw a person/family/dream)
Physical examination including assessment of handedness, motor coordination, or clumsiness

Structured Questionnaire Rating Scales
Provide an overall scale score and problem domain subscale scores

Other Investigations
Psychological tests (e.g., IQ profile)—indicated when there are learning problems, delayed or uneven development, cognitive or perceptual disturbances
Laboratory tests (e.g., chromosome analysis)—indicated when there is the possibility of an associated biological problem, such as fragile X syndrome or thyroid disease
Neuroimaging and electroencephalogram—indicated when there may be associated neurological disorder such as epilepsy

way to observe interactions with parents, caregivers, or others. Several key areas of assessment merit further discussion.

- **Developmental history** includes demographic information, a description of the presenting problem, identification of recent stressors in the family or home, and a history of the child's prenatal, neonatal, and first year of life, including developmental milestones.

The child's general behavior and past and present personality traits should be recorded. Whether a child is seen as shy, timid, unfriendly, aggressive, risk-taking, fearful, or morose are all important.

- **Family history** involves collecting information about all members of the child's family. This will add to understanding the context of the child's current prob-

Table 36-1	Transcultural Psychiatric Nursing Care	
PRINCIPLE OF CARE	**PRACTICE**

A. Assessment
1. The child/adolescent and family can expect to receive an assessment of cultural needs on admission and continuously thereafter.
2. The child/adolescent/family can expect to be an active participant in communicating their mental health needs from their cultural perspective.
	1. The nurse, in partnership with the child/adolescent and family will continuously assess for:
	  a. Culture of origin/significant historical events
	  b. Current cultural conflicts/satisfaction
	  c. Language spoken and understood
	  d. Family kinship network
	  e. Current and memorable experiences that may impact on their view of the environment
	  f. Social, economic, political, technological, educational, and religious views
	  g. Significant values/beliefs
	  h. Food/dress needs or preferences
	  i. Cultural vs. professional health beliefs

B. Diagnosis • Impaired verbal communication related to cultural and/or language differences • Anxiety related to unmet needs • Ineffective coping related to . . . • Noncompliance related to client and provider relationship(s) • Powerlessness related to health care environment • Spiritual distress related to separation from religious and cultural ties • Risk for other-directed violence related to panic state	

C. Planning
1. The child/adolescent/family can expect to participate collaboratively in their health care.
	1. The nurse will strive to be an advocate for the child/adolescent/family within the treatment arena, by promoting:
	  a. Respect and preservation of the individual's cultural orientation.
	  b. Accommodation to client culture within the treatment environment.
	  c. Restructuring of care that innovatively meets the mental health needs of the individual and family without compromising their values.

D. Implementation 1. The child/adolescent/family can expect to receive on-going education related to diagnosis and various therapeutic treatment approaches.	1. The nurse will listen to and ask questions of the client to promote open and responsive communication. 2. Nurse will provide and promote education of child/adolescent/family in all aspects of mental health care.
E. Evaluation 1. The child/adolescent/family can expect on-going timely staff responses to stated cultural health need.	1. The nurse will monitor and evaluate response to treatment in an on-going fashion. 2. The nurse will collaboratively alter treatment approaches to achieve the goal of optimal effective coping and health while preserving cultural values of the client/family.

From International Society of Psychiatric–Mental Health Nurses: *Association of Child and Adolescent Psychiatric Nurses (ACAPN) guidelines for care and practice,* Philadelphia, 1998, Author.

lems. Data about family members' psychiatric diagnoses and psychological and social functioning can be key to determining the child's resources. A family genogram can be a useful tool in gaining an understanding of family issues that span multiple generations (see Chapter 11).

- **Stress and trauma history** is significant to the child's current situation when there has been caretaker absence, abandonment, neglect; physical, sexual, or emotional abuse; placement in a foster home; or parental divorce or separation (Lubit et al, 2003).
- **Strengths of the child** relate to adaptive capacities, resilience, and positive attributes. These can enhance the possible treatment outcomes. A strength-based assessment brings to light the resources the child has available both internally and externally. It focuses on prior and current achievements, no matter how small. Such resources can be identified and reinforced by the nurse and treatment team.

A **mental status examination (MSE)** also should be completed. A standard format is followed with regard to appearance, orientation, general interaction, speech and language, motor ability, intelligence, and memory (see Chapter 7). One also must assess cognitive, reading, and writing abilities; social relatedness; judgment; and insight. For each area of the child MSE, the differences as compared with the adult version are significant. For example, it is critical to observe the child from a developmental perspective (e.g., depression may be confused with shyness). Social relatedness is another important criterion (e.g., observation of personal boundaries and the child's view of the emotional state of others), particularly the observance of behaviors when separating from a parent. Alertness is also significant because sleepiness could be a medication side effect or a symptom of depressive disorder.

Perceptions and hallucinations, if expressed, must be evaluated along with the child's level of concrete thinking. For example, a child may report seeing something the interviewer does not see, which on further clarification, is a picture on the wall behind the interviewer. An evaluation of thought content might reveal suicidality, homocidality, delusions, or unusual preoccupations. Affect must be explored, characterized, and questioned.

Ego Competency Skills

The nursing assessment also should focus on the specific skills that all children need to become competent adults. Regardless of medical diagnosis, a child should be assessed for mastery of the following nine ego competency skills.

Establishing Closeness and Trusting Relationships.
A basic skill for positive growth and development is the child's ability to establish close and trusting relationships with others. Children with the medical diagnosis of generalized anxiety disorder may have difficulty establishing trusting relationships because they are very concerned about their perceived competency. The following questions are used to evaluate this skill:

- Does the child enjoy making friends?
- Does the child often feel picked on by other people?

- Does the child not know what to say when getting to know someone?

Handling Separation and Independent Decision Making.
Children who have separation anxiety have great difficulty tolerating separation from their mother or home. Yet individuation is an important mental health process. Being able to identify and express feelings and make independent decisions is critical to becoming a competent individual. The following questions are used to evaluate this skill:

- Does the child get upset or worry when away from his or her mother?
- Does the child get upset or worry if he or she thinks someone does not like him or her?
- When upset, is there something the child can do to feel better?

Handling Joint Decision Making and Interpersonal Conflict.
Children who have not been allowed to participate in joint decision making or who have not been rewarded for cooperating may be deficient in this skill. A child with oppositional defiant disorder may use aggression instead of negotiation to respond to interpersonal conflict. However, learning the skill of joint decision making is critical for success in interpersonal relationships. The following questions are used to evaluate this skill:

- When the child has a problem, can he or she usually think of several solutions?
- Does the child get angry if he or she does not get his or her way?
- Do other people make the child agitated or easily upset?

Games can be useful in teaching cooperation and compromise to children. What games can you identify that would be particularly helpful in teaching children this important skill? ■

Dealing With Frustration and Unfavorable Events.
Tolerating frustration, although difficult, is critical to becoming a competent adult. Children with conduct disorders often have difficulty understanding a situation from another's perspective. The following questions are used to evaluate this skill:

- Does the child feel bad if he or she has hurt someone's feelings?
- If someone disagrees with the child, does it make him or her angry?
- Does the child not like playing a game if he or she loses?

Do you think that a child's ability to handle frustration and stressful events is influenced by biological makeup? If so, does biology excuse people from being responsible for their actions? ■

Celebrating Good Feelings and Feeling Pleasure.
Healthy children raised in a nurturing environment naturally experience good feelings and pleasure. However, children who are depressed or anxious are not able to celebrate good feelings or experience spontaneous pleasure. Also, in a mal-

adaptive environment, shame is often used to control children's behavior, with the result that they feel guilty for having angry or unacceptable thoughts. Consequently, they may lose the ability to celebrate life and feel pleasure. The following questions are used to evaluate this skill:

- Does the child worry about the future a lot?
- Does the child not like it when people say good things about him or her?
- Does the child feel good about the things he or she does well?

How often and in what ways did your family celebrate good feelings and experience pleasure when you were growing up? How do you incorporate this in your life today? ■

Working for Delayed Gratification. As children grow they are expected to delay needed gratification by following rules and waiting their turn. This skill is often difficult for impulsive children with ADHD or conduct disorder to achieve. The following questions are used to evaluate this skill:

- Does the child believe that most rules are reasonable and does he or she not mind following them?
- Does the child find it difficult to be honest and think that lying is the only thing to do?
- Does the child get angry if his or her mother doesn't give what he or she wants?

Relaxing and Playing. Given the stressful environment of current family life, many children may have little opportunity to learn the skill of relaxing and playing. For children with mood, anxiety, or behavior disorders, learning to relax and play is an important skill. The following questions are used to evaluate this skill:

- Are there some things the child really enjoys doing?
- Can the child have lots of fun?
- Does the child enjoy sitting around and thinking about things?

Cognitive Processing Through Words, Symbols, and Images. Children with psychiatric illnesses may not have developed the important skill of cognitive processing. The following questions are used to evaluate this skill:

- Is it difficult for the child to describe how he or she feels?
- Does the child feel as if he or she never knows how something is going to turn out?
- Can the child identify his or her strengths?

Adaptive Sense of Direction and Purpose. Children who experience symptoms of mental illness may feel hopeless about their purpose in life. As they view adult life from watching those around them, they begin to draw conclusions about themselves in the world. The following questions are used to evaluate this skill:

- Does the child feel that his or her life is going to get better?
- Is the child confused about growing up and doesn't know what to do about it?

- Does the child believe that school is important and see it as his or her job in life at present?

Many people believe that youth in contemporary society lack a sense of hope, direction, and purpose in life. Do you agree with this, and if so, what sociocultural factors might influence the learning of this skill? ■

Brain Imaging

New methods of brain imaging also can be used to assess the child. The goal of assessment in developmental disorders is related to tracking neuronal maturation. Through brain imaging, physiological and developmental brain abnormalities can be identified.

A neuroradiologist may describe the degree of myelinization of an infant or toddler, the relative size of the ventricles, or the presence of atrophy visualized in routine brain MRI protocols. Currently these techniques are being used in the study of ADHD, schizophrenia, anorexia nervosa, obsessive compulsive disorders, autism, affective disorders, and Tourette's syndrome (Hendren, DeBacker, and Pandina, 2000).

Techniques used with proper release signed by a parent include MRI, functional MRI, magnetic resonance spectroscopy, and magnetoencephalography. These tests do not use iodizing radiation or radioactive isotopes (Vujevich, 2003). Positron emission tomography (PET) and single-photon emission computed tomography (SPECT) require the use of isotopes but allow for direct assessment of the biochemistry in the brain.

Scientists have found that ADHD, childhood onset of bipolar disorder, and lead intoxication may have many similarities in presentation, but neurobiological tests can give accurate classification of their important differences. These techniques may provide powerful tools for clinicians to use in following the course and treatment effects and predicting outcomes for children with neuro-developmental disorders.

Significant differences in activation levels of specific brain regions in neuronal activities associated with fundamental biological activities and in defining genetic and environmental aspects of psychiatric, behavioral, and emotional symptoms hold great promise for the future.

■ DIAGNOSIS

Medical Diagnoses

Children with psychiatric illness experience disabling symptoms that are responses to biological alterations, traumatizing situations, or maladaptive learning. A range of efficacious psychosocial and pharmacological treatments can be offered for these disorders (Weisz and Jensen, 1999; USDHHS, 1999; Hoagwood et al, 2001).

The Diagnostic and Statistical Manual of Mental Disorders (DSM-IV-TR) classifies disorders usually first evident in infancy, childhood, or adolescence (American Psychiatric Association, 2000). Children also can experience a number of psychiatric illnesses common to adults. Four of the most common psychiatric disorders in childhood are **anxiety, depression, conduct disorder,** and **attention deficit/hyperactivity disorder (ADHD).** Table 36-2 summarizes the symptoms, assessment,

Table 36-2 Psychiatric Disorders of Children

DISORDER	DESCRIPTION	KEY *DSM-IV-TR* CRITERIA*
Mental Retardation (MR)	Beginning before age 18, MR involves low intelligence and resulting difficulties requiring special help for child in coping with life.	NOTE: MR is the only disorder of infancy, childhood, or adolescence coded on Axis II. Code according to severity.
Pervasive Developmental Disorders (PDD) Autism Rett's disorder Childhood disintegrative disorder Asperger's disorder PDD NOS	Development is slow, sometimes never comes, inability to socialize, to communicate, and to control motor movements.	Impaired social interaction Impaired communication with delays or absence of spoken language Repetitive, restricted, or stereotypical activities, behaviors, and interests
Learning Disorders Reading Mathematics Written expression Academic problem Learning disorder NOS	Child is found to be substantially below expected skill level and has more difficulty than normal in learning specific academic skills. Consideration is given to intelligence level, age, and experience with appropriate education.	Each diagnosis is made based on standardized, individual tests. The deficiency impedes daily living and academic achievement.
Motor Skills Disorders Developmental coordination disorder	A child whose motor coordination is seriously below expectation for intelligence and age. Very young child may have delayed milestones or older child may have fine motor difficulty in sports or handiwork. Cause is unknown.	Incoordination impedes academic achievement or daily living activities.
Communication Disorders Expressive language Mixed receptive/expressive Phonological Stuttering Selective mutism Communication disorder NOS	Impair a child's ability to communicate with others. Most are not commonly known and often go unrecognized.	Child does not use speech sounds expected for age and dialect. Social communication or educational achievement is hindered.
Movement and Tic Disorders Developmental coordination Transient tic Chronic motor or vocal tic disorder Tourette's disorder Stereotypic movement disorder Tic disorder NOS	Tics can be motor or vocal, simple or complex. Simple motor—grimaces, eye muscle twitches, abdominal tensing, or jerking of shoulder, head, or distal extremities. Simple vocal—barks, coughs, throat clearing, sniffs, or single syllables called out. Complex vocals have more organized patterns.	Symptoms begin before age 18, are not generally caused by effects of a medical condition (e.g., Huntington's disease) or substance use, cause notable stress. Generally involuntary movements. Tourette's disorder is usually familial and lasts into adulthood.
Disorders of Intake and Elimination Pica Rumination Feeding disorder of infancy or early childhood Enuresis Encopresis Other eating disorders—anorexia nervosa or bulimia nervosa	Intake: Child eats nonnutrient substances (e.g., dirt, paper), regurgitates and rechews food or fails to eat adequately. Elimination: Urinating on clothes or bed after age 5 years. Repeated passage of feces in inappropriate places after age 4 years. NOTE: Enuresis is most often viewed as physiological condition with physical symptoms, not necessarily mental disorder. It does have emotional sequelae similar to obesity.	Child is at least 4 years and accidentally or purposefully passes feces in inappropriate places (clothing, floor). Occurs at least once a month for 3 months and the behavior is not caused by a laxative or general medical condition.

Data from Morrison J, Anders TF: *Interviewing children and adolescents: skills and strategies for effective DSM-IV diagnosis*, New York, 1999, Guilford Publishing.
*For full *DSM-IV-TR* criteria see American Psychiatric Association: *Diagnostic and statistical manual of mental disorders*, ed 4, text revision, Washington, DC, 2000, American Psychiatric Association.
NOS, Not otherwise specified; ADHD, attention deficit/hyperactivity disorder; MRELD, mixed receptive/expressive language disorder; PTSD, posttraumatic stress disorder.

ASSESSMENT	DEVELOPMENTAL FACTORS	NURSING IMPLICATIONS
Based on intelligence quotient (IQ) Mild, 55-70 Moderate, 40-55 Severe, 25-40 Profound, less than 25 Many causes detected through laboratory studies	Tools to measure IQ and developmental quotient (DQ) vary. A child with associated physical features is diagnosed earlier. Denver and Bayley scales for ages 1-42 months are helpful.	Safety needs must be closely monitored. Self-esteem is usually low and requires frequent reevaluation and enhancement. Higher functioning child generally has a sense of humor and some have a rich fantasy life.
Aspects of these disorders overlap many others. Neurological disorders must be explored with careful attention to gross and fine motor coordination.	The degree of disability varies but the effects on child and family are profound and permanent.	The child may use language inappropriately and ask personal questions which require redirection.
Often some history points to the problem and correct diagnosis. An interview with a child experiencing reading difficulty is also used to examine for accompanying disorders (e.g., ADHD, communication disorder).	Unlikely to be evident until school age.	Take time and support child from a strength-based perspective to assist self-esteem issues. Build on child's achieved communication skills and consult with educational specialist for specific methods.
Physiological, genetic, neurological, or other contributors should be ruled out. Criteria for pervasive developmental disorder do not fit symptoms.	The target symptoms are not from medical condition such as cerebral palsy or muscular dystrophy.	Fit play interventions to age and development. Observation in varied activities gives data to build a care plan.
Encourage child to talk uninterrupted for prolonged periods to get samples of speech rate, repetition, dropped sounds, lack of prosody. Use story telling or have child recount an event as a nonthreatening subject.	Mild case may be missed until teens. Younger MRELD can appear deaf, older child shows confusion. Stuttering begins in early childhood and self-esteem issues are important.	Need a clear sense of use of symbols and ability to comprehend and follow commands given without gestures.
Usually suppressed during sleep, increase in intensity or frequency at times of stress, fatigue, or illness. Present a wide range of symptoms on a continuum from occasional eye blinking to severe motor and vocal tics so severe they preclude normal classroom participation.	Motor tics appear as young as 2 years and usually involve the upper part of the face, vocal occur somewhat later. Transient tics prognosis is better, chronic motor or vocal tics wane within a few years and rarely last into adulthood.	Child with a tic feels out of control of their own body. With Tourette's disorder the child has multiple motor tics in addition to vocal ones and may use socially inappropriate vulgar language (corprolalia). Nursing plan incorporates empathetic care, self-esteem enhancement, supportive environment to improve social relationships, and medication monitoring and teaching.
Symptoms of elimination disorders may be embarrassing. Assess for pain, sensation of need to void. A few years of maturation can separate the pathological situation from the developmental issue.	Normal toddlers put everything in their mouths. Pica should not be considered unless inappropriate eating lasts longer than 1 month in a child developmentally past the toddler stage. Focus on the involuntary nature of the elimination problem, as well as the child's hope for improvement. Build a therapeutic alliance by using child's own words for bodily functions and anatomy.	For eating disorders, direct observation of child and parents at mealtime may help. Most information will come in verbal reports from parent. Watch for other oral behaviors, nail biting and thumb sucking.

Continued

Table 36-2	Psychiatric Disorders of Children—cont'd	
DISORDER	**DESCRIPTION**	**KEY *DSM-IV-TR* CRITERIA***
Attention-Deficit and Disruptive Behavior Disorders ADHD ADHD NOS Conduct disorder Oppositional defiant Child antisocial behavior Disruptive behavior NOS	ADHD: Child's behavior is comprised of either attention deficits or hyperactivity and impulsivity. Develops as a failure of brain mechanisms for self-control and inhibition of impulses or frontal lobe executive functions. Conduct disorder: For 12 months or more child has repeatedly violated rules, age-appropriate societal norms, or rights of others.	Inattention must meet 6 of 10 criteria and hyperactivity must meet 6 of 9 criteria. Some symptoms begin before age 7. Symptoms must be present in two separate situations (school, home, or social functioning). The symptoms do not occur solely in pervasive developmental disorder, or psychotic disorder. Symptoms are not better explained by another disorder, e.g., mood disorder, anxiety, or personality disorder. Conduct disorder: Aggression against people or animals, property destruction, lying, or theft, serious rules violation before age 13 (truancy, run-away).
Mood Disorders Major depressive disorder Bipolar I or II Dysthymic Mixed episode Hypomanic episode Mood disorder due to medical condition Substance-induced mood disorder	A pattern of illness due to abnormal mood. Episode refers to any period of time the child is abnormally happy or sad.	NOTE: Two conditions with mood symptoms but not mood disorders are adjustment disorder with depressed mood or bereavement.
Anxiety Disorders Panic disorder Agoraphobia Specific phobia Social phobia Obsessive-compulsive disorder PTSD Acute stress disorder Generalized anxiety disorder Anxiety due to medical condition Substance-induced anxiety disorder Anxiety disorder NOS	Child presents with prominent anxiety symptoms. Symptoms produce disability or distress. Co-morbidity is the rule. Anxiety symptoms can be found in a child with most any other Axis I disorder, e.g., as part of mood disorder or in response to separation.	Sudden severe fear or discomfort with somatic symptoms. Anxiety about a place and/or situation and avoids them. Either you have disorder or you don't. Most anxious children do not qualify for a well defined DSM-IV anxiety disorder and are diagnosed as anxiety disorder NOS.
Disorders of Relationship Separation anxiety Reactive attachment of infancy or early childhood Parent-child relational problem Sibling relational problem Problems related to abuse or neglect	Inappropriate and excessive anxiety about separation from home or significant person. Parent-child diagnosis (PCD) is relevant when clinically important symptoms or negative effects on functioning are linked with the way a child and parent interact.	Child reports fear of harm to parent. PCD: When two or more individuals have problem getting along and that behavior is current focus of clinical attention or treatment. No Axis I or II disorder can better explain the behavior. Symptoms last less than 6 months after the end of stressor.

developmental factors, and nursing implications for each of these disorders and other psychiatric disorders of children.

Anxiety Disorders. The most common sign of anxiety in children is fear of being separated from parents and home and refusal to attend school. The prevalence of anxiety is highest at times of transition: moving from preschool to primary school, and from primary to secondary school. Children who

refuse to attend school are usually capable but self-critical students, and most have separation anxiety, being frightened to leave home. The prognosis is good with treatment, but persistent anxiety disorder predicts the development of panic disorder in adulthood.

Depression. Contrary to earlier beliefs, persistent depression occurs in children and becomes progressively more common

ASSESSMENT	DEVELOPMENTAL FACTORS	NURSING IMPLICATIONS
Explore problems of inattention, trouble keeping attention on task or play, listening ability, how child responds to and follows instructions, help needed organizing, is easily distracted and avoids tasks requiring mental effort. Appears "on the go," has trouble sitting quietly, talks excessively, consistently squirms or fidgets, inappropriate running or climbing. Greater emphasis is placed on parent and teacher reports of child's behaviors. Conduct disorder: Before age 10 there is at least one problem of conduct.	Can be difficult to sort from normal toddler and pre-school inattentiveness. Older child may report an inner restlessness.	It is important that the nursing plan of care be based on multiple sources of data and reference resources. Talking with child and parent separately is sometimes helpful. Negativistic behaviors are always challenging.
Use of thorough Mental Status Exam to explore current level of functioning. Explore family history of mood disorder. Environmental precipitants in young child. Recurrence or rehospitalization within 2 years.	Very young child expresses depression through irritability, somatic complaints, or refusal to go to school. Manic symptoms are often misread for hyperactivity of ADHD. School age may have somatic complaints (headache, stomachache, abdominal pain). Delusional content depends on developmental stage. Because child has grown up with the disorder, they may not voluntarily discuss symptoms with parents or teacher.	Full assessment for self-harm and contract for safety. Establish safety environment. Monitor sleeping, eating pattern, medications. Educate child about effects for compliance. Work with parents to foster support for child.
Fears are common in children but in 2%-3% they cause a clinical level of distress. Children generally only relive the traumatic incident in dreams (e.g., monsters or frightening images). Children exhibit compulsions more frequently than obsessions. Although equally affected, boy's symptoms begin at an earlier age than girls.	Children often lack the insight that they feel anxious and express symptoms by clinging, crying, or freezing in position. Important to remember that anxiety is a normal, even useful, emotion that will change from one developmental stage to the next. Young children are especially apt to experience PTSD symptoms by talking less, act out their anxieties.	Be specific when interacting with a child, "Are there things that frighten you? What do you worry about most?" The fears can extend to include situations for parents, friends, siblings, or pets. Avoidance and vigilant behaviors may be noted. This child does not volunteer a lot of information about what they are thinking or feeling.
Examine family history for duration and intensity of current problem. Is the interaction difficulty only with one adult (mother, father) and not all adults? All family members involved should be interviewed. A most common occurrence in child mental health practice.	This area of problem is not considered a mental illness but can become the focus of clinical attention. Developmental stage and norms are key to understanding the family or interpersonal dynamics.	When attention span and activity levels are within normal range, ADHD and disruptive disorders can be ruled out. Assess anger, spite, or loss of temper in exchanges with significant others.

after puberty (Luby et al, 2003; Waslick et al, 2003). Up to 14% of children will experience an episode of major depression before age 15 years. It seriously affects social, emotional, and educational development and is the most important predictor of suicidal behavior in young people age 15 to 24 years.

Although the symptoms of depression in children are similar to those seen in adults, they also usually have irritable mood, may fail to make expected weight gain, and tend to keep secret their depressive thoughts and crying. Depression also can occur in combination with another disorder such as anxiety, conduct disorder, or ADHD. The prognosis is good when the depression is secondary to a life stress and responds to psychological treatment.

Suicide is difficult to predict, but does occur in children as young as 8 years of age. Assessment for suicidal ideation, plans, or attempts is paramount. Data from the National

Household Survey on Drug Abuse reveals that almost 3 million youths 12 to 17 years thought about or attempted suicide during the previous year, and more than a third made an actual suicide attempt. Only one third of those at risk received any mental health care (*Am J Nurs*, 2002).

Risk factors for childhood suicide include depression, sexual abuse, prior suicide ideation or plan, substance abuse, impulsive or aggressive behavior, and access to firearms. Research suggests that the suicidal child is not likely to self-refer or seek help, therefore early identification of at-risk youth is critical. Screening approaches should be carefully considered, especially in instances of co-morbidity and a history of suicide in the child's family. A thorough nursing assessment of a child's mood is the first line of prevention of youth suicide.

Do you think a child as young as age 7 can be suicidal? What symptoms would you look for and where would you seek help in a community setting? ▪

Conduct Disorder. Serious and persistent patterns of disturbed conduct and antisocial behavior predominantly affect boys and comprise the largest group of childhood psychiatric disorders. Conduct disturbance may begin early in childhood as oppositional, aggressive, and defiant behavior, becoming established during the primary school years and increasing after puberty.

Conduct disorder occurs in about 16% of boys and 9% of girls. The sources of etiology include family, biological, and psychosocial factors. The presence of other psychological disorders is common in these children, with about 30% showing ADHD and learning problems. Clinical depression is also found in about 20% of young people with conduct disorder.

Conduct disorder is characterized by a longstanding pattern of violation of rules. Other primary features are aggression toward people or animals, theft, vandalism, running away from home, destruction of property, and lying. The child does not appreciate the importance of the welfare of another and has little guilt or remorse about harming others.

Affective aggression (impulsive, uncontrolled, unplanned, or overt) or predatory aggression (goal-oriented, controlled, planned, or hidden) are observed in children with conduct disorder (Weller et al, 1999). The latter type of aggression has a strong basis in bullying behaviors. Approximately 10% of all children attending school are being bullied, and 20% have experienced at least one incident of bullying (Scott, Hague-Armstrong, and Downes, 2003). The consequences of growing up a bully or a victim can be severe with resulting anxiety, depression, self-esteem problems, and deficits in concentration and school achievement.

This childhood disorder requires vigorous early intervention, assessment, and management because, although about a third of children make a reasonable adjustment, there is evidence that at least half of the young people with serious conduct disorder will continue to experience mental health and psychosocial problems in adult life, such as personality disorder, criminality, and alcoholism. As many as 40% of children

with conduct disorder grow into adults with antisocial personality disorder (Searight, Rottnek, and Abby, 2001).

How would you teach parents to deal with a child who is bullying another child at school? What coping skills would you teach a child who is being bullied? ▪

Attention Deficit/Hyperactivity Disorder. Attention deficit disorder has received considerable attention and study (Landgraf, Rich, and Rappaport, 2002; Gonzalez and Sellers, 2002; American Academy of Pediatrics, 2001; Wagner, 2000; Hoagwood et al, 2000; Olfson et al, 2003). Controversy exists regarding the exact nature and extent of this disorder (see Citing the Evidence). It is estimated that 3% to 5% of children have ADHD, and it is more common in boys than girls. A history of difficult and uneven development from infancy is usually noted. It is likely that the disorder has a neurobiological basis that is complicated by social interactions and the progressive consequences of related learning problems.

Another area of controversy is related to medications; questions have been raised as to whether children are being overdiagnosed and overmedicated to ease problematic school behaviors (Dunne, 2002). Family factors and treatment modalities are the focus of multiple studies, publications, and media attention (CHADD, 2003; Barkley, 2000).

Evidence suggests that the young person does not necessarily grow out of the problem. Symptoms tend to persist, although adolescents usually become more goal-directed and less impulsive, channeling activity into sport or work if the opportunity is possible. The outcome is less favorable for those who have an associated conduct disorder. In these cases

---

▎ CITING THE EVIDENCE ON
Attention Deficit/Hyperactivity Disorder

BACKGROUND: The frequency of occurrence of attention deficit/hyperactivity disorder (ADHD) is in dispute. This uncertainty has contributed to the concern that too many children in the United States are being treated with stimulant medication. This was a study to determine the cumulative incidence of ADHD in a population cohort and to estimate the prevalence of pharmacological treatment for children who meet criteria for ADHD.

RESULTS: The highest estimate of the cumulative incidence at age 19 of ADHD was 16%. The lowest estimate was 7.4%. Prevalence of treatment with stimulant medication was 86.5% for definite ADHD, 40% for probable ADHD, and 6.6% for questionable ADHD.

IMPLICATIONS: These results provide insight into the apparent discrepancies in estimates of the occurrence of ADHD, with less stringent criteria resulting in higher cumulative incidence. Children who met the most stringent criteria for ADHD were most likely to receive pharmacological treatment.

Barbaresi WJ et al: *Arch Pediatr Adolesc Med* 156:217, 2002.

the risk of continued mental health, personality, and social adjustment problems is increased.

The comprehensive treatment of children with ADHD is a long-term process because they typically present with a variety of social deficits, learning disabilities, behavior problems, and depression. The approach after a thorough and careful evaluation must be multimodal with the goal of assisting the child to cope with ADHD and the difficulties it brings to family, school, and social functioning.

Nursing Diagnoses

Regardless of the child's medical diagnosis, nursing care must be focused on the child's response to illness with nursing interventions designed to teach and model to the child and family more adaptive coping responses and improved methods of functioning. Thus nursing diagnosis and intervention proceed independently of and concurrently with medical diagnosis and treatment. Although nursing and medicine have collaborative roles, nursing has a critical and distinct contribution to make in the care of the child with psychiatric illness.

Upon completing the assessment, the nurse synthesizes data gathered and arrives at conclusions about the child's needs, formulating a hierarchical problem list for the child. Such a list would start with the **target symptoms** or behaviors that are posing the most problem for the child. Target symptoms such as inattention, distractibility, affective instability, anxious behaviors, impulsivity, thought disorganization, and aggression are common. More complex areas such as **problems with social skills, problem solving, school performance, behavioral inhibition, and communication require ongoing data gathering.** The **strengths, coping abilities,** and **resilience** of the child also should be identified. Nurses caring for children with mental disorders or behavioral problems should refer to the ACAPN Guidelines for Care and Practice for the accepted practice parameters promoting child mental health and improved functioning (International Society of Psychiatric–Mental Health Nurses, 1998).

Nursing diagnoses can be identified for each psychiatric disorder and related behavioral problem. **Risk for self-directed violence** is always assigned the highest priority. Other nursing diagnoses commonly used in working with children include **chronic low self-esteem, situational low self-esteem, ineffective coping, disturbed thought processes, anxiety, risk for other-directed violence,** and **readiness for enhanced family processes.**

Many people believe that families are in crisis in the United States. Describe the evidence for this conclusion, and give specific ways to address these problems. ■

Risk for Self-Directed Violence. A suicidal child requires the same safety precautions one would take with an adult. Interventions include establishing a risk-free environment, close observation, assisting parents to maintain safety if the child is not hospitalized, pharmacotherapy, and supportive coping and problem-solving interventions based on the child's cognitive abilities.

Chronic or Situational Low Self-Esteem. Children with a mental disorder or behavioral problem often have low self-esteem. It may be expressed by infrequent eye contact, lack of motivation, withdrawal, self-deprecating statements, or the use of negative behavior to seek attention. Specific therapeutic activities can be planned to improve a child's self-esteem. Accomplishment of a goal, no matter how small, is very rewarding, and incremental goal setting can be an effective way to provide opportunities for success. The nurse also can provide information and guidance to parents to help them enhance their child's self-esteem (Table 36-3).

Ineffective Coping. A child's coping is directly related to resilience and prevention of further trauma. Interventions for this diagnosis include psychoeducation, problem solving, strengthening self-control mechanisms, and exploration of options and choices. Reviewing past or hypothetical situations that are threatening can help the child explore alternatives. Through practice and decision making in nonstressful situations, the child is able to identify and enact adaptive responses. Behavioral management with use of play, rehearsal, role-play, and group experiences are excellent tools.

Table 36-3	Enhancing a Child's Self-Esteem
TARGETED AREA	STRATEGY
Caregiver expectations	Describe expectations for the child.
	Assess anticipated developmental milestones.
	Review family patterns and influences.
Personal value	Communicate confidence in the child.
	Structure situations to promote success of the child.
	Implement effective ways of praising the child.
	Role model self-value.
Communication	Listen attentively.
	Encourage openness to feelings.
	Avoid using judgmental statements.
	Elicit different points of view.
Discipline	Use effective methods of limit setting.
	Discuss and implement appropriate consequences.
	Review problem-solving techniques.
	Teach that physical punishment should not be used.
Guidance	Encourage open exchanges with the child.
	Know the child's activities away from home.
	Plan family time and activities together.
	Express interest in school events.
	Become familiar with the child's friends.
Autonomy	Demonstrate respect for the child.
	Promote the child's responsible decision making.
	Expect reciprocal respect.

Disturbed Thought Processes. A child with a mood disorder or a psychosis may have disturbed thought processes evidenced by hallucinations, delusions, and disorganized speech and behavior. Anxious or depressed children often have difficulty thinking, identifying options, and making decisions.

Although rare, children may have psychotic episodes. It is important that the psychiatric nurse be able to discriminate between normal and abnormal thought processes in children. Healthy preschool and school-age children typically have vivid imaginations, and their normal fears can become quite intense; however, these responses should not be confused with psychotic delusions or hallucinations.

Psychotic episodes are distinguished by their level of intensity, distress, and duration. They are terrifying and should be treated as psychiatric emergencies. The nurse intervenes to help the child process information from the environment and administers pharmacotherapy and behavioral modification interventions incorporating these into ongoing activities of daily living (Lambert, 2001).

Anxiety. The most common sign of anxiety in children is fear of being separated from parents and home and refusal to attend school. The prevalence of anxiety is highest at times of transition: moving from preschool to primary school and from primary to secondary school.

Cognitive behavioral therapy (see Chapter 31) is an effective nursing intervention for children who have anxiety (Barrett et. al, 2001). The overall prognosis is good with treatment; however, some untreated and persistent anxiety disorders can evolve into the development of more severe anxiety disorders in adulthood.

Risk for Other-Directed Violence. Being able to handle conflict without becoming aggressive toward oneself or others is very important for children to learn. In contemporary American culture, violence is widespread, and children may perceive it to be an acceptable way of dealing with conflict. Also, with extensive media and television coverage of violent events, children may become numb to feelings related to violence. Therefore alternatives such as anger management must be taught so that a child will have a repertoire of solutions to use in conflict situations (see Chapter 30).

A brief time-out may be effective in interrupting behavior that is escalating or becoming out of control. During these periods of being alone, it may be helpful for a child to read a story about a similar conflict or for an older child to write thoughts and feelings in a journal. Another useful strategy is to establish a contract with a child who is capable of understanding, writing, and adhering to it. Such a contract would identify the consequences that the child would face, based on the specific behavior. Contracts allow the child to play an active role in the treatment process and provide immediate and constructive feedback about the child's actions.

What sociocultural changes could be made to curtail the growing violence among the youth of the United States? ■

Readiness for Enhanced Family Processes. Each family has an extensive history that has shaped the development of each family member. This collective family history and its adaptability for change have a powerful influence on a child's prognosis for learning, practicing, and applying new skills. Therefore the family's willingness to participate in the therapeutic process and interest in making change should guide the nursing intervention for the child.

During parent education, a nurse models the effective use of reinforcement, communication, and behavior management techniques identified in Box 36-4. The parents are then expected to practice these techniques with their child during the course of treatment.

Do you think the strategies for behavior management of children described in Box 36-4 are culture bound or culture free? Defend your position. ■

■ PLANNING

The baseline impairment and co-morbid conditions needing to be monitored must be included in the plan of care. The plan is usually multimodal and may involve medications, psychosocial supports (after school programs, big brother mentoring), psychoeducational interventions (e.g., coping skills, problem-solving exercises, role play), and individual or group therapy.

Often a child's maladaptive responses are expressed differently from those of an adult. To develop the nursing plan, the

---

BOX 36-4

Strategies for Behavior Management of Children

- Respond warmly to a child's positive behaviors.
- Communicate approval by facial expression, tone of voice, and touch.
- Express excitement regarding a child's accomplishments.
- Ignore negative behavior whenever appropriate.
- Refrain from giving unnecessary commands.
- Respond calmly but effectively to negative behaviors (e.g., "No yelling," stated in a calm tone of voice).
- Use time-outs when necessary and appropriate (30 to 60 seconds per year of a child's age). This should be done in a nonpunitive manner and presented as a way to help the child gain control or use problem-solving techniques.
- Avoid making unrealistic demands of a child.
- Avoid negative remarks about the child.
- Communicate often, using the following techniques:
  - The parent or staff member telling about personal experiences.
  - The parent or staff member listening, paraphrasing, and asking follow-up questions.
  - Nightly review of positive behaviors noted during the day that the parent wants to be repeated. (Negative behaviors should not be mentioned at this time.)

nurse must learn to recognize and describe symptomatic behavior in children. The nurse should talk with the child about the child's strengths and then discuss the skills that need further development. Strategies used to teach these skills can be explained to the parents, which allows them to become active participants in the planning of nursing care.

Children will be more motivated to cooperate if they are encouraged to sign a copy of their care plan after it has been explained to them. Even if they cannot write, a mark that represents their name is sufficient to signify their participation in the process. Nursing interventions can then be designed to improve the maladaptive responses and teach the accompanying skill.

Leading children to understanding their resilient coping ability is a primary intervention for child psychiatric nurses. A child's effective coping behaviors include several possibilities:

- Withdrawing from the stressful situations
- Postponing an immediate response
- Finding a more manageable situation
- Restructuring (manipulating or shaping) the environment
- Accepting both good and bad as part of everyday life
- Working toward maintaining optimal conditions of adjustment, security, and comfort

The child's resilience and ability to make sense of stressors needs to be the foundation for designing and implementing interventions. Although changed by experiences and sometimes forced to invest enormous energy in surviving and coping, children can and do bounce back. The nurse's task is to find ways to enhance resilience and promote healthy development.

Settings

A variety of settings are available for the delivery of child mental health care. They range from inpatient hospitalization, which is the most restrictive and expensive, to the least restrictive settings of community programs or foster care treatment. These various treatment options are described in Table 36-4.

■ IMPLEMENTATION

Once a thorough assessment has been completed and nursing diagnoses have been formulated, the nurse can implement a variety of individualized interventions that are effective in treating maladaptive responses. Nursing interventions also can be identified for each ego competency skill deficit and developmental stage as summarized in Table 36-5.

Therapeutic Play

Because play is normal and fun for children, it is a very effective tool for nurses to use. Interventions that are enjoyable, arouse curiosity, and stimulate the imagination will capture the child's attention and interest. Many children with psychiatric problems may have lost interest in play or may have never experienced the joy of spontaneous play.

Learning to play is critical not only to a child's development but also to mental health. Therapeutic aspects of play and their beneficial outcomes are listed in Table 36-6. The nurse should keep these elements in mind when incorporating play therapy into the plan of care (Kaduson and Schaefer, 2001).

The first step is for the nurse to develop a therapeutic alliance and trust with the child so that life can be perceived from the child's perspective and the child's concerns can be anticipated. When a child feels understood and safe, participation in therapeutic play with the nurse is common. If the child is anxious, his or her developmental level, which may fluctuate rapidly, should be continuously assessed by the nurse. Care must be taken to ensure that the child does not fail at the activity, either because the developmental level is too advanced or because of the severity of the child's symptoms. Children will become easily frustrated with play that is too difficult and thus feel a sense of failure when their self-esteem is already compromised.

Toys that are age appropriate and imaginative should be offered to a child. These may include blocks, a play-house, family characters, soldiers, trucks, and rescue vehicles. The child is then encouraged to begin play without specific direction from the nurse. The nurse may ask the following clarifying questions:

- What is this person doing?
- How does this little boy feel?
- What is happening now?

The nurse can then follow up with some clarifying and validating statements such as, "This little girl looks afraid." The nurse refrains from guiding the play, making unnecessary remarks, or making interpretations that may link the play to the child's life experience. The play should continue for the allotted time. The nurse can then evaluate the play intervention by considering the following questions:

- What did the play activity communicate about the child's developmental level?
- What emotions and behavioral responses were demonstrated while at play?
- What information can be added to the child's assessment or treatment plan based on observations made during play therapy?

What do you think is meant by the phrase "play is the work of children"? ■

Pharmacotherapy

Experts see psychopharmacology as one among many tools available for treating children with psychiatric disorders. They advocate thoughtfulness and restraint in the prescribing of psychotropic drugs and the judicious use of diagnostic labels. They also encourage conceptualizing all childhood disorders within a developmental framework (Martin et al, 2003).

It is important for nurses to realize that children metabolize and eliminate medications more rapidly than adults. Although initial doses may be low, doses can ultimately be as high as those given to adults, requiring frequent clinical and

Table 36-4 Treatment Options for Children and Adolescents

Treatment Option	Goal	Usual Length of Treatment	Cost	Characteristics
Outpatient treatment	For child and family to receive treatment once or twice a week	Can be short-term (4-6 weeks) or long-term (1-3 years)	One of the least expensive options	Least disruptive to family unit Allows clinician to address ongoing problems related to family and school Keeps child or adolescent in contact with peer group
In-home treatment	To provide brief, intensive mental health services in a specific crisis	Short-term (4-6 weeks) Used mainly for specific periods of crisis or stress	One of the least expensive options	May be slightly disruptive to family life as all members will be asked to attend therapy at specific times Allows clinician to observe how all family members are responding to the crisis
Special education program	To provide the child or adolescent with a positive learning experience with specially trained teachers and to provide an on-site mental health clinician	Long-term (2-5 years)	One of the least expensive options	More intensive than simple outpatient treatment Disrupts normal school environment and possibly peer relationships
Day treatment or partial hospitalization	To provide the child or adolescent with treatment in a structured environment for a portion of the day	Short-term (a few months) or long-term (a couple of years)	Moderately expensive; may be offset by insurance	More intensive than simple outpatient treatment Allows child or adolescent to maintain family and peer group contact Can be an after school program or combined with a special education program May be associated with some stigmatization
Respite care	To provide the parents or caretakers with time off	Short-term (2 weeks-2 months)	Moderately expensive	Provides a break for child or adolescent and parents or caretakers Provides clinician with an opportunity to use intensive individual therapy with the child or adolescent
Foster care	To remove the child or adolescent from a dysfunctional home and to place him/her with foster parents who have been specially trained to work with children	Short-term (a few months during crisis times) or long-term (years)	Moderately expensive	Removal from even the most dysfunctional home can result in a major disruption in the child's life Child or adolescent can continue to attend regular or similar school, or if necessary, a special education program can be incorporated into care Provides the child or adolescent with a more normal, predictable family atmosphere Professional mental health clinicians are available to support the foster parents and reduce burnout

Group home care	To place the child with 10-12 other children who live in a structured, supervised residence	Long-term (several years)	Moderately expensive	Separation from family and peers can result in a major disruption in the child's or adolescent's life Less home-like than foster care Child or adolescent must adapt to group home norms and follow rules established in the home Most group homes have a treatment philosophy, such as behavior modification Usually operated by a childcare agency that is responsible for training the house parents, providing supervision, and providing a full range of mental health services as needed by the children or adolescents
Residential treatment center	To place the child in a center that functions like a therapeutic community in a campus-like, multiple-residence setting	Long-term (several years)	Moderately to very expensive	Separation from family and peers can result in a major disruption in the child's or adolescent's life Less home-like than other options House parents and multidisciplinary teams are available 24 hours Most centers use therapeutic milieu and behavior modification techniques to influence changes in behavior Children or adolescents who are placed in these centers usually have failed at other levels of treatment intervention and have chronic and multiple mental health problems; they are usually know to social services, mental health agencies, or juvenile justice agencies
Inpatient hospitalization	To provide safe mental health care under direct medical and nursing supervision in a secure setting	Short-term (a few days to a couple of weeks; stabilization for inpatient crisis treatment or evaluation)	Most expensive; may be offset by insurance	Results in the most direct disruption of the child's life Many units are locked or geographically very distant from the family Schooling is on-site and is usually a special education program Regimented schedule of daily activities assists in providing a structured environment Usual treatment philosophy is a traditional medical model with behavior modification and therapeutic milieu techniques incorporated Children are placed in these settings when they are considered a potential harm to themselves or others Contact with family members is structured and monitored

Modified from O'Brien PG, Kennedy WZ, Ballard KA: *Psychiatric nursing: an integration of theorist practice*, New York, 1999, McGraw-Hill Nursing Core Series.

Table 36-5 **Ego Competency Skills Summary**

Competency Skill	Developmental Stage	Developmental Tasks	Nursing Care for Skill Deficit
Trusting, closeness, relationship building	Infancy	Trust Attachment Learning to walk, talk, and feed self	Encourage interaction. Use face-to-face positioning. Use touch (when appropriate) and nurturance. Offer food and transitional objects. Be attentive without being unnecessarily intrusive. Offer nurturance to the child's mother. Make attempts to connect family to child. Take time to develop relationship through play.
Handling separation and independence	Toddlers	Autonomy Separation Toilet training Learning right from wrong	Offer frequent exercise and motor activities. Allow child opportunities to make choices. Offer transitional object. Take control if child is out of control; otherwise let child have some control. Set limits and boundaries to help the child feel secure.
Handling joint decisions and interpersonal conflicts	Preschoolers	Initiative Tolerance of others Sexual identity Socialization Developing a conscience	Set up opportunities for problem solving and cooperative thinking. Help child identify fears through books, art, play. Shape appropriate socialization using reinforcement. Become model for conflict resolution.
Dealing with frustration and unfavorable events Celebrating good things, feeling pleasure	Middle childhood	Industry Physical skill development Peer relationships Learning to read, write, and calculate Development of morality and values	Help the child cope with frustration using stories and plays. Model cooperation and reinforce cooperative behavior. Do not use shame or humiliate to gain control. Have fun with the child. Use community meetings for peer support and modeling. Use positive reinforcement for child's strengths and abilities.
Working for delayed gratification	Early adolescence	Identity Role acceptance	Use daily expectations and games to teach delayed gratification. Encourage self-reinforcement.
Relaxing and playing		New relations with peers of both sexes	Encourage playfulness at appropriate times.
Cognitive processing	Later adolescence	Emotional and economic independence from parents	Offer games that use cognitive processing. Discuss abstractions such as the moral of stories or movies.
Adaptive sense of direction and purpose		Preparation for occupation Civic responsibility	Actively listen to and encourage the expression of needs and goals. In community meetings discuss relevant issues and life events. Help the child realistically assess his or her ability and potential.

laboratory follow-up. Pychopharmacological treatment is increasingly being prescribed for children. Some reports indicate significant benefit, but studies of these drugs in children are still relatively few in number. Only limited indications for their use with children have been approved by the Food and Drug Administration (FDA).

Psychiatric disorders are recognized in the pediatric population and evidence exists of substantial use of psychotropic medications in this age-group, including those of preschool age (Zito et al, 2000). Antianxiety, antidepressants, mood stabilizers, and antipsychotics are all used to treat psychiatric disorders in children. These drugs are described in Chapter 27.

Without awareness of the reality of childhood psychiatric illness and the impact it can have on normal growth and de-

velopment, a myth persists that psychotropic drugs should not be used with children. This misperception may, in fact, do harm in delaying parents and professionals from making informed treatment choices for children (Jensen, Edelman, and Nemeroff, 2003).

The regional, professional, and demographic variations are substantial in regard to actual prescribing patterns and practices. Stimulants and antidepressants are the most commonly prescribed psychotropic medications. The most dramatic increase has been in stimulants prescribed primarily for children with ADHD (Jensen, Edelman, and Nemeroff, 2003).

Psychotropics are currently approved for specific syndromes (e.g., conduct disorder, ADHD, major depressive dis-

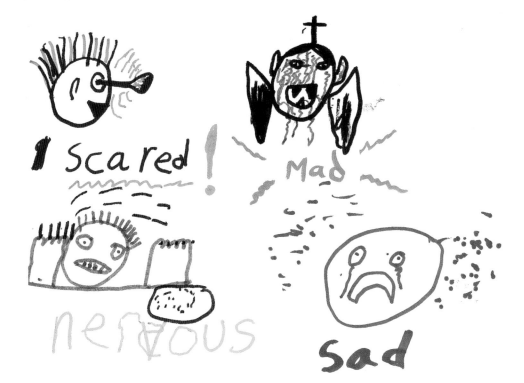

Figure 36-1   Drawing by a hospitalized 6-year-old boy of his different feelings.

Table 36-6	Therapeutic Aspects of Play
THERAPEUTIC FACTOR	BENEFICIAL OUTCOME
Overcoming resistance	Working alliance
Communication	Understanding
Competence	Self-esteem
Creative thinking	Problem solving
Catharsis	Emotional release
Abreaction	Perspective on traumatic event
Role playing	Learning new behaviors
Fantasy	Compensation and sublimation
Teaching through metaphors	Insight
Relationship enhancement	Trust in others
Mastering developmental fears	Growth and development
Game play	Socialization

Modified from Schaefer C: *The therapeutic powers of play*, Northvale, NJ, 1993, Jason Aronson.

order) rather than for nonspecific symptoms (e.g., anxiety, depression, psychosis, or aggression). A major child psychopharmacology challenge is to better define the effectiveness and safety of these medications for the child population.

The psychiatric nurse should consult child psychopharmacology resources (Martin et al, 2003; Green, 2001) for guidance on the safe and effective administration of these medications. Psychiatric nurses must be knowledgeable about these medications and must develop interventions to monitor, educate, and evaluate medication effects with children and their families.

Nurses also should be aware that promoting a child's knowledge of medications can have a positive effect on self-esteem and feelings of control and self-worth, as well as enhance compliance. Thus numerous therapeutic outcomes can be achieved by effective medication teaching.

Expressive Therapies

The term expressive therapy applies to any mode that uses the child's creative process to facilitate self-expression and self-awareness. Any medium can be used, such as painting, singing, dance, movement, or writing. The goal is the process not the product.

This area allows for many creative nursing interventions. A variety of puppet, art, graphics, and audiovisual materials can be used to successfully teach and prepare children for managing their medications and their illness. Peer group participation is particularly effective in helping children describe common experiences, decrease their sense of isolation, and enhance their responses to the teaching materials. Through imaginative but goal-directed nursing interventions, children can learn important information and experience greater control over the treatment of their illness and their future mental health.

Art is particularly useful in assessing a child's therapeutic needs. Drawing is a valuable tool for children to use in describing an event or expressing a feeling (Figure 36-1). Children often do not have the vocabulary to express themselves, and they feel pressured to answer questions they do not understand. Through drawings, a child can provide information about behavior and developmental maturity that the nurse can then use to help the child in preparing for future change.

Children may find that a nondirected art activity helps with stress reduction. With some encouragement they will usually produce an interesting and often revealing picture. The nurse might ask the child what is happening in the picture or to name the people in it. The nurse should make notes about whatever the child reports the people are saying or thinking. This process can be continued over several separate encounters.

In evaluating the effectiveness of this intervention, the nurse should consider the following:

- What was learned about the child's experience, view of the world, and perceptions from this intervention?
- Is there any distortion between the child's perception of personal experience and what was depicted in the exercise?

Bibliotherapy

Bibliotherapy is the use of literature to help children identify and express feelings within the structure and safety of the nurse-patient relationship. Because children actively engage in imaginary thinking, they can easily identify with the fictional characters in a story and gain insight into their own lives.

The child's age, developmental level, and attention span are key factors in selection of reading material. To be effective the story should have illustrations and content that lend to exploring how to cope with everyday problems. The nurse also should think about the child's situation and try to select a book that describes a situation or issue relevant to the child's life situation.

While reading the story, the nurse should be sensitive to the child's response. If the text is wordy, the child may become bored or distracted. If this occurs, paraphrasing the story or asking what the child thinks is happening to the characters may be helpful. In this way the child's imagination becomes engaged, and the experience will have value. It is also important to give the child an opportunity to reflect on the story and discuss any thoughts or feelings about the characters because it is often easier for a child to talk about the feelings of the characters than about his or her own feelings.

After reading the story, the nurse should evaluate the usefulness of the intervention and assess the following:

- Was the story appropriate to the child's developmental age?
- Was the child engaged with the story?
- Did the child enjoy the experience?
- What was learned by the child and about the child as a result of this intervention?

Traditional fairy tales are based on and convey many gender stereotypes. Do you think this is a problem, and how might you go about dealing with this issue in working with children? ▪

Children's Games

Children with behavioral disorders often have difficulty with motor control. Games that teach motor control can be helpful to these children. Such games include Simon Says, Red Light, Musical Chairs, and many others. Games also can be used to increase a child's concentration and frustration tolerance. Games such as Candy Land, Hide and Seek, and Find

the Button can be played with gradually increasing difficulty to teach these skills.

When initiating these activities, the nurse should consider the child's motor development and level of anxiety and choose among games that engage large or small muscle groups. Thought also should be given to the child's tolerance for frustration and competition. Games may then be modified to meet the specific therapeutic needs of the child. Games also can be played in a way that requires the child to use increasing levels of concentration and cognitive processing; however, it is important to stop playing a game when it appears to be too difficult or stressful for a child. The nurse should consider the following questions at the completion of the game:

- Was the game developmentally appropriate for the child?
- Was playing the game a pleasurable experience? If not, why not?
- Was the nurse's therapeutic goal met?
- How should the game be modified in the future to further the child's skill development and adaptive coping responses?

Storytelling

The therapeutic use of storytelling for relieving distress and teaching new coping skills is a valuable intervention. Because children do not separate imaginary experiences from real experiences, stories that teach appropriate problem-solving skills can serve as models for real situations.

Initially the nurse must identify a social skill that the child needs to learn, such as assertiveness. The nurse may make up a story about a character who needs that particular skill, giving the hero or heroine characteristics similar to those of the child. It is important to select an ending to the story that will guide the child in learning the skill. The story should be told using animated facial expressions and expressive voice inflections, and the child should be actively involved in the story as much as possible. At the end of the story, the nurse should ask the child about the story and how it made the child feel. This may then lead to a broader discussion of other aspects of the child's life. In evaluating the outcome of the intervention, the nurse should consider the following questions:

- Could this character be used to teach this child other skills through other stories?
- Could the child add to the story or make up one of his or her own?
- What was the moral of the story, and how did it apply to the child?
- Could the story be used in other creative ways, such as by having the child enact the story or by including others?

Cognitive Behavioral Therapy

Cognitive behavioral therapy (CBT) attempts to correct cognitive distortions, particularly negative conceptions of self (see Chapter 31). It can enhance a child's sense of self-control and begin to nurture healthy problem-solving skills.

Nurses can use cognitive techniques to determine the basis for faulty assumptions, cognitive distortions, or errors in reasoning. For example, a child may describe details of a situation that is taken out of context, being inappropriately blamed for particular events (personalization) or dichotomous thinking that does not allow for intermediate positions.

CBT helps the child test dysfunctional cognitions and change behavior using homework assignments such as structuring time, increasing certain activities, or carrying out exercises related to specific situations. For young children, one can use methods of "the smart thoughts man" or the "bad thoughts monster" to work with distorted perceptions about competence, appearance, or depression (Leahy, 1988).

Milieu Management

An important role of the child psychiatric nurse is the organization, management, and integration of multiple treatment interventions with the child throughout the continuum of care, such as in the inpatient setting, day treatment program, or intensive in-home intervention. The developmental needs of children in a psychiatric milieu are complex and dynamic. The design of the unit and treatment philosophy should provide the context of treatment within a safe, caring environment. A planned program of activities is essential for safe milieu management. Family participation and support from the staff are also essential for successful treatment outcomes.

With escalating aggression among children, the management of a therapeutic milieu in any of these settings is very challenging. The child's day must be organized into manageable time units that are age appropriate, with specific but varied activities being assigned to each time unit. For example, younger children's development requires that they be assigned shorter time units, and large motor activities should be scheduled to follow periods of sitting or after therapy sessions, which might produce anxiety.

Whenever possible, children should be assigned to a small group with specific staff members. A schedule should be set up in advance that is predictable from one day to the next. Staff consistency and predictability are very important.

Transitioning from one activity to the next is often difficult for children; therefore a transitional object such as a reward sheet of stickers that is carried from one activity to the next can be helpful. Before leaving one activity, the child should be prepared for the next activity. Helping children anticipate what is expected of them in the next time period will help them better manage their anxiety.

Anxiety and aggression in any setting can be contagious, and they can escalate abruptly. Nurses should be prepared to act quickly and decisively if a child becomes aggressive. If this occurs, the child who is aggressive or anxious must be separated from children who are in control of their behavior. When nursing interventions structure the environment, aggressive behavior will begin to de-escalate, the child can be helped to regain control, and the process of learning about why this occurred can begin.

A carefully planned milieu schedule anticipates problems, creates solutions, and capitalizes on the strengths and energy of the children. Keeping the milieu safe and therapeutic is a high priority for child psychiatric nursing intervention. Ongoing clinical supervision and peer review improve communication and collaboration among staff members. These activities allow staff to evaluate and refine their therapeutic skills and facilitate goal-directed interactions with children (Delaney, 1999).

Seclusion and Restraint. The use of seclusion and restraint in psychiatric inpatient care is controversial (see Critical Thinking About Contemporary Issues). The debate of ethical appropriateness continues, as do questions about the power and control of adults over children (Mohr and Anderson, 2001). The nurse is directed by the ethical principle of beneficence and the obligation to do no harm and to minimize any unintended adverse consequences of an intervention. Thus alternative, less restrictive interventions are recommended (Allen, 2000).

It is clear that psychiatric nurses encounter children with out-of-control behaviors. If seclusion or restraint is indicated, it is important for the nurse to clearly communicate with the child about the seclusion process, the nurse's intent, and how it will help the child, and alternatives that can be used in the future. The best practice in these situations is to intervene early in the escalation process, allowing the patient to choose

Critical Thinking *About* Contemporary Issues

Is the Use of Seclusion and Restraints With Children Therapeutic?

The use of seclusion and restraint in the care and treatment of children with psychiatric problems has been the subject of considerable debate. Advocates of these techniques cite the widespread problem of violent behavior among psychiatric patients, including children, and describe the clinical efficacy of these interventions.

In fact, seclusion and restraint are used in inpatient settings by nurses who are the front-line professionals responsible for initiating emergency procedures and supervising the actions taken to prevent violent outbursts. However, these interventions also have been associated with punishment, custodial care, and institutional abuse and neglect. Some even view seclusion as a violation of a patient's civil liberties.

A number of alternatives can be used by nurses when dealing with dangerous, inappropriate behavior by children, including aggressive, destructive, and highly disruptive behavior. First, nurses can teach and reinforce acceptable ways for children to express themselves and satisfy their needs. Second, nurses can use less restrictive interventions such as time-outs, therapeutic holding, room programs, or open-door seclusion to reduce inappropriate behavior. Third, nurses should evaluate the effect of these interventions on the child and continuously monitor the efficacy of these interventions in research studies using objective measures and experimental controls.

As with all other nursing interventions, the therapeutic value of seclusion and restraints for children is determined by the treatment goals, context of care, and respect shown by the nurse for the needs of the child and family.

to respond to less restrictive options (Kozub and Skidmore, 2001; ACAPN, 2000).

■ EVALUATION

Evaluation of outcomes is accomplished through child self report, nurse observation, reports from significant others, and the use of behavioral rating scales. Compliance issues can be supported through formal psychoeducation of both child and parents or caregiver. These sessions include such aspects of care as expected and unexpected responses to the treatment, how to access help for unusual responses or concerns, and when symptomatic improvement should be seen.

Finally, it is important for nurses to realize that systems of effective care for children with psychiatric illness do exist but not enough are available to meet the existing need. Thus child psychiatric nurses must continue to carry the advocacy banner for children.

COMPETENT CARING

A Clinical Exemplar of a Psychiatric Nurse
EDILMA L. YEARWOOD, PhD, APRN, BC

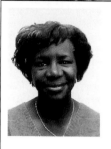

P was 7 years old when he first entered the mental health system. He attempted to set fire to a laundry basket after his mother was hospitalized for a suicide attempt secondary to exacerbation of her symptoms of schizophrenia and depression. P's father abandoned the family when P was 2 years old. His mother had been hospitalized six times by the time he entered the mental health system. Between the ages of 7 and 9, P began having more difficulty concentrating and completing tasks in school, became oppositional at the foster home, was unable to make friends, frequently isolated himself, and talked about feeling "sad." He was described as "under socialized" and "regressed." He was hospitalized after the foster parents became concerned about his preoccupation with morbid thoughts and his overt aggression towards them. He did well while in the hospital and was discharged to a group home on imipramine.

I got to know P while he was in the day hospital treatment program. He was placed in a classroom with eight other children, staffed by two adults. He participated in a boys' socialization group once a week led by a nurse and a psychiatric technician. In addition, I began to see him in individual therapy twice a week. On several occasions during this time he acted out in class and went "on strike" by refusing to do school work. Several behavioral care plans aimed at shaping more socially appropriate behaviors in P were unsuccessful. He was then taken off all medications and sent for a neurological work-up after an episode where he was observed with minor eye blinking and subsequent "staring off" behaviors. His EEG indicated spiking epileptiform changes, and he was placed on divalproex sodium (Depakote).

During this time the content of his conversations became increasingly loose, disorganized, and psychotic. He was passively suicidal, began talking about voices that he had been experiencing, and became increasingly preoccupied with wanting to see his mother. He was then placed on divided doses of risperidone along with Depakote. As the content of his conversations improved, he was paired with other children on the unit for time-limited activities such as board games, cooking activities, and a "managing your feelings" group. At the same time, I began to attend planning meetings with other agencies who had been working with his mother in her treatment. Structured and supervised meetings at the day hospital were set up for P to visit with his mother. After each visit, he appeared brighter, performed better in the classroom, and acted in a more age-appropriate fashion.

Eventually he began to have overnight visits with his mother who was living in the community and attending a sheltered day program herself while receiving support from an intensive case manager. I scheduled home visits to have sessions with P and his mother together during these brief stays in order to more fully evaluate their relationship. I also worked with them to build social skills and better manage their respective psychiatric symptoms. I taught P's mother parenting skills, limit setting, and management of P's medication.

I also continued to meet with the community agencies that would be responsible for supporting and monitoring both of them once they could be permanently reunited. The number of days that P and his mother spent together unsupervised increased as neither displayed any major problems from the increased contact. Although expectations concerning school performance continued to be a struggle for P, he was having fewer episodes of acting out in the classroom and was happy about establishing friendships with several of his peers.

P remained in the day program for 6 months after reuniting with his mother so that he could continue in a known, structured, and supportive environment where the nurse could assess his needs and progress. My own ongoing intensive case management and eventual referral of P to a therapist in his own community allowed this particularly vulnerable child to attain a new, more hopeful place in the world. ■

CHAPTER **FOCUS POINTS**

- Today, 9% to 13% of children have some type of mental disorder, but only 25% to 36% of them receive treatment.
- Psychiatric services are offered to children in a wide variety of settings. Nurses function in these settings by assessing a child's competency skills and providing interventions to teach the skills that are deficient.
- Assessment of the child requires a biopsychosocial approach with a focus on the nine ego skills that all children need to become competent adults.

- Four of the most common medical diagnoses of childhood are anxiety, depression, conduct disorders, and ADHD. Nursing diagnoses relate to each ego competency skill deficit.
- Psychiatric nurses implement a variety of therapeutic treatment modalities when caring for children, including therapeutic play, art therapy, games, bibliotherapy, storytelling, autogenic storytelling, pharmacotherapy, milieu management, and psychotherapy.

KEY TERMS

bibliotherapy, 748
expressive therapy, 747
resilience, 730

CHAPTER REVIEW QUESTIONS

1. Indicate whether the following statements are true (T) or false (F).

_____ A. Mental disorders are rare in children, averaging less than 1% of the population.

_____ B. The first child guidance clinics were established in the United States in the 1930s.

_____ C. Nursing care of children with mental or behavioral disorders is focused on their appropriate developmental level regardless of psychiatric diagnosis.

_____ D. Nurses who take care of children who are suicidal can ignore the child's death statements as being fantasy.

_____ E. Young children who exhibit overt aggressive behavior should be physically restrained in order to not reinforce the behavior.

_____ F. The first goal of communication with a child is to get him or her to respect adults.

2. Fill in the blanks.

A. About _____ of the children who need psychiatric treatment in the United States currently do not receive it.

B. If a child becomes upset when away from his or her mother, it may indicate problems of _____.

C. When completing a mental status examination with a child, reports of hallucinations and suicidal ideation require

_____.

D. _____ is the use of literature to help children identify and express feelings.

E. _____ is a therapeutic activity in which the child participates in developmentally normal activity that stimulates the imagination and captures interest.

F. Reporting child abuse is a _____ and

_____ issue for nurses.

G. The four common psychiatric disorders in childhood are

_____, _____,

_____, and _____.

3. Provide short answers for the following questions.

A. What resiliency characteristics are associated with successful transition from childhood?

B. Identify areas that parents can target to enhance a child's self-esteem.

C. Television networks are now rating television programs for violence and nudity, and new technologies are allowing parents to block the viewing of certain programs. Do you think this will have a significant impact on the upbringing of children? Why or why not?

D. It has been said that children have a low priority in contemporary American society. Learn about how two other countries provide for the health, education, and welfare of their children and compare them to the United States.

Visit Evolve for additional resources related to the content of this chapter.
http://evolve.elsevier.com/Stuart/principles/
• Topical Course Outline • Student Workbook Exercises • Critical Thinking Questions and Activities • Case Studies • Research Topics
• Monthly Content Updates • WebLinks

Student Study CD-ROM

Access the accompanying CD-ROM for animations, interactive exercises, review questions for the NCLEX examination, and an audio glossary.

REFERENCES

American Academy of Pediatrics, Subcommittee on Attention-Deficit/Hyperactivity Disorder and committee on Quality Improvement: Clinical practice guideline: Treatment of school-aged child with attention-deficit/hyperactivity disorder, *Pediatrics* 108:1033, 2001.

American Journal of Nursing: Thoughts of suicide rampant among youths, *Am J Nurs* 102:18, 2002.

Association of Child and Adolescent Psychiatric Nurses (ACAPN): *A position on the rights of children in treatment settings*, Philadelphia, 2001, Author, Division ISPN.

Association of Child and Adolescent Psychiatric Nurses (ACAPN): *Position statement on the use of restraint and seclusion*, Philadelphia, 2000, International Society of Psychiatric–Mental Health Nurses.

Allen JJ: Seclusion and restraint of children: a literature review, *J Child Adolesc Psychiatr Nurs* 13:159, 2000.

American Psychiatric Association: *Diagnostic and statistical manual mental disorders*, ed 4, text revision, Washington, DC, 2000, American Psychiatric Association.

Barkley RA: *Taking charge of ADHD: the complete authoritative guide for parents*, New York, 2000, Guilford Press.

Barrett PM et al: Cognitive-behavioral treatment of anxiety disorders in children: long-term (6-year) follow-up, *J Consult Clin Psychol* 69:135, 2001.

Brazelton TB: *What every child knows*, Boston, 1984, Addison-Wesley.

Children and adults with attention deficit/hyperactivity (CHADD): National Resource Center on AD/HD, www.CHADD.org, 10/10/2003.

Delaney K: Time-out: an overused and misused milieu intervention, *J Child Adolesc Psychiatr Nurs* 12:53, 1999.

Delaney KR, Belmonte-Mann F: Identifying the mental health needs of preschool children, *J School Nurs* 7:222, 2001.

Dunne M: Is Ritalin the answer? Strong clinical skills can prevent misuse of the drug, *Am J Nurs* 102:22, 2002.

Erikson, E: *Identity, youth and crisis*, New York, 1968, WW Norton.

Finke L et al: Survival against drugs: education for school-age children, *J Child Adolesc Psychiatr Nurs* 15:163, 2002.

Gonzalez LO, Sellers EW: The effects of a stress-management program on self-concept, locus of control, and the acquisition of coping skills in school-age children diagnosed with attention deficit hyperactivity disorder, *J Child Adolesc Psychiatr Nurs* 15:5, 2002.

Green WH: *Child and adolescent clinical psychopharmacology*, ed 3, Philadelphia, 2001, Lippincott, Williams & Wilkins.

Hendren RL, DeBacker I, Pandina GJ: Review of neuroimaging studies of child and adolescent psychiatric disorders from the past 10 years, *J Am Acad Child Adolesc Psychiatry* 39:815, 2000.

Hoagwood K et al: Evidence-based practice in child and adolescent mental health services, *Psychiatr Serv* 52:1179, 2001.

Hoagwood K et al: Treatment services for children with ADHD: a national perspective, *J Am Acad Child Adolesc Psychiatry* 39:198, 2000.

International Society of Psychiatric–Mental Health Nurses: *Association of Child and Adolescent Psychiatric Nurses (ACAPN) guidelines for care and practice*, Philadelphia, 1998, Author.

Jensen P, Edelman A, Nemeroff R: Pediatric psychopharmacoepidemiology: who is prescribing? And for who, how, and why? In Martin A et al, editors: *Pediatric psychopharmacology: principles and practice*, New York, 2003, Oxford University Press.

Kaduson HG, Schaefer CE, editors: *101 More favorite play therapy techniques*, New Jersey, 2001, Jason Aronson.

Kohlberg L: Kohlberg's stages of moral development. In Crain WC: *Theories of development: concepts and applications*, ed 4, New York, 1999, Prentice Hall.

Kozub ML, Skidmore R: Least to most restrictive interventions: a continuum for mental health care facilities, *J Psychosoc Nurs* 39:33, 2001.

Lambert LT: Identification and management of schizophrenia in childhood, *J Child Adolesc Psychiatr Nurs* 14:73, 2001.

Landgraf JM, Rich M, Rappaport L: Measuring quality of life in children with attention deficit/hyperactivity disorder and their families: development and evaluation of a new tool, *Arch Pediatr Adolesc Med* 156:384, 2002.

Leahy RL: Cognitive therapy of childhood depression: developmental considerations. In Shirk SR, editor: *Cognitive development and child psychotherapy*, New York, 1988, Plenum Publishing.

Lubit R et al: Impact of trauma on children, *J Psychiatr Pract* 9:128, 2003.

Luby JL et al: The clinical picture of depression in preschool children, *J Am Acad Child Adolesc Psychiatry* 42:340, 2003.

Mandleco B, Peery JC: An organization framework for conceptualizing resilience in children, *J Child Adolesc Psychiatr Nurs* 13:99, 2000.

Martin A et al: *Pediatric psychopharmacology: principles and practice*, New York, 2003, Oxford University Press.

Mohr WK, Anderson JA: Faulty assumptions associated with the use of restraints with children, *J Child Adolesc Psychiatr Nurs* 14:141, 2001.

Morrison J, Anders TF: *Interviewing children and adolescents: skills and strategies for effective DSM-IV diagnosis*, New York, 1999, Guilford Press.

Murray C, Lopez A: *The global burden of disease: a comprehensive assessment of mortality and disability from disease, injuries, and risk factors in 1990 and projected to 2020*, Cambridge, Mass, 1996, Harvard University Press.

Mylant M et al: Adolescent children of alcoholics: vulnerable or resilient? *J Am Psychiatr Nurs Assoc* 8:57, 2002.

Olfson M et al: National trends in the treatment of attention deficit hyperactivity disorder, *Am J Psychiatry* 160:1071, 2003.

Paris J: The primacy of early experience: a critique, an alternative, and some clinical implications, *J Psychiatr Pract* 6:147, 2000.

Piaget J: *The origins of intelligence in children*, New York, 1952, The Norton Library, WW Norton.

Pottick KJ: Children's use of mental health services doubles, new research—policy partnership reports. In *Update: latest findings in children's mental health*, Brunswick, NJ, 2002, Institute for Health, Health Care Policy and Aging Research.

Raphel S: A national action agenda for children's mental health, *J Child Adolesc Psychiatr Nurs* 14:193, 2001.

Scott J, Hague-Armstrong K, Downes K: Teasing and bullying: what can pediatricians do? *Contemp Pediatr* 4:105, 2003.

Searight HR, Rottnek F, Abby SL: Conduct disorder: diagnosis and treatment in primary care, *Am Fam Physician* 63:1579, 2001.

Strayhorn J: *The competent child: an approach to psychotherapy and preventive mental health*, New York, 1989, Guilford Press.

US Department of Health and Human Services (USDHHS): *Mental health: a report of the Surgeon General*. Rockville, Md, 1999, USDHHS, Public Health Service, Office of the Surgeon General.

US Department of Health and Human Services (USDHHS): *Cultural competence standards: in managed mental health care services*, Rockville, Md, 2000a, USDHHS, Substance Abuse and Mental Health Services Administration, Center for Mental Health Services.

US Department of Health and Human Services (USDHHS): *Report of the Surgeon General's conference on children's mental health: a national action agenda*, Rockville, Md, 2000b, USDHHS, Public Health Service, Office of the Surgeon General.

US Department of Health and Human Services (USDHHS): *A national strategy for suicide prevention: goals and objectives for action*, Rockville, Md, 2001a, USDHHS, Public Health Service.

US Department of Health and Human Services (USDHHS): *Youth violence: a report of the Surgeon General*, Rockville, Md, 2001b, USDHHS, Public Health Service, Office of the Surgeon General.

Vujevich KT: Brain imaging for children, *The Clinical Advisor*, 62, June 2003.

Wagner BJ: Attention deficit hyperactivity disorder: current concepts and underlying mechanisms, *J Child Adolesc Psychiatr Nurs* 13:113, 2000.

Waslick B et al: Diagnosis and treatment of chronic depression in children and adolescents, *J Psychiatr Pract* 9:354, 2003.

Weisz Jr, Jensen Ps: Efficacy and effectiveness of child and adolescent psychotherapy and pharmacotherapy, *Ment Health Serv Res* 1:125, 1999.

Weller EB et al: Aggressive behavior in patients with attention-deficit/hyperactivity disorder, conduct disorder, and pervasive developmental disorders, *J Clin Psychiatry* 60(suppl15):5, 1999.

Werner E and Johnson J: The role of caring adults in the lives of children of alcoholics. In Abbott S, editor: *Children of alcoholics*, ed 2, selected readings, pp 119-141, Rockville, Md, 2000, National Association for Children of Alcoholics.

Zauszniewski JA et al: Predictors of resourcefulness in school-aged children, *Issues Ment Health Nurs* 23:385, 2002.

Zito JM et al: Trends in prescribing of psychotropic medications to preschoolers, *JAMA* 283:1025, 2000.

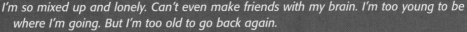
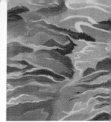

I'm so mixed up and lonely. Can't even make friends with my brain. I'm too young to be where I'm going. But I'm too old to go back again.

JOHN PRINE, *ROCKY MOUNTAIN TIME*

ADOLESCENT PSYCHIATRIC NURSING 37

Audrey Redston-Iselin

LEARNING OBJECTIVES

After studying this chapter, the student should be able to:

1. Identify the developmental tasks of adolescence (I).
2. Compare the various theoretical views of adolescence (II).
3. Discuss the major areas that should be included when assessing adolescents (III).
4. Examine maladaptive responses evident in adolescence (IV).
5. Analyze nursing interventions useful in working with adolescents (V).
6. Evaluate nursing care provided for adolescents (VI).

TOPICAL OUTLINE

evolve   Visit Evolve for additional resources related to the content of this chapter.
http://evolve.elsevier.com/Stuart/principles/

Adolescence is a time of transition—an age when the person is not yet an adult but is no longer a child. The issues raised during adolescence are central to personal development. Psychiatric nurses treating adolescents focus on their movement toward adulthood, considering social, emotional, and physical aspects of their adjustment in their family, school, and peer groups.

■ DEVELOPMENTAL STAGE

Adolescence is a unique stage of development that occurs between ages 11 and 20 years, when a shift in growth and learning occurs. The developmental tasks that emerge during adolescence threaten the person's defenses. They can either stimulate new adaptive ways of coping or lead to regression and maladaptive coping responses. Old problems may interfere with the adolescent's coping abilities, and environmental factors may help or hinder the adolescent's attempts to deal with these issues. Previous coping skills, if used successfully, can promote healthy adaptation and integrated adult functioning.

An earlier, but still popular view of adolescence described it as a time of conflict and upheaval that was necessary for later personality integration. More recent research suggests that this is not true; the complex changes in biological, social, and emotional development do not necessarily lead to psychological conflicts.

During adolescence major events occur, and attempts are made to deal with them. This results in behavior uniquely "adolescent." **Tasks that should be accomplished during adolescence are as follows** (Havighurst, 1972):

- **Achieving new and more mature relations with age mates of both sexes**
- **Achieving masculine or feminine social roles**
- **Accepting physical build and using the body effectively**
- **Achieving emotional independence from parents and other adults**
- **Preparing for marriage and family life**
- **Preparing for a career**

Table 37-1	Summary of Theoretical Views of Adolescence
THEORY	DESCRIPTION
Biological	Emphasis is on physical growth, behavior, and the environment, which influence feelings, thoughts, and actions.
Psychoanalytic	Puberty is called the genital stage in which sexual interest is awakened. Biological changes upset the balance between the ego and id, and new solutions must be negotiated.
Psychosocial	Adolescents attempt to establish and identify within the social environment. They seek to coordinate self-security, intimacy, and sexual satisfaction in their relationships.
Cognitive	Adolescence is an advanced stage of cognition in which the ability to reason goes beyond the concrete to more abstract thinking, described as formal thought.
Moral	Adolescent development is characterized by the ability to take the moral perspective of parents and other members of society into account. Boys' and girls' moral development is different, including responsibility and caring components.
Cultural	Views adolescence as a time when a person believes that adult privileges are deserved but withheld. This stage ends when society gives full power and status of an adult.
Multidimensional	Adolescence is seen as adaptation on a continuum of development. There is less emphasis on age and more on the developmental level and timing of biological, psychological, and environmental influences.

- **Acquiring a set of values and an ethical system as a guide to behavior and developing an ideology**

Different theories describe these developmental tasks and how their positive resolution moves the adolescent toward adulthood. They will be briefly reviewed and are summarized in Table 37-1.

■ THEORETICAL VIEWS OF ADOLESCENCE
Biological Theory

One of the fundamental features of adolescence is the series of biological changes known as puberty. These changes transform the young person physically from a child into a reproductively mature adult. This process is so basic to adolescent development that many people identify puberty as the beginning of adolescence. Puberty involves a set of biological events that produce changes throughout the body. The changes fall into two categories: hormonal and brain development.

In both sexes, **increases in hormone production** lead to the development of reproductive capability and a mature physical appearance. Physical changes include pubic hair growth, breast development, and menarche in girls and genital development, pubic hair growth, voice change, and the emergence of facial hair in boys. A spurt in height and weight occurs in both sexes. Although all adolescents experience the changes of puberty, there are large individual differences in the timing of these changes, as well as the pace at which they take place.

Brain growth continues into adolescence as well. Although the number of neurons does not increase, the support cells that brace and nourish the neurons begin to proliferate. In addition, growth of the myelin sheath around nerve cell axons continues at least until puberty, enabling faster neural processing. Simultaneously, the number of interconnections between adjacent neurons decreases, probably reflecting the disappearance of redundant or inappropriate neural connections. This fine-tuning of the neural system coincides with the development of formal operational thought.

Psychoanalytical Theory

Freud believed that human development was biological and marked by stages. During puberty (age 13 to 18 years), Freud's **genital stage**, a reawakening of sexual interest occurs. The adolescent with new sexual urges looks for gratification outside the home. This renewal comes from physiological maturing, which results in sexual exploration.

Increased drives or impulses due to hormones cause personality reorganization as adolescents attempt to adjust to their new physical status. These increased impulses confront a weak ego. Adolescents therefore return to earlier coping skills in an effort to reestablish mastery over the environment.

Blos (1962) described adolescence as a *normative crisis*, or a normal phase of increased conflict. He defined this developmental period as the **second individuation** process, the first occurring at age 2 years with a defining of one's self. Adolescence individuation is more complex, leading one to self-definition. This is how he accounts for the rebelliousness and stages of experimentation that is characteristic of adolescents.

Psychosocial Theory

Erikson and Sullivan emphasized the effect of social factors on these developmental processes. **Erikson** (1963) described **ego identity,** or the relationship between a person's self-perception and how a person appears to others. To Erikson, adolescence represented an attempt to establish an identity within the social environment.

He described this search as normal adolescent identity crisis and called this stage of adolescence **identity versus identity diffusion**. This stage is followed in young adulthood by the stage of *intimacy versus isolation*. He stressed that identity must be established before intimacy can occur.

For **Sullivan** (1953), psychological growth is driven by a desire to seek **increasingly intimate personal relationships**. He suggested that adolescents try to coordinate needs of self-security and self-esteem, closeness and intimacy, and general activity and satisfaction of sexual strivings. If these needs become conflicting rather than integrated, emotional problems may result.

What problems might adolescents face if they decide to get married as teenagers, and what resources may be helpful to them?

Cognitive Theory

Cognitive theory views adolescence as an advanced stage of cognitive functioning in which the ability to reason goes beyond concrete objects to symbols or abstractions, or what **Piaget** (1968) called **formal thought**. He believed that the adolescent is able to deal with logic, metaphors, and rational thought. This develops continuously from the concrete thinking of childhood to about age 12 years, when the concern with realities, tangible objects, and action is transferred to ideas, allowing for conclusions to be made and for reflection to take place without the reality or object being present.

Moral Development Theory

Kohlberg (Barger, 2000) describes adolescent development in stages similar to Piaget. Adolescent moral development is described as the **conventional stage**. This stage is characterized by the ability to take the moral perspective of one's parents and other important societal members into account.

Gilligan (1982) disputes Freud, Erikson, and Kohlberg's views of adolescent development as being male defined. She believes that boys and girls arrive at puberty with different interpersonal orientations and different social experiences. She disputes Freud's claim that women's moral sense was stunted due to attachment to their mothers and family. Rather, she redefines adolescent development, noting that women are not deficient but different.

According to Gilligan, women develop in adolescence by focusing on connections between people, rather than separation. Girls establish gender identity through attachment and identification with their mothers, whereas boys establish gender identity through separation and individuation from their mothers. Preoccupation with independence, autonomy, achievements, and other traditional male values has overlooked the need for relationship, negotiation, and caring.

Gilligan uses the term "voice" to show that adolescent girls have muted their urge to preserve connectedness, even at the expense of self-expression. The consequences of not speaking in a relationship shows the problems selfless behavior can cause. The absence of voice in a relationship and the loss of responsible choices are often well intended and are a result of concern for others' feelings. However, the lack of the female voice also perpetuates a single male voice civilization.

Her work suggests that the formation of identity and intimacy that occurs in adolescence is defined by two different versions that complement the discovery of maturity. The inclusion of girls' adolescent experiences brings a new perspective to developmental theory by expanding the concept of identity to include **interconnection.** Responsibility and caring are ingredients necessary in adolescent development. The differences between adolescent boys and girls as theorized by Gilligan has allowed present day adolescent girls to be both feminine and assertive.

Cultural Theory

Anthropologists who have studied adolescents in different cultures report that primitive cultures have less stressful periods than those experienced by American teenagers and conclude that adolescent rebellion is culturally determined and not biologically based. They view adolescence as a period when the person believes that adult privileges are deserved but are being withheld. It ends when society gives the person the social status of an adult.

Anthropologists see growth as a continuous process and a cultural phenomenon, with people reacting to social expectations. The more clearly defined these expectations, the less stressful and ambiguous is the adolescent period. The more culture changes, the greater the generation gap becomes.

Several issues in contemporary American society directly influence the support an adolescent can obtain from the environment. Blurring sexual roles is one such issue. Women have less traditional attitudes, expectations, and behaviors, whereas men have become more involved in functions that were previously believed to be women's, and vice versa. So too, adolescents have more overt exposure to sex and violence in society.

Another social issue is the changing job market and the increased costs of higher education, which has resulted in the prolonged economic dependency of youth. Finally, the Internet has become a source of both information and recreation for adolescents, as well as giving them access to material that may not be appropriate to their developmental stage. All of these changes increase the complexity of society and add new pressures to adolescents, who are becoming adults and attempting to define their role in today's cultural milieu.

Multidimensional Theory

Multidimensional theory proposes that there is no one view of adolescent development. Rather, there are three main themes (Meeks, 1990):

- Profiles of ego and moral development are used to characterize adolescents for rates of progression, regression, and stability in age-related development.

- Attention is given to biological, sociological, psychological, and cultural integration. These variables change rapidly during adolescence and affect the adolescent's behavior and view of self.
- The developmental issues of both psychological and biological maturation are viewed as affecting the adolescent's adaptation and functioning. For example, the timing of the adolescent's physical development in relation to a peer group has a direct influence on the teenager's self-esteem.

These issues may vary widely, not only individually but also by culture and society.

The multidimensional view of adolescence sees adaptation on a continuum of development. Less emphasis is placed on specific age and more is put on developmental level and the timing of various biological, psychological, and environmental influences. This theory also proposes that severe family conflict need not necessarily occur. Rather, the degree and nature of conflicts change from childhood through adolescence and reflect both the diversity and the functional and dysfunctional aspects of family life.

■ ASSESSING THE ADOLESCENT

Nursing care of adolescents begins with a thorough assessment of their health status. Data collection by the nurse is based on current and previous functioning in all aspects of an adolescent's life (AACAP, 2001). A variety of approaches

---

BOX 37-1

Components of an Adolescent Assessment

- Present problems and symptoms
- Appearance
- Growth and development (including developmental milestones)
- Parent and family health and psychiatric histories
- Biophysical status (illnesses, accidents, disabilities)
- Emotional status (relatedness, affect, and mental status, including mood and evidence of thought disorder and suicidal or homicidal ideation)
- Cultural, religious, and socioeconomic background
- Performance of activities of daily living (home, school, work)
- Patterns of coping (ego defenses such as denial, acting out, withdrawal)
- Interaction patterns (family, peers, society)
- Sexual behaviors (nature, frequency, preference, sexually transmitted diseases)
- Use of drugs, alcohol, and other addictive substances (tobacco, caffeine)
- Adolescent's perception and satisfaction with health (functional problems or complaints)
- Adolescent's health goals (short- and long-term)
- Environment (physical, emotional, ecological)
- Available human and material resources (friends and school and community involvement)

---

and tools may be used, but data collection should include the information listed in Box 37-1.

These data are collected from adolescents and significant others through interviews, examinations, observations, and reports. In addition, the nurse may ask the following questions of the adolescent's family:

- What concerns you about your adolescent?
- When did these problems start?
- What changes have you noticed?
- Have the problems been noticed in school as well as home?
- What makes the behavior better or worse?
- How have these problems affected your adolescent's relationship with you, siblings, peers, and teachers?
- Has your adolescent's school performance changed?

One outcome of the nursing assessment should be the identification of teenagers at high risk for problems (Champion and Kelly, 2002). Nurses need to understand the difference between constructive and age-appropriate exploration and engagement in activities that are potentially dangerous and threaten the adolescent's physical and emotional well being (see Critical Thinking About Contemporary Issues).

Critical Thinking *About* Contemporary Issues

Are All Adolescents at High Risk for Problems?

Although it is a commonly held belief that adolescence is a time of conflict and turmoil, some dispute the notion that teenagers must experience a difficult adolescence. Nonetheless, nurses should not underestimate the nature of adolescent high-risk behavior and the potential resulting problems. The Youth Risk Behavior Surveillance System conducted a national school-based survey of more than 16,000 students in 151 schools. The data reveal many threats to the health and well-being of teenagers, as follows:

- 19% of students had rarely or never worn seat belts when riding in a car driven by someone else.
- 37% had ridden one or more times with a driver who had been drinking.
- 17% had driven a vehicle one or more times after drinking.
- 88% had rarely or never worn a helmet when riding a bicycle.
- 46% of the male students and 26% of the female students had been involved in at least one physical fight in the past year.
- 28% of the male students and 7% of the female students carried a weapon at least once in the past month.
- 72% of the male students and 54% of the female students participated in vigorous physical activity in the past week.
- 4% of students had missed one or more days of school in the past month because they felt unsafe at school or traveling to and from school.

Each of these findings represents both an area of concern and an opportunity for health education and early intervention by psychiatric nurses.

A profile of the high-risk adolescent is presented in Figure 37-1. Teenage behaviors that contribute to death and injury include smoking, poor diet, lack of physical activities, alcohol and drug abuse, unprotected sex, violence, suicide, homicide, and automobile crashes (CDC, 2003).

A number of factors combine to impact adolescent risk-taking behavior, including age, socioeconomic status, education, race, gender, self-esteem, autonomy, social adaptation, vulnerability, impulsivity, and thrill-seeking activity. Nurses who work in schools and community settings can engage in screening and early nursing intervention with high-risk teenagers to promote adaptive responses and prevent the development of future problems.

In summary, an examination of typical adolescent behaviors reveals that **adolescence is a time of change**. The issues of body image, identity, independence, social role, and sexual behavior can produce adaptive or maladaptive responses as the adolescent attempts to cope with the developmental tasks at hand.

Many nursing students are adolescents themselves. How might this positively and negatively affect their work with adolescent patients? ■

Body Image

Chronological age is not a true guide for physical maturation because growth often occurs in spurts and individual differences exist. Because school classes and extracurricular activities are usually grouped by age, the adolescent must face being with others who vary greatly in physical development and in-

terests. This explains why adolescents often imitate behavior to keep within the expected range of conduct and be compatible with peers. The greater one's difference from the rest of the group, the greater is the adolescent's anxiety. The lack of uniformity of growth often puts great demands on physical and mental adaptability. Growth is uneven and sudden, rather than smooth and gradual, and causes a change in body image.

Adolescents reevaluate themselves in light of these physical changes, particularly the onset of primary and secondary sex characteristics, which are so pronounced. They tend to compare themselves and their physical development to their peers. They are very concerned about the normality of their physical status.

The physical changes of puberty cause adolescents to be self-conscious about their changing bodies. Often they are reluctant to have medical examinations because they fear abnormalities will be found. Examinations may intensify masturbatory conflicts, sexual fantasies, and guilt feelings. The early and middle phases of puberty also may give rise to increased conflict, distance, and dissatisfaction in parental relationships.

Identity

In response to the physical changes of puberty, adolescents experience heightened periods of excitement and tension. They use defenses against these feelings that were helpful in childhood and experiment with new, more adult-like attempts at mastery. Thus in their attempt to cope, adolescents sometimes act like adults and at other times behave like children.

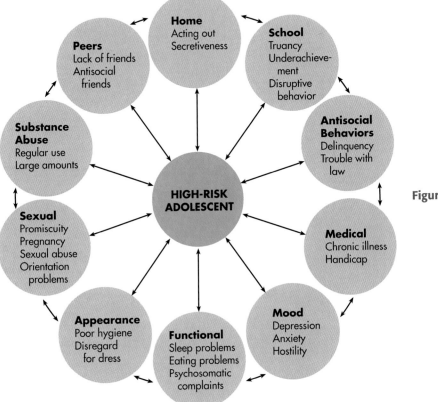

Figure 37-1   Profile of the high-risk adolescent.

For example, adolescents show behavior marked with experimentation and test the self by going to extremes. This can be useful in establishing self-identity. The rebelliousness or negativism of the adolescent shows a movement toward individuation and autonomy that is more complex than but similar to the 2-year-old's "no." Adolescents also may assert themselves by acting in a negative or contrary manner when relating to parents and other authority figures that they believe are not allowing them to be separate and unique. This is seen in the following clinical example.

CLINICAL EXAMPLE

Scottie, an avid football fan for several years, suddenly switched his interest to basketball. He quit his local football team despite his father's urgings to continue. His father, also a football fan, could not understand Scottie's sudden negative attitude toward football and newly found interest in basketball. ■

The individuation process of adolescence is accompanied by feelings of isolation, loneliness, and confusion because it brings childhood dreams to an end and attributes them to fantasy. This realization of childhood's end can create intense fears or panic. Many adolescents attempt to remain in this transitional stage.

The awakening of emotional ties with the family also occurs in the establishment of new, more interdependent relationships. This fearful yet exciting entrance into adulthood is a profound experience that is not resolved in adolescence but is confronted throughout life. Adolescents mourn the loss of childhood, and the feelings of loneliness and isolation that accompany this loss create an intense need for closeness, love, and understanding. If they are unable to obtain support during this struggle, depression may result.

Exploratory behavior allows the adolescent to try on new roles and find what fits as identity is formed. Adolescents with poor identity formation are vulnerable for engaging in high-risk behaviors because of the link between an adolescent's self-concept and the use of adaptive coping responses.

Parenting styles that encourage individuality and relatedness to families are associated with support of adolescent identity exploration. Adolescents expressing high levels of identity exploration have parents who express mutuality and separateness, encourage member differences, and are aware of clear boundaries between themselves and their teenagers. These adolescents are also more likely to have competent approaches to peer and social relationships and more developed skills in initiating, diversifying, sustaining, and deepening peer friendships.

Independence

Adolescents have an unconscious longing to give in to their dependency needs. Adolescence is also a time of movement toward independence. Adolescents show this ambivalence by responding to petty annoyances and irritations with intense outbursts. They see the process of gaining independence as being free of parental control. They do not see gaining independence as a gradual learning process but as an emancipation accomplished by acting "differently."

They believe that if one acts adult, then one is adult. Therefore they expose themselves to situations beyond their capabilities and then become overwhelmed and frightened. They seek reassurance in an attempt to reduce their anxiety by returning to childlike ways and being dependent on those with whom they feel most secure, usually their parents. This accounts for the inconsistency of adolescent behavior.

Well-adjusted adults usually use a problem-solving approach and do not feel as threatened when inexperience requires dependency on others. However, adolescents who are already tempted to give in to dependency needs feel as if they are regressing to childhood, which deflates their self-esteem. They must deny their need for their parents. Sometimes they criticize their parents for treating them as a child and then on other occasions remark that their parents are not helpful enough.

When adolescents seem to be rebelling against their parents, they may be rebelling against their own childhood conscience or superego. They project their ambivalence onto their parents because they were the original source of restrictions. This projection actually reveals a movement toward a more mature standard and also indicates their insecurity about giving up childhood standards. By blaming their parents for their childish actions, they can avoid blows to their fragile self-esteem and protest that their actions result from parental demands, not their own.

The interaction between adolescent changes in autonomy and family relationships is important. Three parenting styles have been described in relation to whether they help or hinder independent functioning in adolescence (Powers, Hauser, and Kilner, 1989):

- **Traditional parents** tend to value a sense of continuity and order. They accept the value judgments that come from previous generations. Adolescents from these families tend to be more attached to their parents, conforming, and achievement oriented. Often they avoid major conflicts in their teenage years.
- **Authoritarian parents** are oriented toward shaping, controlling, and restricting the adolescent to fixed standards. Obedience is seen as a virtue. Power and responsibility are not shared with the adolescent. Harsh discipline is used to curb autonomous strivings that are viewed as willfulness. The approach here is often punitive, and it can result in problems with the adolescent's development of autonomy.
- **Democratic parents** do not believe that their standards are always right. They tend to be supportive and respond to the specific situation with solutions that promote the adolescent's autonomy. They foster stimulation and challenge. This parenting style combines limit setting with negotiation, thus encouraging the teenager's participation in the disciplinary process. It is shown to predict greater independent functioning in adolescents.

Did your parents have a traditional, authoritarian, or democratic parenting style, and what would you do differently in raising children of your own? ■

Social Role

Adolescents respond intensely to people and events. They may be totally invested in one interest and then suddenly change to something different. These intense and unstable feelings can account for their extreme sensitivity to the response of others. They are easily hurt, disappointed, and fearful of others. They have a tendency toward hero worship and crushes, but with little evaluation of the people to whom these feelings are directed.

Adolescent relationships serve many functions. Often adolescents relate to a friend as if neither person were a separate individual. They often mimic each other's dress, speech, language, and thoughts. These relationships help in the development of self-identity and establishment of a social role.

The **peer group is also very important** because within the security of the peer group, adolescents can attempt to resolve conflicts. With peers they can test out their thoughts and ideas. Their thoughts may differ, but through mutual sharing, they can try to find an answer. The peer group also can explore other ways of dealing with problems and offer its members companionship, protection, and security.

In the peer group, adolescents can accept dependency, not as a child but as one of the gang, testing out ideas and trying new values. Within the safety of the peer group, they can observe, comment on, and evaluate the activities of others. Adolescents usually are very loyal to their group of friends. Sometimes group security is so important that it is pursued at all costs, even if it involves destructive behavior.

Adolescents react to many stimuli and drain off the tension created by new drives and impulses by investment in many interests. They do this with great intensity, which is why adolescents are susceptible to fads. This is often seen in their dress, music, or hobbies.

Close relationships with the opposite sex provide adolescents with security (often by "going steady") and a person with whom to discuss problems and evaluate solutions. Often the partner may take on similar characteristics. This reciprocal relationship enhances self-esteem by demonstrating sexual attractiveness to the self and to the world, and it indicates that one is lovable. It also allows for bisexual expression because the girl expresses her partner's feminine parts and her boyfriend represents her masculine parts.

> *Think about a current television program that is a favorite among adolescents and describe why it is popular, based on adolescent norms and developmental tasks.* ∎

Sexual Behavior

Adolescents use fantasy to discharge sexual tension. However, they may feel guilt and shame about sexual feelings or fantasies. Fantasies usually are an attempt to find solutions and evaluate consequences. They may indicate a disturbance if they continually occupy the adolescent's thoughts, are not converted into constructive actions, or are not modified by reality. Then they may disrupt other activities important to adolescent functioning and indicate a withdrawal from reality.

Masturbation is another way in which adolescents discharge sexual tension. The value of masturbation may be lessened if shame and guilt accompany it. Male adolescents often fear discovery of evidence of ejaculation, and females often fear changes in their genitalia as a result of masturbation. Fears are not limited to discovery by others. They also may result from the loss of ego boundaries experienced during orgasm. Mutual masturbation can serve the purposes of tension release and fusing of identity. It can help to dispel anxieties about sexuality by assuring adolescents that they are sexually adequate.

More teens are engaged in sexual activity, including intercourse and oral sex, than ever before and at an earlier age (CDC, 2001b). Some believe that this is a result of increased parental divorce, inattentive parents, and early pubescence. However, most note that society gives very mixed messages to adolescents about sex. Whatever the cause, there is rising concern about the emotional and physical consequences of early sexual activity. Specifically, it is questioned whether the mechanical and dehumanized aspects of early sex may lead to troubled and detached relationships later in life.

Although 5% to 10% of American youth acknowledge homosexual experiences and 5% feel that they could be gay, homosexual experimentation is common during late childhood and early adolescence. Experimentation may include mutual masturbation and fondling of the genitals and does not by itself cause or lead to adult homosexuality. Theories about the cause of homosexuality include genetic, hormonal, environmental, and psychological models (see Chapter 26). Specifically, nurses need to be aware of the following:

- Not all homosexual adolescents are sexually active.
- Many homosexual adolescents are heterosexually active.
- Many heterosexual adolescents are homosexually active.
- The relationship between sexual identity and sexual behavior is variable during adolescence.
- Sexual issues produce stress and anxiety for adolescents of all sexual orientations.

Societal acceptance of homosexuality varies among cultures. The United States lags behind other nations in their attitudes towards homosexuality, often seeing it as "deviant" or "unacceptable." How adolescents cope with their emerging sexuality can be affected by these destructive views. Gay and lesbian adolescents may repress their desires, compartmentalize their experiences, or suppress their sexual impulses by withdrawing and becoming asexual. In such cases the developmental process of identity formation can be jeopardized and healthy emotional adjustment inhibited (SIECUS, 2001).

∎ MALADAPTIVE RESPONSES

Behaviors that impede growth and development may require nursing intervention. The nurse should consider the nature of the adolescent's maladaptive responses and the harm resulting from them. If the difficulty is significant and ongoing, intervention may be needed. Adolescents also may be diagnosed with the various *DSM-IV-TR* psychiatric illnesses described in Chapters 16 through 26 of this text. The nursing interventions described in these chapters can be implemented with adolescents, as well as the various treatment modalities described in Chapters 27 through 33. Evidence-based treatment strategies for adolescents have been identified that take into account the particular developmental issues and the unique challenges of establishing a therapeutic alliance with an adolescent (Weisz and Jensen, 1999).

Inappropriate Sexual Activity

Sexual behaviors can be the cause of many teenage problems. Some of these behaviors are described in Box 37-2. Sexual activity is often not as much an outlet for sexual passion as an attempt to achieve closeness with another person. Adolescents tend to use their sexuality to sublimate other needs, such as those of love and security, and personal anxiety about sexual adequacy, and peer group pressure may lead the adolescent to have inappropriate sexual relations.

For example, some adolescents engage in sexual relations as a means of punishing themselves. Their promiscuity elicits external control and criticism from others. This is especially true when there is an exhibitionistic quality and subtle efforts to "get caught" are seen. This is evident in the following clinical example.

CLINICAL EXAMPLE

Isabel, a 14-year-old girl, had been sexually active since age 12 years. She was brought to the clinic by her parents when a neighbor told them Isabel had bragged of her sexual ventures. Two years before referral, her parents had placed her in a more controlled parochial school because they were concerned she was "acting wild." It became apparent that Isabel wanted her parents to know about and put limits on her behavior. She admitted to not enjoying sexual intercourse very much. She seemed to be trying desperately to get approval from her distant mother. She described her father, who was a policeman, as "a hopeless case," secretly wishing that he would be a better policeman for her. ■

BOX 37-2

Adolescent Sexual Behavior

- 46% of students have had sexual intercourse.
- 7% of students have had sexual intercourse before age 13 years.
- 14% of students have had sexual intercourse with four or more partners.
- 58% of currently sexually active students used a condom during their last sexual intercourse.
- 18% of currently sexually active students used birth control pills before their last sexual intercourse.
- 26% of currently sexually active students used drugs or alcohol during their last sexual intercourse.
- 5% of students had been pregnant or gotten someone else pregnant.
- 89% of students had been taught about HIV/AIDS in school.

From Centers for Disease Control and Prevention: *MMWR* 51(No. SS04), 2002.

However, it is important to differentiate between inappropriate behavior and defects in socialization that may result from the absence of an adequate parental role model, physical disabilities, sexual abuse, and personality temperament.

The additional risk of sexually transmitted diseases, including human immunodeficiency virus (HIV), makes sexual experimentation more problematic because of its potential short-term and long-term effects. Adolescents' needs for exploration and sexual gratification, as well as their feelings of invincibility, put them at great risk for HIV infection and other sexually transmitted diseases.

Despite educational efforts, many adolescents are misinformed about the transmission of these illnesses and effective preventive strategies. Some believe "it can't happen to me" or think that having only one partner ensures their safety. Unprotected sex is the area of highest risk. Oral, anal, and vaginal contacts all pose a risk because they involve the transfer of body fluids that can contain viruses. Alcohol and drug use increases the risk potential of adolescents because they are more likely to have unplanned sex and not use a condom when alcohol and drugs are involved. In the case of drug use, an additional risk is incurred from using contaminated needles.

The nurse must explore the meaning of the adolescent's sexual behavior by asking the following questions:

- Does the adolescent desire sexual gratification or punishment?
- Do the adolescent's goals match the situation, or is self-deception present?
- Is the adolescent demanding adult privileges while acting irresponsibly and dependent?
- To what extent is the sexual behavior experimentation, a defense against depression, or a way of expressing anger toward others?
- Is the sexual behavior a way to avoid anxiety-producing fantasies?
- How close is the relationship to a mature one?

Teen Pregnancy

Pregnancy in adolescence is a complicated issue (Canuso, 2000). Some adolescent girls have low self-esteem and fears of inadequacy. To ease these fears, they may become pregnant. Sometimes being pregnant is an effort to escape a difficult family situation or to force the parents to agree to a marriage that may be inappropriate, as shown in the following clinical example.

CLINICAL EXAMPLE

Susie, a 15-year-old girl, had run away for the second time, only to return home to the same chaos. She had tried to run away with her boyfriend. Her alcoholic mother and angry 19-year-old brother were making life unbearable. Her mother was surprised to learn about 3 months after her return that Susie was pregnant. Susie was delighted because she had hopes that she could get out of the house, knowing her mother would now approve of her marriage to her boyfriend. ■

Occasionally, an emotionally deprived adolescent hopes to give her child what she believes she has never received (or, perhaps more accurately, hopes to receive from the child what she has not been given). Sometimes being pregnant appears to be thought of by the adolescent as an avenue for changing circumstances, a way to change her own parent/child dynamic, such as by forcing her parents to allow her to be more independent or by escaping from a dysfunctional family situation.

Pregnancy in adolescence may have other origins. It can occur accidentally after sexual exploration. The adolescent may be unaware of contraceptive methods or may have delayed obtaining contraceptives. Research suggests that most teenage girls delay seeking contraceptives and become pregnant either because they are unwilling or unable to make conscious decisions about their sexual and contraceptive behavior or because they do not mind becoming pregnant.

Thus regular contraceptive use among sexually active adolescents requires that they believe that they can become pregnant and that using contraceptives is safe and the only way to prevent pregnancy. They also must have access to reliable, affordable contraceptives and must have a positive self-concept that allows them to make conscious decisions about their sexual and contraceptive behavior. Finally, they must want to postpone childbearing. Nurses are in a good position to educate teens about contraception.

Pregnancy for unmarried adolescents also may be associated with sexual promiscuity. If it is, the girl may be ostracized. Sometimes pregnancy occurs within a close, caring relationship. Peer groups can be supportive of a girl who becomes pregnant as a result of a meaningful relationship but intolerant of one whose pregnancy is the result of promiscuity. Both the circumstances and the adolescent's level of maturity need to be assessed. In some cultures, out-of-wedlock pregnancies are an accepted part of adolescence.

The most influential factors that discourage teens from having early intercourse are connection with a parent, especially the mother, and parental attitudes about teenage sex. Mothers who are clear about their values and communicate them to their teenagers in a nonpunitive way have the most influence on teens postponing intercourse (Robert Wood Johnson Foundation, 2002). Childhood sexual abuse is the largest single predictor of teen pregnancy over the last 40 years.

Decisions involving abortion, placement of the baby, and marriage are difficult to make. Attitudes and laws influencing these decisions are diverse. Many believe that to force the adolescent to have the baby and then give the infant up is more traumatic for her than abortion. Others believe that abortion can be more disturbing.

Marriage is another alternative. Forcing adolescents to marry to avoid societal stigma usually adds to their problems, but if the couple is mature, they may do well in marriage. All the alternatives should be presented to the adolescent, with the consequences clearly stated. The adolescent should make her decision with the aid and support of her partner, her family, the nurse, and other involved health care professionals (Logsdon et al, 2002).

Pregnancy among adolescents is increasing in the United States. Why is this, and what, if anything, should be done about it? ■

Depression and Suicide

Adolescent depressive disorders are common and potentially fatal as shown in Box 37-3. The symptoms of depression in adolescence are somewhat different than those seen in adults (Farmer, 2002) (Box 37-4). Adolescents have difficulty describing their emotional or mood states. Young teenagers often do not complain about the way they feel and instead act moody and irritable.

BOX **37-3**

Facts About Depression in Adolescents

- Major depression affects approximately 4% to 8% of adolescents.
- Within 5 years of the onset of major depression, 70% of depressed youths will experience a recurrence.
- Depression in young people often co-occurs with other mental disorders, most often anxiety, disruptive behavior, or substance-abuse disorders.
- Longitudinal follow-up studies estimate that 20% to 25% of depressed adolescents will develop a substance-abuse disorder.
- As many as 5% to 10% of adolescents will complete suicide within 15 years of their initial episode of major depression.
- Although adolescent depression is twice as common in girls as boys, in post-puberty (ages 15-19 years), the male suicide rate is 5 times that of the female rate.

BOX **37-4**

Symptoms of Adolescent Depression

- Frequent, nonspecific physical complaints
- Absences from school
- Poor school performance
- Talk or actions of running away
- Boredom or lethargy
- Outbursts of crying or moody behavior
- Irritable, angry, or hostile demeanor
- Lack of interest in friends
- Alcohol or drug use
- Decreased interaction and communication
- Fears of death
- Lack of interest in usual hobbies, sports, or recreational activities
- Sensitivity to rejection or failure
- Reckless risk-taking behavior
- Relationship problems

Between ages 11 and 15 years the rate of depression in girls rises rapidly, whereas only a slight increase in rate occurs in boys. Girls have been found to worry more than boys, feeling they have less control over their environment and what is happening in their lives. Boys tend to focus more externally on their actions and activities. For both groups, however, symptoms of depression in adolescence strongly predict an episode of major depression in adulthood (Pine et al, 1999).

Those who develop depression between ages 14 and 16 years are at greater risk of major depression later in life. In addition, teens who are depressed often develop anxiety disorders and dependency on nicotine and alcohol. Suicide attempts, educational underachievement, unemployment, and early parenthood also can have a higher expectancy rate in depressed teens (Fergusson and Woodward, 2002).

Adolescents respond differently to medication because they do not show evidence of hypercortisolemia (excessive production of cortisol) as adults often do. Research shows that depressed adolescents do not respond well to the tricyclic antidepressants. The difference in the action between selective serotonin reuptake inhibitors (SSRIs) and tricyclics will contribute to an understanding of the differences in the neurochemistry of depression that has its onset at an early age (Brown, 2002).

Suicide in those ages 15 to 24 years once accounted for 5% of all suicides but now accounts for 14%. **This makes adolescent suicide the third leading cause of death among American teens** (Harvard Mental Health Letter, 2003). Most suicides in adolescents are associated with drug and alcohol use, recent deaths in the family, trouble in school, legal problems, and relationship breakups (Beautrais, 2003). Nearly half of those who commit suicide have experienced a recent personal loss, humiliation, or rejection.

Adolescents who successfully commit suicide use firearms, hanging, jumping, carbon monoxide, and drug overdose. Males age 15 to 19 years are nearly 5 times more likely to kill themselves than females in the same age group, although female adolescents attempt suicide 2 to 3 times more often than their male counterparts (Joe and Marcus, 2003).

Even though completed suicides are more common among white males, attempts are more common among Hispanic Latino girls. This underscores the need for culturally sensitive interventions for this vulnerable population (Rew et al, 2001).

Depression has been shown to be significantly related to suicidal behavior, as have diagnoses of **conduct disorder, bipolar disorder,** and **substance abuse.** As adolescents move away from parental dependency, they increase their isolation and reduce their supervision. Peer problems often add to their sense of distress and alienation. The pressures to deal with intimate relationships, bodily changes, and an unstable sense of self can be overwhelming and lead to hopelessness and helplessness.

One of the most common factors in adolescent suicide is **lack or loss of a meaningful relationship**. It also has been found that suicidal attempts and completion rates appear to be higher in gay, lesbian, and bisexual youth, based perhaps on the stress and loneliness they experience related to their sexual orientation (Fergusson, Horwood, and Beautrais, 1999; Lock and Steiner, 1999).

Suicide is a bid for help that must be recognized. Subtle references, as well as attempts, should always be taken seriously and explored. Suicidal gestures are seen more often in girls; boys often express their depression by acts of bravado that result in accidents, as in the following clinical example. It is often difficult to distinguish between risk-taking behavior and accidents and suicidal gestures, thus the need for careful nursing assessment.

CLINICAL EXAMPLE

John, a 12-year-old depressed adolescent, had just gotten a dirt bike. Six months earlier John's grandfather, his only friend, had died. John's father had died when he was 2 years old, and he had lived with his mother and grandparents ever since. John, feeling hopeless, had ridden his bike into a car. After medical treatment for his broken arm and rib and multiple bruises, John began to receive therapy. He described feeling helpless and lonely, especially without his grandfather. ■

Parent-adolescent relationships can influence suicidal behavior. For example, the adolescent may be prevented from acting on suicidal feelings by parental concern and the establishment of new relationships. In contrast, feelings of helplessness and worthlessness can be engendered by threatened abandonment, by being asked to take on an adult role, and by lack of opportunities to be independent. Sometimes these adolescents perceive themselves to be expendable because they believe that the family unconsciously wishes them dead.

The nurse must make it clear to the adolescent that suicidal behavior is not confidential and that parents must be told. Family involvement is essential if angry, hostile, and hopeless feelings of abandonment are to be quelled and an atmosphere of support and caring is to be fostered.

In working with suicidal adolescents, the nurse should explore the following areas:

- Seriousness of the attempt
- Mental status of the adolescent
- Extent of environmental stress, especially family problems
- Adolescent's wider social environment and the strength of support systems (social isolation, school performance, parental loss, disruption of friendship, or romantic alliance)
- Likelihood of repeated suicidal attempts, especially if conditions remain the same

Nursing interventions related to depression are described in Chapter 19, and interventions related to suicide are described in Chapter 20. Research has shown that school-based prevention programs can help decrease suicidal behavior (Eggert et al, 2002). In addition, a rapid response approach delivered on an out-patient basis, can reduce hospitalization while increasing functioning and decreasing suicidal behaviors (Greenfield et al, 2002). The next two clinical examples illustrate suicide attempts by adolescents.

CLINICAL EXAMPLE

Maria, a 15-year-old girl, was referred to her local community mental health center from the neighborhood emergency room after ingesting pills. Maria had taken five of her mother's "arthritis pills" after an argument with her father about her 17-year-old boyfriend, José. Her father, who came home only on weekends, told her to stay away from him. After he left, the other family members noticed that Maria became sleepy while playing cards in the living room. Maria admitted to taking the pills and was rushed by her mother to the emergency room.

She had performed poorly in school in the year since her father had left the family. Maria had always been her father's favorite. When she reached puberty at age 13 years, that relationship changed. Maria's position as her father's favorite was delegated to a younger female sibling, causing Maria to feel angry and rejected. Her father left the family a year later and returned only for weekend visits, during which he mainly disciplined the children. Maria's attempt to get close to José as a replacement for her father was sabotaged by her father as well. She thought her only recourse was to elicit her father's caring and concern through a suicide attempt. ■

CLINICAL EXAMPLE

Donald, age 13 years, was brought to the emergency department after cutting his wrists one evening when he thought his family was asleep. His mother had awakened and found him bleeding. She rushed him to the local emergency room, where he received medical treatment. It was then revealed that this was Donald's second suicide attempt. The first attempt had occurred a year before, when he had ingested pills. Donald had received therapy for about a month. It was subsequently discontinued when the family moved to a new location, despite recommendations that he continue with a new therapist. Donald was always an isolated child. He was never very close with anyone but had had two friends. Since the move he had become even more withdrawn. He had done well in school in the past but now appeared to have given up and was failing almost every subject. As the youngest of nine children, Donald had little contact with his siblings, who were not at home much. Donald's parents, both approaching old age, seemed not to notice that he had become increasingly withdrawn and upset. Donald was hospitalized because the risk of his attempting suicide again was high. ■

Self-Injury

Deliberately destroying body tissue to change the way one is feeling is becoming more common among adolescents. Forms of self-injury include carving, scratching, burning, cutting, tattooing, excessive body piercing, and picking and pulling at skin (AACAP, 1999b).

Some adolescents hurt themselves to take risks, state their individuality, rebel, or be accepted by their peer group. Others self-mutilate to express their feelings of hopelessness, anger, low self-esteem, and need for attention. Teens who have difficulty verbalizing their feelings may show their emotional pain, physical discomfort, or sense of low self-worth by releasing their perceived psychological distress in the act of self-mutilation. Many times

teens hide their scars and bruises fearing ridicule, rejection, and criticism.

Nurses can help adolescents who mutilate themselves by encouraging them to identify and verbalize their feelings rather than acting them out; use distraction techniques when destructive feelings arise (such as deep breathing, positive imagery, applying ice to the skin, or snapping a rubber band on the wrist); engage in stress management techniques that reduce impulsivity (such as counting to 10, reevaluation, and thought stopping); and develop enhanced social skills. If suicidal ideation is evident, then emergency interventions are necessary.

Conduct Disorders

Adolescents with conduct disorders display behavior that violates the basic rights of others or societal norms and rules (see Citing the Evidence). Examples include fighting, cruelty, lying, truancy, and destroying property. Other behaviors may consist of aggression toward people and animals, bulling and threatening behavior, stealing, forced sexual acts, use of weapons, destruction of property, fire setting, running away, and staying out late (AACAP, 2000).

Conduct-disordered adolescents often have poor relationships with their parents. Antisocial acts allow the adolescent

CITING THE EVIDENCE ON
Bullying Behaviors

BACKGROUND: Although violence among U.S. youth is a current major concern, bullying is infrequently addressed, and no national data on the prevalence of bullying are available. This study measured the prevalence of bullying behavior among U.S. youth and the association of bullying and being bullied with psychosocial adjustment.

RESULTS: A total of 29.9% of the sample reported moderate or frequent involvement in bullying, either as a bully (13%), one who was bullied (10.6%), or both (6.3%). Males were more likely to be both perpetrators and targets of bullying. The frequency of bullying was higher among the 6th through 8th grade students than the 9th and 10th graders. Both perpetrating and experiencing bullying were associated with poorer psychosocial adjustment. Those bullied showed poorer social and emotional adjustment and had greater difficulty making friends, poorer relationships with classmates, and greater loneliness. Those who bullied others were more likely to be involved in other problem behaviors such as drinking alcohol and smoking. They also showed poorer academic achievement and school adjustment but were not socially isolated.

IMPLICATIONS: The prevalence of bullying among U.S. youth is substantial. Given the concurrent behavioral and emotional difficulties associated with bullying, as well as the potential long-term negative outcomes for these youth, the issue of bullying merits serious attention, both for future research and preventive interventions.

Nansel TR et al: JAMA 285:2084, 2001.

to express anger toward parents, who are often punished for the adolescent's acts. Children are socialized mainly by their parents and, it is hoped, learn from their parents' acceptable behaviors that become part of the internalized self or conscience. A good relationship between parent and child facilitates this process.

However, adolescents learn not only from their parents but also from others. The school and peer groups are influencing factors, as are the social, economic, and cultural environments. The self-destructive behaviors seen in conduct-disordered adolescents may indicate the need for punishment, anger at the family, peer group pressure, depression, feelings of self-defeat, a search for opportunities to take what they feel emotionally deprived of, and testing omnipotence through exciting experiences. Alignment with delinquents gives a defeated adolescent a feeling of self-respect and companionship through a sense of belonging to a subculture.

CLINICAL EXAMPLE

Levar, age 13 years, was referred by the juvenile court for therapy because he had been picked up for the second time after breaking into a store with another boy. Levar's parents had been separated for the past 2 years, following his father being incarcerated in jail for possession of drugs. Levar was extremely upset when his parents separated and rarely saw his father. His antisocial acts caused his father to become more involved with him because his father claimed he did not want his son to go through what he had experienced in prison. Levar gained his father's attention during these times, even though his father was angry. His delinquent actions enabled Levar to express his anger at his father's leaving, as well as to fantasize about having his father return. ■

This clinical example illustrates the many factors that may lead to adolescent delinquency. Adolescents may not differentiate between their stealing and their parent's business dealings. Stealing also may be an effective way to rebel against parents. Adolescents may perpetuate childhood by indulging in immediate gratification through stealing rather than working for things. Sometimes adolescents steal in hopes of getting caught and obtaining help. Parents may consciously or unconsciously condone stealing. Adolescents may also act out their anger with the justification that they deserve the stolen items.

Finally, the conflict between dependence and independence may be expressed in poor school adjustment. Some adolescents view teachers as parental surrogates who do not offer help but who merely apply rules of attendance and homework. Dependent feelings are sometimes elicited by these rules, and adolescents, in trying to prove their independence, may react negatively and discount the benefits of learning. They may think that schoolwork is secondary to more important activities they are attempting to master. Daydreaming also may interfere with schoolwork as adolescents concentrate on and fantasize about achieving independence rather than getting an education.

Adolescents may drop out of school for financial reasons, or they may be rebelling against education laws. The adolescent may be part of a peer group that denounces school attendance and involvement. Parents may overtly or covertly discourage education. This is conveyed through lack of support and approval for education or by their making it difficult for the adolescent to follow through with school expectations, as illustrated by the following clinical example.

CLINICAL EXAMPLE

Debbie, a 15-year-old girl, dropped out of school after several years of poor school performance and truancy. She occasionally went shopping with her mother on a school day. Her mother never knew the names of her teachers or guidance counselor and did not provide her with a place or time to study. ■

Violence

Violence among youth in America is on the rise. **Homicide is the second leading cause of death in teens 10 to 19 years of age, and 82% of those who died were killed with guns.** One-third of high school students reported being in a physical fight in the last year, with 4% needing medical attention. Six percent of high school teens report carrying a weapon to school in the last 30 days (Anderson et al, 2001).

Violence may be a learned response to achieve an end, or a habitual, reflexive way of dealing with a stressful environment. Most adolescents displaying aggression have experienced frustration and have had violent role models during their childhood. Aggression is a human impulse that must be channeled constructively by a learned process occurring within a supportive, loving relationship. Under favorable conditions, a child learns the healthy expression of aggression by involvement in activities that result in pleasure and active problem-solving attempts.

Risk factors for adolescent violence include weak bonding with others, ineffective parenting (including excessive or inconsistent punishment and inadequate supervision), exposure to violent acts at home, and social factors (including poverty and an environment that supports aggression). Guns represent the third leading cause of death in 10- to 14-year-olds and the second most common cause of death in teens 15 to 24 years old. Drug abuse, psychiatric problems, and viewing violent television programs promote resolving conflicts by violent means (AACAP, 1999a).

The increase in school-related violence such as the shootings at Columbine High School in Colorado has encouraged the development of efforts by parents and school officials to be more aware of potentially violent children. The National School Safety Center has identified the behaviors listed in Box 37-5 that could indicate a youth's potential for violent behavior. In addition, parents can ask themselves the following questions:

- Do you know your children's friends?
- How are they spending their time?
- What movies, videos, and Internet sites are they watching?
- What music are they listening to?
- Who are their role models and why?

- How are they doing in academics and usual school activities?
- Have they made any threats about hurting another person?

Much anxiety of adolescents is related to the fear that they may be unable to control their destructive aggression. Adolescents often have violent dreams and fantasies that they express overtly in the form of threats, although in some the potential for actual violence is minimal. Pointing out that these thoughts in themselves are harmless may be helpful to adolescents because it informs them that such thoughts are not as powerful as they may fear.

However, some adolescents are genuinely fearful that they will be unable to stop their thoughts from becoming actions. These very real fears must be acknowledged by a trusted adult, and the adolescents should be reassured that external limits are in place. Pointing out to the adolescent the neces-

sity for assuming self-responsibility and control is very important. Their defenses against aggressive outbursts should be reinforced and supported. The focus of counseling should be on the behavior and feared loss of control, not on the roots of the anger. The following clinical example illustrates the management of a violent adolescent.

CLINICAL EXAMPLE

Ricky was a 14-year-old boy referred for treatment because of violent outbursts at home. When frustrated, he would break and destroy objects in his path. Ricky was an only child, adopted shortly after birth by a couple in their forties who were unable to have children. Now Ricky's parents, who were about age 55 years, were increasingly frightened by his aggressive outbursts. They had also felt powerless to deal with his childhood temper tantrums and had consistently responded to his outbursts by attempting to limit frustrating situations. They felt guilty and inadequate about his being an adopted child and continually made attempts to reassure Ricky of their love for him. They consequently reinforced his lack of control by assuming that these outbursts were results of his fear of being unloved and would offer gifts and rewards to make peace. Ricky assumed he was omnipotent, successfully controlling his parents, but was afraid that he could not control his anger.

Acknowledging Ricky's fear of loss of control, applying external controls, and pointing out Ricky's ability to behave responsibly and assume control of aggressive behavior resulted in a gradual decrease in outbursts. ◼

BOX **37-5**

Behavior Checklist for Potentially Violent Youth

_____ Has a history of tantrums and uncontrollable angry outbursts

_____ Characteristically resorts to name calling, cursing, and abusive language

_____ Habitually makes violent threats when angry

_____ Has previously brought a weapon to school

_____ Has a background of serious disciplinary problems at school and in the community

_____ Has a background of drug, alcohol, or other substance abuse or dependency

_____ Is on the fringe of his or her peer group with few or no close friends

_____ Is preoccupied with weapons, explosives, or other incendiary devices

_____ Has previously been truant, suspended, or expelled from school

_____ Displays cruelty to animals

_____ Has little or no supervision and support from parents or a caring adult

_____ Has witnessed or been a victim of abuse or neglect in the home

_____ Has been bullied or bullies or intimidates peers or younger children

_____ Tends to blame others for difficulties and problems caused by self

_____ Consistently prefers television shows, movies, or music expressing violent themes and acts

_____ Prefers reading materials dealing with violent themes and acts

_____ Reflects anger, frustration, and the dark side of life in school essays or writing projects

_____ Is involved with a gang or antisocial group on the fringe of peer acceptance

_____ Is often depressed or has significant mood swings

_____ Has threatened or attempted suicide

From National School Safety Center, Westlake Village, CA, 91362, http://www.nssc1.org/.

Adolescents who have committed extreme acts of violence or homicide are often from families in which violence is condoned in some form. These adolescents may have experienced physical or sexual abuse, as described in Chapter 39, or they may have witnessed violence between their parents. Often these adolescents are encouraged to be violent by the easy access to guns in the home and by family members who extol the virtues of war, hunting, or aggressive activities.

Sometimes parents can predict the adolescent's ability to injure or kill. Often the adolescent has a history of perpetrating dangerous assaults on family members and pets. Other predictors of potentially violent behavior include drug abuse, poor school performance, and a history of fighting (Sege et al, 1999). Severely violent adolescents may exhibit calmness and lack of sorrow or guilt after committing violent acts, or they may claim that outside forces provoked them.

Many homicidal adolescents freely discuss their violent plans or fears. These should be explored and homicidal intent should be evaluated. Does the adolescent have a victim, weapons, or a plan? This information, along with the history, is indicative of the level of success or failure the adolescent has experienced in controlling feelings and delaying gratification.

What do you think society can do to decrease gang violence among adolescents in this country? ◼

Substance Use

Nationwide, substance use and abuse are significant problems for adolescents. They carry serious consequences, causing **50% of the deaths in youth age 15 to 24 years** (CDC, 2001a).

Use of alcohol and drugs also contribute to assaults and rapes perpetrated by adolescents.

Alcohol is the most commonly used and abused substance by youth. Nearly all high school seniors report some experience with alcohol. Although not all youth who drink have a drinking problem, nearly one third of seniors, report being intoxicated in the past 30 days. Higher levels of adolescent alcohol use are associated with the three most common forms of mortality among adolescents: accidental deaths, homicides, and suicides. Nearly 9 out of 10 teenage automobile accidents involve the use of alcohol.

Risk factors for adolescent alcohol use are presented in Table 37-2. Alcohol use also has been characterized as a gateway substance, preceding the use of marijuana and then other illegal substances such as cocaine and heroin (Golub and Johnson, 2001).

The onset of drug use before age 20 years predicts more sustained use over time. From 70% to 90% of males and 50% to 60% of females who abused drugs in adolescence continue to do so in adult life. Chemical dependency is the result of a gradual process.

Table 37-3 presents the stages of adolescent substance abuse. It is important for the nurse to remember that not all adolescents progress through these stages, but the younger the user, the greater the risk for chemical dependency. Specifically, first use of alcohol at age 11 to 14 years greatly increases the risk of the development of an alcohol disorder (DeWit et al, 2000). Substance abuse is discussed in detail in Chapter 24.

The meaning of drug use in adolescence is complex. The adolescent's motivation must be explored. The nurse must keep in mind that it may be an expression of rebelliousness and be supported by of a peer group, as well as a way of obtaining gratification (Kuperman et al, 2001). It also may indicate an effort to come to grips with feelings of vulnerability, victimization, and emptiness (Mainous et al, 2001; Kilpatrick et al, 2000). Repeated and regular use of drugs for recreational purposes can lead to problems of anxiety and depression. Some teenagers use substances to decrease their anxiety, especially when socializing.

Adolescents often report a wish for closeness that is satisfied by sharing a drug experience with friends. Drug users can experience an illusion of closeness because drugs decrease anxiety and users can share anticipation of drug use. Some adolescents fill the void of isolated loneliness with drugs and would otherwise feel suicidally depressed. Drugs can be crippling and delay healthy maturity by promoting the avoidance of developing an adult identity in a real world, as illustrated in the following clinical example.

Table 37-2	**Risk Factors for Adolescent Alcohol Use**
RISK FACTOR	EXAMPLE
Societal-Community	
Laws and normative behavior	Encouragement of youthful drinking in the media, absence of legal enforcement of underage drinking
Availability	Easy access via the home or adults (such as siblings) purchasing liquor for minors
Extreme economic deprivation	Escapist drinking to cope with harsh realities of everyday life
Neighborhood disorganization	Undermine sense of security and purpose in life
School	
Low commitment to school	School expectations and career expectations very low
Academic failure	Poor attendance, poor grades, underachievement
Early persistent behavior problems	High aggression, attention problems
Family	
Family members alcohol users (abusers)	Role modeling influences
Family management practices	Failure to monitor children; inconsistent parenting practices, or harsh discipline
Family conflict	Marital dysfunction or partner violence
Low bonding to family	Lack of reciprocal nurturing and open communication
Peers	
Peer rejection in elementary grades	Rejection or neglect by peers undermines positive self-concept
Associating with alcohol-using peers	Peer selection fosters cycles of negative behaviors
Friends with attitudes favorable to alcohol use	Peer selection fosters cycles of negative attitudes and beliefs
Individual	
Physiological	Genetic susceptibility to alcohol via enhanced tension reduction or misjudgment about level of intoxication
Alienation and rebelliousness	Removed from normative attitudes and values of society and commitments toward societal goals
Early-onset deviant behavior	Early-onset deviant behaviors consolidate and perpetuate negative spiraling cycles
Problem-solving coping skills	Absence of strong problem-solving skills may contribute to adaptation of less desirable negotiating strategies (such as an aggressive coercive interpersonal style)

Table 37-3   The Five Stages of Substance Abuse in Youth

STAGE	DRUGS	SOURCES	FREQUENCY	FEELINGS	BEHAVIOR	TREATMENT
Curiosity	None	Available but not used	—	Curiosity	Risk taking, desire for acceptance	Optimal time, anticipatory guidance to develop good coping skills and strong self-esteem, clear family guidelines on drug and alcohol use, drug education
Experimentation	Tobacco, alcohol, marijuana	House supply, friends, siblings	Weekend use for recreational purposes	Excitement, pleasure, few consequences; learning how easy it is to feel good	Lying, little change	Drug education; attention to societal messages; reduction of supply; strict, loving rules at home; establishment of drug-free alternative activities
Regular use	As above, plus hashish or hash oil, tranquilizers, sedatives, amphetamines	Buying	Progresses to midweek use; purpose is to get high	Excitement followed by guilt	Mood swings, faltering school performance, truancy, changing peer groups, changing style of dress	Drug-free self-help groups (Alcoholics Anonymous or Narcotics Anonymous), family involvement, psychiatric counseling unhelpful unless family therapy and aftercare provided
Psychological or physical dependency	As above, plus stimulants, hallucinogens	Selling to support the habit, possibly stealing or prostitution in exchange for drugs	Daily	Euphoric highs followed by depression, shame, guilt, and perhaps suicidal thoughts	Pathological lying; school failure; family fights; involvement with the law over curfew, truancy, vandalism, shoplifting, driving under the influence, breaking and entering, violence	Inpatient or foster care programs that require family involvement and provide aftercare
Using drugs to feel "normal"	As above; any available drug, including opiates	Any way possible	All day	Euphoria rare and harder to achieve; chronic depression	Drifting, with repeated failures and psychological symptoms of paranoia and aggression; frequent overdosing; blackouts, amnesia; chronic cough, fatigue	Inpatient or foster care programs that require family involvement and provide aftercare

CLINICAL EXAMPLE

Carlos was a 16-year-old boy who had been school phobic since age 10 years. He had been receiving home instruction since that age. Each year he was referred for a yearly assessment, which was required to obtain approval for continuation of home instruction services. During the assessment Carlos proudly spoke of his drug episodes. He and his small group of friends were close and had many exciting experiences induced by various hallucinogens and amphetamines. Carlos had little support in the real world because he had been isolated at home and developed interpersonal relationships with people outside the home primarily by his involvement in obtaining drugs and experiencing their effects. ■

Finally, even though tobacco use has decreased among adults from 40% in 1965 to 25% today, teen smoking has increased. Over 3000 youth start smoking each year, and adolescents account for 85% to 90% of first-time smokers. Smoking usually begins in the 6th to 9th grades, and addiction typically occurs before age 20 years. It has been estimated that 35% of high school students are current tobacco smokers (AACAP, 1999c).

Tobacco can be the first drug adolescents use before expanding the experimentation to other substances. It also has been noted that smoking teens tend to fight more, carry weapons, and engage in risky sexual behaviors. However, simply telling young people the health hazards of smoking does not appear to be an effective smoking cessation strategy. Instead, convincing them that they are being exploited by the tobacco industry seems to be a better approach.

Much work remains to be done in regard to this health issue because only 3% of adolescents who attempt to quit are successful 12 months later (NIH, 2002). Identifying factors that predict teens tendency to smoke would be helpful in developing prevention programs.

You're concerned about your best friend's increasing use of drugs, but she denies that it is a problem. How can you best help her? ■

Weight and Body Image Problems

Eating disorders are another group of problems often seen in adolescence. They include **anorexia nervosa, bulimia nervosa,** and **obesity.** The sociocultural milieu for female adolescents in the United States has precipitated identity and body image confusion and anxiety in this age group. The emphasis on thinness, athletics, and physical attractiveness suggests that these are highly valued achievements for young women. These traits demonstrate self-control and social success and are culturally rewarded. The result is that fear of fat, restrained eating, binge eating, and body image distortion are common problems among teenage girls.

Recent understandings suggest that eating disorders represent a complex of issues related to many possible causes. Psychosocial factors, family characteristics, physiology, and biochemical interactions all play a part in the development and treatment of these disorders. They are discussed in detail in

Chapter 25. The following clinical example illustrates the development of anorexia nervosa in a young girl.

CLINICAL EXAMPLE

Janet, age 15 years, was admitted to the hospital because it was feared that her extreme weight loss was endangering her life. Exploration revealed that Janet was afraid of her sexual feelings and the response of others to her budding sexuality. Her father, provocative and teasing toward Janet, was continually kidding her about her oncoming sexual attractiveness and implied that he really preferred her to her mother. This created panic, and Janet refused to eat in reaction to this. She liked her thinness, which was a protection from sexual desires. In the hospital the area of concentration was not the behavior of not eating, but rather the underlying feelings about her sexuality and her relationship with her father. This provided freedom for normal sexual growth and development. ■

Boys have body image problems as well. They respond to society's pressure to be muscular and virile, and many adolescent boys are ostracized from social groups for being short, overweight, or too thin. Boys also may evaluate their self-worth by the qualities of their bodies. **Body dysmorphic disorder** is a psychiatric illness common in male adolescents in which they are obsessively preoccupied with flaws they perceive in their appearance. Symptoms include continually checking mirrors and attempts to hide perceived, imaginary imperfections. The average age of onset is 15 years.

■ WORKING WITH ADOLESCENTS

Knowledge of normal adolescent development is necessary to differentiate between age-expected behavior and maladaptive responses. When working with an adolescent, it is best if the nurse's initial contact is a one-to-one meeting directly with the adolescent only. Many adolescents are concerned that the nurse is aligned with the parents and not interested in their perspective. Other adolescents take a passive role, preferring to let the adults take responsibility for "straightening things out."

By initiating contact with the adolescent, the nurse is able to align with the patient's independent, mature aspects. Parents asking for advice on how to approach the adolescent about seeking treatment should be advised to be honest, stating the true nature of the visit and their reasons for requesting it. Whatever intervention model is used, working with adolescents incorporates specific considerations.

Health Education

The psychiatric nurse is in an excellent position to educate the adolescent, the parents, and the community. Basic health information can be given in such areas as smoking, drugs, sex and contraception, suicide prevention, and crime prevention. Adolescents want information about what activities are healthy and unhealthy, including facts about exercise, nutrition, dealing with anger, sexuality, conflict resolution, and where they can access help.

Adolescents are preoccupied with their bodies and bodily sensations. They are uncomfortable with their bodies because of the rapid changes in size, shape, and functioning. They therefore respond to bodily sensations with increased intensity. When an adolescent is overly concerned, it may indicate problems with self-image. Hypochondrias occurs when the adolescent has intense anxiety about personal health. The nurse can provide information on healthy emotional functioning, including coping with stress and anxiety and pursuing personally meaningful activities. Successfully coping with stress includes the following elements:

- Skills and motivation to manage acute, major life stressors and recurring daily stressors
- Skills to solve problems (problem-focused coping) and skills for emotion management (emotion-focused coping)
- Personal flexibility and the ability to meet the demands of varying types of stress

Involvement in personally meaningful activities includes the following:

- Skills and motivation to engage in instrumental and expressive activities that are personally meaningful
- Behaviors and activities that are experienced as autonomous and self-determined

By educating them on normal adolescent behavior and by interpreting the underlying conflicts, the nurse prepares parents, teachers, and other community members to support adolescents and encourage healthy independent functioning. Often parents and other adults become frustrated, angry, and confused by the independent strivings of adolescents. Encouraging independence and lessening power struggles can produce a positive change in adolescents' relationships with adults and in their feelings about themselves.

However, adults should still set limits. Setting limits and providing structure can be done in a way that encourages the adolescent's independent functioning. Many parents are conflicted about their children becoming adults. This, together with the adolescent's own ambivalence and fears about independence, can create havoc.

One of the best ways to educate parents on adolescent development is through a parents' group. The nurse can inform parents on normal adolescent functioning and provide them with much needed support from other parents in the same situation. Sharing mutual experiences and searching for solutions in a supportive environment can be extremely helpful to parents.

It is important to remember that parents have nurtured their children up to the stage of adolescence and many believe that "showing them how" is their primary parental responsibility. It is difficult for them to suddenly switch from the "how to" mode of instructing the child to the "try to" mode of guiding the budding adult.

Parents can learn the process of providing increased responsibilities based on a gradual progression of independent functioning. Despite parental fears of their teenagers getting into trouble, they can be educated to promote their child's self-reliance. The next two clinical examples show the need to educate parents and community members.

CLINICAL EXAMPLE

Mr. and Mrs. B came to the attention of the psychiatric nurse as a result of their distressed calls to the community mental health center. Mrs. B tearfully explained that they had lost all control of their 14-year-old daughter. She had become arrogant and hostile, locking herself in her bedroom after an argument they had about her going to the movies with a 14-year-old boy she had met at school. Further exploration revealed that Emily was an honor student at school, maintaining a solid A average. She had many friends at school, was on the volleyball team, and baby-sat regularly on weekends for the neighbors' two children. She had always been pleasant, happy, and friendly. Suddenly this boy that the parents did not know called her at home. After many phone conversations he asked Emily to join him on a weekend evening at the movies. Mr. and Mrs. B felt that Emily was much too young to date, that she could get involved with drugs, sexual promiscuity, and so on. They were sad and worried that they had lost their little girl who always did what she was told. Emily was hurt and furious. She thought her parents were being totally unreasonable and that they did not trust her. It turns out that Mrs. B had gotten into trouble sexually as a young girl. She did not want Emily to make the same mistake. Mrs. B's parents had been very lenient, and she blamed their lack of guidelines for her error. Mrs. B became aware of her overreaction. After discussion with a psychiatric nurse, she was able to understand that dating was a normal part of adolescent development. A compromise was reached when she was able to recognize Emily's competent and responsible functioning. After Mr. and Mrs. B met the boy, Emily was allowed to go to the movies with him and two other friends on a Saturday afternoon. ■

CLINICAL EXAMPLE

Lui Lee, an adolescent girl just starting high school, had always functioned well. However, attending high school would be totally different than any experience she had had previously. She began school in September feeling quite anxious. She felt overwhelmed by the large building, increased academic responsibilities, and complex peer relationships. By October she had succumbed to numerous illnesses that prevented her from attending school. This came to the attention of the school guidance counselor, who had noticed her increased absences. The guidance counselor met with her and, when assessment revealed no medical problems, invited Lui Lee to come to her office whenever she felt sick at school, believing it would be helpful to Lui to have a place of refuge. When this strategy did not help, she suggested that Lui Lee receive instruction at home until she felt less anxious. This validated Lui Lee's fears that she could not handle high school and its increased pressures. Her solution of retreat was supported. Fortunately, her parents sought the help of a psychiatric nurse, who encouraged immediate return to school and involvement in a peer support group, and along with individual sessions initially as needed. This enabled her to talk out her fears and also receive support from her peers. This strengthened her confidence and fostered healthy functioning. She found she could handle high school after all. The nurse educated the guidance counselor on ways to be supportive while encouraging independent functioning. ■

What teaching methods or aids would be particularly effective when implementing a health education program for adolescents? ■

Family Therapy

The nurse needs to assess the level of family functioning and determine how to best interact with and help the family of the adolescent. Family therapy is particularly useful when disturbed family interaction is interfering with the adolescent's development. Sometimes a series of family sessions may be enough, and the adolescent may benefit from either individual or group approaches to support the effort to separate emotionally from the family.

Occasionally, after a few family sessions, it may become clear that the adolescent may not need the intervention directly. Engaging the parents may free the adolescent to progress on the developmental continuum. Whatever modality is selected in working with the adolescent, a family orientation and the adolescent's attempt to separate from the family and become an independent adult should be considered.

Group Therapy

Group therapy addresses adolescents' need for peer support. The conflict between dependence and independence with adults becomes somewhat diluted by the presence of other adolescents. Conflicts, especially about authority, can be detected by peers rather than adults, making group therapy particularly helpful for adolescents. It also is valuable in teaching skills in relating and dealing with others. Group therapy helps fulfill the adolescent's need for a positive, meaningful peer group for ego identity formation.

Adolescent groups, in contrast to other groups, are difficult to manage because many adolescents react to peers defensively. Sibling rivalry often disrupts group cohesion. Many groups suffer from poor attendance, a high dropout rate, antisocial behavior, and a lack of group cohesion. However, group therapy with adolescents has proved to be successful in many community mental health centers, outpatient clinics, and hospital settings.

Often, beginning group sessions with some planned activity provides a stabilizing factor for young adolescents. The number of members to include in the group depends on the type. For example, it may not be feasible to limit an outpatient walk-in group. Because of the age spread among adolescents, it is usually preferable to form at least two groups. One possibility is an early adolescence group consisting of 13- to 15-year-olds who are experiencing conflicts of separation from parents. An older adolescent group, ages 15 to 17 years, would probably focus on issues such as furthering the establishment of identity, beginning to date, sex, experimentation with drugs, handling money, responsibilities of driving, and vocational plans.

Conflict between therapists, if there is an open and honest discussion, can provide a corrective experience because adolescents can see adults disagree without devastating consequences. If therapists are of the opposite sex, a parental similarity is often apparent; members often play on the therapist's feelings and try out tactics as they would with their own parents. Even if both therapists are of the same sex, one is usually more active, and a member may project a good or bad image onto each therapist that corresponds with how the parents are viewed. Group process with adolescents is often similar to that with adults. Specific aspects of working with groups are reviewed in Chapter 32.

When might a same-sex adolescent therapy group be most helpful? Compare this to the value of a mixed male and female group. ■

Individual Therapy

The advanced practice psychiatric nurse does individual therapy. Once the decision to engage in individual therapy is made, a pact or contract between the nurse and adolescent is established and a therapeutic relationship is initiated (see Chapter 2).

Therapeutic Alliance. This contract is a therapeutic alliance in which a nurse aligns herself with the healthy, reality-oriented part of the adolescent's ego and moves toward an honest and critical understanding of the adolescent's thoughts and behaviors. The alliance is a central aspect of individual therapy. Once it is established, a feeling of working together is apparent. Specific ways to establish and maintain this alliance include the following (Meeks, 1990):

- Point out that behavior is motivated by feelings. Often, early in treatment, adolescents express feelings of impatience, helplessness, and failure at having to seek treatment. Defenses are often seen in rebelliousness, passivity, shyness, negativism, and intellectualization. Adolescents generally have a tendency to act out and avoid examining their feelings.
- Limit acting out by pointing out how it interferes with the therapeutic process and that it must be controlled before the process can proceed. Maintain a neutral but interested attitude toward all behavior.
- Point out the adolescent's tendencies to be judgmental and self-critical. This is supportive and helps encourage the adolescent to look for sources of behaviors, attitudes, and feelings.
- Establish that the adolescent's behavior is the result of automatic thoughts and inner feelings that are interfering with the adolescent's happiness. This knowledge strengthens the motivation for therapy and maintains an alignment with the adolescent's wishes for autonomy.
- Point out the adolescent's tendency to see things in extremes; the desire to be complete master opposes the feelings of total helplessness. Reveal areas of strength and competence that are often unrecognized. Avoiding exclusive focus on problems and weaknesses shows neutrality and is supportive. Giving the adolescent as much information as possible to make decisions helps the adolescent work toward self-direction.
- Distinguish among thoughts, feelings, and actions, discouraging impulsiveness. Encourage open expression of strong feeling but not strong action. For example,

anger does not mean killing; sexual feeling does not mean intercourse. Adolescents sometimes confuse discussion with permission to experiment with action, especially with sexual issues.

- Encourage emotional catharsis in sessions by expressing interest in and acceptance of feelings involving the nurse and events outside the session. Point out the importance of feelings.
- Be alert to the defenses of denial and reaction formation. Maintain neutrality and encourage objectivity without directly attacking needed defenses.

Adolescents often act provocatively to force punishment by adults. This puts the nurse in alignment with the self-hatred aspect of the adolescent's conscience and should be avoided. The nurse provides support by continuing therapy even during these difficult periods.

The work of the nurse is to recognize the adolescent's anxiety and assist in finding ways to deal with emerging impulses. Accepting any healthy and adaptive responses of the adolescent strengthens the sense of ego mastery. Adolescents often have wishes that they regard as crazy and frightening. Open discussion of fears helps adolescents realize that these feelings are uncomfortable but harmless thoughts.

Transference. Transference often occurs in adolescent treatment. The nurse must point out that these projections originate in the adolescent's mind and not in reality and that they usually represent a meaningful person such as a parent. It often helps to mention this is a common response. Several common transference patterns include the following:

- **Erotic-sexual**, especially if the nurse is young and of the opposite sex. This transference typically is shown by awkward blushing and agitated confusion on the part of the adolescent. It is usually best to emphasize the mutual work of emotional growth while tactfully establishing the nurse's unavailability as a sexual object. Focusing on origins or encouraging elaboration of these feelings is not helpful and provokes anxiety.
- **Omnipotent**, expecting that the nurse will have answers to all questions. It is easy for the nurse to drift into this pattern because often the adolescent appears to be helpless. The adolescent's secret desire for personal omnipotence is somewhat fulfilled by granting it to the nurse.
- **Negative transference**, usually intense and pervasive. Negative feelings toward the nurse usually represent a negative attitude toward adult authority figures. This transference is often defensive to cover feelings of shame, inadequacy, and anxiety, and it disappears as the adolescent respects the nurse's feelings. The adolescent tries to force the nurse's rejection. Open discussion to explore these feelings objectively and establish their origin is helpful. Sometimes interpretations arouse anger toward the nurse because of the anxiety they create. These are reactions to the realities of therapy and are not to be confused with negative transference. A true negative transference occurs when

situations reactivate early experiences of negative feelings toward important others. The nurse unavoidably will frustrate the adolescent, who often has trouble delaying gratification to reach long-range goals.

Negative transference, like any other resistant behavior, is dealt with through objective exploration, which includes seeking causes of anger and pointing out irrationality. This is often followed by a period of regression and depression. Empathic understanding that the adolescent is mourning a loss is helpful, but it should be emphasized that what was lost was an illusion.

Another common occurrence is for an adolescent to rebel against conscience and then respond to guilt through self-destructive behaviors. Pointing out this pattern helps the adolescent to eventually become aware of this.

Termination. Termination of therapy is an important part of the therapeutic process. Often, leaving therapy symbolizes the process of loosening bonds to parental images and giving up desires to be passive. One therefore expects defensive and regressive behaviors as the adolescent attempts to deal with the anxieties related to the termination process. This can mean the recurrence of emotional crises, symptoms, self-destructive fantasies, and even dependency behavior to provoke rescue.

Termination should be flexible and correctly timed. The decision should be made in line with adolescent norms, not adult ones. Often adolescents verbalize appropriate interest in termination. When this occurs, it is often helpful to open it to discussion without commitment to a set time. This implies that further work needs to be done in a definite time span, and it maintains a focus on the adolescent's responsibility to finish. Gradually supporting and approving of the adolescent's independence and mature functioning prepares for a positive termination.

Sometimes terminations occur prematurely because an alliance has not been established or some external event has occurred. Occasionally terminations are forced because of a nurse's change of location, death, or illness. The adolescent will express anger at the new therapist until the feelings about the lost therapist are accepted and resolved. In working out this attachment, a new therapeutic alliance can be established.

Pharmacotherapy

For adolescents, it is a particular challenge to determine which of the changing and often tumultuous behaviors are target symptoms for psychopharmacological interventions. The treatment strategy is more complex for this age-group because of the following:

- Need for comprehensive family involvement (often optional in adults)
- Developmental differences that affect assessment, treatment alliance, management, compliance, and pharmacokinetics
- Difficulty in diagnosing emerging first episodes versus adjustment disorders in this age-group
- Lack of controlled clinical drug trials in adolescents

In terms of medication management, adolescents are neither children nor adults. They have a metabolism more like adults than like children. Thus dosing regimens for adolescents are usually closer to those of adults. Biologically, it cannot be assumed that drug response will be within the generally expected range for adults.

The current state of the art in adolescent psychiatric practice is to carefully prescribe psychopharmacological agents when they are determined to be appropriate and necessary as part of a comprehensive treatment plan. The increased recognition of psychiatric disorders in adolescents and their resulting negative effects on social, psychological, and emotional development, the increasing efficacy and safety of these drugs in adults, and the increasing evidence of efficacy of these drugs in adolescents have contributed to this practice. Chapter 27 provides comprehensive information about psychopharmacology in general.

- The use of SSRIs is generally preferred over tricyclic antidepressants (TCAs) in the treatment of adolescents because of their lower side effect profile and their relative safety in overdose. Additionally, evidence that indicates they are effective in the treatment of adolescent obsessive compulsive disorder and some anxiety disorders, such as panic disorder, is increasing.
- The use of benzodiazepines for anxiety is generally not recommended in this age-group because of the increase in drug experimentation by adolescents and the negative effects on learning and memory that these drugs may have.
- Lithium is generally well tolerated in this age-group and is effective in the treatment of mania, aggression, and conduct disorder. The other mood stabilizers have not been well studied in adolescents.
- Antipsychotics are the standard treatment for psychotic symptoms in adolescents. Although few studies exist, it appears that children and adolescents respond to lower doses of antipsychotics than adults and are more likely to experience extrapyramidal side effects; particularly teenage males, when conventional rather than atypical drugs are used.
- Adolescents have a positive response to psychostimulants for ADHD, similar to that seen in younger children.

Talking With Adolescents

The following discussion focuses on some important considerations in communicating with adolescents.

Silence. Silence is often effective with adults but frightening to the adolescent, especially in the beginning stages of treatment or evaluation. This anxiety often reflects the adolescent's feelings of emptiness and lack of identity. Brief silences can be creative and productive when the adolescent is engaged in treatment; when the adolescent is able to tolerate them without anxiety, it indicates growth in self-confidence

and acceptance of inner feelings. More often, however, silence is used defensively by adolescents to avoid discovery of hostile feelings or fantasies.

Older adolescents may tolerate interpretive remarks, but with younger adolescents it is usually helpful to suggest an activity to help facilitate discussion and establish a relationship. For some adolescents, silence is a defense of inhibition and withdrawal because they have never learned to communicate in a positive way. In these cases the therapist must be responsible for dialogue.

Confidentiality. Confidentiality is a concern to many, but especially to the adolescent who is fearful of the nurse reporting to parents. A blanket promise to tell nothing to the parents is not advised because the nurse may need to contact the parents if the adolescent reveals suicidal or homicidal behavior or the use of illegal drugs.

It is best to tell the adolescent that the nurse will not give out any information without informing the adolescent in advance. It is also helpful to explain that feelings are confidential but that actions considered dangerous to the adolescent or others must be shared.

 You receive a call from the school guidance counselor of one of your adolescent patients asking what progress is being made in treatment. How would you respond? ■

Negativism. Adolescents often express negative feelings, especially initially, because they are frightened of the implications of coming for treatment. The young adolescent's lack of objectivity and upsurge of impulses, as well as the tendency to confuse fantasy and action, make the discussion of feelings threatening. Usually, gently noting in a supportive way defensive techniques the adolescent uses during the session helps to gain cooperation.

Resistance. Often adolescents begin by testing nurses to see whether they will be authoritarian figures. The rebellious adolescent may deny the need for therapy or help. If the adolescent appears anxious, it is best to be supportive and sympathetic, expressing interest in getting to know the adolescent and then discussing a neutral area.

An angrier, rebellious adolescent may require a direct approach, with the nurse saying openly that the adolescent is opposing the visit because of a false belief that no help is needed. This can lead to a further discussion of feelings about the visit (such as parental coercion to come to the session) or feelings about authority.

Some adolescents are just baiting and testing to see whether the nurse is an anxious, defensive adult. If so, it is best to ignore their comments about not wanting treatment and move on. Often adolescents with an angry facade depend on their omnipotent control of the environment and are successful in manipulating their families. They are angry at attempts to disturb this power, and the anger is expressed in their lack of cooperation in the session.

Arguing. Adolescents often argue and, although they do not admit it, learn from arguments. Often the adolescent goes against the viewpoint of the nurse and then in the next session adopts the nurse's opinion. It is best not to comment on this and accept it as a harmless defense.

Testing. Adolescents often need and want limits. They are confused and cannot set their own limits. Often adolescents test nurses to see how firm and consistent they will be. Controls are effective if there is a basic positive relationship with the nurse. Limits should be set only when they are essential for current and future well-being. Adolescents will dare to be independent if it is conveyed that the nurse will serve as a control against carrying independence too far.

Dreams and Artistic Creations. Adolescents are often creative, and much can be learned from studying their works. As long as the discussion is relevant, it can be a productive source for exploring inner feelings. Along with dreams, these feelings can reveal valuable information about their real concerns, even when the adolescent attempts to avoid them.

Bringing Friends. The adolescent who brings a friend to a session may be attempting to avoid therapy. There is some benefit in sharing the experiences with the peer group because this lowers anxiety. Telling the adolescent that bringing friends is not allowed may not be successful because the nurse cannot always enforce such a rule. The reason for bringing friends may vary, but it should be explored and understood.

Sometimes adolescents want to refer friends. This may be positive but also may focus attention away from the original adolescent. The nurse should insist on exploring motives behind the referral before accepting the new patient because the adolescent may think the nurse's acceptance of another is a betrayal of loyalty. If the friend clearly wants and needs therapy, referral to a colleague is usually best. If a friend is brought late in therapy, it may mean that the adolescent is preparing to terminate.

Embarrassment About Being in Therapy. Embarrassment may occur in any age group, but it is prominent in adolescents, especially during the early stages of treatment. It also can become an issue as therapy progresses because it often reveals the adolescent's embarrassment about a desire for dependency. Therefore adolescents may become uncomfortable in the therapeutic relationship.

This is usually dealt with by indicating that these feelings are normal. Behind the fear of accepting help is the wish for care, and this can be dealt with by pointing out the adolescent's strengths and areas of independence.

Some adolescents, by expressing embarrassment about being in therapy, are actually revealing a fear or social stigma that they have heard from their parents. The adolescent who has feelings of inferiority often focuses these on the therapeutic process, blaming therapy for discomfort. It is best to encourage and support the adolescent, gently refusing to accept blame for this discomfort.

Do you think adolescents can benefit from treatment if their parents deny there is a problem, refuse to be involved, or are opposed to seeking help? ■

Parents of the Adolescent

If group or individual treatment is selected for the adolescent, the nurse must still consider the family. Parents cannot help with the adolescent's treatment if they do not understand and accept it. The nurse can work with the parents without revealing confidential material.

It is helpful for parents to have treatment if the adolescent is asked to assume an inappropriate role at home because this interferes with the adolescent's adaptive responses. If the parents are resistant, the nurse usually must begin with the adolescent and wait until the parents are more receptive.

Telephone contact is a helpful way to ensure cooperation and support by having the parent call when necessary. Parents should tell the adolescent when they call. Parents should be told of normal adolescent behavior they can expect. The nurse should avoid advising the parents about specific actions and focus on attitudes and feelings, especially concerning discipline.

Parents can be helped with understanding the purpose of limit setting. Some parents exclude themselves entirely from their adolescent's life. They have brought the adolescent to treatment to ease their guilt by doing all that is possible. They may want the nurse to take over parenting functions. This should not be permitted, especially during crises. If the adolescent is suicidal or homicidal, the parents are informed and helped to take responsibility for action.

Adolescents often need help in dealing with their parents. Parents should be discussed in an open exploratory way, with emphasis on them having their own feelings and reasons for their actions. Adolescents should be helped to see their parents realistically and to work on their own strengths and weaknesses.

Sometimes adolescents want to leave home because they hope they will feel more adult away from their parents. It is usually best to explore the wish to leave, emphasizing that it must be done in an adult way. If leaving is an impulsive thought with no feasible plan, it will result in failure, parental rescue, and continued dependency.

■ EVALUATING NURSING CARE

Problems presented by adolescents often activate the nurse's own unresolved conflicts. Thus evaluating nursing care must begin with nurses monitoring their own responses, including countertransference reactions. The nurse should watch for alignment with the parents against the adolescent or the adolescent against the parents.

Most adults are resistant to reexperiencing the feelings of adolescence and have repressed these experiences. As a result of anxiety, the nurse occasionally may have trouble listening or may encourage the adolescent (because of unrealized wishes) to do what the nurse never dared to do. The adolescent may be acting as the nurse did during adolescence. The nurse, in an effort to deny this, may see this adolescent behavior as a nonevent.

Identification of the nurse with the adolescent can contribute to delays in exploring areas important for psychological growth. The nurse may relate well to the adolescent but because of unresolved, unrecognized conflicts or resentment toward the nurse's own parents, may be locked into adolescent rebellion. The nurse may overtly or covertly encourage adolescents to express rage toward their families. Both the adolescent and the nurse then avoid facing the reality of adult burdens.

Evaluation of psychiatric nursing care with adolescents also involves objective measurements of the adolescent's and the family's progress toward the goals of treatment. Specifically, the nurse may ask:

- Were the concerns of the adolescent and family addressed?
- Has the problematic behavior decreased and been replaced with more adaptive responses?
- Have the adolescent's relationships with others improved?
- Has school or work performance been enhanced?
- Are the adolescent and family satisfied with the treatment outcome?

By reviewing areas of growth and progress, the adolescent is able to integrate the learning that has been accomplished and gain from the experience a greater sense of self-efficacy and mastery.

COMPETENT CARING   A Clinical Exemplar of a Psychiatric Nurse
Karen M. McHugh, BSN, RN, C

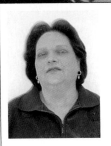

When I graduated with a bachelor's degree in nursing, I never imagined I would be interested in psychiatric nursing. After 1½ years in medical-surgical nursing, I decided I wanted more interpersonal time with my patients rather than being so skill and task oriented. One of my first experiences as a psychiatric nurse was on a 32-bed adolescent unit in North Carolina. There I encountered a 14-year-old girl, S, who was admitted to our inpatient unit for depression. At that time patients typically stayed for about 3 months, which is very different from the current length of stay for adolescents in the hospital, which is most often 5 days.

S had several problems, most occurring within the previous year. She had a history of running away, crying spells, skipping school, failing grades, and suicidal threats. She lived at home with her father and 9-year-old brother. Her mother was no longer involved in her life because she had left the family and given up custody of the children several years before.

S settled into the milieu but had a difficult time engaging with the staff. I began to spend time with her every day to establish a trusting relationship. The first few days we just sat in silence. Eventually we were able to talk about her history of oppositional behavior and low self-esteem. S trusted me more and more over time. Then, about 1 month after admission, she approached me and asked if we could talk again. S asked me if I could promise not to tell anyone (especially her father or doctors) if she confided in me about something. I knew then that something was troubling her, but I had to be honest with her. I told S that I couldn't make that promise because the treatment team works in the best interest of the patient, and I would have to share pertinent information with them. She decided not to confide in me then, but the next day she approached me again.

S began to tell me that the past few months her father had begun to drink and had hit her several times, leaving marks on her legs and arms. She stated that one day she had to stay home from school because her legs were swollen and painful from the bruises. She said that her father always apologized once he was sober and promised that he would never hit her again. I gathered a few more details and was honest with her and informed her that I would have to collaborate with the treatment team and possibly seek help from the Department of Social Services. After meeting with the treatment team the next day, I told S that we had to report her father to Social Services. She began to yell and scream and blame me for telling everyone about her problems. Even though I had been honest with her, she couldn't understand that I was actually helping her.

At this point I had to examine my feelings, and I even questioned my judgment. I went home from work that evening quite upset. I began to ask myself, Did I do the right thing? Will S ever confide in me again or even talk with me? Despite feeling a little guilty, I knew that I had made the right decision because protecting S and her future was of utmost importance. After a few days of cooling off S approached me and was able to express her feelings of relief and even apologized to me. We began to work on identifying and expressing her feelings of guilt, relief, sadness, and concern over the situation with her father. Social Services found no evidence of abuse to her 9-year-old brother, so he remained at home with the father.

At discharge, an aunt assumed foster care of S temporarily until her father could obtain the therapy he needed. S was referred to outpatient therapy as well. Several weeks after her discharge, I saw her at the mall and she thanked me for helping and listening to her even though she didn't see it that way at first. She stated that she was happier now and was doing well in school and that she and her father were continuing therapy.

I had made the right decision. Being a young person's advocate and maintaining a patient's safety during an inpatient stay and after discharge are always a nurse's first priority. As I reflected on this experience, I learned not to take things in my personal life so much for granted, such as a loving and supportive family. I also realized that psychiatric nurses do provide excellence in nursing and that we truly can make a difference. ■

CHAPTER **FOCUS POINTS**

- Adolescence is a unique stage of development that occurs between ages 11 and 20 years and is accompanied by a shift in development and learning.
- Various theories explain the adolescent's resolution of tasks, including biological, psychoanalytical, psychosocial, cognitive, moral development, cultural, and multidimensional.
- Issues that are particularly problematic for adolescents include body image, identity, independence, social role, and sexual behavior.
- Maladaptive responses impede growth and development and require nursing intervention. These are often related to inappropriate

sexual activity, teen pregnancy, depression and suicide, conduct disorders, violence, substance use, and weight and body image problems.
- Nursing interventions useful in working with adolescents include health education, family, group, and individual therapy, and medication management. Special attention should be given to talking with adolescents and working with their parents.
- Evaluation of nursing care requires special focus on countertransference issues and the need for objective measurements of the adolescent's and family's progress toward the treatment goals.

◣ KEY TERMS

adolescence, 753   individuation, 754
delinquency, 764   puberty, 754
identity, 755

◢ CHAPTER REVIEW QUESTIONS

1. Indicate whether the following statements are true (T) or false (F).

_____ A. Brain growth ends before the beginning of adolescence.

_____ B. Chronological age is a good guide for physical maturation during adolescence.

_____ C. A link exists between an adolescent's self-concept and the use of adaptive coping responses.

_____ D. Masturbation can be an effective way for adolescents to discharge sexual tension.

_____ E. When working with adolescents, it is best to have the initial contact with the family to obtain an accurate assessment of the adolescent's problem.

_____ F. Silence is a therapeutic technique that is often frightening to adolescents, especially in the beginning stages of treatment or evaluation.

2. Fill in the blanks.

A. Erikson called the task related to the stage of adolescence

_____.

B. Piaget described adolescence as being characterized by the

cognitive functioning of _____.

C. More _____ than _____ are likely to die by suicide.

D. Drug use is responsible for _____% of the deaths in youth ages 15 to 24 years.

E. When a person is overly preoccupied with flaws perceived in

one's appearance, it is called _____.

F. Two dimensions of positive mental health for adolescents are

_____ and _____.

3. Provide short answers for the following questions.

A. Explain why teenagers delay seeking and using contraceptives.

B. Describe what is meant when tobacco and alcohol are called "gateway drugs."

C. Identify the five stages of substance abuse in adolescence.

D. Give four reasons why medication as a treatment strategy is more complex for adolescents than for adults.

Visit Evolve for additional resources related to the content of this chapter.
http://evolve.elsevier.com/Stuart/principles/
- Topical Course Outline • Student Workbook Exercises • Critical Thinking Questions and Activities • Case Studies • Research Topics
- Monthly Content Updates • WebLinks

Student Study CD-ROM

Access the accompanying CD-ROM for animations, interactive exercises, review questions for the NCLEX examination, and an audio glossary.

REFERENCES

AACAP: "Children and TV violence," *Facts for Families*, #13, 1999a.

AACAP: Comprehensive psychiatric evaluation, *Facts for Families*, #52, 2001.

AACAP: Conduct disorder, *Fact for Families*, #33, 2000.

AACAP: Self-injury in adolescents, *Facts for Families*, #73, 1999b.

AACAP: Tobacco and kids, *Facts for Families*, #68, 1999c.

Anderson MA et al: School-associated violent deaths in the United States, 1994-1999, *JAMA*, 286:2695, 2001.

Barger R: *A summary of Lawrence Kohlberg's stages of moral development*, Notre Dame, Indiana, 2000, University of Notre Dame.

Beautrais AL: Suicide and serious suicide attempts in youth: a multiple-group comparison study, *Am J Psychiatry* 160:1093, 2003.

Blos P: *On adolescence, a psychoanalytic interpretation*, Free Press, 1962, New York.

Blum RW: *Mother's influence on teen sex: connections that promote postponing sexual intercourse*, Center for Adolescent Health and Development, University of Minnesota, 2002.

Brown A: Adolescent depressive disorders, *NARSAD* 1:32, 2002.

Canuso R: A pregnant adolescent: negotiating a difficult journey to adulthood, *J Child Adolesc Psychiatr Nurs* 13:39, 2000.

CDC: Alcohol/Other Drug Use, U.S., *Youth Risk Behavior Surveillance System*, 2001a.

CDC: Sexual Behaviors, U.S., *Youth Risk Behavior Surveillance System*, 2001b.

CDC: Youth Violence, *National Center for Injury Prevention and Control*, 2003.

Champion JD, Kelly P: Protective and risk behaviors of rural minority adolescent women, *Issues Ment Health Nurs* 23:191, 2002.

DeWit DJ et al: Age at first alcohol use: a risk factor for the development of alcohol disorders, *Am J Psychiatry* 157:745, 2000.

Eggert LL et al: Preliminary effects of brief school-based prevention approaches for reducing youth suicide: risk behaviors, depression, and drug involvement, *J Child Adolesc Psychiatr Nurs* 15:48, 2002.

Erikson E: *Childhood and society*, ed 2, New York, 1963, WW Norton.

Farmer TJ: The experience of major depression: adolescents' perspectives, *Issues Ment Health Nurs* 23:567, 2002.

Fergusson DM, Woodward LT: Mental health, educational and social role outcomes of adolescents with depression, *Arch Gen Psychiatry* 59:225, 2002.

Fergusson D, Horwood LJ, Beautrais AL: Is sexual orientation related to mental health problems and suicidality in young people? *Arch Gen Psychiatry* 56:876, 1999.

Gilligan C: *In a different voice, psychological theory and women's development*, Harvard University Press, 1982, Cambridge, Mass.

Golub A, Johnson BD: Variation in youthful risks of progression from alcohol and tobacco to marijuana and to hard drugs across generations, *Am J Public Health* 91:225, 2001.

Greenfield B et al: A rapid-response outpatient model for reducing hospitalization rates among suicidal adolescents, *Psychiatr Serv* 53:1574, 2002.

Harvard Mental Health Letter: Confronting suicide, 19:1, 2003.

Havighurst R: *Developmental tasks and education*, ed 3, New York, 1972, David McKay.

Joe S, Marcus SC: Datapoints: trends by race and gender in suicide attempts among US adolescents, 1991-2001, *Psychiatr Serv* 54:454, 2003.

Kilpatrick DG et al: Risk factors for adolescent substance abuse and dependence: data from a national sample, *J Consult Clin Psychol* 68:19, 2000.

Kuperman S et al: Developmental sequence from disruptive behavior diagnosis to adolescent alcohol dependence, *Am J Psychiatry* 158:2022, 2001.

Lock J, Steiner H: Gay, lesbian, and bisexual youth risks for emotional, physical, and social problems: results from a community-based survey, *J Am Acad Child Adolesc Psychiatry* 38:297, 1999.

Logsdon MC et al: Social support in pregnant and parenting adolescents: research, critique and recommendations, *J Child Adolesc Psychiatr Nurs* 15:75, 2002.

Mainous RO et al: The importance of fulfilling unmet needs of rural and urban adolescents with substance abuse, *J Child Adolesc Psychiatr Nurs* 14:32, 2001.

Meeks J: *The fragile alliance*, ed 4, Malabar, Fla, 1990, Robert Krieger.

NIH: National Heart, Lung and Blood Institute study shows weight concerns increase girl's risk of becoming smokers, *NIH news release*, June 3, 2002.

Piaget J: *Six psychological studies*, New York, 1968, Vintage.

Pine DS et al: Adolescent depressive symptoms as predictors of adult depression: moodiness or mood disorder? *Am J Psychiatry* 156:133, 1999.

Powers SI, Hauser ST, Kilner LA: Adolescent mental health, *Am Psychol* 44:200, 1989.

Rew L et al: Correlates for recent suicide attempts in a triethnic group of adolescents. *J Nurs Scholarsh* 33:361, 2001.

Sege R et al: Ten years after: examination of adolescent screening questions that predict future violence-related injury, *J Adolesc Health* 24:395, 1999.

SIECUS: Lesbian, gay, and bisexual and transgender youth issues, *SIECUS Report*, 29:1, 2001.

Sullivan H: *Interpersonal theory of psychiatry*, New York, 1953, WW Norton.

Weisz JR, Jensen PS: Efficacy and effectiveness of child and adolescent psychotherapy and pharmacotherapy, *Ment Health Serv Res* 1:125, 1999.

Youth is like a fresh flower in May. Age is like a rainbow that follows the storms of life. Each has its own beauty.

DAVID POLIS

GEROPSYCHIATRIC NURSING 38

Georgia L. Stevens

LEARNING OBJECTIVES

After studying this chapter, the student should be able to:
1. Examine the dimensions of mental illness in the elderly and the role of the geropsychiatric nurse (I).
2. Compare the major biopsychosocial theories of aging (II).
3. Discuss the elements of a comprehensive geropsychiatric nursing assessment (III).
4. Formulate nursing diagnoses for geropsychiatric patients (IV).
5. Analyze evidence-based nursing interventions for geropsychiatric patients (V).
6. Evaluate nursing care of geropsychiatric patients (VI).

TOPICAL OUTLINE

evolve   Visit Evolve for additional resources related to the content of this chapter.
http://evolve.elsevier.com/Stuart/principles/

People age 85 years and older comprise the fastest growing age-group in the United States. Changing mortality, fertility, and immigration patterns create some degree of uncertainty when predicting the future size of the elderly population. By the year 2030 older adults will comprise 20% of the population, compared to 13% in 2000. Minority elders will increase from 16% in 1980 to 25% in 2030 (Administration on Aging, 2000).

The future elderly population will be especially diverse. Socioeconomic factors that will affect the elderly's status are advances in health care, changes in the labor force, family structure, and caregiver characteristics. Many of tomorrow's elderly will be better educated, healthier, and wealthier than cohorts at the end of the 20th century, resulting in a rethinking of our concepts of retirement and old age.

Minority groups are projected to have the highest growth rates. Historically, minority groups have had lower socioeco-

nomic status and less access to health care. Thus for many elderly disparity among health, income, and education levels will increase, presenting public health and policy challenges (Administration on Aging, 2001).

Since 1900 the elderly population has doubled approximately three times. Although this group has increased by more than 100% since 1960, the general population has increased by only 50%. This increase in the elderly dependency ratio (the ratio of the elderly to the working-age population) will negatively impact the financial support of social programs such as Medicare, Social Security, and other federal and state health care and disability programs unless functional levels of the oldest old continue to improve (Blazer, 2000).

By the year 2050, the "oldest old" (85 and older) segment of the elderly population is anticipated to increase between 24% and 30%. With projections of 10.8 million to 14 million people requiring long-term care, it is this segment of the population that will drive up the demand for services and programs that address chronic illness and disability.

■ MENTAL ILLNESS IN THE ELDERLY

It is projected that those 65 and older with potentially disabling serious mental illness will increase from 4 million in 1970 to 15 million in 2030. Mortality rates for younger mentally ill patients will decrease, resulting in many mentally ill individuals living into old age. It is also anticipated that aging baby boomers (those born between 1946 and 1964), who number 75 million in the United States, will be at greater risk for substance abuse, anxiety disorders, and depression than the current cohort of elders, and thus the need for these specialty services will increase.

Historically, older adults with mental health problems have relied on their primary care providers for management of all their health needs. The occurrence of mental illness may be underestimated in nonpsychiatric settings, because symptoms may be misattributed to physical disorders, normal aging, cognitive impairment, or the lack of age-appropriate diagnostic criteria. Illnesses such as depression are often misdiagnosed or undertreated. The comorbidity of somatic and psychiatric illnesses makes accurate diagnosis more difficult.

Medicare's restrictive reimbursement policies are especially unsatisfactory for severely mentally ill elderly patients. As of the beginning of the 21st century, Medicare limited inpatient hospital days, imposed restrictions on the number of visits to health care providers, and slowly addressed the need for prescription drug coverage. Similar problems for the elderly mentally ill exist in the recently developed models of managed mental health care. Thus the economic and personal costs of mental disorders of older adults are considerable.

On the other hand, impressive changes in academic and research interests in aging and the elderly have happened in the past few decades. New scientific findings and hypotheses, such as a better understanding of normal aging and the discovery of a cholinergic deficit in Alzheimer's disease, have been combined with the concepts of health promotion and preventive medicine to move studies beyond asking what aging *is*, to what is *possible* with aging. The importance of understanding potential in relation to aging is profound, because doing so will not only enable older people to access latent skills and talents in later life but also challenge today's younger age-groups to think about what is possible for them in their later years in a way they may not have thought about before (Cohen, 2000; Vaillant and Mukamal, 2001).

Helping older adults maximize their potential can be a challenging and rewarding experience for the nurse. Stereotypes and myths often depict the elderly as a homogeneous group. On the contrary, the older adult represents a combination of biological, interpersonal, developmental, and situational experiences. The complexity and interaction of the needs and problems of old age are often understated and misunderstood.

Mental health in late life depends on a number of factors. These include physiological and psychological status, personality, social support system, economic resources, and usual lifestyle. This chapter addresses selected aspects of the psychiatric–mental health needs of geriatric patients and their families.

Role of the Geropsychiatric Nurse

The nurse who works with older adults who have mental illness is challenged to integrate psychiatric nursing skills with knowledge of physiological disorders, the normal aging process, and sociocultural influences on the elderly and their families. Many nurses who work with these patients find that it is useful to combine nurse practitioner and psychiatric nursing skills.

Case management is a particularly effective approach to providing for the biopsychosocial needs of the elderly. Mental health services are provided to this population in a variety of settings, including general and psychiatric hospitals, nursing homes, assisted living residential centers, outpatient mental health clinics, adult day-care programs, senior centers, and the person's own home.

As a primary care provider, the geropsychiatric nurse should be proficient at assessing patients' cognitive, affective, functional, physical, and behavioral statuses, as well as their family dynamics. The nurse also needs knowledge of community resources and how to access them. Planning and nursing intervention may involve collaboration with the patient and family or other caregivers. Providing nursing care to these patients can be complex because they are often involved with a number of agencies, thus the need for coordination of services is great.

As a consultant, the geropsychiatric nurse helps other providers address the behavioral, social, and cognitive aspects of the patient's care. For instance, a nurse may help nursing assistants understand how to respond to a patient who wanders or one who is aggressive. Advanced practice geropsychiatric nurses who have graduate education in this specialty may be employed by agencies to help the entire staff develop therapeutic programs for seniors with psychiatric or behavioral issues (Bartels, Moak, and Dums, 2002b).

Geropsychiatric nurses should be knowledgeable about the effects of psychotropic medication on elderly people. They often work closely with the physician and nurse prescribers to monitor complex medication regimens and help the patient or caregiver with medication management. They may lead a variety of groups, such as orientation, remotivation, bereavement, and socialization groups, whereas nurses with advanced degrees may also provide psychotherapy and medication prescriptions.

Finally, the role of patient advocate is a critical one for the nurse caring for elders with mental illnesses, particularly those with concurrent physical illness. Because of cognitive changes or symptoms of acute or chronic health problems, elders may not be able to effectively voice their wishes or concerns. Sensitivity is required when addressing the families of the seriously mentally ill because they may have been dealing with "caregiving challenges" for many years.

Reviewing legal options such as advance directives or a living will helps in the promotion of the elder's wishes. In cases where conflict exists regarding the elder's care, particularly in long-term care settings, an ombudsman or guardian may be contacted to help resolve these issues. Information about ombudsman or other advocacy programs for the elderly may be obtained by contacting any local office on aging.

■ THEORIES OF AGING

Ways of defining aging and explaining the causes and consequences of the aging process are based on three major theoretical approaches: biological, psychological, and sociocultural theories of aging. The nurse should be well-acquainted with each of these theories of aging to best understand, evaluate, and care for geriatric patients. These theories provide the basis for a number of the evidence-based nursing interventions discussed in this chapter.

Biological Theories

Biological theories of aging are described as follows:

Biological programming theory: The life span of a cell, its "biological clock," is stored within the cell itself; thus the process of aging is programmed by deoxyribonucleic acid (DNA) and is inevitable and irreversible.

Give at least two examples that contradict the biological programming theory of aging. How do you feel about the idea of a biological clock determining life span? ■

Cross-linkage theory: Collagen forms bonds between molecular structures causing increasing rigidity over time.

Error theory: Errors manifested during protein synthesis create error cells that then multiply.

Free radical theory: Free radicals damage cell membranes, causing physical damage and decline.

Gene theories: Harmful genes activate in late life; cell divisions are finite; or failure to produce growth substances stops cell growth and division.

Immunological theory: The immune system becomes less effective in surveillance, self-regulation, and response.

Stress adaptation theory: The positive and negative effects of stress on biopsychosocial development are emphasized; stress may drain a person's reserve capacity physiologically, socially, and economically, increasing vulnerability to illness or injury, accelerating the aging process.

Wear-and-tear theory: Cells wear out from internal and external causes; structural and functional changes may be speeded by abuse and slowed by care; this theory is the basis of many myths and stereotypes ("What can you expect from someone his age?").

Discuss how the wear-and-tear theory of aging compares with the present emphasis on nutrition and physical fitness in American culture. ■

Psychological Theories

The following list details psychological theories of aging:

Erikson's stage of ego integrity: This developmental theory identifies tasks that must be accomplished at each of the eight stages of life. The last stage of development involves reflection about one's life and accomplishments. The result of resolving this conflict between ego integrity and despair is wisdom.

Life review: A universal process of examination and reintegration of memories gives meaning to life and prepares one for death by relieving anxiety and fear.

Stability of personality: One's personality is established by early adulthood and remains fairly stable yet adaptable (rather than being a developmental progression over the life span). Radical changes in personality in old age may be indicative of brain disease.

 Can personality traits be altered in old age? If yes, how? If no, why are we interested in intervening in nonproductive behaviors of older adults? ■

Sociocultural Theories

Sociocultural theories of aging are described in the following list:

Disengagement theory: Older adults and society mutually withdraw from active exchange with each other as part of the normal aging process. This controversial theory assumes this separation to be a sign of psychological well-being and adjustment and has reinforced many stereotypes (such as "older people only enjoy the company of people their own age").

Activity theory: Disputes about the reliability of disengagement theory led to the view that activity produces the most positive psychological climate for older adults and that the aged should remain active as long as possible. It emphasizes the positive influence of activity on the older person's personality, mental health, and life satisfaction.

What type of program would you design for older adults who must stop working or participating in community activities? ■

Family theories: The focus of these theories is on the family as the basic unit of emotional development. Interrelated tasks, problems, and relationships are emphasized within the three-generational family. Physical, emotional, and social symptoms are believed to reflect problems in negotiating the transitions of the family life cycle.

Person-environment fit theory: This approach addresses the relationship of the personal competencies of older adults and their environments. If competencies decrease or change with age, one's capacity to relate to the environment may diminish. Frail older adults are especially vulnerable to perceiving the environment as threatening (environmental demand).

■ ASSESSING THE GERIATRIC PATIENT

Nursing assessment of the geropsychiatric patient is complex. The interplay of biological, psychological, and sociocultural factors related to aging sometimes makes it difficult to clearly identify nursing problems. For example, it can be quite difficult to sort out the behaviors related to the 4 D's of geropsychiatric assessment: **depression, dementia, delirium,** and **delusions** (see Chapter 23). The co-existence of simple medical problems such as a urinary tract infection or dehydration can exacerbate behavioral symptoms.

Aside from major psychotic disorders, delusions are also characteristic of depression in the elderly, and those with dementia may seem delusional because of the trouble they have in interpreting the environment. Delirium may occur as a reaction to physical illness, medications, or sensory deprivation. Behaviors associated with delirium include hallucinations, delusions, confusion, disorientation, and agitation. Delirium may be mistaken for dementia, thereby depriving the patient of treatment that could reverse the problem.

Depressed elders often appear confused and cognitively impaired because of the lethargy and psychomotor retardation related to depression. Patients with dementia also may present with anxiety, agitation, and depression, especially if they are aware of their declining mental functioning. The first episode of depression in later life is associated with greater chronicity, relapse, cognitive dysfunction, and an increased rate of dementia (Paterniti et al, 2002).

Behaviors have been identified that help differentiate between depression and dementia. Depressed patients are oriented and maintain socially appropriate behaviors. They are unlikely to undress in public or be incontinent. In contrast, patients with dementia will try to answer questions but have trouble with logic and relevance. Depressed patients will be annoyed and reject the questioner with silence or short, unresponsive answers. Irritability and hostility are more characteristic of the depressed person.

Careful nursing assessment can be helpful in identifying the primary disorder. Nursing diagnoses are based on observation of patient behaviors and are related to current needs. A comprehensive nursing assessment sets the stage for the rest of the nursing process (Table 38-1).

The Interview

Establishing a supportive and trusting relationship is essential to fostering a positive interview with the geriatric patient. The elderly person may feel uneasy, vulnerable, and confused in a new place or with strangers. Patience and attentive listening promote a sense of security. Comfortable surroundings help the patient relax and focus on the conversation.

Therapeutic Communication Skills. The nurse shows respect by addressing the patient by his or her last name: "Good morning, Mr. Smith." The nurse opens the interview by introducing oneself and briefly orienting the patient to the purpose and length of the interview. Occasionally reinforcing the amount of time left may help direct a wandering discussion and give the patient the security of knowing that the nurse is in control of the situation.

Older people may respond to questions slowly because verbal response slows with age. It is important to give the patient enough time to answer and not assume that a slow response is due to a deficit in knowledge, comprehension, or memory.

The language used by the nurse is important because older people often are unfamiliar with slang, colloquialisms, jargon, abbreviations, or medical terminology. Choice of words should also be based on knowledge of the person's sociocultural background and level of formal education.

Questions should be short and to the point, particularly if the patient has difficulty with abstract thinking and conceptualization. Techniques such as clarification and summarization, described in Chapter 2, are important in validating information. The nurse should rephrase a question if the patient does not answer appropriately or hesitates when answering.

Concentrated verbal interaction may be uncomfortable for the older person. The nurse can demonstrate interest and support by giving nonverbal cues and responses, such as direct eye contact, nodding, sitting close to the patient, and using touch appropriately. Touching the shoulder, arm, or hand of the patient in a firm, purposeful manner conveys support and interest. Avoid stroking or patting the patient. Cultural background and altered tactile perception may result in misinterpretation.

The nurse's ability to collect useful data depends greatly on how comfortable she feels during the interview. Negative feelings toward the aged or ignorance about aging will surface in an interview. Older people are sensitive to others' disregard, lack of interest, and impatience.

Elderly patients have much to tell and may offer more information than the nurse needs at a particular time. The

Table 38-1	Key Components of Geropsychiatric Nursing Assessment	
COMPONENT	KEY ELEMENTS
Interviewing	Therapeutic communication skills
	Comfortable, quiet setting
Mental status	Mini-Mental State Examination
	Mental status examination
	Depression
	Anxiety
	Psychosis
Behavioral responses	Description of behavior and triggers
	Assessment of behavioral change
	Frequently observed challenging behaviors
Functional abilities	Mobility
	Activities of daily living
	Risk for falls
Physiological functioning	General health
	Nutrition
	Substance abuse
Social support	Social support systems past and current
	Family-patient interaction
	Caregiver concerns

nurse should encourage this when possible. Reminiscence and life review may be an excellent source of data about the patient's current health problems and support resources. Even though keeping the patient focused on the topic at hand may be difficult, these formats allow the nurse to assess subtle changes in long-term memory, decision-making ability, judgment, affect, and orientation to time, place, and person.

Many geriatric patients are aware of changes in their physical or psychological functioning. They may hesitate to have their fears confirmed. They may minimize or ignore symptoms, assuming that they are related to age and not to current medical or psychiatric problems. Often these beliefs are reinforced by myths about aging and the false assumption of many health professionals that the problems of older people are irreversible or untreatable.

Contrary to popular myths, most older people do not dwell unrealistically on their health. However, some older people are preoccupied with the physical decline that occurs with age. The nurse should observe carefully for clues that help distinguish whether the patient's preoccupation reflects life-long personality factors or current distress.

The geriatric patient may misunderstand the purpose of the nurse's questions. Questions regarding habits, previous life experience, or social supports may not seem to be related to current concerns. Careful and repeated explanations are necessary to gain the patient's cooperation. The nurse should never assume that the patient understands the purpose or protocol for the assessment interview. It is wiser to overstate than to increase the patient's anxiety and stress by omitting information. The nurse should take cues from the patient's responses by listening carefully and observing constantly.

What special challenges might you face in obtaining informed consent for treatment from a geriatric patient? How might you deal with them? ■

The Interview Setting. The new and unfamiliar surroundings of the health care agency may obstruct the initial interview by distracting the patient and increasing fear of the unknown. If possible, the nurse should assess the patient in a familiar environment to reduce the patient's anxiety. The physical environment should promote comfort. Many older people are unable to sit for long periods because of arthritis or other joint disabilities. Chairs should be comfortable. Changing positions can be encouraged.

Most older people experience some form of sensory deficit, particularly diminished high-frequency hearing or changes in vision as a result of cataracts or glaucoma. The setting should be quiet and without distracting noises. The nurse should speak slowly and in a low-pitched voice. Because fatigue may contribute to diminished mental functioning, morning may be the best time for the interview, as patients may tire as the day progresses.

The reliability of the data obtained from the assessment interview should be carefully evaluated. If there are questions about some of the patient's responses, the nurse should consult family members or other people who know the patient well. The nurse also should consider the impact of the patient's physical condition at the time of the interview and other factors, such as medications, nutrition, or anxiety level.

Mental Status

Mental status should be part of any geropsychiatric assessment for a number of reasons, including the following:

- Increasing prevalence of dementia with age
- Prevalence and reversibility of delirium if recognized and treated
- Close association of clinical symptoms of confusion and depression
- Frequency with which physical health problems present with symptoms of confusion
- Need to identify specific areas of cognitive strength and limitation

An in-depth discussion of the assessment of mental status is presented in Chapter 7.

Depression. Affective status is an essential part of geropsychiatric assessment. The need to include a depression assessment is based on the following:

- Prevalence of depression in the elderly
- Effectiveness of treatment for depression
- Potential negative outcomes of depression (such as suicide or neglect)
- Frequent misdiagnosis of depression as a physical problem
- Tendency to dismiss elders as complainers or demanding
- Necessity of accurately distinguishing between depressive and bipolar disorders
- Tendency for depression to recur with increasing age

General estimates of the prevalence of depression among the elderly are 15% to 20%. The incidence of depression among people of all ages who have disabilities is higher. Because the number of physical disabilities tends to increase with age, this may account for some of the prevalence in the elderly. Prevalence rates for elders residing in the community and those in nursing homes range from 15% to 40% for depressive symptoms and from 1% to 16% for major depressive disorder (Cole and Dendukuri, 2003; Blazer, 2003).

Diagnosis of depression in the elderly is missed 85% of the time, perhaps because it differs in some ways from that in younger populations and thus is assumed to be part of the normal aging process (Bair, 2000). The use of usual diagnostic criteria for psychiatric disorders in the oldest old may be complicated by comorbidity issues and thus geriatric syndromes have been described (Blazer, 2000).

Depression may begin with decreased interest in usual activities and lack of energy. There may be an increased sense of helplessness and dependence on others. Conversation may focus almost entirely on the past. There may be multiple somatic complaints with no diagnosable organic cause. The person may have pain, especially in the head, neck, back, or abdomen with no history or evidence of a physical cause. Other symptoms in the elderly include sleep changes, weight loss, cognitive complaints, irritability/hostility, gastrointestinal distress, and refusal to eat or drink, with potentially life-threatening consequences.

Physical illness can cause secondary depression (see Chapter 19). Some illnesses that tend to be associated with depression include thyroid disorders; cancer, especially lung, pancreas, and brain; Parkinson's disease; stroke; and Alzheimer's disease. Vascular depression has been identified from the association between depression and vascular lesions in the brain.

Many of the medications routinely prescribed for older people can increase depression. Examples include antianxiety drugs and sedative/hypnotics, antipsychotics, cardiotonics (digoxin), and steroids. A medication history is an essential part of patient assessment, especially for the elderly, most of whom tend to take multiple medications.

Anxiety. A thorough assessment of anxiety levels, coping responses, and precipitating stressors provides the nurse with information necessary for planning effective nursing care for the elderly. Anxiety disorders lower the quality of life for many elderly people and increase the burden on family, care providers, and health services.

Anxiety is common and a serious public health concern, with an overall community prevalence of 11.4% for disorders and 17% to 21% for anxiety symptoms. All anxiety disorders affect the elderly: generalized anxiety disorder (17%), phobias (10% to 12%), obsessive compulsive disorder (1.5%), and panic disorder (0.5%) (Administration on Aging, 2001). When combined, their symptom prevalence among older people may be even higher than rates of depression alone.

Untreated or inappropriately treated anxiety among older people also can contribute to sleep problems, cognitive impairments, and decreased quality of life. Comorbid anxiety and depression are common in the elderly and complicate diagnosis and treatment outcomes.

Psychosis. Although the prevalence of schizophrenia is estimated to be 0.6% of older adults, the prevalence of psychotic disorders increases with age and is estimated to be between 4% and 23% in the elderly (Administration on Aging, 2001). Therefore the nurse may frequently find prominent psychotic features during the assessment of older adults. Psychosis may be associated with delirium, dementia, depression with psychosis, substance abuse, or problems with reality testing.

It is important for the nurse to be familiar with the clinical risk factors for developing psychosis in later life. These include cognitive impairment, sensory impairments (vision and hearing), social isolation, female gender, confinement to bed with a conflictual caregiver relationship, somatic comorbidity, multiple medications, or underlying medical disorders. Patients with a psychiatric diagnosis of psychosis may respond to supportive therapy and low doses of atypical antipsychotic drugs (see Chapter 27).

Behavioral Responses

A thorough behavioral assessment is especially important as a basis for planning nursing care for an elderly person. Behavioral changes may be the first sign of many physical and mental disorders. It is important to identify who is bothered by the behavior—the patient, the family, peers, or unrelated caregivers. Behaviors are variously referred to as behavior problems, disruptive behaviors, disturbing behaviors, and challenging behaviors (Edberg, Gerdner, and Buckwalter, 2003). The latter term is thought to be the most effective because it reinforces the nurse's role in understanding what the behavior is communicating.

If possible, the initial assessment should be completed in a familiar environment. This will capitalize on environmental factors that reduce the elder's anxiety. It will also give the nurse a chance to observe possible triggers of disruptive behavior. Family members or other caregivers can be asked about their usual responses to the patient's behavior, especially what is helpful and unhelpful. This may provide further clues about the source of the behavior.

It is also helpful to know why the behavior is bothersome. Elders and their families may be frightened by changes in behavior because they associate them with deterioration and the possible onset of dementia. Based on the assessment, the cause of the problem may be treated and the person returned to prior levels of function.

For instance, a woman who is agitated because of an undiagnosed urinary tract infection returns to her usual, calm self after the infection is treated. In other cases it may not be possible to remove the cause of the behavior, but nursing intervention can help the patient and family adapt to it. For example, a man is irritable because he is becoming forgetful. Early Alzheimer's disease is diagnosed. The patient becomes less irritable after the nurse teaches him and his family ways to maximize his memory. Behavioral changes related to declining cognitive functioning are often difficult to manage and necessitate creative treatment.

Behavioral assessment involves defining the behavior; its frequency; duration; and precipitating factors or triggers, including the environment. When a behavioral change occurs, it is important to analyze the underlying meaning. For instance, the person may be experiencing a threat to self-esteem or a change in sensory input. A complete physical examination is needed after any abrupt behavioral change to rule out delirium (Salzman, 2004). Caregiver response to behavior must also be assessed because it may reinforce or increase challenging behavior. Common challenging behaviors (behavioral excesses) in the elderly are listed in Box 38-1.

Mr. Jones, an elderly patient, strikes out at the staff every morning when he is approached at bath time. Describe the steps you would take to assess this behavior. What questions might you ask his family? What advice would you give to the staff who work with him? ∎

Functional Abilities

Assessment of the geropsychiatric patient is not limited to indicators of mental health. Rather, mental status can depend greatly on the older person's overall functional ability. This discussion emphasizes the aspects of the functional assessment that have the greatest impact on mental and emotional status.

BOX 38-1

Behavioral Challenges Observed in Geropsychiatric Patients

Agitation	Intrusiveness
Apathy	Isolating self
Biting	Kicking
Catastrophic reaction	Negativity
Complaining	Pacing
Confusion	Rapid speech
Constant talking	Refusal to eat/drink
Delusions	Repetitive movement
Disinhibition	Resistiveness
Emotional lability	Restlessness
Fatigue	Scolding
Forgetting	Sexual disinhibition
Hallucinations	Spitting
Hand wringing	Suspiciousness
Hitting	Swearing/racial slurs
Hoarding and hiding	Threats of harm
Incontinence	Throwing things
Indifference	Wandering

Table 38-2 Assessment of Risk for Falls

RISK FACTORS	ASSESSMENT FACTORS
Environmental hazards	Excessive stimulation (noise)
	Poor lighting
	Slippery or wet surfaces
	Stairs (no handrails, steep, poorly lit)
	Loose objects on the floor
	Throw rugs
	Small pets underfoot
Patient variables	History of falls
	Diurnal alertness level
	Familiarity with surroundings
	Emotional state (agitated, angry, etc.)
	Willingness to request help
	Confusion
	Usual activity level
	Type of activity
Assistive devices	Presence and adequacy of:
	Eyeglasses
	Hearing aid
	Ambulation aids (cane, tripod, walker)
	Prostheses
	Environmental aids (grab bars, hand rails)
	Uncluttered surroundings
Medications	Taking medications (prescribed or over-the-counter) that cause:
	Drowsiness
	Confusion
	Orthostatic hypotension
	Incoordination
	Decreased sensation
	Polypharmacy
Physical or mental disorders	Cardiovascular
	Orthopedic
	Neuromuscular
	Perceptual
	Cognitive
	Affective
	Altered nutritional status
	Fatigue and weakness
	Unsteady gait/mobility problems

Mobility. Mobility and independence are important to the elder's perception of personal health. Three aspects of mobility should be assessed:

1. **Moving within the environment**
2. **Participating in necessary activities**
3. **Maintaining contact with others**

In assessing ambulation the nurse would address motor losses, adaptations made, use of assistive devices, balance, eyesight, and the amount and type of help needed. Factors that influence ambulation include restriction of joints caused by degenerative diseases, orthostatic hypotension, and the type and fit of footwear. Motor ability of the arms can be tested by observing the patient comb the hair, shave, dress, and eat.

Many medications taken by geriatric patients alter perception, making ambulation and mobility difficult and thus contributing to falls. This is particularly so with sedative-hypnotics, antianxiety, cardiovascular, and hypertensive drugs. Patients should be cautioned about side effects of medications and should be encouraged to take time when ambulating and moving from one position to another.

The incidence of falls and negative outcomes increases with age; 30% of people over 65 fall every year, with women falling at twice the rate of men. Falls result in physical injuries, such as hip fractures, as well as psychological effects, such as fearfulness. Risk factors should be assessed and are summarized in Table 38-2.

Activities of Daily Living. The assessment of self-care needs and activities of daily living (ADLs) is essential for determining the patient's potential for independence. Activity may be limited because of physical dysfunction or psychosocial impairment. Although geriatric patients should be encouraged to become more independent in self-

care, it is unrealistic to expect all patients to function independently. This is particularly so for people who are in a hospital or long-term–care setting. Conforming to the routines and procedures of the institutional environment fosters dependence in the patient. Because such behavioral deficits or excess disability are associated with premature comorbidity and mortality, institutional environments present the nurse with opportunities for creative intervention and care planning.

ADLs (bathing, dressing, eating, grooming, and toileting) are concrete and task-oriented. They provide an opportunity for purposeful nurse-patient interaction. Encouraging patients to be as independent as possible in performing their own ADLs is important. This helps elders meet their needs for safety, security, personal space, self-esteem, autonomy, and personal identity.

Physiological Functioning

General Health. Assessment of physical health is especially important with elderly patients because of the interaction of multiple chronic conditions, the presence of sensory deficits, the taking of many medications, and the behavioral presentation of many physical health problems. Diagnostic procedures that may be useful include blood and urine chemistry values; the electrocardiogram; and for some patients, the electroencephalogram, lumbar puncture, and brain visual imaging techniques, such as the computed tomography scan and magnetic resonance imaging.

In addition to these physiological factors, nutritional status and substance use should be assessed. A complete medication profile that includes all prescription and over-the-counter drugs, drugs "borrowed" from another, and all herbal remedies (including teas) and dietary supplements is essential.

Evidence documents a direct relationship among stress, immune system functioning, and mood. Clinical observations have identified a failure-to-thrive syndrome, especially in the final phase of life. This includes weight loss, decreased appetite, poor nutrition, fatigue, weakness, and inactivity. It is often accompanied by dehydration, depressive symptoms, impaired immune functions, and a low serum cholesterol level. Failure to thrive in the elderly occurs in both acute and chronic forms, leading to impaired functional status, morbidity from infection, pressure wounds, and increased mortality.

Nutrition. Many elderly patients do not require help to eat or plan a nutritious diet. However, some geropsychiatric patients do have psychosocial problems that create a need for help with eating and monitoring dietary intake. These problems include the following:

- Depression or loneliness, resulting in decreased appetite
- Changes in cognition, such as confusion, agnosia, or apraxia
- Suicidal tendencies
- Removal from familiar ethnic and cultural eating patterns
- Fear of institutional routines or procedures

The range of physical problems varies greatly. The following areas should be assessed:

- Whether the patient has enough mobility and strength to open cartons of milk, cut meat, and handle utensils
- Presence of neurological or joint conditions that interfere with hand and arm coordination
- Presence of vision problems
- Missing teeth and other losses of chewing ability
- Problems in swallowing or breathing
- Presence of ulcerations on the tongue or elsewhere in the mouth
- Periodontal disease
- Dry mouth because of medications

The nurse should routinely evaluate the patient's dietary needs. Nutritional deficiencies are one of the most significant problems of the institutionalized elderly and can cause other problems, such as skin breakdown, inadequate absorption of medications, and impaired wound healing.

Nutritional assessment also should explore personal preferences, including prior routines (such as having largest meal at lunchtime), time of day for meals, portion sizes, and food likes and dislikes. Serum cholesterol and albumin levels provide additional information about the person's nutritional status.

Substance Abuse. Most studies of alcoholism have focused on a younger population, so the prevalence of alcohol abuse by elders has not been well documented. There is a risk of developing alcoholism in later life if there has been habitual drinking in the past. A second group begins drinking in later life (Lantz, 2002). Significant loss and role changes or increased anxiety and concern over health add to the risk. **Alcohol is the most commonly abused substance by the elderly** because it is readily available and not usually perceived as a drug.

The abuse of **prescription drugs**, particularly sedative-hypnotic and antianxiety medications, is also common and may not be seen as an addiction. Alcohol and substance abuse can lead to increased morbidity and mortality. Abuse of alcohol or any substance may be a means of attaining distance from painful issues such as loss and loneliness.

Social Support

Positive support systems are essential for maintaining a sense of well-being throughout life. This is especially important for the geropsychiatric patient. With age, close family members and friends are lost. As a person's significant contacts decrease in number, it is important that the remaining support systems be consistent and meaningful.

Caring behaviors among elderly nursing home residents have been found to be a major way in which residents maintain their personal identity, sense of value, and continuation of personhood. This demonstrates that support systems that develop among patients are beneficial to those who give and receive care. Such relationships should be fostered.

Health behaviors, such as acceptance of outside interventions and self-efficacy, are guided by cultural beliefs and life experiences. For example, access to services has been limited for the poor, frail, and members of ethnic minority groups. These groups may have depended more on informal caregivers, such as the extended and immediate family, and informal support networks.

The nurse should be sensitive to the individual's belief system and should assess the support systems available to the patient while at home, in the hospital, or in another health care setting. Family and friends can help reduce the shock and stress of hospitalization and offer reassurance and comfort to the distressed elder.

Family-Patient Interaction. Family demographics are changing. Increased life expectancy, declining birth rate, and higher life expectancy for women all affect the availability of family to participate in caregiving and support of the elder.

The majority of elders have a minimum of weekly contact with their children.

Discuss the ways in which changing demographics in American society are affecting the social support systems of elderly people. What is the impact on their families? ■

Family expectations about caring for older members vary. The decision to care for an aging member at home or to include extended family members in the household is discussed over time within the family unit. The majority of caregiving in the United States is provided by family members. Significant issues that affect families in late adulthood are retirement, widowhood, grandparenthood, and illness.

Nurses should become more comfortable and knowledgeable about dealing with issues of sexuality, marital discord, cohabitation, spousal abuse, and elder abuse. The cultural norms that previously placed elderly people in a position of respect as pivotal members of the community appear to have eroded in much of American society. Social and organizational structures have not developed supports to replace those previously available through extended family networks.

A great deal of discussion can be found in the literature concerning abuse of elderly people, but more research is needed to establish its prevalence and the factors related to it. The nurse should be aware of changing trends and be alert for the possibility of elder abuse, which is addressed in more detail in Chapter 39.

When assessing the older adult, the nurse should note previous success in dealing with life issues. The elder's adjustment to losses and changes associated with aging is affected by earlier life experiences. Challenging behaviors in the elderly may result from the family's inability to deal with the losses and increasing dependence of an older member. Reliable and valid measurement tools, along with a careful diagnosis, help strengthen the nursing process, moving it from intuitive to evidence-based assessment (Bartels et al, 2002a).

■ DIAGNOSIS OF THE GERIATRIC PATIENT

Although older adults may experience a wide range of psychiatric problems, the nursing diagnosis of greatest significance to the nurse and patient in promoting a therapeutic outcome is altered thought processes.

Disturbed Thought Processes

Impaired Memory. **Memory loss is one of the most distressing and frustrating aspects of aging.** Although memory loss may be caused by organic brain disease or depression, it is not necessarily related to a disease process. **With age, loss of short-term memory (recall of recent events) is more likely to occur than loss of long-term memory (recall of events that occurred in the distant past).** Speed of access to memories appears to slow with increasing age. Failure in retrieval of information, original acquisition, or learning may cause memory impairment (Ebersole and Hess, 2001).

Many factors contribute to altered memory in older adults. Stress or crisis, depression, a sense of worthlessness, loss of interest in present events, cerebrovascular changes that affect cerebral function, loss of neural cells because of disease or trauma, and sensory deprivation or social isolation all may occur with advancing age. Impaired memory for recent events may actually be a result of decreased vision or hearing. This may lead the older person to seek comfort in old memories and experiences, which replace the need to remain in touch with the present.

Institutionalized elderly people appear to have more difficulty with memory than those who live at home or in other community settings. Psychosocial, functional, and environmental approaches to nursing intervention can counteract and often reverse decline and withdrawal in the elderly psychiatric patient. As the person becomes more comfortably involved in relationships and activities, memory and function may improve.

Confusion. Confusion is a constellation of behaviors, including inattention and memory deficits; challenging behaviors such as aggressiveness, combativeness, and delusions (called *behavioral excesses*); and inability or failure to perform ADLs (called *behavioral deficits*) (Mehta, Yaffe, and Covinsky, 2002). Often, confusion is a nonspecific term used by staff to label apathetic, withdrawn, or uncooperative patients.

Several categories of patients are likely to be labeled as confused: the problem patient, the patient with communication problems (slurred speech, expressive dysphasia), the patient who challenges staff members' personal values, the depressed patient, and the patient who does not get well. It is important for the nurse to be specific when referring to a patient as "confused."

Institutionalized elders are at particular risk of confusion. From 40% to 80% suffer from some degree of organic brain disease, with disorientation to time, place, and person; remote and recent memory loss; and inability to do simple calculations. In many long-term care facilities, more than 30% of the patients have severe confusion (Ebersole and Hess, 2001). The precipitating factors depend on both the physiological and psychological condition of the patient.

Early morning confusion, sometimes called sunrise syndrome, may result from the hangover effects of sedative-hypnotics or other nighttime medications that interact with drugs for sleep. Sleep problems and insomnia are common in the elderly. Adverse reactions to drugs prescribed for sleep often occur.

Increasing disorientation or confusion at night, resulting from loss of visual accommodation and other factors, is known as sundowning syndrome. The nurse should take special precautions to prevent falls at these times.

The most logical cause of sundowning is the deterioration of the suprachiasmatic nucleus in the hypothalamus. This major pacemaker of circadian rhythms regulates the sleep-wake cycle (see Chapter 6) and has been found to be deteriorated in demented people. Assessing and then minimizing or eliminating any environmental and underlying physiological causes of afternoon or evening confusion or irritability would be important activities for the nurse. These include the following:

- Elimination of psychosocial, toxic, infectious, metabolic, or pharmacological causes of delirium
- Elimination of underlying physiological causes of agitation and confusion such as pain, febrile illnesses, and incontinence
- Minimization or elimination of daytime sleep
- At least minimal exposure to direct sunlight each day, particularly in the morning, to reset the circadian pacemaker
- Increase in mild activity, such as walking
- Increase in conversations and other social interactions with staff and others
- Assessing for appropriateness of short-term use of low-dose antipsychotic drugs

A nurse's aide tells you that a patient is "wandering down the hall, staggering, pajama top unbuttoned." It is early morning, and the other patients are asleep. What would you do in this situation? ■

The nurse should never assume that confusion and disorientation are natural results of changes in cognitive or physiological status. Confusion is reversible in more than half the patients who experience it. It is usually transient or short term. The nurse has primary responsibility for intervening in this problem. Well-planned nursing care can be a significant factor in preventing and intervening in this distressing condition.

Although the term **disorientation** is often used interchangeably with **confusion**, they are different. A disoriented patient is not necessarily confused, and a confused patient does not necessarily experience complete disorientation. Mental status tests differentiate disorientation to place, person, and time from components of confusion, such as alterations in memory, judgment, decision making, and problem solving. Cognitive responses are discussed in detail in Chapter 23.

Paranoia. Some older people react to loss, isolation, and loneliness with paranoia and fear. Classic paranoia, involving a well-organized and elaborate delusional system, is rare in older people. Delusions and disturbances in mood, behavior, and thinking may be caused by sensory deprivation or sensory loss, social isolation, medications, deliriums, dementias, and early- and late-onset schizophrenia (Ebersole and Hess, 2001).

Paranoid symptoms may be general or specific. The geriatric patient may feel threatened by certain people (such as unfamiliar staff, or even by family, friends, or neighbors) or at certain times (such as night). Relocation to a new home, new room, or strange environment may cause fears; anxiety; and for some, paranoid ideation. It is ineffective to invalidate a person's paranoid ideation, although the provision of a sense of safety and security is helpful.

The personality of aging paranoid patients is characterized by withdrawal, aloofness, fearfulness, oversensitivity, and often secretiveness. As long as patients do not call attention to themselves or threaten themselves or others, their paranoia

may remain hidden. Once they become a potential threat to themselves or others, institutionalization may be needed. Older people who have transient or chronic paranoia are at high risk for victimization by others as well as self-neglect and abuse (such as refusal to eat, take prescribed medications, or attend to hygiene needs).

Affective Responses

Disturbances in mood, mood swings, or oversensitive emotional reactions are common to people of all ages. An older person's reaction to physical limitations or disabilities, psychological loss (particularly of a spouse or other close person), or the possibility of institutionalization depends on past coping styles, support systems (especially family), and present psychological and physiological strength.

Extreme or sudden mood changes occur in response to stress or as inadequate coping mechanisms in people facing progressive loss or dependency. When this behavior is seen in elderly people who have been content and happy, physiological factors, including side effects of medications, should be considered. Reassurance and support are given to reduce the patient's anxiety and diminish the perceived threat.

Dysfunctional Grieving and Hopelessness. Depression and sadness are sometimes viewed as a natural part of aging. In fact, depression, grief, and loss are common in later life. Prolonged grief and mourning over a real or imagined loss should be recognized and treated as depression (Talerico, 2003). Common symptoms include weight loss; appetite loss; fatigue; apathy; loss of interest in friends, family, and usual activities; and psychomotor retardation. None of the symptoms is caused by increasing age; all are problems that can be effectively treated (see Chapter 19).

Death of a life partner can compound the cumulative loses of aging. Key points from research on grief responses in the elderly for the nurse to remember when caring for a grieving elder are as follows (Hegge and Fischer, 2000):

- Elderly widow(er)s are likely to have multiple cumulative losses of aging, which complicate the grieving process.
- Coping strategies of elderly widow(er)s include faith, flexibility, participation in activities, and support of family or friends.
- Symptoms of grief such as disruptions in sleeping and eating patterns can lead to false labels of dementia.
- Peaks and valleys of grief are less intense in the eldest widow(er)s because they are more at peace with their own mortality.

The loss of hope expressed by some older people, particularly those with increasing disabilities, may cause or result from a depressive reaction. Undiagnosed depression may have serious effects on the elderly because depression always involves physical symptoms.

The person's attitude toward aging, dying, and death influences whether the depression can be treated successfully. The old differ from the young in their attitudes toward death in several ways: Older people tend to (1) integrate attitudes toward death with their religious beliefs; (2) have experienced the death of significant others; (3) be more accepting of death; and (4) approach problems primarily from an internal focus. The state of the older person's health, in addition to what he or she has learned from seeing people die, may signal that his or her life may be ending. Awareness of the older person's "stage of dying" is important to understanding his or her needs and concerns.

Risk for Self-Directed Violence.

Intentional deaths among the elderly are common. **Older people in the United States have the highest suicide rate of any age-group.** The suicide rate of white males older than 65 is especially high (Administration on Aging, 2001).

Others at high risk include isolated elderly people who have lost family or friends through death; those with changes in body function and decreased independence because of pain, weakness, immobility, or shortness of breath; those with changes in body function because of surgery or stroke; and those who are terminally ill (see Citing the Evidence). Suicide in elderly people is strongly associated with depression, physical illness, loss of adaptive coping mechanisms, and neurobiological alteration.

Elderly suicide victims use more violent and lethal means to take their lives, resulting in a higher ratio of completed-to-attempted suicides, suggesting that effective treatment must include prevention. Sadly, the majority (70%) of elderly suicide victims have seen their primary care provider in the month before death, but their suicidal intentions were not detected and they were not treated for their depression (Morris, 2001).

Finally, other examples of intentional deaths include excessive risk-taking; lack of caution in the management of ordinary affairs; refusal to eat; overuse or misuse of alcohol or drugs; and noncompliance with life-sustaining medical regimens, such as refusal to take insulin or digoxin (Abrams et al, 2002). Suicidal behavior is discussed in detail in Chapter 20.

> *Were you surprised to learn that the elderly have the highest suicide rate? How would you increase public awareness of this important public health problem?* ∎

Situational Low Self-Esteem.

Low self-esteem in the elderly is often expressed through preoccupation with physical and emotional health and expression of concern through body complaints. This may be labeled hypochondriasis but really represents the person's insecurity.

One of the problems encountered by elders with a history of somaticizing is health professionals' tendency to dismiss their complaints, assuming there is no real illness. All symptoms should be taken seriously and investigated thoroughly. Ways in which to promote self-esteem are discussed in Chapter 18.

As a sign of the geriatric patient's sense of deterioration, somaticism communicates the distress that accompanies decreased self-worth. The sick role is a legitimate and socially acceptable way to deal with stress and anxiety. The patient receives support, concern, and interest and experiences a sense of control. Unfortunately, caregivers may reinforce the elder's dependency by providing care that discourages the pa-

CITING THE EVIDENCE ON
Suicide in Late Life

BACKGROUND: Despite the fact that people age 65 and older have the highest rates of suicide of any age-group, late-life suicide has a low prevalence, making it difficult to conduct prospective studies. The authors examined risk factors for late-life suicide on the basis of general information collected directly from older subjects participating in a community-based prospective study of aging.

RESULTS: Of the 14,456 people surveyed, 21 committed suicide over the 10-year observation period. Depressive symptoms, perceived poor health status, poor sleep quality, and absence of a relative or friend to confide in predicted late-life suicide. Suicide victims did not have greater alcohol use and did not report more medical illness or physical impairment.

IMPLICATIONS: This study provides additional information about the context of late-life depression that also contributes to suicidal behavior. Because both depression and social support are amenable to intervention, this study provides further evidence for the possible effectiveness of such strategies to reduce suicides among older adults.

Turvey C et al: *Am J Geriatrc Psychiatry*, 10:398, 2002.

tient from doing for himself or herself. This vicious cycle sets the stage for behavioral deficits, excess disability, and decreased self-worth (Bruce et al, 2002).

Somatic Responses

Disturbed Sleep Pattern.

Insomnia may be a symptom or a problem in itself for the geropsychiatric patient. Many older adults experience chronic or intermittent sleep problems. Persistent insomnia, a risk factor for major depression, occurs among 5% to 10% of elders. Complaints of interrupted sleep; loss of sleep; or poor sleep, with frequent awakenings and morning exhaustion, are common. Daytime napping and drowsiness add to the problem. Nonetheless, sleep disorders in the elderly can be systematically diagnosed and treated (Salzman, 2001).

Opinions vary regarding normal sleep patterns in older adults. Some researchers suggest that people need less sleep as they age. However, chronic fatigue, physical illness, pain, and decreased mobility may cause a need for more sleep. Geriatric patients often express distress over their inability to sleep well. Perceived lack of sleep becomes a cyclical reaction. Worry about lack of sleep prevents falling asleep. Fatigue is the most common physical complaint of adults older than 75. Lack of exercise, limited mobility, and side effects of drugs also may contribute to insomnia.

Imbalanced Nutrition: Less Than Body Requirements.

Appetite loss is common in patients with depression. Inadequate dietary intake also occurs in confused or disoriented patients. Forgetting to eat or being unable to prepare meals may add to the problem of appetite loss. Side effects of some drugs (such as dry mouth or change in taste) contribute to lack of interest in food. The toothless patient or someone with gum disease avoids chewing when possible. The interaction of appetite loss and emotional dysfunction should always be considered in the nutritional evaluation. Poor nutrition contributes to fatigue, listlessness, and immobility.

Stress Responses

Progressively Lowered Stress Threshold (PLST). Nurses should know the competencies and capacities for environmental mastery of cognitively impaired patients. For instance, as cognitive responses slow, the stress threshold decreases and capacities deteriorate. Staff often overwhelm sensory processing and coping abilities of elderly patients, leading to catastrophic reactions and other challenging behaviors. Finding a better fit between the patient's stress threshold and the demands of the environment can strengthen patient competencies and reduce behavioral excesses (Garand et al, 2002).

Relocation Stress Syndrome. This condition involves physical or psychosocial disturbances related to transfer from one environment to another. Since 1950 the care of many elderly mentally ill has shifted from state psychiatric hospitals to nursing homes. In fact, the number of mentally ill elderly residing in nursing homes greatly exceeds that in state psychiatric hospitals. This shift in treatment sites drew attention to the process and consequences of relocation.

Risk factors related to relocation stress syndrome include the following (NANDA, 2003):

- Impaired psychosocial or physical health status
- Other recent losses
- Losses associated with the move
- Inadequate preparation for the move
- Feelings of powerlessness
- Moderate to great difference between the old and new environments
- Prior relocation experiences
- Inadequate support system

Behaviors associated with relocation stress syndrome are listed in Box 38-2.

The stress of relocation should be anticipated for all geriatric patients. Intervention should be planned to reduce the impact. In transfers between institutions, it may be helpful to arrange for the patient to visit the new location before the actual move. This allows the patient to meet other residents and staff, see the physical surroundings, and ask questions about the program. Post-transfer visits by staff from the transferring agency also ease the transition, as does offering staff from both agencies the opportunity to communicate about nursing approaches.

Allowing the patient to have personal belongings, liberal visiting hours for family or friends, and careful explanations of the purpose and routines of the institution are a few of the ways in which the stress of change can be minimized. Establishing an effective support system within the new setting may prevent the challenging behaviors often observed in isolated elders: apathy, depression, aggression, or hostility.

Risk for Caregiver Role Strain. Disabled elderly people who live in the community rely on support and care from family members. As the percentage of elderly people in the population grows, family resources will be increasingly important to keep elders in the community and provide care that is less expensive than professional care.

This role is stressful for people who care for frail elders. Providing elder care can result in emotional, physical, interpersonal, and occupational problems. Research also has demonstrated that stress to the caregiver increases over time. A caregiver under stress is at risk for problems in performing the caregiver role. Risk factors for caregiver role strain are listed in Table 38-3.

Table 38-3	**Risk Factors for Caregiver Role Strain**
CATEGORY	**RISK FACTORS**
Pathophysiological	Severe illness of elder
	Unpredictable illness course
	Addiction or co-dependency
	Elder discharged with serious home-care needs
	Caregiver health impairment
Psychosocial	Caregiver is female
	Psychosocial/cognitive problems in care receiver
	Family problems before caregiving
	Marginal caregiver coping patterns
	Poor relationship between caregiver and receiver
	Caregiver is spouse
	Care receiver has deviant or bizarre behavior
Situational	Abuse or violence
	Other sources of stress on family
	Need for long-term caregiving
	Inadequate physical environment
	Family/caregiver isolation
	Lack of caregiver respite or recreation
	Inexperience
	Competing role commitments
	Complex/demanding caregiving tasks

BOX 38-2

Behaviors Associated With Relocation Stress Syndrome

- Anxiety, apprehension, restlessness, and verbalization of being concerned/upset about transfer
- Vigilance, dependency, increased verbalization of needs, insecurity, and lack of trust
- Increased confusion
- Depression, sad affect, withdrawal, and loneliness
- Sleep disturbance
- Change in eating habits, gastrointestinal disturbances, and weight changes
- Unfavorable comparison of posttransfer and pretransfer staff

In addition, several other factors affecting the caregiver are predictors of institutionalization of the elder, including the following (Kelley, Buckwalter, and Mass, 1999; Ducharme and Trudeau, 2002):

- Safety concerns
- Incontinence
- Erratic sleep patterns of care recipient
- Critical health events (e.g., falls, wandering, hospitalization)

Nurses are in a unique position to identify and address the caregiver's needs for education, intervention, and support services. Such support can decrease caregiver role strain and premature institutionalization of the elder.

Behavioral Responses

Social Isolation. Multiple social losses or fear of loss may lead to social isolation. Prolonged grief after the loss of a spouse, sibling, child, or close friend may make the elder hesitant to become involved in other close relationships. The person who has been close to only a few family members or friends will have even more difficulty with loss.

Elderly patients experiencing organic cognitive impairment (such as Alzheimer's disease and related disorders) often withdraw from social contacts, daily routines, and ADLs. They may deny having a problem or fear the consequences of memory changes. Social isolation can become a defense mechanism, reinforcing denial of perceived disability, yet worsening the cognitive deficits. Sensory deficits such as hearing or vision impairment also can contribute to isolation for the elderly (Jervis, 2002).

Self-Care Deficit/Behavioral Deficit. Chronic illness is one aspect of aging that may result in the inability to care for oneself. With increasing years comes a greater chance of multiple chronic health problems. Affective illnesses such as major depression or bipolar disorder may cause psychomotor retardation, preventing elders from meeting their basic needs. Medications may cause forgetfulness, lethargy, and physical impairment.

Because of increasing frailty or cognitive impairment, many elders are unable to converse or complete basic self-care activities such as bathing, toileting, grooming, and feeding. The underlying cause of the deficit must be determined and appropriate nursing interventions planned.

Aphasia, agnosia, and apraxia contribute to self-care deficits. Admission to a nursing home often results in dependency in ADLs among those who previously were independent in such basic activities (Jervis, 2002). Nurses are in a unique position to reduce the incidence of behavioral deficits and excess disability by enhancing self-efficacy and environmental competence.

Challenging Behaviors/Behavioral Excess. The high incidence of challenging behaviors is very troubling to caregivers. Even one resident displaying such behaviors can disrupt an inpatient unit or nursing home floor, setting off a chain reaction in other residents, and contributing significantly to caregiver stress. Nurses can assist staff to assess and intervene effectively using a variety of behavioral and environmental strategies, thus reducing use of physical and chemical restraints. Enhancing the self-efficacy of staff in perceiving and coping with behaviors seen as challenging decreases negative feelings of stress and vulnerability to burnout (Evers, Tomic, and Brouwers, 2001).

■ PLANNING AND INTERVENTION

Expected outcomes related to the nursing care of the geropsychiatric patient should be realistically based on the person's potential to change. If the person's challenging behaviors result from a treatable disorder, expected outcomes and short-term goals may reflect a return to pre-illness functioning. For example, a goal for a patient with depression who is neglectful of personal hygiene might be:

> *The patient will bathe, dress, and brush his teeth independently.*

Empirically validated treatments for depression and anxiety in the aged are summarized in Box 38-3.

If the condition is chronic and either no change or progressive deterioration is expected and current treatments do not effect change in target behaviors, then the outcomes of care focus on adaptation to the situation. For example, a goal for a patient with Alzheimer's disease who neglects personal hygiene might be:

> *The patient will help with bathing, dressing, and brushing his teeth.*

If the patient's condition is not expected to improve, the expected outcomes and goals may focus on the caregiver as

BOX **38-3**	SUMMARIZING THE EVIDENCE ON Depression and Anxiety in the Aged
Disorder	Depression and anxiety in the aged
Treatment	◆ The primary classes of antidepressant medications (SSRIs and TCAs) were effective in both the acute and maintenance phases of late-life depression, although the latter has a heightened risk of adverse side effects. ◆ Electroconvulsive therapy (ECT) has shown its effectiveness and safety in the short-term management of late-life, severe psychotic depression and mania. ◆ Psychosocial interventions were efficacious, especially cognitive, behavioral, and cognitive-behavioral therapy, in treating major depressive disorder in the aged.

From Bartels SJ et al: *Psychiatr Serv* 53:1419, 2002.
SSRIs, Selective serotonin reuptake inhibitors; *TCAs,* tricyclic antidepressants.

well as the patient. For example, a goal for a caregiver of a person with Alzheimer's disease might be:

> At least once a week the caregiver will participate in a recreational activity outside of the home while the home health aide is with the patient.

The plan of care must be developed with the active participation of the patient and the caregiver. It also must be reviewed often to ensure that it is relevant to the patient's current needs. Caregiver education is an important part of the plan.

Older adults respond well to both individual and group interventions. They need the opportunity to talk, be supported in their efforts to deal with day-to-day problems, and plan for a meaningful future. The type of nursing intervention selected depends on the nursing care problems identified, the interests and preferences of the elder, and the setting in which the care is to be provided. In the past, most geropsychiatric care was provided in state psychiatric hospitals.

Nurses also will find older patients with mental illness in acute psychiatric units, nursing homes, emergency rooms, and increasingly in community settings. Nursing care for cognitively impaired patients in inpatient settings is addressed in Chapter 23, including approaches to behaviors such as wandering, aggression, agitation, falls, and confusion.

Therapeutic Milieu

Whether in a hospital, nursing home, community program, or at home, the care environment should support effective interventions. There are several basic characteristics of a therapeutic milieu for the elderly.

Cognitive Stimulation. Activities should be planned to maintain or improve the patients' cognitive functioning. Discussion groups help patients focus on topics of interest to them while they socialize. Projects can reinforce skills and offer an opportunity for success. Patients with dementia can participate in a wide variety of activities. The nurse can collaborate with the rehabilitation therapist in planning interesting and appropriate activities.

Promote a Sense of Calm and Quiet. Elders often do best in a setting that is designated for their care. In particular, inpatient units that admit all age-groups may be too stimulating for confused elder patients. In general, the geropsychiatric setting should be decorated in soft colors. If music is played, it should be soothing and preferably familiar to the elderly. Bright lights that create glare should be avoided.

Although the environmental background should be subdued, planned periods of increased activity help maintain interest and alertness. For elders who are not in their own home, personal articles such as family pictures, religious objects, favorite books, afghans, or decorative objects are reassuring and offer a sense of security.

Consistent Physical Layout. In residential or inpatient settings, room changes should be avoided as much as possible. Furniture arrangements should be stable; this helps disoriented people orient themselves and adds to their security. Environmental barriers should be removed for wandering patients.

Structured Routine. The daily schedule should be as predictable as possible. Bedtime, waking time, nap times, and mealtimes should not vary. For elders who have recently moved to a new setting, it is helpful to give them and their families copies of the weekly schedule. Time should be allowed for reviewing the schedule with patients. Periodic reinforcement of the routines may be needed until patients adjust to the environment. A predictable routine can enhance an elder's capacity to function at his or her maximum level.

Focus on Strengths and Abilities. Most elders have strengths related to their past accomplishments. If the person is unable to communicate, family members can give information about the patient's life and suggest activities that are likely to be successful. Nursing creativity can be used to find ways to capitalize on elders' strengths by planning opportunities for them to help staff and other patients or participate in activities based on their abilities. Successful experiences can enhance perceptions of self-efficacy and control, decreasing premature dependency.

Minimize Challenging Behavior. Understanding the patient's behavioral patterns can help reduce agitation and behavioral crises. Observation reveals situations that lead to challenging behaviors. Adhering to the person's usual lifestyle as closely as possible reduces conflicts.

For instance, a person who has always taken a bath in the evening before bed should not be forced to shower before breakfast. Patients who agitate each other should be kept apart as much as possible. Distraction often can interrupt a conflict before it gets out of control. Understanding challenging behaviors or behavioral excesses from the perspective of the elder will strengthen the nurse's ability to design interventions that affect underlying causes (Cody, Beck, and Svarstad, 2002).

Minimal Demands for Compliant Behavior. Elders who are cognitively impaired often resist demands from others. They may not understand what is being asked of them or they may be frightened of an unexpected change in activity. Some older adults resent being under the control of others and feel the need to assert themselves. It is best to avoid pressuring the patient to comply. Reapproaching the person after a few minutes is often successful. If the patient needs to be in control, it is helpful to negotiate a time of voluntary compliance.

How would the therapeutic milieu differ if most patients were elderly and (a) depressed, (b) demented, (c) delusional, or (d) cognitively intact? ■

Providing Safety. Safety is fundamental to a therapeutic milieu; thus safety needs must always be considered. The nurse should be alert for safety hazards and remove them. Because falls are a concern, floors should be free from slippery spots, obstacles, uneven surfaces, and loose rugs. Thresholds should be flush with the surrounding floor. Hand rails and grab bars are helpful for frail elders. Fire is also a concern. Open flames should be avoided. If smoking is allowed, it may be necessary to provide supervision in an area of the facility that permits smoking.

In many facilities restraints are still used in the mistaken notion that they enhance the patient's safety or control challenging behavior. Physical restraints include a variety of devices such as mitts, posey vests, and geri chairs applied with a physician's order, although nurses are the professionals most intimately involved in decisions to restrain patients. Although such devices may help staff, they limit patient freedom of choice and movement, as well as threaten dignity. Six myths related to physical restraint of elderly patients are summarized in Table 38-4.

To limit the use of restraints and to incorporate more appropriate methods to address safety concerning the elderly, nurses, in collaboration with other health care professionals, should develop a hospital or facility policy and protocol related to the use of restraints (Chien, 2000). National nursing efforts to expose these myths and realities led to federal regulations to implement less-restrictive alternatives, resulting in a decreased use of restraints (Administration on Aging, 2001).

Somatic Therapies

Electroconvulsive Therapy. Electroconvulsive therapy (ECT) has been found to be very effective in the treatment of depression in the older adult. Chapter 28 has a detailed discussion of ECT. Contraindications for this type of therapy are an intracranial space-occupying lesion with increased intracranial pressure, arrhythmias, and myocardial infarction within the last 3 months.

Psychotropic Medications. The addition of psychotropic medications to the care regimen of elders must be approached carefully and competently. Basic guidelines for medication administration for elders include the slow initiation of medications, preferably one at a time, using lower dosages: "start low and go slow," although treatment must be maintained at a therapeutic level for an appropriate duration to be effective.

Special consideration must be given to psychotropic medications and elders because drugs that affect behavior also affect the central nervous system. Also, elderly patients are especially vulnerable to developing side effects, with sedation, orthostatic hypotension, agitation, extrapyramidal symptoms, and anticholinergic effects being especially troublesome.

The nurse should remember that age-related pharmacokinetic and pharmacodynamic changes affect drug response and increase the risk for side effects in the elderly, making the atypicals the first-line treatments for psychosis in the elderly because of their more favorable side effect profile (Yeung et al, 2000; Masand, 2000). Table 38-5 describes recommended dosages of psychotropic medications for the elderly (Jacobson et al, 2002). (See Chapter 27 for a thorough discussion of psychopharmacology.)

Special attention must be given to the older adult when assessing medication use. Four factors place the elder at risk for drug toxicity and should be included in any assessment: **advanced age, polypharmacy, decreased medication adherence**, and **comorbidity**. Misuse of drugs by the elderly is also a factor in the rising cost of health care for this population.

Age. As a person ages, physiological responses to medications change. In the older-than-65 age-group, drug dosages must be monitored carefully for continuing effectiveness. A medication dosage that is safe and effective at age 65 may be toxic at age 75. Gastrointestinal absorption, hepatic blood flow and metabolism, and renal clearance may all decline.

Also, the ratio of fat to lean muscle mass increases with age. Many psychoactive medications are **lipophilic** (attach to fat), which increases the risk of drugs building up in fatty tissue and causing toxicity (Schatzberg et al, 2003). Experimental drugs are often tested on nonelderly adult populations. This does not allow evaluation of the differing effects of newly approved drugs on older people before they are made available in the marketplace.

Polypharmacy. Several surveys report that older adults take an average of 8 to 10 medications daily. It is also suggested that the use of over-the-counter medicines is underreported because they are not thought to be significant. Drugs such as alcohol and acetaminophen (Tylenol) are not always reported but can be toxic in combination with other drugs.

Table 38-4	**Myths and Realities About Physical Restraint**
MYTH	REALITY
Restraints reduce the risk of injury related to falls.	Restraints do not reduce the risk of injury from falls and may increase it. Falls do increase the likelihood of future restraint.
Restraining meets the nurse's moral duty to protect the patient from harm.	Restraints may increase the risk of injury and lead to problems related to immobility, confusion, aggression, depression, and incontinence.
Failure to restrain results in legal liability.	Federal and state laws and regulations prohibit the unnecessary use of restraint.
Older people do not mind being restrained.	Older people do not wish to be restrained. They feel angry, hurt, and embarrassed by the experience.
Inadequate staffing justifies restraining patients.	Federal and state laws and regulations forbid restraining patients for staff convenience. Providing adequate nursing care to a restrained patient takes at least as much time as caring for an unrestrained one.
There are no adequate alternatives to physical restraint.	Nursing care alternatives have been identified in several categories: Physical care: comfort, relief of pain, positioning Psychosocial care: remotivation, communication, attention Activities Environmental manipulation: improved lighting, removal of restraint devices, redesigned furniture Administrative support and staff training

Table 38-5	Psychoactive Medications
CATEGORY	**RECOMMENDED DAILY DOSAGE RANGE FOR OLDER ADULTS**
Selective Serotonin Reuptake Inhibitors (SSRIs) and Other Newer Antidepressants	
Escitalapram (Lexapro) (SSRI)	10-20 mg/day
Fluoxetine (Prozac) (SSRI)	5-40 mg/day
Citalopram (Celexa) (SSRI)	10-40 mg/day
Fluvoxamine (Luvox) (SSRI)	50-150 mg/day
Sertraline (Zoloft) (SSRI)	12.5-150 mg/day
Paroxetine (Paxil) (SSRI)	5-20 mg/day
Venlafaxine (Effexor) (SNRI)	12.5-225 mg/day
Nefazodone (Serzone) (SARI)	50-200 mg/day
Mirtazapine (Remeron) (NaSSA)	7.5-45 mg/day
Bupropion (Wellbutrin) (NDRI)	75-300 mg/day
Trazodone/Desyrel (SARI)	25-150 mg/day (sleep) 25-200 mg/day (antidepressant)
Tricyclic Antidepressants (TCAs)	
Desipramine (Norpramin)	10-150 mg/day
Nortriptyline (Aventyl, Pamelor)	10-100 mg/day
Monoamine Oxidase Inhibitors (MAOIs)	
Phenelzine (Nardil)	7.5-45 mg/day
Tranylcypromine (Parnate)	5-30 mg/day
Mood Stabilizers	
Lithium	25-1200 mg tid/qid
Carbamazepine (Tegretol)	50-1200 mg/day
Valproate (Depakote)	125-1800 mg/bid; titrate up slowly
Gabapentin (Neurontin)	150-1200 mg qd or bid
Anxiolytic Agent	
Buspirone (BuSpar)	5-80 mg/day, divided doses
Anxioltyic Benzodiazepines	
Clonazepam (Klonopin)	10-45 mg/day
Oxazepam (Serax)	0.25-2 mg (divided in 3-4 doses)
Lorazepam (Ativan)	0.25-2 mg bid to tid
Sedative/Hypnotic Benzodiazepines	
Zolpidem (Ambien)	5-10 mg qhr
Temazepam (Restoril)	7.5-30 mg qhr
Estazolam (ProSom)	0.5-2 mg qhr
Antipsychotics: Atypical (Novel)	
Risperidone (Risperdal)	0.25-2 mg/day
Olanzapine (Zyprexa)	2.5-10 mg/day
Quetiapine (Seroquel)	25-100 mg/day
Clozapine (Clozaril)	10-100 mg/day
Aripiprazole (Abilify)	15-20 mg/day
Antipsychotics: Typical (Conventional)	
Haloperidol (Haldol)	0.25-4 mg/day
Fluphenazine (Prolixin)	0.25-4 mg/day
Thioridazine (Mellaril)	10-200 mg/day
Chlorpromazine (Thorazine)	10-200 mg/day

Data from Jacobson S et al: *Handbook of geriatric psychopharmacology*, Washington, DC, 2002, AP Publishing.

Adherence. Many drugs take up to 6 weeks to effect a change in affective disorders. In the interim, elders may see no benefit to continued adherence and may abandon their medication regimen. Education regarding the time to effectiveness, the purpose, therapeutic value, and side effects (and their treatments) of medications should be provided to elders to enhance medication adherence and awareness.

Comorbidity. Acute and chronic illnesses and their treatments can alter the body's response to psychotropic medications. This includes chronic renal or liver failure, congestive heart failure, and structural and functional changes in the central nervous system. These conditions may result in heightened sensitivity to psychotropic drugs.

Interpersonal Interventions

Psychotherapy. Elderly patients can benefit from both individual and group psychotherapy sessions. Nurses who have advanced degrees in psychiatric nursing are qualified to provide these services (see Critical Thinking About Contemporary Issues). The following therapeutic approaches have demonstrated effectiveness in treating a variety of psychiatric problems:

- **Interpersonal psychotherapy** has been demonstrated to be effective in treating depression. The foci of treatment include grief, role changes, multiple losses, bereavement, social isolation, and helplessness (Cole and Dendukuri, 2003).

Critical Thinking *About* Contemporary Issues

Is Psychotherapy an Appropriate Intervention for Geropsychiatric Patients?

Some believe that psychotherapy for elderly patients is inappropriate and not helpful. Psychotherapy requires confronting and working through basic personality traits. It is argued that the elderly do not have the capacity, stamina, or interest to take on such a challenging task. Is this based on an accurate estimate of the elder's cognitive ability and interpersonal potential? Psychotherapy may be a long-term process. Is it reasonable to ask a person who is nearing the end of life to make a commitment to an effort that might not be completed? People in therapy often change their relationships with others. Should the elderly be put in the position of possibly jeopardizing their support systems by changing their expectations of themselves and others?

Geropsychiatric nurse specialists have begun to document their experiences in providing psychotherapy to elders (Bourbonniere and Evans, 2002). These nurses believe that elderly patients benefit from this intervention. They describe the elder's ability to change and grow. Psychotherapists have noted that older patients are more focused on therapeutic work, perhaps because they know they do not have unlimited time to achieve their goals. Elders have a wealth of life experiences to bring to therapy and a need to find meaning in their lives that is often aided by therapeutic intervention. In groups, they also benefit from the mutuality and cohesion they find. Thus reflecting on these considerations sheds new light on the question: Is it worth the investment to improve the life experience of one who may or may not have enough time left to experience long-term rewards of psychotherapy?

- **Cognitive therapy** has a focus on identifying and changing thoughts and underlying belief systems and supports higher-level defense mechanisms such as rationalization and intellectualization. It encourages active participation of patients in the therapy and reinforces positive change within a time-limited framework.
- **Cognitive-behavioral therapy** has several goals, which include changing thoughts and behaviors, improving skills, and modifying emotional states.

Problem-solving therapy is also an effective treatment for elders with mild depression. Problem-solving therapy involves helping patients in identifying issues that are critical in their lives. These issues should be described in a measurable and observable format, appropriate solutions to these issues should be devised, and possible consequences should be predicted.

Life Review Therapy. Life review therapy has a positive psychotherapeutic function, providing an opportunity for the person to reflect on life and resolve, reorganize, and reintegrate troubling or disturbing areas (Jones and Beck-Little, 2002). Life review works well with groups or individuals. In a group, members may positively reinforce each other and stimulate mutual learning. Developing individual autobiographies to share with the group is one way to introduce common experiences and interests among the members and put them at ease. The group cohesion and sharing can build self-esteem and a feeling of belonging, in addition to the positive effect of the review itself.

Life review therapy is different from reminiscence. Both are planned interventions that are led by a mental health professional. Reminiscence is usually a pleasant experience in which the patient reviews life events without any particular structure and talks about meanings and feelings. The nurse listens and responds but does not try to interpret or probe for deeper meanings.

The life review is structured, with the emphasis on analyzing life events. The nurse helps the patient look for the meaning of experiences and resolve conflicts and lingering feelings. Life review helps the elder achieve the ego integrity and wisdom identified by Erikson (1963), in his classic work decades ago, as the goal of the last stage of life.

Reality Orientation. Both 24-hour and structured reality orientation can prevent confusion and keep patients oriented to time, place, person, and situation. Reality orientation discussion is not meant to be a "do you know test" but rather an orienting conversational aide. The environment, when it is kept simple and focused, reinforces contact with reality, the here and now. Helpful physical props include pictures, photos, clocks, directional signs, calendars, and orientation boards (season of the year, weather, and so on).

Reality orientation groups can provide an opportunity to reinforce time, place, and person orientation with patients who have short attention spans and need extra verbal and visual stimulation. Reality orientation, along with a discussion of current events, stimulates patients to maintain contact with the real world and their place in it. Current events discussions, used alone, may be structured in various ways, such as sharing of newspaper articles or group viewing of television news programs. The scope of the group depends on the patients' abilities and the other therapeutic modalities at hand.

Validation Therapy. Although reality orientation is effective for many institutionalized and community-based elderly with confusion or disorientation, some evidence indicates that for some older adults, especially those with minimal organic impairment, disorientation may be a form of denial of unpleasant realities. These elders may become more anxious or agitated if constantly reminded of environmental realities.

An alternate approach to confused and disoriented older adults was developed several decades ago by Feil (1984) in relation to working with the patient who does not respond to reality orientation. This approach involves searching for the emotion and meaning in the patient's disoriented or confused words and behavior (such as wandering) and validating them verbally with the patient.

A series of verbal cues or steps are involved that allow the patient to focus on key words or phrases in the confused interaction, and the nurse validates by asking for description, more detail, or clarification. What is sometimes identified as meaningless or incoherent conversation may often have significant meaning for the patient and can be related to current or past events. Validation is being used successfully with both mild and moderately impaired elders, providing an effective avenue for reaching older adults experiencing cognitive dysfunction.

Cognitive Training. Much research is under way using cognitive training and stimulation (see Chapter 31). Problem-solving situations, formal or didactic memory training, and selected memory exercises have been effective in increasing attention span, efficiency of recall, and the ability to learn new skills (such as mathematical calculations and vocabulary).

Intelligence does not decline with age but may be dulled by depression, drugs, or lack of use. Cognitive training can keep older adults active mentally, which in turn enhances emotional well-being and positive engagement, while decreasing passive behaviors. The "use it or lose it" adage is as true for maintenance of intelligence as it is for physical functioning. Research suggests that cognitive retraining activities can be effective with demented elderly patients and compare with the efficacy of drug treatment (Camp et al, 2002; Spector et al, 2003). Such strategies can reduce behavioral deficits and excess disability.

Stimulating cognitive skills can challenge the nurse's creativity in relating to geropsychiatric patients. To be able to capitalize on the patient's interests and skills, the nurse must be familiar with the patient's past occupation, hobbies, and leisure activities. The nursing interview should focus on gathering as much of that information as possible on admission and adding it to the database as the nurse builds a trusting relationship with the patient and family.

Relaxation Therapy. Besides promoting a sense of physical well-being, relaxation can release tension and reduce stress, reducing barriers to communication. Additional information about relaxation therapy is presented in Chapters 16, 29, and 32. Relaxation, combined with mild isometric exercises, increases cardiovascular output, energy, and mobility and reduces stress.

Relaxation and exercise strategies, used in group or individual contexts, do not require advanced skills of the nurse or the patient. They may begin with simple tension-releasing muscle exercises, coupled with verbal instructions about breathing and concentration. Other sensory stimulation strategies include music, aromatherapy, and therapeutic touch. Meaningful activity programs are increasingly being used to meet patients' physical activity and social needs while reducing the incidence of behavioral challenges such as wandering (Camp et al, 2002).

Supportive and Counseling Groups. Geropsychiatric patients respond well to both supportive and counseling groups. These interventions may use either a nondirective or unstructured format or a more structured, didactic approach. Group members can ventilate feelings, try out problem-solving approaches, and resolve conflict in a rational, systematic manner. These groups may incorporate some aspects of cognitive training or reminiscence, described earlier in this chapter. Older adults respond well to a supportive group structure, which increases self-esteem, self-confidence, risk-taking, and empathy (Cole and Dendukuri, 2003).

Humor may be an effective way to reach the nonverbal or withdrawn elder. The ability to laugh at oneself and see the irony in everyday events provides an effective outlet for frustration, anger, stress, and anxiety. Promoting humor by telling jokes and stories and watching cartoons or situation comedies can be therapeutic in a group or with individual patients. Expressions of humor and active laughter allow older adults to step out of their situations, releasing some of the tension related to coping with changes accompanying aging.

Patient Education. Older adults often question the physiological and cognitive changes that occur naturally in aging. Slowed response time, benign memory loss, altered gait, and interrupted sleep patterns are a few of the normal changes of aging that elders may interpret as pathological. The nurse has an opportunity to teach patients about their own developmental changes during the assessment phase of the nurse-patient relationship.

Dispelling myths and stereotypes related to aging is a primary goal for patient education. Exercises for promoting positive thoughts and images, visualization, and repetitive cognitive games can be used as a basis for teaching new patterns of behavior. Cognitive training, relaxation, and life review approaches are well-suited to patient education formats.

Your friend's grandfather is 85 years old and constantly complains of feeling tired and forgetful. He has been to many physicians and still feels no better. Your friend asks what she should do next. How would you respond? ∎

Family Education and Support. Because 80% of the elders living at home are cared for by a spouse, sibling, their adult child or that child's spouse, education and support groups for family caregivers are essential. Many community agencies, clinics, and senior citizen centers are responding to the needs of family caregivers with special activities, classes, and support groups. Extensive nursing research for more than a decade demonstrates the effectiveness of nursing interventions in educating and empowering family caregivers (Kelley, Buckwalter, and Mass, 1999; Ducharme and Trudeau, 2002).

Family members often view nurses as the most approachable health care professionals in regard to understanding family relationships, conflicts, needs, and resources. Family education about aging processes, family dynamics, problem solving, behavioral management, the caregiving trajectory, and stresses inherent in the caregiver role need to be integrated into counseling sessions with family members regardless of the setting.

A more formal approach to family education can be developed using the numerous books available that address caring for older adults. These materials provide practical, step-by-step guidelines to handling common care issues of the frail elderly, including agitation, wandering, withdrawal, resistance, anxiety, insomnia, incontinence, anorexia, and restlessness.

These books, which have been written specifically for the consumer, supply the text for nurse-family teaching sessions and are excellent resource materials for use in the home (Mace and Rabins, 2001). Families genuinely want to provide good caregiving for as long as possible. Increasingly, nurses need to support family caregivers of geropsychiatric patients to help them be successful and feel less burdened (Horton-Deutsch et al, 2002; Mignor, 2000).

EVALUATING CARE OF THE GERIATRIC PATIENT

Implementing evidence-based care designed to promote optimum cognitive function and emotional well-being has been considered the role of the geropsychiatric nurse. Increasingly, research is being initiated to determine the most appropriate approach to meet the needs of patients and family caregivers and the most effective interventions to use.

Evaluation of patient care should be based on a model that explains the progression of behavior from adaptive to maladaptive. The type of care and the evaluation of outcome would be directly related to the level of behavior targeted for intervention.

The goal of nursing intervention is to promote maximum independence of the older adult, based on capacity and functional abilities. Evaluation of outcomes of nursing care would not be based on reversal of behaviors or elimination of patient needs but on the change the patient demonstrates based on individual abilities. This approach reinforces the emphasis on the individual as a unit for evaluation and allows for patient differences and for the process of change over time.

The effectiveness of family caregiver interventions also must be evaluated. Important dimensions include the caregiver's health and stress level, family coping strategies, caregiver knowledge and competence, status of the elder, and freedom from abuse.

Community geropsychiatric programs will become increasingly important in regard to addressing the impending demographic shift. Important evaluative criteria will include accessibility and coordination of services; patient, family, and systems outcomes and satisfaction; staff training; compliance with patient-centered regulatory systems; program goals; and cost-effectiveness.

In the final analysis, the most important evaluation criterion is the feedback from the patient and caregivers that nursing care was helpful and growth producing. The challenge to the nurse is to be creative in producing a positive experience for each elderly patient.

COMPETENT CARING   **A Clinical Exemplar of a Psychiatric Nurse**
SHARON CORWELL, RN, NHA

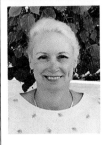

I have been working in the same nursing home for 35 years, first as a nursing assistant, then as a nurse, then as the Director of Nursing, and now as the Administrator. In a facility such as this (22 beds in a converted home), things are a lot more informal than at other care settings, we feel more like a family. We've had a lot of residents transfer here from the state hospital since the 1980s. In assessing our ability to provide care, I look at the total person and consider all of his or her needs; it doesn't matter whether these are psychiatric or somatic. I contemplate can we give adequate care to the resident and help make a good life for him or her. By that I mean preventing decompensation as long as possible while we treat people as individuals, meeting them where they are, and not trying to change them.

J came to us when she was 63. She had been in an acute psychiatric unit because of verbal and physical threats and inappropriate behavior secondary to her early-onset dementia. She also had chronic obstructive pulmonary disease (COPD), depression, hypertension, and Parkinson's disease. Her daughter lived 2½ hours away; J had been turned down by three other facilities closer to where her daughter lived when she was placed in our care. Caring for J also meant caring for her daughter; we did this by giving her emotional support, reassurance, focusing on the positive, and sometimes by just listening. J's daughter was an only child who was devoted to her mom. She made a visit every month for the 2½ years J was with us.

When J first came to stay with us, she could barely feed herself and needed help even to stand up. Yet she would say things like: "I'm going to kill you" or "I'm going to cut you up." You could say her behavior was inappropriate, but you had to look at J the person. Because she couldn't understand what we were saying, her actions were based on fear. Her striking out was a protective instinctual reaction, the same as anyone's normal reaction. As J continued to deteriorate, she was no longer able to express what she was feeling inside, but you could tell from her eyes that she was still there.

J required a lot of physical care as she deteriorated. She would tense up during care and pull back. Nonetheless we had her up everyday. We would clean her, keep her comfortable, and feed her. It often took an hour and a half to feed her a single meal. She was evaluated for surgical insertion of a feeding tube and was cleared to have the procedure, but soon after she developed shortness of breath and was hospitalized with a viral infection. She died 2 weeks later. During those last weeks, when I'd look into her eyes, it was as though they were saying "enough is enough."

We received the nicest note from her daughter that really reflected what we try to do in our facility:

"Watching a loved one deteriorate is one of the hardest things a family can go through. There are so many worries and heartbreaks along the way. The genuine caring and individual attention you gave to my mother went beyond a job. It speaks of your true love, caring, and dedication for the people you protect and nurture. You remembered there was someone beneath her shell who had lived and loved and was still loved deeply by everyone who knew her. You treated her with dignity and care. There will never be enough words to express my feelings of gratitude for the care you gave to my mother and the peace of mind you gave my family and me." ∎

CHAPTER FOCUS POINTS

- The demographics of aging continue to expand. The 21st century will see increasing longevity, geropsychiatric disability, and the need for evidence-based, accessible, cost-effective programs.
- The role of the geropsychiatric nurse includes providing primary mental health nursing care, including intervening with caregivers, providing case management, and consulting with other care providers. Advanced practice nurses provide individual and group psychotherapy, take leadership in program development, and prescribe medications in most states.
- Biological, psychological, and sociocultural theories of aging guide the development of evidence-based nursing practice.
- A comprehensive geropsychiatric nursing assessment includes application of interviewing skills. The areas to be assessed include mental status, behavioral responses, functional abilities, physiological functioning, and social support.
- NANDA nursing diagnoses for geropsychiatric patients are related to disturbed thought processes and affective, somatic, stress, and behavioral responses.
- Nursing interventions with geropsychiatric patients include creation of a therapeutic milieu, involvement in somatic therapies, and interpersonal interventions. Caregivers should be involved in planning, implementing, and evaluating nursing interventions.
- Evaluation of geropsychiatric nursing care focuses on the patient's ability to reach maximum independence.

KEY TERMS

life review, 793
reality orientation, 793
reminiscence, 793

sundowning syndrome, 785
sunrise syndrome, 785

CHAPTER REVIEW QUESTIONS

1. **Match each term in Column A with the correct description in Column B.**

Column A

_____ Activity theory
_____ Cross-linkage theory
_____ Person-environment fit theory
_____ Biological programming theory
_____ Disengagement theory
_____ Life review theory
_____ Stability of personality
_____ Stress adaptation theory

Column B

A. The life span of a cell is stored within the cell itself.
B. Older adults and society mutually withdraw from active exchange.
C. Past experiences return to consciousness, and memories are examined and reintegrated.
D. Personality is viewed as unchanging from early adulthood through old age.
E. Collagen forms more rigid molecular bonds over time.
F. Older adults should find substitutes for work or participation in community organizations if they must stop these activities.
G. Positive and negative effects of stress on biopsychosocial development.
H. If capacities decrease, the environment may be threatening.

2. Fill in the blanks.

A. Increasing disorientation or confusion at night resulting from loss of visual accommodation is called _____.

B. Mitts, posey belts, and geri chairs are examples of _____ that should be used with caution with the elderly.

C. Contraindications for _____ therapy are increased intracranial pressure, arrhythmias, and a myocardial infarction within the last 3 months.

D. When older patients need antipsychotic medications, atypicals are usually prescribed because of their _____.

E. _____ orientation can prevent confusion and keep patients oriented to time, place, person, and situation.

F. Intelligence is dulled by depression, drugs, or lack of use, but is stimulated by _____ therapy.

G. Evaluation of geropsychiatric nursing care focuses on the patient's ability to reach _____.

H. Doses of psychopharmacological drugs for older patients are usually _____.

3. Provide short answers for the following questions.

A. Highlight important communication factors to consider when interviewing older patients.
B. List the risk factors for falls with older patients.
C. Some believe that the lack of regard shown by health care professionals for living wills and advance directives of the elderly is related to their high suicide rate. Explore the many aspects of this complex issue.

Visit Evolve for additional resources related to the content of this chapter.
http://evolve.elsevier.com/Stuart/principles/
• Topical Course Outline • Student Workbook Exercises • Critical Thinking Questions and Activities • Case Studies • Research Topics
• Monthly Content Updates • WebLinks

Student Study CD-ROM

Access the accompanying CD-ROM for animations, interactive exercises, review questions for the NCLEX examination, and an audio glossary.

REFERENCES

Abrams RC et al: Predictors of self-neglect in community-dwelling elders, *Am J Psychiatry* 159:1724, 2002.

Administration on Aging: *A profile of older Americans: 2000*, Washington, DC, 2000, US Department of Health and Human Services.

Administration on Aging: *Older adults and mental health*, Washington, DC, 2001, US Department of Health and Human Services.

Bair BD: Presentation and recognition of common psychiatric disorders in the elderly, *Clin Geriatr* 8:26, 2000.

Bartels SJ et al: Evidence-based practices in geriatric mental health care, *Psychiatr Serv* 53:1419, 2002a.

Bartels SJ, Moak GS, Dums AR: Models of mental health services in nursing homes: a review of the literature, *Psychiatr Serv* 53:1390, 2002b.

Blazer DG: Depression in late life: review and commentary, *Am J Psychiatry* 58A:249, 2003.

Blazer DG: Psychiatry and the oldest old, *Am J Psychiatry* 157:1915, 2000.

Bourbonniere M, Evans LK: Advanced practice nursing in the care of frail older adults, *J Am Geriatr Soc* 50:2062, 2002.

Bruce ML et al: Major depression in elderly home health care patients, *Am J Psychiatry* 159:1367, 2002.

Camp CJ et al: Use of nonpharmacologic interventions among nursing home residents with dementia, *Psychiatr Serv* 53:1397, 2002.

Chien W: Use of physical restraints on hospitalized psychogeriatric patients, *J Psychosoc Nurs* 38:13, 2000.

Cody M, Beck C, Svarstad BL: Challenges to the use of nonpharmacologic interventions in nursing homes, *Psychiatr Serv* 53:1402, 2002.

Cohen GD: Aging at a turning point in the 21st century, *Am J Geriatr Psychiatry* 8:1, 2000.

Cole MG, Dendukuri N: Risk factors for depression among elderly community subjects: a systematic review and meta-analysis, *Am J Psychiatry* 160:1147, 2003.

Ducharme F, Trudeau D: Qualitative evaluation of a stress management intervention for elderly caregivers at home: a constructivist approach, *Issues Ment Health Nurs* 23:691, 2002.

Ebersole P, Hess P: *Geriatric nursing and healthy aging*, St Louis, 2001, Mosby.

Edberg A, Gerdner L, Buckwalter K: Behavioral and psychological symptoms of dementia: nursing module 10. In Finkel SI, editor: *The BPSD IPA Education Pack*, Cheshire, 2003, Gardiner-Caldwell Communications, Ltd.

Erikson E: *Childhood and society*, New York, 1963, WW Norton.

Evers W, Tomic W, Brouwers A: Effects of aggressive behavior and perceived self-efficacy on burnout among staff of homes for the elderly, *Issues Ment Health Nurs* 22:439, 2001.

Feil N: Communicating with the confused elderly patient, *Geriatrics* 39:131, 1984.

Garand L et al: A pilot study of immune and mood outcomes of a community-based intervention for dementia caregivers: the PLST intervention, *Arch Psychiatr Nurs* 16:156, 2002.

Hegge M, Fischer C: Grief responses of senior and elderly widows: practice implications, *J Gerontol Nurs* 26:35, 2000.

Horton-Deutsch SL et al: The PLUS intervention: a pilot test with caregivers of depressed older adults, *Arch Psychiatr Nurs* 16:61, 2002.

Jacobson S et al: *Handbook of geriatric psychopharmacology*, Washington, DC, 2002, AP Publishing.

Jervis L: Contending with "problem behaviors" in the nursing home, *Arch Psychiatr Nurs* 16:32, 2002.

Jones ED, Beck-Little R: The use of reminiscence therapy for the treatment of depression in rural-dwelling older adults, *Issues Ment Health Nurs* 23:279, 2002.

Kelley LS, Buckwalter KC, Mass ML: Access to health care resources for family caregivers of elderly persons with dementia, *Nurs Outlook* 47:8, 1999.

Lantz MS: Alcohol abuse in the older adult, *Clin Geriatrics* 10:40, 2002.

Lenze EJ et al: Comorbid anxiety disorders in depressed elderly patients, *Am J Psychiatry* 157:722, 2000.

Mace N, Rabins R: *The 36-hour day*, New York, 2001, Warner Books.

Mehta KM, Yaffe K, Covinsky KE: Cognitive impairment, depressive symptoms and functional decline in older people, *J Am Geriatr Soc* 50:1045, 2002.

Masand PS: Side effects of antipsychotics in the elderly, *J Clin Psychiatry* 61(suppl 8):43, 2000.

Mignor D: Effectiveness of use of home health nurses to decrease burden and depression of elderly caregivers, *J Psychosoc Nurs* 38:34, 2000.

Morris D: Geriatric mental health: an overview, *J Am Psychiatr Nurses Assoc* 7:S2, 2001.

North American Nursing Diagnosis Association: *NANDA nursing diagnosis, definitions and classification 2003-2004*, Philadelphia, 2003, NANDA.

Paterniti S et al: Depressive symptoms and cognitive decline in elderly people: longitudinal study, *Br J Psychiatry* 181:406, 2002.

Salzman C: *Psychiatric medications for older adults: the concise guide*, New York, 2001, The Guilford Press.

Salzman C: Treatment of agitation and aggression in the elderly. In Schatzberg A, Nemeroff C: *Textbook of psychopharmacology*, ed 3 Washington, DC, 2004, AP Publishing.

Schatzberg A et al: *Manual of clinical psychopharmacology*, ed 4, Washington, DC, 2003, American Psychiatric Publishing.

Spector A et al: Efficacy of an evidence-based cognitive stimulation therapy programme for people with dementia: randomized controlled trial, *Br J Psychiatry* 183:248, 2003.

Talerico K: Grief and older adults: differences, issues and clinical approaches, *J Psychosoc Nurs* 41:12, 2003.

Vaillant GE, Mukamal K: Successful aging, *Am J Psychiatry* 158:839, 2001.

Yeung P et al: Quetiapine for elderly patients with psychotic disorders, *Psychiatric Annals* 30:197, 2000.

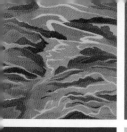

When I was a laddie I lived with my granny
And many a hiding my granny di'ed me.

Now I am a man and I live with my granny
And do to my granny what she did to me.

TRADITIONAL RHYME, ANONYMOUS

39 CARE OF SURVIVORS OF ABUSE AND VIOLENCE

Nancy Fishwick ▪ *Barbara Parker* ▪ *Jacquelyn C. Campbell*

LEARNING OBJECTIVES

After studying this chapter, the student should be able to:

1. Define family violence, its possible causes, and characteristics of violent families (**I**).
2. Describe behaviors and values of nurses related to survivors of family violence (**I**).
3. Examine physiological, behavioral, and psychological responses of survivors of family violence (**I**).
4. Discuss primary, secondary, and tertiary prevention nursing actions related to family violence (**I**).
5. Analyze nursing assessment and intervention in abuse and violence among specific populations (**II**).
6. Evaluate issues and nursing care related to survivors of sexual assault (**III**).

TOPICAL OUTLINE

I. Dimensions of Family Violence
  A. Characteristics of Violent Families
  B. Nursing Attitudes toward Survivors of Violence
  C. Responses of Survivors
  D. Preventive Nursing Interventions
II. Special Populations
  A. Child Abuse
  B. Intimate Partner Violence
  C. Elder Abuse
III. Rape and Sexual Assault
  A. Definition of Sexual Assault
  B. Marital Rape
  C. Nursing Care of the Sexual Assault Survivor

evolve   Visit Evolve for additional resources related to the content of this chapter.
http://evolve.elsevier.com/Stuart/principles/

Nurses encounter survivors of abuse and violence in many settings. However, because experiencing violence is generally devastating, survivors of abuse and violence are often seen in psychiatric settings. At times the violence is openly discussed and recognized as a precipitating factor for the current health care visit, as when a survivor of sexual assault is treated in an emergency room. Often, however, violence is disclosed only after a trusting nurse-patient relationship is formed.

Although there are various forms of violence, such as gang behavior and drug-related violence, the types most often described by psychiatric patients are family violence and non-family rape and sexual assault. Because the dynamics of these two forms of violence are different, they are covered in two separate sections of this chapter. Rape and sexual assault also can be forms of family violence. In addition, attention is given to populations that are particularly at risk for abuse: children, intimate partners, and the elderly.

The words used to describe people who have experienced violence are important. Traditionally the word **victim** has been used, along with discussions of syndromes. These labels distance nurses from the person who has been abused as they search for differences between themselves and the victims to decrease their own feelings of vulnerability. In this chapter the word **survivor** is used to emphasize that the person who

has experienced abuse has many strengths and coping strategies that can be incorporated into the plan of care.

Do you agree with the use of the word survivor instead of victim in this chapter? What do you think of when you hear the words victim and survivor? ▪

■ DIMENSIONS OF FAMILY VIOLENCE

Family violence is a range of harmful behaviors that occur between family and other household members. It includes physical and emotional abuse of children, child neglect, abuse between adult intimate partners, marital rape, and elder abuse. Although each family is unique, some characteristics appear to be common to most violent families. Furthermore, regardless of the type of abuse occurring within a family, all members, including the extended family, are affected. Family violence, although often unnoted, is at the core of many family disturbances. Violence may be a family secret and often continues through generations.

Although many research studies and theories have been directed toward the causes, treatment, and prevention of family violence, more questions are still unanswered than answered. Some believe that the family is the training ground for violence and ask why the social group that is supposed to provide love and support is also the most violent group to which most people belong. Behaviors that would be unacceptable between strangers, co-workers, or friends are often tolerated within families.

Violence and abuse are caused by an interaction of personality, demographic, biological, situational, and sociocultural factors. Many of the unique characteristics of the family as a social group—time spent together, emotional involvement, privacy, and in-depth knowledge of each other—can lead to both intimacy and violence. Thus a given family can be loving and supportive as well as violent.

To understand violence in American families, the influence of society on the family must be examined. The United States has a high level of violence compared with other Western nations. Many believe that society's willingness to tolerate violence sets the stage for family violence.

Social norms are sometimes used to justify violence to maintain the family system. For example, a husband's use of violence may be considered legitimate if the wife is having an extramarital affair. Historical attitudes toward women, children, and the elderly; economic discrimination; the nonresponsiveness of the criminal justice system; and the belief that women and children are property are social factors that promote violence. Changing norms about family privacy and when the government should intervene in family matters have also influenced the definition and recognition of family violence.

Why do you think more violence occurs in American society than in other Western nations? What societal factors influence the use of violence? ■

Characteristics of Violent Families

Factors common to violent families include the multigenerational family process, social isolation, the use and abuse of power, and the effect of alcohol and drug abuse.

Multigenerational Transmission. Multigenerational transmission means that family violence is often perpetuated through generations by a cycle of violence (Ehrensaft et al, 2003). Figure 39-1 shows the multigenerational transmission of family violence. Social learning theory related to violence states that a child learns this behavior pattern in a family setting by taking a violent parent as a role model. In this case, violence and victimization are behaviors learned through childhood experience. The child learns both the means and the approval of violence. Children who witness violence not only learn specific aggressive behaviors but also come to believe that violence is a legitimate way to solve problems. When frustrated or angry as an adult, the person relies on this learned behavior and responds with violence.

Experiencing abuse as a child does not totally determine an adult's later behaviors. Many people who were abused as children are able to avoid violence with their own children. A key factor may be the age at which the child was abused or which parent was abusive. Experiencing abuse from a father at age 4 years may be totally different from experiencing abuse from a mother as an adolescent.

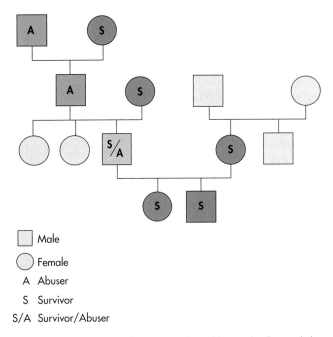

	Male
	Female
A	Abuser
S	Survivor
S/A	Survivor/Abuser

Figure 39-1 Genogram demonstrates the multigenerational transmission of family violence.

The incidence of violence in the families of both the survivors of wife abuse and their abusers also supports multigenerational transmission. A classic literature review identified witnessing parental violence during childhood or adolescence as one of the strongest risk factors for the abuse of wives in adulthood (Hotaling and Sugarman, 1986). It is less clear that women learn to tolerate wife abuse from childhood experiences with violence.

To date, the evidence of multigenerational transmission of violence in elder abuse is limited. Abuse, neglect, and exploitation of older adults is generally perpetrated by the person's primary caregiver. The caregiver may be a family member, such as a spouse or adult child, but also may be a nonfamily personal care attendant in the home or in a residential facility.

Many treatment modalities, especially cognitive-behavioral approaches, are based on the social learning model that violent reactions can be unlearned and replaced with constructive responses to conflict.

Social Isolation. Violent families are also socially isolated. One reason may be that some types of violence are considered abnormal or illegitimate and become a family secret. Exposure of family violence can result in both formal and informal sanctions from other family members, neighbors, the police, or the judicial system; therefore, the abuser often purposely keeps the family isolated. Social isolation is a factor in elder abuse, intimate partner violence, and child abuse.

Use and Abuse of Power. Another common factor within the various forms of family violence is the use and abuse of power. In almost all forms of family violence, the abuser has some form of power or control over the victim. For example,

BOX **39-1**

Forms of Abuse Within Families Reflecting Struggles for Power and Control

Physical
- **Inflicting or attempting to inflict physical injury or illness**—for example, grabbing, pinching, shoving, slapping, hitting, hair-pulling, biting, arm-twisting, kicking, punching, hitting with blunt objects, stabbing, shooting.
- **Withholding access to resources necessary to maintain health**—for example, medication, medical care, wheelchair, food or fluids, sleep, hygienic assistance.
- **Forcing alcohol or other drug use.**

Sexual
- **Coercing or attempting to coerce any sexual contact without consent**—for example, marital rape, acquaintance rape, forced sex after physical beating, attacks on the sexual parts of the body, bestiality, forced prostitution, unprotected sex, fondling, sodomy, sex with others, use of pornography.
- **Attempting to undermine the victim's sexuality**—for example, treating her or him in a sexually degrading manner, criticizing sexual performance and desirability. Also, accusations of infidelity, withholding sex.

Psychological
- **Instilling or attempting to instill fear**—for example, intimidation, threatening physical harm to self, victim, or others, threatening to harm or kidnap children, menacing, blackmail, harassment, destruction of pets and property, mind games.

- **Isolating or attempting to isolate victim from friends, family, school, or work**—for example, withholding access to phone or transportation, undermining victim's personal relationships, harassing others, constant "checking up," constant accompaniment, unfounded accusations, forced imprisonment.

Emotional
- **Undermining or attempting to undermine victim's sense of self-worth**—for example, constant criticism, belittling victim's abilities and competency, name calling, insults, put-downs, silent treatment, manipulating victim's feelings and emotions to induce guilt, subverting a partner's relationship with the children, repeatedly making and breaking promises.

Economic
- **Making or attempting to make the victim financially dependent**—for example, maintaining total control over financial resources, including victim's earned income or resources received through public assistance or social security, withholding money or access to money, forbidding attendance at school, forbidding employment, on-the-job harassment, requiring accountability and justification for all money spent, forced welfare fraud, withholding information about family finances, running up bills for which the victim is responsible for payment.

From New York State Office for the Prevention of Domestic Violence.

with the sexual abuse of children, the abuser is usually a male in an authority position victimizing a child in a subordinate position (USDHHS, 2000; Lawson, 2003).

Power issues appear to be a central factor in intimate partner abuse and violence. For example, in marriage, abusers may justify the use of violence for trivial events such as not having a meal ready or not keeping the house tidy. However, the controlling behaviors and violence often are related to the husband's need for total domination of his wife. Wife abuse often begins or escalates when the woman behaves more independently by working or attending school. Box 39-1 describes five forms of abuse within families that reflect domestic struggles for power and control.

Alcohol and Drug Abuse. Survivors of violence often report concurrent substance abuse by the abuser (Torres and Han, 2003). However, one behavior is not necessary for the other to occur. That is, people who abuse alcohol are not consistently violent, and people who are violent are not always intoxicated. Instead, it has been suggested that the person uses alcohol as a socially acceptable explanation for the behavior. Family and friends may attribute the conduct to the effects of alcohol, which to some extent may decrease the degree of blame. The use of alcohol or drugs also may increase violent behavior by reducing fear or inhibitions and decreasing sensitivity to the impact of the behavior.

Connections between drug abuse and family violence have been less well researched. Research on aggressiveness and illicit drugs has established that marijuana and heroin use are not related to violence. In contrast, drugs such as crack cocaine, amphetamines, mescaline, "angel dust" (PCP), and steroids have been associated with increased violence in general. The current use of "date-rape drugs" such as flunitrazepam (Rohypnol) clearly places people, primarily young women, in danger of sexual exploitation and physical harm.

Nursing Attitudes Toward Survivors of Violence

It can be difficult and frustrating to provide nursing care for survivors of violence. The attitudes nurses bring to these situations shape their responses. Studies of health care professionals' attitudes indicate that myths about battered women are accepted even though there is sympathy toward the survivor. Table 39-1 describes common myths about survivors of abuse.

Although most nurses do not actually blame survivors for what has happened to them, research reveals that they are less tolerant of certain behaviors. For example, nurses are more apt to blame a rape survivor if the woman had gone out late at night, not locked her car doors, gone shopping for beer rather than milk for the baby, or did not resist the assault "enough." They have difficulty understanding abused chil-

Table 39-1	Beyond the Myths: Recognizing Abuse Survivors
MYTH	REALITY
Family violence is most common among families living in poverty.	Family violence occurs at all levels of society without regard to age, race, culture, status, education, or religion. It may be less evident among the affluent because they can afford private physicians, attorneys, counselors, and shelters. In contrast, people with less money must turn to public agencies for help.
Violence rarely occurs between dating partners.	Estimates vary among studies, but violence occurs in a large percentage of dating relationships.
Abused spouses can end the violence by divorcing their abuser.	According to the U.S. Department of Justice, about 75% of all spousal attacks occur between people who are separated or divorced. In many cases, the separation process brings on an increased level of harassment and violence.
The victim can learn to stop doing things that provoke the violence.	In a battering relationship, the abuser needs no provocation to become violent. Violence is the abuser's pattern of behavior and the victim cannot learn how to control it. Even so, many victims blame themselves for the abuse, feeling guilty—even responsible—for doing or saying something that seems to trigger the abuser's behavior. Friends, family, and service providers reinforce this by laying the blame and the need to change on the shoulders of the victim.
Alcohol, stress, and mental illness are major causes of physical and verbal abuse.	Abusive people—and even their victims—often use those conditions to excuse or minimize the abuse. But abuse is a learned behavior, not an uncontrollable reaction. People are abusive because they have acquired the belief that violence and aggression are acceptable and effective responses to real or imagined threats. Fortunately, because violence is a learned behavior, abusers can benefit from counseling and professional help to alter their behavior. But dealing only with the perceived problem (for example, alcohol, stress, or mental illness) will not change the abusive tendencies.
Violence occurs only between heterosexual partners.	Gay and lesbian partners experience violence for varied but similar reasons as heterosexual partners do.
Being pregnant protects a woman from battering.	Battering often begins or escalates during pregnancy. According to one theory, the abuser who already has low self-esteem views his wife as his property. As a result, he resents the intrusion of the fetus as well as the extra attention his wife gets from friends, family, and health care providers.
Abused women tacitly accept the abuse by trying to conceal it, not reporting it, or failing to seek help.	Many women, when they do try to disclose their situation, are met with denial or disbelief. This only discourages them from persevering.

dren who want to return to abusive parents and battered women who do not leave their abusers.

Studies describe how survivors find the health care system to be unhelpful and even traumatizing when they go for help. Nurses often use a paternalistic and individualistic model of helping battered women. The **paternalistic model** may be contrasted with the **empowerment model**. Table 39-2 compares the characteristics of these models. When the paternalistic model is used, the nurse is more likely to be frustrated because the survivor does not follow the nurse's advice. Therefore the empowerment model is not only more helpful to the survivor but also more professionally satisfying for the nurse.

Origins of Negative Attitudes. Several theories can help in understanding nurses' attitudes. The **just world hypothesis** proposes that people believe that others generally get what they deserve: Good things happen to good people and bad things happen to bad people. This belief helps one feel safe because one sees oneself as basically good and therefore protected.

When a person is victimized by violence, people feel a need to make sense of this horrible circumstance. The easiest way is not to see it at all, which explains some of the lack of

Table 39-2	A Comparison of the Paternalistic and Empowerment Models of Intervention With Battered Women	
PATERNALISTIC MODEL	EMPOWERMENT MODEL
Nurse is perceived to be more knowledgeable than the survivor.	There is mutual sharing of knowledge and information.
Responsibility for ending the violence is placed on the survivor.	The nurse strategizes with the survivor. Survivors are helped to recognize societal influences.
Advice and sympathy are given rather than respect.	The survivor's competence and experience are respected.

recognition. However, when family violence is unmistakable, one needs to understand why that particular person is the victim. If bad things happen to bad people, the victimized person must have done something wrong or at least something stupid, something different from what oneself would have done.

The whole process of victim blaming is easier if the survivor is of "a type" who is already the focus of bias. It is easier to blame and distance oneself from women or minority groups if there is already bias against them. Conversely, the more the person resembles oneself, the harder it is to recognize the violence. An example of this is society's focus on the "collusive" mother in cases of the sexual abuse of her child. Because it is difficult to blame the child, the blame is shifted to the mother rather than trying to understand the mother's normal responses to such a horrible dilemma.

Even though some of the societal forces that lead to incest have been exposed, they are generally not addressed in recommendations for clinical interventions. The focus is often misplaced on the "dysfunctional family unit" rather than on the real issue: a criminal who has violated the safety and health of a child in a society uncomfortable with the attitudes that may encourage such behavior.

Yet another perspective is that of **deviance theory**, which proposes that making the survivors and perpetrators of violence into objects to be studied or diagnostic categories creates further distance between them and the nurse (May et al, 2003). This is the problem with a psychiatric diagnosis specific to survivors of violence. If adults receive diagnoses only because they were abused sometime in their past, the assumption of pathology becomes concrete. The survivor of family violence is officially sick and has the responsibility to become well. There is no chance that the person's responses will be seen as survival strategies or normal reactions; they become symptoms. Survivors become a "deviant group" to be studied and "fixed."

Because the nursing profession remains a predominantly female group, more nurses have been victimized by violence than other groups, which might explain nurses' negative attitudes toward other survivors. Regardless of the specific violence experience of nurses, power, control, and exploitation

issues certainly have shaped the history of the nursing profession and continue to influence nurses' daily reality.

Overcoming Negative Attitudes. The first step in providing effective nursing care is exploring one's own attitudes toward survivors of family violence. Understanding the mechanisms that help create such attitudes is also helpful. Nurses who have had clinical experience with survivors may be less blaming than nurses who have not. Therefore, it is important to gain this experience through educational programs or as a volunteer in programs such as rape crisis centers, battered women's shelters, or child protection programs.

Formal continuing and in-service education on family violence should be directed toward recognizing and changing feelings as well as learning facts about violence. Nurses also can increase their own understanding and appreciation of the experience of survivors by reading books and watching media programs about these issues (see Citing the Evidence).

Many television shows and movies explore the issues of family abuse and violence. Do you think they have helped change attitudes or reinforced fears and stereotypes? ■

Responses of Survivors

A growing body of knowledge describes how people respond to violence from other family members.

Physical Responses to Family Violence. A characteristic pattern of injuries, especially to the head, neck, face, throat, trunk, and sexual organs has been seen in all forms of family violence. For all groups experiencing family violence, sexual abuse often accompanies physical abuse. This has been best documented in battered women; several studies have found that approximately 40% were also sexually assaulted by their partners. All survivors of family violence tend to have injuries at multiple sites in various stages of healing.

Survivors of family violence often experience a range of physical symptoms not obviously related to their injuries, such as headaches, menstrual problems, chronic pain, and digestive and sleeping disturbances. Symptoms such as headaches and other forms of chronic pain may be the result of repetitive blows to the head or other parts of the body. In addition, the stress experienced from past or on-going family violence may negatively affect the immune system, putting the individual at risk for a variety of health problems.

Although the physical manifestations of family violence have often been diagnosed as evidence of somatization, they may be more accurately identified as part of a physical stress reaction that is common to those who have experienced various types of emotional trauma.

Behavioral Responses to Family Violence. Many attempts have been made to understand the behavior of survivors of family violence, especially their continued involvement with an abuser. This has been especially damaging in literature addressing the question of why battered women remain in the relationship. It is assumed that she should leave

---

■ CITING THE EVIDENCE ON
Nurses' Perceptions of Interpersonal Violence

BACKGROUND: Research shows that education related to interpersonal violence varies greatly among nursing programs. Two hundred and fifty-one nurses were surveyed to determine their screening and intervention practices, knowledge of the legal requirements, time devoted to educational preparation, and perceived educational needs regarding interpersonal violence.

RESULTS: The findings support the reports of other studies that indicate there is disparity in nursing education regarding interpersonal violence and a need among practicing nurses for further assistance to help them become comfortable with and effective in assessment and intervention in cases involving interpersonal violence.

IMPLICATIONS: This study suggests that an opportunity to intervene and respond more effectively to interpersonal violence by providing curricula that are ongoing and disseminated to direct care providers does exist.

Glaister J, Kesling G: *Nurs Outlook* 50:137, 2002.

rather than stay. In actuality, when a battered woman leaves, she is in the most danger of being stalked and killed by a partner obsessed with power and control (Spitzberg, 2003; Morewitz, 2003). At the other end of the continuum, some battered women are able to end the violence but maintain their relationships using a variety of strategies.

However, family violence usually escalates in severity and frequency. In cases where the violence does not end, it is normal and healthy for a battered woman to consider her entire existence and that of her significant others for a long time before ending her most important attachment relationship.

Constraints that make it difficult to leave include cultural sanctions, perceived stigma, strong emotional attachment to her partner, and lack of resources. It has been observed that women usually make moral decisions by weighing the consequences to others more heavily than consequences to themselves (Gilligan, 1982). Thus concern for her children is a major issue in the woman's decision making.

Most women eventually leave a relationship that is continuously violent, but there is often a pattern of leaving and returning many times before making a final break. Rather than being a sign of weakness, this can be seen as a normal process. It is influenced by the quality of social support and assistance to the woman and the batterer's behavior rather than the woman's psychological factors. Leaving and returning are purposeful and meant to pressure the abuser into meaningful change, test external and internal resources, or evaluate how the children react without their father.

Similar long processes of ending attachment relationships are seen with spouses of alcoholics, divorced and separated women, and people experiencing anticipatory grief. In addition, grief can explain the denial that is often seen in battered women. Clinical reports also describe the reluctance of abused children and elderly family members to view their families as pathological rather than normal. These responses seem more understandable and healthy if they are related to normal grief and fear of abandonment and possible placement in foster homes or nursing homes.

Discuss the issue of women remaining in abusive relationships. What factors keep them in these relationships? How do health professionals usually respond to a woman who has remained in an abusive relationship? What approach would be helpful to her? ∎

Psychological Responses to Family Violence. It has been shown that an emotionally abusive family environment, the experience of physical and sexual abuse, and the witnessing of maternal battering have a negative impact on one's mental health (Edwards et al, 2003; Ray, 2001; Kendler et al, 2000). More work has been done to explore psychological responses to intimate partner violence than to either child abuse or elder abuse.

What is known about the emotional responses to incest are reports of delayed reactions rather than immediate ones. In addition, the question of "false memories" has complicated the diagnosis and treatment process (see Critical Thinking About Contemporary Issues). Psychological responses studied most often include the cognitive responses of attribution and problem solving and the emotional responses of depression and lowered self-esteem.

It is also known, however, that some women who have been battered are able to display remarkable adaptability in the wake of such trauma and do *not* develop serious psychological sequelae. This may be due to the woman's resilience, a pattern of successful outcomes in individuals despite challenging or threatening circumstances (Humphreys, 2003).

Attributions. Attributions are the reasoning processes people use to explain events. Attributions affect how people feel about their behavior and interpret life events. Some believe that self-blaming attributions may be adaptive for survivors of violence as a way of maintaining control over their lives. Others think that self-blame may contribute to long-term depression.

To date, the evidence is insufficient to assume that self-blame is either widespread among survivors or always patho-

---

Critical Thinking *About* Contemporary Issues

Can Adults Remember Repressed Episodes of Child Abuse or Are These Part of a "False Memory Syndrome"?

Considerable controversy has been generated concerning the validity of memories of childhood abuse. Some people have reported delayed recall of forgotten abuse that occurred during childhood, many years earlier. These reports of delayed recall of abuse have been challenged on a number of fronts, and in some cases people have retracted their allegations. Some experts claim that psychotherapists practicing "recovered memory therapy" created false memories of abuse through leading questions or excessive insisting. These therapists reportedly believe that psychopathology is related to childhood trauma and that the goal of therapy is to help patients remember incidents of previously forgotten abuse from childhood in order to get well.

That many people forget episodes of childhood abuse is well established. As many as 38% of trauma survivors who experienced abuse severe enough to result in a visit to a hospital emergency room had no memory of the event 20 or more years later. At issue is the meaning of these findings. Some investigators have explained the loss of memory of abuse as secondary to "repression" or dissociative amnesia: Memories of abuse, although present in the mind, may not be available to consciousness. The opposite viewpoint holds that the loss of memories of abuse is a process of "normal forgetting," arguing that believing that forgotten memories exist somewhere in the brain and are only awaiting the proper stimulus to bring them to consciousness again is a popular misconception.

Neuropeptides and neurotransmitters released during stress can modulate memory function, acting in the limbic system at the level of the hippocampus (responsible for turning short-term memory into long-term memory), amygdala (responsible for emotion), and other brain regions involved in these functions. Such release may interfere with the accurate laying down of memory traces for incidents of childhood abuse. Also, childhood abuse may result in long-term alterations in the function of these neuromodulators. Nurses can help these patients by keeping up to date with the neuroscientific research in this area and with the impact of these findings on the controversy surrounding these issues.

logical. Nurses who use the empowerment model when working with survivors believe it will help the person identify his or her attributions and how they effect that person's feelings and relationships.

Problem-solving techniques. Problems with academic performance and school behavior have been reported in abused children. In addition, some studies have found that women in abusive relationships have trouble with problem solving. However, recent research has revealed that women use a variety of approaches to achieve and maintain safety for themselves and their children, suggesting logical problem solving and appropriate decision making. Undoubtedly, some battered family violence survivors are so frequently and severely beaten and controlled that their ability to solve problems is compromised.

Extreme difficulty in problem solving could be explained by posttraumatic stress disorder, with its symptoms of memory impairment and difficulty concentrating. Problem-solving difficulties noted in widows and divorcees have been explained as normal responses to loss. Such problems also could be explained as one of the cognitive aspects of depression.

Depression. Depression is common among women in abusive relationships, adult survivors of incest, abused children, and survivors of other forms of violence (Dienemann et al, 2000). Depression is discussed in detail in Chapter 19.

In summary, responses to family violence can be interpreted either as symptoms of pathology or as a way in which normal people respond to incredible physical and emotional trauma and yet survive. Research regarding this latter approach is beginning to document survivor mechanisms and a recovery process from abuse.

Preventive Nursing Interventions

Psychiatric–mental health nurses have important roles to play in the primary prevention of family violence. They do this through educating the public, detecting risk factors for or actual experience of family violence early on to facilitate timely intervention, and preventing complications and recurrence of abuse or violence for survivors.

Primary Prevention. Primary prevention is an activity that stops a problem before it occurs. Changing society's acceptance of violence and abuse is an important first step in prevention. Effective primary prevention includes eliminating cultural norms and values that accept and glamorize violence. This can begin by limiting the amount of violence permitted on television and in other media.

The prevalence of violence on television, in movies, and in advertising plays a role in creating a social climate that says violence is exciting and appropriate. The average child watches television 20 hours a week. It has been estimated that American children observe 18,000 killings before they graduate from high school. Violent content in children's video and computer games and on the internet also are of great concern.

A related area of primary prevention is the elimination of pornography, especially violent pornography, which has been associated with sexual violence. Concerned parents and law enforcement are also challenged by the increasing ease of sexual exploitation of children through child pornography on the Internet.

Primary prevention of abuse also includes strengthening individuals, families, and communities so they can cope more effectively with stress and resolve conflict nonviolently. Working collaboratively with school nurses, community health nurses, social services, law enforcement, and other community stakeholders, psychiatric–mental health nurses can help develop and implement educational programs in a variety of community arenas such as schools, workplaces, and senior citizen centers. Programs can focus on healthy growth and development across the lifespan, healthy intimate relationships, preparation for parenting, ways to discipline children nonviolently, safe storage of firearms in the home, and raising awareness of the ways in which people can become controlled, manipulated, and potentially exploited by others.

Nurses can be involved in teaching family life and sex education courses in elementary and middle schools. Child sexual abuse can be prevented or detected when children are taught about inappropriate sexual contact and what they should do if it occurs. Middle school students need information about how to have relationships in which jealousy is not viewed as a sign of love and domination of one partner over the other is not expected.

Family violence prevention also includes anticipatory guidance while working with families. For example, respite care is needed for families with chronically ill or incapacitated members, including the elderly and children. Planning in advance for relief from responsibility will prevent strained relationships and potential violence or abuse.

Families also need to anticipate the difficult developmental stages of children. Parents need to know that infants are not intentionally frustrating to parents, that toddlers' obstinacy is necessary for independence in later childhood, and that bed-wetting is a signal for the need of increased positive attention, not punishment (Banks, 2002).

A society must develop programs and policies that support families and reduce stresses and inequities. This includes adequate and appropriate day care for children and incapacitated elders, equity in salary and wages to make women less financially dependent, public education that ensures an adequate foundation for full employment of all, and sufficient financing of prevention and treatment programs.

 Go to a computer store and search for the most popular games. Evaluate them for level of violence, sexual roles, and issues related to power and control. ■

Secondary Prevention. Secondary prevention efforts involve identification of families at risk for abuse, neglect, or exploitation of family members as well as early detection of those who are beginning to use violence. Assessing the health and well-being of women during their pregnancies affords an ideal opportunity to identify women at risk for becoming battered or those who may be involved in the early stages of an abusive relationship.

Box 39-2 lists indicators of actual or potential abuse that should be included in a nursing assessment. Availability and

BOX 39-2

Indicators of Actual or Potential Abuse

Nursing History
Primary reason for contact
Vague information about cause of problem
Discrepancy between physical findings and description of cause
Minimizing injuries
Inappropriate delay between time of injury and treatment
Inappropriate family reactions (such as lack of concern, overconcern, threatening demeanor)
Information from family genogram
Family violence in history (child, spouse, elder)
History of violence outside of home
Incarcerations
Violent deaths in extended family
Alcoholism/drug abuse in family history
Health history
History of traumatic injuries
Spontaneous abortions
Psychiatric hospitalizations
History of depression
Substance abuse
Sexual history
Prior sexual abuse
Use of force in sexual activities
Venereal disease
Child with sexual knowledge beyond that appropriate for age
Promiscuity
Personal/social history
Access to firearms or other weapons
Unwanted or unplanned pregnancy
Adolescent pregnancy
Social isolation (difficulty naming people available for help in a crisis)
Lack of contact with extended family
Unrealistic expectations of relationships or age-appropriate behavior
Extreme jealousy by spouse
Rigid traditional sex-role beliefs
Verbal aggression
Belief in use of physical punishment
Difficulties in school
Truancy, running away
Psychological history
Feelings of helplessness/hopelessness
Feeling trapped
Difficulty making plans for future
Tearfulness
Chronic fatigue, apathy
Suicide attempts
Financial history
Poverty
Finances rigidly controlled by one family member

Unwillingness to spend money on health care or adequate nutrition
Complaints about spending money on family members
Unemployment
Use of elders' finances for other family members
Family beliefs/values
Belief in importance of physical discipline
Autocratic decision making
Intolerance of differing views among members
Mistrust of outsiders
Family relations
Lack of visible affection or nurturing between family members
Extreme dependency between family members
Autonomy discouraged
Numerous arguments
Temporary separations
Dissatisfaction with family members
Lack of enjoyable family activities
Extramarital affairs
Role rigidity (inability of members to assume nontraditional roles)

Physical Examination
General appearance
Fearful, anxious, hyperactive, or hypoactive
Poor hygiene, careless grooming
Inappropriate dress
Increased anxiety in presence of abuser
Looking to abuser for answers to questions
Inappropriate or anxious nonverbal behavior (such as giggling at serious questions or questions related to abuse)
Flinching when touched
Vital statistics
Overweight or underweight
Hypertension
Skin
Bruises, welts, edema
Presence of scars and indications of injuries in various stages of healing
Cigarette burns
Head
Bald patches on scalp from pulling hair
Subdural hematoma
Eyes
Subconjunctival hemorrhage
Swelling
Black eyes
Ears
Hearing loss from prior injury or untreated infections

Mouth
Bruising
Lacerations
Untreated dental caries
Venereal infection
Abdomen
Intraabdominal injuries
Abdominal injuries during pregnancy
Extremities
Bruising to forearms from attempts to protect self from blows
Broken arms
Radiological indications of previous fractures
Neurological
Developmental delays
Difficulty with speech or swallowing
Hyperactive reflex response
Genital/urinary
Genital lacerations or bruising
Urinary tract infections
Sexually transmitted disease
Rectal
Rectal bruising
Bleeding
Edema
Tenderness
Poor sphincter tone

Nursing Observations
General observations
Observations that differ significantly from history
Family members inadequately clothed or groomed
Home environment
Inadequate heating
Inappropriate sleeping arrangements
Total household disorganization
Inadequate food
Spoiled food not discarded
Family communication pattern
One parent answers all questions
Looking for approval of other family members before answering questions
Members continually interrupt each other
Negative nonverbal behavior in other members when one member speaking
Members do not listen to each other
Taboo topics (family secrets)
Emotional climate
Tense, secretive atmosphere
Unhappiness
Lack of affection
Apparent fear of other family members
Verbal arguing

storage of firearms or other deadly weapons in the home needs to be addressed because easy access has played a role in intentional injuries to family members as well as in communities and schools. Other early indicators of families at risk include violence in the family of origin of either partner, communication problems, and excessive family stress such as an unplanned pregnancy, unemployment, or inadequate family resources.

When the nurse becomes aware of an indication of risk, immediate nursing intervention is required. Taking the time to explore the risk factors, discuss perceptions and attitudes, and create a safety planning checklist with the patient is time well spent (Box 39-3).

Tertiary Prevention. Tertiary prevention efforts refer to those nursing activities that address the immediate and long-term needs of victims and survivors as they recover from their experiences in order to ameliorate negative effects. Tertiary prevention also is focused on stopping the current abuse and preventing the recurrence of abuse.

For example, if the victim-survivor is a child or dependent older adult, that individual may need to be removed from the home for safety. In some cases, such as abuse of an older adult by a personal care attendant in the home, it may be possible to remove the perpetrator from the home, rather than disrupt the security of the older adult. Legal recourse against the perpetrator may be mandated in the case of abuse of a child or older adult and may be voluntarily pursued by an adult survivor of intimate partner violence.

It is important for nurses to know the mandatory reporting laws in their state. **All 50 states mandate reporting of child abuse and neglect, and most states have some form of mandatory reporting of abuse, neglect, or exploitation of the elderly.** At this time, however, reporting of domestic violence is mandated only in California, Connecticut, Colorado, Kentucky, and Tennessee. Many nursing and medical organizations are opposed to mandatory reporting of domestic violence because it violates an individual's autonomy and violates patient confidentiality.

High rates of family violence and low rates of detection, reporting, and therapeutic intervention by health care professionals are well documented. The lack of educational content on child abuse, intimate partner violence, and elder abuse in professional training programs for physicians, nurses,

---

BOX **39-3**

Safety Planning Checklist for Victims of Domestic Violence

During a Violent Argument
Move to a space where you are least likely to be injured.
Avoid the kitchen, bathroom, garage, and rooms without an outside door.

Plan Ahead
Keep emergency numbers posted.
Work out a signal with a neighbor to call for help.
Plan with your children. Work out a code word or signal and teach them how to call 911.
Practice ways to get out safely.
Park your car so that you are not blocked in.
Make an extra set of car keys and keep your gas tank full.
Even if you don't think there will be a next time, plan three places you can go to be safe.
Find out about legal options and protective orders before you need them.
Open your own savings account at a separate bank.

Put Things in Their Place
Keep extra cash and clothes where you can access them safely (at a friend's home, at your workplace).
Make copies of important documents and keep them somewhere safe.

If You Have a Protective Order
Keep a copy with you at all times.
Give copies to your children's school or daycare facility and to your employer.
Report all violations to the police.

If Your Partner No Longer Lives With You
Change the locks.
Install additional locks.
Plan escape routes.
Get caller ID.
Work out a signal with a neighbor to call for help.
Notify police so they know your situation.

Safety at Work
Use voice mail or have someone screen your calls.
Notify security or your supervisor.
Make a safety plan with co-workers to deal with your particular situation.

Build a Network of Support
Connect with old friends.
Join a support group.
Call the local domestic violence hotline.

Alcohol and Drugs
The use of alcohol or drugs reduces awareness and the ability to act quickly to protect yourself and your children. Batterers often use alcohol or drugs as an excuse for their violent behavior.

Break the Silence
Tell your family members, friends, neighbors, co-workers, and physician about the abuse.
Remember that isolation increases your risk.

From Little K: *Postgraduate Med* 108:135, 2000.

psychologists, social workers, and dentists underscores the need for educators to expand curricula on family violence and for students' clinical mentors to model effective ways to screen for and respond to indicators of family violence.

Do you think it should be mandatory to report cases of domestic violence? Why or why not? ■

■ SPECIAL POPULATIONS
Child Abuse

The earliest form of family violence recognized in the health professional literature was physical abuse to children. Although violence to children was identified as a social problem in the nineteenth century, it was not until the 1940s that it became a medical problem, even a unique "syndrome." By the end of the 1960s, every state had enacted legislation mandating the report of suspected child abuse and neglect.

There are many forms of child abuse, including physical abuse or battering, emotional abuse, sexual abuse, and neglect. Children who witness family violence and abuse are themselves victimized. Although they are often overlooked, they can be affected in myriad ways as a result of this abuse (Box 39-4). Much is still unknown about the causes, treatment, or prevention of child abuse. In addition, research has failed to identify any factors that are present in all abusing and absent in all nonabusing parents.

BOX **39-4**
Effects of Witnessing Violence in Childhood

Infant
Disrupted attachment
Disrupted routines (sleeping, eating)
Risk of physical injury
Eating and sleeping problems in 50%
Decreased responsiveness to adults, increased crying

Preschool
Feeling that world is not safe or stable
Yelling, irritability, hiding, stuttering; signs of terror
Many somatic complaints and regressive behaviors
Anxious attachment behaviors: whining, crying, clinging
Increased separation and stranger anxiety
Insomnia, sleepwalking, nightmares, bed-wetting

School-Age
Greater willingness to use violence
Holding self responsible for violence at home
Shame and embarrassment of the family secret
Distracted and inattentive, labile, and hypervigilant
Limited range of emotional responses
Psychosomatic complaints
Uncooperative, suspicious, guarded behavior

Adolescent
Feelings of rage, shame, betrayal
School truancy, early sexual activity, substance abuse, delinquency
Unresponsiveness
Little memory of childhood
Defensiveness
Short attention

Sexual Abuse of Children and Adolescents. Sexual abuse is the involvement of children and adolescents in sexual activities they do not fully comprehend and to which they do not, or cannot, freely consent because of physical, cognitive, and psychological immaturity. When this occurs within families, the perpetrator is a relative or surrogate relative who exploits the child for his or her sexual gratification. Sexual assault of children and adolescents by nonfamily members is discussed later in this chapter.

Sexual abuse within families violates a child's trust in an adult who is supposed to love and protect them. Threats of harm to the child or to other family members, pets, or cherished possessions and threats of humiliation effectively keep the child from disclosing the abusive experiences to others. Subsequent feelings of confusion, helplessness, and shame can profoundly affect a child's mental health, both at the time and for the rest of his or her life. As an adult, sexual problems, difficulty trusting others, and the development of depression and anxiety disorders may, in fact, be rooted in the earlier trauma of sexual abuse.

Although sexual abuse within families is usually a well-guarded secret, which is never openly disclosed, nurses may observe behavioral signals from the child that may be indicative of past or current sexual abuse from a family member.

Observable signs of sexual abuse include sexual acting-out, physical aggression, excessive masturbation, social withdrawal, expressions of low self-esteem, impaired school performance, and disturbed sleep. Children also may develop a variety of physical problems related to sexual abuse including sexually transmitted infections; bleeding, soreness, or itching in or around the genitals, perineum, or rectal area; recurrent urinary tract infections; chronic pain syndromes; or unintended pregnancy.

School Violence. Violence in American schools has been highlighted in the media recently, but it is not a new phenomenon. Abuse and violence, including homicide, have long occurred in urban schools, often involving adolescents of color with few resources and usually based on an interpersonal dispute and a single victim. School violence received little public attention until the 1997-1998 school year in which massacres by means of firearms were committed by middle-class, white adolescents from small towns and suburbs who had no prior criminal record (Garbarino, 2001).

In spite of these large scale tragedies, school-associated homicides remain rare. School is, in general, a much safer environment for children and adolescents than their neighborhoods and family homes. A variety of risk factors for school violence have been identified. The most explanatory factors seem to be drug use, carrying a weapon, antisocial and impulsive behavior, and family and community disorganization and unresponsiveness (Strawhacker, 2002).

According to a 2001 national survey, bullying, verbal harassment, and intimidation are pervasive behaviors that students experience in middle school and high school. The same survey found that 6% of high school students (10% of male students) said they had carried a weapon to school in the last month; nearly 7% of the students had missed at least 1 day of school in the last month because they felt unsafe at school or unsafe traveling to or from school (Kaufman et al, 2002).

Identify two ways in which school nurses can intervene to help prevent school violence. ■

Abduction of Children. The vast majority of cases of child abduction involve a family member, usually a parent, taking or keeping the child in violation of a custody order or other legitimate custodial right. Cases in which a child or adolescent is kidnapped by a stranger or slight acquaintance remain relatively rare, with an estimated 115 cases in the United States in 1999 (Finkelhor, Hammer, and Sedlak, 2002).

A survey of family abductions found that children under age 6 were particularly vulnerable to abduction, and abduction was more likely to occur in families in which the child did not live with both parents. The majority of children abducted by a family member were abducted by their biological father; 25% were abducted by their biological mother (Finkelhor, Hammer, and Sedlak, 2002).

In a series of studies in the San Francisco area, researchers developed profiles of parents at risk for abducting their children. Key characteristics of parents at risk for abducting their children include parents who (a) have made a prior threat of or actual abduction; (b) suspect that the other parent is abusing, molesting, or neglecting the child and feels that authorities have not investigated adequately; (c) are paranoid and markedly irrational, believing that they have been betrayed by their former partner and they therefore must protect themselves and the child; (d) are sociopathic and use the child as an instrument of revenge or punishment or as a trophy in their fight with the former partner; or (e) are from another country and want the child to be raised in the home country of origin (Johnston et al, 2001).

Nursing Assessment. Nursing assessment of actual or potential child abuse begins with a thorough history and physical examination. Gathering a history of child abuse can be a stressful experience for both the nurse and the family. It is essential for the nurse to examine personal values and past experiences to maintain a therapeutic and nonjudgmental clinical approach.

It is important to use an honest, open approach that does not punish or shame either the child or the parent. Most abusive parents are genuinely embarrassed about their behavior and would like help in developing alternative approaches to discipline. This knowledge can be used by the nurse to establish an environment that will facilitate honesty and sharing. The setting for the interview must be quiet, private, and uninterrupted.

In general, the child and the adults should be separated for the initial interview. However, deciding whether to do this decision depends on the child's age and other factors. The nurse should honestly state the purpose of the interview and the type of questions being asked, and describe the subsequent

physical examination. The approach must be calm and supportive because both the child and the family will be uneasy.

The interview with the parent can begin with a discussion of the problem that first brought the child to a health care facility. During this discussion the nurse should pay particular attention to the parent's understanding of the problem, discrepancies in the stories, and the parent's emotional responses. The interview can then be expanded to discussions of how the parent "disciplines" or spanks the child. Nurses should be alert to risk factors for child abduction such as ongoing divisive custody disputes between the child's parents. The initial interview is not the time to confront a suspected abuser directly because measures must be taken to document and report the abuse in a way that will ensure the child's safety.

Nursing Interventions. When child abuse is suspected, the nurse must report it to protective services. An investigation by the state protective service agency is legally mandated and also reinforces to the family the seriousness of the problem. When protective services are involved, the nurse should explain to the family precisely what will happen in an investigation and the amount of time involved. The nurse should maintain frequent contact with the assigned worker to ensure a comprehensive, consistent approach.

Nurses who work with violent families need to know exactly how protective services in their community operate. Ongoing professional relationships with colleagues at the agency will enable the nurse to remain informed about policies and reporting protocols and ensure successful coordination and continuity. In cases of separated or divorced parents, all staff involved in the care of the child must be clear about custody and visitation arrangements for that child and about any restrictions placed on one or both parents' access to their child.

Intimate Partner Violence

The term *intimate partner violence* refers to a pattern of assaultive and coercive behaviors, including physical, sexual, and psychological abuse and violence, that adults or adolescents use against their intimate partners. *Intimate partnerships* include current or former dating, married, or cohabiting relationships of heterosexuals, lesbian women, or gay men. It is purposeful behavior, directed at achieving compliance from, or control over, the targeted person (Family Violence Prevention Fund, 2002). The violence is part of a system of coercive control that may also include financial coercion, threats against children and other family members, and destruction of property.

Abuse of female partners is the most widespread form of family violence (Box 39-5). One in three adult women experience at least one physical assault by a partner during adulthood. Sexual abuse, or marital rape, is part of the violence against female partners in almost half the cases. Although women do hit men, female violence is much more likely to be in self-defense. It seldom takes the intentional repeated, serious, and controlling form characteristic of abuse against female partners.

One of the most frightening realities of intimate partner violence is the potential for homicide of the victim or abuser, or for homicide-suicide in which the abuser kills his partner and sometimes kills their children and then commits suicide. The majority of female homicide victims in the United States are killed by a husband, lover, or ex-husband or ex-lover. The majority of these murders are preceded by extensive abuse.

There is evidence that **a woman is in most danger of homicide when she leaves her abusive partner or makes it clear to him that she is ending the relationship. Risk factors for this degree of danger include having a handgun in the house, a history of suicide threats or attempts in either partner, battering during pregnancy, sexual abuse, substance abuse, and extreme jealousy and controlling behavior.** A frequent statement made by potentially lethal abusers is, "If I can't have you, no one can."

Some women kill their abusive partners, usually after repeated and extensive abuse and after repeated inadequate responses from police and other helpers. Interestingly, the number of women who kill their abusers has decreased significantly as the availability of community-based domestic violence programs and effective law enforcement responses have increased.

Do you endorse the "battered woman" legal defense? ■

Nursing Assessment. The most prevalent cause of trauma in women treated in emergency rooms is abuse by an intimate partner. It is also a common cause of female visits to mental health treatment centers. Thus a nursing assessment for all forms of violence is critical. **Assessment for intimate partner violence should be mandatory in mental health settings, as well as in emergency rooms, prenatal settings, and primary care facilities** (Poirier, 2000).

When no injuries are obvious, assessment for abuse is best included with the history about the patient's primary intimate attachment relationship. Answers to general questions on the quality of that relationship should be assessed for feelings of being controlled or needing to control. A relationship characterized by excessive jealousy (of possessions, children, jobs, friends, and other family members, as well as potential sexual partners) is more likely to be violent.

The patient can be asked about how the couple solves conflicts; one partner needing to have the final say or frequent and forceful verbal aggression also can be considered risk factors. Finally, the patient should be asked whether arguments ever involve "pushing or shoving." Questions about minor violence within a couple relationship help to normalize the woman's experience and to lessen the stigma of disclosure. If the patient hesitates, looks away, displays other uncomfortable nonverbal behavior, or reveals risk factors for abuse, she or he can be asked again later in the interview about physical violence.

BOX 39-5

Fact Sheet on Domestic Violence (DV)

- 31% of American women report being physically or sexually abused by a husband or boyfriend at some point in their lives.
- 30% of Americans say they know a woman who has been physically abused by her husband or boyfriend in the past year.
- Although women are less likely than men to be victims of violent crimes overall, women are 5 to 8 times more likely than men to be victimized by an intimate partner.
- 37% of all women who sought care in hospital emergency departments for violence-related injuries were injured by a current or former spouse, boyfriend, or girlfriend.
- DV leads to long-term health problems including arthritis, chronic neck or back pain, migraine and other frequent headaches, stammering, visual and hearing loss, sexually transmitted diseases, chronic pelvic pain, stomach ulcers, spastic colon, and frequent indigestion, diarrhea, or constipation.
- Emotional health effects: 56% of women in DV relationships are diagnosed with a psychiatric disorder; 29% of all women who attempt suicide are battered; 37% of battered women are depressed; 46% have anxiety disorders; and 45% experience post traumatic stress disorder.
- 92% of women who were battered did not discuss these incidents with their physicians; 57% did not discuss this with anyone.
- 70% to 81% of patients report that they would like their health care providers to ask them privately about intimate partner violence.

If abuse is revealed, the nurse's first response is critical. It is important that an abused woman realize that she is not alone; important affirmation can be given with a statement about the frequency of abuse. The extent and types of the abuse must be identified and described in the record. Careful documentation using a body map identifying the locations of bruises, contusions, or cuts is necessary for potential legal actions, which are often child custody suits as well as criminal actions related to the violence.

The woman's responses to the violence are a critical area for mental health assessment. It is important to interpret these responses to the woman as normal within the circumstances. Signs of posttraumatic stress disorder, depression, and low self-esteem must be assessed and recorded. Attribution regarding the abuse is also important. The nurse must carefully assess the woman's beliefs regarding the abuse and responsibility for the abuse. Because many abusive male partners find an excuse for the violence, the woman may be unnecessarily accepting the blame for his actions.

If the patient is an abuser, mental state is also important, and the potential for further violence must be assessed carefully. The safety of the abused partner is a concern, as is treatment for the abuser. Consultation with legal advisors about the nurse's duty to warn may be needed (see Chapter 10).

Nursing Interventions. Most communities have treatment programs for abusive men. They have been found to be most effective when the court has ordered treatment, with punishment for noncompliance. Severely abusive men seldom admit they have a problem and often need to be mandated to enter and remain in treatment. The nurse needs to confront the violence and clarify that the responsibility lies with the abuser. A combination of strategies may be needed to get the abuser into treatment if he is not involved with the court.

The type of referral chosen is extremely important. Long-lasting change is more likely if the treatment combines behavioral therapy centered on anger control along with a program designed to change attitudes toward women. Traditional marriage therapy or couple counseling as the only treatment is potentially dangerous to the woman because of the unequal power in the relationship and the possibility of retaliatory violence.

Several themes expressed by women who have been in abusive relationships with men have been identified (Hall, 2003; Smith, 2003). These themes, outlined in Box 39-6, can help the nurse in assessing and intervening with women who have been in abusive relationships.

To empower an abused woman, one must first make sure she has accurate information on which to base her difficult decisions. This includes knowledge of the related state and local laws and ordinances. She also needs to be aware of community resources such as domestic violence programs that provide ad-

vice, support, group participation, and if needed immediately or in the future, safe shelter for herself and her children.

Mutual goal setting is particularly important when working with abused women. Nurses can be frustrated if they impose their goals on the women, who may not be ready for drastic action. Ideally they will have an established relationship during which the nurse and patient can work through the normal denial and minimization that takes place when the primary attachment relationship is threatened.

The nurse and patient can then consider all the options the woman has thought about and devise others. Dealing with an abusive situation is a recovery process that takes time and ongoing support. The nurse can help the patient mobilize natural, social, and professional support so that both her economic and emotional needs are addressed.

Evaluation of nursing interventions is based on mutual goals, not on a preconceived notion of what a battered woman should do. Because most abused women eventually leave a seriously violent situation or end the violence in some other way and seek help when the violence becomes severe, the nurse can be optimistic about the eventual outcome. Interventions may not result in an immediately happy ending, but they can plant the seeds of empowerment that facilitate the woman's recovery process.

Elder Abuse

Estimates of the numbers of older Americans who are abused, neglected, or exploited vary widely because the problem is underreported. The U.S. Senate Special Committee on Ag-

---

BOX **39-6**

Themes of Women Who Have Been in Abusive Relationships

Themes of Dysfunction While in the Relationship

- **Lack of relational authenticity:** The women never felt emotionally real, never established relationships with themselves as individuals, and were uncertain about their own identities. This increased their perceived threat of rejection and their efforts to please the abuser in order to maintain the relationship. Leaving the abusive relationship was seen as a threat to one's personal identity.
- **Immobility:** Abuse permeated every aspect of the life of women in the study. Living in constant fear for their own well-being and that of their children created an appearance to outsiders that they were scattered, incapable, and indecisive. This fear created a barrier to others that increased their sense of isolation and decreased their ability to seek help.
- **Emptiness:** These women experienced multiple losses in their lives, including problems maintaining relationships with others, self-esteem, pride, a sense of control, and a sense of accomplishment. They eventually escaped the pain of abuse by having no feelings, not thinking, just constantly "doing" an intense schedule of the routines of daily living. This created a numbing effect that allowed them to continue to the next day.
- **Disconnection:** The women's sense of sexuality was adversely affected. They equated sex with love, so being sexually active was the only way they felt connected to another person.

They lacked support from extended family members, who disapproved of the relationship. The abuse created physical illnesses because of the stress of the relationship. Many had indirect self-destructive behaviors (such as alcoholism and eating disorders), and some had suicidal or homicidal ideation as a means of escaping the abuse.

Themes of Healing While Recovering

- **Flexibility:** Women reported a readiness to alter the course of their lives in response to changing conditions and the acquiring of new behaviors. This included an acknowledgment of the past, resiliency with everyday events, increased self-awareness, and establishment of appropriate boundaries.
- **Awakening:** A turning point occurred within each woman when she realized there were choices and meaning in her life. This resulted in a sense of inner strength, hope, spirituality, and inner peace.
- **Relationship:** Women described an integration of all aspects of self, a sense of trust and connectedness between self and others, a feeling of harmony and contentment, and a linkage between internal and external events.
- **Empowerment:** Women related a new ability to make choices in their lives, which resulted in a valuing of the self, self-determination, and a sense of accomplishment.

ing estimates that there may be as many as five million victims each year. Older adults are primarily abused, neglected, or exploited by their caregivers, most of whom are spouses, adult children, or other family members.

Because much of the abuse is committed by spouses, spouse abuse and elder abuse are often overlapping categories. Older persons who are socially isolated, cognitively impaired, or dependent on others for daily personal needs seem to be most vulnerable to abuse and neglect. Social isolation also puts an older person at risk for financial exploitation by a family member or by scams perpetrated by nonfamily members (Quinn, 2002; Shugarman et al, 2003). Characteristics of the abuser, such as having mental and emotional problems including substance abuse, create a family situation at risk for elder abuse.

Nursing Assessment. It is important to assess for elder abuse in families where an emotionally ill person is financially dependent on aging parents. Family interviews should not focus exclusively on the patient but should also assess the interactions among family members for indications of verbal and physical aggression.

It is difficult for abused elders to admit being physically hurt by an adult child, spouse, or caregiver. Gentle inquiry about the family's usual approach to resolving interpersonal difficulties is useful. At least part of this assessment must take place with the elder alone. An elder may be reluctant to disclose abuse because of fear of being abandoned to a nursing home or a life of total isolation. Only by establishing a trusting relationship over time or using an already established relationship with someone else can the nurse completely explore the abusive situation.

Assessment is even more difficult when the elder is mentally or emotionally impaired. In those cases, physical assessment and careful attention to nonverbal behavior are critical. Bruises to the upper arms from shaking are especially common in elder abuse. Although bruises from abuse are difficult to differentiate from those normally seen in aging, bilateral upper outer arm bruises are definitive. Bruises from being tied into a chair or bed may be found on the wrists or ankles. Lacerations, especially to the face, are not usually caused by falls and should be regarded with suspicion. Vaginal lacerations or bruises and twisting bone fractures are particularly indicative of abuse.

Signs of neglect are more common than those of physical abuse. Neglect may be manifested by poor hygiene, breakdown of the skin, malnutrition, dehydration, or underdosing or overdosing of prescriptive medications. Determining whether the neglect is intentional is the key to planning a nursing course of action.

Whenever a dependent elderly person is being cared for by another, their interaction will give important clues about the relationship. Flinching or shrinking away by the elder and rough physical treatment accompanied by verbal denigration by the caretaker are possible indicators of abuse. As with all types of family violence, the nurse needs to analyze the data from the history, physical examination, and direct observations to make an assessment of abuse.

The decision to report is difficult, especially if it appears likely that the outcome will be a nursing home placement unwanted by the elder. However, most states have laws that require nurses to report suspected elder abuse.

You are providing home care services to an elderly person who shows evidence of physical abuse. The patient's caregiver handles her roughly and is impatient with her. The patient denies that she is unhappy or abused. Describe your response to this situation. What is your obligation to report your suspicions? ∎

Nursing Interventions. When the nurse must report elder abuse, it is usually less damaging to the therapeutic relationship to inform the family first. Deciding whether to discuss reporting beforehand is influenced by the likelihood of the abusing family member disappearing and the severity of the abuse.

If the abuse is less severe or mainly a neglectful or caretaker stress situation, discussing the intent to report first makes the action seem less a condemnation, allows protective services to be perceived as a helping agency rather than a punitive one, and increases the chances that the nurse will be seen as a continuing source of help. Respite care or other stress relievers may be the key interventions for an overburdened caretaker.

In other cases the primary intervention may be therapeutic assistance for the abusers. This may include counseling, therapy for mental disorders, or substance abuse treatment. The success of various interventions for elder abuse is not yet known because research into this issue is scant. However, one should assume that the treatment will need to involve specific components aimed at the violence as well as at whatever other problems are involved.

∎ RAPE AND SEXUAL ASSAULT

Rape and sexual assault are concerns for individuals, families, and the community. Sexual assaults against women and children (the most common survivors) result in physical trauma, psychic and spiritual disruptions, and deterioration of social relationships. In addition, fear of rape and sexual assault has major effects on women because as a result they restrict their activities in attempts to ensure their safety.

Survivors of sexual assaults include women and men of all ages, social classes, races, and occupations. Sexual assault disrupts every aspect of the survivor's life, including social activities, interpersonal relationships, employment, and career.

How would you respond to a roommate who returned from a date tearful and saying that her boyfriend forced her to have sex even though she refused? Would it make any difference if she had been sexually active with him in the past? Why or why not? ∎

Definition of Sexual Assault

Sexual assault is the forced perpetration of an act of sexual contact with another person without consent. Lack of consent could be related to the victim's cognitive or personality development, feelings of fear or coercion, or the offender's physical or verbal threats. **Sexual assault is not a sexual act** but is instead motivated by a desire to humiliate, defile, and dominate the victim. It has occurred for centuries but is now recognized as a social and public health problem.

A sexual assault occurs once every 6.4 minutes in the United States. One in every six women will be raped in her lifetime. Although a woman is 4 times more likely to be assaulted by someone she knows than by someone she does not know, the majority of these crimes go unreported even though rape is a felony.

Sexual consent can be thought of as a continuum, as seen in Box 39-7. This continuum demonstrates degrees of coercion, including bribery, taking advantage of one's position of power or trust in a relationship, or the victim's inability to consent freely.

Marital Rape

Marital rape is legally recognized in most states and is often reported along with physical abuse. Many husbands of abused women believe it is their right to have sex whenever they want. Victims of marital rape describe forced vaginal intercourse; anal intercourse; being hit, burned, or kicked during sex; having objects inserted into their vagina and anus and other degradations while being threatened with weapons or beaten if they refuse to take part in these activities.

Marital rape is especially devastating for the survivor who often must continue to interact with the rapist because of her dependence on him. In addition, many survivors do not seek health care or the support of family members or friends because of embarrassment or humiliation.

Nursing Care of the Sexual Assault Survivor

Nursing Assessment. The initial assessment is an important phase of the treatment of rape and sexual assault survivors. Although most nurses would quickly recognize the woman brought to the emergency department by the police after an attack by a stranger, many survivors of sexual assault are not so easily identified. Therefore, **all nursing assessments must include questions to determine current or past sexual abuse.**

Because people have different definitions of rape, the assessment question must be broadly stated, such as "Has anyone ever forced you into sex that you did not wish to participate in?" This question may uncover other types of sexual trauma such as incest, date rape, or childhood sexual abuse. If the answer is yes, it can be gently followed with broad questions, such as "Can you tell me more about it?" or "How often has it happened?"

Often the response may be hesitation, questioning, or an embarrassed laugh. When this occurs, the nurse can increase the patient's comfort by explaining that the question is routine because sexual assault is common.

Nursing Interventions. When it is determined that abuse has occurred, it cannot be ignored. Disclosing sexual abuse is an indication of trust. If nurses immediately refer the patient elsewhere, they communicate that the problem is too distasteful or delicate to handle or that there are serious psychological implications. Therefore, **an immediate response of nonjudgmental listening and psychological support is essential.**

In addition, if a recent attack is disclosed, **physical evidence** will be needed if the victim chooses to take legal action against the perpetrator. Evidence collection is an appropriate nursing responsibility and requires special training. Later interventions may include referrals to survivors' groups, shelters for battered women, or legal services. The organizations listed in Box 39-8 may be useful when helping survivors of abuse and violence organize their resources.

People respond to sexual assault differently depending on their past experiences, personal characteristics, and the

---

BOX 39-7

Sexual Behavior: the Force Continuum

1. **Freely consenting.** Partners with equal power mutually choosing sexual activity. Equal power means each partner has equal status, knowledge, and ability to consent. This includes one partner agreeing to engage in sexual activity, even if not aroused, as an expression of love and caring for the other person.
2. **Economic partnership.** One person agrees to sexual activity as part of an economic agreement. The types of sexual behavior permitted are mutually determined as part of the economic agreement.
3. **Seduction.** One party attempts to persuade the other to engage in sexual activities.
4. **Psychic rape.** Assault to another person's dignity and self-respect, such as verbal abuse, street harassment, or the portrayal of violence or pornography in the media.
5. **Bribery or coercion.** The use of emotional or psychological force to persuade the other to take part in sexual activities. This includes situations of unequal power, especially when one person is in a position of authority.
6. **Acquaintance rape.** Sexual assault occurring when one party abuses the trust of a relationship and forces the other into sexual activities.
7. **Fear rape.** When one party engages in sexual activities out of fear of potential violence if she resists.
8. **Violent rape.** When violence is threatened or occurs. This includes forced sexual activity between spouses, acquaintances, or strangers.

BOX 39-8

Hotline Numbers for Survivors of Abuse Violence

National Center for Victims of Crime
1-800-FYI CALL (394-2255)
Provides immediate referrals to the closest, most appropriate services in the victim's community (includes sexual assault)

National Domestic Violence Hotline
1-800-799-7233 (TDD: 1-800-787-3224)
Provides crisis intervention, information, and referrals

National Organization for Victim Assistance (NOVA)
1-800-TRY-NOVA (879-6682)
Provides advocacy, information, and referrals for crime victims (including sexual assault)

amount and type of support received from significant others, health care providers, and the criminal justice system. **The acute stage, immediately after the attack, is characterized by extreme confusion, fear, disorganization, and restlessness.** However, some survivors may mask these feelings and appear to be outwardly calm or subdued.

The second phase involves the long-term process of reorganization. It generally begins several weeks after the attack. This phase may include intrusive memories of the traumatic event during the day and while asleep, fears, or phobias such as extreme fears of being alone, being in a crowd, or traveling. Survivors often have a sense of living in a dangerous, unpredictable world and may become preoccupied with feelings of victimization and vulnerability. They may encounter difficulties in sexual relationships or in their ability to relate comfortably to persons of the same sex as the perpetrator. Some survivors develop secondary phobic reactions to people, places, or situations that remind them of the attack.

> *How do you think the woman's movement and feminist thinking have influenced society's views on family violence? On rape and sexual assault? On pornography?* ■

Coping strategies may include changing one's phone number or residence, talking with friends or family, or taking classes in self-defense. Nursing actions to help the survivor of sexual assault include active listening, empathic responses, active concern and caring, assistance in problem solving, and referral to sexual assault crisis centers. Table 39-3 presents a sample Nursing Treatment Plan Summary for survivors of sexual assault.

Table 39-3	**NURSING TREATMENT PLAN SUMMARY**	Survivors of Abuse and Violence

Nursing Diagnosis: Rape-trauma syndrome
Expected Outcome: The patient will resume his or her usual lifestyle and social relationships.

SHORT-TERM GOAL	INTERVENTION	RATIONALE
The patient will express feelings related to the assault, including guilt, fear, and vulnerability.	Allow patient to discuss feelings regarding assault. Communicate knowledge and understanding of emotional responses to sexual assault to help in identification of feelings. Provide anticipatory guidance regarding common physical, psychological, and social responses.	Women often experience various feelings, including guilt, shame, anger, and embarrassment. It is necessary to identify and express these feelings to develop coping skills. Knowing what to expect reassures the patient that her reactions are normal and can be managed.
The patient will identify supportive people to help in dealing with this crisis.	Explore relationships with significant others. Encourage the patient to discuss the situation with trusted and supportive people.	According to the principles of crisis intervention, it is important for the person in crisis to identify and use a social support system.
The patient will seek medical care for physical problems related to the assault.	Advise patient of the potential for sexually transmitted diseases or pregnancy. Help in identifying a medical care provider. Offer to accompany to the medical examination.	Early identification of physical problems provides the patient with the maximum number of treatment choices. Many women relive the assault during a gynecological examination. Support from a trusted person can be helpful.
The patient will be actively involved in mobilizing systems.	Support decision making and active problem solving. Provide written information about community services and encourage use of them. Plan for a follow-up phone contact within a few days.	Active involvement in seeking resources gives the patient a sense of control over life, counteracting the helplessness related to the assault.

COMPETENT CARING **A Clinical Exemplar of a Psychiatric Nurse**
PAT ENGDAHL, RN, C

When thinking about how I may have made a difference in a patient's life, I remembered an experience I had with a young woman just over 30 years of age who was admitted to the unit in a state of extreme panic, hardly able to process a simple request such as "I need you to please move away from the door." She told me this later, saying her first memories of being on our floor included a voice saying the above words "in the kindest, firmest, most caring tones" she had ever heard—and she felt safe. She said she didn't want to move away from the locked door, but she did it anyway and she said, "I think it was your voice."

We worked very hard together. She was a survivor of childhood sexual and physical abuse and, as often happens, married a man who also abused her. She talked; I listened. She said she had shed enough tears and wasn't going to cry anymore. I replied she needed to "cry a river" for the therapeutic process to begin. We role-played. We practiced handling verbal abuse and daring to express anger—the latter frightened her more than the former. But she was

Continued

not able to deal with issues related to her abusive husband and her angry feelings of being victimized in the marriage.

The night before her discharge she began to discuss these feelings, as they had suddenly risen to the surface during a group meeting. In this meeting a male patient had boasted that he never struck his wife except when he was drunk, and then he "only slapped her around a few times, not enough to send her to the hospital or such—nothing like that." When my patient heard this, she got up in a rage and ran out of the group. Several hours later, during our one-on-one, she was finally able to discuss the episode. She berated herself for being "gutless" and not being able to say something right

then. She paced and questioned whether she really was ready to go home and said that maybe she wasn't as strong as she thought.

We continued exploring her feelings of childhood helplessness. She talked until her rage was spent, but she did not seem to reach closure in her thoughts or feelings. She was discharged the next morning before I came to work for my evening shift. However, in my mailbox, I found a powerful note in which, among other things, she simply wrote, "I was able to confront that male patient in group today. . . . I guess I was ready for discharge after all. Thanks." It was now my turn to become a little emotional as my eyes filled with tears and I whispered, "You're welcome, you'll never know how welcome." ■

CHAPTER **FOCUS POINTS**

- Family violence refers to a range of behaviors occurring between family members and includes physical and emotional abuse of children, child neglect, intimate partner violence, marital rape, and elder abuse. Characteristics of violent families include multigenerational transmission, social isolation, abuse of power, and substance abuse.
- Many nurses have a negative response to survivors of violence. It is important to identify and overcome these attitudes.
- Physical responses to family violence include a characteristic pattern of injuries and the occurrence of a variety of stress-related symptoms.
- Behavioral responses to family violence include reluctance to leave the violent situation.

- Psychological responses to violence include attributions, problem-solving techniques, and depression.
- Nursing actions related to the prevention of family violence include strategies to change norms and values, preventive education, identification of families and individuals at high risk for abuse and violence, and early detection of family violence for timely and appropriate interventions.
- Nursing interventions can be focused on special populations including children, intimate partners, and the elderly.
- Nursing care of survivors of sexual assault include nonjudgmental listening, psychological support, evidence collection, and mobilization of community support such as rape response programs, domestic violence programs, and legal services.

◄ KEY TERMS

attributions, 803
child abuse, 807
elder abuse, 811

family violence, 798
multigenerational transmission, 799

sexual abuse, 807
sexual assault, 811

■ CHAPTER REVIEW QUESTIONS

1. Match each term in Column A with the correct definition in Column B.

Column A

_____ Attributions
_____ Sexual assault
_____ Multigenerational transmission
_____ Myth about abuse
_____ Paternalistic model of health care
_____ Psychological abuse
_____ The force continuum
_____ Intimate partner violence
_____ Just world view
_____ Primary prevention

Column B

A. Family violence is often perpetuated from grandparents, to parents, to children.
B. Others generally get what they deserve in life.
C. Advice and sympathy are given rather than respect for a patient's competence and experience.
D. Reasoning processes people use to explain why certain events happen.
E. An intervention that stops an action before it occurs.
F. A view of sexual behavior that ranges from free consent to violent rape.
G. The victim can learn to stop doing things that provoke the violence.
H. A pattern of coercive and assaultive behaviors toward a partner in an ongoing intimate relationship.
I. Forced act of sexual contact with another person without consent.
J. Instilling fear or isolating victim from family, friends, school, or work.

2. Indicate whether the following statements are true (T) or false (F).

_____ A. Many nurses have a negative response to survivors of violence.
_____ B. Children who only witness family violence are usually safe from its effects.
_____ C. Family violence is most prevalent among families living in poverty.
_____ D. Witnessing parental violence during childhood or adolescence is one of the strongest risk factors for becoming an abuser in adulthood.
_____ E. Abusive people and their victims often excuse the abuse by blaming alcohol, stress, or drugs.

3. Provide short answers for the following questions.

A. Briefly describe the four characteristics of violent families.
B. Compare the paternalistic model with the empowerment model used by nurses to help battered women.
C. Each culture and society has a different attitude toward and tolerance of violence. Compare the United States with another country in this regard.

Visit Evolve for additional resources related to the content of this chapter.
http://evolve.elsevier.com/Stuart/principles/
• Topical Course Outline • Student Workbook Exercises • Critical Thinking Questions and Activities • Case Studies • Research Topics
• Monthly Content Updates • WebLinks

Student Study CD-ROM

Access the accompanying CD-ROM for animations, interactive exercises, review questions for the NCLEX examination, and an audio glossary.

REFERENCES

Banks JB: Childhood discipline: challenges for clinicians and parents, *Am Fam Physician* 66:1447, 2002.

Dienemann J et al: Intimate partner abuse among women diagnosed with depression, *Issues Ment Health Nurs* 21:499, 2000.

Edwards VJ et al: Relationship between multiple forms of childhood maltreatment and adult mental health in community respondents, *Am J Psychiatry* 160:1453, 2003.

Ehrensaft MK et al: Intergenerational transmission of partner violence: a 20-year prospective study, *J Consul Clin Psychol* 71:741, 2003.

Family Violence Prevention Fund: *National consensus guidelines on identifying and responding to domestic violence victimization in health care settings*, San Francisco, 2002, FVPF.

Finkelhor D, Hammer H, Sedlak AJ: *Nonfamily abducted children: National estimates and characteristics*, Washington, DC, 2002, US Department of Justice, Office of Justice Programs, Office of Juvenile Justice and Delinquency Prevention.

Garbarino J: Making sense of school violence: Why do kids kill? In Shafii M, Shafii SL, editors: *School violence: assessment, management, and prevention*, Washington, DC, 2001, American Psychiatric Publishing.

Gilligan C: *In a different voice*, Cambridge, Mass, 1982, Harvard University Press.

Hall JM: Positive self-transitions in women child abuse survivors, *Issues Ment Health Nurs* 24:647, 2003.

Hotaling GT, Sugarman DB: An analysis of risk markers in husband to wife violence: the current state of knowledge, *Violence Vict* 1:101, 1986.

Humphreys J: Resilience in sheltered battered women, *Issues Ment Health Nurs* 24:137, 2003.

Johnston JR et al: *Early identification of risk factors for parental abduction*, Washington, DC, 2001, Department of Justice, Office of Justice Programs, Office of Juvenile Justice and Delinquency Prevention.

Kendler KS et al: Childhood sexual abuse and adult psychiatric and substance use disorders in women, *Arch Gen Psychiatry* 57:953, 2000.

Kaufman, P et al: *Indicators of school crime and safety: 2001*, Washington, DC, 2002, US Departments of Education and Justice.

Lawson L: Isolation, gratification, justification: offenders' explanations of child molesting, *Issues Ment Health Nurs* 24:695, 2003.

May B et al: Are abused women mentally ill? *J Psychosoc Nurs* 41:21, 2003.

Morewitz S: *Stalking and violence: new patterns of trauma and obsession*, New York, 2003, Plenum Publishers.

Poirier N: Psychosocial characteristics discriminating between battered women and other women psychiatric inpatients, *J Am Psychiatr Nurs Assoc* 6:144, 2000.

Quinn MJ: Undue influence and elder abuse: recognition and intervention strategies, *Geriatric Nurs* 23:11, 2002.

Ray S: Male survivors' perspectives of incest/sexual abuse, *Perspect Psychiatr Care* 37:49, 2001.

Shugarman LR et al: Identifying older people at risk of abuse during routine screening practices, *J Am Geriatr Soc* 51:24, 2003.

Smith ME: Recovery from intimate partner violence: a difficult journey, *Issues Ment Health Nurs* 24:543, 2003.

Spitzberg B: Reclaiming control in stalking cases, *J Psychosoc Nurs* 41:38, 2003.

Strawhacker MT: School violence: an overview, *J School Nurs* 18:68, 2002.

Torres S, Han HR: Women's perceptions of their male batterers' characteristics and level of violence, *Issues Ment Health Nurs* 24:667, 2003.

U.S. Department of Health and Human Services (USDHHS): *Child maltreatment: reports from the states to the National Child Abuse and Neglect Data System*, Washington, DC, 2000, US Government Printing Office.

40

PSYCHOLOGICAL CARE OF PATIENTS WITH LIFE-THREATENING ILLNESS

Penelope Chase

LEARNING OBJECTIVES

After studying this chapter, the student should be able to:

1. Deliver effective and compassionate care to persons with a life-threatening illness (I).
2. Provide psychosocial and mental health care to patients who have life-threatening illness and their families (II).
3. Implement palliative care approaches for managing symptoms to promote a comfortable, dignified death (III).
4. Analyze issues related to transitioning patients and families to end-of-life care (IV).
5. Assist patients and families in preparing for death (V).
6. Become aware of one's personal responses to caring for persons who may not survive their illness (VI).

TOPICAL OUTLINE

I. Working With Patients and Families With Life-Threatening Diagnoses
   A. Time of Uncertainty
   B. Concerns of Patients and Family Members
II. Psychosocial and Mental Health Care
   A. Anxiety
   B. Depression
   C. Caregiver Stress, Anger, and Sleep Deprivation
III. Symptom Management and Palliative Care
   A. Pain
   B. Constipation and Diarrhea
   C. Nausea and Vomiting
   D. Hiccups and Other Troublesome Symptoms
IV. Transitioning to End-of-Life Care
   A. Advocating for the Patient
   B. The Changing Focus of Hope
   C. Making Decisions
   D. Withholding and Withdrawing Life-Sustaining Treatment
   E. Medically Ineffective Treatment
   F. Hospice
V. Preparing for Death
   A. Anticipatory Grieving
   B. The Dying Process
VI. Concerns of Nurses Working With Life-Threatening Illness
   A. Deaths of Infants and Children
   B. Identifying With the Patient or Family
   C. Medically Provided Nutrition and Hydration
   D. Professional Integrity

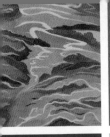 Visit Evolve for additional resources related to the content of this chapter.
http://evolve.elsevier.com/Stuart/principles/

The Latin origin of the word compassion means "to suffer with." Another definition is "the deep feeling of sharing the suffering of another, together with the inclination to give aid or support or to show mercy" (American Heritage Dictionary, 1991). Nurses working in many different settings may find themselves caring for a person with a life-threatening illness. Doing so with compassion is part of the art of nursing.

WORKING WITH PATIENTS AND FAMILIES WITH LIFE-THREATENING DIAGNOSES

Many illnesses or chronic diseases can threaten life. Box 40-1 lists some of the most common life-threatening illnesses. These illnesses affect all patient populations including neonatal, pediatric, young adult, adult, and elders.

Besides providing comfort, one of the most skillful and valued interventions a nurse can make while caring for

BOX 40-1

Common Life-Threatening Illnesses or Conditions

- Various types of cancer
- End-stage renal disease (ESRD)
- Congestive heart failure (CHF)
- End-stage cardiomyopathy (CM)
- End-stage liver disease (ESLD)
- Cerebral vascular accident (CVA)
- Hepatitis C
- Certain congenital anomalies in newborns or infants
- Severe burns or trauma
- Amyotrophic lateral sclerosis (ALS or Lou Gehrig's disease)
- Acquired immunodeficiency syndrome (AIDS)
- Alzheimer's disease
- Chronic obstructive pulmonary disease (COPD)
- Multiple sclerosis
- Parkinson's disease
- Severe asthma
- Complications of diabetes mellitus
- Scleroderma
- Persistent vegetative state (PVS)

CITING THE EVIDENCE ON

Patient Attitudes Toward Advance Directives

BACKGROUND: The purpose of this study was to explore hospitalized patients' attitudes toward advance directives, their reasons for completing or not completing advance directive forms, and demographic differences between patients who did and did not complete advance directive forms.

RESULTS: The overwhelming majority of participants had received information on advance directives, and they were moderately positive about them. The majority who had completed advance directives were white, female, over age 65, had less than a high school education, and perceived their health as poor. Most believed that an advance directive would ensure they received the treatment they desired at the end of life.

IMPLICATIONS: Patients' attitudes alone did not determine who will and who will not complete advance directives. Most participants who completed advance directives had specific reasons for doing so. Nurses have responsibility for discussing advance directives with patients, families, and physicians to ensure adequate education about their completion.

Douglas R, Brown H: *J Nurs Scholarsh* 34: 61, 2002.

these patients and families is the use of presence. Presence is a term used to describe the therapeutic, healing, respectful, watchful, and compassionate experience of being in relationship with another human being in a state of empathy and positive regard (Geller and Greenberg, 2002; Hines, 1992). It is an essential part of the therapeutic relationship (see Chapter 2). Presence is also described as 'being with' rather than 'doing to' (Frisch, 2001). The therapeutic use of presence involves centering, using intuition, openness, and active listening, and being at ease with silence (Du-Mont, 2003).

Time of Uncertainty

Between the development of symptoms and a definitive diagnosis, patients and their family members or loved ones have to endure a time of uncertainty. Uncertainty is anxiety producing. During this time the nurse should assess for any hopes, worries, fears, or anxieties a patient or family member may be experiencing, manifesting, or projecting. Often the best way to begin the intervention is to tell the person what behavior or emotion you are observing and give it a name (such as shock, disbelief, fear, or sadness). It is important to validate and seek the person's agreement with or refinement of this perception.

Nursing interventions should be designed to help patients separate issues and decisions over which they have control from those they cannot change or control. This is an appropriate time to ask about any advance directives the patient may have, such as a living will, health care power of attorney, preference about cardiopulmonary resuscitation (CPR), intubation for ventilatory support, or organ donation (see Citing the Evidence).

The nurse may suggest to patients that they discuss their wishes regarding life-sustaining treatment with their surrogate decision maker or someone close to them. This is very important, in the event that patients become unable to speak for themselves in the future. Instances when a health care surrogate may be called upon to make a treatment decision include when the patient is demented, experiencing delirium, in a coma, or is intubated on a ventilator or sedated (Scanlon, 2003).

Concentrating is often difficult while waiting for a diagnosis. Providing distraction sometimes helps alleviate anxiety while waiting. Some patients find a simple task such as working with a crossword puzzle book helps distract them from distressing and intrusive thoughts. Age-appropriate activities for seriously ill pediatric patients and their families should be identified. Many children's services have specialists and unique settings where play therapy or counseling is provided.

Have you or one of your family or friends experienced the "time of uncertainty," waiting for diagnostic test results? If so, what was helpful during this time? ■

Concerns of Patients and Family Members

If a diagnostic test or tumor biopsy is reported as normal or benign, patients and their family members usually experience relief. The nurse may experience elation along with the patient and family. At this point families may be open to education regarding healthy behaviors. They may now see the vital importance of making changes in unhealthy habits, such as quitting smoking, sticking to an exercise program, complying with medication regimes, or changing unhealthy eating patterns.

However, if the diagnosis shows pathology, patients and families immediately have concerns, whether or not they express them. Many patients are afraid that verbalization of these fears may upset family members and therefore avoid voicing them. Nurses should ask questions about hopes and fears. Acknowledging these concerns with patients and families helps normalize them, and in naming the fears they become less formidable and then can be addressed.

Concerns that patients frequently have include the following:

- How long do people with this illness usually live?
- Will I be able to pay for treatment and other financial obligations?
- How will my family and friends be emotionally affected or inconvenienced?
- Will I be a burden or become dependent on others?
- Will surgery leave me with disfigurement?
- Will I suffer pain as I have heard others have suffered?
- Will I die all alone?
- Is God punishing me with this illness?
- Why can't I be in control of what is happening to me?
- How can I die when I still have so much left to do in my life?

Patients and family members may project anger and helplessness onto nurses or the medical team, complaining about such things as poor care, lack of communication, delay in call bells being answered, and substandard food preparation or choices. Many patient and family complaints are valid. However, some complaints are maladaptive responses to the stressful situation.

It is important for nurses to acknowledge complaints and respond to them with patience and without defensiveness. There is so much that patients and those who care for them have no control over that family members tend to feel calmer, more satisfied, and more in control when problems they identify are attended to promptly and respectfully.

Ways in which the nurse can respond to patient or family concerns include the following:

- **Listen without interrupting or defending.** This allows the person to ventilate and feel a bit more in control. Ask yourself if there is anything you can do to resolve the situation. Be creative. Use your available resources.
- **Provide what is asked for, if possible**, such as asking a dietician to see the patient about food preferences, getting a broken room thermostat or television fixed, and so forth.
- **Explain the process of how you dispense medications** and suggest the patient allow as "normal" a certain amount of time between request and delivery before asking again.
- **Express genuine regret with the reality of the situation**, such as the need to remain fasting for still another test or procedure, despite hunger or thirst.
- **Use prn medications as ordered.** Teach patients what prn medications have been ordered for them and how to request them. Ask the treating team to write orders for symptom management as needed.

- **Make time to simply sit with the patient or family members.** Let them initiate conversation or speak of nonmedical matters. Patients often come to associate nurse visits to their bedside as always being task oriented and may welcome nontreatment-related presence. Plan this time into your busy schedule. You may discover something significant that could be used in care planning or care delivery that the patient thought was not relevant or important to the team. Active listening may uncover worries about a physical symptom, a death anniversary, a robbery or house fire, another family member who is ill, or a missed birthday or special event.

The nurse may ask patients open-ended questions to identify their support system and help the patient or family member cope with or clarify their immediate concerns.

Box 40-2 lists some sample questions that may help disclose concerns at the time of diagnosis. The nurse's language should be adapted to the developmental level, culture, spiritual beliefs, and educational level of the patient, and to the personal communication style of the nurse.

Patients often seek information about their illness from friends or relatives, books or magazines. Patients or family members also seek out information on medical conditions and treatments on the Internet. Nurses should direct their patients to reputable and accurate websites, such as the National Institutes of Health (http://www.nih.gov) or the National Cancer Institute (http://www.cancer.gov). Other reputable websites for patient families and nurses about various diseases and conditions are listed in the WebLinks for this chapter on the Evolve website. Many of these sites have information in Spanish or other languages.

A patient tells you he is confused by the many sites on the Internet with information about his illness. What guidelines would you give him on how to select and evaluate the quality of a website? ■

BOX 40-2

Questions To Ask at Time of Diagnosis

- What has the doctor told you about your/your child's illness?
- How can I help you understand what the doctors told you?
- What seems to be worrying you just now?
- How do you usually deal with stress?
- Do you have any religious beliefs that might help you now?
- Who do you usually talk with about how you're feeling?
- Would you like me to call a therapist, social worker, chaplain, or dietician to talk with you now?
- What is the best that you are hoping for?
- What is the worst that you are afraid of?
- Do you know someone who's been through something like this?
- What can I do for you right now to help ease your mind?
- Who can I contact to come visit you now or this weekend?

■ PSYCHOSOCIAL AND MENTAL HEALTH CARE

Patients being treated for life-threatening illness are often anxious, depressed, or angry. Nurses should be vigilant for these conditions and seek help or counseling for their patients. Treating the emotional responses that may accompany life-threatening illness helps to improve the patient's quality of life and provides comfort and relief to worried family members and nursing staff alike (see Critical Thinking About Contemporary Issues).

A psychiatric consultation liaison nurse can be very helpful in addressing the mental health needs of these patients. A psychiatric consultation liaison nurse (PCLN) is an advanced practice nurse who practices psychiatric and mental health nursing in a medical setting, providing consultation and education to patients, families, the health care team, and the community. A PCLN may provide assessment, recommendations, and/or supportive therapy to patients who are anxious, depressed, or experiencing other psychological problems or emotional distress (Chase et al, 2000).

Anxiety

The patient's symptoms of anxiety need not meet criteria for a formal psychiatric diagnosis in order to be treated. Pharmacological treatment with benzodiazepines is common practice and nurses should initiate requests for an order if the patient does not already have one. Clinical indicators of anxiety in the medically ill include expressions of fear or dread, persistent tachycardia or hypertension, hyperventilation, frightening dreams, difficulty sleeping, anorexia, or debilitating worry. If a family member appears overly anxious, the nurse may suggest he or she ask his or her primary care provider for a short-term prescription to help him or her cope with the stress.

Nonpharmacological interventions for anxiety reduction, such as soothing music, progressive muscle relaxation, and visualization exercises are readily available on compact disk (CD), video, or audiocassette. Nurses may suggest that visitors bring a radio, cassette, or CD player for individual patients if the facility does not provide them.

Sometimes patient education materials designed to inform and change mistaken beliefs can allay anxiety. At other times these materials may increase anxiety, thus the nurse should carefully assess the patient's needs and wishes. Some institutions have a list of former patients who are happy to meet with newly diagnosed patients to describe their coping experience.

Depression

Several of the salient symptoms of major depression are also symptoms of life-threatening illness. Medically ill people may experience fatigue, have trouble sleeping, lose their appetite, or find it difficult to concentrate (Paice, 2002).

A persistent myth proposes that if a person "has a reason" to be depressed, no treatment is needed because this "functional depression" is a "normal" response. However, this myth denies the patient needed and effective treatment. With the advent of selective serotonin reuptake inhibitors (SSRIs) and new classes of antidepressants with their favorable side effect profiles, clinicians have no valid reason to forego prescribing antidepressants for seriously ill patients.

If a patient's "prominent and persistent" depressed mood is believed to be related to the medical condition, antidepressant therapy is indicated. The *DSM-IV-TR* medical diagnosis would be **mood disorder due to general medical condition** (American Psychiatric Association, 2000). If patients show vegetative symptoms that interfere with self-care or if the able patient refuses to get out of bed or ignores meals, psychostimulants (such as methylphenidate or pemoline) may improve appetite and provide energy and motivation (Bowers and Boyle, 2003; Lenz, 2003). Patients who have had life-sustaining surgery that radically alters their physical appearance are especially prone to depression and lowered self-esteem and may have second thoughts about their choice to have future surgery.

The nurse who observes a patient who is frequently tearful, irritable, apathetic, has a depressed mood, is socially withdrawn, wants the room kept dark, expresses hopelessness, or refuses to participate in rehabilitation efforts such as physical therapy should suspect depression. If the individual is hospitalized, the nurse should request a psychiatric evaluation by a PCLN or psychiatrist. For an outpatient or long-term care facility resident, the nurse should make a referral to an available mental health provider.

The following questions are helpful in assessing a medically ill patient who appears depressed.

- How would you describe your mood these past few weeks?
- Are you feeling sad, "blue," "down," or depressed?
- Do you find yourself tearful or crying sometimes?

Critical Thinking *About* Contemporary Issues

What Is the Evidence Base for End-of-Life Care?

Providers of palliative and end-of-life care consider the psychological needs of patients and the provision of support and counseling to be an important part of their work. Yet very few outcome studies exist that have evaluated the usefulness of psychotherapy for palliative care patients (Spiess et al, 2002). Some work has been done that examined therapy for oncology patients with pain, and group therapy has been found to be helpful for patients with metastatic breast carcinoma. Cognitive-behavioral and relaxation techniques also have been shown to be effective. Life review, interpersonal therapy, and supportive therapy all appear to have a role in helping palliative care patients and their families.

A clear understanding of what patients, families, and health care practitioners view as important at the end of life is integral to the success of improving care of dying patients. Yet empirical evidence defining these factors also is lacking (Steinhauser et al, 2000). It is evident that more work is needed to provide better understanding of which patients can be helped and by which interventions in their end-of-life care. Studies also need to examine the factors considered to be important at the end of life by seriously ill patients, recently bereaved families, and health care providers.

- Do you ever feel you or others would be better off without you?
- If yes, how long have you felt this way?
- Have you ever thought of helping yourself to die?
- Are you feeling suicidal now?
- Have you been treated for depression in the past?
- Would you like some help to feel more like your old self?

In addition to pharmacotherapy, patients may find comfort with a visit from a minister, pastor, rabbi, imam, or priest if the patient uses faith to cope. Some patients may experience spiritual distress and have doubts, fears, or other concerns involving their religious faith, beliefs, or practice. Others may feel guilty for being angry with their God or believe their illness is punishment. Although the nurse may uncover these concerns, they are best addressed by a spiritual advisor.

Caregiver Stress, Anger, and Sleep Deprivation

Caregiver stress is the emotional and physical strain experienced by a person caring for someone with a chronic debilitating disease or life-threatening condition. Caregivers may become patients themselves, especially if they neglect meeting their own needs. Nurses should inquire whether caregivers are remembering to eat, rest, or take prescribed medications, and encourage them to take care of their own needs as part of caring for the person who is ill.

It is not unusual for caregivers to express feelings of anger. This is especially true for caregivers who have been used to being able to control circumstances in their occupations or professions. Those caregivers who have not developed the coping skills needed for situations in which they are powerless to change the process or outcome may exhibit behavior nurses sometimes label as "controlling." Family members tend to feel there should be something they can do to comfort or to heal their loved one. Skillful nurses offer choices whenever possible to lessen the patient's or family's feelings of powerlessness and helplessness and to help them feel more "in control."

Caregiver stress often manifests as criticism or complaints. It is helpful for nurses to recognize this and not take these grievances personally or react with defensiveness or controlling behavior in response to them. Patients or family members may react with anger when a diagnostic procedure is delayed or postponed, a second or third round of chemotherapy is not working, the patient's symptoms are troublesome despite attempts to allay them, or simply that the room floor has not been mopped that day.

Stress becomes magnified and unmanageable when the family member has sleep deprivation. Sleep deprivation is a state of physical and mental exhaustion brought on by lack of sleep in which the abilities to concentrate and reason are disturbed and judgment is diminished. Nursing strategies for helping patients and family members with stress, anger, and sleep deprivation are outlined in Box 40-3.

The spouse of your patient is constantly calling for nurses and complaining about how "no one is here to help." She threatens to report you to the State Board of Nursing. How might you best respond to her? ■

SYMPTOM MANAGEMENT AND PALLIATIVE CARE

When patients are undergoing treatment for cure and recovery, and when the goal of care changes to preserving dignity while dying, patients will experience symptoms that require management. Nurses have the opportunity and obligation to patients and their families to help ensure freedom from unnecessary suffering. Palliative care is the medical and nursing care that provides comfort to a moribund person without prolonging the dying process.

Pain

One of the symptoms most feared by patients and their families is unrelieved pain. Pain is the "fifth vital sign" and should be assessed regularly and managed appropriately as identified in Box 40-4 (JCAHO, 2003). Pain medicine can be administered by mouth, buccal or sublingual routes, intramuscular injection, via gastroscopy or jejunostomy tubes, intravenous transfusion, intrathecal or epidural infusion, rectal suppository, by dermal patch, and by patient-controlled anesthesia (PCA) pumps (Lenz, 2003). Intensive care units (ICUs) have laminated cards with pictures that an intubated patient

---

BOX 40-3

Helping Patients and Family Members Who Are Stressed, Angry, or Sleep Deprived

- Do not promise something that you may not be able to do. State what you intend to do and qualify why you may not be able to do it. Patients often perceive what you say through their filters of pain, fear, or anxiety, and misinterpret or misunderstand what they are told. They may translate messages into either what they wish to hear or are afraid they will hear. Ask them to repeat back to you what they have heard. You may need to repeat information several times.
- Set limits if the patient repeatedly puts on the call bell after you have just been in the room and asked before leaving if the patient had any other needs. State firmly a length of time when you will check on him or her (15 to 30 minutes) and keep to that schedule. For consistency, document your approach in the care plan.
- Although it is helpful if family members stay with the ill person to provide moral support, it may pose a problem to either the patient or the nurse. Many caregivers are afraid that if their loved one dies while they are not there, they will be somehow negligent or may be perceived as unloving. Empathize with the caregiver who may not have felt able to leave the hospital for days, but remind the person that she or he needs to get some sleep as well. Suggest to family members that they find a substitute caregiver for a night or weekend so that they can go to a motel or hotel or go home to sleep in their own bed or to take care of pets, plants, laundry, get a haircut, or pay bills. If the caregiver is reluctant to leave a critically ill patient but is beginning to decompensate emotionally, this may be a good time to ask the PCLN to intervene.

can point to and indicate whether he or she is experiencing pain or other symptoms.

The nurse needs to reassess the pain level after administering pain medication to check the effectiveness of the medication and ensure adequate dosing. Adult patients are asked to rate pain on a 1 to 10 scale, with 10 being the most excruciating pain.

Using the Wong-Baker FACES Pain Rating Scale, pediatric patients 3 years and older can be asked to choose the face that best describes their pain—from a smiley face to a tearful one (Figure 40-1). The Wong-Baker Scale instructions are available in translation in Spanish, French, Italian, Portuguese, Romanian, Bosnian, Vietnamese, Japanese, Chinese, and German.

Adjuvant analgesics may be given to augment opioid or nonsteroidal anti-inflammatory drugs (NSAIDs). Some commonly used adjuvant medications include tricyclic antidepressants (e.g., amitriptyline, venlafaxine), anticonvulsants (e.g., gabapentin), corticosteroids, benzodiazepines, and ket-

amine (in refractory pain). Patients who are sedated and receiving paralytic drugs while on a ventilator or who are in a comatose state may experience pain and be unable to indicate this. The ICU nurse learns to recognize restlessness, agitation, grimacing, moaning, or increasing tachycardia as signs of pain in the unconscious patient.

Why do you think that pain is referred to as the "fifth vital sign"? ■

Constipation and Diarrhea

Constipation occurs in as many as two thirds of patients receiving palliative care. Patients taking narcotic pain medications on a regular basis should have prophylactic treatment for constipation, such as a bowel regimen, stool softeners, and laxatives as needed. Bowel hygiene is very important in preventing painful constipation or opioid-induced bowel obstruction (Lenz, 2003).

Medications, treatments, diet, infection, or intestinal obstruction may cause diarrhea. Besides discomfort, diarrhea may lead to painful skin breakdown or electrolyte imbalance. Frequent loose stools should be reported to the physician so that diagnostic testing and treatment can be initiated.

Nausea and Vomiting

Nausea and vomiting are common, unwelcome side effects of life-sustaining treatment. Antiemetic medications provide the first line of relief. Lorazepam may relieve some chemotherapy-related nausea, as well as the anxiety evoked by anticipating nausea or vomiting (Cope, 2003). Other measures that provide psychological comfort to patients experiencing nausea are management of odors in the sick room, provision of only foods tolerated by the patient in this state, and careful mouth care.

Hiccups and Other Troublesome Symptoms

Persistent or intractable hiccups are disturbing to both patients and their families. Some of the conditions that may precipitate hiccuping are advanced HIV, uremia of end-stage renal disease, fever, hyponatremia, and gastric distension. Breath-holding, swallowing a spoonful of sugar, breathing into a paper bag, rapidly drinking a glass of water, and nasopharynx stimulation are some conservative measures

---

BOX 40-4

JCAHO Concepts for Pain Management

- Recognize the right of patients to appropriate assessment and management of pain.
- Assess the existence, nature, and intensity of pain in all patients.
- Record the results of the pain assessment in a way that facilitates regular reassessment and follow-up.
- Determine and assure staff competency in pain assessment and management, and address pain assessment and management in the orientation of all new staff.
- Establish policies and procedures that support the appropriate prescription or ordering of effective pain medications.
- Educate patients and their families about effective pain management.
- Address patient needs for symptom management in the discharge planning process.
- Maintain a pain control performance improvement plan.

Adapted from *Pain standards*, Joint Commission on Accreditation of Healthcare Organization (JCAHO), 2003.

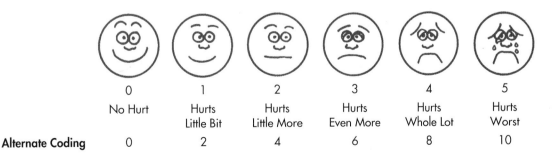

	0	1	2	3	4	5
	No Hurt	Hurts Little Bit	Hurts Little More	Hurts Even More	Hurts Whole Lot	Hurts Worst
Alternate Coding	0	2	4	6	8	10

Figure 40-1   Wong-Baker FACES Pain Rating Scale. Brief word instructions: Point to each face using the words to describe the pain intensity. Ask the child to choose the face that best describes own pain and record the appropriate number. (From Wong DL et al: *Wong's essentials of pediatric nursing*, ed 6, St Louis, 2001, p 1301. Copyrighted by Mosby, Inc. Reprinted by permission.)

used to interrupt hiccups. Chlorpromazine (Thorazine) is the most often used medication and is approved by the U.S. Food and Drug Administration (FDA) for treating hiccups. Baclofen, valproic acid, and nifedipine are other drugs that may provide relief.

Itching or tingling may be caused by the elevated bilirubin of jaundice, various rashes, or as an allergic reaction to a new medication. Antihistamines are the treatment of choice and may help the patient get some rest as well. Chemotherapy-induced mucositis affects both the mouth and the anal-rectal area. The nurse should provide numbing medicines and gentle mouth or peri-anal care.

Mental status changes are not uncommon with high doses of pain medications or in the dying. Family members are often dismayed by the patient's audio-visual hallucinations or the inability to process information or remember names and faces (Hendry and Douglas, 2003). Some causes of delirium at the end of life are fever, brain metastases, encephalopathy, and pain medications. Providing explanations of altered mental status and reassurance to both patient and family is comforting. Treating the underlying organic condition with antipsychotic drugs such as haloperidol, olanzapine, risperidone, or ziprasidone is the first step in clearing the sensorium.

Dyspnea occurs in many chronic and end-stage diseases such as obstructive lung disease, progression of lung cancer, heart failure, pleural effusion, pneumonia, and obstruction caused by ascites. Nurses can assist the patient with shortness of breath or "air hunger" to find a comfortable elevated position for sitting or sleeping. Bronchodilators and anxiolytic medication may provide some relief (Inzeo and Tyson, 2003). The presence of calm and reassuring nurses and family members, guided imagery, music, massage, and prayer are examples of nonpharmacological treatments. Nasal or facemask oxygen may be provided for comfort in the event of terminal dyspnea and will not prolong the dying process. In addition, morphine, nebulized fentanyl, and anticholinergic medications may be used to relieve dyspnea associated with end-stage disease (Coyne, 2003; Lance, 2002; Westphal and Campbell, 2002).

▪ TRANSITIONING TO END-OF-LIFE CARE
Advocating for the Patient

When recovery is in doubt or no longer thought to be possible, planning should begin for end-of-life care. **End-of-life is generally accepted as the probable last 6 months of life.** The bedside nurse is often the first to become aware of the need for a family conference—one in which all involved parties can express their thoughts, feelings, wishes, and rationale for advocating a particular approach. As an advocate, the nurse's primary commitment is to the patient, whether an individual or family (ANA, 2001b). The purpose of the meeting would be to improve communication, explore options, and clarify the new goals of treatment.

If an inclusive meeting fails to improve communication and resolve a dilemma, the nurse may initiate an ethics consultation. Every institution certified by the Joint Commission

on Accreditation of Healthcare Organizations (JCAHO) is required to have a mechanism for addressing ethical concerns. The institution should also ensure that anyone who requests an ethics consultation may do so without fear of intimidation or reprisal (JCAHO, 2003).

It is essential that the nurse be culturally competent, especially when caring for families whose ethnic identity differs from that of the treatment team (see Chapter 8). Studies have shown, for example, that many African Americans, Mexican Americans, and other ethnic minority groups distrust the health care system or have values that may not fit with standard practices of Western medicine. Some non-Western cultures believe the welfare of the group takes precedence over individual autonomy and in those cultures health care decisions may be made by family consensus rather than by the patient alone (Hopp and Duffy, 2000; Mazanec and Tyler, 2003).

The Changing Focus of Hope

Patients, family members, nurses, and other clinicians often find it emotionally difficult and painful to acknowledge that the illness does not appear to be responding to treatment as hoped. When, for example, cancer is discovered at a late, metastatic stage, human nature sometimes offers a secret hope that a "miracle cure" will occur.

This "hope against hope" may not mean that the patient or family is in denial, but rather that they are using denial as an adaptive defense mechanism. Nurses uncomfortable with the patient's or family's lack of acknowledgment of the poor prognosis or imminence of death should ask themselves what purpose confrontation would serve at this point in time. Forcing patients and families to acknowledge blunt statistical medical predictions or probabilities may be devastating to those who are struggling to maintain a sense of hope and ego integrity.

However, neither should the nurse reinforce false beliefs or unrealistic hopes. Simply ignoring or discouraging such statements at first, then later reassessing and gently asking about the patient's plans and reframing the self-deception or reality distortion may be a skillful way to deal with this defense. Often it is the patient who first understands the finality of the situation; sometimes it is someone close to the patient, sometimes it is the clinical team.

The transition from hope for recovery to hope for a peaceful, pain-free, dignified death usually happens gradually (Hahn, 2002). The new focus of hope is for a "good death." Quality of life issues may lead to the switch from cure to end-of-life care, as problems arise in more than one organ system and no longer respond to therapies. Patients begin to question their present or projected quality of life, based on their personal values, especially when proposed or repeated treatments are uncomfortable and have unpleasant side effects, or when multiple organ systems begin to fail (Virani and Sofer, 2003).

Do you believe that patients should never give up hope? Why or why not? ▪

Making Decisions

Before patients or surrogates can make decisions and give informed consent or informed refusal, certain conditions must be met (see Chapter 10). First the person must possess decision-making capacity. This is sometimes mistakenly referred to in health care as competence, which is a legal term that can only be determined in a court of law. Two physicians, however, can determine decisional capacity for health care decisions. The other conditions required are that the decision-maker be given information about the disease process, prognosis, including risks and benefits of each choice, and the likely effect of no treatment. Finally, the consent must be voluntary and free from coercion.

When hope for recovery has diminished, palliative care should be explained to the patient and family. Palliative care includes pain medications, stomach ulcer prevention, skin and mouth care, and other comfort measures. These will not prolong the dying process. Rather they help ensure that the patient is allowed to die with comfort and dignity.

When patients lack decisional capacity, their surrogate is morally obligated to choose as the patient would choose if able, which is the **substituted-judgment standard**. Lacking that knowledge, a surrogate must decide what is best for the patient, using the **best interests standard**, based on what would promote the welfare of the "average" patient. The best interests standard is also used when making treatment decisions for infants, children, and those who never were able to make their own decisions, such as patients with severe mental retardation.

A combination of both standards may be used for emancipated minors or "mature minor" patients, depending on the case and the decision at hand. Although teenagers younger than 18 years old may not be judged to have legal competence to make non–health care decisions, most ethicists argue that they do indeed have the right to informed consent or informed refusal in treatment decisions, based on their ability to reason and deliberate concerning the decision (Derish and Huevel, 2000). Mature minors who have been ill for some time, have spent time in an intensive care unit, and have seen fellow patients dying may ethically and legally be allowed to give significant input into deciding whether to forego further life-sustaining medical treatment.

Which standard is a family using when they direct care based upon the advance directive of their loved one? ■

Withholding and Withdrawing Life-Sustaining Treatment

Life-sustaining treatment is medical treatment designed to keep a person alive when vital organ systems are failing or have failed. It includes **renal dialysis, most medications, chemotherapy,** and **medically provided nutrition and hydration**.

Although withholding and withdrawing life-sustaining treatment carry equal moral and ethical weight, deciding to terminate treatments already begun is often more difficult emotionally. A justification for not starting a treatment is also sufficient justification for ceasing it (President's Commission, 1982). Noticing family or surrogate discomfort when a decision about withholding or withdrawing treatment is being considered, the nurse may reflect that, "This decision seems very hard for you. Can you tell me more about that" (Scanlon, 2003).

Withholding or withdrawing life-sustaining treatment is always an option when the patient, surrogate, or physician believes that the burdens of treatment exceed the benefits. If a patient wishes to forego further aggressive treatment, but is not ready for withdrawal of treatment, such things as renal dialysis, artificial nutrition, and hydration may provide additional quality time for the patient. Goals of sustaining life may be to see a child graduate or marry, to see an expected grandchild, to take a dream vacation, go fishing, work in the garden, or to take time to say good-bye and enjoy being surrounded by family and friends.

Deciding to forego or stop tube feedings or dialysis may be more difficult for family members than patients (National Kidney Foundation, 1999; Paice, 2002). Deciding to withhold or withdraw treatment for infants and children is psychologically very difficult for nurses and parents alike. Pediatric treatment dilemmas are discussed in more depth in pediatric literature such as "When the Bough Breaks: Parental Perceptions of Ethical Decision-Making in the NICU" (Pinch, 2002).

Medically Ineffective Treatment

Treatments that, in the best professional judgment of the physician, are medically ineffective or do not have a reasonable chance of benefiting the patient should not be offered (American Medical Association, 2003). Such treatment is thought to be more burdensome to the patient than beneficial and to prolong suffering. Treatment that will not bring about cure is often referred to as "futile care." Bioethicists tend to agree that the term *futility* is difficult to define. Organizations usually have policies regarding "futile" or medically ineffective treatment that provide guidance and practice standards.

A family may demand treatment that offers little or no hope of benefiting the patient. This is especially true when a patient is in a permanent vegetative state and is having brain stem reflex movements that the family mistakenly interprets as signs of neurological recovery or when they do not comprehend the meaning of "brain dead." If the family or surrogate does not agree with the physician's recommendation to allow the dying process to transpire, an ethics consultation may facilitate an acceptable resolution.

Life-prolonging treatments that may be withheld or withdrawn include the following:
- Chemotherapy or radiation (unless for comfort)
- Diagnostic tests
- Invasive procedures
- Blood pressure stabilizing medications
- Antibiotics
- Artificial hydration and nutrition
- Renal dialysis
- Admittance to an intensive care unit

Once a decision has been made to withdraw life-sustaining treatment, the family is given time to gather and say good-bye. Family members may or may not choose to be present at the time of withdrawal. The nurse's reassurance that either choice is acceptable will help each family member decide. Many ICUs waive usual visiting restrictions so that families can keep vigil at the bedside. In an ICU, monitors may be turned off or left on depending on the preference of family or staff. The presence of a spiritual counselor is usually requested and provided if the family wishes.

Extubating a dying or brain dead patient from a ventilator is called *terminal weaning*. Families need to be made aware that patients may linger hours or occasionally days after life-sustaining treatment is withdrawn. In this case patients will be kept comfortable and may be moved from the ICU to a conventional hospital room.

Morphine or other opioid agonists prevent gasping for air or terminal dyspnea during terminal weaning or ventilator withdrawal. The American Medical Association's Code of Medical Ethics states: "Physicians have an obligation to relieve pain and suffering and to promote the dignity and autonomy of dying patients in their care. This includes effective treatment even though it may foreseeably hasten death" (AMA, 2003, p. 66).

When morphine is used with the intent of relieving suffering, enough should be administered to provide relief of symptoms. Patients who have chronic pain often become medically dependent upon opioids and develop tolerance, requiring more frequent and higher dosing to achieve effective pain relief. The nurse should feel comfortable with very high doses of narcotics not used elsewhere in practice when providing end-of-life care to terminally ill patients (Pitorak, 2003; Scanlon, 2003).

Hospice

Hospice care offers an alternative to dying in a health care facility. A little more than a decade ago three-fourths of new hospice patients had cancer diagnoses. By 2000, only 51% of new hospice patients had a diagnosis of cancer (Hospice Association of America, 2003). Eligibility requires the patient to have a prognosis of 6 months or less of life remaining. If dying patients are stable enough to leave the hospital, they may choose hospice services in the home or a special facility. Services that hospice provides to adult and pediatric patients and their families include the following:

- Pain and symptom management
- Nutritional counseling
- Physical, occupational, and speech therapies
- Home health services for personal care
- Psychosocial emotional support
- Grief counseling
- Crisis care during medical emergencies

Unfortunately many patients are not referred to hospice until their condition is well advanced. One study showed the median length of stay for hospice patients was 19 days (Hospice Association of America, 2003). Early referral to a hospice program improves quality of life for both patients and their families at the end of life (Cramer et al, 2003).

Why do you think that more patients are not referred to a hospice for end-of-life care? What might help families take greater advantage of this resource?

■ PREPARING FOR DEATH

Anticipatory Grief

Anticipatory grief is emotional work begun before the actual loss of a valued person, object, or concept. Anticipatory grief is an adaptive response to an expected loss and helps prepare both patients and families for the actual moment of death. As family members come to the understanding that the patient is in the process of dying they will begin to "let go." Adult patients may grieve the loss of their plans for the future, such as seeing a grandchild born, relaxing in retirement, or taking a long-postponed dream vacation. Family members start adapting to their loss by beginning to say good-bye and trying to imagine how their lives will be changed by their loved one's absence.

Parents of dying infants and children may grieve the loss of their child's potential. Siblings of a dying child should be made aware of the severity of the illness in a manner and at a time appropriate for their developmental age. Below the age of 6, attitudes toward death are often a matter of fact rather than emotion.

Siblings should be offered the choice of whether or not to see the patient one last time to say good-bye, and whether or not they wish to attend a funeral, burial, or memorial service. Older children should be told that they have permission to change their minds about a last visit or attending a service for a sibling, parent, or grandparent. Many areas have grief support groups for parents and siblings. Nurses should know local grief resources and how to refer surviving family members to them.

The nurse may facilitate anticipatory grieving by asking adult patients to reminisce or family members to recall milestones in their lives, such as where they grew up, how they met, the birth of children, pets they have had, or how they have dealt with other losses in their lives (Webster and Haight, 2002). It may be helpful to ask how the deaths of pets have been explained to young children or to inquire about religious beliefs.

Children may benefit from play therapy or counseling both before and after an anticipated death. They may express grief by altered behavior as well as altered emotions. The nurse can coach a responsible adult to alert the child's school guidance teacher about the situation in the family, and remind family members that public libraries offer books for helping children understand and deal with death. It is most important to let children and adults know that sadness and grief are a normal response to the loss of a loved one.

The Dying Process

Patients and family members alike are curious and want to know what to expect of the dying process. As death approaches they will notice certain physiological changes as body systems shut down. Patients may lose their appetites. Keeping lips moistened or giving small amounts of favorite foods provides comfort if the patient requests this. Patients who are near death may imagine they see or hear loved ones who have died before them. Other signs of imminent death are difficulty arousing the person, restlessness, and altered breathing patterns with periods of apnea (Pitorak, 2003).

Unfortunately, families at home may panic if patients are moaning or have labored breathing and call for emergency assistance. Hospice nurses usually provide counseling about ways to manage situations that are frightening to caregivers in the home or long-term care facility. Dying at home is not the choice or option for some. Patients who do not die in an ICU cannot be considered for organ donation because life-support for the vital organs cannot be initiated.

CONCERNS OF NURSES WORKING WITH PATIENTS WITH LIFE-THREATENING ILLNESS
Deaths of Infants and Children

Many nurses find it particularly difficult to deal with the deaths of infants and children. When an infant or child is born with devastating anomalies, suffers a significant loss of oxygen perfusion to the brain, is diagnosed with a life-threatening disease or condition, or is rescued from a motor vehicle collision, near drowning, or fire, the parent or parents face difficult choices. Decisions made at this time affect not only the child's possible future and life but also the parent or family's future quality of life.

Witnessing the death of a child elicits a feeling of injustice and a loss of possibilities for that child's life. If a nurse finds it difficult to accept a decision a parent has made, professional ethics preclude the nurse from discussing these personal concerns with the parents. If a nurse believes a treatment decision is not in the best interests of a child and discussions with physicians and peers fail to reassure, an ethics consultation may be requested.

Identifying With the Patient or Family

When a patient is near the same age as the nurse or the nurse's child, parent, partner, or grandparent, or has the same condition as a loved one who has died, it may be challenging for the nurse to maintain professional boundaries. If a nurse finds himself or herself in this position, it is advisable to discuss the conflict with an experienced nurse or supervisor, or to seek reassignment until the nurse has learned to adapt emotionally.

Nurses who notice potential boundary violations in themselves or others may request an in-service consultation to help put compassion into perspective with professional behavior. Shedding tears with the family upon the death of a patient with whom the nurse has worked over time may not violate boundaries. In fact, families often express appreciation for this show of emotion and perceive the nurse's tears as a sign of true compassion.

Medically Provided Nutrition and Hydration

The consensus in the bioethics community is that medically provided nutrition and hydration are life-sustaining treatments. As such they may ethically be withheld or withdrawn in patients who are no longer receiving curative medical treatment. Research has shown that patients who are dying do not experience hunger or thirst (Zerwekh, 1997). However, a compelling psychological attachment to providing nourishment often makes withdrawal of artificial feeding emotionally difficult for caregivers.

Professional Integrity

If due to religious or other beliefs nurses feel participating in any aspect of patient care would compromise their personal or professional integrity, they should address their conscientious objections through appropriate channels. Whenever possible, the nurse's objections should be made known in advance so that alternative arrangements can be made for patient care (ANA, 2001b).

Nurse participation in euthanasia **(actively causing a death) and physician-assisted suicide (such as aiding a patient to take an intentionally lethal dose of prescribed medication) is prohibited by the Code of Ethics for Nurses** (ANA, 2001b). However, no positions or guiding principles on rational suicide are available from either the American Medical Association or the American Nurses Association (Fontana, 2002).

A study in Australia of terminally ill patients reported that 14% had a high wish to hasten their death (Kelly et al, 2003). Patients with life-threatening or terminal illness may suffer in three dimensions: psychological, social, and physical. Some of the reasons why patients may wish to hasten death are as follows:

- Loss of autonomy
- Lack of dignity
- Unrelieved pain
- Fatigue
- Anorexia
- Fear of the future
- Untreated depression

When pain and depression are adequately treated, patient requests to hasten death diminish (Bowers and Boyle, 2003; Kelly et al, 2003; Paice, 2002). When patients say they would prefer death to their current emotional or physical suffering, nurses should seek adequate pain relief and treatment for depression before clinicians consider a request for withdrawal of treatment (ANA, 2001a; Chase, 2003).

Table 40-1 presents a summary of aspects of care for patients with life-threatening illness. Working with patients whose life expectancy is suddenly in doubt or who are dying may be one of the most satisfying experiences of one's nursing career. Helping patients and family members in their transition from hope for recovery to hope for a peaceful, dignified death is both challenging and rewarding, and perhaps the ultimate act of compassion. This is reflected in the words of two different families. The first is the parent of a 30-year-old patient who had leukemia and a bone marrow transplant and who spent the last weeks of his life in an intensive care unit.

At first when we got the diagnosis I thought, "This has to be a bad dream." Then I felt overwhelmed, very, very sad, and I prayed a lot. Other emotions I felt during those 13½ months were helplessness, fear, shock, anxiety, and determi-

Table 40-1 Aspects of Care for Patients With Life-Threatening Illness

PHASE	EMOTION OR ATTITUDE	NURSE INTERVENTION
Symptoms or suspicious diagnostic test results	Shock	Help refocus on present
	Fear	Provide presence
	Disbelief	Suspend judgment
	Curiosity	Be watchfully aware
	Hope	Offer website information
Waiting for diagnosis	Anxiety	Treat anxiety as needed
	Worry	Focus on what patient can control
	Hope	Help deal with uncertainty
	Fear	Provide distraction
Benign diagnosis or resolution of threat	Relief	Educate
		Celebrate
Life-threatening diagnosis	Determination to fight	Give information about the disease and treatment
	Fear	Provide presence
	Denial	Ask about advance planning
	Hopefulness	Help balance hope with pragmatism
	Hopelessness	Discuss options and choices
		Encourage positive attitude
	Anger	Explore expressions of anger with patient and family
	Guilt	Offer spiritual advisor
	Depression	Assess for depression
	Not being in control	Help patient maintain some control over situation
Attempt for recovery or cure	Feeling more in control	Answer questions honestly
	Courage	Give positive feedback for coping skills
	Hope for cure	Teach patient about lab values and their significance
	Faith	Ask about spiritual beliefs
	Discouragement	Remain cautiously optimistic
		Offer to help patient decorate room
	Depression	Treat depression
		Keep window blinds open
Palliation/dying process	Denial	Introduce "what if" ideas
	Anticipatory grief	Begin life review
	Anger	Address anger
		Inquire about family or pastoral support
		Reframe hope
	Acceptance	Gently teach about DNR order and "No ICU" options
		Discuss hospice and dying at home options/choices
	Appreciation of comfort	Offer palliative measures and relieve bothersome symptoms
	Hope for a "good death"	Explain to patient and family what to expect in the final days and moments
		Do not avoid discussion of who needs to be notified, funeral arrangements, autopsy, or organ donation

DNR, Do not resuscitate; *ICU,* intensive care unit.

nation to beat the leukemia. The nursing care I found most compassionate was the kindness shown towards my son. Their words and actions showed that the nurses really did care, such as by moving him carefully when he was in pain, or trying to find some food that appealed to him when he was able to eat. My husband and I appreciated positive explanations for things that were happening in the ICU. We also valued when the nurses took a few minutes to talk with our son about something he cared about—such as his dog or his college football team's performance in the latest game. Small actions perhaps, but they had a major impact on our son and his family.

The second note was written to a PCLN by the daughter of a patient admitted to the hospital with a life-threatening illness.

You are someone I will never forget. When I was going through the agony of seeing my mother near death, you were there to talk to when I could not talk to my Dad. Now surely I didn't agree with you when you said I may have to face the fact that my mother was very ill and could possibly die. But I knew in my heart that she was not going to die that time, in that hospital. Actually, my mother is still with us today. She is a functional, sporty woman. If you never believed in miracles...well she is one! Yes, things appeared to be gloomy, however, God kept her with me. She was able to see me graduate from college and launch into my professional career. So I just wanted to let you know that your stress ball and listening skills impacted my life. I am currently working as a care coordinator for the disabled, elderly population. I am able to give hope to people who are in need and bring a level of empathy to those I serve because of you. Thank you so very much.

COMPETENT CARING

A Clinical Exemplar of a Psychiatric Nurse
Penelope Chase, MSN, MEd, RN, CS

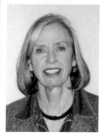

This letter was written to "Dear Abby," the noted newspaper columnist.

Dear Abby,

I am a clinical ethics consultant and an advanced practice psychiatric nurse. I work in a medical hospital counseling patients and families with their emotional responses to their physical illnesses. All too often I am asked to help family members of unconscious and dying people make choices about withholding or withdrawing life-sustaining treatments. All too often these otherwise loving and caring family members find that they have never talked with each other about "what if" so the surrogate or substitute decision maker has to guess what the patient would want. This usually comes when the family member is in the height of shock or despair, and is often sleep-deprived and not able to think or process clearly.

So please tell your readers to make sure that they tell several people they love and trust to speak up should the time come, and tell the nurses and doctors what they would want or not want in terms of life- or death-prolonging treatment in a hospital. Better yet, write down your instructions in case you cannot speak for yourself, and put a copy in your kitchen drawer or in your wallet with your driver's license. Don't hide this vital information in an office file with a mound of other papers or in a safe deposit box where it is inaccessible when most needed. Sadly, young and healthy people can have life threatening or fatal accidents, so everyone needs to have these discussions. A written living will and durable power of attorney are even better.

And don't just think about resuscitation and breathing or feeding tubes, or when to ask the doctor for a DNR (do not resuscitate) order. Rather talk about kidney dialysis, special tests, and even antibiotics. Also let them know your preference about being an organ donor. Some people hope for a miracle when a person has been kept "alive" on a breathing machine (ventilator) and with drugs for a long time. I have seen a couple of miracles, but those were after the man-made machines were turned off.

A young widow said to me in a grief follow-up phone call, "I miss him so much. I know that he loved me, but I wish he could have told me just one more time before he died." So be sure to tell those you care about that you love them today...and each and every day thereafter.

Finally, I encourage everyone to make a copy of this letter, share it with others and set aside a time and place to talk about these issues with those you love while you still can. Keep a written, dated, and witnessed record of what was said and requested. I call this "vital tough love," and it may be the most loving act of your life.

Sincerely,
Penelope Chase ∎

CHAPTER **FOCUS POINTS**

- Nurses working in many different settings may find themselves caring for a person with a life-threatening illness. Doing so with compassion is part of the art of nursing.
- Working with patients who have life-threatening illness and with their families requires sensitivity to issues of uncertainty, the importance of advance directives, and respectful responses to patient and family fears, emotions, and requests for information.
- Treating the emotional responses, such an anxiety, depression, and anger, that may accompany life-threatening illness helps improve the patient's quality of life, provide comfort to worried family members, and relieve caregiver stress.
- A psychiatric consultation liaison nurse (PCLN) can be very helpful in addressing the mental health needs of these patients.
- Mental health care includes medications and psychosocial interventions.
- Palliative care is the medical and nursing care that provides comfort to a moribund person without prolonging the dying process.
- When patients are undergoing treatment for cure and recovery, and when the goal of care changes to preserving dignity while dying,

patients will experience symptoms that require management. Nurses have the opportunity and obligation to patients and their families to help ensure freedom from unnecessary suffering.

- Transitioning to end-of-life care involves advocating for the patient, refocusing issues of hope, and enhancing decision making of the patient and family related to withholding and withdrawing life-sustaining treatment, resisting medically ineffective treatment, and considering hospice placement.
- Anticipatory grief is an adaptive response to an expected loss and helps prepare both patients and families for the dying process and the actual moment of death.
- Nurses may have difficulty dealing with the dying patient and maintaining professional boundaries. If a nurse finds himself or herself in this position, it is advisable to discuss the conflict with an experienced nurse or supervisor, or to seek reassignment.
- Nurse participation in euthanasia (actively causing a death) and physician-assisted suicide (such as aiding a patient in taking an intentionally lethal dose of prescribed medication) is prohibited by the Code of Ethics for Nurses.

KEY TERMS

CHAPTER REVIEW QUESTIONS

1. Indicate whether the following statements are true (T) or false (F).

_____ A. Clinicians have no valid reason to forego prescribing antidepressants for seriously ill patients.

_____ B. Every institution certified by the Joint Commission on Accreditation of Healthcare Organizations (JCAHO) is encouraged to have a mechanism for addressing ethical concerns.

_____ C. The best interests standard is employed when patients lack decisional capacity, and their surrogate is morally obligated to choose as the patient would choose if able.

_____ D. Families need to be made aware that patients may linger hours or occasionally days after life-sustaining treatment is withdrawn.

2. Fill in the blanks.

A. A term used to describe the therapeutic, healing, respectful, watchful, and compassionate experience of being in a relationship with another human being in a state of empathy and positive regard is _____.

B. A _____ is an advanced practice nurse who practices psychiatric and mental health nursing in a medical setting, providing consultation and education to patients, families, the health care team, and the community.

C. Nonpharmacological interventions for anxiety reduction include

_____, _____,

and _____.

D. If a patient's "prominent and persistent" depressed mood is believed to be related to the medical condition,

_____ is indicated.

E. _____ is the medical and nursing care that provides comfort to a moribund person without prolonging the dying process.

F. One of the symptoms most feared by patients and their

families is _____.

G. _____ can determine decisional capacity for health care decisions.

H. Actively causing the death of a patient is called

_____.

3. Provide short answers for the following questions.

A. Identify four concerns that patients with life-threatening illness often express.

B. What is the best way for a nurse to respond to the complaints of a patient or family member?

C. What are some of the common causes of delirium at the end of life?

Visit Evolve for additional resources related to the content of this chapter.

 http://evolve.elsevier.com/Stuart/principles/
• Topical Course Outline • Student Workbook Exercises • Critical Thinking Questions and Activities • Case Studies • Research Topics
• Monthly Content Updates • WebLinks

 ### Student Study CD-ROM

Access the accompanying CD-ROM for animations, interactive exercises, review questions for the NCLEX examination, and an audio glossary.

REFERENCES

American heritage dictionary, 2nd College ed, Boston, 1991, Houghton Mifflin Company.

American Nurses Association (ANA): *A compendium of position statements on the nurse's role in end-of-life decisions*, Washington, DC, 2001a, American Nurses Publishing.

American Nurses Association (ANA): *The code of ethics for nurses with interpretive statements*, Washington, DC, 2001b, American Nurses Publishing.

American Medical Association (AMA): *Code of medical ethics: current opinions with annotations*, Futile care: 2.035, Council on Ethical and Judicial Affairs, Chicago, 2003, American Medical Association Press.

American Psychiatric Association: *Diagnostic and statistical manual of mental disorders*, fourth edition, text revision. Washington, DC, 2000, American Psychiatric Association.

Bowers L, Boyle DA: Depression in patients with advanced cancer, *Clin J Oncol Nurs* 7:281, 2003.

Chase P: Applying the 2001 Code of Ethics for Nurses in practice, *South Carolina Nurse* 9:11, 2003.

Chase P et al: The psychiatric consultation/liaison nurse role in case management, *Nurs Case Manag* 5:73, 2000.

Cope D: Oncology Patient Evidence-Based Notes (OPEN): antiemetics for chemotherapy-induced nausea and vomiting, *Clin J Oncol Nurs* 7:461, 2003.

Coyne PJ: The use of nebulized fentanyl for the management of dyspnea, *Clin J Oncol Nurs* 7:334, 2003.

Cramer LD et al: Nurses' attitudes and practice related to hospice care, *J Nurs Scholarsh* 35:249, 2003.

Derish MT, Heuvel KV: Mature minors should have the right to refuse life-sustaining medical treatment, *J Law Med Ethics* 28:109, 2000.

Du Mont PM: *The concept of therapeutic presence in nursing*. Paper presented at the 5th annual conference of the International Society of Psychiatric–Mental Health Nurses, Charleston, SC, 2003.

Fontana J: Rational suicide in the terminally ill, *J Nurs Scholarsh* 34:147, 2002.

Frisch N: Nursing as a context for alternative/complementary modalities, *Online J Issues Nurs* 6(2): Manuscript 2, 2001. Available at: www.nursingworld.org/ojin/topic/tpc15_2.htm

Geller SM, Greenberg LS: Therapeutic presence: therapists' experience of presence in the psychotherapy encounter [On line], *J World Assoc Person-Centered Experiential Psychother Counseling* 1: Abstract, 2002.

Hahn TN: No death, no fear: comforting wisdom for life, New York, 2002, Riverhead Books.

Hendry KC, Douglas DH: Promoting quality of life for clients diagnosed with dementia, *J Am Psychiatr Nurs Assoc* 9:96, 2003.

Hines DR: Presence: Discovering the artistry in relating, *J Holistic Nurs* 10: 294, 1992.

Hopp FP, Duffy SA: Racial variations in end-of-life care, *J Am Geriatr Soc* 48:658, 2000.

Hospice Association of America: *Hospice facts and statistics*, retrieved August 9, 2003, from the World Wide Web: http://www.nahc.org/consmer/hpcstats.html

Inzeo D, Tyson L: Nursing assessment and management of dyspneic patients with lung cancer, *Clin J Oncol Nurs* 7:332, 2003.

Joint Commission on Accreditation of Healthcare Organizations (JCAHO): Pain assessment and management: an organizational approach, Oakbrook, Ill, 2003, JCAHO.

Kelly B et al: Factors associated with the wish to hasten death: a study of patients with terminal illness, *Psychol Med* 33:75, 2003.

Lance MM: Terminal weaning: how to make ethical choices for your patients and their families, *Adv Nurses Carolinas/Georgia*, May 27, pp 33-34, 2002.

Lenz K L: The pharmacology of symptom control. In Taylor GJ, Kurent JE, editors: A clinicians guide to palliative care, Malden, Mass, 2003, Blackwell Science.

Mazanec P, Tyler MK: Cultural considerations in end-of-life care: how ethnicity, age, and spirituality affect decisions when death is imminent, *Am J Nurs* 103:50, 2003.

National Kidney Foundation: *When stopping dialysis treatment is your choice*, New York, 1999 edition, National Kidney Foundation.

Paice JA: Managing psychological conditions in palliative care, *Am J Nurs* 102:36, 2002.

Pinch WJ: Moral voices of parents. In Pinch WJ: *When the bough breaks: parental perceptions of ethical decision-making in the NICU*, Lanham, Md, 2002, University Press of America.

Pitorak EF: Care at the time of death: How nurses can make the last hours of life a richer, more comfortable experience. *Am J Nurs* 103:42, 2003.

President's Commission for the Study of Ethical Problems in Medicine and Biomedical and Behavioral Research: *Making health care decisions*, Washington, DC, 1982, US Government Printing Office.

Scanlon C: Ethical concerns in end-of-life care, *Am J Nurs* 103:48, 2003.

Spiess JL et al: Palliative care: something else we can do for our patients, *Psychiatr Serv* 53:1525, 2002.

Steinhauser KE et al: Factors considered important at the end of life by patients, family, physicians, and other care providers, *JAMA* 284:2476, 2000.

Virani R, Sofer D: Improving the quality of end-of-life care, *Am J Nurs* 103:52, 2003.

Webster JD, Haight BK: *Critical advances in reminiscence work: from theory to application*, New York, 2002, Springer Publishing Company.

Westphal CG, Campbell ML: Nebulized morphine for terminal dyspnea: a treatment option in chronic obstructive pulmonary disease or end-stage congestive heart failure, *Am J Nurs* (Suppl):11, 2002.

Zerwekh JV: Do dying patients really need IV fluids? *Am J Nurs* 97:26, 1997.

NANDA-Approved Nursing Diagnoses

Activity intolerance
Activity intolerance, Risk for
Adjustment, Impaired
Airway clearance, Ineffective
Allergy response, Latex
Allergy response, Risk for latex
Anxiety
Anxiety, Death
Aspiration, Risk for
Attachment, Risk for impaired parent/infant/child
Autonomic dysreflexia
Autonomic dysreflexia, Risk for

Body image, Disturbed
Body temperature, Risk for imbalanced
Bowel incontinence
Breastfeeding, Effective
Breastfeeding, Ineffective
Breastfeeding, Interrupted
Breathing pattern, Ineffective

Cardiac output, Decreased
Caregiver role strain
Caregiver role strain, Risk for
Communication, Impaired verbal
Communication, Readiness for enhanced
Conflict, Decisional
Conflict, Parental role
Confusion, Acute
Confusion, Chronic
Constipation
Constipation, Perceived
Constipation, Risk for
Coping, Ineffective
Coping, Defensive
Coping, Readiness for enhanced
Coping, Ineffective community
Coping, Readiness for enhanced community
Coping, Compromised family
Coping, Disabled family
Coping, Readiness for enhanced family

Death syndrome, Risk for sudden infant
Denial, Ineffective
Dentition, Impaired
Development, Risk for delayed
Diarrhea
Disuse syndrome, Risk for
Diversional activity, Deficient

Energy field, Disturbed
Environmental interpretation syndrome, Impaired

Failure to thrive, Adult
Falls, Risk for
Family processes: alcoholism, Dysfunctional
Family processes, Interrupted
Family processes, Readiness for enhanced
Fatigue
Fear
Fluid balance, Readiness for enhanced
Fluid volume, Deficient
Fluid volume, Excess
Fluid volume, Risk for deficient
Fluid volume, Risk for imbalanced

Gas exchange, Impaired
Grieving, Anticipatory
Grieving, Dysfunctional
Growth and development, Delayed
Growth, Risk for disproportionate

Health maintenance, Ineffective
Health-seeking behaviors
Home maintenance, Impaired
Hopelessness
Hyperthermia
Hypothermia

Identity, Disturbed personal
Incontinence, Functional urinary
Incontinence, Reflex urinary
Incontinence, Stress urinary
Incontinence, Total urinary
Incontinence, Urge urinary
Incontinence, Risk for urge urinary
Infant behavior, Disorganized

From North American Nursing Diagnosis Association: *NANDA nursing diagnoses: definitions and classification 2003-2004*, Philadelphia, 2003, NANDA.

Infant behavior, Risk for disorganized
Infant behavior, Readiness for enhanced organized
Infant feeding pattern, Ineffective
Infection, Risk for
Injury, Risk for
Injury, Risk for perioperative-positioning
Intracranial adaptive capacity, Decreased

Knowledge, Deficient
Knowledge, Readiness for enhanced

Loneliness, Risk for

Memory, Impaired
Mobility, Impaired bed
Mobility, Impaired physical
Mobility, Impaired wheelchair

Nausea
Neglect, Unilateral
Noncompliance
Nutrition: less than body requirements, Imbalanced
Nutrition: more than body requirements, Imbalanced
Nutrition, Readiness for enhanced
Nutrition: more than body requirements, Risk for imbalanced

Oral mucous membrane, Impaired

Pain, Acute
Pain, Chronic
Parenting, Readiness for enhanced
Parenting, Impaired
Parenting, Risk for impaired
Peripheral neurovascular dysfunction, Risk for
Poisoning, Risk for
Post-trauma syndrome
Post-trauma syndrome, Risk for
Powerlessness
Powerlessness, Risk for
Protection, Ineffective

Rape-trauma syndrome
Rape-trauma syndrome: compound reaction
Rape-trauma syndrome: silent reaction
Relocation stress syndrome
Relocation stress syndrome, Risk for
Role performance, Ineffective

Self-care deficit, Bathing/hygiene
Self-care deficit, Dressing/grooming

Self-care deficit, Feeding
Self-care deficit, Toileting
Self-concept, Readiness for enhanced
Self-esteem, Chronic low
Self-esteem, Situational low
Self-esteem, Risk for situational low
Self-mutilation
Self-mutilation, Risk for
Sensory perception, Disturbed
Sexual dysfunction
Sexuality pattern, Ineffective
Skin integrity, Impaired
Skin integrity, Risk for impaired
Sleep deprivation
Sleep pattern, Disturbed
Sleep, Readiness for enhanced
Social interaction, Impaired
Social isolation
Sorrow, Chronic
Spiritual distress
Spiritual distress, Risk for
Spiritual well-being, Readiness for enhanced
Suffocation, Risk for
Suicide, Risk for
Surgical recovery, Delayed
Swallowing, Impaired

Therapeutic regimen management, Effective
Therapeutic regimen management, Ineffective
Therapeutic regimen management, Readiness for enhanced
Therapeutic regimen management, Ineffective community
Therapeutic regimen management, Ineffective family
Thermoregulation, Ineffective
Thought processes, Disturbed
Tissue integrity, Impaired
Tissue perfusion, Ineffective
Transfer ability, Impaired
Trauma, Risk for

Urinary elimination, Impaired
Urinary elimination, Readiness for enhanced
Urinary retention

Ventilation, Impaired spontaneous
Ventilatory weaning response, Dysfunctional
Violence, Risk for other-directed
Violence, Risk for self-directed

Walking, Impaired
Wandering

APPENDIX B

Diagnostic Criteria for Mental Disorders (*DSM-IV-TR*)

DSM-IV-TR Classification

NOS = Not Otherwise Specified.

An *x* appearing in a diagnostic code indicates that a specific code number is required.

An ellipsis (. . .) is used in the names of certain disorders to indicate that the name of a specific mental disorder or general medical condition should be inserted when recording the name (e.g., 293.0 Delirium Due to Hypothyroidism).

If criteria are currently met, one of the following severity specifiers may be noted after the diagnosis:

Mild
Moderate
Severe

If criteria are no longer met, one of the following specifiers may be noted:

In Partial Remission
In Full Remission
Prior History

▌DISORDERS USUALLY FIRST DIAGNOSED IN INFANCY, CHILDHOOD, OR ADOLESCENCE

Mental Retardation

NOTE: *These are coded on Axis II.*

317	Mild Mental Retardation
318.0	Moderate Mental Retardation
318.1	Severe Mental Retardation
318.2	Profound Mental Retardation
319	Mental Retardation, Severity Unspecified

Learning Disorders

315.00	Reading Disorder
315.1	Mathematics Disorder
315.2	Disorder of Written Expression
315.9	Learning Disorder NOS

Motor Skills Disorder

315.4	Developmental Coordination Disorder

From American Psychiatric Association: *Diagnostic and statistical manual of mental disorders*, ed 4, text revision, Washington, DC, 2000, American Psychiatric Association.

Communication Disorders

315.31	Expressive Language Disorder
315.32	Mixed Receptive-Expressive Language Disorder
315.39	Phonologic Disorder
307.0	Stuttering
307.9	Communication Disorder NOS

Pervasive Developmental Disorders

299.00	Autistic Disorder
299.80	Rett's Disorder
299.10	Childhood Disintegrative Disorder
299.80	Asperger's Disorder
299.80	Pervasive Developmental Disorder NOS

Attention-Deficit and Disruptive Behavior Disorders

314.xx	Attention-Deficit/Hyperactivity Disorder
.01	Combined Type
.00	Predominantly Inattentive Type
.01	Predominantly Hyperactive-Impulsive Type
314.9	Attention-Deficit/Hyperactivity Disorder NOS
312.xx	Conduct Disorder
.81	Childhood-Onset Type
.82	Adolescent-Onset Type
.89	Unspecified Onset
313.81	Oppositional Defiant Disorder
312.9	Disruptive Behavior Disorder NOS

Feeding and Eating Disorders of Infancy or Early Childhood

307.52	Pica
307.53	Rumination Disorder
307.59	Feeding Disorder of Infancy or Early Childhood

Tic Disorders

307.23	Tourette's Disorder
307.22	Chronic Motor or Vocal Tic Disorder
307.21	Transient Tic Disorder
	Specify if: Single Episode/Recurrent
307.20	Tic Disorder NOS

Elimination Disorders

	Encopresis
787.6	With Constipation and Overflow Incontinence
307.7	Without Constipation and Overflow Incontinence
307.6	Enuresis (Not Due to a General Medical Condition)

Specify type: Nocturnal Only/Diurnal Only/Nocturnal and Diurnal

Other Disorders of Infancy, Childhood, or Adolescence

309.21	Separation Anxiety Disorder
	Specify if: Early Onset
313.23	Selective Mutism
313.89	Reactive Attachment Disorder of Infancy or Early Childhood
	Specify type: Inhibited Type/Disinhibited Type
307.3	Stereotypic Movement Disorder
	Specify if: With Self-Injurious Behavior
313.9	Disorder of Infancy, Childhood, or Adolescence NOS

DELIRIUM, DEMENTIA, AND AMNESTIC AND OTHER COGNITIVE DISORDERS

Delirium

293.0	Delirium Due to . . . *[Indicate the General Medical Condition]*
___.___	Substance Intoxication Delirium (*refer to Substance-Related Disorders for substance-specific codes*)
___.___	Substance Withdrawal Delirium (*refer to Substance-Related Disorders for substance-specific codes*)
___.___	Delirium Due to Multiple Etiologies (*code each of the specific etiologies*)
780.09	Delirium NOS

Dementia

294.xx	Dementia of the Alzheimer's Type, With Early Onset (*also code 331.0 Alzheimer's disease on Axis III*)
.10	Without Behavioral Disturbance
.11	With Behavioral Disturbance
294.xx	Dementia of the Alzheimer's Type, With Late Onset (*also code 331.0 Alzheimer's disease on Axis III*)
.10	Without Behavioral Disturbance
.11	With Behavioral Disturbance
290.xx	Vascular Dementia
.40	Uncomplicated
.41	With Delirium
.42	With Delusions
.43	With Depressed Mood

Specify if: With Behavioral Disturbance

Code presence or absence of a behavioral disturbance in the fifth digit for Dementia Due to a General Medical Condition:

0 = Without Behavioral Disturbance
1 = With Behavioral Disturbance

294.1x	Dementia Due to HIV Disease (*also code 042 HIV on Axis III*)
294.1x	Dementia Due to Head Trauma (*also code 854.00 head injury on Axis III*)
294.1x	Dementia Due to Parkinson's Disease (*also code 332.0 Parkinson's disease on Axis III*)
294.1x	Dementia Due to Huntington's Disease (*also code 333.4 Huntington's disease on Axis III*)
294.1x	Dementia Due to Pick's Disease (*also code 331.1 Pick's disease on Axis III*)
294.1x	Dementia Due to Creutzfeldt-Jakob Disease (*also code 046.1 Creutzfeldt-Jakob disease on Axis III*)
294.1x	Dementia Due to . . . *[Indicate the General Medical Condition not listed above]* (*also code the general medical condition on Axis III*)
___.___	Substance-Induced Persisting Dementia (*refer to Substance-Related Disorders for substance-specific codes*)
___.___	Dementia Due to Multiple Etiologies (*code each of the specific etiologies*)
294.8	Dementia NOS

Amnestic Disorders

294.0	Amnestic Disorder Due to . . . *[Indicate the General Medical Condition]*
	Specify if: Transient/Chronic
___.___	Substance-Induced Persisting Amnestic Disorder (*refer to Substance-Related Disorders for substance-specific codes*)
294.8	Amnestic Disorder NOS

Other Cognitive Disorders

294.9	Cognitive Disorder NOS

MENTAL DISORDERS DUE TO A GENERAL MEDICAL CONDITION NOT ELSEWHERE CLASSIFIED

293.89	Catatonic Disorder Due to . . . *[Indicate the General Medical Condition]*
310.1	Personality Change Due to . . . *[Indicate the General Medical Condition]*
	Specify type: Labile Type/Disinhibited Type/Aggressive Type/Apathetic Type/Paranoid Type/Other Type/Combined Type/Unspecified Type
293.9	Mental Disorder NOS Due to . . . *[Indicate the General Medical Condition]*

■ SUBSTANCE-RELATED DISORDERS

The following specifiers may be applied to Substance Dependence as noted:

[a]With Physiologic Dependence/Without Physiologic Dependence

[b]Early Full Remission/Early Partial Remission/Sustained Full Remission/Sustained Partial Remission

[c]In a Controlled Environment

[d]On Agonist Therapy

The following specifiers apply to Substance-Induced Disorders as noted:

[I]With Onset During Intoxication/[W]With Onset During Withdrawal

Alcohol-Related Disorders

Alcohol Use Disorders

303.90	Alcohol Dependence[a,b,c]
305.00	Alcohol Abuse

Alcohol-Induced Disorders

303.00	Alcohol Intoxication
291.81	Alcohol Withdrawal
	Specify if: With Perceptual Disturbances
291.0	Alcohol Intoxication Delirium
291.0	Alcohol Withdrawal Delirium
291.2	Alcohol-Induced Persisting Dementia
291.1	Alcohol-Induced Persisting Amnestic Disorder
291.x	Alcohol-Induced Psychotic Disorder
.5	With Delusions[I,W]
.3	With Hallucinations[I,W]
291.89	Alcohol-Induced Mood Disorder[I,W]
291.89	Alcohol-Induced Anxiety Disorder[I,W]
291.89	Alcohol-Induced Sexual Dysfunction[I]
291.89	Alcohol-Induced Sleep Disorder[I,W]
291.9	Alcohol-Related Disorder NOS

Amphetamine (or Amphetamine-Like)– Related Disorders

Amphetamine Use Disorders

304.40	Amphetamine Dependence[a,b,c]
305.70	Amphetamine Abuse

Amphetamine-Induced Disorders

292.89	Amphetamine Intoxication
	Specify if: With Perceptual Disturbances
292.0	Amphetamine Withdrawal
292.81	Amphetamine Intoxication Delirium
292.xx	Amphetamine-Induced Psychotic Disorder
.11	With Delusions[I]
.12	With Hallucinations[I]
292.84	Amphetamine-Induced Mood Disorder[I,W]
292.89	Amphetamine-Induced Anxiety Disorder[I]
292.89	Amphetamine-Induced Sexual Dysfunction[I]
292.89	Amphetamine-Induced Sleep Disorder[I,W]
292.9	Amphetamine-Related Disorder NOS

Caffeine-Related Disorders

Caffeine-Induced Disorders

305.90	Caffeine Intoxication
292.89	Caffeine-Induced Anxiety Disorder[I]
292.89	Caffeine-Induced Sleep Disorder[I]
292.9	Caffeine-Related Disorder NOS

Cannabis-Related Disorders

Cannabis Use Disorders

304.30	Cannabis Dependence[a,b,c]
305.20	Cannabis Abuse

Cannabis-Induced Disorders

292.89	Cannabis Intoxication
	Specify if: With Perceptual Disturbances
292.81	Cannabis Intoxication Delirium
292.xx	Cannabis-Induced Psychotic Disorder
.11	With Delusions[I]
.12	With Hallucinations[I]
292.89	Cannabis-Induced Anxiety Disorder[I]
292.9	Cannabis-Related Disorder NOS

Cocaine-Related Disorders

Cocaine Use Disorders

304.20	Cocaine Dependence[a,b,c]
305.60	Cocaine Abuse

Cocaine-Induced Disorders

292.89	Cocaine Intoxication
	Specify if: With Perceptual Disturbances
292.0	Cocaine Withdrawal
292.81	Cocaine Intoxication Delirium
292.xx	Cocaine-Induced Psychotic Disorder
.11	With Delusions[I]
.12	With Hallucinations[I]
292.84	Cocaine-Induced Mood Disorder[I,W]
292.89	Cocaine-Induced Anxiety Disorder[I,W]
292.89	Cocaine-Induced Sexual Dysfunction[I]
292.89	Cocaine-Induced Sleep Disorder[I,W]
292.9	Cocaine-Related Disorder NOS

Hallucinogen-Related Disorders

Hallucinogen Use Disorders

304.50	Hallucinogen Dependence[b,c]
305.30	Hallucinogen Abuse

Hallucinogen-Induced Disorders

292.89	Hallucinogen Intoxication
292.89	Hallucinogen Persisting Perception Disorder (Flashbacks)
292.81	Hallucinogen Intoxication Delirium
292.xx	Hallucinogen-Induced Psychotic Disorder
.11	With Delusions[I]
.12	With Hallucinations[I]
292.84	Hallucinogen-Induced Mood Disorder[I]
292.89	Hallucinogen-Induced Anxiety Disorder[I]
292.9	Hallucinogen-Related Disorder NOS

Inhalant-Related Disorders

Inhalant Use Disorders
304.60 Inhalant Dependence[b,c]
305.90 Inhalant Abuse

Inhalant-Induced Disorders
292.89 Inhalant Intoxication
292.81 Inhalant Intoxication Delirium
292.82 Inhalant-Induced Persisting Dementia
292.xx Inhalant-Induced Psychotic Disorder
.11   With Delusions[I]
.12   With Hallucinations[I]
292.84 Inhalant-Induced Mood Disorder[I]
292.89 Inhalant-Induced Anxiety Disorder[I]
292.9 Inhalant-Related Disorder NOS

Nicotine-Related Disorders

Nicotine Use Disorder
305.1 Nicotine Dependence[a,b]

Nicotine-Induced Disorder
292.0 Nicotine Withdrawal
292.9 Nicotine-Related Disorder NOS

Opioid-Related Disorders

Opioid Use Disorders
304.00 Opioid Dependence[a,b,c,d]
305.50 Opioid Abuse

Opioid-Induced Disorders
292.89 Opioid Intoxication
        Specify if: With Perceptual Disturbances
292.0 Opioid Withdrawal
292.81 Opioid Intoxication Delirium
292.xx Opioid-Induced Psychotic Disorder
.11   With Delusions[I]
.12   With Hallucinations[I]
292.84 Opioid-Induced Mood Disorder[I]
292.89 Opioid-Induced Sexual Dysfunction[I]
292.89 Opioid-Induced Sleep Disorder[I,W]
292.9 Opioid-Related Disorder NOS

Phencyclidine (or Phencyclidine-Like)–Related Disorders

Phencyclidine Use Disorders
304.60 Phencyclidine Dependence[b,c]
305.90 Phencyclidine Abuse

Phencyclidine-Induced Disorders
292.89 Phencyclidine Intoxication
        Specify if: With Perceptual Disturbances
292.81 Phencyclidine Intoxication Delirium
292.xx Phencyclidine-Induced Psychotic Disorder
.11   With Delusions[I]
.12   With Hallucinations[I]
292.84 Phencyclidine-Induced Mood Disorder[I]

292.89 Phencyclidine-Induced Anxiety Disorder[I]
292.9 Phencyclidine-Related Disorder NOS

Sedative-, Hypnotic-, or Anxiolytic-Related Disorders

Sedative, Hypnotic, or Anxiolytic Use Disorders
304.10 Sedative, Hypnotic, or Anxiolytic Dependence[a,b,c]
305.40 Sedative, Hypnotic, or Anxiolytic Abuse

Sedative-, Hypnotic-, or Anxiolytic-Induced Disorders
292.89 Sedative, Hypnotic, or Anxiolytic Intoxication
292.0 Sedative, Hypnotic, or Anxiolytic Withdrawal
        Specify if: With Perceptual Disturbances
292.81 Sedative, Hypnotic, or Anxiolytic Intoxication Delirium
292.81 Sedative, Hypnotic, or Anxiolytic Withdrawal Delirium
292.82 Sedative-, Hypnotic-, or Anxiolytic-Induced Persisting Dementia
292.83 Sedative-, Hypnotic-, or Anxiolytic-Induced Persisting Amnestic Disorder
292.xx Sedative-, Hypnotic-, or Anxiolytic-Induced Psychotic Disorder
.11   With Delusions[I,W]
.12   With Hallucinations[I,W]
292.84 Sedative-, Hypnotic-, or Anxiolytic-Induced Mood Disorder[I,W]
292.89 Sedative-, Hypnotic-, or Anxiolytic-Induced Anxiety Disorder[W]
292.89 Sedative-, Hypnotic-, or Anxiolytic-Induced Sexual Dysfunction[I]
292.89 Sedative-, Hypnotic-, or Anxiolytic-Induced Sleep Disorder[I,W]
292.9 Sedative-, Hypnotic-, or Anxiolytic-Related Disorder NOS

Polysubstance-Related Disorder
304.80 Polysubstance Dependence[a,b,c,d]

Other (or Unknown) Substance-Related Disorders

Other (or Unknown) Substance Use Disorders
304.90 Other (or Unknown) Substance Dependence[a,b,c,d]
305.90 Other (or Unknown) Substance Abuse

Other (or Unknown) Substance-Induced Disorders
292.89 Other (or Unknown) Substance Intoxication
        Specify if: With Perceptual Disturbances
292.0 Other (or Unknown) Substance Withdrawal
        Specify if: With Perceptual Disturbances
292.81 Other (or Unknown) Substance–Induced Delirium
292.82 Other (or Unknown) Substance–Induced Persisting Dementia

292.83 Other (or Unknown) Substance–Induced Persisting Amnestic Disorder

292.xx Other (or Unknown) Substance–Induced Psychotic Disorder
   .11 With Delusions[I,W]
   .12 With Hallucinations[I,W]

292.84 Other (or Unknown) Substance–Induced Mood Disorder[I,W]

292.89 Other (or Unknown) Substance–Induced Anxiety Disorder[I,W]

292.89 Other (or Unknown) Substance–Induced Sexual Dysfunction[I]

292.89 Other (or Unknown) Substance–Induced Sleep Disorder[I,W]

292.9 Other (or Unknown) Substance–Related Disorder NOS

SCHIZOPHRENIA AND OTHER PSYCHOTIC DISORDERS

295.xx Schizophrenia

The following Classification of Longitudinal Course applies to all subtypes of Schizophrenia:

Episodic With Interepisode Residual Symptoms (*specify if:* With Prominent Negative Symptoms)/Episodic With No Interepisode Residual Symptoms

Continuous (*specify if:* With Prominent Negative Symptoms)

Single Episode in Partial Remission (*specify if:* With Prominent Negative Symptoms)/Single Episode In Full Remission

Other or Unspecified Pattern
   .30 Paranoid Type
   .10 Disorganized Type
   .20 Catatonic Type
   .90 Undifferentiated Type
   .60 Residual Type

295.40 Schizophreniform Disorder
Specify if: Without Good Prognostic Features/With Good Prognostic Features

295.70 Schizoaffective Disorder
Specify type: Bipolar Type/Depressive Type

297.1 Delusional Disorder
Specify type: Erotomanic Type/Grandiose Type/Jealous Type/Persecutory Type/Somatic Type/Mixed Type/Unspecified Type

298.8 Brief Psychotic Disorder
Specify if: With Marked Stressor(s)/Without Marked Stressor(s)/With Postpartum Onset

297.3 Shared Psychotic Disorder

293.xx Psychotic Disorder Due to . . . [*Indicate the General Medical Condition*]
   .81 With Delusions
   .82 With Hallucinations

___.___ Substance-Induced Psychotic Disorder (*refer to Substance-Related Disorders for substance-specific codes*)

Specify if: With Onset During Intoxication/ With Onset During Withdrawal

298.9 Psychotic Disorder NOS

MOOD DISORDERS

Code current state of Major Depressive Disorder or Bipolar I Disorder in fifth digit:

   1 = Mild
   2 = Moderate
   3 = Severe Without Psychotic Features
   4 = Severe With Psychotic Features
      Specify: Mood-Congruent Psychotic Features/Mood-Incongruent Psychotic Features
   5 = In Partial Remission
   6 = In Full Remission
   0 = Unspecified

The following specifiers apply (for current or most recent episode) to Mood Disorders as noted:
[a]Severity/Psychotic/Remission Specifiers/[b]Chronic/[c]With Catatonic Features/[d]With Melancholic Features/[e]With Atypical Features/[f]With Postpartum Onset

The following specifiers apply to Mood Disorders as noted:
[g]With or Without Full Interepisode Recovery/[h]With Seasonal Pattern/[i]With Rapid Cycling

Depressive Disorders

296.xx Major Depressive Disorder
   .2x Single Episode[a,b,c,d,e,f]
   .3x Recurrent[a,b,c,d,e,f,g,h]

300.4 Dysthymic Disorder
Specify if: Early Onset/Late Onset
Specify: With Atypical Features

311 Depressive Disorder NOS

Bipolar Disorders

296.xx Bipolar I Disorder
   .0x Single Manic Episode[a,c,f]
      Specify if: Mixed
   .40 Most Recent Episode Hypomanic[g,h,i]
   .4x Most Recent Episode Manic[a,c,f,g,h,i]
   .6x Most Recent Episode Mixed[a,c,f,g,h,i]
   .5x Most Recent Episode Depressed[a,b,c,d,e,f,g,h,i]
   .7 Most Recent Episode Unspecified[g,h,i]

296.89 Bipolar II Disorder[a,b,c,d,e,f,g,h,i]
Specify (current or most recent episode): Hypomanic/Depressed

301.13 Cyclothymic Disorder

296.80 Bipolar Disorder NOS

293.83 Mood Disorder Due to . . . [*Indicate the General Medical Condition*]
Specify type: With Depressive Features/With Major Depressive-Like Episode/With Manic Features/With Mixed Features

___.___ Substance-Induced Mood Disorder (*refer to Substance-Related Disorders for substance-specific codes*)

Specify type: With Depressive Features/With Manic Features/With Mixed Features
Specify if: With Onset During Intoxication/With Onset During Withdrawal

296.90 Mood Disorder NOS

ANXIETY DISORDERS

300.01 Panic Disorder Without Agoraphobia
300.21 Panic Disorder With Agoraphobia
300.22 Agoraphobia Without History of Panic Disorder
300.29 Specific Phobia
    Specify type: Animal Type/Natural Environment Type/Blood-Injection-Injury Type/Situational Type/Other Type
300.23 Social Phobia
    Specify if: Generalized
300.3 Obsessive-Compulsive Disorder
    Specify if: With Poor Insight
309.81 Posttraumatic Stress Disorder
    Specify if: Acute/Chronic
    Specify if: With Delayed Onset
308.3 Acute Stress Disorder
300.02 Generalized Anxiety Disorder
293.84 Anxiety Disorder Due to . . . [*Indicate the General Medical Condition*]
    Specify if: With Generalized Anxiety/With Panic Attacks/With Obsessive-Compulsive Symptoms
___.__ Substance-Induced Anxiety Disorder (*refer to Substance-Related Disorders for substance-specific codes*)
    Specify if: With Generalized Anxiety/With Panic Attacks/With Obsessive-Compulsive Symptoms/With Phobic Symptoms
    Specify if: With Onset During Intoxication/With Onset During Withdrawal
300.00 Anxiety Disorder NOS

SOMATOFORM DISORDERS

300.81 Somatization Disorder
300.82 Undifferentiated Somatoform Disorder
300.11 Conversion Disorder
    Specify type: With Motor Symptom or Deficit/With Sensory Symptom or Deficit/With Seizures or Convulsions/With Mixed Presentation
307.xx Pain Disorder
 .80 Associated With Psychologic Factors
 .89 Associated With Both Psychologic Factors and a General Medical Condition
    Specify if: Acute/Chronic
300.7 Hypochondriasis
    Specify if: With Poor Insight

300.7 Body Dysmorphic Disorder
300.82 Somatoform Disorder NOS

FACTITIOUS DISORDERS

300.xx Factitious Disorder
 .16 With Predominantly Psychologic Signs and Symptoms
 .19 With Predominantly Physical Signs and Symptoms
 .19 With Combined Psychologic and Physical Signs and Symptoms
300.19 Factitious Disorder NOS

DISSOCIATIVE DISORDERS

300.12 Dissociative Amnesia
300.13 Dissociative Fugue
300.14 Dissociative Identity Disorder
300.6 Depersonalization Disorder
300.15 Dissociative Disorder NOS

SEXUAL AND GENDER IDENTITY DISORDERS
Sexual Dysfunctions

The following specifiers apply to all primary Sexual Dysfunctions:
 Lifelong Type/Acquired Type
 Generalized Type/Situational Type
 Due to Psychologic Factors/Due to Combined Factors

Sexual Desire Disorders
302.71 Hypoactive Sexual Desire Disorder
302.79 Sexual Aversion Disorder

Sexual Arousal Disorders
302.72 Female Sexual Arousal Disorder
302.72 Male Erectile Disorder

Orgasmic Disorders
302.73 Female Orgasmic Disorder
302.74 Male Orgasmic Disorder
302.75 Premature Ejaculation

Sexual Pain Disorders
302.76 Dyspareunia (Not Due to a General Medical Condition)
306.51 Vaginismus (Not Due to a General Medical Condition)

Sexual Dysfunction Due to a General Medical Condition
625.8 Female Hypoactive Sexual Desire Disorder Due to . . . [*Indicate the General Medical Condition*]
608.89 Male Hypoactive Sexual Desire Disorder Due to . . . [*Indicate the General Medical Condition*]
607.84 Male Erectile Disorder Due to . . . [*Indicate the General Medical Condition*]

625.0	Female Dyspareunia Due to . . . *[Indicate the General Medical Condition]*
608.89	Male Dyspareunia Due to . . . *[Indicate the General Medical Condition]*
625.8	Other Female Sexual Dysfunction Due to . . . *[Indicate the General Medical Condition]*
608.89	Other Male Sexual Dysfunction Due to . . . *[Indicate the General Medical Condition]*
___.__	Substance-Induced Sexual Dysfunction (*refer to Substance-Related Disorders for substance-specific codes*) *Specify if:* With Impaired Desire/With Impaired Arousal/With Impaired Orgasm/With Sexual Pain *Specify if:* With Onset During Intoxication
302.70	Sexual Dysfunction NOS

Paraphilias

302.4	Exhibitionism
302.81	Fetishism
302.89	Frotteurism
302.2	Pedophilia *Specify if:* Sexually Attracted to Males/Sexually Attracted to Females/Sexually Attracted to Both *Specify if:* Limited to Incest *Specify type:* Exclusive Type/Nonexclusive Type
302.83	Sexual Masochism
302.84	Sexual Sadism
302.3	Transvestic Fetishism *Specify if:* With Gender Dysphoria
302.82	Voyeurism
302.9	Paraphilia NOS

Gender Identity Disorders

302.xx	Gender Identity Disorder
.6	In Children
.85	In Adolescents or Adults *Specify if:* Sexually Attracted to Males/Sexually Attracted to Females/Sexually Attracted to Both/ Sexually Attracted to Neither
302.6	Gender Identity Disorder NOS
302.9	Sexual Disorder NOS

■ EATING DISORDERS

307.1	Anorexia Nervosa *Specify type:* Restricting Type; Binge-Eating/Purging Type
307.51	Bulimia Nervosa *Specify type:* Purging Type/Nonpurging Type
307.50	Eating Disorder NOS

■ SLEEP DISORDERS
Primary Sleep Disorders

Dyssomnias

307.42	Primary Insomnia
307.44	Primary Hypersomnia *Specify if:* Recurrent
347	Narcolepsy
780.59	Breathing-Related Sleep Disorder
307.45	Circadian Rhythm Sleep Disorder *Specify type:* Delayed Sleep Phase Type/Jet Lag Type/Shift Work Type/Unspecified Type
307.47	Dyssomnia NOS

Parasomnias

307.47	Nightmare Disorder
307.46	Sleep Terror Disorder
307.46	Sleepwalking Disorder
307.47	Parasomnia NOS

Sleep Disorders Related to Another Mental Disorder

| 307.42 | Insomnia Related to . . . *[Indicate the Axis I or Axis II Disorder]* |
| 307.44 | Hypersomnia Related to . . . *[Indicate the Axis I or Axis II Disorder]* |

Other Sleep Disorders

780.xx	Sleep Disorder Due to . . . *[Indicate the General Medical Condition]*
.52	Insomnia Type
.54	Hypersomnia Type
.59	Parasomnia Type
.59	Mixed Type
___.__	Substance-Induced Sleep Disorder (*refer to Substance-Related Disorders for substance-specific codes*) *Specify type:* Insomnia Type/Hypersomnia Type/Parasomnia Type/Mixed Type *Specify if:* With Onset During Intoxication/ With Onset During Withdrawal

■ IMPULSE-CONTROL DISORDERS NOT ELSEWHERE CLASSIFIED

312.34	Intermittent Explosive Disorder
312.32	Kleptomania
312.33	Pyromania
312.31	Pathologic Gambling
312.39	Trichotillomania
312.30	Impulse-Control Disorder NOS

■ ADJUSTMENT DISORDERS

309.xx	Adjustment Disorder
.0	With Depressed Mood
.24	With Anxiety

.28   With Mixed Anxiety and Depressed Mood
.3   With Disturbance of Conduct
.4   With Mixed Disturbance of Emotions and
       Conduct
.9   Unspecified
       Specify if: Acute/Chronic

■ PERSONALITY DISORDERS

NOTE: *These are coded on Axis II.*

301.0	Paranoid Personality Disorder
301.20	Schizoid Personality Disorder
301.22	Schizotypal Personality Disorder
301.7	Antisocial Personality Disorder
301.83	Borderline Personality Disorder
301.50	Histrionic Personality Disorder
301.81	Narcissistic Personality Disorder
301.82	Avoidant Personality Disorder
301.6	Dependent Personality Disorder
301.4	Obsessive-Compulsive Personality Disorder
301.9	Personality Disorder NOS

■ OTHER CONDITIONS THAT MAY BE A FOCUS OF CLINICAL ATTENTION

Psychologic Factors Affecting Medical Condition

316   . . . [*Specified Psychologic Factor*] *Affecting* . . .
       [*Indicate the General Medical Condition*]
       Choose name based on nature of factors:
       Mental Disorder Affecting Medical
         Condition
       Psychological Symptoms Affecting Medical
         Condition
       Personality Traits or Coping Style Affecting
         Medical Condition
       Maladaptive Health Behaviors Affecting
         Medical Condition
       Stress-Related Physiological Response Affect-
         ing Medical Condition
       Other or Unspecified Psychological Factors
         Affecting Medical Condition

Medication-Induced Movement Disorders

332.1	Neuroleptic-Induced Parkinsonism
333.92	Neuroleptic Malignant Syndrome
333.7	Neuroleptic-Induced Acute Dystonia
333.99	Neuroleptic-Induced Acute Akathisia
333.82	Neuroleptic-Induced Tardive Dyskinesia
333.1	Medication-Induced Postural Tremor
333.90	Medication-Induced Movement Disorder NOS

Other Medication-Induced Disorder

995.2   Adverse Effects of Medication NOS

Relational Problems

V61.9   Relational Problem Related to a Mental
         Disorder or General Medical Condition

V61.20	Parent-Child Relational Problem
V61.10	Partner Relational Problem
V61.8	Sibling Relational Problem
V62.81	Relational Problem NOS

Problems Related to Abuse or Neglect

V61.21	Physical Abuse of Child
	(*code 995.5 if focus of attention is on victim*)
V61.21	Sexual Abuse of Child
	(*code 995.5 if focus of attention is on victim*)
V61.21	Neglect of Child
	(*code 995.5 if focus of attention is on victim*)
___.___	Physical Abuse of Adult
V61.12	(if by partner)
V62.83	(if by person other than partner) (*code 995.81 if focus of attention is on victim*)
___.___	Sexual Abuse of Adult
V61.12	(if by partner)
V62.83	(if by person other than partner) (*code 995.83 if focus of attention is on victim*)

Additional Conditions That May Be a Focus of Clinical Attention

V15.81	Noncompliance With Treatment
V65.2	Malingering
V71.01	Adult Antisocial Behavior
V71.02	Child or Adolescent Antisocial Behavior
V62.89	Borderline Intellectual Functioning
	NOTE: *This is coded on Axis II.*
780.9	Age-Related Cognitive Decline
V62.82	Bereavement
V62.3	Academic Problem
V62.2	Occupational Problem
313.82	Identity Problem
V62.89	Religious or Spiritual Problem
V62.4	Acculturation Problem
V62.89	Phase of Life Problem

■ ADDITIONAL CODES

300.9	Unspecified Mental Disorder (nonpsychotic)
V71.09	No Diagnosis or Condition on Axis I
799.9	Diagnosis or Condition Deferred on Axis I
V71.09	No Diagnosis on Axis II
799.9	Diagnosis Deferred on Axis II

■ AXIS II: PERSONALITY DISORDERS

301.0	Paranoid Personality Disorder
301.20	Schizoid Personality Disorder
301.22	Schizotypal Personality Disorder
301.7	Antisocial Personality Disorder
301.83	Borderline Personality Disorder
301.50	Histrionic Personality Disorder
301.81	Narcissistic Personality Disorder
301.82	Avoidant Personality Disorder
301.6	Dependent Personality Disorder

| 301.4 | Obsessive-Compulsive Personality Disorder |
| 301.9 | Personality Disorder NOS |

AXIS III: ICD-9-CM GENERAL MEDICAL CONDITIONS

Infectious and Parasitic Diseases (001-139)

Neoplasms (140-239)

Endocrine, Nutritional, and Metabolic Diseases and Immunity Disorders (240-279)

Diseases of the Blood and Blood-Forming Organs (280-289)

Diseases of the Nervous and Sense Organs (320-389)

Diseases of the Circulatory System (390-459)

Diseases of the Respiratory System (460-519)

Diseases of the Digestive System (520-579)

Diseases of the Genitourinary System (580-629)

Complications of Pregnancy, Childbirth, and the Puerperium (630-676)

Diseases of the Skin and Subcutaneous Tissue (680-709)

Diseases of the Musculoskeletal System and Connective Tissue (710-739)

Congenital Anomalies (740-759)

Certain Conditions Originating in the Perinatal Period (760-779)

Symptoms, Signs, and Ill-Defined Conditions (780-799)

Injury and Poisoning (800-999)

AXIS IV: PSYCHOSOCIAL AND ENVIRONMENTAL PROBLEMS

Problems with Primary Support Group (Childhood [V61.9], Adult [V61.9], Parent-Child [V61.2])—e.g., death of a family member; health problems in family; disruption of family by separation, divorce, or estrangement; removal from the home; remarriage of parent; sexual or physical abuse; parental overprotection; neglect of child; inadequate discipline; discord with siblings; birth of sibling

Problems Related to the Social Environment (V62.4)—e.g., death or loss of friend, inadequate social support, living alone, difficulty with acculturation, discrimination, adjustment to life cycle transition (such as retirement)

Educational Problems (V62.3)—e.g., illiteracy, academic problems, discord with teachers or classmates, inadequate school environment

Occupational Problems (V62.2)—e.g., unemployment, threat of job loss, stressful work schedule, difficult work conditions, job dissatisfaction, job change, discord with boss or co-workers

Housing Problems (V60.9)—e.g., homelessness, inadequate housing, unsafe neighborhood, discord with neighbors or landlord

Economic Problems (V60.9)—e.g., extreme poverty, inadequate finances, insufficient welfare support

Problems with Access to Health Care Services (V63.9)—e.g., inadequate health care services, transportation to health care facilities unavailable, inadequate health insurance

Problems Related to Interaction with the Legal System/Crime (V62.5)—e.g., arrest, incarceration, litigation, victim of crime

Other Psychosocial and Environmental Problems (V62.9)—e.g., exposure to disasters, war, other hostilities; discord with non-family caregivers such as counselor, social worker, or physician; unavailability of social service agencies

AXIS V: GLOBAL ASSESSMENT OF FUNCTIONING (GAF) SCALE

Consider psychological, social, and occupational functioning on a hypothetical continuum of mental health–illness. Do not include impairment in functioning due to physical (or environmental) limitations.

Code (NOTE: Use intermediate codes when appropriate, e.g., 45, 68, 72.)

100 **Superior functioning in a wide range of activities, life's problems never seem to get out of hand, is sought out by others because of his many positive qualities. No symptoms.**

91

90 **Absent or minimal symptoms** (e.g., mild anxiety before an exam), **good functioning in all areas, interested and involved in a wide range of activities, socially effective, generally satisfied with life, no more than everyday problems or concerns** (e.g., an occasional argument with family members).

81

80 **If symptoms are present, they are transient and expectable reactions to psychosocial stressors** (e.g., difficulty concentrating after family argument); **no more than slight impairment in social, occupational, or school functioning** (e.g., temporarily falling behind in schoolwork).

71

70 **Some mild symptoms** (e.g., depressed mood and mild insomnia) **OR some difficulty in social, occupational, or school functioning** (e.g., occasional truancy, or theft within the household), **but generally functioning pretty well, has some meaningful interpersonal relationships.**

61

The rating of overall psychological functioning on a scale of 0-100 was operationalized by Luborsky in the Health-Sickness Rating Scale (Luborsky L: Clinicians' judgments of mental health, *Arch Gen Psychiatry* 7:407-417, 1962). Spitzer and colleagues developed a revision of the Health-Sickness Rating Scale called the Global Assessment Scale (GAS) (Endicott J et al: The global assessment scale: a procedure for measuring overall severity of psychiatric disturbance, *Arch Gen Psychiatry* 33:766-771, 1976). A modified version of the GAS was included in *DSM-III-R* as the Global Assessment of Functioning (GAF) Scale.

60 **Moderate symptoms** (e.g., flat affect and circumstantial speech, occasional panic attacks) **OR moderate difficulty in social, occupational, or school functioning** (e.g, few friends, conflicts with peers or co-workers).

51

50 **Serious symptoms** (e.g., suicidal ideation, severe obsessional rituals, frequent shoplifting) **OR any serious impairment in social, occupational, or school functioning** (e.g., no friends, unable to keep a job).

41

40 **Some impairment in reality testing or communication** (e.g., speech is at times illogical, obscure, or irrelevant) **OR major impairment in several areas, such as work or school, family relations, judgment, thinking, or mood** (e.g., depressed man avoids friends, neglects family, and is unable to work; child frequently beats up younger children, is defiant at home, and is failing at school).

31

30 **Behavior is considerably influenced by delusions or hallucinations OR serious impairment in communication or judgment** (e.g., sometimes incoherent, acts grossly inappropriately, suicidal preoccupation) **OR inability to function in almost all areas** (e.g., stays in bed all day; no job, home, or friends).

21

20 **Some danger of hurting self or others** (e.g., suicide attempts without clear expectation of death, frequently violent, manic excitement) **OR occasionally fails to maintain minimal personal hygiene** (e.g., smears feces) **OR gross impairment in communication** (e.g., largely incoherent or mute).

11

10 **Persistent danger of severely hurting self or others** (e.g., recurrent violence) **OR persistent inability to maintain personal hygiene OR serious suicidal act with clear expectation of death.**

1

0 Inadequate information.

Outline for Cultural Formulation

The following outline for cultural formulation is meant to supplement the multiaxial diagnostic assessment and to address difficulties that may be encountered in applying DSM-IV criteria in a multicultural environment. The cultural formulation provides a systematic review of the individual's cultural background, the role of the cultural context in the expression and evaluation of symptoms and dysfunction, and the effect and cultural differences they may have on the relationship between the individual and the clinician.

It is important that the clinician take into account the individual's ethnic and cultural context in the evaluation of each of the DSM-IV axes. In addition, the cultural formulation suggested below provides an opportunity to describe systematically the individual's cultural and social reference group and ways in which the cultural context is relevant to clinical care. The clinician may provide a narrative summary for each of the following categories:

Cultural identity of the individual. Note the individual's ethnic or cultural reference groups. For immigrants and ethnic minorities, note separately the degree of involvement with both the culture of origin and the host culture (where applicable). Also note language abilities, use, and preference (including multilingualism).

Cultural explanations of the individual's illness. The following may be identified: the predominant idioms of distress through which symptoms or the need for social support are communicated (e.g., "nerves," possessing spirits, somatic complaints, inexplicable misfortune), the meaning and perceived severity of the individual's symptoms in relation to norms of the cultural reference group, any local illness category used by the individual's family and community to identify the condition, the perceived causes or explanatory models that the individual and the reference group use to explain the illness, and current preferences for and past experiences with professional and popular sources of care.

Cultural factors related to psychosocial environment and levels of functioning. Note culturally relevant interpretations of social stressors, available social supports, and levels of functioning and disability. This would include stresses in the local social environment and the role of religion and kin networks in providing emotional, instrumental, and informational support.

Cultural elements of the relationship between the individual and the clinician. Indicate differences in culture and social status between the individual and the clinician and problems that these differences may cause in diagnosis and treatment (e.g., difficulty in communicating in the individual's first language, in eliciting symptoms or understanding their cultural significance, in negotiating an appropriate relationship or level of intimacy, in determining whether a behavior is normative or pathological).

Overall cultural assessment for diagnosis and care. The formulation concludes with a discussion of how cultural considerations specifically influence comprehensive diagnosis and care.

Appendix C

Behavioral Rating Scales

■ GENERAL HEALTH

Clarity Health Assessment Scales Index Version
Clarity Well-Being Scales Comprehensive Version
Freidman Quality of Life Scale
Freidman Well-Being Scale
Functional Activities Questionnaire
General Health Questionnaire (GHQ)
Katz Index of Activities of Daily Living
MOS Health Survey (SF-36)
MOS Health Survey (SF-12)
Older Americans Resources and Services (OARS) Social
    Resources Scale
Sickness Impact Profile
Social Skills Inventory
Tennessee Self-Concept Scale: Second Edition (TSCS:2)

■ GENERAL PSYCHIATRIC

Acculturation Scale
Acuity of Psychiatric Illness, Adult Version
Behavior and Symptom Identification Scale (BASIS-32)
Behavior Rating Scale
Brief Psychiatric Rating Scale (BPRS)
Brief Symptom Inventory (BSI)
Brown Assessment of Beliefs Scale
Clinical Global Impression (CGI)
Colorado Client Assessment Record (CCAR)
Columbia Impairment Scale (CIS)
Community-Oriented Programs Environmental Scale
    (COPES)
Compass Treatment Assessment System
Conners' Adult ADHD Rating Scales (CAARS)
COPE Inventory
Derogatis Psychiatric Rating Scale (DPRS)
Employee Assistance Program Index
Functional Assessment Rating Scale (FARS)
Functional Status Questionnaire (FSQ)
Goal Attainment Scale
Global Assessment Scale (GAS)
Global Assessment of Functioning Scale (GAF)
Independent and Living Skills
Menninger Revision of Role Functioning Scale
Million Clinical Multiaxial Inventory III (MCMI-III)
Multnomah Community Ability Scale
Neuropsychological Impairment Scale (NIS)

Nurse Observation Scale for Inpatient Evaluation (NOSIE)
Personal Adjustment and Role Skills (PARS)
Personal Problem Scale (PPS) and Personal Functioning
    Index (PFI)
Profile of Adaptation to Life (PAL Scale)
PsychSentinel 3.2
Quality of Life Interview (QOLI)
Quality of Life Inventory (QOLI)
Quality of Well-Being Scale (QWB)
Role Functioning Scale
Self-Perception Profile for Adults
Sheehan Disability Scale
Social Adjustment Scale II
Social Behavior Schedule
Social Dysfunction Rating Scale
Social Functioning Scale
Social Readjustment Scale
Stress Response Scale (SRS)
Structured Clinical Interview for the DSM-IV
Symptom Checklist-90 (SCL-90)
Treatment Events Checklist (TEC)
Treatment Outcome Package (TOP)
Treatment Outcome Profile
Young Adult Behavior Checklist
Young Adult Self-Report (YASR)

■ AFFECTIVE DISORDERS

Apparent Affect Rating Scale (AARS)
Beck Depression Inventory (BDI)
Beck Depression Inventory II (BDI-II)
Carroll Self-Rating Scale
Center for Epidemiologic Studies Depression Scale (CES-D)
Dementia Mood Assessment Scale (DMAS)
Depression Arkansas Scale (D-ARK Scale)
Depression Outcome Module (DOM)
Geriatric Depression Scale (GDS)
Hamilton Depression Scale (Ham-D)
Inventory for Depressive Symptomatology (IDS)
Manic State Rating Scale (MSRS)
Montgomery-Asberg Depression Rating Scale (MADRS)
Profile of Mood States
Raskin Depression Scale
Young Mania Scale
Zung Self-Rating Depression Scale (ZSRDS)

■ AGGRESSION

Brown-Goodwin Assessment for Life History of Aggression
Buss-Durkee Hostility Inventory
Hostility and Direction of Hostility Questionnaire
Overt Aggression Scale

■ ANXIETY DISORDERS

Beck Anxiety Inventory (BAI)
Brief Social Phobia Scale
Covi Anxiety Scale
Dissociative Experience Scale
Dissociative Disorders Interview Schedule (DDIS)
Hamilton Rating Scale for Anxiety (Ham-A)
Maudsley Obsessional Compulsive Inventory
Panic Disorder Outcomes Module (PDOM)
Panic Disorder Severity Scale
Phobic Avoidance Rating Scale
Posttraumatic Distress Disorder (PTSD) Inventory
Spielberger State-Trait Anxiety Inventory (STAI)
Taylor Anxiety Scale
Yale-Brown Obsessive Compulsive Scale (YBOCS)
Zung Anxiety Scale

■ EATING DISORDERS

Body Attitudes Test
Diagnostic Survey for Eating Disorders (DSED)
Eating Behaviors Diary
Eating Disorders Inventory 2 (EDI-2)
Eating Habits Checklist

■ ORGANIC MENTAL DISORDERS

Alzheimer's Disease Assessment Scale (ADAS)
Behavior Pathology in Alzheimer's Disease
Blessed Dementia Scale
Brief Cognitive Rating Scale
Clinical Dementia Rating Scale
Cognitive Abilities Screening Instrument (CASI)
Cohen-Mansfield Agitation Inventory
Confusion Assessment Method
Cornell Scale for Depression in Dementia
Delirium Index
Delirium Rating Scale
Delirium Symptom Interview
Disruptive Behavior Scale
Face-Hand Test
Haycox Dementia Behavioral Scale
Memory and Behavior Problems Checklist
Mini-Mental State Examination (MMSE)
Multidimensional Observation Scale for Elderly Subjects
Neecham Confusion Scale
Neurobehavioral Rating Scale for Dementia (NRS)
Overt Agitation Severity Scale
Short Portable Mental Status Questionnaire (SPMSQ)

■ PSYCHOTIC DISORDERS

Behavioral Observation Schedule
Brief Psychiatric Rating Scale (BPRS)
Life Skills Profile: Schizophrenia (LSP)
Positive and Negative Syndrome Scale (PANSS)
Scale for Assessment of Negative Symptoms (SANS)
Scale for Assessment of Positive Symptoms (SAPS)
Schizophrenia Outcomes Module (SOM)
University of Washington Paranoia Scale

■ SUBSTANCE USE DISORDERS

Addiction Severity Index (ASI)
Alcohol Dependence Scale (ADS)
Alcohol/Substance Abuse Questionnaire (ASAQ)
Alcohol Use Disorders Identification Test (AUDIT)
Alcohol Use Inventory (AUI)
Alcohol Use Scale (AUS)
Brief Drug Abuse Screening Test (B-DAST)
CAGE Questionnaire
Chemical Use, Abuse, and Dependence Scale (CUAD)
Children of Alcoholics Screening Test (CAST)
Clinical Institute Narcotic Assessment (CINA)
Clinical Institute Withdrawal Assessment–Alcohol, Revised (CIWA–AR)
Drug Abuse Screening Test (DAST)
Drug Use Scale (DUS)
Drug Use Screening Inventory (revised) (DUSI)
Family Alcohol and Drug Survey (FADS)
Follow-up Drinker Profile
Inventory of Drinking Situations (IDS)
Michigan Alcoholism Screening Tool (MAST)
Rapid Alcohol Problems Screen (RAPS)
Rutgers Alcohol Problem Index (RAPI)
Substance Abuse Outcome Module (SAOM)
Substance Abuse Subtle Screening Inventory (SASSI)
Substance Abuse Treatment Schedule (SATS)
Treatment Services Review (TSR)

■ SUICIDALITY

Assessment of Suicidal Potentiality
Beck Scale for Suicidal Ideation
Suicide Risk Scale

■ ANTIPSYCHOTIC MEDICATION SIDE EFFECTS

Abnormal Involuntary Movement Scale (AIMS)
Barnes Akathesia Scale
Simpson-Angus Extrapyramidal Symptoms Scale

■ CHILD

ADHD Rating Scale–IV
Ansell-Casey Life Skills Assessment 2.0 (ACLSA)
Brief Psychiatric Rating Scale (BPRS) for Children

Caregiver-Teacher Report Form for Ages 2-5 (C-TRF/2.5)

Child and Adolescent Adjustment Profile (CAAP)

Child and Adolescent Functional Assessment Scale (CAFAS)

Child Assessment Schedule (CAS)

Child Behavior Checklist (CBCL)

Child Depression Inventory

Children's Depression Rating Scale, R (CDRS-R)

Children's Global Assessment Scale (CGAS)

Columbia Impairment Scale

Competency Skills Questionnaire (CSQ)

Conners' Parent and Teacher Rating Scale—Home and School Questionnaire

Developmental Behavior Checklist

Devereux Rating Scale School Form (DSF)

Direct Observation Form and Profile for Ages 5-14 (DOF)

Ohio Youth Problems, Functioning, and Satisfaction Scales

Revised Behavior Problem Checklist

Severity of Psychiatric Illness: Child and Adolescent Version

Self-Control Rating Scale

Tennessee Self-Concept Scale: Second Edition (TSCS-2)

Vanderbilt Functioning Inventory (VFI)

Yale-Brown Obsessive Compulsive Scale (YBOCS) for Children

Youth Outcome Questionnaire (YOQ)

■ ADOLESCENT

Adolescent Drinking Index (ADI)

Adolescent Treatment Outcomes Module (ATOM)

Ansell-Casey Life Skills Assessment 2.0 (ACLSA)

Child and Adolescent Adjustment Profile (CAAP)

Child and Adolescent Functional Assessment Scale (CAFAS)

Devereux Rating Scale School Form (DSF)

Devereux Scales of Mental Disorders (DSMD)

Million Adolescent Clinical Inventory (MACI)

Million Adolescent Personality Inventory (MAPI)

Ohio Youth Problems, Functioning, and Satisfaction Scales

Revised Behavior Problem Index (RAPI)

Severity of Psychiatric Illness: Child and Adolescent Version

Tennessee Self-Concept Scale: Second Edition (TSCS-2)

Vanderbilt Functioning Inventory (VFI)

Youth Outcome Questionnaire (YOQ)

Youth Self Report (YSR)

■ FAMILY

Assessment of Strategies in Families Effectiveness Scale

Conflict Tactics Scale

Family APGAR

Family Burden Interview Schedule (FBIS)

Family Empowerment Scale

Family Environment Scale (FES)

Family Functioning Measures

Zarit Burden Interview

■ HEALTH SERVICES

Beginning Services Syndrome (BSS)

Behavioral Healthcare Rating of Satisfaction (BHRS)

Client Experience Questionnaire (CEQ)

Client Satisfaction Questionnaire (CSQ)

Client Satisfaction Survey (CSS)

Consumer Satisfaction Index (CSI)

Inpatient Patient Satisfaction Survey System

Managed Care Organization Satisfaction Survey (MCO-SS)

Older Adults Resources and Services (OARS)

Outpatient Patient Satisfaction Survey System

Patient Satisfaction Survey IV (PSS-IV)

Perceptions of Care (Inpatient and Outpatient)

Process of Care Review Form

Satisfaction Survey (SS)

Service Satisfaction Scale (SSS-30)

Treatment Satisfaction Survey

Youth Satisfaction Questionnaire

APPENDIX **D**

Answers to Chapter Review Questions

Chapter 1

1. A. Linda Richards
   B. Hildegard Peplau
   C. direct care, communication, management
   D. Basic (RN); advanced (APRN)
   E. American Psychiatric Nurses Association
2. A. True   C. True
   B. True   D. True
   E. False: More than 82,000 psychiatric nurses are working in mental health organizations.
   F. False: Few studies have been conducted in this important area of psychiatric nursing.
3. A. The development of psychotropic drugs allowed patients to become more treatable, and fewer environmental constraints were needed to contain patient behavior. Also, the introduction of medications gave new hope to psychiatric patients and allowed psychiatric nurses to spend more time engaging patients in therapeutic activities.
   B. The five core mental health disciplines are psychiatric nursing, marriage and family therapy, psychiatry, psychology, and social work.
   C. The six dimensions of the nurse-patient partnership are clinical competence, patient-family advocacy, fiscal responsibility, interdisciplinary collaboration, social accountability, and legal-ethical parameters.
   D. Individual answers will vary.

Chapter 2

1. A. Preinteraction   F. Orientation
   B. Orientation   G. Preinteraction
   C. Orientation   H. Working
   D. Termination   I. Working
   E. Working   J. Termination
2. A. incongruent
   B. validation
   C. empathy
   D. boundary violation
3. A. Will the self-disclosure enhance the patient's (1) cooperation, (2) learning, (3) catharsis, or (4) support?
   B. Names of individuals, roles of nurse and patient, responsibilities of nurse and patient, expectations of nurse and patient, purpose of the relationship, meeting location and time, conditions for termination, confidentiality

   C. Use of feelings
         Social: Variable
         Therapeutic: Patient encouraged to share feelings
      Content of interaction
         Social: Social and spontaneous
         Therapeutic: Goal-directed and purposeful
      Confidentiality
         Social: Not an issue
         Therapeutic: Protection for the patient
      Termination
         Social: Open-ended
         Therapeutic: Mutually predetermined and honored
   D, E. Individual answers will vary.
4. G. Altruism
   B. Catharsis
   F. Confrontation
   D. Countertransference
   E. Resistance
   C. Role-playing
   A. Transference

Chapter 3

1. D. Freud
   F. Rockland
   A. Ellis
   C. Spitzer
   B. Sullivan
   E. Szasz
2. A. difficulty in earlier stages of development
   B. Free association
   C. faulty interpersonal relationships
   D. satisfaction; security
   E. social conditions that culturally define what is acceptable
   F. social
   G. one is out of touch with one's self or the environment
   H. encounter
   I. problems in living from biopsychosocial causes
   J. active; partner
   K. disorders of the central nervous system
   L. continuous learning about the brain and nervous system using the scientific process
   M. *DSM-IV-TR*

3. A. Psychoanalysis proposes that dreams provide insight into areas of unresolved conflict in thoughts or feelings. Dream analysis or dream work is a common notion in contemporary society, and dreams play an important role in the belief system of various cultures.

   B. Stranger, resource person, teacher, leader, surrogate, counselor

   C, D. Individual answers will vary.

Chapter 4

1. A. True
   B. False: One out of every two people will do so.
   C. True
   D. False: The sympathetic division is stimulated.
   E. True
   F. True

2. A. reality perception/reality testing
   B. resilience
   C. psychological
   D. Social attribution
   E. harm/loss; threat; challenge
   F. II
   G. culture-bound syndromes

3. A. The three parts of a hardy personality are commitment, challenge, and control. They help people cope with stress by transforming events to their advantage and reframing problems as opportunities for growth and learning.

   B. The three types of coping mechanisms are problem-focused, cognitive-focused, and emotion-focused.

   C. Nurses assess risk factors and look for vulnerabilities; physicians assess disease states and look for causes. Nursing diagnoses focus on the adaptive-maladaptive coping continuum of human responses; medical diagnoses focus on the health-illness continuum of health problems. Nursing intervention consists of caregiving activities; medical intervention consists of curative treatments.

   D. The four stages of psychiatric treatment and related level of prevention are crisis, secondary prevention; acute, secondary prevention; maintenance, tertiary prevention; and health promotion, primary prevention.

Chapter 5

1. A. True
   B. False: Randomized controlled clinical trials are the gold standard.
   C. True
   D. False: Practice guidelines vary greatly in clinical orientation, clinical purpose, complexity, format, and intended users.
   E. True
   F. False: Studies show that very few psychiatric nurses routinely use behavioral rating scales in their practice.

2. A. research; receive
   B. 1, Defining the clinical question; 2, finding the evidence; 3, analyzing the evidence; 4, using the evidence; and 5, evaluating the outcome
   C. meta-analysis
   D. practice guidelines
   E. Algorithms
   F. clinical; functional; satisfaction; financial

3. A. Central to this accountability is the ability to examine nursing practice patterns, evaluate the nature of the data supporting them, and demonstrate sound clinical decision making in a way that can be empirically supported. This is the essence of evidence-based practice.

   B. There are four bases for nursing practice. The lowest level is the **traditional basis** for practice, which includes rituals, unverified rules, anecdotes, customs, opinions, and unit culture. The second level is the **regulatory basis** for practice, which includes state practice acts and reimbursement and other regulatory requirements. The third level is the **philosophical** or **conceptual basis** for practice, which includes the mission, values and vision of the organization, professional practice models, untested conceptual frameworks, and ethical frameworks and professional codes. The fourth and highest level is **evidence-based practice,** which includes research findings, performance data, and consensus recommendations of recognized experts. Apart from situations requiring a philosophical or regulatory basis, the best basis to substantiate clinical practice is the evidence of well-established research findings. Such evidence reflects verifiable, replicable facts and relationships that have been exposed to stringent scientific criteria.

   C. Individual answers will vary.

Chapter 6

1. H. Basal ganglia
   I. Eugenics
   B. Hippocampus
   A. Hypothalamus
   E. Locus ceruleus
   G. PET
   D. REM
   C. Synapse
   F. Tryptophan

2. A. blood-brain; blood-CSF
   B. neurotransmission
   C. neurosciences
   D. circadian rhythms

3. A. False: The interval timer acts like a stopwatch. It is flexible and can easily be turned on or off.
   B. True
   C. True
   D. False: CT scans have found enlargement of ventricles.
   E. True

4. A. Axon: Presynaptic cell; stores and releases neurotransmitter. Dendrite: Postsynaptic cell; contains
receptor cells. Receptor cell: Recognizes the neurotransmitter, receives it, and reacts to it. Second messengers: Chemicals within the cell that continue the
process of neurotransmission. Reuptake: Neurotransmitter is taken back up into the presynaptic cell.
Enzymatic degradation: Neurotransmitter is metabolized and inactivated.

   B. It is the emotional brain, concerned with both subjective emotional experiences and body functions
associated with emotional states, such as aggressive
and submissive behavior, sexual behavior, pleasure,
memory, learning, mood, motivation, and sensations,
all central to preservation.

   C. Stage one, falling asleep; stage two, sleep (50% of sleep
time); stages three and four: deep sleep (15% of sleep
time); stage five, rapid eye movement (REM) sleep, or
dream sleep (20% to 25% of sleep time). REM latency
is the period of time (60 to 90 minutes) it usually takes
the normal person to enter the first REM period.
Decreased REM latency (5 to 30 minutes) is a biological marker for depression that occurs in approximately
90% of people with depression, thus indicating that
there is sleep dysregulation in depression.

Chapter 7

1. C. Affect
   A. Delusion
   E. Flight of ideas
   F. Hallucinations
   B. Illusions
   H. Insight
   D. Loose associations
   G. Mood
2. A. flat affect
   B. command hallucinations
   C. sound or hearing
   D. confabulation
3. A. The major categories of information in a mental status
examination are general description, emotional state,
experiences, thinking, and sensorium and cognition.
   B. Person (What is your name?), place (Where are you
today?), and time (What is today's date?)
   C. To measure the extent of the patient's problem, make
an accurate diagnosis, track patient progress over
time, and document the efficacy of treatment
   D, E. Individual answers will vary.

Chapter 8

1. F. Disadvantagement
   D. Discrimination
   G. Intolerance
   B. Prejudice
   E. Racism
   A. Stereotype
   C. Stigma

2. A. culture counts
   B. ethnicity
   C. Substance abuse; antisocial personality
   D. Affective; anxiety
   E. schizophrenia, manic depression
   F. increase; decrease
   G. awareness; skill; knowledge; encounters; desire
3. A. True
   B. False: Ethnicity can be either a risk or protective
factor depending on the situation and individual
characteristics.
   C. True
   D. True
4. A. Cultural competency is the ability to view each
patient as a unique individual, fully considering the
patient's cultural experiences within the context of
the common developmental challenges faced by all
people.
   B, C. Individual answers will vary.

Chapter 9

1. A. Access
   F. Capitation
   E. Case rate
   B. Clinical appropriateness
   D. Outcomes
   C. Utilization review
2. A. behavioral
   B. person; population
   C. Medicaid
   D. primary care providers
   E. employee assistance programs
   F. equal
   G. Telepsychiatry
3. A. HMOs are organized delivery systems that provide
care to a defined population, usually for a predetermined fixed amount (capitation rate). Consumers
enrolled in HMOs are restricted to using HMO
providers.
      IPOs are a network of providers who serve
enrollees but who can also participate in other
networks.
      POSs are plans that contract with a limited
number of clinicians, most often physicians,
and hospitals that provide care at discounted
rates.
      PPOs allow consumers to choose between delivery
systems at the time they seek care.
   B. Medicare and Medicaid were designed to help
those who were medically in need. The law passed
in 1996 implies that chemical dependency problems are not medical conditions but rather the
result of personal choice or weakness. In this way
it further stigmatizes people with these debilitating
conditions.
   C. Individual answers will vary.

Chapter 10

1. A. True
   B. False: The police power is currently emphasized.
   C. False: Mental Health Courts keep those who are mentally ill and commit minor offenses from being put in jail and allow them to get treatment instead.
   D. False: People with mental illness are not more violent or more dangerous than people in the general population.
   E. True
   F. True
   G. False: The patient's right of confidentiality does not allow police or lawyers access to information about patients without the patient's expressed consent.
   H. True
   I. False: Patient records belong to the treatment facility or clinician, and the original should remain on file and never be given to patients.
   J. False: Fairness is based on the concept of justice and benefit to the least advantaged in society.
   K. False: Three states—Montana, Idaho, and Utah—have abolished the insanity defense.
2. A. 48 to 72
   B. history of violent behavior; noncompliance with medications; current substance abuse; psychosis; antisocial personality
   C. Outpatient commitment
   D. informed; competent; voluntary
   E. Protection and Advocacy
   F. advance directives
   G. ethic
3. A. Dangerous to self or others, mentally ill and in need of treatment, and unable to provide for own basic needs
   B. Confidentiality involves the disclosure of certain information to another person, but it is limited to authorized people. It applies to all patients at all times. Privilege or testimonial privilege applies only in court-related proceedings, and it exists only if established by law.
   C. The duty to warn obliges the clinician to assess the threat of violence to another, identify the person being threatened, and implement some affirmative and preventive action.
   D. Individual answers will vary.

Chapter 11

1. A. strengths, resources, or competencies; deficits, pathological states, and dysfunction
   B. educate; support
   C. National Alliance for the Mentally Ill (NAMI)
2. Individual answers will vary.

Chapter 12

1. C. Data collection   E. Nursing diagnosis
   A. Evaluation   D. Outcome identification
   B. Implementation   F. Planning

2. A. Specific
   B. Measurable
   C. Attainable
   D. Current
   E. Adequate
   F. Mutual
   G. psychotherapy; prescription of medications; consultation
   H. health promotion; maintenance; acute; crisis
   I. develop insight; change behavior
   J. patient
   K. costs/disadvantages; benefits/advantages
   L. Accountability
   M. autonomy
   N. Internet
   O. interdisciplinary
3. A. *DSM-IV-TR* diagnoses are used in most mental health settings to describe and classify the symptoms of mental disorders. Nurses should use both NANDA and *DSM-IV-TR* diagnoses to conceptualize patient problems, needs, and treatment strategies.
   B. Goal setting with psychiatric patients can be difficult for a number of reasons, including issues such as resistance, confusion, lack of insight, denial, vagueness about problem areas, and inability to articulate ideas. The nurse needs to clarify the reason and develop specific strategies to address it, which is part of the therapeutic process.
   C. The aim of supervision is to teach psychotherapeutic skills. The goal of therapy is to alter a person's patterns of coping to enable the person to function more effectively in all areas of life.
   D. Individual answers will vary.

Chapter 13

1. A. Primary prevention
   B. Secondary prevention
   C. Tertiary prevention
2. A. work with people to avoid or better cope with stressors; change the resources, policies, or agents of the environment to enhance individual functioning
   B. competence building or self-efficacy
   C. public health model
   D. stigma
   E. environmental change
   F. all three (primary, secondary, and tertiary)
3. A. The medical prevention model focuses on mental illness prevention and the importance of biological and brain research to discover the specific causes of mental illness. The nursing prevention model assumes that problems are multicausal, that everyone is vulnerable to stressful life events, and that any disability can arise in response to them. It focuses on intervention based on stressful events and vulnerable groups with known risk factors.

B. Universal interventions are targeted to the general population without consideration of risk factors. Selective interventions are targeted to individuals or groups with a significantly higher risk of developing a particular disorder. Indicated interventions are targeted to high-risk individuals who indicate a predisposition for developing the disorder.

C. Increasing a person's awareness of issues related to health and illness; increasing understanding of potential stressors and adaptive and maladaptive coping responses; increasing knowledge of where and how to acquire needed resources; and increasing the actual abilities such as the problem-solving skills, social skills, or self-esteem of the individual or group

D, E. Individual answers will vary.

Chapter 14

1. G. Catharasis
   A. Clarification
   D. Reinforcement of behavior
   C. Exploration of solutions
   E. Raising self-esteem
   F. Suggestion
   B. Support of defenses
2. A. crisis
   B. precipitating events
   C. precrisis
   D. assessment
   E. health educator
3. A. True
   B. False: A crisis is a short-term event requiring short-term treatment.
   C. True
   D. False: The patient's perception of the precipitating event is critically important.
   E. False: The generic approach is the correct answer.
4. A. Maturational crises are social and biological developmental events requiring role changes. These types of crises can be influenced by role models, interpersonal resources, and the acceptance of others. Situational crises occur when a life event upsets an individual's or a group's psychological equilibrium. This can cause feelings of inadequacy, bereavement, role change, financial stress, fear of loss, and feelings of helplessness and guilt. They can also be accidental, uncommon, and unexpected events.
   B. Cultural factors to be considered in crisis intervention are migration and citizen status, gender and family roles, religious belief systems, child-rearing practices, and use of extended family and support systems.
   C. Identify your own behaviors, precipitating events, perception of the event, support systems and coping resources, and previous strengths and coping mechanisms.

Chapter 15

1. A. True
   B. False: The career potential of people with mental illness, as with anyone else, depends on the person's talents, abilities, experience, motivation, and health status.
   C. True
   D. False: Consumers of mental health services can be productive as providers of mental health services. They can provide positive staff-recipient relationships, good knowledge of mental health resources and ways to overcome barriers, and positive role modeling.
   E. True
2. A. rehabilitation
   B. family burden
   C. recovery
   D. Social skills training
   E. psychoeducation
3. A. Grief, guilt, anger, powerlessness, and fear
   B. Helping people develop their strengths and potential, learn living skills, manage their illness, and access environmental support
   C. Ways in which nurses can share power with families include clarifying mutual goals, not expecting families to fit a specific model, acknowledging one's own limitations, pointing out family strengths, working with families as a team, learning to respond to intense feelings, encouraging family enrichment, providing psychoeducation, offering practical advice, making a personal commitment, acknowledging diverse beliefs, and developing one's own supports.

Chapter 16

1. G. Affective responses
   A. Anxiety
   C. Cognitive responses
   I. Ego-oriented reactions
   F. Fear
   J. Moderate anxiety
   E. Neurosis
   D. Panic
   H. Psychosis
   B. Task-oriented reactions
2. A. anxiety, depression
   B. obsessions
   C. GABA system; norepinephrine system; serotonin system
   D. physical integrity; self-esteem
   E. benzodiazepines; antidepressants
3. A. Conflict is the clashing of two opposing interests. The person experiences two competing drives and must choose between them. A reciprocal relationship exists between conflict and anxiety. Conflict produces anxiety, and anxiety increases the perception of conflict by producing feelings of helplessness.

B. Allow the patient to determine the amount of stress he can handle at any given time. Do not force the patient into situations that he is not able to handle. Do not attack the patient's coping mechanisms or try to strip him of these. Do not ridicule the nature of his defense. Do not argue with the patient or try to talk him out of the defense. Do not reinforce the defense by focusing too much attention on it. Know when to eventually place some limits on the defense as more adaptive coping mechanisms fall into place. Assess for suicidal ideation as appropriate.

C. Individual answers will vary.

Chapter 17

1. E. Body dysmorphic disorder
    C. Conversion disorder
    H. Hypersomnia
    D. Hypochondriasis
    I. Insomnia
    F. Pain disorder
    G. Parasomnia
    J. Sleep pattern disturbance
    A. Somatization disorder
    B. Somatoform disorders
2. A. alarm; resistance; exhaustion
    B. repression; denial; compensation; regression
    C. verbally; physical
    D. conversion disorder
    E. Psychoneuroimmunology
3. A. Supportive therapy, insight therapy, group therapy, cognitive-behavioral strategies, stress reduction, and relaxation training
    B. Secondary gain is an indirect benefit, usually obtained through an illness or disability. Such benefits may include personal attentions, release from unpleasant situations and responsibilities, or monetary and disability benefits.
    C. Individual answers will vary.

Chapter 18

1. A. True
    B. False: Research indicates that self-esteem has a genetic component.
    C. True
    D. False: The development of insight is not the desired outcome; the ultimate goal is to take action to effect lasting behavioral changes.
    E. False: Sympathetic responses by the nurse do not help patients assume responsibility for their own behavior. In fact, they can reinforce the patient's self-pity.
2. A. self-ideal
    B. self-esteem
    C. Roles
    D. identity
    E. Depersonalization
    F. child abuse
    G. reminiscence

3. A. Provide the child with success, instill ideas, encourage the child's aspirations, and help the child build defenses against attacks to one's self-perceptions
    B. In adolescence, the crisis of identity versus identity diffusion occurs. The task is one of self-definitions as the adolescent strives to integrate previous roles into a unique and reasonably consistent sense of self.
    C. Positive and accurate body image, realistic self-ideal, positive self-concept, high self-esteem, satisfying role performance, clear sense of identity
    D. Individual answers will vary.

Chapter 19

1. C. Behaviors related to emotional responses
    A. Coping mechanisms
    D. *DSM-IV-TR* diagnoses
    B. Precipitating stressors
    E. Predisposing factors
    F. Seasonal affective disorder
2. A. electroconvulsive therapy (ECT)
    B. serotonin
    C. bipolar; unipolar
    D. risk
    E. prefrontal cortex
    F. anxiety; substance abuse
    G. 75; 85
    H. response; 6; 12; remission
    I. recovery; relapse; 4; 9
    J. recurrence; indefinitely
3. A. Emotional responsiveness: The person is affected by and is an active participant in both internal and external worlds. Uncomplicated grief reaction: The person is facing the reality of the loss and is immersed in the work of grieving. Suppression of emotions: This is the denial of feelings, detachment from them, or the internalization of all aspects of one's affective world. Delayed grief reaction: This is a prolonged suppression of emotion that ultimately interferes with effective functioning. Depression/mania: The most maladaptive emotional responses, recognized by their intensity, pervasiveness, persistence, and interference with usual functioning.
    B. To increase the patient's sense of control over goals and behavior, increase the patient's self-esteem, and help the patient modify negative thinking patterns
    C, D. Individual answers will vary.

Chapter 20

1. A. False: The highest rate of suicide is among white men older than 65 years.
    B. True
    C. False: All suicidal behavior is serious and, whatever the intent, must be given full consideration.
    D. True
    E. True
    F. False: The tricyclics have the higher rate of death by overdose.

G. True

H. False: A person already has the suicidal idea, and asking about it gives the person an opportunity to talk about how he or she feels.

2. A. psychological autopsy

B. mood disorders; substance abuse; schizophrenia; anxiety disorders

C. serotonin (5-HT)

D. Communicating hope

E. hostility; impulsivity; depression

F. Surgeon General

3. A. Patients often appear less depressed immediately before attempting suicide because they feel relief at having made a decision and developed a plan to carry out the suicide.

B. Psychiatric diagnosis, personality traits and disorders, psychosocial and environmental factors, genetic and familial variables, biochemical factors

C. Suicidal patients can be treated in a variety of settings. Factors that should be considered in deciding on the best setting relate to your assessment of overall risk and should include whether the patient is resolute or ambivalent about suicide, has impaired judgment, and has dependable social supports available in the home.

D. Individual answers will vary.

Chapter 21

1. C. Attention

D. Perception

E. Hallucinations

G. Mood

A. Cognition

H. Anhedonia

I. Affect

J. Decision making

B. Memory

F. Soft signs

2. A. cognition, perception; emotion; behavior and movement; socialization

B. apraxia

C. dysregulation hypothesis

D. Symptom triggers

E. overextension; restricted consciousness; disinhibition; psychotic disorganization; psychotic resolution

3. A. True

B. False: The majority are auditory.

C. False: Atypical antipsychotics often provide a better response and fewer side effects and should be considered first-line treatments.

D. True

E. False: It is called Family to Family.

4. A. Nursing interventions should address the positive symptoms of schizophrenia, which include delusions, hallucinations, thought disorders, and bizarre behaviors, as well as the negative symptoms of flat affect, alogia, avolition, anhedonia, and attentional impair-

ment. Positive symptoms respond well to typical and atypical antipsychotic medications. Negative symptoms respond best to atypical antipsychotic medications.

B. The specific genetic defects that cause schizophrenia have not been identified yet, but family studies show increased risk for the disease and other psychiatric illnesses in people with a first-degree relative with schizophrenia. Children with a biological parent with schizophrenia have a 15% risk of developing the disorder. If both of the child's parents have schizophrenia, the risk increases up to 35%.

C. Things you may notice are facial expressions, style of dress, mannerisms, tone of voice, behaviors, use of language, and body contact with others.

Chapter 22

1. B. Antisocial personality disorder

C. Avoidant personality disorder

B. Borderline personality disorder

C. Dependent personality disorder

B. Histrionic personality disorder

B. Narcissistic personality disorder

C. Obsessive-compulsive personality disorder

A. Paranoid personality disorder

A. Schizoid personality disorder

A. Schizotypal personality disorder

2. A. adolescence; adulthood

B. borderline personality disorder

C. serotonin

D. splitting

E. Projective identification

F. countertransference

3. A. Distinguishing characteristics of personality disorders include chronic and long-standing, not based on a sound personality structure, and difficult to change.

B. Two levels of evaluation necessary when working with patients with personality disorders are evaluation of the nurse and the nurse's participation in the relationship and evaluation of the patient's behavior and the behavioral changes that the nurse works to facilitate.

C, D, E. Individual answers will vary.

Chapter 23

1. C. Delirium   H. Sundown syndrome

D. Denial   A. Amygdala

F. Dementia   G. Aphasia

B. Agnosia   J. Apraxia

E. Pseudodementia   I. Excess disability

2. A. neurotic plaques; neurofibrillary tangles

B. Alzheimer's disease

C. catastrophic reaction

D. Delirium

3. A. Working memory, the ability to keep in mind recent events or the moment-to-moment results of mental processing, is mediated by the prefrontal cortex, which is responsible for executive functions. Long-term memory: Declarative memory (facts and events)

is mediated by the hippocampus (in the limbic system), which consolidates new memories into long-term memories. Procedural memory (skills and procedures) is mediated by several brain structures: the striatum, motor cortex, and cerebellum (skills and habits); the amygdala (emotional associations); and the cerebellum (conditional reflexes).

B. Understand the possible causes of the cognitive impairment, adjust communication approaches to the person who is cognitively impaired, assist with self-care of the individual as needed, obtain available community services, engage in stress reduction activities, use respite care, participate in a peer support group, access social supports

C. Individual answers will vary.

Chapter 24

1. A. False: Substance abuse affects all races.
   B. False: Only 1 in 10 people progress from use to abuse to dependence.
   C. True
   D. False: In the addicted population, prevalence of psychiatric illness is no greater than in the general population.
   E. False: In the addicted population, prevalence of psychiatric illness is no greater than in the general population.
   F. True
   G. False: Shorter half-lives result in more withdrawal.
   H. True
   I. False: Most people have one or more slips in their attempt at recovery.
   J. True
2. A. substitution of a medication from the same drug class for gradual tapering
   B. dual diagnosis
   C. gateway
   D. CAGE questionnaire
   E. breathalyzer
   F. Co-dependence
   G. endorphins or enkephalins
   H. CNS depressant
   I. detoxification
   J. Antabuse; naltrexone
3. A. Patients in maintenance methadone programs may object to the following: (1) they must remain on stable doses of the drug for years—some even for the rest of their lives, and (2) they must report to the clinic daily or they may be given take-home doses for certain days if they qualify.
   B. The advantages of having treatment programs staffed by counselors who have also recovered from substance abuse include that they may have a heightened sense of empathy for the patient population, a greater understanding of the realities of the abuse, and provide positive recovery-based role modeling. There is controversy in the field, however, about

what proportion of the staff should be recovered individuals. Some believe that a critical number of staff who have not been substance abusers is necessary to provide a professional balance to the treatment program. More research is needed in this area.

C, D, E. Individual answers will vary.

Chapter 25

1. C. Maladaptive eating regulation responses
   D. SSRIs
   A. Adaptive eating regulation responses
   E. Predisposing factors
   B. Serotonin
2. A. females; 1; 4
   B. Binge eating
   C. avoidance; intellectualization; isolation of affect; denial
   D. cognitive distortion
   E. cognitive behavioral therapy
3. A. Weight loss: Severe with anorexia; less weight loss with bulimia
      Hunger: Hunger denied with anorexia; hunger experienced with bulimia
      Personality features: Obsessional and perfectionistic with anorexia; avoidant, dependent, and borderline with bulimia
   B. The patient will restore healthy eating patterns and normalize physiological parameters related to body weight and nutrition.
   C, D, E. Individual answers will vary.

Chapter 26

1. I. Bisexuality
   B. Gender identity
   J. Gender role
   A. Genetic identity
   G. Heterosexuality
   F. Homophobia
   H. Homosexuality
   E. Orgasm
   L. Pedophilia
   K. Sexual orientation
   C. Transsexualism
   D. Transvestism
2. A. cognitive dissonance
   B. XX, XY
   C. Oedipus/Electra
   D. childhood sexual abuse
   E. Education
   F. acceptance
3. A. Between two consenting adults, mutually satisfying to both, not psychologically or physically harmful to either party, lacking in force or coercion, and conducted in private
   B. Safe sex practices include using condoms, reducing the number of sexual partners, and promoting sexual behaviors that decrease the exchange of body fluids.
   C, D. Individual answers will vary.

Chapter 27

1. J. Barbiturates
    H. Selective serotonin reuptake inhibitors
    I. Antianxiety drugs
    K. Cytochrome P-450 inhibition
    L. Anti-parkinsonian drugs
    E. Tricyclics
    A. Serotonin syndrome
    D. Sedative-hypnotics
    B. Atypical antidepressants
    C. Hypertensive crisis
    G. Typical antipsychotics
    F. Mood stabilizers
2. H. H$_1$ receptor blockade
    A. DA reuptake inhibition
    F. Alpha$_2$ receptor blockade
    G. NE reuptake inhibition
    B. ACh receptor blockade
    C. 5-HT reuptake inhibition
    D. Alpha$_1$ receptor blockade
    E. 5-HT$_2$ receptor blockade
3. A. role of the nurse
    B. drug co-administration
    C. Pharmacokinetics
    D. dysregulation hypothesis
    E. neurosciences; psychopharmacology; clinical management
4. A. False: Serotonin syndrome is a life-threatening emergency caused by combining 5-HT-enhancing drugs.
    B. False: With NMS, all drugs should be discontinued.
    C. True
    D. True
    E. True
5. A. Positive symptoms include delusion, hallucinations, formal thought disorder, and bizarre behavior. Negative symptoms include affective flattening, alogia, avolition/apathy/anhedonia, asociality, and attentional impairment. These symptoms respond better to the atypical antipsychotics than they do to the typical or conventional neuroleptic antipsychotics.
    B. Reuptake inhibition occurs when drugs such as TCAs and SSRIs prevent the presynaptic cell from reabsorbing the neurotransmitter after it has been released into the synapse. It is thought that this strategy produces an antidepressant effect by making more neurotransmitter available to the receptors in illnesses such as depression, in which increasing the effects of some neurotransmitters appears to exert a therapeutic effect.

    Receptor blockade occurs when drugs such as antipsychotics prevent a postsynaptic receptor from receiving a neurotransmitter after it has been released into the synapse. It is thought that this strategy produces an antipsychotic effect by making less neurotransmitter available to receptors in illnesses such as schizophrenia, in which decreasing the effects of some neurotransmitters appears to exert a therapeutic effect.

    C. When receiving antidepressants for the treatment of depression, patients begin to look better and sleep and eat better, and they feel more energy and motivation before the remission of subjective depressive feelings and suicidal thoughts. Objectively, they appear to be less depressed at a time when their safety must still be assessed because they now have the energy to act on suicidal impulses that have not responded to treatment.

Chapter 28

1. A. True
    B. False: ECT may be followed by antidepressant medication to prevent relapse.
    C. False: There is no evidence that ECT causes brain damage.
    D. True
    E. True
    F. False: The long-term efficacy of light therapy has not been fully evaluated.
    G. False: Light therapy appears to be insufficient for severely ill patients.
    H. True
    I. False: TMS is a noninvasive procedure using magnetic fields.
2. A. 6; 12
    B. 20; 30
    C. major depression
    D. 80%
    E. surgical
    F. headache; muscle soreness; nausea
    G. 50; 60
    H. mania
    I. mood
    J. Vagus nerve stimulation
3. A. ECT is a treatment in which a grand mal seizure is artificially induced in an anesthetized patient by passing an electrical current through electrodes applied to the patient's temples.
    B. Avoiding medications is often recommended for women who are in their first trimester of pregnancy. ECT allows the depression of the woman to be treated while avoiding the need to expose the fetus to antidepressant medications.
    C, D. Individual answers will vary.

Chapter 29

1. A. False: Use of CAM therapies is increasing.
    B. True
    C. True
    D. False: Drug interactions have been reported, and it should not be taken with other antidepressants.
    E. True
    F. False: Most studies on the use of acupuncture for cocaine and other substance use disorders have failed to detect differences between experimental (real) and control (sham) acupuncture groups.

2. A. Complementary and alternative medicine (CAM)
   B. St. John's wort
   C. melatonin
   D. Progressive muscle relaxation
   E. Therapeutic touch
   F. Kava-kava
   G. Ginko biloba
3. A. Enhanced public health education had heightened health care awareness and interest in making lifestyle changes. CAM therapies often seem to be more available, accessible, and therefore more appealing to the health care consumer. In addition, the benefits of CAM therapies may include less cost, more convenience, fewer side effects, more individualized care, and more contact with practitioners.
   B. Ethical concerns about CAM therapies include issues of safety and effectiveness, as well as the expertise and qualifications of the practitioner. Of equal importance is the communication between the CAM and traditional health care provider. Other concerns are related to effective symptom management, potential for drug interactions, possible side effects, and the lack of regulation of herbal products for purity and potency.
   C. It is believed that acupuncture may stimulate the synthesis and release of endorphins, serotonin, and norepinephrine.

Chapter 30

1. A. Assertive behavior
   E. Debriefing
   G. Limit-setting
   D. Passive behavior
   F. Restraint
   C. Seclusion
   B. Token economy
2. A. False: Research suggests that this intervention may actually increase the patient's potential for aggressive behavior.
   B. True
   C. False: A patient's diagnosis is complicated by many factors and is at best merely suggestive of potentially violent behavior.
   D. True
   E. True
3. A. Areas of the brain include the limbic system, frontal lobe, and temporal lobe.
   B. Preventive strategies include self-awareness, patient education, and assertiveness training. Anticipatory strategies include communication, environmental change, behavioral action, and psychopharmacology. Containment strategies include crisis management, seclusion, and restraint.
   C. You should assume a supportive stance at least one leg length or 3 feet away from the patient. You should be at an angle to the patient, with hands kept open and out of pockets.
   D. Individual answers will vary.

Chapter 31

1. B. Behavior
   G. Biofeedback
   F. Contingency contracting
   H. Extinction
   D. Flooding
   A. Punishment
   E. Shaping
   J. Social skills training
   C. Systematic desensitization
   I. Reframing
2. A. classical conditioning
   B. operant conditioning or negative reinforcement
   C. punishment; response cost; extinction
   D. perception or interpretation
   E. Hierarchy
   F. direct patient care; planning treatment programs; teaching others cognitive behavior therapy techniques
   G. homework
3. A. A cognitive behavioral assessment would include collecting data about a patient's actions, thoughts, and feelings; identifying problems from the data, defining the problem behavior, deciding how to measure the problem behavior, and identifying environmental variables that influence the problem behavior. It includes a review of the patient's strengths and deficits and minimizes the use of assumptions and unvalidated inferences.
   B. The ABCs of behavior are **antecedent, behavior,** and **consequence.** The ABCs of treatment are **affective, behavioral,** and **cognitive.**
   C. Use of the form allows patients to distinguish between thoughts and feelings and to identify adaptive responses that would be alternatives to the situation.
   D. Individual answers will vary.

Chapter 32

1. E. Follower
   C. Moralist
   H. Truant
   A. Gatekeeper
   J. Encourager
   G. Questioner
   B. Facilitator
   I. Leader
   F. Complainer
   D. Summarizer
2. A. Power
   B. orientation
   C. 60-120 minutes; 20-40 minutes
   D. forming; storming; norming; performing
   E. universality; altruism
3. A. A group is a collection of individuals who have a relationship with one another, are independent, and may have common norms. Eight components of small groups are structure, size, length of sessions, communication, roles, power, norms, and cohesion.

B. Psychoeducational groups are designed to teach symptom identification, symptom management, and recovery planning skills.

Intensive problem-solving groups are designed for 6 to 10 patients, each working on the identification and resolution of specific target problems, goals, and problem-solving strategies identified in an individual treatment plan.

Activity groups are designed to enhance the psychological and emotional well-being of psychiatric patients. These groups are a combination of group psychotherapy and remotivation therapy that stimulates interaction among members by focusing on simple tasks that encourage members to focus on group rather than individual goals.

C. Group norms facilitate the accomplishment of the group's goals or tasks, control interpersonal conflict, interpret social reality, and foster group interdependence.

D, E. Individual answers will vary.

Chapter 33

1. A. True
   B. False: Family therapists from any discipline should have advanced training at the graduate level.
   C. False: There are many theoretical approaches to working with families. Current approaches are integrative and draw upon several theories.
   D. True
2. A. deinstitutionalization; blaming the parents
   B. National Alliance for the Mentally Ill (NAMI); the Federation for Families for Children's Mental Health; and the National Mental Health Association (NMHA)
   C. relational problems
   D. youth with serious mental health problems
   E. firearms, medications, and other means of suicide
   F. Strengthening Families Program
3. Individual answers will vary.

Chapter 34

1. C. Allows for predictable organization of time, place, and person
   E. Affirming the patient's worldview
   D. Offering education and encouragement
   B. Promoting the patient's attention and interaction with the social environment
   A. Provision of food, shelter, medical care, and safety from harm
   D. Unconditional acceptance, nurturance, and promotion of self-esteem
   C. Use of contracts, token economies, and required meetings
   E. Use of individualized treatment plans and showing respect for patients' rights
   B. Use of open doors, open rounds, and patient-led groups
   A. Use of time-outs and room programs

2. A. crisis; stabilization
   B. institutionalism
   C. multidisciplinary
   D. therapeutic community
   E. Florence Nightingale
   F. Joint Commission on Accreditation of Healthcare Organizations (JCAHO)
3. A. Crisis stabilization and intermediate-term treatment
   B. The exact nature of the crisis bed concept depends on the structure of the health system in which it operates. Common goals include a focus of issues of suicidality, homicidality, and violence; assessment; rapid resolution of the crisis; decreased dependency on the hospital; prevention of regressive behaviors; and improved functioning of the inpatient environment.
   C, D, E. Individual answers will vary.

Chapter 35

1. A. False: The attempt to move patients into community care as a result of deinstitutionalization was considered by mental health experts to be a failure.
   B. True
   C. True
   D. False: About one-third of the estimated 600,000 homeless people in the United States have a severe mental illness, but as few as 5% to 7% of these need to be institutionalized.
   E. False: The rate of serious mental illness in the incarcerated population is about 3 to 4 times that of the general U.S. population.
2. A. inpatient; emergency; partial hospitalization; outpatient; consultation and education
   B. Assertive Community Treatment
   C. multisystemic therapy
   D. forensic
   E. Medicare
3. A. Common elements of ACT and MST include use of a social-ecological framework, pragmatic treatment approaches, home-based interventions, individualized treatment goals and emphasis on outcomes and innovation.
   B, C, D. Individual answers will vary.

Chapter 36

1. A. False: 9% to 13% of all children have some type of mental disorder.
   B. True
   C. True
   D. False: Young children exhibiting suicidal behaviors may be at high risk for self-harm or death. The nurse must evaluate the disparities between child and caretaker statements.
   E. False: The nurse should employ a policy of least restrictive intervention and explore alternatives to replace the current reactive crisis.
   F. False: The first goal is to establish trust.

2. A. 75%-80%
   B. separation anxiety
   C. follow-up questions and assessment of safety
   D. Bibliotherapy
   E. Play
   F. legal and ethical
   G. anxiety; depression; conduct disorder; attention deficit/hyperactivity disorder (ADHD)
3. A. Positive individual characteristics are cognitive competence, experiences of self-efficacy resulting in self-confidence, temperament characteristics that elicit positive responses from others, parenting in a way that fostered competence, positive self-esteem, supportive adults who fostered trust and acted as gatekeepers, opportunities in major life transitions that allowed them to reinforce and reward their own competencies.
   B. Parents can enhance child's self-esteem by having realistic expectations, being consistent in caring and discipline, demonstrating positive personal values, and communicating clearly.
   C, D. Individual answers will vary.

Chapter 37

1. A. False: Brain growth continues into adolescence, and there is also additional fine tuning of the neural system.
   B. False: Chronological age is not a good indicator of physical maturation during adolescence because growth often occurs in spurts and individual differences exist.
   C. True
   D. True
   E. False: It is best for the nurse to have the initial contact directly with the adolescent because he or she is often concerned that the nurse will be aligned with the parents rather than with the adolescent.
   F. True
2. A. identity versus identity diffusion
   B. formal operational thought
   C. males; females
   D. 50
   E. body dysmorphic disorder
   F. coping with stress and anxiety; involvement in personally meaningful activities
3. A. Female teenagers delay seeking and using contraceptives either because they are unwilling or unable to make conscious decisions about their sexual and contraceptive behavior or because they either do not mind becoming pregnant or do not think it will happen to them.
   B. They are called gateway drugs because their use often precedes the use of marijuana and other illegal substances.
   C. Curiosity, experimentation, regular use, psychological or physical dependence, and using drugs to feel "normal"

D. Medicating adolescents necessitates comprehensive family involvement; developmental differences in adolescence affect psychopharmacological assessment, treatment alliance, management, and compliance; difficulty in diagnosing emerging first episodes versus adjustment disorders in adolescents; and lack of controlled clinical drug trials in adolescents

Chapter 38

1. F. Activity theory
   E. Cross-linkage theory
   H. Person-environment fit theory
   A. Biological programming theory
   B. Disengagement theory
   C. Life review theory
   D. Stability of personality
   G. Stress adaptation theory
2. A. sundown syndrome
   B. physical restraints
   C. electroconvulsive
   D. more favorable side effects profile
   E. Reality
   F. cognitive
   G. maximal independence
   H. lower than for younger patients
3. A. Show respect by addressing the patient by his or her last name, reinforce the amount of time left in the interview, give sufficient time for response, tie the interview to historical events, choose words that are based on the sociocultural background of the patient, use touch to convey support and interest, and give careful and repeated explanations to increase understanding and cooperation.
   B. Environmental hazards, patient variables, assistive devices, medications, and physical or mental disorders
   C. Individual answers will vary.

Chapter 39

1. D. Attributions
   I. Sexual assault
   A. Multigenerational transmission
   G. Myth about abuse
   C. Paternalistic model of health care
   J. Psychological abuse
   F. The force continuum
   H. Intimate partner violence
   B. Just world view
   E. Primary prevention
2. A. True
   B. False: Children who witness abuse are also victimized.
   C. False: Family violence occurs at all levels of society regardless of income, age, race, education, or religion.
   D. True
   E. True

3. A. Violent families have the following characteristics: multigenerational transmission (family violence is often perpetuated through generations within a family by a cycle of violence), social isolation (violent families are often isolated by the abuser to keep the "family secret," thus avoiding formal and informal sanctions from others in the community), use and abuse of power (the abuser almost always has some form of power or control over the victim), and alcohol and drug abuse (survivors often report concurrent substance abuse by the abuser, although one behavior is not necessary for the other to occur).

B.
Paternalistic model	*Empowerment model*
Nurse is perceived to be more knowledgeable than the survivor.	There is a mutual sharing of knowledge and information.
Responsibility for ending the violence is placed on the survivor.	The nurse strategizes with the survivor. Survivors are helped to recognize societal influences.
Advice and sympathy are given rather than respect.	The survivor's competence and experience are respected.

C. American social norms that maintain violence include historical attitudes toward women, children, and the elderly; the belief that violence is justified to maintain the family system; economic discrimination; the nonresponsiveness of the criminal justice system; and the belief that women and children are property.

Chapter 40

1. A. True
   B. False: This is a requirement of JCAHO.
   C. False: This is the substituted-judgment standard.
   D. True
2. A. presence
   B. psychiatric consultation liaison nurse (PCLN)
   C. soothing music; progressive muscle relaxation; visualization exercises
   D. antidepressant therapy
   E. Palliative care
   F. unrelieved pain
   G. Two physicians
   H. euthanasia
3. A. How long do people with this illness usually live? Will I be able to pay for treatment and other financial obligations? How will my family and friends be emotionally affected or inconvenienced? Will I be a burden or become dependent on others? Will I suffer pain as I have heard others have? Will I die alone?
   B. It is important for nurses to acknowledge complaints and respond to them with patience and without defensiveness.
   C. Some causes of delirium at the end of life are fever, brain metastases, encephalopathy, and pain medications.

GLOSSARY

access The degree to which services and information about health care are easily obtained.

accountability To be answerable to someone for something, focusing responsibility on the individual for personal actions or lack of actions.

acupuncture Involves the insertion of needles into acupoints located along the body's meridians (energy channels that run throughout the body) for the purpose of restoring energy balance.

addiction The biological and/or psychosocial behaviors related to substance dependence.

adolescence The period from the beginning of puberty to the attainment of maturity. The transitional stage during which the youth is becoming an adult man or woman.

advance directives Documents, written while a person is competent, that specify how decisions about treatment would be made if the person were to become incompetent.

advanced practice registered nurse (APRN) A licensed RN who has a master's degree and a depth of knowledge of psychiatric nursing theory, supervised clinical practice, and competence in advanced psychiatric nursing skills.

advocacy Helping people to receive available services and influencing providers to improve existing services and develop new ones.

affect Feeling, mood, or emotional tone.

agnosia Difficulty recognizing well-known objects.

agonist In pharmacology, a substance that acts with, enhances, or potentiates a specific chemical activity.

agoraphobia Anxiety disorder characterized by a fear of being in open, crowded, or public spaces.

agranulocytosis A significant decrease in the white blood cell count that does not return to normal.

AIDS dementia complex Subcortical encephalopathy characterized by progressive dementia; believed to result primarily from direct infection with HIV.

alexithymia Difficulty naming and describing emotions.

altruism A concern for the welfare of others that can be expressed at the level of the individual or the larger social system.

amnesia Significant memory impairment in the absence of clouded consciousness or other cognitive symptoms.

amotivational syndrome A cluster of symptoms apparently related to prolonged marijuana use that includes apathy, lack of energy, loss of desire to work or be productive, diminished concentration, poor personal hygiene, and preoccupation with marijuana.

anhedonia Inability or decreased ability to experience pleasure, joy, intimacy, and closeness.

anorexia nervosa An eating disorder in which the person experiences hunger but refuses to eat because of a distorted body image, leading to a self-perception of fatness. Starvation ensues.

antagonist In pharmacology, a substance that blocks or inhibits a specific chemical activity.

antecedent The stimulus or cue that occurs before behavior that leads to its occurrence.

anticipatory grief Emotional work begun before the actual loss of a valued object or concept.

antisocial personality disorder A disorder occurring in adult patients; characterized by poor work record, disregard for social norms, aggressiveness, financial irresponsibility, impulsiveness, lying, recklessness, inability to maintain close relationships or to meet responsibilities for significant others, or a lack of remorse for harmful behavior.

anxiety A diffuse apprehension vague in nature and associated with feelings of uncertainty and helplessness. It is an emotion without a specific object, is subjectively experienced by the individual, and is communicated interpersonally. It occurs as a result of a threat to the person's being, self-esteem, or identity.

apathy Lack of feelings, emotions, interests, or concern.

aphasia Difficulty finding the right word.

appraisal of a stressor An evaluation of the significance of an event for one's well-being that takes place on the cognitive, affective, physiological, behavioral, and social levels.

apraxia Inability or difficulty in performing a purposeful organized task or similar skilled activities.

assertive community treatment (ACT) An evidence-based psychiatric rehabilitation practice designed to provide intensive community supports to individuals who have serious mental illnesses. The goal is to prevent hospitalization and support the individual in achieving the highest possible level of functioning.

assertiveness The midpoint of a continuum that runs from passive to aggressive behavior. Assertive behavior conveys a sense of self-assurance but also communicates respect for the other person.

ataxia Difficulty walking.

attention The ability to focus on one activity in a sustained, concentrated manner.

attributions Reasoning processes used to explain events.

augmentation The addition of another class of medication to supplement the effectiveness of the primary medication.

autonomy Self-determination that fosters independence and self-regulation; the condition that allows for definition of and control over a domain.

aversion therapy Reduces unwanted but persistent maladaptive behaviors by applying an aversive or noxious stimulus when that maladaptive behavior occurs.

avolition Lack of energy and drive.

axon The presynaptic part of a neuron.

B

behavior Any observable, recordable, and measurable act, movement, or response.

behavioral health A term used to describe both mental health and addiction services.

bibliotherapy Use of literature to help patients identify and express feelings within the structure and safety of the nurse-patient relationship.

binge eating The rapid consumption of large quantities of food in a contained period of time.

bioavailability How much of a drug reaches systemic circulation unchanged.

biofeedback The use of a machine to communicate physical changes; used to train a person to reduce anxiety and modify behavioral responses.

bipolar disorder A subgroup of the affective disorders characterized by at least one episode of manic behavior, with or without a history of episodes of depression.

bisexuality A sexual attraction to people of both sexes and the engagement in both homosexual and heterosexual activity.

blood levels The concentration of a drug in the plasma, serum, or blood. In psychiatry the term is most often applied to levels of lithium or some tricyclic antidepressants. Maximum clinical responses to these agents have been correlated with specific ranges of blood levels.

body dysmorphic disorder A somatoform disorder characterized by a normal-appearing person's belief that he or she has a physical defect.

body image Sum of the conscious and unconscious attitudes the person has toward his or her body. It includes present and past perceptions, as well as feelings about size, function, appearance, and potential.

borderline personality disorder A disorder with the essential features of unstable mood, interpersonal relationships, and self-image; characteristic behaviors may include unstable relationships, exploitation of others, impulsive behavior, labile affect, problems expressing anger appropriately, self-destructive behavior, and identity disturbances.

boundary violation When a nurse goes outside the limits of the therapeutic relationship and establishes a social, economic, or personal relationship with a patient.

brain electrical activity mapping (BEAM) Images brain activity and function by using CT techniques to display data derived from EEG recordings of brain electrical activity that has been sensory evoked by specific stimuli or cognitive evoked by specific mental tasks.

bulimia nervosa An eating disorder characterized by uncontrollable binge eating alternating with vomiting or dieting.

C

caregiver stress Emotional and physical strain experienced by a person caring for someone with a chronic debilitating disease or condition, especially if the caregiver neglects meeting his or her own needs simultaneously.

case management Providing services aimed at linking the service system to the patient and coordinating the service components so that the patient can achieve successful community living.

catatonia A stuporous state.

catharsis Release that occurs when the patient is encouraged to talk about things that bother him or her most. Fears, feelings, and experiences are brought out into the open and discussed.

chemical restraints Medications used to restrict the patient's freedom of movement or for emergency control of behavior but are not a standard treatment for the patient's medical or psychiatric condition.

child abuse The physical abuse or battering, emotional abuse, sexual abuse, or neglect of a child.

chromosome The self-replicating genetic structure of cells containing the cellular DNA that bears in its nucleotide sequence the linear array of genes. In prokaryotes chromosomal DNA is circular, and the entire genome is carried on one chromosome. Eukaryotic genomes consist of a number of chromosomes whose DNA is associated with different kinds of proteins.

circadian rhythms The correlation between human activities and behaviors and external environmental stimuli for a 24-hour period.

circumstantial Thought and speech of a person associated with excessive and unnecessary detail that is usually relevant to a question; an answer is eventually provided.

classical conditioning A theory describing the process by which involuntary behavior is learned, in which an event occurs when one stimulus, by being paired with another stimulus, comes to produce the same response as the other stimulus.

clinical algorithms These focus on treatment or medications and take practice guidelines to a greater level of specificity by providing step-by-step recommendations on issues such as treatment options, treatment sequencing, preferred dosage, and progress assessment.

clinical appropriateness The degree to which the type, amount, and level of clinical services are delivered to promote the best clinical outcomes.

clinical pathway A shortened version of the plan of care for a particular patient that lists key nursing and medical processes and corresponding time lines to which the patient must adhere to achieve standard outcomes within a specified period.

clinical supervision A support mechanism for practicing professionals within which they can share clinical, organizational, developmental, and emotional experiences with another professional in a secure, confidential environment to enhance knowledge and skills.

cognition The mental process characterized by knowing, thinking, learning, and judging.

cognitive dissonance Arises when two opposing beliefs exist at the same time.

cognitive distortions Positive or negative distortions of reality that might include errors of logic, mistakes in reasoning, or individualized views of the world that do not reflect reality.

cohesion The strength of group members' desire to work together toward common goals.

collaboration The shared planning, decision making, problem solving, goal setting, and assumption of responsibilities by people who work together cooperatively and with open communication.

collegiality An essential aspect of professional practice that requires that nurses view their peers as collaborators in the caregiving, research, or educational process who are valued and respected for their unique contributions.

command hallucinations Hallucinations that tell the patient to take some specific action, such as to kill oneself, harm another, or join someone in afterlife.

commitment Involuntary admission in which the request for hospitalization did not originate with the patient. When committed, the patient loses the right to leave the hospital when he or she wishes. It is usually justified on the ground that the patient is dangerous to self or others and needs treatment.

community support systems Systems developed by community mental health centers to provide patients with necessary specialized mental health service. Includes such community-based components as crisis response services, health and dental care, rehabilitation services, and protection and advocacy.

compensation Process by which a person makes up for a deficiency in self-image by strongly emphasizing some other feature that the person regards as an asset.

complementary and alternative medicine (CAM) Term commonly used to describe a broad range of healing philosophies, approaches, and therapies that focus on the whole person, including biopsychosocial and spiritual aspects.

completed suicide Self-inflicted death. Also see *suicide*.

compulsion A recurring irresistible impulse to perform some act.

computed tomography (CT) Depicts brain structure with a series of radiographs that is computer-constructed into "slices" of the brain that can be stacked by the computer, giving a three-dimensional view.

concreteness Use of specific terminology rather than abstractions in the discussion of the patient's feelings, experiences, and behavior.

confabulation A confused person's tendency to make up a response to a question when he or she cannot remember the answer.

confidentiality Nondisclosure of specific information about another unless authorized by that person.

confrontation An expression by the nurse of perceived discrepancies in the patient's behavior. It is an attempt by the nurse to bring to the patient's awareness the incongruence in feelings, attitudes, beliefs, and behaviors.

congruent communication A communication pattern in which the sender is communicating the same message on both the verbal and the nonverbal levels.

consequence The effect (positive, negative, or neutral) of a behavior on the individual.

contingency contracting A formal contract between the patient and the therapist defining what behaviors are to be changed and what consequences follow the performance of these behaviors.

conversion disorder A somatoform disorder characterized by a loss or alteration of physical functioning without evidence of organic impairment.

coping mechanism Any effort directed at stress management. It can be problem, cognitive, or emotion focused.

coping resources Characteristics of the person, group, or environment that help people adapt to stress.

countertransference An emotional response of the nurse that is generated by the patient's qualities and is inappropriate to the content and context of the therapeutic relationship or inappropriate in the degree of emotional intensity.

crisis A disturbance caused by a stressful event or a perceived threat to self.

crisis intervention Short-term therapy focused on solving the immediate problem and allowing the patient to return to a precrisis level of function.

cultural competency The ability to view each patient as a unique individual, fully considering the patient's cultural experiences within the context of the common developmental challenges faced by all people.

culture-bound syndrome Recurrent, locality-specific patterns of aberrant behavior and troubling experience that may or may not be linked to a particular *DSM–IV–TR* diagnostic category.

cyclothymia A disorder resembling bipolar disorder with less severe symptoms, characterized by repeated periods of nonpsychotic depression and hypomania for at least 2 years.

cytochrome P-450 inhibition Some drugs, such as some SSRIs and TCAs, inhibit this liver enzyme, causing potentially dangerous changes in the metabolism of many drugs.

D

debriefing Therapeutic intervention that includes reviewing the facts related to an event and processing the response to them.

decatastrophizing Helping patients to evaluate whether they are overestimating the catastrophic nature of a situation.

decision-making capacity The determination of mental, emotional, and intellectual ability to make health care decisions, depending on the requirement of the task at hand.

decision making Arriving at a solution or making a choice.

defense mechanisms Coping mechanisms of the ego that attempt to protect the person from feelings of inadequacy and worthlessness and prevent awareness of anxiety. They are primarily unconscious and involve a degree of self-deception and reality distortion.

deinstitutionalization At the patient level, the transfer to a community setting of a patient hospitalized for an extended time, generally many years; at the mental health care system level, a shift in the focus of care from the large, long-term institution to the community, accomplished by discharging long-term patients and avoiding unnecessary admissions.

delinquency A minor violation of legal or moral codes, especially by children or adolescents. Juvenile delinquency is such behavior by a young person (usually younger than 16 or 18 years of age) that brings him or her to the attention of a court.

delirium The medical diagnostic term that describes an organic mental disorder characterized by a cluster of cognitive impairments with an acute onset and the identification of a specific precipitating stressor.

delusion A false belief that is firmly maintained even though it is not shared by others and is contradicted by social reality.

dementia The medical diagnostic term that describes an organic mental disorder characterized by a cluster of cognitive impairments that are generally of gradual onset and irreversible. The predisposing and precipitating stressors may or may not be identifiable.

dendrite The postsynaptic part of a neuron.

denial Avoidance of disagreeable realities by ignoring or refusing to recognize them.

deoxyribonucleic acid (DNA) The molecule that encodes genetic information. DNA is a double-stranded molecule held together by weak bonds between base pairs of nucleotides. The four nucleotides in DNA contain the bases adenine (A), guanine (G), cytosine (C), and thymine (T).

depersonalization A feeling of unreality and alienation from oneself. One has difficulty distinguishing self from others, and one's body has an unreal or strange quality about it. The subjective experience of the partial or total disruption of one's ego and the disintegration and disorganization of one's self-concept.

depression An abnormal extension or overelaboration of sadness and grief. The word depression can denote a variety of phenomena (e.g., a sign, symptom, syndrome, emotional state, reaction, disease, or clinical disorder).

depressive disorder An illness characterized by depressed mood and loss of interest or pleasure in life.

DNA sequence The relative order of base pairs, whether in a DNA fragment, gene, chromosome, or an entire genome.

detoxification The removal of a toxic substance from the body, either naturally through physiological process, such as hepatic or renal functions, or medically by the introduction of alternative substances and gradual withdrawal.

direct self-destructive behavior (DSDB) Suicidal behavior.

disadvantagement The lack of socioeconomic resources that are basic to biopsychosocial adaptation.

discrimination Differential treatment of individuals or groups not based on actual merit.

displacement Shift of an emotion from the person or object toward which it was originally directed to another usually neutral or less dangerous person or object.

dissociation The separation of any group of mental or behavioral processes from the rest of the person's consciousness or identity.

drug interaction The effects of two or more drugs being taken simultaneously, producing an alteration in the usual effects of either drug taken alone. The interacting drugs may have a potentiating or additive effect, and serious side effects may result.

DSM–IV–TR Commonly used abbreviation for the *Diagnostic and Statistical Manual of Mental Disorders,* which contains standard nomenclature of emotional illness used by all health-care practitioners. *DSM–IV–TR* is a text revision of the version published in 1994; it updates and classifies mental illnesses and presents diagnostic criteria for various mental disorders.

dual diagnosis Simultaneous occurrence of a mental illness and a substance abuse disorder.

dyspareunia Recurrent or persistent genital pain occurring before, during, or after intercourse (male or female).

dysthymia A milder form of depression lasting 2 or more years.

E

echopraxia Purposeless imitation of other's movements.

ego defense mechanisms See *defense mechanisms.*

elder abuse A variety of behaviors that threaten the health, comfort, and possibly the lives of elderly people, including physical and emotional neglect, emotional abuse, violation of personal rights, financial abuse, and direct physical abuse.

electroconvulsive therapy (ECT) Artificial induction of a grand mal seizure by passing a controlled electrical current through electrodes applied to one or both temples. The patient is anesthetized, and the seizure attenuated by administration of a muscle relaxant medication.

empathy Ability to view the patient's world from his or her internal frame of reference. It involves the nurse's sensitivity to the patient's current feelings and the verbal ability to communicate this understanding in a language attuned to the patient.

employee assistance programs (EAPs) Worksite-based programs designed to help identify and resolve behavioral, health, and productivity problems that may affect employees' well-being or job performance.

enabler The role that is often assumed by the significant others of substance abusers, characterized by covert support of the substance-abusing behavior.

ethic A standard of behavior or a belief valued by an individual or group.

ethical dilemma Exists when moral claims conflict with one another, resulting in a difficult problem that seems to have no satisfactory solution because of the existence of a choice between equally unsatisfactory alternatives.

ethnicity A person's racial, national, tribal, linguistic, or cultural origin or background.

eugenics The study of improving a species by artificial selection; usually refers to the selective breeding of humans.

euthanasia Deliberately bringing about the death of a person who is suffering from an incurable disease or illness.

evidence-based practice The ability to examine clinical practice patterns, evaluate the nature of the data supporting them, and demonstrate sound clinical decision making in a way that can be empirically supported.

exhibitionism Intense sexual arousal or desire and acts, fantasies, or other stimuli involving exposing one's genitals to an unsuspecting stranger.

existential (therapy) A school of philosophical thought that focuses on the importance of experience in the present and the belief that humans find meaning in life through their experiences.

extinction The process of eliminating the occurrence of a behavior by ignoring or not rewarding that behavior.

expressive therapy Any therapeutic mode that uses a person's creative process to facilitate self-expression and self-awareness.

extended family Includes people other than parents and children who are related by blood or marriage.

extrapyramidal syndrome (EPS) A variety of signs and symptoms, including muscular rigidity, tremors, drooling, shuffling gait (Parkinsonism); restlessness (akathisia); peculiar involuntary postures (dystonia); motor inertia (akinesia); and many other neurological disturbances. Results from dysfunction of the extrapyramidal system. May occur as a reversible side effect of certain psychotropic drugs, particularly antipsychotics.

eye movement desensitization and reprocessing (EMDR) An intervention that requires the patient to generate a number of rapid lateral eye movements while engaging in imaginal recall of significant aspects of a particular traumatic memory or feared stimuli.

F

family A group of people living in a household who are attached emotionally, interact regularly, and share concerns for the growth and development of individuals and the family.

family burden The impact of a family member's mental illness on the entire family.

family therapy Refers to both specific family interventions and a broader conceptual framework for intervention, which includes family-centered treatment, family/couples psychotherapy, family skills building, multiple family groups, and in-home support.

family violence A range of behaviors occurring between family members, including physical and emotional abuse of children, child neglect, spouse battering, marital rape, and elder abuse.

fetishism Intense sexual arousal or desire and acts, fantasies, or other stimuli involving nonliving objects by themselves.

flat affect The absence of emotional expression as seen by a patient who reports significant life events without any emotional response.

flight of ideas Overproductive speech characterized by rapid shifting from one topic to another and fragmented ideas.

flooding Exposure therapy in which the patient is immediately exposed to the most anxiety-provoking stimuli.

Food and Drug Administration (FDA) One of a number of health administrations under the assistant Secretary of Health of the U.S. Department of Health and Human Services to set standards for, to license the sale of, and in general to safeguard the public from the use of dangerous drugs and food substances.

forensic nursing A subspecialty of nursing that has as its objective to assist the mental health and legal systems in serving individuals who have come to the attention of both.

free association The verbalization of thoughts as they occur, without any conscious screening or censorship.

frotteurism Intense sexual arousal or desire and acts, fantasies, or other stimuli involving rubbing against a nonconsenting person.

functional family therapy (FFT) A family therapy approach that integrates systems, behavioral, and cognitive views of dysfunction with the goal of modifying interaction and communication patterns to foster more adaptive family functioning.

G

gender identity A person's perception of one's maleness or femaleness.

gender identity disorder Also known as *gender dysphoria*, it is a profound discomfort with one's own sex and a strong and persistent identification with the opposite gender.

gene therapy An experimental procedure aimed at replacing, manipulating, or supplementing nonfunctional or misfunctioning genes with healthy genes.

genes The fundamental physical and functional unit of heredity. A gene is an ordered sequence of nucleotides located in a particular position on a particular chromosome that encodes a specific functional product (i.e., a protein or RNA molecule).

genetic map A map of the relative positions of genetic loci on a chromosome, determined on the basis of how often the loci are inherited together. Distance is measured in centimorgans (cM).

genetic testing Analyzing an individual's genetic material to determine predisposition to a particular health condition or to confirm a diagnosis of genetic disease.

genogram A structured method of gathering family information and graphically symbolizing factual and emotional relationship data.

genome   All the genetic material in the chromosomes of a particular organism; its size is generally given as its total number of base pairs.

genuineness   A quality of the nurse characterized by openness, honesty, and sincerity. The nurse is self-congruent and authentic and relates to the patient without a defensive facade.

glial cells   Support cells that form myelin sheaths; thought to remove excess transmitters and ions from the extracellular spaces in the brain, provide glucose to some nerve cells, and direct the flow of blood and oxygen to various parts of the brain.

grief   A person's subjective response to the loss of a person, object, or concept that is highly valued. Uncomplicated grief is a healthy, adaptive, reparative response.

group   A collection of people who have a relationship with one another, are interdependent, and may have common norms.

H

habeas corpus   A right retained by all psychiatric patients that provides for the release of a person who claims that he or she is being deprived of liberty and detained illegally. The hearing for this determination takes place in a court of law, and the patient's sanity is at issue.

half-life   The amount of time it takes the body to excrete approximately half of an ingested drug; after this time the effects of the drug usually begin to deteriorate.

hallucination   Perceptual distortion arising from any of the five senses.

hallucinogens   A class of abused drugs that cause a psychotic-like experience.

hardiness   A measurement of a person's psychological capability to resist illness when faced with a stressful life event.

heterosexuality   Sexual attraction to members of the opposite sex.

homophobia   Persistent and irrational fear of homosexuals along with a negative attitude and hostility toward them.

homosexuality   Sexual attraction to members of the same sex.

household   A residence consisting of an individual living alone or a group of people sharing a common dwelling and cooking facilities.

Human Genome Project   Collective name for several projects begun in 1986 by the U.S. Department of Energy (DOE) to create an ordered set of DNA segments from known chromosomal locations, develop new computational methods for analyzing genetic map and DNA sequence data, and develop new techniques and instruments for detecting and analyzing DNA. This DOE initiative is now known as the Human Genome Program. The joint national effort, led by DOE and the National Institutes of Health (NIH), is known as the Human Genome Project.

hypersomnia   Disorders of excessive somnolence.

hypochondriasis   A somatoform disorder characterized by the belief that one is ill without evidence of organic impairment, involving somatic overconcern with and morbid attention to details of body functioning.

hypomania   A clinical syndrome that is similar to but less severe than that described by the term *mania* or *manic episode*.

hypoxia   Inadequate oxygen at the cellular level, characterized by cyanosis, tachycardia, hypertension, peripheral vasoconstriction, dizziness, and mental confusion.

I

ideas of reference   Incorrect interpretation of casual incidents and external events as having direct personal references.

identification   Process by which a person tries to become like someone else whom he or she admires by taking on the thoughts, mannerisms, or tastes of that person.

identity   Organizing principle of the personality system that accounts for the unity, continuity, uniqueness, and consistency of the personality. It is the awareness of the process of being oneself that is derived from self-observation and judgment. It is the synthesis of all self-representations into an organized whole.

identity diffusion   A person's failure to integrate various childhood identifications into a harmonious adult psychosocial identity.

identity foreclosure   Premature adoption of an identity that is desired by significant others without coming to terms with one's own desires, aspirations, or potential.

illusions   False perceptions of or false responses to a sensory stimulus.

immediacy   State that occurs when the current interaction of the nurse and the patient is the focus.

incidence   The number of new cases of a disease or disorder in a population over a specified period of time.

incompetency   A legal status that must be proved in a special court hearing. As a result of the hearing, the person is determined incapable of making important decisions about himself or herself and can thus be deprived of many civil rights. Incompetency can be reversed only in another court hearing that declares the person competent.

incongruent communication   A communication pattern in which the sender is communicating a different message on the verbal and nonverbal levels and the listener does not know to which level he or she should respond.

indirect self-destructive behavior (ISDB)   Any activity that is detrimental to the person's well-being and could cause death, accompanied by lack of conscious awareness of the self-destructive nature of the behavior.

individuation   A process that leads one to self-definition.

informed consent   Disclosure of a certain amount of information to the patient about the proposed treatment and the attainment of the patient's consent, which must be competent, understanding, and voluntary.

insight   The patient's understanding of the nature of the problem or illness.

insomnia   Disorder of initiating or maintaining sleep.

intellectualization   Excessive reasoning or logic used to avoid experiencing disturbing feelings.

interdisciplinary team   A team with members of different disciplines involved in a formal arrangement to provide patient services while maximizing educational interchange.

interoceptive exposure   A technique used to desensitize a patient to catastrophic interpretations of internal bodily cues such as tachycardia, blurred vision, and shortness of breath.

intolerance   Unwillingness to accept different opinions or beliefs from people of different backgrounds.

introjection   An intense type of identification in which one incorporates qualities or values of another person or group into one's own ego structure.

isolation   An ego defense mechanism that involves the splitting off of emotional components of a thought.

K

kindling   An increased biochemical responsiveness to stable, low doses of stimulation (chemical or environmental) over time.

L

learned helplessness   A behavioral state and personality trait of people who believe they are ineffectual, their responses are futile, and they have lost control over the reinforcers in the environment.

learning   Any relatively permanent change in behavior that results from experience.

life review   Guided progressive return to consciousness of past experiences.

limit setting   Nonpunitive, nonmanipulative act in which the patient is told what behavior is acceptable, what is not acceptable, and the consequences of behaving unacceptably.

loose associations   Lack of a logical relationship between thoughts and ideas that renders speech and thought inexact, vague, diffuse, and unfocused.

M

magical thinking   Belief that thinking equates with doing, characterized by lack of realistic understanding of cause and effect.

magnetic resonance imaging (MRI)   Depicts brain structure using a magnetic field that surrounds the head and induces brain tissues to emit radio waves that are then computerized for clear and detailed construction of sections of the brain.

magnetic seizure therapy (MST)   Developed based on the ECT model, MST uses a magnetic stimulus to produce a seizure.

malingering   Deliberate feigning of an illness.

malpractice   Failure of a professional person to give the type of proper and competent care provided by other members of his or her profession. This failure causes harm to the patient.

managed care   A defined group of people receive treatment services that are clinically necessary, medically appropriate, within defined benefit parameters, for a set amount of time, in compliance with quality standards, and with outcomes that are anticipated and measurable.

mania   A condition characterized by a mood that is elevated, expansive, or irritable. It is a component of bipolar illness.

manipulation   A maladaptive social response in which people treat others as objects, enter relationships that are centered around control issues, and are self-oriented or goal oriented rather than other oriented.

marital therapy   Treatment of the distress in a committed relationship or education about relationships, such as communication skills.

maturational crisis   A developmental event requiring a role change.

Medicaid   A health-care entitlement program for Aid to Families with Dependent Children (AFDC) recipients; Supplemental Security Income (SSI) recipients; low-income, disabled, elderly people; low-income pregnant women, infants, and children; and medically needy recipients.

medical diagnosis   A physician's or advanced practice nurse's independent judgment of the patient's health problems or disease states.

memory   The retention or storage of knowledge learned about the world.

mental health   Indicators of mental health include positive attitudes toward self, growth, development, self-actualization, integration, autonomy, reality perception, and environmental mastery.

mental status examination   Represents a cross-section of the patient's psychological life and the sum total of the nurse's observations and impressions at the moment, serving as a basis for future comparison to track the progress of the patient.

methadone maintenance   A treatment program in which methadone is given to a patient recovering from heroin abuse to prevent the characteristic withdrawal symptoms, since methadone substitutes for the heroin without causing withdrawal symptoms or impaired functioning.

mindfulness meditation   A technique for gaining control over emotions by intentionally suspending awareness of the present-moment experience without reaction, judgment, or partiality.

modeling   Strategy used to form new behavior patterns, increase existing skills, or reduce avoidance behavior in which the patient observes a person modeling adaptive behavior and is then encouraged to imitate it.

mood   The patient's self-report of prevailing emotional state and a reflection of the patient's life situation.

mourning   Includes all the psychological processes set in motion by a loss. The process of mourning is resolved only when the lost object is internalized, bonds of attachment are loosened, and new object relationships are established.

multidisciplinary team   A team with members of different disciplines, each providing specific services to the patient.

multigenerational transmission The repetition of relationship patterns and anxiety associated with toxic issues passed through generations in a family.

multiple personality disorder   The existence within an individual of two or more distinct personalities or personality states, with each having its own pattern of perceiving, feeling, and thinking.

multisystemic therapy (MST)   A highly flexible treatment approach that addresses the multiple, interrelated needs of youths with serious behavioral and emotional problems and their families. It is usually delivered through the family preservation model of service delivery to provide interventions in home, school, and neighborhood settings.

myelin sheath   Provides insulation to the cells of the nervous system. See *glial cells*.

N

narcissism   A maladaptive social response characterized by egocentric attitude, fragile self-esteem, constant seeking of praise and admiration, and envy.

narcissistic personality disorder   A disorder having the essential features of a pattern of grandiosity, lack of empathy, and hypersensitivity to the evaluation of others, beginning in early adulthood; characteristic behaviors may include rageful reactions to criticism, exploitation of others, inability to recognize how others feel, sense of entitlement, envy, belief that one's problems are unique, preoccupation with grandiose fantasies, and search for constant attention and admiration.

negative identity   Assumption of an identity that is at odds with the accepted values and expectations of society.

negative reinforcement   Increases the frequency of a behavior by reinforcing the behavior's power to control an aversive stimulus.

neologisms   New word or words created by the patient; often a blend of other words.

neuroleptic malignant syndrome   A potentially fatal side effect of antipsychotic medications.

neurons   The basic functional unit of the brain structures of the nervous system.

neurosis   Category of health problems distinguished by the following characteristics: recognized by the person as unacceptable, reality testing intact, behavior overall consistent with social norms, problem enduring or recurrent, and no apparent organic cause.

neurotransmission   The process whereby neurons communicate with each other through chemical messengers called neurotransmitters.

neurotransmitters   Chemical messengers of the nervous system, manufactured in one neuron, released from the axon into the synapse, received by the dendrite of the next neuron.

nihilistic ideas   Thoughts of nonexistence and hopelessness.

noncompliance   The failure of a patient to carry out the self-care activities prescribed in a health care plan.

nonverbal communication   Transmission of a message without the use of words. It involves all five senses.

norms   Standards of behavior.

nuclear family   Refers to parents and their children.

nursing diagnosis   A nurse's judgment of the patient's behavioral response to stress. It is a statement of the patient's problems, which may be overt, covert, existing, or potential, and includes the behavioral disruption or threatened disruption, the contributing stressors, and the adaptive or maladaptive health responses.

nursing process   An interactive, problem-solving process; a systematic and individualized way to achieve the outcomes of nursing care. The phases of the nursing process as described by the *Scope and Standards of Psychiatric–Mental Health Nursing Practice* are assessment, diagnosis, outcome identification, planning, implementation, and evaluation.

nystagmus   Involuntary rhythmic movement of the eyeball.

O

obsession   An idea, emotion, or impulse that repetitively and insistently forces itself into consciousness; unwanted, but cannot be voluntarily excluded from consciousness.

operant conditioning   A theory concerned with the relationship between voluntary behavior and the environment that states that behaviors are influenced by their consequences and that operant behaviors are cued by environmental stimuli.

orgasm   Peaking of sexual pleasure and the release of sexual tension accompanied by rhythmic contractions of the perineal muscles and pelvic reproductive organs.

outcomes   The extent to which health care services are cost-effective and have a favorable effect on the patient's symptoms, functioning, and well-being.

outpatient commitment   The process by which the courts can order patients committed to a course of outpatient treatment specified by their clinicians.

P

pain disorder   A preoccupation with pain in the absence of physical disease to account for its intensity.

palliative care   Medical and nursing care that provides comfort to a moribund person without prolonging the dying process.

panic   A state of extreme anxiety that involves the disorganization of the personality. Distorted perceptions, loss of rational thought, and inability to communicate and function are evident.

panic attacks   A discrete period of intense fear or discomfort in which symptoms peak within 10 minutes.

paraphilia   A condition in which one experiences sexually arousing fantasies, sexual urges or sexual acts involving nonhuman objects, the suffering or humiliation of one's partner, or children or other nonconsenting persons.

parasomnia   Disorder associated with sleep stages, such as sleepwalking, night terrors, nightmares, and enuresis.

pedophilia   Intense sexual arousal or desire and acts, fantasies, or other stimuli involving children 13 years of age or younger.

perception   Identification and initial interpretation of a stimulus based on information received through the five senses of sight, hearing, taste, touch, and smell.

perseveration   Involuntary, excessive continuation or repetition of a single response, idea, or activity; may apply to speech or movement, but most often verbal.

personality disorder   A set of patterns or traits that hinder a person's ability to maintain meaningful relationships, feel fulfilled, and enjoy life.

personality fusion   A person's attempt to establish a sense of self by fusing or belonging to someone else.

pharmacodynamics   The study of the effects of the drug on the body, particularly the interaction of the drug on the targeted receptor site.

pharmacogenetics   The discipline that blends pharmacology with genomic capabilities.

pharmacogenomics   The study of the interaction of an individual's genetic makeup and response to a drug.

pharmacokinetics   The study of the process and rates of drug absorption, metabolism, distribution, and excretion in the organism.

phobia   A morbid fear associated with extreme anxiety.

phototherapy   Light therapy that consists of exposing patients to artificial therapeutic lights about 5 to 20 times brighter than indoor lighting and more consistent with the light spectrum of natural sunlight.

physical dependence   A characteristic of drug addiction that is present when withdrawal of the drug results in physiological disruptions.

physical restraints   Any manual method or physical or mechanical device attached to or adjacent to the patient's body that he or she cannot easily remove that restricts freedom of movement or normal access to one's body, material, or equipment.

polypharmacy   Use of combinations of psychoactive drugs in a patient at the same time without determining whether one drug by itself is effective; can cause drug interactions and may increase the incidence of adverse reactions.

positive reinforcement   Increases the frequency of a behavior by reinforcing the behavior's power to achieve a rewarding stimulus.

positron emission tomography (PET)   Depicts brain activity and function using an injected radioactive substance that travels to the brain and shows up as a bright spot on the scan; different substances are taken up by the brain in different amounts, depending on the type of tissue and activity level.

postvention   Therapeutic intervention with the significant others of a person who has committed suicide.

potency   The amount of drug dose required to achieve certain effects.

power   The member's ability to influence the group and its other members.

practice guidelines   In psychiatric care, practice guidelines are strategies for mental health care delivery that are developed to facilitate clinical decision making and provide patients with critical information about their treatment options.

preadmission certification   A process related to admission for psychiatric treatment that takes into account the patient's medical and psychiatric status, level of functioning, socioenvironmental factors, and procedural issues related to treatment.

precipitating stressors   Stimuli that the person perceives as challenging, threatening, or harmful. They require the use of excess energy and produce a state of tension and stress.

predisposing factors   Risk factors that influence both the type and the amount of resources that the person can elicit to cope with stress. They may be biological, psychological, or sociocultural.

prejudice   A preconceived, unfavorable belief about individuals or groups that disregards knowledge, thought, or reason.

premature ejaculation   Ejaculation that occurs with minimal sexual stimulation or before, on, or shortly after penetration and before the person wishes it.

presence   The active, respectful, watchful compassionate experience of being with a person in a state of empathy and positive regard. It involves "being with," and not "doing to" the person.

prevalence   The number of existing cases of a disease or disorder in a population at a specified point in time.

priapism   Sustained and painful penile erection.

primary prevention   Biological, social, or psychological intervention that promotes health and well-being or reduces the incidence of illness in a community by altering the causative factors before they have an opportunity to do harm.

prodromal phase   The time between the onset of symptoms and the need for treatment.

progressive muscle relaxation (PMR)   A systematic technique of tensing and releasing groups of muscles starting from facial muscles and moving down the body to the muscles in the feet in order to gain control over anxiety-provoking thoughts and muscle tension.

projection   Attributing one's own thoughts or impulses to another person. Through this process the person can attribute intolerable wishes, emotional feelings, or motivations to another person.

protective factors   Characteristics of a person that can significantly decrease the potential for developing a psychiatric disorder, increase the potential for recovery, or both.

protein A large molecule composed of one or more chains of amino acids in a specific order; the order is determined by the base sequence of nucleotides in the gene that codes for the protein. Proteins are required for the structure, function, and regulation of the body's cells, tissues, and organs; and each protein has unique functions. Examples are hormones, enzymes, and antibodies.

proteome Proteins expressed by a cell or organ at a particular time and under specific conditions.

proteomics The study of the full set of proteins encoded by a genome.

pseudodementia A depressive condition of the elderly characterized by impaired cognitive function.

psychiatric consultation liaison nurse (PCLN) An advanced practice nurse who practices psychiatric and mental health nursing in a medical setting and provides consultation and education to patients, families, the health care team, and the community.

psychiatric nursing An interpersonal process that strives to promote and maintain patient behavior that contributes to integrated functioning. It uses the theories of human behavior as its science and the purposeful use of self as its art. Psychiatric nursing is directed toward both preventive and corrective effects on mental disorders and their sequelae and is concerned with the promotion of optimum mental health for society, the community, and individuals.

psychoanalysis A therapeutic approach based on the belief that behavioral disorders are related to unresolved, anxiety-provoking childhood experiences that are repressed into the unconscious. The goal of psychoanalysis is to bring repressed experiences into conscious awareness and to learn healthier means of coping with the related anxiety.

psychoeducation The teaching of a patient and family about the mental illness and the coping skills that will help with successful community living.

psychological autopsy A retrospective review of the person's behavior for the time preceding death by suicide.

psychological dependence A characteristic of drug addiction that is manifested in a craving for the abused substance and a fear that it will not be available in the future.

psychoneuroimmunology The scientific field exploring the relationship between psychological states and the immune response.

psychopharmacogenetics Deals with genetic and environmental factors that control or influence psychotropic drug-metabolizing enzymes.

psychopharmacology Drugs that treat the symptoms of mental illness and whose actions in the brain provide us with models to better understand the mechanisms of mental disorders.

psychosis A category of health problems that are distinguished by regressive behavior, personality disintegration, reduced level of awareness, great difficulty in functioning adequately, and gross impairment in reality testing.

puberty A series of biological changes that transform the young person physically from a child into a reproductively mature adult.

punishment Decreases the frequency of a behavior by causing an aversive stimulus to occur after that behavior.

purging A variety of maladaptive behaviors intended to prevent weight gain, including vomiting; excessive exercise; and use of diuretics, diet pills, laxatives, and steroids.

R

racism The belief that inherent differences among races determine individual achievement and that one race is superior over others.

rationalization Offering a socially acceptable or apparently logical explanation to justify or make acceptable otherwise unacceptable impulses, feelings, behaviors, and motives.

reaction formation Development of conscious attitudes and behavior patterns that are opposite to what one really would like to have.

reality orientation Formal process of keeping a person alert to events in the here and now.

receptor A specialized area on a nerve membrane, blood vessel, or muscle that receives the chemical stimulation that activates or inhibits normal action of the nerve, blood vessel, or muscle.

recovery The consumer-centered rehabilitation philosophy that is characterized by awareness of the illness and what is needed to recover; management of one's own mental health; interconnectedness with others; and the combination of internal strengths with interconnectedness to provide self-help, advocacy, and caring about what happens to oneself and to others.

recurrence Return of a new episode of illness.

regression A retreat in the face of stress to behavior that is characteristic of an earlier level of development.

rehabilitation The process of enabling a mentally ill person to return to the highest possible level of functioning.

relapse Return of symptoms.

relaxation training Training a person to relax and thus reduce anxiety. Procedures include rhythmic breathing, reduced muscle tension, and an altered state of consciousness.

reminiscence Thinking about or relating past experiences, especially those that are personally significant.

remission Occurs when a patient is symptom free at the end of a phase of preillness functioning.

repression Involuntary exclusion of a painful or conflictual thought, impulse, or memory from awareness. It is the primary ego defense, and other mechanisms tend to reinforce it.

resilience The personal and community qualities that enable us to rebound from adversity, trauma, tragedy, threats, or other stresses—and to go on with life with a sense of mastery, competence, and hope.

resistance   Attempt of the patient to remain unaware of anxiety-producing aspects within the self. Ambivalent attitudes toward self-exploration in which the patient both appreciates and avoids anxiety-producing experiences that are a normal part of the therapeutic process.

respect   An attitude of the nurse that conveys caring for, liking, and valuing the patient. The nurse regards the patient as a person of worth and accepts the patient without qualification.

response cost   Decreases the frequency of a behavior through the experience of a loss or penalty following the behavior.

response prevention   Patient is encouraged to face a particular fear or situation without engaging in the accompanying behavior.

reuptake   The process of neurotransmitters returning to the presynaptic cell after communication with receptor cells.

risk factors   Characteristics of a person that can significantly increase the potential for developing a psychiatric disorder, decrease the potential for recovery, or both.

role playing   Acting out of a particular situation. It functions to increase the person's insight into human relations and can deepen one's ability to see a situation from another point of view.

role strain   Stress associated with expected roles or positions and experienced as frustration.

roles   Set of socially expected behavior patterns associated with one person's function in various social groups. Roles provide a means for social participation and a way to test identities for consensual validation by significant others.

room program   A titration of the amount of time patients are allowed in the unit milieu, with patients asked to stay in their rooms for certain lengths of time and conversely allowed out of their rooms for a specific amount of time.

S

seasonal affective disorder (SAD)   Depression that comes with shortened daylight in fall and winter that disappears during spring and summer.

seclusion   Separating the patient from others in a safe, contained environment with minimal stimulation.

secondary gain   A related benefit that a patient experiences as a result of one's illness. For example, the development of the illness may result in the patient experiencing favorable environmental, interpersonal, monetary, or situational changes. Specific types of secondary gain include financial compensation, avoiding unpleasant situations, increased sympathy or attention, escape from work or other responsibilities, attempted control of people, and lessening of social pressures.

secondary prevention   A type of prevention that seeks to reduce the prevalence of illness by interventions that provide for early detection and treatment of problems.

self-concept   All the notions, beliefs, and convictions that constitute a person's knowledge of self and influence relationships with others.

self-disclosure   Revelation that occurs when a person reveals information about self, ideas, values, feelings, and attitudes.

self-efficacy   A belief in one's personal capabilities, that one has control over the events in his or her life, and that one's actions will be effective.

self-esteem   The person's judgment of personal worth obtained by analyzing how well his or her behavior conforms to self-ideal.

self-help groups   Groups composed of members who organize to solve their own problems; the members share a common experience, work together toward a common goal, and use their strengths to gain control over their lives.

self-ideal   The person's perception of how he or she should behave on the basis of certain personal standards. The standard may be either a carefully constructed image of the type of person one would like to be or merely various aspirations, goals, or values that one would like to achieve.

self-injury   The act of deliberate harm to one's own body.

serotonin syndrome   Hyperserotonergic state (confusion, autonomic dysfunction, muscle rigidity, ataxia) that occurs when SSRIs are given concurrently with other serotonin-enhancing drugs, causing an excess of serotonin in the system.

sexual abuse   The involvement of children, adolescents, and adults in sexual activities that they do not fully comprehend and/or to which they cannot or do not fully consent.

sexual assault   Forced perpetration of an act of sexual contact with another person without consent.

sexual orientation   The gender to which one is romantically attracted.

shaping   Introduces new behaviors by reinforcing behaviors that approximate the desired behavior.

single photon emission computed tomography (SPECT)   Permits the study of brain metabolism and cerebral blood flow.

situational crisis   Occurs when a life event upsets an individual's or group's psychological equilibrium.

sleep deprivation   A state of physical and mental exhaustion brought on by lack of sleep in which the abilities to concentrate and reason are disturbed and judgment is diminished.

sleep deprivation therapy   A possible therapy for depressed and bipolar patients based on reports that as many as 60% of depressed patients improve immediately after a night of sleep deprivation.

social skills training   Teaching smooth social functioning to those who do not manifest social skills, using the principles of guidance, demonstration, practice, and feedback, resulting in the acquisition of behaviors that will support community living.

somatization disorder   A somatoform disorder characterized by multiple physical complaints with no evidence of organic impairment.

somatoform disorder   A category of psychophysiological disruptions with no evidence of organic impairment.

somatoform pain disorder   A preoccupation with pain in the absence of physical disease to account for its intensity.

spiritual distress A state where people have doubts, fears, guilt, or other concerns involving their religious faith, beliefs, or practice.

splitting Viewing people and situations as either all good or all bad. Failure to integrate the positive and negative qualities of oneself and objects.

steady state Exists when the body has reached a state of drug level equilibrium: a drug has been taken long enough that the amount of drug excreted equals the amount ingested. This occurs in approximately four to six half-lives.

stereotype A depersonalized conception of individuals within a group.

stigma An attribute or trait deemed by the person's social environment as negative, different, and diminishing.

sublimation Acceptance of a socially approved substitute goal for a drive whose normal channel of expression is blocked.

substance abuse The use of any mind-altering agent to such an extent that it interferes with the person's biological, psychological, or sociocultural integrity.

substance dependence A severe condition of addictive behaviors often resulting in physical problems, as well as serious disruptions of work, family life, and social life; usually considered a disease.

suicide Self-inflicted death. Also see *completed suicide*.

suicide attempt A deliberate action that, if carried to completion, will result in death.

suicide ideation The thought of self-inflicted death, either self-reported or reported to others.

suicide threat A warning—direct or indirect, verbal or nonverbal—that the person plans to attempt suicide.

sundowning syndrome Cognitive ability diminishing in the late afternoon or early evening.

sunrise syndrome Unstable cognitive ability on rising in the morning.

suppression A process that is the conscious analogy of repression. It is the intentional exclusion of material from consciousness.

surrogate decision maker The person designated by law or advance directive to make health care decisions for a person who does not have the decisional capacity to make his or her wishes known.

synapse The gap between the membrane of one neuron and that of another. The synapse is the point at which the transmission of nerve impulses occurs.

systematic desensitization Designed to decrease avoidance behavior linked to a specific stimulus by helping the patient change the response to a threatening stimulus.

T

tangential Thought and speech of a person that strays from the original discussion, never returns to the central point, and never answers the original question.

tardive dyskinesia Literally, "late-appearing abnormal movements," a variable complex of choreiform or athetoid movements developing in patients exposed to antipsychotic drugs. Typical movements include tongue writhing or protrusion; chewing; lip puckering; choreiform finger movements; toe and ankle movements; leg jiggling; and movements of neck, trunk, and pelvis.

target symptoms Symptoms of an illness that are most likely to respond to a specific treatment such as a particular psychopharmacological drug.

telepsychiatry Connects people by audiovisual communication and is seen as one means of providing expert health care services to patients distant from a source of care.

teratogenicity The adverse effects of a drug on the fetus.

tertiary prevention Rehabilitative measures designed to reduce the severity, disability, or residual impairment resulting from illness.

testimonial privilege A term used in court-related proceedings to refer to the communication between two parties. The right to reveal information belongs to the person who spoke, and the listener cannot disclose the information unless the speaker gives permission. This includes communication between husband and wife, attorney and patient, and clergy and church member.

themes Underlying issues or problems experienced by the patient that emerge repeatedly during the course of the nurse-patient relationship.

therapeutic community An inpatient environment described as a community in which each patient is an active participant in one's own care and is involved in the daily problems and activities of the unit.

therapeutic impasses Roadblocks in the progress of the nurse-patient relationship. They arise for a variety of reasons and may take different forms, but they all create stalls in the therapeutic relationship.

therapeutic index A relative measure of the safety and toxicity of a drug.

therapeutic milieu The controlled environment of treatment facilities that shelters patients from what they perceive to be painful and frightening stressors, thus providing them with a stable and coherent social environment that facilitates the development and implementation of treatment.

therapeutic nurse-patient relationship A mutual learning experience and corrective emotional experience for the patient in which the nurse uses self and specified clinical techniques in working with the patient to bring about behavioral change.

therapeutic touch The nurse's laying of hands on or close to the body of an ill person for the purpose of helping or healing.

thought blocking Sudden stopping in the train of thought or in the midst of a sentence.

thought broadcasting The belief that one's thoughts are being aired to the outside world.

thought insertion The belief that one's thoughts are being placed into one's mind by outside people or influences.

thought stopping Teaching a patient to interrupt dysfunctional thoughts.

time-out Short-term removal of the patient from overstimulating and sometimes reinforcing situations.

token economy A form of positive reinforcement in which patients are rewarded for performing desired target behaviors with tokens that they can use for desired purchases or activities.

tolerance A characteristic of some potentially addictive drugs that refers to the progressive need for more of the drug to achieve the desired effect.

transactional analysis A model of communication developed by Eric Berne that consists of the study of the communication or transactions between people and the sometimes unconscious and destructive ways ("games") in which people relate to each other.

transcranial magnetic stimulation (TMS) A noninvasive procedure in which a changing magnetic field is introduced into the brain to influence the brain's activity.

transference An unconscious response of patients in which they experience feelings and attitudes toward the nurse that were originally associated with significant figures in their early life.

transsexual A person who is anatomically a male or female but who expresses, with strong conviction, that he or she has the mind and emotions of the opposite sex, lives as a member of the opposite sex part time or full time, and seeks to change his or her sex legally and through hormonal and surgical sex reassignment.

transvestism Condition in which a male (less often a female) has a sexual obsession for or addiction to women's (men's) clothes.

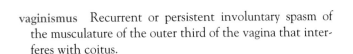

U

undoing An act or communication that partially negates a previous one.

unidisciplinary team A team with members of the same discipline.

V

vaginismus Recurrent or persistent involuntary spasm of the musculature of the outer third of the vagina that interferes with coitus.

vagus nerve stimulation (VNS) A somatic treatment for depression which involves surgically implanting a small generator into the patient's chest with an electrode threaded subcutaneously from the generator to the vagus nerve on the left side of the patient's neck. The end of the electrode is wrapped around the nerve, and the generator is programmed for the frequency and intensity of the stimulus.

validation Reflection of the content of the patient's communication back to the patient.

values The concepts that a person holds worthy in personal life. They are formed as a result of one's life experiences with family, friends, culture, education, work, and relaxation.

values clarification process A method whereby a person can assess, explore, and determine personal values and how they influence their own thoughts, attitudes, and behaviors.

verbal communication Occurs through words spoken or written.

vestibular desensitization training An exposure therapy for patients whose panic attacks are provoked by environmental cues that cause them to have symptoms of motion sickness.

visualization The conscious programming of desired change with positive images.

voyeurism Intense sexual arousal or desire and acts, fantasies, or other stimuli involving the observation of unsuspecting people who are naked, in the act of disrobing, or engaging in sexual activity.

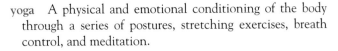

W

withdrawal symptoms Result from a biological need that develops when the body becomes adapted to having an addictive drug or substance in the system. Characteristic symptoms occur when the level of the substance in the system decreases.

word salad Series of words that seem totally unrelated.

Y

yoga A physical and emotional conditioning of the body through a series of postures, stretching exercises, breath control, and meditation.

INDEX

871